Atlas of
Head & Neck Surgery—
Otolaryngology

197 Contributors

Illustrated by Anthony Pazos
with assistance from Natalie Johnson

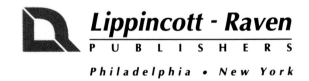

Lippincott · Raven
P U B L I S H E R S
Philadelphia • New York

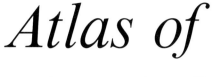

Atlas of
Head & Neck
Surgery—
Otolaryngology

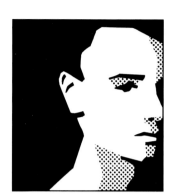

Byron J. Bailey, MD, FACS
Wiess Professor and Chairman
Department of Otolaryngology
University of Texas Medical Branch
Galveston, Texas

Karen H. Calhoun, MD, FACS
Professor and Vice Chair
Department of Otolaryngology
University of Texas Medical Branch
Galveston, Texas

Amy R. Coffey, MD
Assistant Professor
Department of Otorhinolaryngology
University of Texas Southwestern Medical Center
Dallas, Texas

J. Gail Neely, MD, FACS
Professor and Director
Otology/Neurotology/Base of Skull Surgery
Director of Research
Professor, Occupational Therapy Program
Washington University School of Medicine
Department of Otoloaryngology—Head and Neck Surgery
St. Louis, Missouri

Acquisitions Editor: James D. Ryan
Developmental Editor: Susan R. Skand
Associate Managing Editor: Elizabeth A. Durand
Production Manager: Caren Erlichman
Senior Production Coordinator: Kevin P. Johnson
Design Coordinator: Doug Smock
Indexer: Alexandra Nickerson
Compositor: Tapsco, Incorporated
Printer: Quebecor/Kingsport

Library of Congress Cataloging-in-Publication Data

Atlas of head and neck surgery—otolaryngology/[edited by] Byron J.
  Bailey . . . [et al.]; 197 contributors; illustrated by Anthony
Pazos with assistance from Natalie Johnson.
      p.   cm.
    Companion v. to: Head and neck surgery—otolaryngology/[edited
by] Byron J. Bailey . . . [et al.]. Philadelphia: Lippincott, © 1993.
    Includes bibliographical references and index.
    ISBN 0-397-51315-1 (alk. paper)
    1. Otolaryngology, Operative—Atlases.   2. Head—Surgery—Atlases.
3. Neck—Surgery—Atlases.   I. Bailey, Byron J., 1934–   .
II. Pazos, Anthony.
    [DNLM: 1. Otorhinolaryngologic Diseases—surgery—atlases.
2. Otolaryngology—atlases.   3. Head—surgery—atlases.   4. Neck—
surgery—atlases.   WV 17 A8807 1996]
RF51.A774   1996
617.5′ 1059—dc20
DNLM/DLC
for Library of Congress   95-25057
                                                                                    CIP

9   8   7   6   5   4   3   2   1

DEDICATION

"If we were to start all over again and there were no surgical specialties, the ideal would be to create a single specialty of head and neck surgery to include everything above the clavicles with the exception probably of the eye and brain. It is still the ideal, but we are not permitted to start all over again and must accept some sort of compromise, men still being jealous of their own prerogatives, which they only seldom are willing to sacrifice for the common good. We, therefore, need to plan our teaching approach to the problem upon the spirit of compromise. First, we will not succeed at all if we follow a policy of exclusion. To create a well rounded teaching program we need to include teachers in fields other than Otolaryngology rather than exclude them. We will not succeed by trying to exclude anyone with a legitimate right to teach or operate in this area." (Joel J. Pressman, MD)

May we always keep our focus on the best that we have within ourselves and the best in those whom we strive to emulate as we study, learn, and practice the science and art of surgery.

BYRON J. BAILEY

Dedicated to our patients, who are our greatest teachers, and to our willingness to ask the same question again and again until we find an answer that helps these patients.

KAREN H. CALHOUN

Dedicated to those from whom I have learned so much—my patients, professors, fellow residents, students and colleagues. I am especially grateful to Dr. Bailey, who had faith in my abilities—Ken and Marianna Rasco for their love, guidance, and example—Dr. Allen Coffey for his encouragement and cooperation—and Dr. Golda Leonard, mentor and dear friend.

AMY R. COFFEY

Dedicated to my father, El Roy C. Neely, whose hunger for knowledge and its application continues to inspire me, and, I hope, others through me, even after his death. Also dedicated to the young men and women who have the courage and tenacity to think.

J. GAIL NEELY

Foreword

As President of the American Academy of Otolaryngology—Head and Neck Surgery in 1995, I gave Byron J. Bailey, MD, a Presidential Citation that read, "To Byron J. Bailey, MD, a skilled surgeon, a fine leader, and a consummate educator who has served many organizations with great distinction and always left them better than he found them." This textbook, *Atlas of Head and Neck Surgery—Otolaryngology,* certainly is a product of the qualities that typify Dr. Bailey.

This atlas is complementary to Dr. Bailey's very well received multi-volume textbook and study guide, *Head and Neck Surgery—Otolaryngology.* The atlas is detailed, comprehensive, and will suit the needs of surgeons operating in the head and neck region, whether they are otolaryngologists or surgeons from overlapping disciplines.

The book is divided appropriately with subspecialty areas of otology, head and neck, paranasal sinus, and plastic and reconstructive surgery. To me, the comprehensive nature of this book is typified by the first segment, "Salivary Glands," which includes eight procedures described in detail by experts in this field. Dr. Bailey has selected experts whose names are indelibly linked with these procedures, thereby lending a great deal of authenticity to the text.

Each chapter is very well organized, providing not only the indications, instrumentation, and management of pitfalls and complications, but an enormously detailed step-by-step, in fact almost millimeter-by-millimeter, description of the surgical procedure which, on the facing page, is extraordinarily well illustrated. Tony Pazos, who provided illustrations for the entire text, has worked with Dr. Bailey previously and is a gifted medical artist who draws with great clarity using a form that is lean yet also aesthetically pleasing.

Dr. Bailey has written and edited many textbooks, and this experience together with his ten years as editor of the *AMA Archives of Otolaryngology* and now as editor of *The Laryngoscope* brings to this book a unique background and understanding of the editorial process. His experience as department chairman and as a member of the RRC and American Board of Otolaryngology have also provided an insight into the educational process of an otolaryngologist.

Eugene N. Myers, MD, FACS

Preface

As we approached the completion of the task of developing the multivolume textbook and study guide *Head and Neck Surgery— Otolaryngology,* we decided to launch a companion volume in the form of a comprehensive surgical atlas. After giving the matter considerable thought, we realized that there are many potential approaches to the illustration of core elements of our surgical specialty. Several surgical atlases are already available, including volumes by renowned surgeons and books that deal in depth with a particular subspecialty such as neurotology or facial plastic surgery. There are regional surgical atlases dealing with a particular anatomical zone such as the skull base, and there are other atlases centered around important surgical concepts such as functional endoscopic sinus surgery. Other examples grow out of a novel technology such as laser surgery.

We finally settled on a different, more comprehensive theme. In this surgical atlas we seek to compose a comprehensive overview of the array of surgical procedures performed by head and neck surgeons, facial plastic surgeons, reconstructive surgeons, otologists, pediatric otolaryngologists, general otolaryngologists, and endoscopists. We want to display in one volume the broad range of surgery in our specialty, yet we recognize the practical limits that prevent us from going into every detail of each subspecialty.

We settled on the approach of identifying an expert in each procedure or related group of procedures. We adopted a standard format for the text and artwork and we selected a single artist to present the basics of each procedure.

This surgical atlas is organized around 160 surgical procedures that are central to a training of a head and neck surgeon. These are the core procedures that are tracked by the Residency Review Committee for Otolaryngology in the process of residency program ac-

creditation and by the American Board of Otolaryngology in the application process for Board Certification.

Each procedure is presented in the *Atlas* with a left-hand page of descriptive text and a right-hand page of illustrations. The text page is organized using consistent headings including the definition of the procedure, indications, contraindications, complications and their avoidance, pitfalls, special instruments, and a narrative description of the operation itself.

Operative procedures have been assigned either two or four pages in the *Atlas,* based on their complexity or the space required to present the relevant surgical concepts in a manner that will be clearly understood and easily learned and remembered.

We are understandably proud of the success of the two primary volumes in this group. The *Atlas* will serve to enhance and complete the original concept, which we described as "More than a textbook— it's a learning system."

Surgical training is challenging by its nature. Because of the human elements at the core of the surgeon and the patient, surgery continues to be both an art and a science. To facilitate the acquisition of the knowledge base required to perform a surgical procedure, we have tried to boil vast amounts of information down so that we can present you with the essence of years of experience in small, digestible, and memorable bites. Our goals in developing this *Atlas* have been to make it clear, be concise, keep it practical, and emphasize the key clinical information.

We hope that you will conclude that we have accomplished our mission and achieved our goals.

Byron J. Bailey, MD, FACS

Acknowledgments

Developing this surgical atlas has been an exercise that has brought us great joy and satisfaction. The mundane tasks of reminding authors and facilitating the communication between contributors and our artist have been overshadowed by the sense of accomplishment that we feel as we conclude our pre-production work. I appreciate beyond words the time and effort that have been given to this project by my coeditors, Karen Calhoun, M.D., Gail Neely, M.D., and Amy Coffey, M.D. Their oversight of their respective sections has been outstanding in every way. They have worked with the section editors and the individual contributors to assemble a valuable learning tool that has no equal in our specialty.

I congratulate Tony Pazos on the excellent quality of the artwork that he has produced. Tony has spent hundreds of hours in operating rooms in various parts of the country, and the blend of his skill as an artist with his surgical knowledge has produced illustrations of remarkable clarity and insight. He sought the answers to questions and pursued information above and beyond the call of duty and without personal compensation other than expanding his own knowledge of surgical techniques and anatomy.

Once again I have the great pleasure of expressing my gratitude and appreciation to several other very special people:

To Margi, my partner for life and my editorial associate of many years

To Marilyn Streck, my Administrative Assistant, who continues to provide support and encouragement through the years that we have shared

To Rebecca Fisher, the Project Coordinator in our office, who has given generously of her time to develop reports, answer questions, keep after contributors, keep track of our artwork budget, and keep everyone's morale at a high level as she radiates laughter and happiness to everyone around her

To James Ryan, Kimberly Cox, Elizabeth Durand, Caren Erlichman, Kevin Johnson, Susan Skand, Doug Smock, and the other fine professionals at Lippincott-Raven who have guided many decisions along the path to publication and who have encouraged the timely preparation of excellent education material.

My heartfelt thanks to each and every one of you.

Byron J. Bailey, MD, FACS

Section Editors and Managers

Section I—HEAD AND NECK
Section Editor—Byron J. Bailey

Section Managers

Dale H. Rice
Los Angeles, California

Lanny G. Close
Dallas, Texas

Christopher H. Rassekh
Galveston, Texas

Jonas T. Johnson
Pittsburgh, Pennsylvania

Robert H. Miller
New Orleans, Louisiana

Jesus E. Medina
Oklahoma City, Oklahoma

Michael D. Maves
Alexandria, Virginia

Gayle E. Woodson
Memphis, Tennessee

George H. Petti, Jr.
Loma Linda, California

Gary L. Schechter
Norfolk, Virginia

Charles M. Stiernberg
Houston, Texas

Steven D. Schaefer
New York, New York

Section II—OTOLOGY
Section Editor—J. Gail Neely

Section Managers

Mitchell K. Schwaber
Nashville, Tennessee

Sam E. Kinney
Cleveland, Ohio

Jeffrey T. Vrabec
Galveston, Texas

Newton J. Coker
Houston, Texas

Richard T. Miyamoto
Indianapolis, Indiana

Herbert H. Silverstein
Sarasota, Florida

John P. Leonetti
Maywood, Illinois

Paul R. Lambert
Charlottesville, Virginia

Section III—PLASTIC AND RECONSTRUCTIVE SURGERY
Section Editor—Karen H. Calhoun

Section Managers

Karen H. Calhoun
Galveston, Texas

Section IV—ENDOSCOPY
Section Editor—Amy R. Coffey

Section Managers

Amy R. Coffey
Dallas, Texas

Harold C. Pillsbury
Chapel Hill, North Carolina

Section V—PEDIATRIC AND GENERAL OTOLARYNGOLOGY
Section Editors—Byron J. Bailey and Amy R. Coffey

Section Managers

Amy R. Coffey
Dallas, Texas

Harold C. Pillsbury
Chapel Hill, North Carolina

Contributors

Robert F. Aarstad, MD
Assistant Professor and Vice Chief
Department of Otolaryngology/Head and
  Neck Surgery
Louisiana State University Medical School
Shreveport, Louisiana

Peter A. Adamson, BSc, MD, CCFP, FRSC,
  FACS
Associate Professor
Department of Otolaryngology
University of Toronto
Active Staff
The Toronto Hospital
The Hospital for Sick Children
Toronto, Ontario
Canada
New York General Hospital
Consultant Staff
New York, New York

Eugene L. Alford, MD
Assistant Professor
Department of Otolaryngology and
  Communicative Science
Department of Dermatology
Division of Plastic Surgery
Baylor College of Medicine
The Methodist Hospital
Houston, Texas

Ossama Al-Mefty, MD
Professor and Chairman
University of Arkansas for Medical
  Sciences
University Hospital of Arkansas
Little Rock, Arkansas

I. Kaufman Arenberg, MD, FACS
Associate Clinical Professor
Otolaryngology (Otology-Neurotology)
University of Colorado Medical School
  and Health Sciences Center
Denver, Colorado
Program Director
International Meniere's Disease Research
  Institute (IMDRI) at Colorado
  Neurologic Institute
Swedish Medical Center (Health ONE)
Englewood, Colorado

William B. Armstrong, MD
Assistant Clinical Professor
University of California, Irvine
University of California, Irvine Medical
  Center
Long Beach Veterans Hospital
Irvine, California

Robert J. Backer, MD
Staff Neurosurgeon
St. John's Mercy Medical Center
St. Louis, Missouri

Byron J. Bailey, MD, FACS
Wiess Professor and Chairman
Department of Otolaryngology
University of Texas Medical Branch,
  Galveston
Galveston, Texas

William R. Blythe, MD
Resident, Division of Otolaryngology-
  Head and Neck Surgery
University of North Carolina Hospitals
Chapel Hill, North Carolina

Derald E. Brackmann, MD
Clinical Professor of Otolaryngology and
  Neurological Surgery
University of Southern California
House Ear Clinic
Los Angeles, California

Linda Brodsky, MD
Associate Professor
Otolaryngology and Pediatrics
State University of New York at Buffalo
School of Medicine and Biomedical
  Sciences
Director, Department of Pediatric
  Otolaryngology
Children's Hospital of Buffalo
Buffalo, New York

Orval E. Brown, MD
Associate Professor
University of Texas Southwestern Medical
  Center at Dallas
Attending Physician
Children's Medical Center of Dallas
Dallas, Texas

John E. Buenting, MD, MPH
Resident
Division of Otolaryngology-Head and
  Neck Surgery
University of North Carolina, Chapel Hill
  School of Medicine
University of North Carolina Hospitals
  and Clinics
Chapel Hill, North Carolina

Robert M. Bumsted, MD
Professor, Department of Otolaryngology
 and Bronchoesophagology
Rush Medical College
Rush-Presbyterian-St. Luke's Medical
 Center
Chicago, Illinois

Karen H. Calhoun, MD
Professor and Vice Chair
Department of Otolaryngology
University of Texas Medical Branch
John Sealy Hospital
Galveston, Texas

C. Ron Cannon, MD
Clinical Associate Professor, Division of
 Otolaryngology
Clinical Associate Professor, Department
 of Family Medicine
Clinical Associate Professor, School of
 Dentistry
Division of Diagnostic Sciences
University of Mississippi School of
 Medicine
Jackson, Mississippi

Vincent N. Carrasco, MD
Assistant Professor
University of North Carolina at Chapel
 Hill School of Medicine
University of North Carolina Hospitals
Chapel Hill, North Carolina

Ricardo L. Carrau, MD, FACS
Assistant Professor
Department of Otolaryngology-Head and
 Neck Surgery
University of Pittsburgh School of
 Medicine
University of Pittsburgh Medical Center
Pittsburgh, Pennsylvania

William R. Carroll, MD, FACS
Bozeman Otolaryngology Associates
Bozeman Deaconess Hospital
Bozeman, Montana

Nicholas J. Cassisi, DDS, MD
Professor and Chairman
Department of Otolaryngology-Head and
 Neck Surgery
University of Florida College of Medicine
Attending Physician
Shands Hospital at the University of
 Florida
Gainesville, Florida

George D. Chonkich, MD
Director, Residency Program
Division of Otolaryngology-Head and
 Neck Surgery
Associate Professor
Loma Linda University Medical Center
Loma Linda, California

William D. Clark, MD, DDS
Assistant Professor of Surgery
Uniformed Services
University of the Health Sciences
Clinical Assistant Professor of
 Otolaryngology
University of Texas Medical Branch,
 Galveston
Director of Residency and Chief of
 Pediatric Otolaryngology
Department of Otolaryngology
Wilford Hall Medical Center
Lackland AFB, Texas

Lanny Garth Close, MD
Howard W. Smith Professor and
 Chairman
Department of Otolaryngology-Head and
 Neck Surgery
College of Physicians and Surgeons
Columbia University
Director
Otolaryngology-Head and Neck Surgery
 Service
Columbia-Presbyterian Medical Center
New York, New York

Mark A. Clymer, MD
Resident Physician
Department of Otolaryngology
Vanderbilt University Medical Center
Nashville, Tennessee

Amy R. Coffey, MD
Assistant Professor
University of Texas Southwestern Medical
 Center
Pediatric Otolaryngology
Presbyterian Hospital of Plano and
 Children's Medical Center
Dallas, Texas

Noel L. Cohen, MD
Professor and Chairman
Department of Otolaryngology
New York University School of Medicine
Attending and Director
Department of Otolaryngology
New York University Medical Center
New York, New York

Newton J. Coker, MD
Professor
Department of Otorhinolaryngology and
 Communicative Sciences
Baylor College of Medicine
Houston, Texas

Jack A. Coleman, Jr., MD, FACS
Assistant Professor
Department of Otolaryngology
Vanderbilt University Medical Center
Vanderbilt University Hospital
Nashville, Tennessee

Thomas V. Conley, MD
University of Kentucky
Louisville, Kentucky

Minas S. Constantinides, MD
Assistant Professor of Otolaryngology
New York University Medical School
Director, Facial Plastic and Reconstructive
 Surgery
New York University Medical Center
New York, New York

Paul R. Cook, MD
Assistant Professor of Surgery
 (Otolaryngology)
University of Missouri School of Medicine
University of Missouri Hospitals and
 Clinics
Columbia, Missouri

David A. Cottrell, DMD
Assistant Professor and Director of
Resident Research
Department of Oral and Maxillofacial
Surgery
Boston University School of Graduate
Dentistry
Assistant Visiting Oral and Maxillofacial
Surgeon
Boston University Medical Center
Boston, Massachusetts

Mark S. Courey, MD
Assistant Professor
Department of Otolaryngology
Vanderbilt University Medical Center
Nashville, Tennessee

Dennis M. Crockett, MD
Associate Professor
Department of Otolaryngology-Head and
Neck Surgery
University of Southern California School
of Medicine
University of Southern California
University Hospital
Children's Hospital of Los Angeles,
Los Angeles County
University of Southern California Medical
Center
Los Angeles, California

R. Kim Davis, MD, FACS
Beckstrand Professor and Chairman
Division of Otolaryngology-Head and
Neck Surgery
University of Utah School of Medicine
University of Utah Health Sciences Center
Salt Lake City, Utah

Douglas D. Dedo, MD, FACS
Assistant Clinical Professor of
Otolaryngology-Head and Neck Surgery
University of Miami Medical School
Attending, Good Samaritan Hospital
St. Mary's Hospital
Wellington Regional Hospital
Miami, Florida

Lawrence W. DeSanto, MD
Professor, Mayo Medical School
Department of Otolaryngology-Head and
Neck Surgery
Chairman Emeritus
Mayo Clinic Scottsdale
Department of Otolaryngology-Head and
Neck Surgery
Scottsdale, Arizona

Ronald W. Deskin, MD, FAAP
Chief, Division of Pediatric
Otolaryngology
Associate Professor of Otolaryngology and
Pediatrics
University of Texas Medical Branch
Chief, Division of Pediatric
Otolaryngology
Department of Otolaryngology
Children's Hospital-University of Texas
Medical Branch
Galveston, Texas

Eric J. Dierks, MD, DMD, FACS
Clinical Associate Professor of Oral and
Maxillofacial Surgery
Oregon Health Sciences University
Chairman
Department of Head and Neck Surgery
Legacy Portland Hospitals
Portland, Oregon

Karen Jo Doyle, MD, PhD
Assistant Professor in Residence
Department of Otolaryngology-Head and
Neck Surgery
University of California, Irvine
Attending Otolaryngologist-Head and
Neck Surgeon
University of California, Irvine, Medical
Center
Veterans Affairs Medical Center, Long
Beach
Irvine, California

Amelia F. Drake, MD, FACS
Associate Professor
Otolaryngology-Head and Neck Surgery
Departments of Surgery and Pediatrics
University of North Carolina School of
Medicine
Surgeon/Attending Physician
University of North Carolina Hospitals
and Clinics
Chapel Hill, North Carolina

David W. Eisele, MD, FACS
Associate Professor
Departments of Otolaryngology-Head and
Neck Surgery and Oncology
Director, Division of Head and Neck
Surgery
Department of Otolaryngology-Head and
Neck Surgery
The Johns Hopkins Hospital
Baltimore, Maryland

Ramon M. Esclamado, MD
Associate Professor and Director
Division of Head and Neck Surgery
Department of Otolaryngology-Head and
Neck Surgery
University of Michigan
Associate Professor, Department of
Otolaryngology-Head and Neck Surgery
University of Michigan Medical Center
Ann Arbor, Michigan

Jay B. Farrior, MD
Clinical Faculty at University of South
Florida
Chairman, Ear, Nose, and Throat
Department
St. Joseph's Hospital
Tampa, Florida

Charles N. Ford, MD
Professor and Chairman
Division of Otolaryngology-Head and
Neck Surgery
University of Wisconsin, Center for Health
Sciences
Madison, Wisconsin

Marvin P. Fried, MD, FACS
Associate Professor of Otology and
    Laryngology
Harvard Medical School
Otolaryngologist-in-Chief
Beth Israel Hospital
Otolaryngologist-in-Chief
Brigham and Women's Hospital
Boston, Massachusetts

Ellen M. Friedman, MD
Professor
Department of Otorhinolaryngology and
    Communicative Sciences
Baylor College of Medicine
Chief of Service, Pediatric Otolaryngology
Texas Children's Hospital
Houston, Texas

John L. Frodel, MD, FACS
Associate Professor
Johns Hopkins Medical Institute
The Johns Hopkins Hospital
Baltimore, Maryland

Richard R. Gacek, MD
Professor of Otolaryngology, Department
    of Oral Health Sciences Center
Research Professor of Anatomy, Health
    Sciences Center
Attending Surgeon, Department of
    Otolaryngology
University Hospital
Syracuse, New York

Linda Gage-White, MD, PhD
Associate Clinical Professor
Louisiana State University Medical School
Shreveport, Louisiana

Steven L. Garner, MD
Private Practice
Plastic and Reconstructive Surgery
Santa Cruz, California

C. Gaelyn Garrett, MD
Assistant Professor
Department of Otolaryngology
Vanderbilt University Medical Center
Nashville, Tennessee

Gerard J. Gianoli, MD
Assistant Professor
Department of Otolaryngology-Head and
    Neck Surgery
Tulane University School of Medicine
New Orleans, Louisiana

F. Brian Gibson, MD
Clinical Instructor, Department of
    Otolaryngology
Vanderbilt University School of Medicine
Nashville, Tennessee
Active Staff
Presbyterian Hospital
Carolina Medical Center
Charlotte, North Carolina

Hayes B. Gladstone, MD
Research Fellow
University of California, San Francisco
San Francisco, California

Michael E. Glasscock III, MD, FACS
Clinical Professor of Surgery
University of North Carolina School of
    Medicine
Chapel Hill, North Carolina
Clinical Professor of Surgery (Otology and
    Neurotology)
Vanderbilt University School of Medicine
Baptist Hospital
Nashville, Tennessee

Michael G. Glenn, MD
Associate Professor
Department of Otolaryngology-Head and
    Neck Surgery
University of Washington School of
    Medicine
University Hospital and Medical Center
Seattle, Washington

Jack L. Gluckman, MD
Professor and Chairman
Department of Otolaryngology-Head and
    Neck Surgery
University of Cincinnati Medical Center
Professor and Chairman
University Hospital
Cincinnati, Ohio

Andrew N. Goldberg, MD, FACS
Assistant Professor
Department of Otorhinolaryngology-Head
    and Neck Surgery
University of Pennsylvania Medical Center
Philadelphia, Pennsylvania

Richard L. Goode, MD
Professor of Otolaryngology-Head and
    Neck Surgery
Stanford University School of Medicine
Stanford University Medical Center
Stanford, California

Harsha V. Gopal, MD
Instructor in Otology and Laryngology
Harvard Medical School
Associate Surgeon
Beth Israel Hospital
Associate Surgeon
Brigham and Women's Hospital
Boston, Massachusetts

Gerald S. Gussack, MD
Associate Professor of Otolaryngology-
    Head and Neck Surgery
Director of Residency Education
Emory University School of Medicine
Attending Physician
Emory University Hospital
Henrietta Egleston Children's Hospital
Grady Memorial Hospital
Crawford-Long Hospital
Atlanta, Georgia

Richard E. Hayden, MD, CM, FACS
Professor
University of Pennsylvania
Department of Otorhinolaryngology
Director
Center for Head and Neck Cancer
Hospital of the University of Pennsylvania
Philadelphia, Pennsylvania

Gerald B. Healy, MD
Professor of Otology and Laryngology
Harvard Medical School
Otolaryngologist-in-Chief
Surgeon-in-Chief
Boston Children's Hospital
Boston, Massachusetts

James A. Heinrich, MD
Assistant Professor and Director
Facial Plastic and Reconstructive Surgery
Division of Otolaryngology-Head and
  Neck Surgery
Loma Linda University School of
  Medicine
Loma Linda, California

Douglas E. Henrich, MD
Resident
Department of Otolaryngology-Head and
  Neck Surgery
University of North Carolina
University of North Carolina Hospitals
  and Clinics
Chapel Hill, North Carolina

Denis K. Hoasjoe, MD, FRCSC
Assistant Professor
Department of Otolaryngology-Head and
  Neck Surgery
Louisiana State University
Louisiana State University Medical Center
Shreveport, Louisiana

Henry T. Hoffman, MD, FACS
Associate Professor
University of Iowa College of Medicine
Director, Head and Neck Oncology
Director, Voice Clinic
University of Iowa Hospitals and Clinics
Associate Professor
Iowa City, Iowa

G. Richard Holt, MD, MSE, MPH
Clinical Professor of Otolaryngology-Head
  and Neck Surgery
The University of Texas Health Science
  Center at San Antonio
San Antonio, Texas

Jean Edwards Holt, MD, FACS
Clinical Professor
Department of Ophthalmology
University of Texas Health Science Center
Resident-Elect Medical Executive Board
Baptist Memorial Hospital System
San Antonio, Texas

J.V.D. Hough, MD
Clinical Professor
Otolaryngology-Head and Neck Surgery
University of Oklahoma Health Sciences
  Center
Oklahoma City, Oklahoma
Baptist Medical Center
University of Oklahoma Health Sciences
  Center

William F. House, MD
Hoag Hospital
Newport Beach, California

Robert K. Jackler, MD
Associate Professor of Otolaryngology and
  Neurological Surgery
University of California, San Francisco
San Francisco, California

C. Gary Jackson, MD, FACS
Clinical Professor
Department of Surgery
Division of Otolaryngology-Head and
  Neck Surgery (Otology and
  Neurotology)
University of North Carolina School of
  Medicine
Chapel Hill, North Carolina
Clinical Professor of Hearing and Speech
  Sciences
Vanderbilt University School of Medicine
Nashville, Tennessee

Ivo P. Janecka, MD, FACS
Professor, Departments of Otolaryngology
  and Neurological Surgery
University of Pittsburgh School of
  Medicine
Director, Center for Cranial Base Surgery
University of Pittsburgh Medical Center
Pittsburgh, Pennsylvania

Jonas T. Johnson, MD, FACS
Professor, Departments of Otolaryngology
  and Radiation Oncology
Vice Chairman, Department of
  Otolaryngology
Director, Division of Head and Neck
  Surgery and Immunology
University of Pittsburgh School of
  Medicine
University of Pittsburgh Medical Center
Presbyterian University Hospital
The Eye and Ear Hospital
Pittsburgh, Pennsylvania

Frank M. Kamer, MD
Medical Corporation
Beverly Hills, California

Jennifer Keir-Garza, MD
Resident, Otolaryngology-Head and Neck
  Surgery
University of Texas Health Science Center
Houston, Texas

Daniel J. Kelley, MD
Chief Resident
Otolaryngology-Head and Neck Surgery
University of Cincinnati Medical Center
Cincinnati, Ohio

Robert M. Kellman, MD
Professor
State University of New York, Health
  Science Center
Department of Otolaryngology
Chairman, Department of Otolaryngology
University Hospital
Syracuse, New York

David W. Kennedy, MD
Professor and Chair
Department of Otorhinolaryngology-Head
  and Neck Surgery
University of Pennsylvania
Attending Physician
Chair of the Medical Board
University of Pennsylvania Medical Center
Philadelphia, Pennsylvania

Sam E. Kinney, MD
Head, Section of Otology/Neurotology
Department of Otolaryngology
Cleveland Clinic Foundation
Clinical Associate Professor of
    Otolaryngology-Head and Neck Surgery
Case Western Reserve School of Medicine
Cleveland Clinic Foundation
Cleveland, Ohio

John B. Kinsella, FRCS (Ed)
Head and Neck Oncologic Surgery Fellow
University of Texas Medical Branch
Galveston, Texas

Cynthia L. Kish, MD
Otolaryngology-Head and Neck Surgery
Indiana University School of Medicine
Indianapolis, Indiana
Parkview Hospital
Ft. Wayne, Indiana

G. Robert Kletzker, MD, FACS
Clinical Instructor
Otolaryngology-Head and Neck Surgery
Washington University School of
    Medicine
Attending Surgeon
St. John's Mercy Medical Center
Barnes Hospital
St. Louis, Missouri

Robert I. Kohut, MD, FACS
James A. Harrill Professor and Chairman
The Bowman Gray School of Medicine of
    Wake Forest University
Professor and Chairman
Department of Otolaryngology
North Carolina Baptist Hospital
Winston-Salem, North Carolina

Peter J. Koltai, MD, FACS, FAAP
Professor of Surgery and Pediatrics
Chief, Section of Pediatric Otolaryngology
Albany Medical College
Albany Medical Center
Albany, New York

John F. Kveton, MD
Associate Professor of Surgery
Section of Otolaryngology
Yale University School of Medicine
Attending Physician
Yale-New Haven Hospital
New Haven, Connecticut

Paul R. Lambert, MD
Professor, Department of Otolaryngology-
    Head and Neck Surgery
Director, Division of Otology-Neurotology
University of Virginia Health Sciences
    Center
Charlottesville, Virginia

Donald C. Lanza, MD, FACS
Assistant Professor
Department of Otorhinolaryngology-Head
    and Neck Surgery
University of Pennsylvania
Assistant Professor
University of Pennsylvania Medical Center
Philadelphia, Pennsylvania

Wayne F. Larrabee, Jr., MD, FACS
Clinical Professor
Department of Otolaryngology-Head and
    Neck Surgery
University of Washington, Seattle
Staff
Swedish Hospital
Seattle, Washington

Arthur M. Lauretano, MD
Instructor in Otology and Laryngology
Harvard Medical School
Associate Surgeon
Beth Israel Hospital
Associate Surgeon
Brigham and Women's Hospital
Boston, Massachusetts

Peter F. Lawrence, MD
Professor of Surgery
Chief, Vascular Surgery
University of Utah Health Sciences Center
Salt Lake City, Utah

Rande H. Lazar, MD
Director, Pediatric Otolaryngology
    Fellowship Program
Le Bonheur Children's Medical Center
Memphis, Tennessee

John P. Leonetti, MD
Associate Professor
Loyola University Medical Center
Foster G. McGaw at Loyola University
    Medical Center
Maywood, Illinois

Paul A. Levine, MD
Professor
Department of Otolaryngology-Head and
    Neck Surgery
University of Virginia School of Medicine
Acting Chairman and Director of Head
    and Neck Surgical Oncology
Department of Otolaryngology-Head and
    Neck Surgery
University of Virginia Health Sciences
    Center
Charlottesville, Virginia

Eric O. Lindbeck, MD
Assistant Professor of Otolaryngology-
    Head and Neck Surgery
East Carolina University School of
    Medicine
Pitt County Memorial Hospital
Greenville, North Carolina

**Christopher J. Linstrom, MD, CM, FACS,
    FRCSC**
Assistant Professor of Otolaryngology
New York Medical College
Valhalla, New York
Director of Otology, Neurotology, and
    Skull Base Surgery
New York Eye and Ear Infirmary
New York, New York

Neal M. Lofchy, MD, FRCSC
Fellow, Department of Otolaryngology/
    Bronchoesophagology
Rush Medical College
Clinical Instructor, Department of
    Otolaryngology/Bronchoesophagology
Rush-Presbyterian-St. Luke's Medical
    Center
Chicago, Illinois

Thomas C. Logan, MD
Resident Physician
Otolaryngology-Head and Neck Surgery
University of North Carolina at Chapel
    Hill School of Medicine
University of North Carolina Hospitals
    and Clinics
Chapel Hill, North Carolina

Frank E. Lucente, MD, FACS
Professor and Chairman
Department of Otolaryngology
Senior Associate Dean for Graduate
  Medical Education
State University of New York-Health
  Science Center at Brooklyn
Chairman, Department of Otolaryngology
Long Island College Hospital
University Hospital of Brooklyn
Brooklyn, New York

Elizabeth S. Luken, MS, CCC-SLP
Independent Consultant
Ohio State University
Columbus, Ohio

John D. Macias, MD
Private Practice
Phoenix, Arizona

Scott C. Manning, MD
Associate Professor and Chief
Department of Pediatric Otolaryngology-
  Head and Neck Surgery
University of Washington
Children's Hospital and Medical Center
Seattle, Washington

Andrew Marc Marlowe, MD
Assistant Professor
Medical College of Pennsylvania and
  Hahnemann University
Philadelphia, Pennsylvania

Michael D. Maves, MD, MBA
Adjunct Professor
Department of Otolaryngology-Head and
  Neck Surgery
Georgetown University
Washington, DC
Adjunct Professor
Department of Otolaryngology-Head and
  Neck Surgery
St. Louis University
St. Louis, Missouri
Georgetown University Medical Center
Washington, DC

John S. May, MD
Assistant Professor of Surgical Sciences
Department of Otolaryngology
Bowman Gray School of Medicine of
  Wake Forest University
Winston-Salem, North Carolina

Toby G. Mayer, MD, FACS
Indiana University School of Medicine
Clinical Professor
Otolaryngology-Head and Neck Surgery
  Division of Facial Plastic and
  Reconstructive Surgery
University of Southern California
Staff Membership, Cedars-Sinai Medical
  Center
Los Angeles, California

John A. McCurdy, Jr., MD
Oahu, Hawaii

Michael McGee, MD
Associate Professor of Otolaryngology
University of Oklahoma Health Science
  Center
Otologic Medical Clinic
Baptist Medical Center
Oklahoma City, Oklahoma

Becky L. McGraw-Wall, MD, FACS
Assistant Professor and Vice-Chairman
Department of Otolaryngology-Head and
  Neck Surgery
University of Texas Medical School
Houston, Texas

Chapman T. McQueen, MD
Resident, Otolaryngology-Head and Neck
  Surgery
University of North Carolina School of
  Medicine
University of North Carolina Hospitals
Chapel Hill, North Carolina

Jesus E. Medina, MD, FACS
Professor and Chairman, Department of
  Otorhinolaryngology
College of Medicine
The University of Oklahoma Health
  Sciences Center
Chief of Otorhinolaryngology
The University Hospital
Children's Hospital of Oklahoma
Veterans Affairs Medical Center
Oklahoma City, Oklahoma

Scott D. Meredith, MD
Assistant Professor of Otolaryngology-
  Head and Neck Surgery
University of North Carolina School of
  Medicine
Attending Physician, Department of
  Ear, Nose, and Throat/Head and Neck
  Surgery
Wake Area Health Education Center
Wake Medical Center
Charlottesville, Virginia

Alan G. Micco, MD
Assistant Professor
Department of Otolaryngology-Head and
  Neck Surgery
Northwestern University Medical School
Associate Staff
Northwestern Memorial Hospital
Chicago, Illinois

Robert H. Miller, MD, FACS
Professor and Chairman
Department of Otolaryngology-Head and
  Neck Surgery
Adjunct Professor
Department of Pediatrics
Vice Chief of Staff
Tulane University Hospital
New Orleans, Louisiana

Richard T. Miyamoto, MD
Arilla Spence DeVault Professor
Department of Otolaryngology-Head and
  Neck Surgery
School of Medicine
Chairman, Department of Otolaryngology-
  Head and Neck Surgery
Indiana University Medical Center
Indiana University
Indianapolis, Indiana

Juan F. Moscoso, MD
Assistant Professor, Department of
  Otolaryngology
The Mount Sinai School of Medicine
Attending, Department of Otolaryngology
Mount Sinai Medical Center
New York, New York

Jacqueline F. Mostert, MD
Chief Resident, Department of
    Otolaryngology/Head and Neck Surgery
The University of Texas Health Science
    Center at Houston
Houston, Texas

Harlan R. Muntz, MD
Associate Professor
Otolaryngology-Head and Neck Surgery
Washington University School of
    Medicine
St. Louis Children's Hospital
St. Louis, Missouri

Eugene N. Myers, MD
Professor and Chairman
Department of Otolaryngology
University of Pittsburgh School of
    Medicine
Professor
Department of Diagnostic Services
University of Pittsburgh School of Dental
    Medicine
Chairman
Department of Otolaryngology
University of Pittsburgh Medical Center
The Eye and Ear Institute of Pittsburgh
Pittsburgh, Pennsylvania

H. Bryan Neel III, MD, PhD
Professor of Otorhinolaryngology
Mayo Medical Center
Rochester Methodist Hospital
St. Mary's Hospital
Rochester, Minnesota

J. Gail Neely, MD, FACS
Professor and Director
Otology/Neurotology/Base of Skull
    Surgery
Director of Research, Department of
    Otolaryngology
Washington University School of
    Medicine
Professor, Program in Occupational
    Therapy
Washington University School of
    Medicine
Barnes Hospital
Jewish Hospital
St. Louis Children's Hospital
St. Louis, Missouri

James L. Netterville, MD
Associate Professor
Director, Division of Head and Neck
    Surgery
Department of Otolaryngology Head and
    Neck Surgery
Vanderbilt Medical Center
Nashville, Tennessee

Kerry D. Olsen, MD, FACS
Professor, Otorhinolaryngology-Head and
    Neck Surgery
Mayo Medical School
Consultant, Otorhinolaryngology-Head
    and Neck Surgery
Mayo Clinic
Rochester, Minnesota

Robert H. Ossoff, DMD, MD
Guy M. Maness Professor and Chairman
Department of Otolaryngology
Vanderbilt University Medical Center
Vanderbilt University Hospital
Nashville, Tennessee

Tapan A. Padhya, MD
University of Louisville
Division of Otology-Head and Neck
    Surgery
Louisville, Kentucky

Ira D. Papel, MD, FACS
Assistant Professor
Division of Facial Plastic and
    Reconstructive Surgery
Department of Otolaryngology-Head and
    Neck Surgery
The Johns Hopkins Medical Institutions
Baltimore, Maryland

Lorne S. Parnes, MD, FRCSC
Associate Professor, Department of
    Otolaryngology
University of Western Ontario
Chief, Department of Otolaryngology
University Hospital
London, Ontario
Canada

Steven M. Parnes, MD, FACS
Professor and Head
Division of Otolaryngology-Head and
    Neck Surgery
Albany Medical Center
Albany, New York

David S. Parsons, MD, FAAP, FACS
Professor of Surgery and Pediatrics
University of Missouri School of Medicine
The Children's Hospital
University Hospitals and Clinics
Columbia, Missouri

Bruce W. Pearson, MD, FACS, FRCSC
Serene M. and Francis C. Durling
    Professor of Otorhinolaryngology
Mayo Medical School
Chief of Otorhinolaryngology
St. Luke's Hospital
Jacksonville, Florida

Myles L. Pensak, MD
Professor
University of Cincinnati College of
    Medicine
Department of Otolaryngology-Head and
    Neck Surgery
University of Cincinnati Hospital
Cincinnati, Ohio

Rodney C. Perkins, MD
Professor of Surgery, Stanford School of
    Medicine
California Ear Institute at Stanford
Stanford, California

Guy J. Petruzzelli, MD, PhD
Assistant Professor
Head and Neck Surgical Oncology
Loyola Cancer Center
Loyola University Medical Center
Maywood, Illinois

George H. Petti, Jr., MD
Professor, Division of Otolaryngology-
    Head and Neck Surgery
Chief, Division of Otolaryngology-Head
    and Neck Surgery
Loma Linda University Medical Center
Loma Linda, California

Harold C. Pillsbury III, MD, FACS
Thomas J. Dark Distinguished Professor of
   Surgery
Professor and Chief
Otolaryngology/Head and Neck Surgery
Department of Surgery
University of North Carolina School of
   Medicine
Surgeon/Attending Physician
University of North Carolina Hospitals
   and Clinics
Chapel Hill, North Carolina

Robert L. Pincus, MD
Associate Professor of Otolaryngology
New York Medical College
Attending
Beth Israel Medical Center
New York, New York

Louis G. Portugal, MD
Assistant Professor of Otolaryngology-
   Head and Neck Surgery
University of Illinois College of Medicine
Attending Physician
Department of Otolaryngology-Head and
   Neck Surgery
Veterans Administration Medical Center
   (West Side)
Chicago, Illinois

Aaron J. Prussin, MD
Chief Resident
University of Tennessee
Department of Otolaryngology-Head and
   Neck Surgery
Memphis, Tennessee

Christopher H. Rassekh, MD
Assistant Professor
Chief, Division of Head and Neck Surgery
Department of Otolaryngology
University of Texas Medical Branch
Galveston, Texas

James S. Reilly, MD
Chief, Pediatric Otolaryngology
Professor of Otolaryngology and Pediatrics
Jefferson Medical College
Philadelphia, Pennsylvania
Chief, Division of Pediatric
   Otolaryngology
Alfred I. DuPont Institute Children's
   Hospital
Wilmington, Delaware

Gregory J. Renner, MD
Associate Professor of Surgery/Division of
   Otolaryngology
American Cancer Society Professor of
   Clinical Oncology
University of Missouri School of Medicine
Attending Physician
University of Missouri Hospital and
   Clinics
Ellis Fischel Cancer Center
Consulting Physician
Truman Memorial Veterans Hospital
Columbia, Missouri

Dale H. Rice, MD
Tiber/Alpert Professor and Chair
Department of Otolaryngology-Head and
   Neck Surgery
University of Southern California School
   of Medicine
Los Angeles, California

Wm. Russell Ries, MD
Assistant Professor
Vanderbilt University Medical Center
Nashville, Tennessee

K. Thomas Robbins, MD, FRCS, FACS
Professor and Chairman
Department of Otolaryngology-Head and
   Neck Surgery
University of Tennessee
Memphis, Tennessee

Thomas Romo III, MD, FACS
Director of Facial Plastic and
   Reconstructive Surgery
Department of Otolaryngology at the New
   York Eye and Ear Infirmary
Director of Facial Plastic and
   Reconstructive Surgery
Department of Otolaryngology at Lenox
   Hill Hospital
New York, New York

Seth I. Rosenberg, MD, FACS
Clinical Assistant Professor
Department of Otorhinolaryngology
University of Pennsylvania
Philadelphia, Pennsylvania
Director of Medical Education
Ear Research Foundation
Sarasota, Florida

Steven D. Schaefer, MD
Professor and Chair
Department of Otolaryngology and
   Communicative Sciences
New York Eye and Ear Infirmary
New York Medical College
Chair, Department of Otolaryngology
New York Eye and Ear Infirmary
St. Vincent Medical Center of New York
Westchester County Medical Center
New York, New York

David G. Schall, MD, MPH, FACS
Chief/Program Director
Otolaryngology-Head and Neck Surgery
Madigan Army Medical Center
Tacoma, Washington

Gary L. Schechter, MD, FACS
Chairman, Department of Surgery
Professor and Chairman, Otolaryngology-
   Head and Neck Surgery
Eastern Virginia Medical School
Norfolk, Virginia

Victor L. Schramm, Jr., MD
Assistant Clinical Professor
Department of Otolaryngology
University of Colorado Health Sciences
   Center
Director
The Center for Head and Neck and
   Craniofacial Skull Base Surgery
Presbyterian/St. Luke's Hospital
Denver, Colorado

Harold F. Schuknecht, MD
Walter Augustus LeCompte Professor
   Emeritus
Department of Otology and Laryngology
Harvard Medical School
Emeritus Chief Otolaryngology
Massachusetts Eye and Ear Infirmary
Boston, Massachusetts

Mitchell K. Schwaber, MD
Associate Professor
Vanderbilt University Medical Center
Nashville, Tennessee

Bruce A. Scott, MD
Assistant Clinical Professor
University of Louisville
Louisville, Kentucky

Frank W. Shagets, MD, FACS
Assistant Clinical Professor
University of Missouri
St. John's Region Medical Center
Freeman Health Care System
Joplin, Missouri

Aaron L. Shapiro, MD
Clinical Instructor
Department of Otolaryngology
Thomas Jefferson University Hospital
Philadelphia, Pennsylvania

John J. Shea, Jr., MD
Clinical Professor
Department of Otolaryngology
University of Tennessee School of
 Medicine
Shea Clinic
Memphis, Tennessee

William W. Shockley, MD, FACS
Associate Professor
Division of Otolaryngology/Head and
 Neck Surgery
University of North Carolina School of
 Medicine
Attending Physician/Surgeon
University of North Carolina Hospitals
 and Clinics
Chapel Hill, North Carolina

Kevin A. Shumrick, MD, FACS
Associate Professor of Clinical
 Otolaryngology
University of Cincinnati College of
 Medicine
Director, Division of Facial Plastic Surgery
 and Maxillofacial Trauma
University Hospital
Cincinnati, Ohio

William E. Silver, MD
Clinical Instructor
Emory University School of Medicine
Atlanta, Georgia
Associate Clinical Professor
Department of Surgery (Otolaryngology)
Medical College of Georgia
Augusta, Georgia

Herbert H. Silverstein, MD, FACS
Clinical Professor
Department of Otorhinolaryngology
University of Pennsylvania
Philadelphia, Pennsylvania
Clinical Professor of Surgery, Division of
 Otolaryngology
University of South Florida
President of the Florida Ear and Sinus
 Center and Ear Research Foundation
Active Staff
Sarasota Memorial Hospital
Doctors Hospital
Tampa, Florida

Lane F. Smith, MD
Institute of Facial and Cosmetic Surgery
Murray, Utah

Peter G. Smith, MD, PhD
Associate Clinical Professor of
 Otolaryngology-Head and Neck Surgery
Washington University School of
 Medicine
Attending Surgeon
St. John's Mercy Medical Center and
 Barnes Hospital
St. Louis, Missouri

Richard J. H. Smith, MD
Professor, Pediatric Otolaryngology
Director, Molecular Otolaryngology
 Research Laboratories
Director, Pediatric Otolaryngology
University of Iowa Hospitals and Clinics
Iowa City, Iowa

Timothy L. Smith, MD
Resident
Department of Otolaryngology-Head and
 Neck Surgery
University of North Carolina Hospitals
Chapel Hill, North Carolina

Kweon I. Stambaugh, MD, FACS
Colonel, Medical Corps
Associate Professor of Clinical Surgery
Uniformed Services University of Health
 Sciences
Bethesda, Maryland
Chief, Otolaryngology-Head and Neck
 Surgery
Walter Reed Army Medical Center
Washington, DC

Robert B. Stanley, Jr., MD, DDS
Professor, Department of Otolaryngology-
 Head and Neck Surgery
University of Washington School of
 Medicine
Chief, Department of Otolaryngology-
 Head and Neck Surgery
Harborview Medical Center
Seattle, Washington

C. Richard Stasney, MD, FACS
Clinical Associate Professor of
 Otolaryngology/Head and Neck Surgery
Baylor College of Medicine
Senior Attending Physician
The Methodist Hospital
Houston, Texas

Charles M. Stiernberg, MD, FACS
Professor and Chairman,
Department of Otolaryngology-Head and
 Neck Surgery
Assistant Dean for Continuing Medical
 Education
University of Texas Health Science Center
Chief of Service, Otolaryngology
Hermann Hospital
Houston, Texas

Fred J. Stucker, MD, FACS
Professor, Department of Otolaryngology-
 Head and Neck Surgery
Louisiana State University School of
 Medicine
Department Head
Louisiana State University Medical Center
Shreveport, Louisiana

Thomas A. Tami, MD
Associate Professor
Department of Otolaryngology-Head and
 Neck Surgery
University of Cincinnati
Cincinnati, Ohio

M. Eugene Tardy, Jr., MD, FACS
Professor of Clinical Otolaryngology-Head
  and Neck Surgery
Director, Division of Facial Plastic and
  Reconstructive Surgery
University of Illinois School of Medicine
  at Chicago
Professor of Clinical Otolaryngology-Head
  and Neck Surgery
Department of Otolaryngology
Indiana University
Bloomington, Indiana
Instructor in Otolaryngology-Head and
  Neck Surgery
Northwestern University
Chicago, Illinois

J. Regan Thomas, MD, FACS
Assistant Clinical Professor, Department
  of Otolaryngology
Washington University School of
  Medicine
St. Louis, Missouri
Director, The Facial Plastic Surgery Center
St. Louis, Missouri

Dean M. Toriumi, MD, FACS
Associate Professor
University of Illinois at Chicago College of
  Medicine
Division of Facial Plastic and
  Reconstructive Surgery
Department of Otolaryngology-Head and
  Neck Surgery
University of Illinois at Chicago Hospital
Chicago, Illinois

Jeffrey T. Vrabec, MD
Assistant Professor
Otology/Neurotology, Department of
  Otolaryngology
University of Texas Medical Branch
Galveston, Texas

David Van Wagner, MD
Fellow, Head and Neck Oncologic Surgery
Facial Plastic and Reconstructive Surgery
  in the Department of Otolaryngology-
  Head and Neck Surgery
University of Iowa
Iowa City, Iowa
Private Practice
Sioux City, Iowa

Tom D. Wang, MD
Associate Professor
Section of Facial Plastic and
  Reconstructive Surgery
Department of Otolaryngology/Head and
  Neck Surgery
Oregon Health Sciences University
Portland, Oregon

Roger E. Wehrs, MD
Clinical Professor
University of Oklahoma College of
  Medicine at Tulsa
Active Staff
Saint Francis Hospital
Tulsa, Oklahoma

Raymond L. Weiss, Jr., MD
Clinical Instructor
University of Texas Medical Branch
Galveston, Texas
Ocean Springs Hospital
Ocean Springs, Mississippi

Mark C. Weissler, MD
Associate Professor
Division of Otolaryngology
University of North Carolina
University of North Carolina Hospitals
Chapel Hill, North Carolina

Tracey G. Wellendorf, MD
Jennie Edmundson Hospital
Mercy Hospital
Council Bluffs, Iowa

Jay A. Werkhaven, MD
Assistant Professor
Vanderbilt University Medical Center
Nashville, Tennessee

Stephen J. Wetmore, MD
Professor and Chairman
Department of Otolaryngology-Head and
  Neck Surgery
School of Medicine
West Virginia University
Active Staff
West Virginia University Hospitals, Inc.
Morgantown, West Virginia

Ernest A. Weymuller, Jr., MD
Professor, Otolaryngology-Head and Neck
  Surgery
University of Washington School of
  Medicine
Professor and Chairman
Department of Otolaryngology-Head and
  Neck Surgery
University of Washington Medical Center
Seattle, Washington

Michael J. Wheatley, MD
Assistant Professor of Surgery
Division of Plastic and Reconstructive
  Surgery
Oregon Health Sciences University
Attending Physician
Oregon Health Sciences University
Portland Veterans Administration
  Hospital
Portland, Oregon

Mark H. Widick, MD
Clinical Assistant Professor
Nova Southeastern University
Staff Physician
North Broward Medical Center
Boca Raton, Florida

Richard J. Wiet, MD, FACS
Professor of Clinical Otolaryngology and
  Neurosurgery
Director of Fellowship Program
  (Neurotology, Skull Base Surgery)
Northwestern University Medical School
Chicago, Illinois
Attending Medical Staff
Northwestern Memorial Hospital
Chicago, Illinois
Hinsdale Hospital
Hinsdale, Illinois

Jeffrey L. Wilson, MD
Assistant Professor
Indiana University Medical Center
Indianapolis, Indiana

S. Anthony Wolfe, MD
Clinical Professor of Plastic Surgery
University of Miami School of Medicine
Miami, Florida

Brian R. Wong, MD
Assistant Professor
Director, Ophthalmic Plastic and
    Reconstructive Surgery
University of Texas Medical Branch
John Sealy Hospital
Galveston, Texas

Frank S. H. Wong, MD
Associate Professor
The University of Tennessee, Memphis
Department of Otolaryngology-Head and
    Neck Surgery
Memphis, Tennessee

Robert E. Wood, MD, PhD
Professor of Pediatrics
University of North Carolina-Chapel Hill
Director, UNC Center for Pediatric
    Bronchology
University of North Carolina Hospitals/
    North Carolina Children's Hospital
Chapel Hill, North Carolina

Gayle Ellen Woodson, MD, FACS, FRCSC
Professor of Otolaryngology
University of Tennessee, Memphis
Director, University of Tennessee
    Methodist Voice Institute
Methodist Hospital
Staff Surgeon, Le Bonheur Children's
    Hospital
Memphis, Tennessee

Wendell G. Yarbrough, MD
Fellow, Surgical Oncology
University of North Carolina School of
    Medicine
Division of Otolaryngology
University of North Carolina Hospitals
Chapel Hill, North Carolina

Ramzi T. Younis, MD
Chief of Pediatric Otolaryngology
Assistant Professor of Surgery and
    Pediatrics
Yale University School of Medicine
Yale-New Haven Hospital
New Haven, Connecticut

Steven M. Zeitels, MD, FACS
Assistant Professor
Department of Otology and Laryngology
Harvard Medical School
Assistant Surgeon and Associate Medical
    Director of Voice and Speech
    Laboratory
Massachusetts Eye and Ear Infirmary
Boston, Massachusetts

Contents

Section I. **HEAD AND NECK** 1
Byron J. Bailey

■ **Salivary Glands** 2

1. Parotid Superficial Lobectomy 2
   Kerry D. Olsen

2. Parotid Deep Lateral Lobectomy With
   Nerve Sparing 4
   Kerry D. Olsen

3. Intraoral Salivary Gland Tumor Removal (Parotid
   Intraoral Deep-Lobe Tumor Excision) 6
   Kerry D. Olsen

4. Total Parotidectomy With the Seventh
   Nerve Spared 8
   Dale H. Rice

5. Total Parotidectomy With Nerve Resection
   and Graft 10
   Dale H. Rice

6. Submandibular Salivary Gland Excision 12
   Kerry D. Olsen

7. Sublingual Salivary Gland Tumor Excision 14
   Dale H. Rice

8. Salivary Gland Trauma Management 16
   Dale H. Rice

■ **Nose and Maxilla** 18

9. Total Rhinectomy 18
   Lanny G. Close

10. Midline Forehead Flap Nasal Reconstruction 20
    Lanny G. Close

11. Lateral Rhinotomy 22
    Lanny G. Close

12. Medial Maxillectomy 24
    Lanny G. Close

13. Weber-Ferguson Approach With Subtotal
    Maxillectomy and Total Maxillectomy
    With Orbital Preservation 26
    Lanny G. Close

14. Radical Maxillectomy With Orbital
    Exenteration 30
    Ivo P. Janecka and Guy J. Petruzzelli

15. Craniofacial Resection, Including the Ethmoid
    Labyrinth and Cribriform Plate 34
    Guy J. Petruzzelli and Ivo P. Janecka

16. Facial Translocation for Nasopharyngeal
    Angiofibroma Resection 38
    Ivo P. Janecka and Guy J. Petruzzelli

■ **Lips** 42

17. Vermilionectomy 42
    John B. Kinsella

18. Vermilionectomy Plus Wedge Excision 44
    John B. Kinsella

19. Lip Excision: W-Excision and Pentagonal
    Shield Pattern 46
    John B. Kinsella

20. Abbe-Estlander Reconstruction of the Lips
    (Lip Switch Flap) 48
    Tom D. Wang and H. Bryan Neel III

21. Gillies Fan Flap 50
    Christopher H. Rassekh

22. Karapandzic Flap Lip Reconstruction 52
    Ricardo L. Carrau

23. Check Advancement Flaps for
    Lip Reconstruction 54
    Christopher H. Rassekh

24. Pectoralis Major Flap and Deltopectoral Flap
    Reconstruction of the Lips 58
    Frank W. Shagets

25. Nasolabial Flap for Upper Lip 60
    Christopher H. Rassekh

26. Reconstruction of the Upper Lip: Advancement
    Flaps with Modified Burow's Technique 62
    Ricardo L. Carrau

27. Lateral Commissure Repair 64
    David V. Wagner and Henry T. Hoffman

■ **Oral Cavity** 66

28. Surgical Approaches 66
    C. Ron Cannon

29. Partial Anterior Glossectomy 70
    C. Ron Cannon

30. Partial Posterior Glossectomy of the
    Tongue Base 72
    C. Ron Cannon

31. Partial Midline Glossectomy of the
    Tongue Base 76
    Jonas T. Johnson

32. Near-Total Glossectomy 78
    Jonas T. Johnson

33. Total Glossectomy 82
    Jonas T. Johnson

34. Anterior Floor of Mouth Resection 84
    Eugene N. Myers

35. Lateral Floor of Mouth Resection **86**
Eugene N. Myers

36. Floor of Mouth Resection With Anterior
Mandible Invasion **88**
Eugene N. Myers

37. Floor of Mouth Resection With Lateral
Mandible Invasion **90**
Eugene N. Myers

38. Marginal Resection of Posterior Floor of Mouth
with Mandibular Invasion **92**
C. Ron Cannon

39. Alveolar Ridge Resection **94**
Robert H. Miller and Gerard J. Gianoli

40. Resection of the Hard Palate **96**
Robert H. Miller and Gerard J. Gianoli

41. Resection of the Soft Palate **98**
Robert H. Miller and Gerard J. Gianoli

42. Partial-Thickness and Full-Thickness
Buccal Resection **100**
Robert H. Miller and Gerard J. Gianoli

43. Midline, Paramedian, Lateral, and Ascending Ramus
Mandibular Osteotomy **102**
Robert H. Miller

44. Tongue Flaps for Reconstruction **104**
Lawrence W. DeSanto and Kerry D. Olsen

45. Intraoral Skin Grafting **106**
Lawrence W. DeSanto

46. Segmental Resection for Mandibular Cysts
and Tumors **108**
Robert H. Miller and Gerard J. Gianoli

47. Superficial and Plunging Ranula Excision **110**
William W. Shockley and C. Gaelyn Garrett

48. Resection of Tonsil and Retromolar Trigone With
and Without Mandibular Involvement **112**
William W. Shockley

49. Vestibuloplasty **116**
William W. Shockley and William R. Blythe

50. Mandibular Reconstruction **118**
William W. Shockley

■ **Ear 124**

51. Auriculectomy **124**
Steven D. Schaefer

52. Pinna Reconstruction: Regional, Wedge, and
Stellate Excision **126**
Steven D. Schaefer and Thomas Romo III

53. Pinna and Conchal Reconstruction With
Composite Grafts **130**
Steven D. Schaefer and Thomas Romo III

54. Local Excision and Skin Graft **132**
Steven D. Schaefer and Christopher J. Linstrom

55. Superficial, Intermediate, and Radical Temporal
Bone Resection **134**
J. Gail Neely and Harold C. Pillsbury III

■ **Neck 138**

56. Various Incisions for Neck Surgery **138**
K. Thomas Robbins

57. Radical Neck Dissection **140**
Jesus E. Medina

58. Supraomohyoid Neck Dissection **144**
Jesus E. Medina

59. Modified Radical Neck Dissection Preserving the
Spinal Accessory Nerve **148**
Jesus E. Medina

60. Modified Radical Neck Dissection Preserving the
Spinal Accessory Nerve, the Internal Jugular Vein
and the Sternocleidomastoid Muscle **150**
Jesus E. Medina

61. Transsternal Mediastinal Node Dissection **154**
Michael D. Maves

62. Cervical Node Biopsy **158**
Michael D. Maves

63. Scalene Node Biopsy **160**
Michael D. Maves

64. Posterolateral Neck Dissection **162**
Jesus E. Medina

65. Excision of Supraclavicular Space Masses **164**
Michael D. Maves

66. Drainage of Deep Neck Space Abscesses **166**
Michael D. Maves

67. Management of Penetrating Injuries
to the Neck **168**
Michael D. Maves

■ **Larynx 170**

68. Endoscopic Partial Laryngectomy for
Supraglottic Disease **170**
Steven M. Zeitels

69. Endoscopic Partial Laryngectomy at the
Glottic Level **172**
Robert H. Ossoff and Mark S. Courey

70. Laryngofissure and Cordectomy **174**
Christopher H. Rassekh

71. Vertical Partial Laryngectomy, Including the
Thyroid Cartilage **176**
Harsha V. Gopal and Marvin P. Fried

72. Anterior Commissure and Anterolateral Vertical
Partial Laryngectomy **180**
Harsha V. Gopal and Marvin P. Fried

73. Vertical Partial Laryngectomy **184**
Byron J. Bailey

74. Vertical Partial Laryngectomy With Excision
(Subtotal or Three-Quarter Laryngectomy) **188**
Arthur M. Lauretano and Marvin P. Fried

75. Supraglottic Laryngectomy (Horizontal
Hemilaryngectomy) **190**
Frank Wong

76. Extended Supraglottic Partial Laryngectomy **194**
Frank Wong

77. Near-Total Laryngectomy **196**
Bruce W. Pearson

78. Total Laryngectomy **200**
Frank Wong

79. Total Laryngectomy With Extension **204**
Frank Wong

80. Total Pharyngolaryngectomy 206
Frank Wong

81. Tracheoesophageal Shunt
(Voice Rehabilitation) 210
Aaron J. Prussin

82. Recurrent Laryngeal Nerve Section
and Avulsion 212
James L. Netterville

83. Laryngeal Diversion 214
Gayle E. Woodson

84. Arytenoidectomy 216
Gayle E. Woodson

■ **Thyroid and Parathyroid 218**

85. Thyroid Lobectomy and Isthmusectomy 218
Robert H. Ossoff and Mark S. Courey

86. Subtotal Thyroidectomy 222
Robert H. Ossoff and Mark S. Courey

87. Mediastinal (Retrosternal) Goiter 224
Robert H. Ossoff and Mark S. Courey

88. Total Thyroidectomy 228
Jack L. Gluckman and Louis G. Portugal

89. Total Thyroidectomy With Paratracheal and
Superior Mediastinal Node Dissection 230
Jack L. Gluckman and Louis G. Portugal

90. Total Thyroidectomy With Tracheal Resection for
Malignant Invasion 232
Jack L. Gluckman and Louis G. Portugal

91. Parathyroidectomy 236
George H. Petti

92. Total Parathyroidectomy
and Autotransplantation 240
George H. Petti

93. Recurrent Hyperparathyroidism and Cancer
of the Parathyroid 242
George H. Petti

■ **Pharynx, Trachea, and Parapharyngeal
Space 246**

94. Tracheostomy 246
Nicholas J. Cassisi

95. Tracheal Reconstruction 248
Nicholas J. Cassisi

96. Tracheal Resection and Reanastomosis 250
Nicholas J. Cassisi

97. Cervical Esophagostomy 254
Gary L. Schechter

98. Pharyngeal Pouches (Zenker's Diverticulum) 256
Nicholas J. Cassisi

99. Mediastinal Exploration and Dissection 258
Gary L. Schechter

100. Cricopharyngeal Myotomy and Myectomy 262
Gary L. Schechter

101. Revision of Stenotic Tracheostomy 264
Nicholas J. Cassisi

102. Partial and Total Pharyngectomy 266
Gary L. Schechter

103. Pharyngeal Reconstruction 270
Gary L. Schechter

■ **Cysts, Abscesses, Vessels 274**

104. Thyroglossal Duct Cyst 274
Charles M. Stiernberg

105. Branchial Cleft Cysts 276
Charles M. Stiernberg

106. Lymphangioma 278
Charles M. Stiernberg

107. Dermoid Cyst of the Neck 280
Charles M. Stiernberg

108. Excision of Laryngocele 282
Robert L. Pincus

109. Carotid Body Tumor Resection 284
R. Kim Davis

110. External Carotid Artery Ligation 286
Robert L. Pincus

111. Lipoma Excision or Liposuction 288
Charles M. Stiernberg

112. Drainage of Neck Abscesses 290
Robert L. Pincus

113. Major Vessel Repair 292
Peter F. Lawrence and R. Kim Davis

Section II. **OTOLOGIC PROCEDURES 295**
J. Gail Neely

■ **External Auditory Canal
and Tympanic Membrane 296**

114. Meatoplasty and Canaloplasty 296
Myles L. Pensak and Daniel J. Kelley

115. Excision of Exostoses or Osteoma 298
John F. Kveton

116. Soft Tissue Canal Stenosis 300
Jay B. Farrior

117. Myringotomy Tube Placement and Removal 302
Jay A. Werkhaven

118. Tympanomeatal Flap for Exploratory
Tympanotomy 304
Jay B. Farrior

119. Myringoplasty and Tympanoplasty Type I 308
Mitchell K. Schwaber

120. First Branchial Cleft Fistula
and Cyst Excision 312
William B. Armstrong

■ **Middle Ear and Ossicular Chain 314**

121. Tympanoplasty Type II 314
Roger E. Wehrs

122. Type III Tympanoplasty 318
Sam E. Kinney

123. Type IV Tympanoplasty 322
Harold F. Schuknecht

124. Reconstruction of Large Tympanic
Membrane Perforations 324
Rodney C. Perkins

125. Cholesteatoma Removal from the Middle Ear   328
Sam E. Kinney

126. Stapedotomy and Stapedectomy   330
Richard J. Wiet and Alan G. Micco

127. Perilymphatic Fistula Repair   332
Robert I. Kohut

128. Office Repair of Tympanic Membrane Perforations   336
Robert K. Jackler and Hayes B. Gladstone

129. Tympanic Neurectomy   338
Sam E. Kinney

■ Mastoid   340

130. Simple Mastoidectomy   340
Jeffrey T. Vrabec

131. Modified Radical Mastoidectomy   344
Michael E. Glasscock III, David G. Schall, John D. Macias, and Mark H. Widick

132. Mastoidectomy: Radical Cavity and Middle Ear Obliteration   348
Vincent N. Carrasco

133. Implantation of an Audiant Bone Conductor Hearing Device   352
J. V. D. Hough and Michael McGee

134. Glomus Tympanicum   354
Jeffrey T. Vrabec

135. Petrous Apicectomy   356
J. Gail Neely

136. Facial Recess Approach   358
Jeffrey T. Vrabec

137. Management of Brain Herniation and Cerebrospinal Fluid Leak Repair   360
J. Gail Neely

■ Facial Nerve   362

138. Facial Nerve Grafting   362
Newton J. Coker

139. Hypoglossal—Facial Cranial Nerve Crossover Techniques   366
Newton J. Coker

140. Facial Nerve Decompression   368
J. Gail Neely

141. Tarsorrhaphy   372
Eugene L. Alford

142. Eyelid Reanimation Procedures   374
Eugene L. Alford

■ Cochlea, Labyrinth   376

143. Labyrinthectomy   376
Richard T. Miyamoto and Cynthia L. Kish

144. Cochlear Implants   380
Richard T. Miyamoto

145. Endolymphatic Sac Exposure, Decompression, or Shunt   382
I. Kaufman Arenberg

146. Posterior Semicircular Canal Occlusion   384
Lorne S. Parnes

147. Singular Neurectomy   386
Richard R. Gacek

148. Streptomycin Perfusion of the Labyrinth   388
John J. Shea, Jr.

■ Transtemporal Skull Base   390

149. Vestibular Neurectomy   390
Herbert H. Silverstein and Seth I. Rosenberg

150. Translabyrinthine Approach to Acoustic Neuroma   394
William F. House and Karen Jo Doyle

151. Middle Fossa Resection of Acoustic Neuroma   398
Derald E. Brackmann

152. Acoustic Neuroma Resection (Retrosigmoid Approach)   402
Noel L. Cohen

■ Lateral Skull Base   406

153. Extensive Glomus Tumor Excision   406
C. Gary Jackson

154. Extreme Lateral Transcondylar Approach   410
Peter G. Smith, G. Robert Kletzker, and Robert J. Backer

155. Access to the Nasopharynx   414
Victor L. Schramm, Jr. and Andrew M. Marlowe

156. Petrosal Approach   418
John P. Leonetti and Ossama Al-Mefty

■ Congenital Aural Atresia   422

157. Repair of Congenital Aural Atresia   422
Paul R. Lambert

Section III.   PLASTIC AND RECONSTRUCTIVE SURGERY   427
Karen H. Calhoun

■ Otoplasty and External Ear   428

158. Otoplasty for the Deep Conchal Bowl   428
Peter A. Adamson and Minas S. Constantinides

159. Otoplasty for the Antihelical Fold   430
Peter A. Adamson and Minas S. Constantinides

160. Otoplasty Refinement Techniques   434
Peter A. Adamson and Minas S. Constantinides

161. Partial and Total Avulsions of the Auricle   436
F. Brian Gibson

162. Auricular Hematoma   440
F. Brian Gibson

■ Rhinoplasty   442

163. Nasal–Facial Analysis   442
Becky L. McGraw-Wall

164. Local Anesthesia for Nasal Surgery   444
Bruce A. Scott

165. Nasal Septoplasty and Submucous Resection   446
Richard L. Goode and Lane F. Smith

166. Rhinoplasty   450
Karen H. Calhoun

167. Osteotomies   452
Karen H. Calhoun

168. Nasal Tip Procedures   454
*M. Eugene Tardy, Jr., Eric O. Lindbeck,
and James A. Heinrich*

169. Nasal Base Procedures   458
*M. Eugene Tardy, Jr., Eric O. Lindbeck,
and James A. Heinrich*

170. Nasal Dorsal Changes   462
Frank M. Kamer

171. Major Nasal Reconstruction   464
Kevin A. Shumrick

172. Outline Revision Rhinoplasty   466
Frank M. Kamer

173. Nasal Valve Surgery   470
Richard L. Goode and Lane F. Smith

174. Cleft-Lip Nasal Repair   472
G. Richard Holt

175. Rhinophyma Surgical Techniques   476
Fred J. Stucker and Denis K. Hoasjoe

176. Non-Caucasian Rhinoplasty   478
Fred J. Stucker and Robert F. Aarstad

■ **Mentoplasty and Malarplasty   480**

177. Mentoplasty Outline   480
Kweon I. Stambaugh

178. Chin Implant   482
Kweon I. Stambaugh

179. Genioplasty: Horizontal Position Changes   484
Eric J. Dierks

180. Genioplasty: Vertical Position Changes   486
Eric J. Dierks

181. Malar Implants   488
William E. Silver

■ **Rhytidectomy and Related Procedures   490**

182. Rhytidectomy Incisions   490
Frank M. Kamer

183. Rhytidectomy Using Superficial
Musculoaponeurotic System Plication
and a Short Flap or Long Flap   492
Ira D. Papel

184. Liposuction of the Neck With
Facelift Pretunneling   496
Douglas D. Dedo

185. Submental Tuck for the Aging Neck   498
Douglas D. Dedo

186. Analysis of the Upper One Third of the
Face and Neck   500
Wayne F. Larrabee, Jr.

187. Browlifts: Coronal, Trichophytic,
Pretrichal   502
Wayne F. Larrabee, Jr.

188. Browlifts: Direct, Indirect, Midforehead   504
Wayne F. Larrabee, Jr.

189. Injections of Collagen or Fat   506
Douglas D. Dedo

190. Dermabrasion   508
Wayne F. Larrabee, Jr.

191. Chemical Peels   510
F. Brian Gibson

■ **Blepharoplasty   512**

192. Upper Lid Blepharoplasty   512
G. Richard Holt

193. Lower Lid Blepharoplasty   514
John A. McCurdy, Jr.

194. Upper Lid Blepharoplasty for the Asian Eye   518
John A. McCurdy, Jr.

195. Eyelid Laceration Repair   520
Jean Edwards Holt

196. Upper Eyelid Defect Repair   522
Jean Edwards Holt

197. Lower Eyelid Defect Repair   526
Jean Edwards Holt

198. Surgical Treatment of Lower Lid Malposition
After Blephasoplasty   528
John A. McCurdy, Jr.

■ **Facial Trauma   530**

199. Closed Reduction of Nasal Fractures   530
Stephen J. Wetmore

200. Nasal Septal Fracture-Dislocation   532
Stephen J. Wetmore

201. Zygomatic Arch Reduction   534
Thomas A. Tami

202. Zygomatic-Trimalar Reduction and Fixation   536
Thomas A. Tami

203. Wiring and Plating of a Palatal Fracture   538
Robert M. Kellman

204. LeFort I Fracture Repair (Guerin's
Fracture Repair)   540
Wm. Russell Ries and Mark A. Clymer

205. LeFort II Repair of Pyramidal Fracture   542
Wm. Russell Ries and Mark A. Clymer

206. LeFort III Fracture Repair (Craniofacial
Disjunction)   544
Wm. Russell Ries and Mark A. Clymer

207. Orbital Blowout Fracture   548
Wm. Russell Ries and Mark A. Clymer

208. Nasoethmoid Fracture   550
John L. Frodel

209. Medial Canthal Tendon Repair   552
John L. Frodel

210. Nasolacrimal System Evaluation and Repair   554
Jean Edwards Holt

211. Anterior Wall Frontal Sinus Fracture **558**
Gerald S. Gussack

212. Posterior Wall Frontal Sinus Fracture **560**
Gerald S. Gussack

213. Frontonasal Duct Injury **562**
Gerald S. Gussack

214. Late Repair of Traumatic Enophthalmous **564**
John L. Frodel

215. Pediatric Facial Fracture **566**
Gerald S. Gussack

216. Intermaxillary Fixation **568**
William D. Clark

217. Mandibular Fractures: Open Reduction and Internal Fixation With Compression Plating **570**
Robert M. Kellman

218A. Mandibular Fracture: Open Reduction and Internal Fixation With Noncompression Plating **572**
Robert M. Kellman

218B. Mandibular Fracture: Open Reduction and Internal Fixation With Lag Screws **574**
Robert M. Kellman

219. Mandibular Fractures: External Fixation With a Biphase Apparatus **576**
Robert M. Kellman

220. Mandibular Fractures: Use of Dentures and Splints **578**
William D. Clark

221. Mandibular Fractures: Special Problems in Children **580**
William D. Clark

■ **Laryngoplasty and Tracheoplasty** **582**

222. Anterior Laryngotracheal Decompression (Anterior Cricoid Split) **582**
Gerald B. Healy

223. Posterior Glottic Split With Cartilage Graft **584**
Richard J. H. Smith

224. Anterior and Posterior Laryngotracheal Reconstruction **586**
Richard J. H. Smith

225. Laryngeal Webs **590**
C. Richard Stasney

226. Stroboscopy **592**
Elizabeth S. Luken and James L. Netterville

227. Thyroplasty (Phonosurgery) Type I **594**
C. Richard Stasney

228. Thyroplasty (Phonosurgery) Type II **598**
Charles N. Ford

229. Thyroplasty (Phonosurgery) Type III **600**
Charles N. Ford

230. Thyroplasty (Phonosurgery) Type IV **602**
Charles N. Ford

231. Vocal Cord Injection for Paralysis **604**
Charles N. Ford

232. Laryngeal Fracture Repair **606**
Charles N. Ford

■ **Local and Regional Flaps** **608**

233. Nasolabial Flap **608**
Paul A. Levine and Scott D. Meredith

234. Bilobed Flap **610**
Jacqueline F. Mostert

235. Median Forehead Flap **612**
Dean M. Toriumi

236. Glabellar Flaps **614**
Linda Gage-White

237. Cheek–Neck Rotation Flap **616**
Ramon M. Esclamado

238. Rhomboid Flap **618**
Ira D. Papel

239. Deltopectoral Flap **620**
David W. Eisele

240. A to T Flap **622**
Karen H. Calhoun

241. Z-plasty **624**
Ira D. Papel

242. Advancement Flaps **626**
Linda Gage-White

243. Triple Rhomboid Flaps **628**
Karen H. Calhoun

244. Pericranial Flap **630**
Paul A. Levine and Scott D. Meredith

245. Tissue Expansion **632**
Richard E. Hayden

246. Pectoralis Major Myocutaneous Flap **636**
Ernest A. Weymuller, Jr. and Michael G. Glenn

247. Superior Trapezius Flap **640**
James L. Netterville

248. Lateral Island Trapezius Flap **642**
James L. Netterville

249. Lower Island Trapezius Flap **644**
James L. Netterville

250. Latissimus Dorsi Myocutaneous Flap **648**
James L. Netterville

251. Temporoparietal Fascia Flap **652**
Steven L. Garner and S. Anthony Wolfe

252. Temporalis Muscle Flap **654**
Steven L. Garner and S. Anthony Wolfe

253. Platysma Flap **656**
Steven L. Garner and S. Anthony Wolfe

254. Sternocleidomastoid Flap **658**
Steven L. Garner and S. Anthony Wolfe

■ **Grafts and Free Flaps** **660**

255. Skin Grafts, Dermal Grafts, and Mucosal Grafts **660**
Bruce A. Scott and Thomas V. Conley

256. Cartilage Grafts from the Septum **664**
Bruce A. Scott

257. Ear Cartilage Grafts **666**
M. Eugene Tardy, Jr., Eric O. Lindbeck and James A. Heinrich

258. Composite Grafts from the Ear   668
     Bruce A. Scott and Tapan A. Padhya

259. Harvesting Rib Grafts   670
     John L. Frodel

260. Harvesting Calvarial Bone Grafts   672
     John L. Frodel

261. Nerve Grafts Using the Greater Auricular
     and Sural Nerves   674
     Steven M. Parnes

262. Microvascular Surgery   678
     Eugene L. Alford

263. Scapular Free Flap, With and Without Bone   680
     Juan F. Moscoso

264. Iliac Crest Internal Oblique Free Flap   684
     Juan F. Moscoso

265. Radial Forearm Flap   688
     Juan F. Moscoso

266. Lateral Arm Free Flap   690
     Ramon M. Esclamado and William R. Carroll

267. Fibular Osteocutaneous Free Flap   692
     William R. Carroll and Ramon M. Esclamado

268. Inferior Rectus Abdominis Free Flap   694
     Eugene L. Alford

269. Free Jejunal Transfer   696
     Eugene L. Alford

■ Facial Reanimation and Fascial Sling   698

270. Cross Facial Nerve Graft   698
     Steven M. Parnes

271. Nerve-Muscle Pedicle   700
     Steven M. Parnes

272. Static Slings   702
     G. Richard Holt

273. Dynamic Temporalis and Masseter
     Muscle Transposition   706
     G. Richard Holt

■ Mandibular Surgery, Cleft Lip/Palate,
   TMJ Surgery   710

274. Sagittal Osteotomy of the Mandibular
     Ramus   710
     Eric J. Dierks

275. LeFort I Osteotomy and Advancement   712
     Eric J. Dierks

276. Transnasal Repair of Choanal Atresia   714
     Richard J.H. Smith

277. Transpalatal Repair of Choanal Atresia   716
     Richard J.H. Smith

278. Unilateral Cleft Lip Repair Using a Rotation-
     Advancement Technique   720
     Tom D. Wang

279. Bilateral Cleft Lip Repair   724
     Tom D. Wang

280. Complete Secondary Palatal Cleft Repair (Two-Flap
     Palatoplasty With Intravelar Veloplasty)   726
     Becky L. McGraw-Wall

281. Incomplete Secondary Palatal Cleft Repair   728
     Becky L. McGraw-Wall

282. Complete Unilateral Cleft Palate Repair (Two-Flap
     Palatoplasty With Intravelar Veloplasty)   730
     Becky L. McGraw-Wall

283. Oronasal and Oroantral Fistula Repair   732
     Becky L. McGraw-Wall and Jennifer Keir-Garza

284. Superiorly Based Pharyngeal Flap   734
     Tom D. Wang

285. Surgical Approaches to the
     Temporomandibular Joint   736
     David A. Cottrell

286. Temporomandibular Joint Articular Disc
     Repositioning   738
     David A. Cottrell

287. Bone Graft Reconstruction of the
     Temporomandibular Joint   740
     David A. Cottrell

288. Skeletal Correction of Hemifacial
     Microsomia   742
     Michael J. Wheatley

■ Excision of Skin Lesions and Scar Revision   744

289. Aesthetic Facial Subunits   744
     Aaron L. Shapiro and J. Regan Thomas

290. Local Excision and Primary Closure   746
     Aaron L. Shapiro and J. Regan Thomas

291. Scar Excision   748
     Dean M. Toriumi

292. Complex Facial Laceration Repair   752
     Dean M. Toriumi

■ Aesthetic Reconstruction   754

293. Grafts for Hair Transplantation   754
     Toby G. Mayer

294. Fleming-Mayer Flap Procedure   758
     Toby G. Mayer

295. Scalp Reduction   762
     Toby G. Mayer

296. Tissue Expansion   766
     Toby G. Mayer

Section IV.   **ENDOSCOPY**   769
           Amy R. Coffey

■ Laryngoscopy   770

297. Direct Laryngoscopy With
     and Without Biopsy   770
     Ronald W. Deskin

298. Nasopharyngoscopy   772
     Ellen M. Friedman

299. True Vocal Cord Injection for Paralysis   774
     Amelia F. Drake and Wendell G. Yarbrough

300. Laser Laryngoscopy for Papilloma Removal **776**
Ronald W. Deskin

301. Laser Arytenoidectomy **780**
Harold C. Pillsbury III and Timothy L. Smith

302. Microsuspension Laryngoscopy and Laser Excision of Early-Stage Vocal Cord Carcinoma **782**
Harold C. Pillsbury III and John E. Buenting

303. Microsurgery for Vocal Cord Polyps, Cysts, and Nodules **784**
Douglas E. Henrich and Harold C. Pillsbury III

■ Esophagoscopy **786**

304. Esophagoscopy **786**
Orval E. Brown

305. Esophagoscopy for Foreign Body Removal **788**
Ellen M. Friedman

306. Esophagoscopy for Caustic Ingestion **790**
Ellen M. Friedman

307. Esophagoscopic Dilation Under Direct Vision **792**
Orval E. Brown

308. Antegrade Esophageal Dilation **794**
Orval E. Brown

309. Retrograde Esophageal Dilation **796**
Orval E. Brown

■ Bronchoscopy **798**

310. Diagnostic Bronchoscopy **798**
C. Gaelyn Garrett and Amelia F. Drake

311. Bronchoscopy for a Foreign Body **800**
Ronald W. Deskin

312. Bronchoscopic Stricture Dilation **804**
Amelia F. Drake and Tracey G. Wellendorf

313. Laser Techniques for Bronchoscopy **806**
Amelia F. Drake and Jeffrey L. Wilson

314. Flexible Bronchoscopy **808**
Amelia F. Drake and Robert E. Wood

Section V. **PEDIATRIC AND GENERAL OTOLARYNGOLOGY 811**
Byron J. Bailey and Amy R. Coffey

■ Tonsillectomy, Adenoidectomy, UPPP **812**

315. Tonsillectomy **812**
Byron J. Bailey

316. Lingual Tonsillectomy **814**
Linda Brodsky

317. Adenoidectomy **816**
Linda Brodsky

318. Uvulopalatopharyngoplasty **818**
Jack A. Coleman, Jr. and James S. Reilly

319. Extended Uvulopalatopharyngoplasty **820**
Jack A. Coleman, Jr. and James S. Reilly

320. Hyoid Myotomy Suspension and Genioglossus Advancement **822**
Jack A. Coleman, Jr. and James S. Reilly

■ Nasal Polypectomy, Septal Surgery **824**

321. Nasal Polypectomy **824**
Frank E. Lucente

322. Endoscopic Excision of Antrochoanal Polyps **826**
Andrew N. Goldberg and Donald C. Lanza

323. Submucous Resection of the Nasal Septum **828**
Frank E. Lucente

324. Septoplasty **830**
Harold C. Pillsbury III and Mark C. Weissler

325. Extracranial Closure of Cerebrospinal Fluid Rhinorrhea Using a Mucoperiosteal Flap **832**
Donald C. Lanza and Andrew N. Goldberg

326. Septal Dermoplasty **836**
Harold C. Pillsbury III and Jeffrey L. Wilson

327. Repair of Septal Perforation **838**
Harold C. Pillsbury III and Chapman T. McQueen

328. Septal Resection for Benign and Malignant Neoplasia **840**
Harold C. Pillsbury III and Thomas C. Logan

329. Nasal Cavity Examination With Nasal Biopsy or Foreign Body Removal **842**
Ronald W. Deskin

330. Submucous Resection of the Turbinate **844**
Frank E. Lucente

331. Endoscopic Management of Nasal Encephaloceles and Meningoceles **846**
Donald C. Lanza and David W. Kennedy

332. Nasal Congenital Dermoid Cyst and Sinus Opening **850**
Peter J. Koltai

333. Sublabial and Septal Incisions **852**
Gregory Renner

■ Maxillary, Ethmoid, and Sphenoid Sinuses **854**

334. Intranasal Antrostomy Through the Inferior Meatus **854**
Rande H. Lazar and Ramzi T. Younis

335. Sublabial Antrostomy (Caldwell-Luc Procedure) **856**
Rande H. Lazar and Ramzi T. Younis

336. Transantral Ligation of the Internal Maxillary Artery **858**
John S. May

337. Vidian Neurectomy **860**
Robert M. Bumsted and Neal M. Lofchy

338. Intranasal Ethmoidectomy **864**
Rande H. Lazar and Ramzi T. Younis

339. External Ethmoidectomy **866**
Harlan R. Muntz

340. External Frontoethmoidectomy **868**
Christopher H. Rassekh

341. Transantral Ethmoidectomy **870**
George D. Chonkich

342. Intranasal Sphenoidectomy **872**
Peter J. Koltai

343. Transethmoidal Sphenoidectomy **874**
Raymond L. Weiss

344. Transsphenoidal Hypophysectomy **876**
Peter J. Koltai

345. Ligation of the Anterior Ethmoid Artery **878**
John S. May

346. Maxillary Decompression for Exophthalmus **880**
Scott C. Manning

347. Midfacial Degloving Procedure **882**
Dennis M. Crockett

348. Endoscopic Maxillary, Ethmoid, Sphenoidectomy **886**
Rande H. Lazar and Ramzi T. Younis

349. Endoscopic Frontal Sinusectomy **890**
Ramzi T. Younis and Rande H. Lazar

350. Management of Orbital Hemorrhage With Lateral Canthotomy and Cantholysis **894**
Brian R. Wong

■ Frontal Sinus **896**

351. Frontal Sinus Trephination **896**
Ramzi T. Younis and Rande H. Lazar

352. Osteoplastic Frontal Sinusectomy Procedure and Fat Obliteration **898**
Ramzi T. Younis and Rande H. Lazar

353. Frontal Sinus Ablation and Collapse **902**
Ramzi T. Younis and Rande H. Lazar

354. Endoscopic Sinus Surgery in Children **904**
David S. Parsons and Paul R. Cook

355. Frontal Defect Reconstruction **906**
Robert B. Stanley, Jr.

356. Dacryocystorhinostomy **908**
Brian R. Wong

■ Miscellaneous **910**

357. Incisional and Excisional Biopsy **910**
Harlan R. Muntz

358. Needle Biopsy **912**
Amy R. Coffey

359. Endoscopic Biopsy **914**
Amy R. Coffey

360. Punch Biopsy **916**
Amy R. Coffey

361. Common Injection Sites for Local Anesthesia **918**
John S. May

Figure Credits **920**

Index **921**

Atlas of
Head & Neck
Surgery—
Otolaryngology

Atlas of Head and Neck Surgery–Otolaryngology,
edited by Byron J. Bailey, J. Gail Neely, Karen H. Calhoun, and Amy R. Coffey.
Lippincott-Raven Publishers, Philadelphia © 1996.

Section One
Head and Neck

Section Editor:

Byron J. Bailey

Salivary Glands
Nose and Maxilla
Lips
Oral Cavity
Ear
Neck
Larynx
Thyroid and Parathyroid
Pharynx, Trachea, and Parapharyngeal Space
Cysts, Abscesses, and Vessels

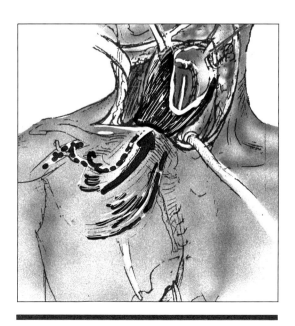

■ 1. PAROTID SUPERFICIAL LOBECTOMY

Removal of the parotid gland lateral to the facial nerve

Indications

1. Benign and low-grade malignant parotid neoplasms
2. Recurrent parotid sialadenitis or sialolithiasis
3. Cosmetic reduction of enlarged glands secondary to sialosis or other conditions
4. Removal of parotid lymph nodes in an area of suspected or known metastasis

Contraindications

1. Treatment of moderate or high-grade parotid gland neoplasms
2. Benign parotid gland neoplasms located in the inferior-most portion of the parotid gland with only a narrow glandular connection

Special Considerations

1. Preoperative imaging studies if the tumor is not freely mobile or if the deep component is not easily palpated
2. Fine-needle aspiration is occasionally helpful.
3. Sialography generally is not helpful.
4. Tumor histology is important, and the availability of frozen-section diagnosis is essential.

Special Instruments, Positions, and Anesthesia

1. General anesthesia with oral uplead endotracheal tube
2. Reverse Trendelenburg 30° position, with the ear, neck, parotid, corner of mouth, and corner of eye exposed
3. Preoperative typing and crossmatching of blood unnecessary
4. Bipolar cautery
5. Curved mosquito and fine mosquito clamps

Tips and Pearls

1. Use of a facial nerve stimulator is unnecessary except in reoperations.
2. Reoperating in the parotid bed should be done with the aid of intraoperative facial nerve monitoring.
3. Key landmarks for identifying the facial nerve include the cartilaginous pointer, the mastoid tip, and the posterior belly of the digastric muscle.
4. Tympanomastoid suture line is generally not a helpful landmark for identifying the facial nerve.
5. Be prepared to perform a retrograde parotidectomy if the tumor position prevents safe isolation of the main trunk of the facial nerve.
6. Postauricular artery or its branch crosses the main trunk of the facial nerve and can be a source of significant bleeding if it is not properly identified and ligated; avoid injury to the main trunk of the facial nerve.
7. Observation by an assistant and notation of facial twitching and motion and its location generally are more helpful than the use of a facial nerve stimulator.
8. Avoid making the posterior portion of the flap in the infraauricular area too thin or too long to prevent skin necrosis.
9. Infection after parotidectomy is rare; preoperatively, antibiotics are only needed with a preexisting history of sialadenitis.

Pitfalls and Complications

1. Facial paresis or paralysis often results from poor technique and failure to preserve small nerve branches.
2. Bleeding and hematoma formation can significantly compromise the airway.
3. Rare persistent salivary leakage or sialocele formation
4. Frey syndrome
5. Skin-flap necrosis

Postoperative Care Issues

1. Hemovac drain usually in place for 24 hours
2. Place a conforming pressure dressing, inspect the wound, and reapply a new dressing for an additional 24 hours the day after operations.

Operative Procedure

An incision in front of the ear curves behind the angle of the mandible and extends anteriorly two fingerbreadths beneath the lower border of the jaw (Fig. 1-1). The incision is made with a #10 blade, and the first few centimeters of the parotid flap are elevated with the knife. Rakes are placed in the skin flap, and while an assistant uses countertraction, the surgeon places sponges for countertraction and hemostasis. The parotid flap is raised over the parotid capsule with a Jones scissors. The scissors spread in a direction perpendicular to the capsule of the gland. Numerous small, filamentous structures coming from the capsule of the parotid gland to the skin flap can be ignored and cut. The facial nerve branches leave the gland at the periphery and do not enter the skin overlying the parotid gland. Dissection continues to the anterior portion of the gland until the fascia overlying the masseter muscle is identified.

A posterior skin flap is raised, separating the skin from the parotid gland back to the posterior and inferior portion of the parotid gland. Two Kocher clamps are placed in the lower portion of the parotid gland. The gland is elevated off of the sternocleidomastoid muscle. The greater auricular nerve is divided. If a posterior branch is identified, it often can be preserved. A small rake is placed on the tragus, and Kocher clamps are placed on the portion of the parotid gland opposite the tragal cartilage. A scissors is directed parallel to the ear cartilage, and the parotid gland is separated from the cartilaginous ear canal. The dissection continues until the cartilaginous pointer is clearly seen. A small bridge of tissue remains between the plane established at the level of the sternocleidomastoid muscle and the cartilaginous ear canal. This bridge of tissue can be divided as the parotid gland is retracted anteriorly. Several veins in this bridge of tissue may require suture ligation or cauterization. Bipolar cautery is used for the remaining portion of the operation.

The posterior belly of the digastric muscle is identified, and the gland is separated from this muscle (Fig. 1-2). The cartilaginous pointer, the most superior portion of the posterior belly of the digastric muscle, and the level of the mastoid process are readily identified. These three landmarks identify the location of the facial nerve (Fig. 1-3). Working on a broad front, the surgeon uses a small curved mosquito clamp to elevate and separate progressively the remaining parotid gland tissue from the mastoid tip, the cartilaginous ear canal, and the posterior belly of the digastric muscle. The dissection proceeds from an inferior to a superior direction, with countertraction on the gland, and from a posterior to an anterior direction. The assistant keeps the patient's face in view and reports any sign of muscular activity.

The main trunk of the facial nerve (cranial nerve VII) is readily visible as a white structure approximately 2 mm in diameter. It is easily seen and should not be confused with other structures, such as connective tissue fibers or blood vessels. A branch of the postauricular artery usually overlies the main trunk of the facial nerve, and identification and division of this artery helps to control nuisance bleeding. Dissection with a mosquito clamp proceeds on top of the nerve until the pes anserinus is identified.

Depending on the location of the tumor, removal of the gland can proceed from a superior to an inferior or an inferior to a superior direction (Fig. 1-4). A mosquito clamp or the closed end of a Jones scissors is used to separate the gland from the nerve. Working on a broad front, the surgeon follows the facial nerve branches to the periphery of the gland. The parotid duct is divided at the periphery of the specimen, and the specimen is removed (Fig. 1-5). The wound is irrigated with saline solution. Hemostasis is attained with bipolar cautery and selective ligation of any branches of the deep venous system. A Hemovac drain is inserted, and the parotid incision is closed in layers with chromic sutures and 6-0 mild chromic sutures in the skin.

KERRY D. OLSEN

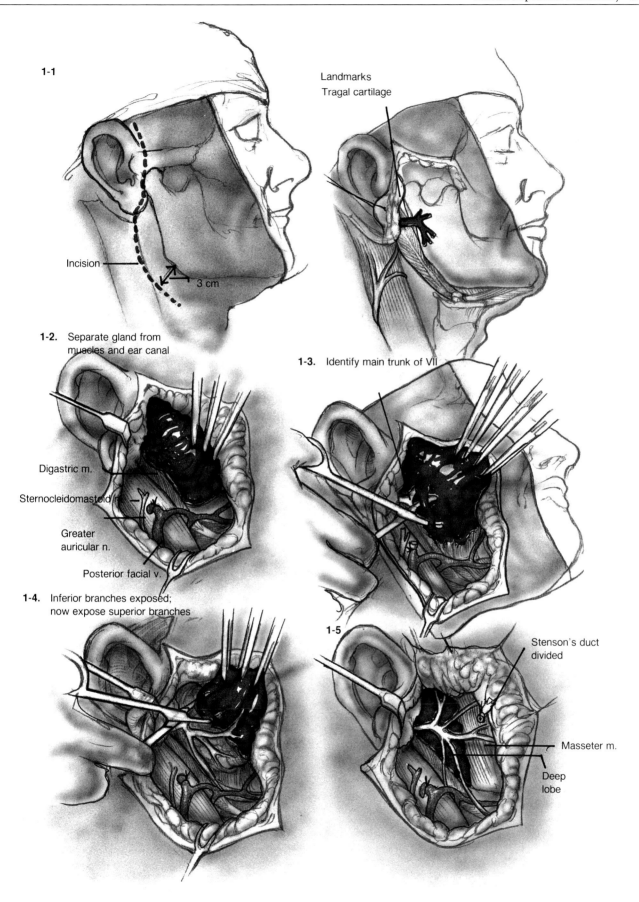

1-1

Landmarks
Tragal cartilage

Incision ——

3 cm

1-2. Separate gland from muscles and ear canal

Digastric m.

Sternocleidomastoid m.

Greater auricular n.

Posterior facial v.

1-3. Identify main trunk of VII

1-4. Inferior branches exposed; now expose superior branches

1-5

Stenson's duct divided

Masseter m.

Deep lobe

2. PAROTID DEEP LATERAL LOBECTOMY WITH NERVE SPARING—Removal of that portion of the parotid gland deep to the level of the facial nerve

Indications
1. Benign and malignant deep-lobe parotid tumors
2. Removal of the deep portion of the parotid gland for moderate and high-grade malignancies found in the superficial portion of the parotid gland
3. Chronic sialadenitis
4. Dumbbell-shaped, deep-lobe parapharyngeal and parotid tumors

Contraindications
1. Bleeding disorder
2. Failure to obtain preoperative computed tomography or magnetic resonance imaging studies

Special Considerations
1. In most cases, a superficial parotidectomy is done first.
2. Unless there is direct invasion or proximity of a high-grade tumor to the facial nerve, the facial nerve can be preserved in most cases of malignant disease.
3. The extent of tissue that comprises the deep lobe of the parotid gland varies greatly among individuals.
4. The possibility of performing a neck dissection should be discussed with the patient preoperatively.
5. Frozen-section pathologic examination should be available.
6. Deep-lobe tumors can displace the facial nerve considerably, altering the typical position and appearance of the nerve.

Special Instrumentation, Position, and Anesthesia
1. Nerve hooks
2. Bipolar cautery

Tips and Pearls
1. Key to the total removal of the deep lobe of the parotid gland is identification and isolation of the main regional vessels.
2. For malignant parotid neoplasms, removal of the deep lobe of the parotid gland also removes the nodes found in the deep lobe and parapharyngeal region.
3. Many deep-lobe, benign neoplasms may not require the complete removal of the parotid deep lobe.
4. For parapharyngeal extension of the deep-lobe parotid tumors, key points in safe removal without tumor rupture include identification of the upper neck vessels and nerves, division of the stylomandibular ligament, retraction of the mandible, and identification and retraction of the facial nerve.
5. A deep-lobe parotid tumor is often removed beneath, above, or between the branches of the facial nerve.
6. It may be helpful to remove the styloid process if a deep-lobe tumor extends around the structure.

Pitfalls and Complications
1. Mobilization of the facial nerve generally causes temporary paresis, especially in the elderly; eye protection postoperatively is important.
2. Loss of superficial or deep portions of the parotid glands or of the complete glands can cause a cosmetic deformity, especially if the regional musculature is removed; reconstruction with a gracilis free flap should be considered.
3. Bleeding, hematoma, and airway compromise can occur; meticulous hemostasis and Hemovac drainage are important.
4. The surgeon should be aware of the possibility of a tortuous loop in the internal carotid artery, extending within the musculature of the bed of the parotid gland.

Postoperative Care Issues
1. Hemovac drain
2. Compression dressing
3. Postoperative surgical film to identify sponges

Reference
Beahrs OH. Parotidectomy. Surgical techniques 1976;1(1):43.

Operative Procedure
After completion of a superficial parotidectomy, the deep portion of the parotid gland can be removed (Fig. 2-1). Nerve hooks are used to elevate the facial nerve, and a small, sharp scissors is used to cut the fascial connections from the gland to the nerve, completely freeing and isolating the entire course of the facial nerve from the main trunk at the level of the styloid foramen to the periphery over the masseter muscle.

The portion of the parotid gland located beneath the nerve and overlying the masseter muscle is retracted and elevated off the fascia of the masseter muscle back beyond the angle of the jaw (Fig. 2-2). Inferiorly, the gland is elevated off the stylohyoid muscle. The posterior facial vein is divided, and the external carotid artery is identified as it passes deep to the digastric and stylohyoid muscles and enters the deep portion of the parotid gland beneath the angle of the mandible and lies above the remaining styloid muscles. The external carotid artery is divided (Fig. 2-3). The superficial temporal artery and vein are divided. The superior portion of the deep lobe is reflected inferiorly off the temporomandibular joint, bony ear canal, and condyle of the mandible (Fig. 2-4). The gland is completely freed from the main trunk of the facial nerve and elevated off the styloglossus and stylopharyngeus muscles that form the remaining portion of the bed of the deep lobe of the parotid gland.

By working beneath and between the branches of the facial nerve, the surgeon progressively mobilizes the gland, ligating and cauterizing several venous branches that enter the pterygoid musculature. The final attachment of tissue includes the internal maxillary artery and its associated veins. These vessels are ligated (Fig. 2-5). The entire deep lobe and tumor can then be removed inferior to the facial nerve or between the branches as necessary (Fig. 2-6). Meticulous hemostasis is achieved. The wound is irrigated and closed over a Hemovac drain. A conforming pressure dressing is applied.

KERRY D. OLSEN

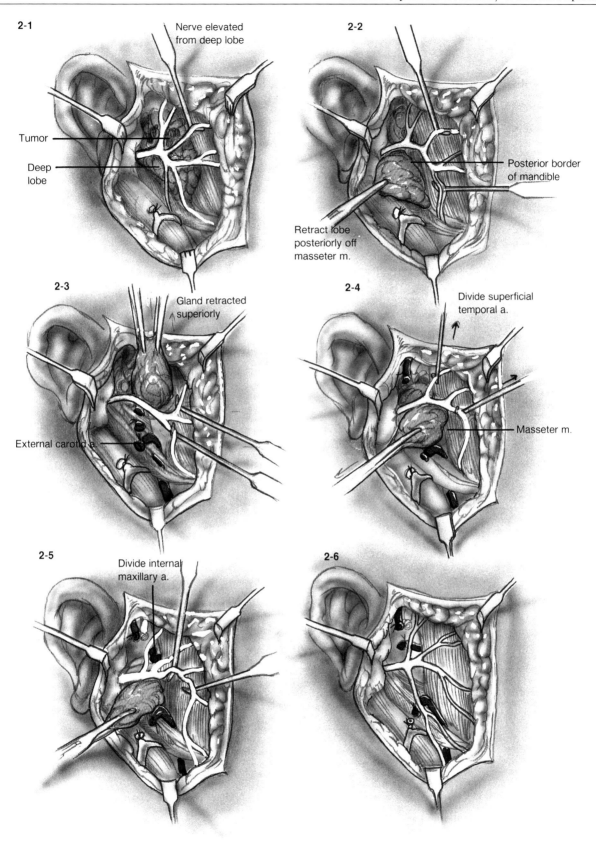

2-1

Nerve elevated
from deep lobe

Tumor

Deep
lobe

2-2

Posterior border
of mandible

Retract lobe
posteriorly off
masseter m.

2-3

Gland retracted
superiorly

External carotid a.

2-4

Divide superficial
temporal a.

Masseter m.

2-5

Divide internal
maxillary a.

2-6

■ *3.* INTRAORAL SALIVARY GLAND TUMOR REMOVAL (PAROTID INTRAORAL DEEP-LOBE TUMOR EXCISION)—Removal of select benign salivary gland neoplasms using a transoral approach

Indications
1. Benign minor salivary gland parapharyngeal tumors
2. Tumor smaller than 5 cm
3. Superior and medial benign parapharyngeal tumors that are nonvascular, nonmalignant, and not parotid in origin

Contraindications
1. Parotid deep-lobe salivary gland tumors with parapharyngeal extension
2. Dumbbell-shaped, deep-lobe parotid tumors
3. Malignant salivary gland tumors
4. Parapharyngeal tumors of indeterminate histology
5. Vascular parapharyngeal tumors
6. Parapharyngeal tumors with extension into the cervical vertebral bodies or base of skull
7. Bleeding disorder

Special Considerations
1. The transoral approach is rarely used for parapharyngeal tumors.
2. A fat plane must be visible between the tumor and the deep lobe of the parotid gland on imaging studies to confirm the minor salivary gland origin.

Preoperative Preparation
1. Computed tomography scan with contrast medium or magnetic resonance imaging scan with gadolinium enhancement
2. Fine-needle aspiration through the transoral route confirms the presence of a benign tumor.
3. The patient should be aware the intraoral operation may be extended to include a cervical-parotid approach and possible mandibulotomy.

Special Instrumentation, Position, and Anesthesia
1. General anesthesia
2. Rose position
3. McIver or Dingman mouth gag
4. Bipolar and monopolar cautery
5. Headlight
6. Tonsillectomy instrumentation

Tips and Pearls
1. Adhere strictly to appropriate criteria for operating.
2. Adequate incision and external pressure on the neck should help remove the tumor bluntly without rupture.
3. Do not clamp the capsule of the tumor with instruments.

Pitfalls and Complications
1. Tumor rupture
2. Incomplete removal
3. Uncontrolled hemorrhage

Postoperative Care Issues
1. Leave the midportion of the wound open to heal secondarily.
2. Patient can eat and be dismissed 1 to 2 days postoperatively.
3. Long-term follow-up for possible tumor recurrence is essential.

Reference
Goodwin WJ, Chandler JR. Transoral excision of lateral parapharyngeal space tumors presenting intraorally. Laryngoscope 1989;98:266.

Operative Procedure
With the patient in the Rose position and an endotracheal tube in the down position, a McIver or Dingman mouth gag is inserted to expose the palate and tonsillar region. The tumor should be easily visible, displacing the superior portion of the tonsil and soft palate medially (Fig. 3-1). An incision is made over the most prominent aspect of the swelling in the tonsil and palate area and extends above and below the apparent location of the tumor (Fig. 3-2). The initial incision can be made with cautery or knife, but meticulous hemostasis should be maintained throughout the procedure.

Dissection continues through the thinned constrictor muscle. Generally, the initial incision runs in the palate and in front of the anterior tonsillar pillar. The constrictor muscle is identified. A curved clamp is placed in a plane deep to the constrictor muscle and on top of the tumor, and the constrictor muscle is divided well above and below the apparent extent of the tumor and in a controlled, meticulous manner.

The tumor capsule should be visible (Fig. 3-3). No retractors are placed on the tumor capsule, and pressure on the neck often assists in removal of the tumor. A blunt instrument, such as a suction tip or a curved clamp, commonly is used to separate slowly any fascial connections from the tumor to its adjacent bed (Fig. 3-4). The tumor is progressively delivered into the mouth, from which it is removed.

Any vascular connections to the tumor can be cauterized as the tumor is removed. Meticulous hemostasis is achieved with bipolar cautery. The superior and inferior portions of the wound are closed with interrupted 2-0 chromic sutures. The midportion of the wound is left open to heal secondarily (Fig. 3-5).

KERRY D. OLSEN

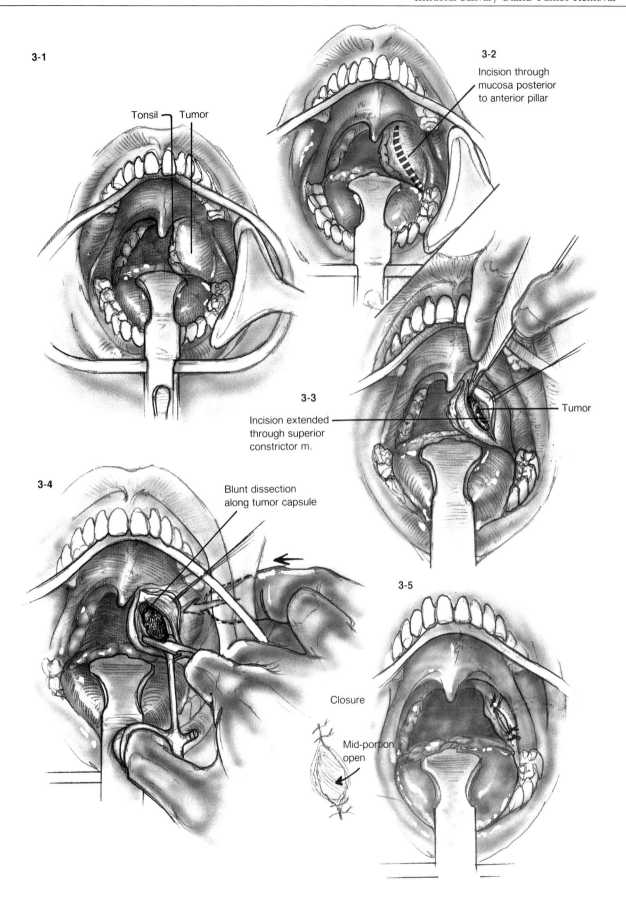

3-1

Tonsil — Tumor

3-2

Incision through
mucosa posterior
to anterior pillar

3-3

Incision extended
through superior
constrictor m.

Tumor

3-4

Blunt dissection
along tumor capsule

3-5

Closure

Mid-portion
open

■ 4. TOTAL PAROTIDECTOMY WITH THE SEVENTH NERVE SPARED—Excision of all of the parotid gland while sparing the seventh cranial nerve

Indications
1. Large benign or malignant neoplasm
2. Deep-lobe neoplasm
3. Chronic or chronic recurrent sialadenitis
4. Some cases of metastatic disease to the parotid gland and its lymph nodes

Special Considerations
1. Extent of disease
2. Proximity of the disease to the facial nerve
3. Multiply recurrent pleomorphic adenomas or recurrent malignant tumors

Preoperative Preparation
1. Routine laboratory studies for general anesthetic
2. Bleeding and clotting studies
3. Consider facial nerve monitoring.

Special Instruments, Position, and Anesthesia
1. Headlight
2. Face covered with transparent drape to monitor motion
3. Orbital or Cummings retractors
4. Hypotensive anesthesia
5. Bipolar cautery

Tips and Pearls
1. Wide exposure before identifying the facial nerve
2. Meticulous dissection on the nerve at all times
3. Minimal use of a nerve stimulator

Pitfalls and Complications
1. Attempting to identify the facial nerve without wide exposure and excellent visualization
2. Attempting to identify the facial nerve with poor hemostasis
3. Inadvertent incision into the tumor while dissecting out the facial nerve

Postoperative Care Issues
1. Suction drainage for 24 hours
2. Pressure dressing for 24 hours
3. Careful monitoring of eye protection if facial nerve is weak

References
Rankow RM, Polayes IM. Diseases of the salivary glands. Philadelphia: WB Saunders, 1976.
Rice DH. Surgery of the salivary glands. Philadelphia: BC Decker, 1982.

Operative Procedure

After the removal of the superficial lobe as previously described and illustrated, the facial nerve should have been dissected out in its entirety, with the remaining deep lobe below (Fig. 4-1). The next step is to free the individual branches of the facial nerve from the residual parotid tissue. This is best done with a combination of sharp and blunt dissection with *gentle* retraction on the nerve branches. The part of the parotid gland remaining between the posterior border of the mandible and the mastoid can be removed with a combination of sharp and blunt dissection. This is largely done with blunt dissection, particularly in benign disease, with care taken to identify the terminal branches of the external carotid artery and the accompanying veins (Fig. 4-2).

After this is accomplished, the only remaining gland is usually between the cervicofacial and temporofacial trunks overlying the masseter muscle. This tissue can generally be easily removed from the surface of the masseter muscle with gentle superior and interior retraction of the appropriate nerves. During this portion of the dissection, the posterior facial vein may need to be clamped, divided, and ligated, if this has not been previously performed (Fig. 4-3).

Rarely, a mandibulotomy may be necessary to gain access to extensive involvement of the deep lobe medially. If so, the mandible is usually transected across the angle (Fig. 4-4).

Some surgeons prefer to transect the mandible anterior to the mental foramen to preserve nerve function. Before the mandibulotomy, an appropriate reconstruction plate should be placed across this area, with the holes drilled and the screws set before the plate is removed. This ensures correct reestablishment of occlusion at the end of the procedure when the plate is attached to realign the mandibular segments. This always results in a slight spread of the mandible at the mandibulotomy site. No attempt should be made to approximate the two ends if the patient has normal dentition, because disturbance will cause malocclusion. In the edentulous patient, this probably will not be a problem, but it is still unnecessary (Fig. 4-5).

DALE H. RICE

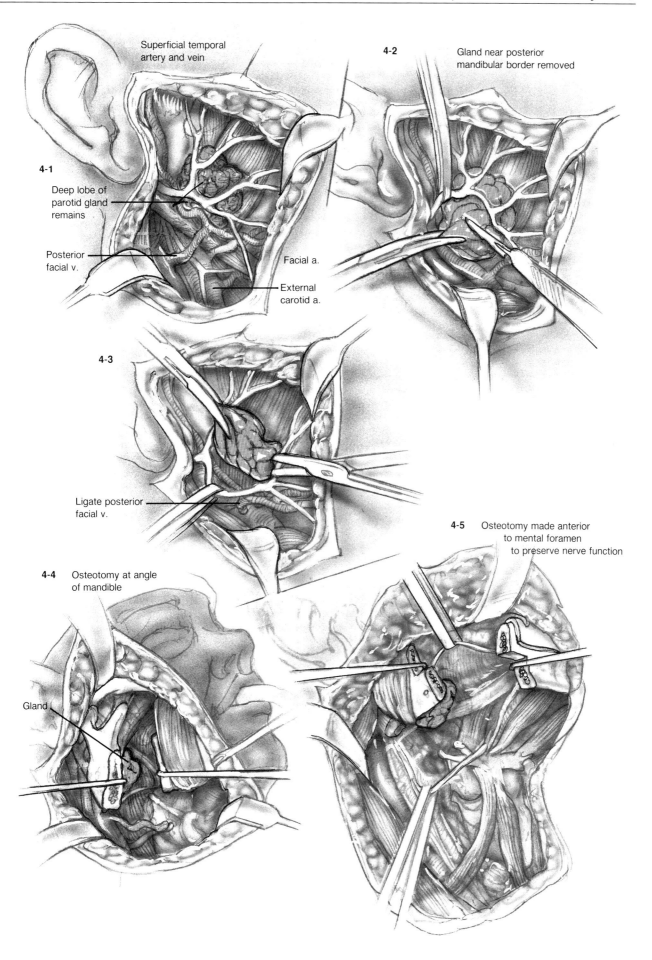

Superficial temporal artery and vein

4-1

Deep lobe of parotid gland remains

Posterior facial v.

Facial a.

External carotid a.

4-2   Gland near posterior mandibular border removed

4-3

Ligate posterior facial v.

4-4   Osteotomy at angle of mandible

Gland

4-5   Osteotomy made anterior to mental foramen to preserve nerve function

■ 5. TOTAL PAROTIDECTOMY WITH NERVE RESECTION AND GRAFT—Total excision of the parotid gland and facial nerve with repair of the nerve by grafting

Indications
1. Malignant neoplasms involving the facial nerve
2. Rarely, the multiply recurrent pleomorphic adenoma after all else has failed

Special Considerations
1. Extensive involvement of the facial nerve, because spread may go proximally into the temporal bone

Preoperative Preparation
1. Routine laboratory studies
2. Bleeding and clotting studies

Special Instruments, Position, and Anesthesia
1. Headlight
2. Hypotensive anesthesia
3. Operating microscope
4. Orbital or Cummings retractors
5. Microinstruments for nerve repair
6. Prep and drape expected nerve donor site

Tips and Pearls
1. Wide exposure before identification of the main trunk of the facial nerve
2. Careful tagging of the distal branches of the facial nerve as they are identified

Pitfalls and Complications
1. Tumor may have extended medially along the nerve into the temporal bone.
2. Level two lymph nodes should be examined.

Postoperative Care Issues
1. Underflap suction for 24 hours
2. Pressure dressing for 24 hours
3. Tarsorrhaphy should be performed to protect the eye.

References
Rankow RM, Polayes IM. Diseases of the salivary glands. Philadelphia: WB Saunders, 1976.
Rice DH. Surgery of the salivary glands. Philadelphia: BC Decker, 1982.

Operative Procedure
During parotidectomy, the facial nerve usually is resected en bloc with the parotid gland, with the main trunk transected somewhere proximal to the pes anserinus and the distal branches resected where appropriate, usually where they emerge from the gland. For some tumors, the resection may involve only one branch, such as the temporofacial or cervicofacial. In this setting, the procedure often is begun as a nerve-sparing procedure, and nerve involvement is encountered, although, originally unsuspected.

Several donor nerves are available for nerve grafting. The most commonly used are the anterior branch of the great auricular, the sural, and the lateral femoral cutaneous nerves. The great auricular nerve may be used on the ipsilateral side, unless there is a chance that it may be involved with tumor as well. If this is the case, and it often is, the contralateral nerve should be used. The fascia should be stripped from the nerve, as is done in a neck dissection, if there is any chance of lymphatic spread in that area. The nerve can be used with or without branching, as is appropriate to the situation (Fig. 5-1).

The sural nerve also can be used. A vertical incision 2 to 3 cm long is made between the lateral malleolus and the Achilles tendon. The distal nerve lies in the subcutaneous fatty tissue at this level, in intimate association with the saphenous vein. The vein should be retracted laterally and the nerve mobilized to obtain the length and branching necessary. Additional incisions can be made up the calf if necessary (Fig. 5-2).

A third nerve can be used particularly for fine or distal branches. This is the lateral femoral cutaneous nerve. This nerve lies along the anterior thigh approximately 10 cm inferior to the anterosuperior iliac spine (Fig. 5-3).

The ends of the recipient and donor nerves are freshly cut with a very fine scalpel or razor blade. In general, the approximation is better done under the microscope with the appropriate suture for the diameter of the nerve involved. A careful epineural repair usually should be performed with suture from 7-0 to 10-0 nylon (Figs. 5-4 and 5-5).

DALE H. RICE

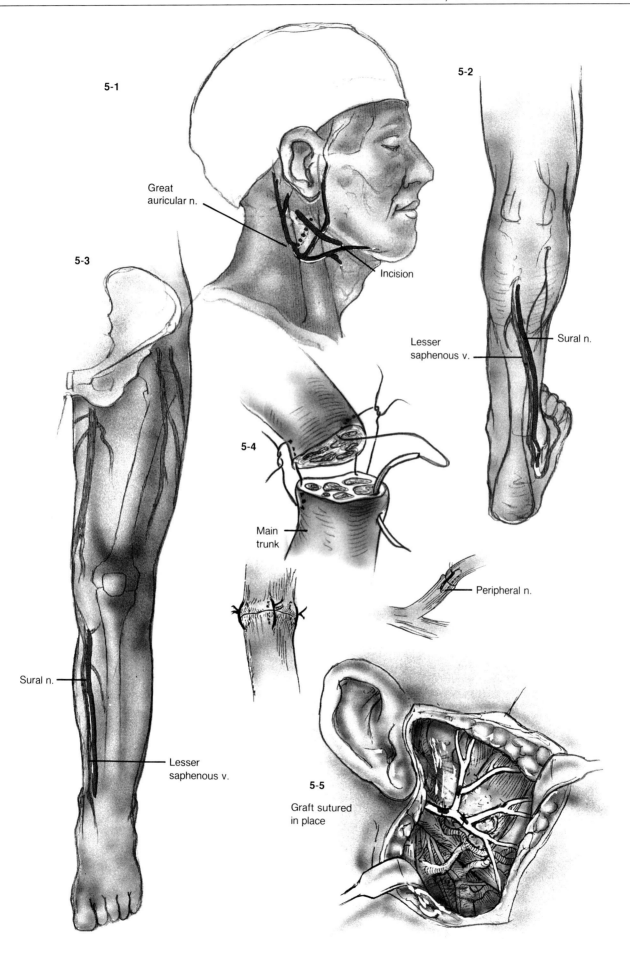

5-1

Great auricular n.

Incision

5-2

Sural n.

Lesser saphenous v.

5-3

Sural n.

Lesser saphenous v.

5-4

Main trunk

Peripheral n.

5-5

Graft sutured in place

■ 6. SUBMANDIBULAR SALIVARY GLAND
EXCISION—Surgical removal of the submandibular salivary gland

Indications
1. Recurrent sialadenitis
2. Sialolithiasis
3. Benign submandibular gland tumors
4. Malignant submandibular gland tumors
5. As part of a select, modified, radical neck dissection to remove lymph nodes in area 1 of the neck

Contraindications
1. Known high-grade malignancy
2. Bleeding disorder
3. Acute infection
4. Stones confined to the distal portion of Wharton's duct

Special Considerations
1. Approximately 50% of neoplasms are benign, and 50% are malignant.
2. Sialography is not helpful.
3. Ultrasound helps to differentiate ptotic glands from tumor.
4. Frozen-section diagnosis is necessary.
5. The surgeon should be prepared to proceed with neck dissection if indicated.
6. Dental mandibular occlusal radiographic views are helpful in determining number and location of stones in Wharton's duct.

Special Instrumentation, Position, and Anesthesia
1. General anesthesia with oral uplead endotracheal tube
2. Head of bed elevated 30° (ie, reverse Trendelenburg position)
3. Draping should be done for a complete neck dissection in case it is necessary.
4. Bipolar cautery
5. Routine neck dissection instrumentation

Tips and Pearls
1. Identify the marginal branch of the mandibular nerve in all cases.
2. Before clamping the postganglionic attachments from the lingual nerve and dividing Wharton's duct, visualize the hypoglossal nerve.
3. Always remove the tumor with the gland; never perform an enucleation.
4. Multiple prior infections can cause significant scarring in a region of the duct and lingual and hypoglossal nerves; dissection in these scarred areas should be done carefully.
5. Remove the facial nodes with the gland if they are enlarged.

Pitfalls and Complications
1. Marginal nerve injury
2. Lingual nerve injury
3. Hypoglossal nerve injury
4. Bleeding and hematoma
5. Retained stone in the distal portion of Wharton's duct
6. Infections are rare; antibiotics should only be used preoperatively if there has been a history of sialadenitis.

Postoperative Care Issues
1. Hemovac drain generally in place for 24 hours
2. Pressure neck dressing
3. Dismissal from the hospital generally occurs 1 day after surgery if there is no evidence of hematoma or other complications.

Reference
Beahrs OH, Kiernan PO, Hubert JP Jr. An atlas of the surgical techniques of Oliver H. Beahrs. Philadelphia: WB Saunders, 1985.

Operative Procedure
An incision approximately 10 cm long is made approximately two fingerbreadths (3 cm) beneath the mandible over the submandibular gland. The incision is extended through the subcutaneous tissues until the platysma muscle is identified. Hemostasis is achieved and the muscle is divided. Rakes are placed by an assistant for retraction superiorly, and the thin fascia beneath the platysma muscle is slowly divided.

The surgeon identifies the facial vein and carefully preserves the marginal mandibular branch of the facial nerve. The anterior facial vein and facial artery are ligated (Fig. 6-1). The facial nodes are reflected inferiorly with the submandibular gland. The fascial attachments from the gland to the free border of the mandible are bluntly divided to expose the free border of the mandible. This dissection continues back to the level of the posterior facial vein and anteriorly to the level of the digastric muscle. Inferiorly, the neck flaps are elevated over the remaining portion of the gland to the level of the digastric muscle.

The submandibular gland is separated from the mylohyoid muscle (Fig. 6-2). The mylohyoid pedicle is isolated and divided. The gland is retracted laterally, and the free border of the mylohyoid muscle is identified. A ribbon retractor is placed beneath the mylohyoid muscle to reflect it medially. The gland is retracted inferiorly with a sponge. This provides excellent visualization of the lingual nerve (Fig. 6-3). Blunt dissection with a curved clamp inferior to the lingual nerve permits identification of the submandibular duct and the hypoglossal nerve. A natural bend in the course of the lingual nerve is readily apparent, and in this location, the postganglionic parasympathetic fibers that extend from Langley's ganglion to the submandibular gland are divided. This tissue often includes several small veins. With the hypoglossal nerve visible, the remaining gland surrounding Wharton's duct is isolated. The duct is divided, and the gland is reflected off the hyoglossus muscle (Fig. 6-4). Inferiorly, a terminal branch of the anterior jugular vein may enter the region of the gland and can be divided.

The gland is progressively isolated from the tendon and posterior belly of the digastric muscle. The common facial vein is divided (Fig. 6-5). The gland is progressively freed from any other facial connections until the only remaining connection is the facial artery. This artery is ligated with a silk suture, and the specimen is removed (Fig. 6-6). Meticulous hemostasis is attained. The wound is irrigated, and a Hemovac drain is inserted. The incision is closed in layers by using chromic sutures in the subcutaneous tissues and 6-0 fast-absorbing chromic sutures in the skin. A pressure dressing is applied.

KERRY D. OLSEN

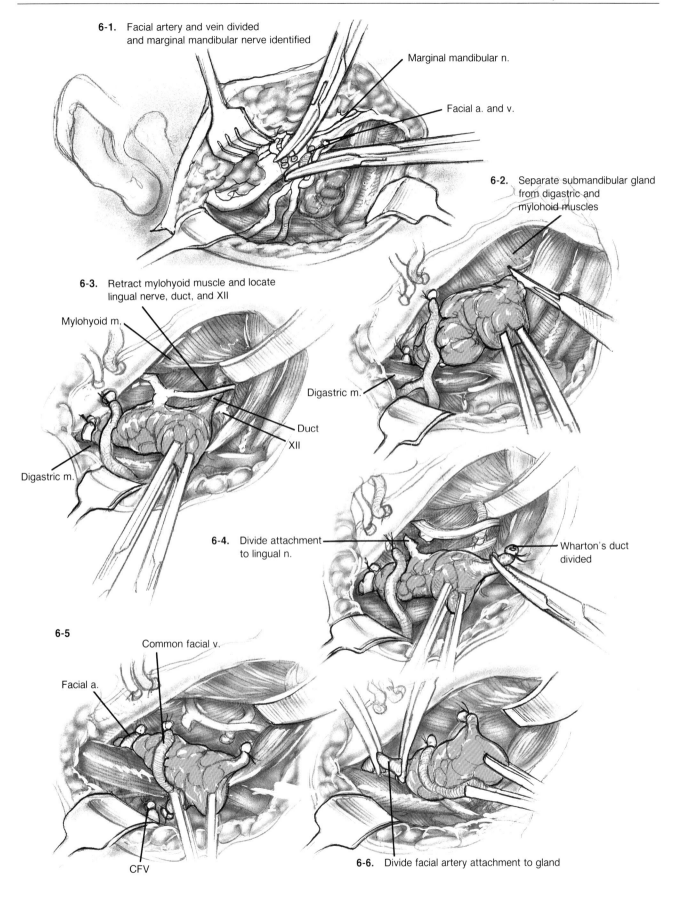

6-1. Facial artery and vein divided and marginal mandibular nerve identified

Marginal mandibular n.

Facial a. and v.

6-2. Separate submandibular gland from digastric and mylohoid muscles

6-3. Retract mylohyoid muscle and locate lingual nerve, duct, and XII

Mylohyoid m.

Digastric m.

Duct

XII

Digastric m.

6-4. Divide attachment to lingual n.

Wharton's duct divided

6-5

Common facial v.

Facial a.

CFV

6-6. Divide facial artery attachment to gland

■ **7. SUBLINGUAL SALIVARY GLAND TUMOR EXCISION**— Surgical removal of the sublingual salivary gland

Indications
1. Benign or malignant tumor involving the sublingual gland
2. Anterior floor of mouth squamous cell carcinoma

Special Considerations
1. Proximity of the submandibular duct
2. Possible involvement of the mandible
3. Possible involvement of the lingual nerve

Preoperative Preparation
1. Routine laboratory studies
2. Bleeding and clotting studies
3. Mandibular series if there is a question of bone involvement

Special Instruments, Position, and Anesthesia
1. Headlight
2. McIvor or Dingman retractor
3. Hypotensive anesthesia

Tips and Pearls
1. Retract the tongue posteriorly and superiorly.
2. Cannulate the submandibular duct if necessary to identify its exact position.

Pitfalls and Complications
1. Inadvertent injury to the submandibular duct or lingual nerve
2. Postoperative bleeding into the floor of mouth

Postoperative Care Issues
1. Careful monitoring for bleeding in floor of mouth
2. Delay oral feedings for 24 to 48 hours.

Reference
Rankow RN, Mignogna F. Cancer of the sublingual gland, 1969. Am J Surg 1969;118:790.

Operative Procedure
A sublingual salivary gland tumor usually occurs as a submucosal bulge in the floor of the mouth anteriorly. Generally, it is lateral to the opening of Wharton's duct (Fig. 7-1). An incision is made over the bulging mass of the sublingual gland and mucosal flaps elevated anteriorly and posteriorly with a combination of sharp and blunt dissection. The gland is usually intimately associated with Wharton's duct, and cannulation of the duct may aid in its preservation (Fig. 7-2). Care should be taken to identify the lingual nerve as well. Depending on the disease process, the excision can take one of several forms. For benign disease, the gland can merely be removed by a combination of blunt and sharp dissection from the surrounding structures, particularly the submandibular duct and the lingual nerve (Fig. 7-3). For malignant disease, a more extensive excision should be done; for an adenoid cystic carcinoma, the excision should include the overlying mucosa, the submandibular duct, and the lingual nerve. For extensive disease, the excision may also include the alveolar ridge of the mandible in that location (Figs. 7-4 and 7-5). After the excision, the mucosa is closed primarily, or if there is insufficient mucosa, a mucosal or skin graft is applied and covered with a bolster (Fig. 7-6).

DALE H. RICE

7-2

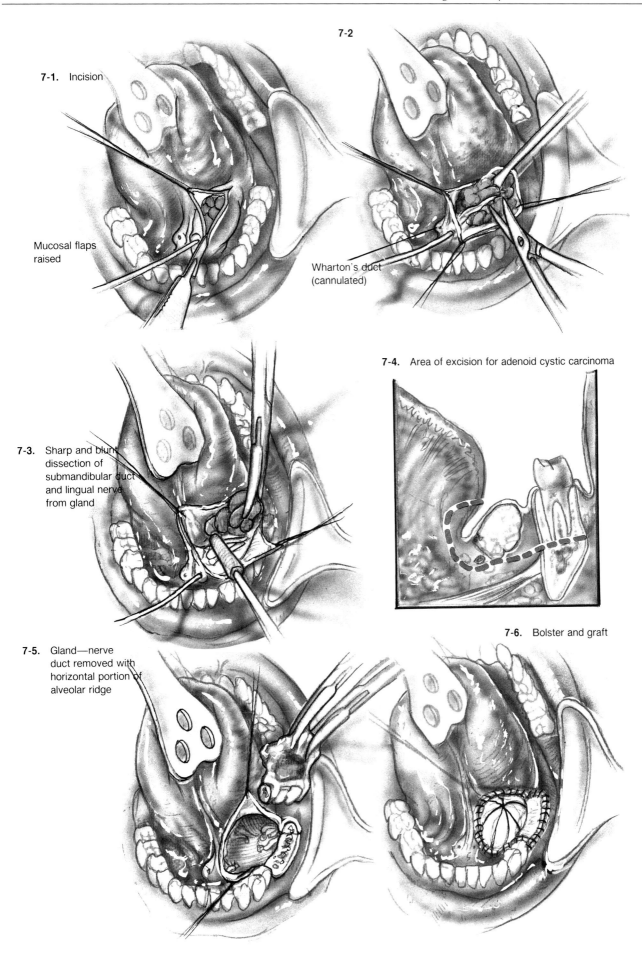

7-1. Incision

Mucosal flaps
raised

Wharton's duct
(cannulated)

7-3. Sharp and blunt
dissection of
submandibular duct
and lingual nerve
from gland

7-4. Area of excision for adenoid cystic carcinoma

7-6. Bolster and graft

7-5. Gland—nerve
duct removed with
horizontal portion of
alveolar ridge

■ 8. SALIVARY GLAND TRAUMA MANAGEMENT—

Various structures may require management during the care of patients who have suffered blunt or penetrating trauma to the major salivary glands.

Indications
1. Penetrating injury to the face in the area of the parotid gland
2. Penetrating injury in the area of the submandibular triangle

Special Considerations
1. Type of penetrating injury
2. Associated injuries
3. Preoperative assessment, especially the function of the facial nerve and the parotid duct

Preoperative Preparation
1. Routine laboratory studies
2. Bleeding and clotting studies
3. Careful assessment of the facial nerve, parotid duct, lingual nerve, Wharton's duct and hypoglossal nerve

Special Instruments, Position, and Anesthesia
1. Headlight
2. Operating microscope
3. Microinstruments
4. Orbital or Cummings retractors
5. Hypotensive anesthesia
6. Nerve stimulator

Tips and Pearls
1. When possible, explore the injury through the penetrating injury site directly.
2. If additional exposure is necessary, consider a formal incision, as for parotidectomy or submandibular gland excision.

Pitfalls and Complications
1. Perform a careful check for associated vascular injuries.
2. Carefully assess for possible injury to adjacent bony structures.

Postoperative Care Issues
1. Perform a tarsorrhaphy if eye function is not completely normal.
2. Consider perioperative antibiotics.
3. Monitor for postoperative hematoma.

References
May M. The facial nerve. New York: Thieme, 1986.

Morel AS, Firestein A. Repair of traumatic fistula of the duct. Arch Surg 1963;87:623.

Olsen NR. Traumatic lesions of the salivary glands. Otolaryngol Clin North Am 1977;10:345.

Operative Procedure

Blunt trauma to the parotid gland or to the submandibular gland generally requires no treatment other than occasional evacuation of the hematoma. Rarely is there significant damage to the structure of the gland or to an adjacent nerve. Penetrating injury, however, may potentially injure a number of structures of the parotid gland. The structures at risk include the parenchyma, facial nerve, and Stensen's duct (Fig. 8-1). Penetrating injuries to the parotid parenchyma alone generally require little or no treatment. The wound should be inspected and cleaned. The physician should be certain that neither a branch of the facial nerve nor a main trunk of the duct system has been injured. In the absence of these injuries, the parenchyma may be closed with one or two loose sutures and the wound drained and closed. The same is true for injury to the submandibular parenchyma.

Treatment for injury to the facial nerve depends on the branch involved and the area in which the injury occurs. If the injury is medial to the anterior border of the masseter muscle, which approximates a vertical line from the lateral canthus, repair is generally unnecessary, because satisfactory healing usually occurs. Injuries proximal to this require exploration and repair. This should be done as early as possible, consistent with the proper care of other injuries. The injury can usually be explored through the wound causing the injury, although it may need to be enlarged for adequate exposure. Some surgeons prefer performing a lateral parotidectomy first, through the usual incision. Both ends of the nerve should be identified and repaired as mentioned in the section on nerve resection and grafting. Identification of the distal segment with a nerve stimulator is usually easy in acute injury. The proximal segment usually is found in proximity to it and can be readily identified with blunt dissection. If the nerve cannot be found, a parotidectomy should be performed and the facial nerve traced out. The ends should be freshened and then approximated under the microscope (Fig. 8-2).

It is possible for Stensen's duct to be injured without injury to the facial nerve. The injury can be found by exploring the wound directly. The proximal end of the duct can be readily identified by passing a probe from intraorally (Fig. 8-3). The more distal end may be more difficult to identify. Often, it can be found if the wound is dried carefully and the appropriate area watched as the gland is massaged, looking for a drop of saliva. Once found, a polyethylene tube should be passed intraorally across the line of transection and into the proximal duct. The ends should then be approximated under the microscope with 7-0 or 8-0 nylon (Fig. 8-4). Polyethylene tubing should be left in place for approximately 10 to 14 days by suturing it to the buccal mucosa and taping it to the cheek (Fig. 8-5).

The same general principles apply for the submandibular gland. Parenchymal injuries usually require simple closure. Injuries to Wharton's duct are extremely rare because of the projective coverage of the mandible; if injured, the duct should be repaired as for Stensen's duct. An alternative is excision of the gland to obviate future problems. If the lingual nerve or the hypoglossal nerve is injured, it should be explored and repaired. This type of injury is rare because of the protection afforded by the mandible. This is especially true of the lingual nerve. The hypoglossal nerve can be injured by penetrating injuries below the level of the gland near the digastric muscle (see Fig. 8-5).

DALE H. RICE

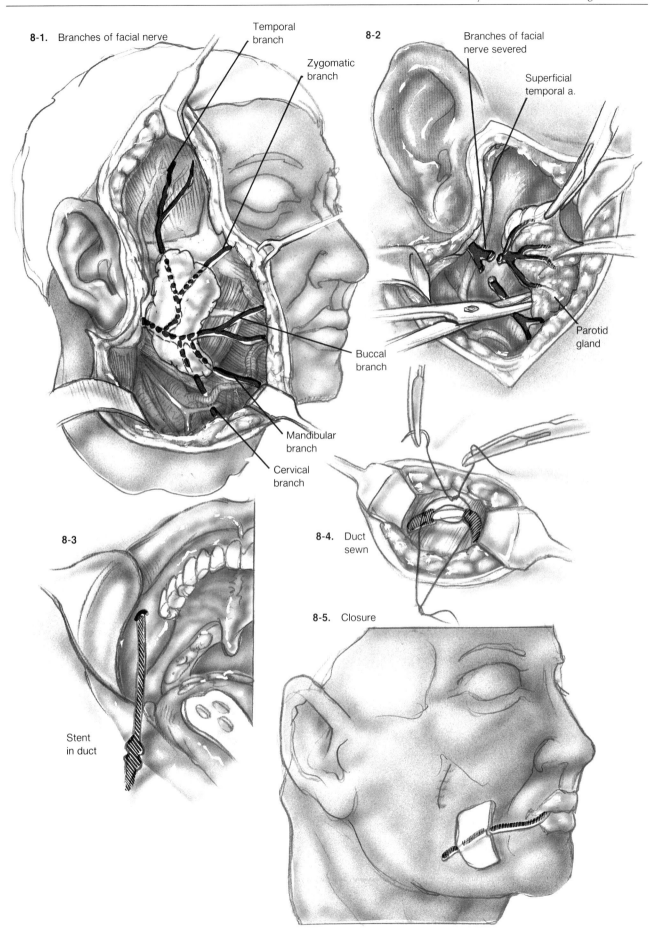

8-1. Branches of facial nerve

Temporal branch

Zygomatic branch

Buccal branch

Mandibular branch

Cervical branch

8-2

Branches of facial nerve severed

Superficial temporal a.

Parotid gland

8-3

Stent in duct

8-4. Duct sewn

8-5. Closure

■ 9. TOTAL RHINECTOMY

Total surgical removal of the skin, soft tissue, and framework of the external nose

Indications

1. Invasive cancer of the nasal skin
2. Cancer of the nasal septum and columella with or without the nasal framework

Special Considerations

1. Skin cancers arising in the nasal area are equally distributed between squamous cell carcinoma (SCCA) and basal cell carcinoma (BCCA).
2. Ninety percent of cancers occurring in the nasal cavity are SCCA.
3. Regional node metastases are unusual at the time of presentation.

Preoperative Preparation

1. Routine lab studies
2. Computed tomography or magnetic resonance imaging of the nasal and paranasal area
3. Biopsy to confirm histopathologic diagnosis

Special Instruments, Position, and Anesthesia

1. Headlight
2. Orotracheal intubation in midline to avoid misalignment if primary reconstruction performed

Tips and Pearls

1. Resect the tumor with wide margins and send margin strips for frozen-section confirmation of the adequacy of the excision to avoid local recurrence.
2. Leaving the base of the columella and one or both alae improves reconstructed appearance of nose (unnecessary if a prosthesis used).
3. Preservation of nasal bones allows seating of a nasal prosthesis.
4. Extension of cancer into the premaxilla, upper lip, palate, or anterior cranial fossa is best treated by an incontinuity resection.

Pitfalls and Complications

1. Recurrence of cancer
2. Bleeding

Postoperative Care Issues

1. Cancer recurs in approximately 33% of patients. Close follow-up by examination and radiologic studies is recommended.
2. Because about 67% of recurrences occur within 2 years of surgery, delayed reconstruction (>2 yr) should be strongly considered.
3. A custom-fitted prosthesis allows the best follow-up examination for recurrence while providing a satisfactory cosmetic and functional result.

References

Harrison DFN. Total rhinectomy—a worthwhile operation? J Laryngol Otol 1982;96:1113.

Teichgraeber JF, Goepfert H. Rhinectomy: timing and reconstruction. Otol Head Neck Surg 1990;102:362.

Operative Procedure

For a total rhinectomy, the patient is placed on the operating table in a supine position. A skin incision begins along the lateral edge of one naris (Fig. 9-1). The incision is then carried out along that side of the external nose (Fig. 9-2). After a through-and-through incision has been accomplished, retraction of the ipsilateral soft tissues of the nose allows adequate visualization of the internal extent of the neoplasm (Fig. 9-3). After both lateral walls of the nose have been sectioned, the columella and septal incisions are made (Fig. 9-4). Stay sutures or double sharp hooks are used to retract the edges of the lateral wall margins, avoiding the use of clamps and forceps, which may fragment the tumor resulting in tumor implantation. Cartilaginous margins are easily obtained using a knife. Bony margins may require the use of a cutting bur, chisel, or bone-cutting forceps. Packing the nose may or may not be necessary to control bleeding. Normally, the blood vessels in jeopardy include the alveolar and septal branches of the facial artery as well as the ophthalmic and maxillary arteries. Bleeding from these vessels normally is easily controlled by direct clamping or cauterization.

Primary closure is usually possible using the surrounding skin and soft tissue of the area (Fig. 9-5). The use of split-thickness skin grafts is rarely necessary. An adequate cosmetic result can usually be achieved using a prosthesis or a forehead flap reconstruction (see Procedure 10).

LANNY G. CLOSE

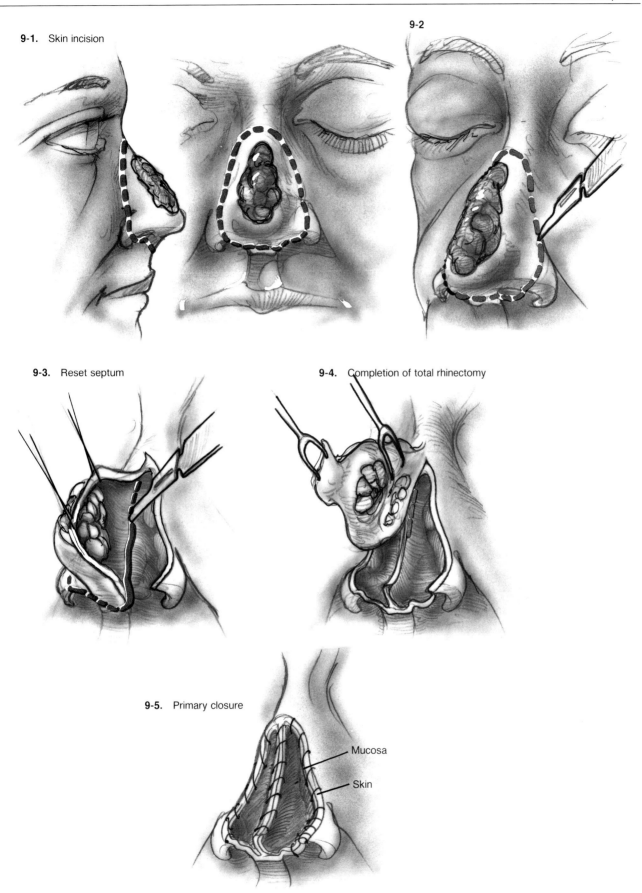

9-1. Skin incision

9-2

9-3. Reset septum

9-4. Completion of total rhinectomy

9-5. Primary closure

Mucosa

Skin

10. MIDLINE FOREHEAD FLAP NASAL RECONSTRUCTION— Reconstruction of the skin, soft tissue, and framework of the external nose using local tissue and regional skin and soft tissue of the forehead

Indications
1. Large defects of the external nose after trauma or surgical resection for cancer

Contraindications
1. Skin cancer (ie, condemned skin) of the forehead

Special Considerations
1. A forehead flap provides excellent color and texture match for nasal reconstruction.
2. A prosthetic nose may be preferable for two reasons: superior postoperative inspection of the cavity and superior cosmesis.
3. If flap reconstruction is planned after resection of a cancer, a delay of as long as 2 years is recommended to allow detection of a recurrence.

Preoperative Preparation
1. Routine laboratory studies
2. A tissue expander can be placed in the subgaleal plane of the forehead donor site for more than 3 weeks before reconstruction with several potential, but controversial, advantages: increased flap length, easier donor-site closure, and decreased flap thickness.

Special Instruments, Position, and Anesthesia
1. Headlight
2. Small, delicate plastic surgery instruments
3. Bipolar cautery

Tips and Pearls
1. A superiorly based mucoperichondrial-septal cartilage flap provides septal framework for the reconstructed nose.
2. Inner epithelial lining (ie, inverted local flaps) are essential for optimal results.
3. Onlay cartilage grafts (eg, auricle donor site) can be used to replace lower lateral cartilages.
4. The pericranium should not be included in forehead flap.
5. The blood supply of the flap (ie, supratrochlear artery) should be maintained until all flap revisions are completed.
6. Large defects may require free-flap reconstruction for the inner lining.
7. Bone grafts (eg, calvarial, rib, iliac crest) may be necessary for skeletal support.

Pitfalls and Complications
1. Unsatisfactory appearance (eg, bulbous, asymmetric tip)
2. Nasal airway obstruction
3. Absorption of cartilage grafts and loss of tip support

Postoperative Care Issues
1. All flap revisions (eg, thinning of flap, placement of cartilage or bone grafts) should be completed before vascular pedicle is divided.

References
Adamson JE. Nasal reconstruction with the expanded forehead flap. Plast Reconstr Surg 1988;81:12.

Kroll SS, Rosenfield L. Delayed pedicle separation in forehead flap nasal reconstruction. Ann Plast Surg 1989;23:327.

Operative Procedure

For midline forehead flap nasal reconstruction, the patient is positioned on the operating table in a supine position. After the onset of adequate general anesthesia, the nasal defect is inspected. If structural support is needed, a hinged, superiorly based nasal septal cartilage flap lined on each side by mucoperichondrium can be rotated forward to buttress the reconstructed columella and septal dorsum (Fig. 10-1). The cartilage flap is secured to the nasal spine periosteum or adjacent caudal septal cartilage with one or two horizontal mattress through-and-through sutures of 3-0 polydioxane (PDS) or 3-0 chromic catgut. Turn-in flaps—two nasal labial and one inferiorly based nasal dorsal flap (see Fig. 10-1)—are then elevated, made as thin as possible, and reflected into the nasal defect and sutured to one another with 4-0 chromic or 4-0 PDS suture. These turn-in flaps are essential to provide inner lining for the reconstructed nose.

Further structural support for the reconstructed nasal tip is provided by onlay cartilage grafts placed over the turn-in flaps to simulate the lateral crura of the lower lateral cartilages. These cartilage grafts are also designed to replace the fatty subcutaneous tissue of the nasal alae. The cartilage grafts, which are usually obtained from the auricle, can each be secured in position with a single horizontal mattress suture of 4-0 chromic catgut with the knot placed on the inner surface of the turn-in flap. The donor sites for the turn-in nasal labial flaps are closed primarily with 4-0 chromic catgut to the soft tissue and 5-0 nylon to the skin. The donor site for the turn-in nasion flap is left open to receive the forehead flap (Fig. 10-2).

A sea-gull-designed forehead flap based on the supratrochlear artery is outlined, sized, and raised in the subgaleal plane. As shown in Figure 10-2, this flap can be incised over a 400-cc rectangular tissue expander, which is placed in the subgaleal plane of the forehead donor site several weeks before reconstruction. Although placement of the tissue expander in the forehead is controversial (ie, some think the expanded flap constricts over time), the expander does offer several advantages, which are listed under Preoperative Preparation. The distal end of the forehead flap is raised superficial to the frontalis muscle to allow thinning of the flap, avoiding excessive bulbosity of the reconstructed nose. The forehead donor site is closed primarily using 3-0 chromic catgut sutures to the deep tissues and 4-0 nylon to the skin. The increased length of the sea-gull flap secondary to the use of the tissue expander can be demonstrated at this time by laying the flap over the forehead donor site after closure of this area (Fig. 10-3). The forehead flap is brought into position. The distal end is shaped and contoured to form the reconstructed tip as shown (Fig. 10-4). Special care must be taken to avoid touching or crossing the ipsilateral eye with the flap; it is recommended that the flap pedicle remain attached until all revision work on the reconstructed nose is completed. Closure of the flap to the recipient site is performed meticulously using 3-0 or 4-0 absorbable suture to the deep soft tissues and 4-0 or 5-0 nylon to the skin.

LANNY G. CLOSE

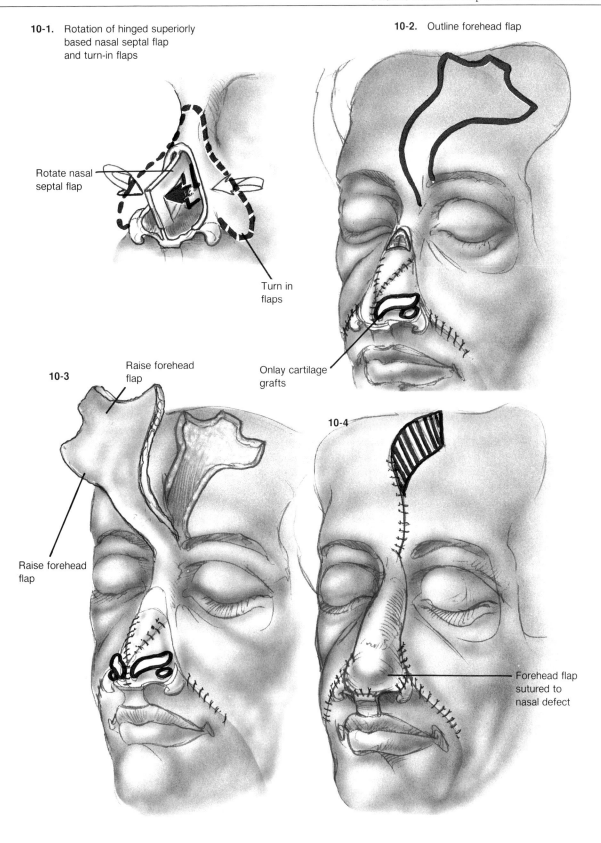

10-1. Rotation of hinged superiorly based nasal septal flap and turn-in flaps

Rotate nasal septal flap

Turn in flaps

10-2. Outline forehead flap

Onlay cartilage grafts

10-3

Raise forehead flap

Raise forehead flap

10-4

Forehead flap sutured to nasal defect

■ *11.* LATERAL RHINOTOMY

An incision along one side of the nose that, when combined with division of the nasal ala, provides limited access to the anterior cavity

Indications

1. Exposure for removal of lesions limited to the anterior nasal cavity and adjacent medial third of the maxilla and ethmoid sinuses
2. Exposure for repair of anteriorly placed nasal septal perforations

Contraindications

1. Exposure required lateral to the infraorbital foramen
2. Exposure required for resection of tumors involving the palate, infratemporal fossa, nasopharynx, or anterior cranial fossa
3. Exposure for salvage surgery after failed high-dose irradiation to the nasal or paranasal area, in which case facial incisions should be avoided

Preoperative Preparation

1. Routine laboratory studies
2. Computed tomography or magnetic resonance studies of nasal and paranasal areas

Special Instruments, Position, and Anesthesia

1. Headlight
2. Orotracheal intubation in the midline to avoid misalignment of closure
3. Electrosurgical cutting knife

Tips and Pearls

1. The medial canthal ligament should be reattached 1 to 2 mm anterior and superior to its normal position to counter the tendency to slide inferiorly after closure.
2. If a brow extension is used, the incision should parallel the hair follicles to avoid hair loss.
3. The frontal sinus floor should be exposed in the subperiosteal plane to avoid injury to the trochlea.
4. If septal resection is performed, caudal and septal struts should be left to avoid a saddle deformity.

Pitfalls and Complications

1. Transient diplopia
2. Epiphora
3. Nasocutaneous fistula
4. Telecanthus
5. Nasal collapse
6. Vestibular stenosis
7. Facial neuralgia (eg, infraorbital nerve injury)

Postoperative Care Issues

1. Sutures in nonirradiated patients should be removed from the skin on the fifth postoperative day.

References

Bernard PJ, Lawson W, Biller HF, LeBenger J. Complications following rhinotomy. Ann Otol Rhinol Laryngol 1989;98:684.

Mertz JS, Pearson BW, Kern EB. Lateral rhinotomy. Arch Otolaryngol 1983;109:235.

Operative Procedure

For a lateral rhinotomy, the patient is stationed on the operating table in a supine position. After the induction of general anesthesia, a tarsorrhaphy suture of 5-0 silk is placed to approximate the upper and lower eyelids. A curvilinear incision is then made, beginning just below the medial aspect of the eyebrow and extending inferiorly in a plane approximately one-half the distance between the medial canthus and the nasion. A broken line at the medial canthal level is used to prevent postoperative webbing (Fig. 11-1).

The incision then continues downward in or just anterior to the nasomaxillary sulcus, curving laterally to fall within the alar sulcus and ending within the nostril. Hatch marks may be placed at the alar rim to allow exact skin realignment at closure. The incision is then deepened in layers, with hemostasis obtained by electrocautery or ligature of the angular vessels and their branches. The incision is carried down to the underlying bone, barring soft tissue involvement by the neoplasm to be removed. A precise periosteal cut is made, and the periosteum is elevated in one layer over the bone of the maxilla and its frontal process. The medial canthal ligament is detached from the anterior and posterior lacrimal crests in this same periosteal plane, and the lacrimal sac is carefully displaced from its fossa and retracted laterally (Fig. 11-2). The sac is not transected unless a medial subtotal or total maxillectomy is being performed. If necessary, the periorbita can be elevated superiorly and posteriorly to allow lateral retraction of the orbital contents.

The nasal ala is detached and mobilized by completing the alar sulcus incision by dividing the vestibular lining with a knife or scissors (see Fig. 11-2). A lateral osteotomy of the nasal pyramid is then performed low, along the frontal process of the maxilla, using a curved Nivert chisel or oscillating saw (Fig. 11-3). The corresponding nasal mucosa is incised using the electrocautery, and the bone is out-fractured, rotated, and retracted to the opposite side with a 2-0 silk suture or double hook through the ala to allow maximum exposure of the anterior septum and nasal cavity. The periosteum of the anterior face of the maxilla can then be elevated laterally, avoiding injury to the infraorbital nerve.

Bone cuts of the facial skeleton may be required at this point according to the procedure performed (see Procedures 13 and 14). Additional skin incisions may be made for further exposure of the nasal cavity or facial skeleton (see Fig. 11-1, *dotted line*).

Wound closure after lateral rhinotomy is performed by approximating the deep periosteal layer with multiple, interrupted 4-0 catgut sutures. Special care should be exercised in reattaching the periosteum of the medial canthal area to ensure proper orientation of the structure. Closure of the subcutaneous layer in the area of the ala should be reinforced by a deep suture from the alar soft tissues into the cheek tissues. Skin closure is then accomplished using a 5-0 or 6-0 nylon suture (Fig. 11-4).

LANNY G. CLOSE

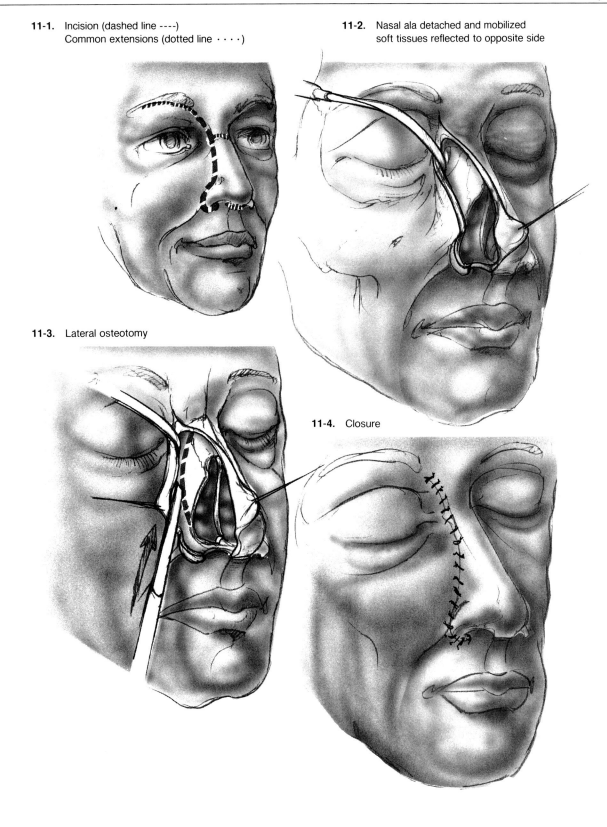

11-1. Incision (dashed line - - - -)
Common extensions (dotted line · · · ·)

11-2. Nasal ala detached and mobilized
soft tissues reflected to opposite side

11-3. Lateral osteotomy

11-4. Closure

12. MEDIAL MAXILLECTOMY

En bloc resection of the medial maxillary sinus wall and ipsilateral ethmoid sinus, including the lamina papyracea, lacrimal bone, and medial orbital floor

Indications
1. Benign tumors and low-grade malignancies confined to the lateral nasal wall, maxillary antrum, and ethmoid sinus

Contraindications
1. Invasive malignancies of the maxillary or ethmoid sinus area
2. Tumors with palatal, pterygoid, or extensive orbital bone involvement
3. Tumors with intracranial (ie, dural) extension

Special Considerations
1. Can be combined with craniofacial resection for benign tumors or low-grade malignancies involving the lateral nasal wall and floor of the anterior cranial fossa

Preoperative Preparation
1. Routine laboratory studies
2. Computed tomography or magnetic resonance studies of nasal and paranasal areas

Special Instruments, Position, and Anesthesia
1. Headlight
2. Orotracheal intubation in the midline to avoid misalignment of closure
3. Electrosurgical cutting knife
4. Bipolar cautery
5. Large right-angled scissors (eg, Foman)

Tips and Pearls
1. Intraoperative blood loss can be diminished by bipolar coagulation of the anterior and posterior ethmoid arteries before sectioning.
2. Blood loss can also be reduced by performing the posterior osteotomy last, removing the specium and exposing the sphenopalatine vessels for clamping or cauterization.
3. Marsupialization of the bisected end of the lacrimal sac to the surrounding tissue of the nose provides adequate lacrimal drainage in most cases.
4. A split-thickness skin graft is needed only if extensive resection of the periorbita results in herniation of orbital fat.

Pitfalls and Complications
1. Epiphora and dacrocystitis
2. Transient diplopia
3. Telecanthus
4. Nasal collapse
5. Mucocele
6. Facial neuralgia (eg, infraorbital nerve injury)

Postoperative Care Issue
1. Twice-daily saline lavages should be started within 1 week of surgery to avoid drying and crusting of the cavity.

References
Osguthorpe JD, Weisman RA. "Medial maxillectomy" for lateral nasal wall neoplasms. Arch Otolaryngol Head Neck Surg 1991;117:751.
Sessions RB, Humphreys DH. Technical modifications of the medial maxillectomy. Arch Otolaryngol 1983;109:575.

Operative Procedure

For medial maxillectomy, the patient is in the supine position on the operating table. Exposure can be provided by a facial degloving approach (see Procedure 353), a lateral rhinotomy (see Procedure 11), or a Weber Ferguson incision (see Procedure 13). After the underlying bone is exposed, the periosteum is elevated in one layer over the bone of the maxilla, including the frontal process, with a Freer elevator (Fig. 12-1). The medial canthal ligament is detached from the anterior and posterior lacrimal crest in the subperiosteal plane, and the dissection is continued posteriorly over the lacrimal fossa and lamina papyracea, allowing lateral retraction of the lacrimal sac and orbital contents. The lacrimal sac is then transected tangentially along its widest segment to allow a subsequent decrocystorhinostomy (see Fig. 12-1). Transection of the lacrimal sac facilitates lateral retraction of the orbital contents and identification of the anterior and posterior ethmoid arteries.

The subperiosteal elevation is then extended laterally along the floor of the orbit to a point just lateral to the plane of the infraorbital nerve. An extensive removal of the anterior wall of the maxillary sinus, including that portion medial to the infraorbital foramen, is performed under direct vision. An osteotomy of the adjacent nasal process of the maxilla is made low, along the face of the maxilla, allowing retraction of the lateral wall of the nose toward the opposite side of the face (see Fig. 12-1). The initial bone cut for removal of the specimen is made along the floor of the nose, sharply incising the medial wall of the maxillary sinus from its most anterior aspect posteriorly to the posterior wall of the maxillary sinus or the pterygoid plate (see Fig. 12-1).

A second bone cut is then made through the maxillary antrostomy. This cut extends from the floor of the nasal cavity superiorly in the most anterior point of the maxillary sinus, extending superiorly to end at the lacrimal fossa (Fig. 12-2).

The third bone cut is made using the medial canthal approach, with the orbital contents retracted laterally. The cut extends just below the frontoethmoidal suture line identified by the plane of the anterior and posterior ethmoid arteries, beginning anteriorly at the lacrimal fossa and extending posteriorly to the posterior ethmoid artery. The bone cut should not extend beyond the posterior ethmoid artery foramen, avoiding injury to the optic nerve. A bone cut along the floor of the orbit extending from the anterior lacrimal crest to the plane of the infraorbital nerve joins this cut to the previously made anterior bone cut (Fig. 12-3).

The fourth bone cut is made along an imaginary line drawn along the orbital floor, beginning anteriorly just medial to the infraorbital nerve and extending diagonally and posteriorly across the lamina papyracea to join the posterior extent of the previously performed superior bone cut (Fig. 12-3).

The final bone cut is performed to divide the only remaining bony attachments of the lateral nasal wall, the portion of the palatine bone lying just anterior to the pterygoid process of the sphenoid bone. Transection of this bone, which extends from the floor of nose up to the posterior tip of the superior turbinate, is best performed using a large, right-angled scissor (ie, Foman) (Fig. 12-4). The most superior extent of the cut cannot be completed with this instrument; this bony attachment is thin and best released by using a bimanual maneuver employing the index finger of both hands, one in the maxillary sinus and the other in the nasal cavity. A dacryocystorhinostomy is performed and the medial canthal tendon is then secured in position. Closure of the facial incision or the degloving approach is accomplished in the usual fashion (see Procedures 11, 13, and 353).

LANNY G. CLOSE

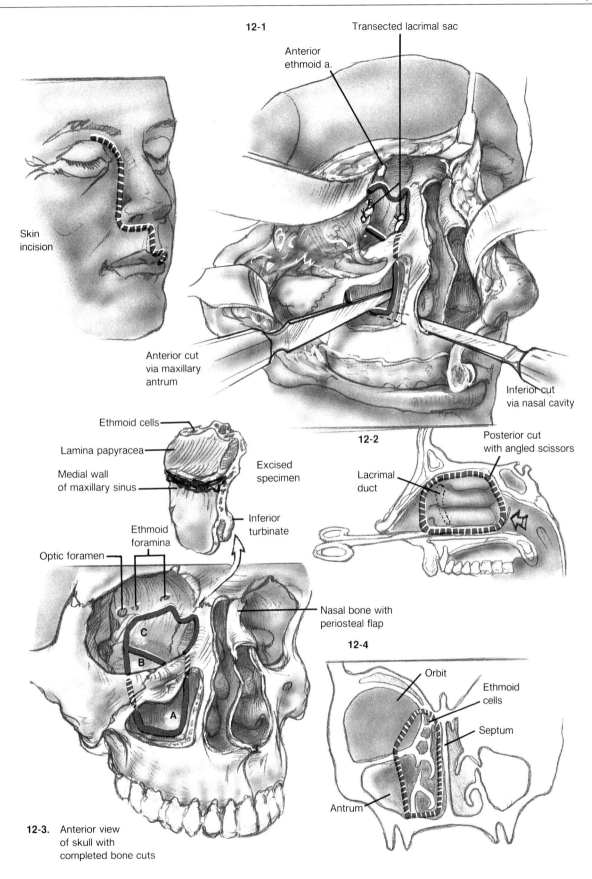

12-1

Transected lacrimal sac

Anterior ethmoid a.

Skin incision

Anterior cut via maxillary antrum

Inferior cut via nasal cavity

Ethmoid cells

Lamina papyracea

Medial wall of maxillary sinus

Excised specimen

Optic foramen

Ethmoid foramina

Inferior turbinate

12-2

Lacrimal duct

Posterior cut with angled scissors

Nasal bone with periosteal flap

C

B

A

12-3. Anterior view of skull with completed bone cuts

12-4

Orbit

Ethmoid cells

Septum

Antrum

▪ 13. WEBER-FERGUSON APPROACH WITH SUBTOTAL MAXILLECTOMY AND TOTAL MAXILLECTOMY WITH ORBITAL PRESERVATION

13a. **Weber-Ferguson Approach**—An extension of the lateral rhinotomy incision that includes splitting the upper lip

Indications
1. Exenteration of the maxilla for a total or subtotal maxillectomy (splitting the upper lip releases the facial flap for adequate lateral retraction and adds transoral exposure of the palate and teeth)

Special Instruments, Position, and Anesthesia
1. Headlight
2. Delicate plastic surgery instruments

Tips and Pearls
1. Stair-stepping the incision at the vermilion border and performing a Z-plasty as part of the mucosal incision reduces contracture.

Pitfalls and Complications
1. Necrosis of the flap is more likely when salvage surgery is performed for a high-dose irradiation failure.

Postoperative Care Issues
1. Routine cleaning and application of antibiotic ointment.

Reference
Sobol SM, Wood B, Levine H. An approach to total maxillectomy with emphasis on orbital preservation. Plast Reconstr Surg 1982;69:945.

Subtotal (Partial) Maxillectomy—En bloc resection of a segment of the maxilla, preserving one or more bony buttresses or perimeters normally resected in a total maxillectomy

Indications
1. Benign or malignant neoplasms confined to the medial wall or floor of the maxillary sinus

Contraindications
1. Tumors with pterygoid or extensive orbital bone involvement
2. Tumors with intracranial (ie, dural) extension
3. Tumors with lateral extension or palatal involvement
4. Tumors with orbital floor or malar involvement

Special Considerations
1. Medial subtotal maxillectomy can be combined with craniofacial resection for tumors involving the lateral nasal wall and floor of the anterior cranial fossa.

Preoperative Preparation
1. Computed tomography (CT) or magnetic resonance (MR) studies of nasal and paranasal areas
2. Imaging should precede a biopsy to avoid surgical artifacts.
3. Tumors that appear vascular or that are close to major vessels should be evaluated by arteriography.
4. Vascular tumors should be biopsied in the operating room.

Pitfalls and Complications
1. Epiphora or dacryocystitis
2. Transient diplopia
3. Facial neuralgia (eg, infraorbital nerve injury)

Postoperative Care Issues
1. Careful inspection of the maxillectomy cavity must be performed at appropriate intervals to detect recurrent or residual tumor.
2. Follow-up CT or MR imaging of the cavity at 6- to 12-month intervals can facilitate detection of recurrent disease.

References
Barton RT. Management of carcinoma arising in the lateral nasal wall. Arch Otolaryngol 1980;106:685.

Operative Procedure
The upper lip incision begins in the ipsilateral nasal vestibule (Fig. 13-1). It is brought just lateral to the base of the nasal columella, across to the midline of the upper lip, and then extended down to the vermilion border. The incision can be brought straight down through the vermilion or, as shown, along the vermilion border to the contralateral edge of the Cupid's bow of the upper lip and then down through the vermilion (see Fig. 13-1).

The infraorbital portion of the Weber-Ferguson incision begins at the lateral canthus and extends medially in the subciliary level, 3 to 4 mm below the ciliary line. The orbicularis oculi muscle is incised tangentially in an inferior direction, exposing but protecting the integrity of the orbital septum. A gingival-buccal incision is begun in the midline at the end of the lip splitting incision and extended laterally to the ipsilateral maxillary tuberosity. A 1- to 1.5-cm cuff of mucosa should be preserved on the dental side to facilitate closure.

Extensions of the Weber-Ferguson incision (see Fig. 13-1) include a superior extension from the medial canthus parallel and just inferior to the eyebrow. If this incision is employed, it is carried down to the underlying bone. Periosteum is then elevated over the frontal process of the maxilla and the roof of the orbit.

The facial flap is then elevated laterally in a subperiosteal plane over the maxilla and around the infraorbital nerve, which is preserved (Fig. 13-2). The dissection is then carried laterally over the lateral buttress of the maxilla. The orbital contents are dissected from the medial and inferior walls of the orbital cavity in the subperiosteal plane, exposing the lacrimal sac and the anterior and posterior ethmoid arteries. These structures are managed as described for a medial maxillectomy (see Procedure 12). The anterior wall of the maxillary antrum is penetrated by creating a window of bone using a 4-mm chisel. This antrostomy is enlarged using a Kerrison rongeur, preserving a rim of bone around the infraorbital nerve and extending the window superiorly toward the lamina papyracea.

If a medial subtotal maxillectomy is to be performed, the first osteotomy begins at the floor of the piriform aperture and extends posteriorly at the level of the nasal floor until the osteotome perforates the posterior wall of the antrum (Fig. 13-3). The orbital contents are retracted laterally, and a second osteotomy is performed at the frontoethmoid suture line, extending posteriorly to a point 1 to 2 mm posterior to the posterior ethmoid artery. A bony rim is left around the optic foramen to protect the optic nerve from injury. A third bone cut in the thin bone of the medial orbital floor extends from the posterior end of the second or superior osteotomy to a point just medial to the infraorbital nerve (see Fig. 13-3).

The final bone cut is difficult and can require up to three steps. First, a small (2–4-mm) osteotome is introduced through the antrostomy and directed toward the most posterior extent of the medial antral wall, cutting this mucosa and bone from a point corresponding to the most posterior end of the superior osteotomy down to the most posterior extension of the inferior osteotomy. Second, a wide osteotome is introduced into the ipsilateral nose, impacted against the anterior wall of the sphenoid sinus, and displaced laterally. The third step requires the use of a heavy right-angle scissors, which is guided through the inferior osteotomy with one blade in the nose and the other in the antrum, cutting through bone just posterior to the turbinates. The specimen can then be removed by anterior and inferior traction.

LANNY G. CLOSE

Subtotal Maxillectomy

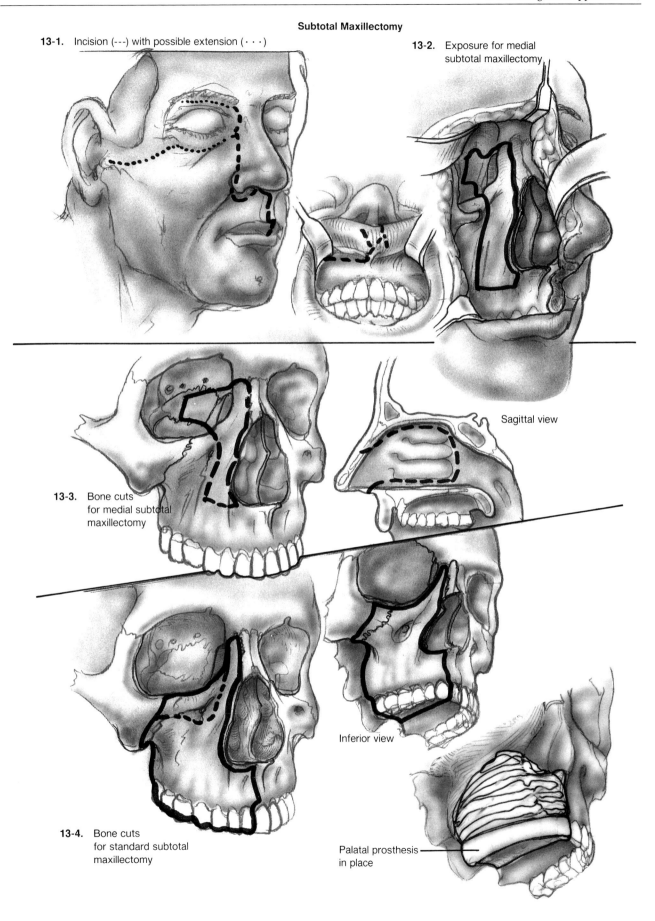

13-1. Incision (---) with possible extension (· · ·)

13-2. Exposure for medial subtotal maxillectomy

Sagittal view

13-3. Bone cuts for medial subtotal maxillectomy

13-4. Bone cuts for standard subtotal maxillectomy

Inferior view

Palatal prosthesis in place

■ *13.* WEBER-FERGUSON APPROACH WITH SUBTOTAL MAXILLECTOMY AND TOTAL MAXILLECTOMY WITH ORBITAL PRESERVATION *(continued)*

13b. Total Maxillectomy With Orbital Preservation—
En bloc resection of the entire maxilla, preserving the ipsilateral orbital contents

Indications
1. Malignant or benign aggressive tumors involving the maxillary sinus without erosion of the orbital floor

Contraindications
1. The orbital contents cannot be preserved (ie, orbital exenteration indicated) because of erosion of the bony floor or medial wall of the orbit; because of invasion of the periorbita, orbital apex, or infraorbital nerve; or because of the need for postoperative irradiation to the orbit for close or positive margins (irradiation usually results in a nonfunctional eye).
2. Tumors with intracranial (ie, dural) extension (see cranial facial resection, Procedure 15).

Special Considerations
1. The surgical treatment of lesions approximating the posterior wall of the maxillary antrum should include resection of the pterygoid plates and surrounding pterygoid muscles.

Preoperative Preparation
1. Computed tomography or magnetic resonance studies of nasal and paranasal areas
2. Imaging should precede a biopsy to avoid surgical artifacts.
3. Tumors that appear vascular or that are close to major vessels should be evaluated by arteriography.
4. Vascular tumors should be biopsied in the operating room.
5. If a lymphoreticular tumor is suspected, fresh tissue for imprinting and immunohistochemical analysis is necessary.

Special Instruments, Position, and Anesthesia
1. Electrosurgical cutting knife
2. Bipolar cautery

Tips and Pearls
1. Marsupialization of the bisected end the lacrimal sac to the surrounding tissue of the nose provides adequate lacrimal drainage in most cases.
2. Enophthalmos can occur after resection of the orbital floor. In addition to an intact periorbita, suspension with a skin graft, fascia lata graft, or temporalis muscle flap can minimize this problem.

Pitfalls and Complications
1. Epiphora or dacryocystitis
2. Diplopia or enophthalmos
3. Facial neuralgia (eg, infraorbital nerve injury)

Postoperative Care Issues
1. An open, epithelium-lined cavity is preferred to facilitate cleaning and inspection of the cavity. Packing the cavity holds grafts or flaps in position and prevents excessive bleeding.
2. Regional or microvascular free flaps are indicated to provide support to the eye or brain, to isolate the intracranial contents from the UADT, for patients who are unable to care for a prosthesis, or for large skin defects.
3. A well-designed prosthesis is generally superior to a tissue flap for function and cosmesis.

References
Sisson GA, Toriumi DM, Atiyah RA. Paranasal sinus malignancy: a comprehensive update. Laryngoscope 1989;99:143.

Stern SJ, Goepfert H, Clayman G, Byers R, Kian Ang K, El-Naggar AK. Squamous cell carcinoma of the maxillary sinus. Arch Otolaryngol Head Neck Surg 1993;119:964.

Operative Procedure
A tracheotomy is always indicated in a total maxillectomy if there is any question regarding the oral airway during surgery. After the onset of general anesthesia, a Weber-Ferguson incision (see Procedure 13a) is performed. A subciliary extension of the incision is joined to the lateral rhinotomy limb near the medial canthus (Fig. 13-5). This incision begins at the lateral canthus and extends medially at a level 3 to 4 mm below the ciliary line. A transconjunctival incision may be substituted if desired. The eye is protected by a temporary tarsorrhaphy stitch. The orbicularis oculi muscle is incised tangentially in an inferior direction, exposing but protecting the integrity of the orbital septum. The gingivobuccal incision is extended laterally to the ipsilateral maxillary tuberosity (see Fig. 13-5). The soft palate is incised at the hard-soft palate junction, transecting its bony attachments. The mucoperiosteum of the hard palate is incised following a paramedian line ipsilateral to the lesion. If the floor of the maxillary sinus is not involved by cancer, this incision my be brought laterally through the tooth socket of the ipsilateral canine or first premolar, which has been extracted. Saving the ipsilateral lateral incisor and canine along with the adjacent anterior hard palate lends greater stability to a palatal prosthesis. Otherwise, the incision is joined to the gingivobuccal incision through a gingival defect created by the extraction of an upper incisor on the side of the lesion. The paramedian strip of mucoperiosteum is preserved for later imbrication over the bony edge of the hard palate to facilitate subsequent fitting of a prosthesis.

The facial flap is then elevated laterally in a subperiosteal plane to expose the surgical area. Involvement of the anterior wall of the maxillary antrum necessitates elevation of the flap in a subcutaneous plane, including the facial musculature in the specimen. Involved skin may also be resected en bloc if necessary. The dissection is then carried laterally, over the lateral buttress of the maxilla, identifying and clipping the internal maxillary artery at the pterygomaxillary fissure (Fig. 13-6). The orbital septum is dissected from the medial, inferior, and lateral walls of the orbital cavity, exposing the lacrimal sac, the anterior and posterior ethmoid arteries and the infraorbital fissure. These structures are managed as described for a subtotal maxillectomy. Osteotomies and removal of the specimen follow. The body and frontal process of the zygoma are divided with a nitrogen-powered oscillating saw. A bone cut is made, separating the maxilla from the nasal bones, and the osteotomy is extended superiorly to the frontal ethmoidal suture line (Fig. 13-7). From this point, the osteotomy is carried posteriorly, just inferior to the level of anterior and posterior ethmoid arteries, to a point 1 to 2 mm posterior to the posterior ethmoid artery (ie, 1–2 mm anterior to the optic foramen). An osteotomy is then performed, connecting the lateral and medial orbital wall osteotomies across the inferior orbital fissure. The hard palate is then transected near the midline with an oscillating or Gigli saw (see Fig. 13-7).

The maxilla can then be disattached from the skull by tapping a chisel placed in pterygomaxillary fissure in the posterior superior direction. If tumor involves the posterior wall of the maxilla, the pterygoid plates can be transected with a chisel as shown (see Fig. 13-7). The superior attachments of the turbinate are sharply divided as described for the medial subtotal maxillectomy. Anteroinferior traction and gentle rocking allows removal of the specimen. The ethmoidectomy can be completed under direct visualization. The coronoid process of the mandible can be removed to avoid subsequent displacement of the maxillary prosthesis when opening and closing the jaw. Routine closure and reconstruction after a total maxillectomy with orbital preservation includes lining the exposed facial soft tissues, pterygoid muscles, and periorbita with a split-thickness skin graft that is 0.35 to 0.45 mm thick (Fig. 13-8). A prefabricated obturator or palatal prosthesis is then wired to the remaining upper arch dentition or suspended from the zygomatic arch and piriform aperture. Closure of the soft tissue and skin is performed as described for the Weber-Ferguson incision (see Procedure 13a).

LANNY G. CLOSE

Total Maxillectomy With Orbital Preservation

13-5

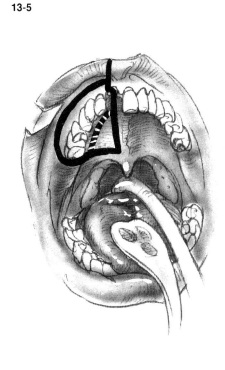

13-6. Operative field after flap raised

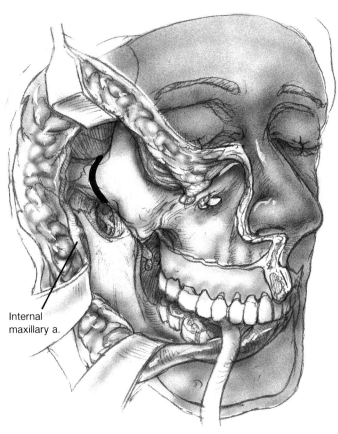

Internal
maxillary a.

13-7. Bone cuts for total maxillectomy

Optic
foramen

Ethmoid
foramina

13-8. Split-thickness skin graft placement
following removal of specimen

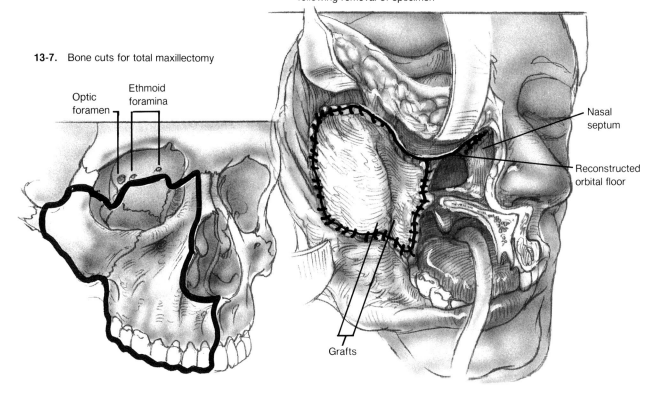

Nasal
septum

Reconstructed
orbital floor

Grafts

■ 14. RADICAL MAXILLECTOMY WITH ORBITAL EXENTERATION—Radical en bloc resection of the maxilla, ethmoid labyrinth, anterior zygoma, and the orbit and adnexal structures

Indications

1. Malignant tumor of the maxillary sinus or maxilla with superior extension into the orbit
2. Aggressive infection of the maxillary sinus (invasive mucormycosis) in the immunocompromised host

Special Considerations

1. Involvement of the orbit of the only seeing eye
2. Retrograde involvement of intracranial structures or the cavernous sinus
3. Extension of the tumor into the cavernous sinus or nasopharynx

Preoperative Preparation

1. Comprehensive imaging evaluation (computed tomography with contrast, and gadolinium-enhanced magnetic resonance imaging) to evaluate three-dimensional extent of tumor
2. Obtain and review preoperative biopsy. The Caldwell-Luc procedure or endoscopic antrostomy may be needed to obtain adequate tissue sample.
3. Preoperative neuroophthalmology consultation
4. Review patient at multidisciplinary tumor board, and obtain input from radiation oncology and medical oncology.
5. Maxillofacial prosthetic evaluation for postoperative surgical obturator and prosthesis.
6. Type and crossmatch patient for 4 units of packed red blood cells. The use of autologous blood transfusion may depend on institutional guidelines.

Special Instruments, Position, and Anesthesia

1. Mayfield or horseshoe head holder
2. Headlight
3. Reciprocating saw with thin (<1-mm) blade
4. Automatic vascular clip applier
5. Armored endotracheal tube wired to mandibular dentition of the mandible (if edentulous)

(continued)

Operative Procedure

The patient is placed in the supine position, with the head on a Mayfield head holder. General anesthesia is carried out in the usual fashion using orotracheal intubation and intravenous control. Before making any incisions, the skin and subcutaneous tissue can be infiltrated with a 0.25% solution of lidocaine with 1:400,000 epinephrine. A tarsorrhaphy suture is placed.

The skin is incised from the medial canthus inferiorly along the lateral nasal wall, nasal-alar groove, and nasal sill and is completed with a lip split through the philtrum. Notching the incision at the philtrum-vermilion border facilitates closure and prevents scar contracture of the lip. The superior aspect of the skin incision is continued laterally from the medial canthus, excising the lid margin from the upper and lower eyelids. At the lateral canthus, the incision is extended laterally an additional 2 cm (Fig. 14-1). A mucosal incision is made in the gingivobuccal sulcus from the anterior midline laterally to the maxillary tuberosity (Fig. 14-2).

Using electrocautery, an incision is made posteriorly at the hard-soft palate junction and extended anteriorly in the midline of the palate. An incisor tooth can be extracted at this time. The mucoperiosteum of the hard palate is elevated to expose palatal bone. The nasal cavity is then entered by incising the nasal mucosa at the piriform aperture (see Fig. 14-2).

Facial flaps are elevated in the subperiosteal plane, unless there is clinical or radiographic evidence of soft tissue invasion. A more superficial dissection may be required if tumor has eroded the anterior wall of the maxillary antrum (Fig. 14-3).

Bone cuts are made with a reciprocating saw using a narrow (<1-mm) blade. Laterally, on osteotomy is made at the junction of temporal process of the zygoma and the zygomatic process of the temporal bone. Superiorly, an osteotomy is made from above malar eminence to the inferior orbital fissure (Figs. 14-4 and 14-5). Intraoperative bradycardia may occur when the optic nerve is transected (Fig. 14-6).

(continued)

14-1. Incisions with possible extensions

14-2. Hard–soft palate incision

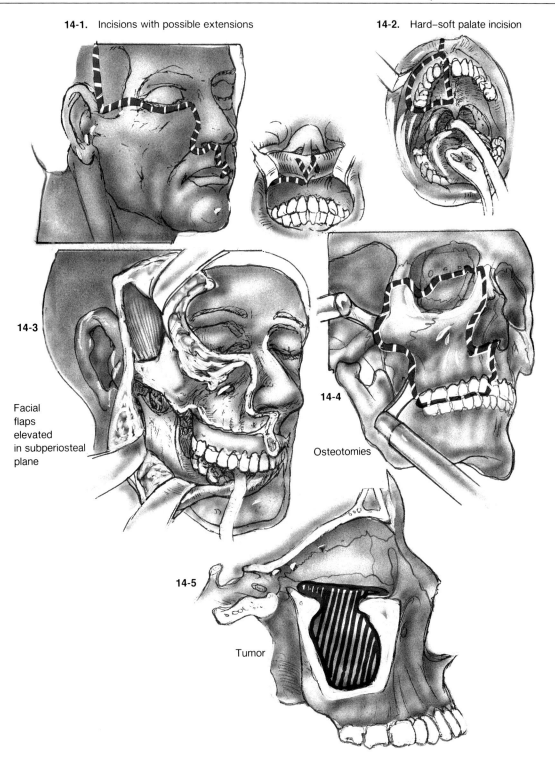

14-3

Facial
flaps
elevated
in subperiosteal
plane

14-4

Osteotomies

14-5

Tumor

■ *14.* RADICAL MAXILLECTOMY WITH ORBITAL EXENTERATION *(continued)*

Tips and Pearls

1. Removal of the zygoma results in a smoothing of the contour of the exenteration defect and may facilitate prosthetic rehabilitation.
2. The temporalis muscle may be transposed into defect and obviate the need for free-flap reconstruction.
3. If the eyelids are free of tumor, they can be used to resurface the defect.

Pitfalls and Complications

1. Intraoperative bradycardia when the optic nerve is transected
2. Unanticipated involvement of the anterior cranial base (superiorly) or cavernous sinus (posteriorly)
3. Incomplete tumor resection, as indicated by tumor-positive margin

Postoperative Care Issues

1. Maintenance of good oral hygiene and care of the maxillectomy defect
2. Special attention to protection of the contralateral, unoperated eye
3. Paresthesia in the V_1 and V_2 distributions

References

Janecka IP. Cranial base surgery for paranasal sinus cancer: indications. Head Neck Cancer 1993;3:945.

Rice DH, Stanley RB. Surgical therapy of nasal cavity, ethmoid sinus, and maxillary sinus tumors. In: Thawley SE, Panje WR, Batsakis JG, Lindberg RD, eds. Comprehensive management of head and neck tumors. Philadelphia: WB Saunders, 1987:368.

Sessions DG, Cummings CW, Weymuller EA, et al. Atlas of access and reconstruction in head and neck surgery. St. Louis: Mosby-Year Book, 1992

Sisson G, Snyderman NL, Becker S. Cancer of the nasal cavity and paranasal sinuses. In: Myers EN, Suen JY, eds. Cancer of the head and neck. 2nd ed. New York: Churchill Livingstone, 1989:311.

Optimum reconstruction of the radical maxillectomy–orbital exenteration defect should be single staged, rapid, and allow early return of deglutition and articulation (Fig. 14-7). The temporalis muscle flap is frequently used for dead space obliteration and restoration of facial contour. A palatal obturator facilitates oronasal separation.

To harvest the temporalis muscle flap, the scalp is incised in a hemicoronal fashion. Scalp flaps are undermined posteriorly and anteriorly. The borders of the temporalis muscle are delineated with the electric cautery. The muscle is elevated in the subperiosteal plane. The superficial temporal artery is unnecessary, but preservation of the internal maxillary artery system is essential for flap survival. Removal of the zygomatic arch greatly facilitates the transposition of the muscle anteriorly. A greater arch of rotation can be achieved by removal of the coronoid process of the mandible. Care should be taken to preserve the deep temporal arteries during removal of the coronoid process (Fig. 14-8).

The muscle is transposed anteriorly and sutured to the periphery of the defect. The soft tissues of the cheek flap are rotated medially and over the temporalis muscle. This obliterates the dead space of the orbit, ethmoid, and maxillary sinuses. Removal of the zygoma and some lateral orbital wall prevents the formation of a deep orbital socket and provides for a smooth contour of the defect (Fig. 14-9).

A circumferential dressing may be applied to facilitate coaptation between the cheek flap and the underlying temporalis muscle.

IVO P. JANECKA
GUY J. PETRUZZELLI

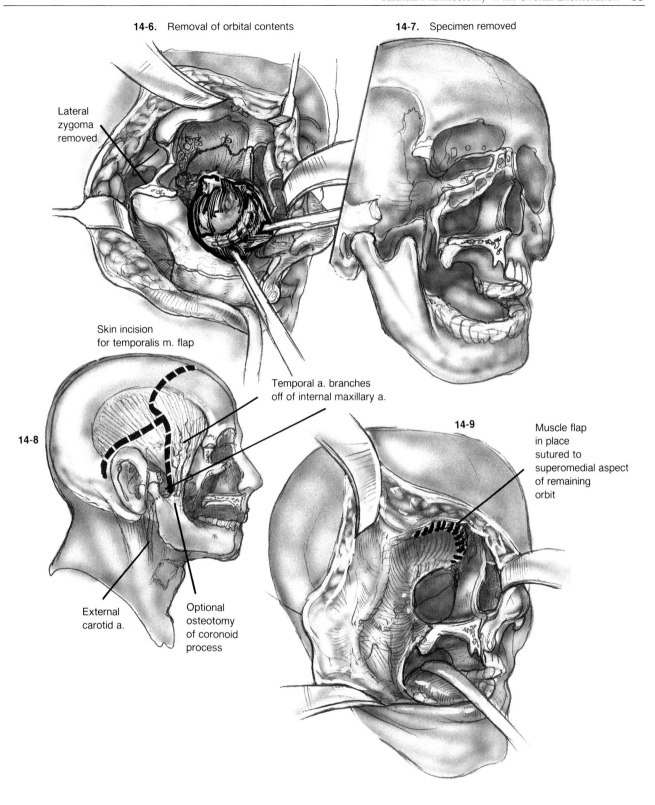

14-6.   Removal of orbital contents

14-7.   Specimen removed

Lateral
zygoma
removed

Skin incision
for temporalis m. flap

Temporal a. branches
off of internal maxillary a.

14-8

14-9

Muscle flap
in place
sutured to
superomedial aspect
of remaining
orbit

External
carotid a.

Optional
osteotomy
of coronoid
process

■ *15.* CRANIOFACIAL RESECTION, INCLUDING THE ETHMOID LABYRINTH AND CRIBRIFORM PLATE—En bloc resection of the floor of the central and paracentral cranial base, including the cribriform plate, medial aspects of the fovea ethmoidalis, superior nasal septum, and ethmoid labyrinth

Indications

1. Benign or malignant neoplasms (eg, olfactory neuroblastoma, olfactory groove meningioma) of the cribriform plate or olfactory tracts
2. Advanced paranasal sinus malignancies with involvement of the superior ethmoid or cribriform plate

Special Considerations

1. Involvement of the dura and brain parenchyma
2. Extension of the tumor into the cavernous sinus or clivus

Preoperative Preparation

1. Preoperative ophthalmologic evaluation
2. Neurosurgery consultation to review preoperative planning and evaluation
3. Evaluation of the patient by a neuroanesthesiologist
4. Obtain and review the biopsy of the lesion. If it is a malignant tumor, the case should be presented at the multidisciplinary tumor conference to review treatment options and the eligibility for protocols.
5. Evaluation by radiation oncologist
6. Review preoperative imaging, including axial and direct coronal computed tomography (CT) scans and T1- and T2-weighted magnetic resonance images, with the neurosurgeon and neuroradiologist. Special attention should be directed to dural involvement by the tumor, extension of the tumor into the brain parenchyma, presence of fluid or secretions, and tumor involvement of the paranasal sinuses.
7. Crossmatch 4 units of packed red blood cells.
8. Notify the blood bank to have cryoprecipitate tissue adhesive (ie, fibrin glue) available.
9. Use antithromboembolism sequential compression devices on the lower extremities.
10. Administer prophylactic anticonvulsant medication.
11. Administer a prophylactic antibiotic with known penetration into cerebrospinal fluid.

Special Instruments, Position, and Anesthesia

1. Place a lumbar subarachnoid drain for brain decompression.
2. Be prepared to decompress the brain with furosemide or mannitol intraoperatively.
3. Miniplating and microplating systems for rigid fixation of the craniofacial skeleton
4. Headlights
5. Mayfield (horseshoe) head holder
6. Reciprocating saw with a thin (<1 mm) blade
7. Separate surgical setup, prepping, and draping for harvesting the tensor fascia lata graft

(continued)

Operative Procedure

Surgical access to the cribriform plate–anterior cranial base region is best accomplished by a combination of superior and inferior approaches. The superior exposure can be obtained through a bifrontal craniotomy encompassing the frontal sinus or through a more limited transfrontal sinus approach. The inferior exposure can be accomplished by a lateral rhinotomy, midface degloving, open rhinoplasty, or transseptal approach. The bifrontal craniotomy–lateral rhinotomy approach for resection of cribriform plate or anterior cranial base neoplasms is outlined.

The patient is positioned in the supine position on a Mayfield or other horseshoe head holder, and general endotracheal anesthesia is administered. Perioperative parenteral antibiotics with good CSF penetration should be administered. A lumbar subarachnoid drain should be placed preoperatively. Furosemide or mannitol should be available to reduce CSF volume intraoperatively.

If the patient's head is not to be fully shaved, the hair should be carefully washed with povidone-iodine (Betadine) or other surgical scrub solution. The patient's hair should be parted along the path of the proposed bicoronal incision. The scalp is incised parallel to the direction of the hair follicles to prevent alopecia. The incision is carried down to the bone, and the flap is elevated deep to the periosteum. Careful attention is paid to preserving the supraorbital and supratrochlear vessels. The flap is elevated anteriorly to the supraorbital ridge of the frontal bone, after which the supraorbital vessels can be identified in the notch or foramen. Additional length on the flap can be gained by gently opening the bony notch or foramen with an osteotome and freeing the neurovascular bundle. This maneuver facilitates the dissection of the roof of the orbit and frees the periorbita superiorly (Fig. 15-1).

With the flap secured anteriorly, the neurosurgical team proceeds with a bifrontal craniotomy. The inferior extent of the bone cut should be close to the supraorbital rim. The frontal lobes are then dissected from the internal aspect of the frontal bone, and the anterior dural attachment to the crista galli with the olfactory nerves is divided (Figs. 15-1*B* and 15-2).

Subfrontal removal of the supraorbital rim helps to increase exposure and reduce brain retraction. Using malleable retractors, the frontal lobes and orbital contents are protected (Fig. 15-3). A reciprocating saw is used extracranially to divide the frontal bone at the nasion. This cut transects the nasofrontal ducts. The supraorbital rims are divided with vertical saw cuts. The lateral position of this cut depends on the location of the tumor and amount of bone to be removed. Intracranially, the vertical osteotomy is continued with a bone cut across the roof of the orbits. A final vertical osteotomy is made intracranially anterior to the crista galli (Fig. 15-4). This frees this central bony segment containing the supraorbital rims and nasion. The frontal sinus is then cranialized by removing all mucosa and the posterior bony wall of the sinus.

After removal of the frontal bone and central supraorbital segment, the dura can be more easily elevated posteriorly to the planum sphenoidale. The extent of dural invasion is assessed at this time, and a resection of the dura can be performed.

(continued)

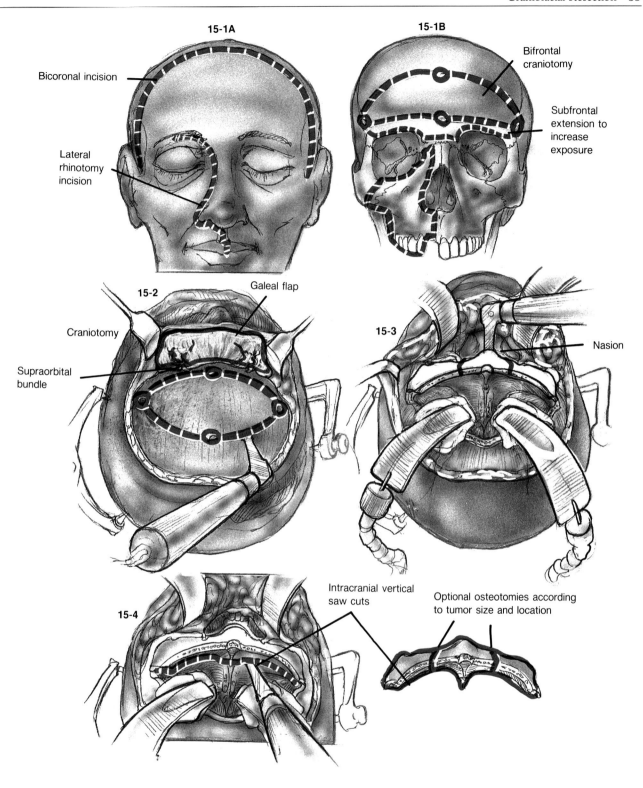

15-1A

Bicoronal incision

Lateral rhinotomy incision

15-1B

Bifrontal craniotomy

Subfrontal extension to increase exposure

15-2

Galeal flap

Craniotomy

Supraorbital bundle

15-3

Nasion

15-4

Intracranial vertical saw cuts

Optional osteotomies according to tumor size and location

■ *15.* CRANIOFACIAL RESECTION, INCLUDING THE ETHMOID LABYRINTH AND CRIBRIFORM PLATE *(continued)*

Tips and Pearls

1. Wide transfacial exposure to deliver tumor from below
2. Supraorbital rim removal to reduce brain retraction
3. Elevate the pericranial flap just before the graft inset to reduce flap desiccation or excessive traction on vessels.

Pitfalls and Complications

1. Bilateral hypesthesia of supraorbital and supratrochlear nerves
2. Brain injury, hematoma, subdural, or intraparenchymal hemorrhage
3. Failure of the dural repair, with cerebrospinal fluid (CSF) leak and meningitis
4. Osteomyelitis of the frontal bone flap
5. Excessive frontal lobe retraction, causing alteration in sensorium and personality changes
6. Coagulopathy
7. Syndrome of inappropriate antidiuretic hormone secretion or diabetes insipidus
8. Seizures
9. Stress peptic ulcer

Postoperative Care Issues

1. Perioperative monitoring in the neurosurgical intensive care unit, with frequent neurologic assessment of the level of consciousness, pupil responses, cranial nerves, and extremities
2. CT scan without contrast on the morning after surgery
3. Monitor serum and urine osmolarity for 48 hours postoperatively.
4. Intravenous fluid administered below maintenance dose
5. Scalp drain to bulb suction or closed passive drain if at high risk for CSF leak

References

Janecka IP, Sekhar LN. Anterior and anterolateral craniofacial resection. In: Sekhar LN, Janecka IP, eds. Surgery of cranial base tumors. New York: Raven Press, 1993:147.

Sekhar LN, Nanda N, Sen CN, et al. The extended frontal approach to tumors of the anterior, middle, and posterior skull base. J Neurosurg 1992;76:198.

Snyderman CH, Janecka IP, Sekhar LN, et al. Anterior cranial base reconstruction: role of galeal and pericranial flaps. Laryngoscope 1990;100:607.

The brain is protected by self-retaining retractors, and the floor of the anterior cranial fossa is widely visualized. Using a reciprocating saw, parallel bone cuts are made lateral to the margin of the cribriform plate (Fig. 15-5). The posterior osteotomy is made in the region of the planum sphenoidale (Fig. 15-6). The operating microscope is useful when making the posterior cut to avoid damage to the optic nerves or chiasm. This completes the superior aspect of the dissection and releases the specimen from above.

The extent of the tumor dictates the size and degree of transnasal exposure necessary for tumor removal. Options include limited or complete medial maxillectomy, maxillectomy with palate preservation, total maxillectomy, and radical maxillectomy with orbital exenteration.

A commonly used approach is through a lateral rhinotomy incision, respecting the aesthetic units of the nose. The nasal sill can be incised and the nose reflected medially to provide greater exposure (Fig. 15-7*A*). The periosteum is elevated over the face of the maxilla and the medial wall of the orbit (Fig. 15-7*B*). The frontoethmoidal suture is identified and followed posteriorly to the anterior ethmoid artery, which is cauterized. The lacrimal sac is identified and elevated from the lacrimal fossa. The sac can be transected low. Subsequently, it may be incised and the edges sutured open to prevent epiphora.

Using the reciprocating saw, facial osteotomies are made as dictated by the three-dimensional extent of the tumor. These usually include horizontal cuts through the nasal septum and lateral walls of the nose and vertical cuts through the medial orbital walls. The posterior-superior cut across the nasal septum can be made with a right-angle rhinoplasty scissors (Fig. 15-8).

The specimen is delivered from below. Removal of the specimen creates a large defect, producing direct communication among the paranasal sinuses, nasopharynx, and anterior cranial fossa (Fig. 15-9). Additional margins can be obtained from the patient at this time. Bleeding encountered from branches of the sphenopalatine artery at the posterior attachment of the middle turbinate can be controlled with bipolar cautery (see Fig. 15-2).

After complete tumor removal, meticulous hemostasis, and assessment of the surgical margins with frozen-section control (if necessary), the cranial and nasal cavities are separated with a pericranial flap.

The avascular plane between the pericranium and galea is developed, with sharp dissection beginning at the free edge of the bicoronal incision. The flap is dissected to the level of the supraorbital rim. However, care should be taken not to extend the dissection too far anteriorly, which could compromise the supraorbital or supratrochlear feeding vessels.

The flap is then transposed intracranially and sutured posteriorly to dural attachments or suture holes placed in the region of the planum sphenoidale. Care must be taken to avoid the optic chiasm or optic nerves when securing the posterior aspect of the flap (Fig. 15-10). Any additional dead space can be obliterated with free fat grafts.

The supraorbital rim is replaced over the pericranial flap and secured with plate fixation, as is the craniotomy.

GUY J. PETRUZZELLI
IVO P. JANECKA

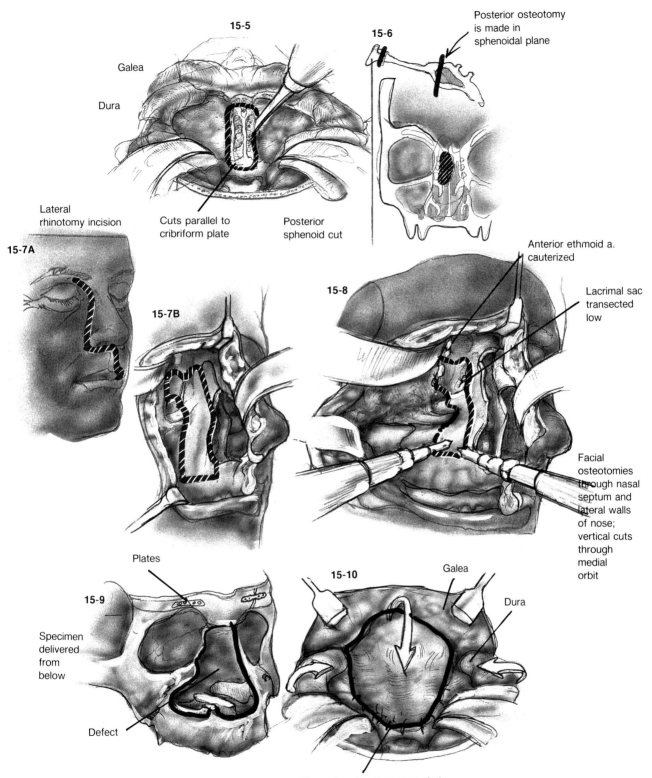

15-5

Galea

Dura

Lateral rhinotomy incision

Cuts parallel to cribriform plate

Posterior sphenoid cut

15-6

Posterior osteotomy is made in sphenoidal plane

15-7A

15-7B

15-8

Anterior ethmoid a. cauterized

Lacrimal sac transected low

Facial osteotomies through nasal septum and lateral walls of nose; vertical cuts through medial orbit

Plates

15-9

Specimen delivered from below

Defect

15-10

Galea

Dura

Flap sutured to dura posteriorly

■ 16. FACIAL TRANSLOCATION FOR NASO-PHARYNGEAL ANGIOFIBROMA RESECTION—

Temporary disarticulation of the craniofacial skeleton to increase access to the nasopharynx, clivus, and cavernous sinus, with immediate reinsertion and fixation of the bony elements and reconstruction of the soft tissue components

Indications

1. Benign or malignant tumors of the nasopharynx (eg, carcinoma, angiofibroma, adenocarcinoma)
2. Tumor of the clivus (eg, chordoma, chondrosarcoma)
3. Tumors of the cavernous sinus (eg, meningioma, hemangioma)

Special Considerations

1. Intracranial extension of tumor requiring combined neurosurgical procedure, such as a middle or anterior fossa craniotomy
2. Cavernous sinus involvement

Preoperative Preparation

1. Carotid arteriography with balloon occlusion testing for neoplasms of the cavernous sinus
2. Review preoperative imaging, including axial and direct coronal computed tomography scans and T1- and T2-weighted magnetic resonance images, with the neurosurgeon and neuroradiologist. Special attention should be directed to dural involvement by tumor, extension of the tumor into the brain parenchyma, presence of fluid or secretions, and tumor involvement in the paranasal sinuses.
3. Preoperative ophthalmologic evaluation
4. Schedule intraoperative monitoring of the frontal branches of the facial nerve
5. Appropriate preoperative consultation with neurosurgeon if the tumor extends intracranially
6. Preoperative embolization, if technically feasible, for vascular tumors

(continued)

Operative Procedure

The patient is positioned in the supine position on a Mayfield or other horseshoe head holder, and general endotracheal anesthesia is administered. A hemicoronal incision from the vertex to the tragus is made, staying superficial to the temporoparietal fascia (Fig. 16-1). Using magnification and a facial nerve monitor, several twigs of the frontal branch of the facial nerve are identified, tagged for later neurorrhaphy, and divided. The anterior scalp flap is then undermined to the level of the supraorbital rim. The zygoma is skeletonized, and the attachment of the masseter muscle is divided.

An inferiorly based cheek flap based on the facial and labial vascular pedicle is developed as a separate layer or as a composite layer with the underlying fascial skeleton. A lip-splitting incision may be made, beginning at the vermilion border and extending superiorly into the alar groove along the lateral nose, to the midpoint of the lateral crus of the lower lateral cartilage. The incision is extended vertically, respecting the aesthetic units of the nose, into the medial canthus. A horizontal limb is then carried into the medial canthal area, and the attachment of the medial canthal tendon onto the lacrimal bone is marked before performing a medial canthotomy. A transconjunctival incision is carried into the lateral canthus, and a lateral canthotomy is performed. This incision is extended horizontally across the temple to join the preauricular component of the scalp incision.

Several craniofacial osteotomies are performed: a LeFort I from the piriform aperture laterally to the pterygoid buttress, horizontally at the junction of the medial and inferior orbital walls, laterally from the inferior orbital fissure through the zygomaticomaxillary buttress, and using the right-angle oscillating blade, across the orbital floor (Fig. 16-2). A frontotemporal craniotomy is added as needed for exposure of the middle cranial base.

At this point, the surgeon can see the posterior nasal septum, the contralateral nasopharynx and eustachian tube, posterior wall of the ipsilateral maxillary sinus and pterygoid plates, and the ipsilateral infratemporal fossa. The three-dimensional extent of the tumor can be appreciated, and the tumor can be removed in a well-controlled fashion (Fig. 16-3).

(continued)

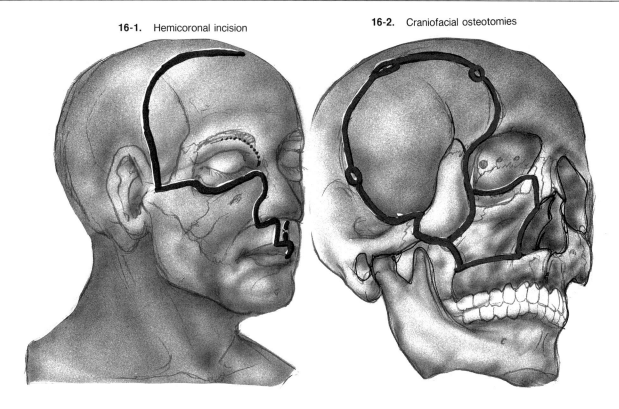

16-1. Hemicoronal incision

16-2. Craniofacial osteotomies

Forehead flap

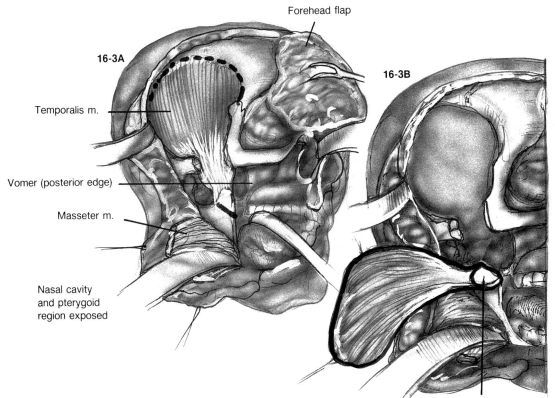

16-3A

Temporalis m.

Vomer (posterior edge)

Masseter m.

Nasal cavity
and pterygoid
region exposed

16-3B

Out-fracture of coronoid process,
reflected inferiorly with the
temporalis m.

■ 16. FACIAL TRANSLOCATION FOR NASO-PHARYNGEAL ANGIOFIBROMA RESECTION
(continued)

Special Instruments, Position, and Anesthesia

1. Facial nerve stimulator and nerve monitor to facilitate identification of frontal branches
2. Reciprocating saw with a thin (<1 mm) blade
3. Oscillating blade with 90° bend for intraorbital osteotomy
4. Miniplating and microplating systems for rigid fixation of the craniofacial skeleton
5. The anesthesia team should avoid muscle relaxants during the initial phase of the procedure.
6. Mayfield (horseshoe) head holder
7. Prophylactic perioperative antibiotics
8. Antiembolism sequential pneumatic compression device
9. Headlight

Tips and Pearls

1. Temporary lateral tarsorrhaphy
2. Magnification (loupes) for facial nerve neurorrhaphy
3. Intubation of the lacrimal system can help to prevent canalicular stenosis.

Pitfalls and Complications

1. Epiphora
2. Ectropion
3. Loss of temporalis muscle flap due to excessive traction or ligation of the internal maxillary artery
4. Nasal stenosis
5. Temporary weakness of the ipsilateral forehead branches of the facial nerve and the need for temporary tarsorrhaphy
6. Hypesthesia of the ipsilateral infraorbital nerve

Postoperative Care Issues

1. Attention to eye care for ipsilateral eye, which may need a temporary eye patch
2. Frequent saline irrigations of the nasal cavity to prevent crusting

References

Arriaga MA, Janecka IP. Facial translocation approach to the cranial base: the anatomic basis. Skull Base Surg 1991;1:26.

Janecka IP, Sen CN, Sekhar LN, Arriaga MA. Facial translocation: a new approach to the cranial base. Otolaryngol Head Neck Surg 1990;103:413.

After confirmation of tumor removal by frozen-section analysis, reconstruction is begun by repairing the dura. The temporalis muscle can be transposed anteriorly to reconstruct the nasopharynx, pterygoid, or infratemporal fossa regions (Figs. 16-4, 16-5, and 16-6). The craniofacial skeleton is reconstructed by means of rigid fixation using microplates. The orbital floor can be reconstructed with split calvarial bone grafts or micromesh (Fig. 16-7). The medial and lateral canthal ligaments must be reattached to reestablish the normal position of the globe. The lacrimal system is reconstructed by intubation of the superior and inferior canaliculi with thin Silastic tubing, which is drawn into the nose and left in place for 4 to 6 weeks. The inferior lid fornix is closed, and the previously tagged stumps of the frontal branches of the facial nerve are reapproximated. A temporary lateral tarsorrhaphy is performed and remains in place for 7 to 10 days. A nasopharyngeal airway is placed to prevent nasopharyngeal stenosis and is removed 7 to 10 days postoperatively.

IVO P. JANECKA
GUY J. PETRUZELLI

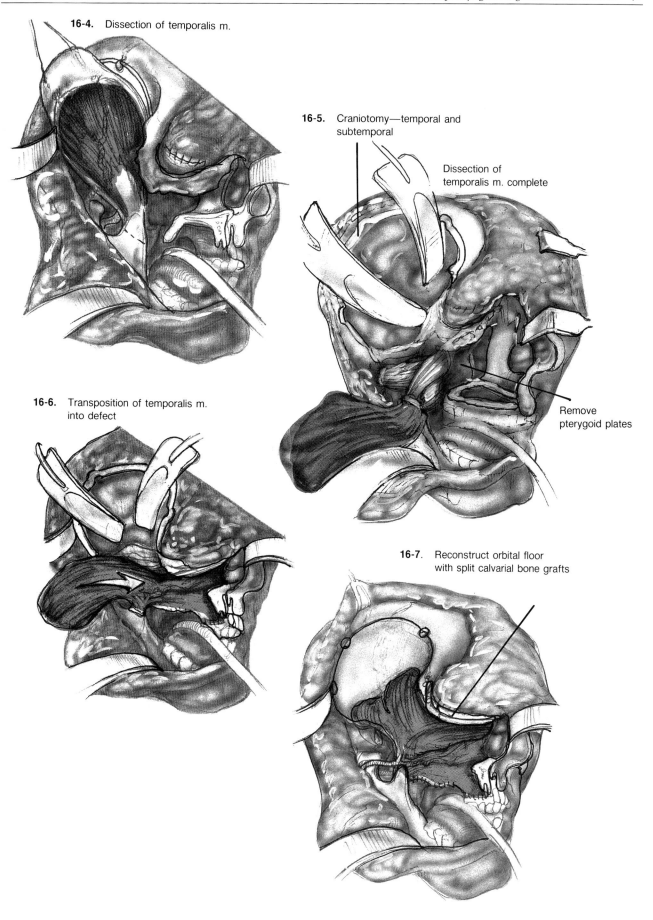

16-4.   Dissection of temporalis m.

16-5.   Craniotomy—temporal and subtemporal

Dissection of temporalis m. complete

Remove pterygoid plates

16-6.   Transposition of temporalis m. into defect

16-7.   Reconstruct orbital floor with split calvarial bone grafts

■ *17.* VERMILIONECTOMY

Partial or total excision of the exposed vermilion area of the lip

Indications

1. Chronic actinic cheilitis
2. Dysplasia
3. Carcinoma in situ
4. Microinvasive carcinoma

Contraindications

1. Frankly invasive carcinoma

Special Considerations

1. Gross dental infection
2. Nasal sepsis
3. Prior treatment, if any
4. Neck node status

Preoperative Preparation

1. Routine lab studies
2. Diagnostic biopsy

Special Instruments, Position, and Anesthesia

1. Headlight (optional)
2. Skinhooks, toothed Adson forceps, fine Metzenbaum scissors, measuring calipers
3. Table in neutral position, head turned toward the surgeon
4. Local anesthesia by lip infiltration or bilateral mental nerve block, if the patient is unfit for general anesthesia

Tips and Pearls

1. Frozen-section control
2. Excise down to orbicularis oris muscle for microinvasive carcinoma
3. Adequate buccal mucosal advancement is essential to preserve labial bulk. However, advancement further forward than the original vermilion-cutaneous junction causes a feminizing effect
4. Undermine buccal mucosa for a distance of 1.5 times the maximum diameter of excised vermilion
5. Undermine skin for a distance equal to the maximum diameter of the excised vermilion
6. Tensionless closure

Pitfalls and Complications

1. Edema and ecchymosis
2. Postoperative bleeding
3. Persistent paresthesia
4. Pruritus
5. Prickling sensation in upper lip of male patients, caused by upward projection of hairs from lower lip
6. Flattening of lip
7. Excessive fullness of lip, with feminizing.

Postoperative Care Issues

1. Antibiotic ointment during healing phase
2. Decrease sun exposure and quit tobacco
3. Five-year cancer follow-up.

References

Bailey BJ, Nichols ML. Small defects (vermilion, mucosa, and less than one third lower lip). In Calhoun KH, Stiernberg CM, eds. Surgery of the lip. New York: Thieme Medical Publishers, 1992:24.

Freeman MS, Thomas JR. Vermilionectomy. In Bailey BJ (ed). Surgery of the oral cavity. Chicago: Year Book Medical Publishers, 1989:1.

Operative Procedure

The patient is placed on the operating table in a supine position, with the head turned toward the surgeon.

The proposed excision is outlined with methylene blue. The outer incision usually corresponds to the vermilion border, but should include 5 mm of skin if lip disease extends to the cutaneous margin. The lip is gently steadied with the fingers of the surgeon's nondominant hand. Using a #15 blade scalpel, the outer incision is extended from commissure to commissure, staying superficial to the orbicularis oris musculature. A corresponding elliptical incision is made on the mucosal aspect of the lip, including a margin of approximately 5 mm of normal appearing mucosa. The inner and outer incisions are connected at the commissures (Fig. 17-1). The surgical specimen is then grasped at the left commissure with a toothed Adson forceps, and retracted. The diseased mucosa is elevated with the scalpel from left to right commissure, in a submucosal plane immediately superficial to the orbicularis, and excised (Figs. 17-2 and 17-3) Care must be exercised to avoid buttonholing the diseased mucosa. Bleeding tends to be brisk during this phase of the operation; it can be controlled by judicious use of needletip electrocautery. Some minor salivary glands will be included in the specimen. Protruding salivary glands left behind on the musculature should be trimmed with Metzenbaum scissors.

Mucosal and deep margins are sent for frozen section. When margins are clear, reconstruction of the vermilion can begin.

The edge of the remaining normal labial mucosa is grasped with a toothed Adson forceps and retracted. This mucosa is undermined with a Metzenbaum scissors for a distance of approximately 1.5 times the maximum width of the excised specimen. The skin edge is similarly undermined but only for a distance corresponding to the maximum width of the specimen. Further undermining will be necessary, on both sides, if there is excessive tension.

Always check for adequate hemostasis before final closure.

The skin is sutured to the labial mucosal flap with a single layer of interrupted 5-0 Prolene (Figs. 17-4 and 17-5). This must be done in a very meticulous fashion, ensuring accurate and symmetrical approximation of skin and mucosal edges, at the level of the original vermilion-cutaneous junction.

Finally, a thin layer of antibiotic ointment is applied to the "new" lip. This is maintained during the postoperative healing phase.

Alternatively, a carbon dioxide laser, at a power setting of 5 to 10 watts, may be used to carry out a vermilionectomy. This method vaporizes the diseased mucosa and does not provide the pathologist with a specimen for microscopic analysis. Therefore, it is not recommended for microinvasive disease. Healing is by secondary intention. Antibiotic ointment should be applied until reepithelialization has occurred.

JOHN B. KINSELLA

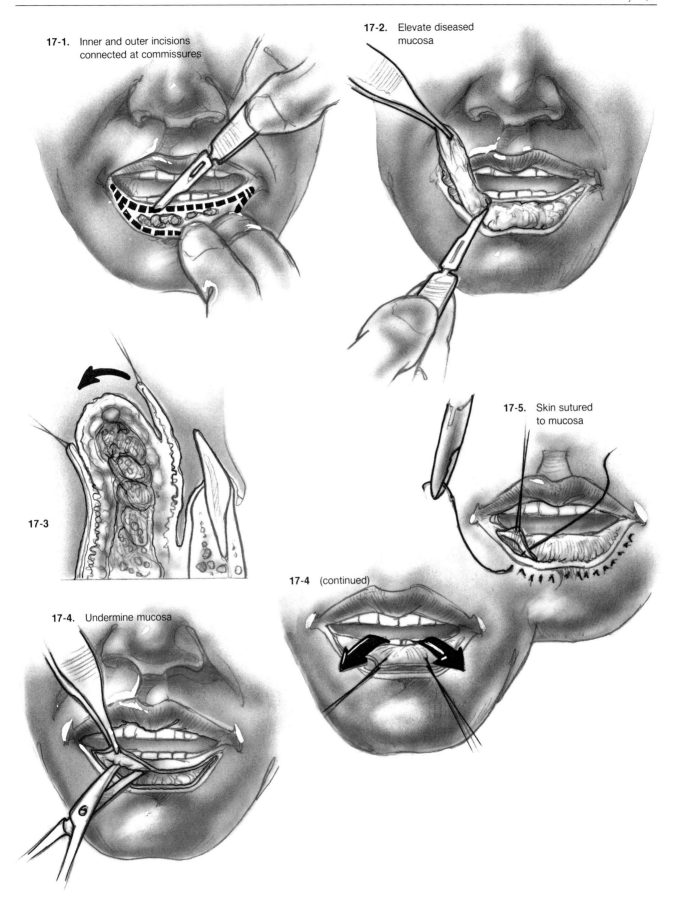

17-1. Inner and outer incisions connected at commissures

17-2. Elevate diseased mucosa

17-3

17-4. Undermine mucosa

17-4 (continued)

17-5. Skin sutured to mucosa

■ *18.* VERMILIONECTOMY PLUS WEDGE
EXCISION—Partial or total excision of the exposed vermilion of the lip, plus a through-and-through excision of a V-shaped area of the same lip

Indications
1. Invasive carcinoma combined with chronic actinic cheilitis
2. Invasive carcinoma combined with chronic dysplasia
3. Invasive carcinoma combined with carcinoma in situ

Contraindications
1. Lesions larger than 1.5 cm (ie, vermilion defects larger than 3 cm)
2. Lesions involving the oral commissure
3. Lesions extending deep into the oral cavity
4. Lesions extending deep into the lip musculature

Special Considerations
1. Gross dental infection
2. Nasal sepsis
3. Prior treatment
4. Neck node status

Preoperative Preparation
1. Routine laboratory studies
2. Diagnostic biopsy

Special Instruments, Position, and Anesthesia
1. Headlight (optional)
2. Skin hooks, toothed Adson forceps, fine Metzenbaum scissors, measuring caliper
3. Table in neutral position, head turned toward the surgeon
4. Local anesthesia by lip infiltration or bilateral mental nerve block if the patient is unfit for general anesthesia

Tips and Pearls
1. Design the wedge so that its central axis is orientated favorably with the relaxed skin tension lines.
2. Avoid carrying excision lines across mental crease, wherever possible.
3. Send frozen sections to confirm the adequacy of the excision.
4. Careful, three-layer closure with eversion of mucosa and skin edges
5. Accurate reapproximation of the vermilion edges at either end of the V-shaped excision avoids notching.

Pitfalls and Complications
1. Step deformity, if vermilion-cutaneous margins are realigned incorrectly
2. Microstomia, if wedge diameter is greater than 3 cm

Postoperative Care Issues
1. Splint the wound to decrease tension and movement.
2. Antibiotic ointment during healing phase
3. Counsel to decrease sun exposure and quit tobacco
4. Five-year cancer follow-up

References
Bailey BJ, Nichols ML. Small defects (vermilion, mucosa, and less than one third lower lip). In: Calhoun KH, Stiernberg CM, eds. Surgery of the lip. New York: Thieme Medical Publishers, 1992:24.

Calhoun KH. Reconstruction of small- and medium-sized defects of the lower lip. Am J Otolaryngol 1992;13:16.

Renner GJ, Zitsch RP. Reconstruction of the lip. Otolaryngol Clin North Am 1990;23:975.

Operative Procedure
The patient is placed on the operating table in a prone position, with the head turned toward the surgeon. Nasal endotracheal intubation keeps the airway out of the operative field. The proposed excision lines are marked with methylene blue (Fig. 18-1). A V-shaped excision centered at the site of the palpable carcinoma is outlined and added to the markings for a standard vermilionectomy, as previously described.

The following description applies to a carcinoma located near the center of the lower lip. The vermilionectomy is performed initially. The outer incisions usually correspond to the vermilion-cutaneous junction. A #15 blade scalpel is used to make these incisions, beginning at the commissures and extending as far as the borders of the wedge. Corresponding elliptical mucosal incisions are made, including 5 mm of normal tissue. These mucosal incisions connect with the outer incisions at the commissures. Beginning at each commissure, the diseased mucosa is then elevated off the orbicularis oris musculature as far as the edges of the wedge using Adson forceps and a scalpel (Fig. 18-2).

At this point, the skin of the V is incised with the same #15 blade scalpel. The orbicularis muscle and internal labial mucosa are then incised, creating a through-and-through wedge defect (Fig. 18-3). The labial artery requires ligation at both ends of the V when connecting the lip shave to the wedge excision.

The margins are sent for frozen-section analysis to confirm adequate surgical excision.

The defect is closed if the margins are clear and hemostasis is satisfactory. The orbicularis muscle layer of the wedge defect is approximated first, starting at the apex and using 3-0 Dexon or Vicryl suture (Fig. 18-4).

Attention is then turned to reconstruction of a new vermilion surface. The remaining normal labial mucosa and skin edges are undermined and mobilized with a fine Metzenbaum scissors. The labial flap is then advanced over the exposed musculature of the lip and carefully approximated to the mobilized skin edges with a single layer of everted and interrupted vertical mattress sutures of 5-0 silk (Fig. 18-5).

Three-layer closure of the wedge defect is completed using 4-0 Dexon or Vicryl for the subcutaneous tissue and 5-0 silk for skin. These skin sutures should be interrupted and vertically mattressed to provide strong and accurate approximation, with eversion.

Antibiotic ointment is applied to the suture lines during the healing phase. Splinting the wound protects it from movement and excessive wound tension, which helps to prevent notching and scarring. To create a splint, the skin adjacent to the closure line of the wedge is painted with tincture of benzoin. A piece of one inch tape is then applied over this, on each side of the wound. A large safety pin is then placed through the mesial end of each piece of tape. An elastic band wrapped around the safety pins helps to counterbalance distraction forces tending to pull the wound edges apart (Fig. 18-6).

JOHN B. KINSELLA

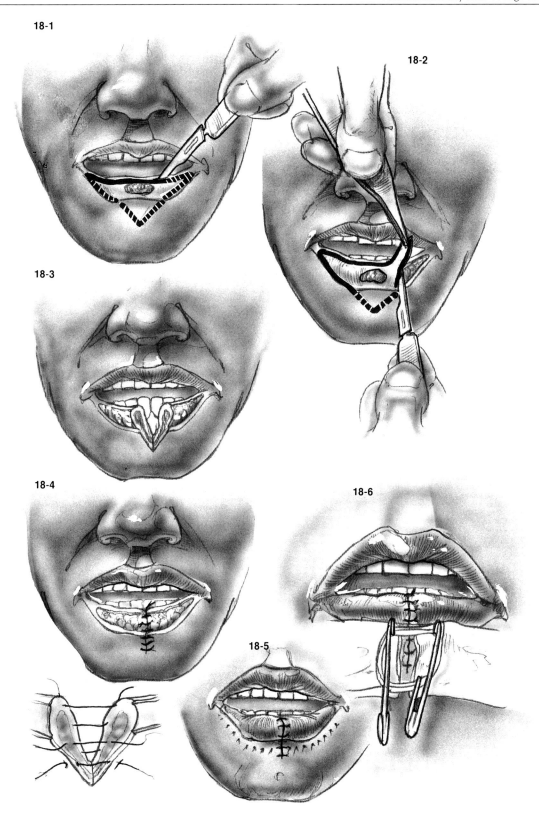

18-1

18-2

18-3

18-4

18-5

18-6

■ 19. LIP EXCISION: W-EXCISION AND PENTAGONAL SHIELD PATTERN—Full-thickness excision of the lip, producing a W- or pentagon-shaped defect, with primary closure, which are variations on the simple wedge pattern. The W pattern allows excision of a long horizontal portion of vermilion, without requiring a long vertical component, which would cross the mental crease. The pentagonal pattern excises a broader surgical specimen beyond the vermilion-cutaneous junction than that of the wedge or W variations.

Indications

1. W-pattern excision may be suitable for tumors 16 to 20 mm long (ie, 26–30-mm defect), with limited invasion beyond vermilion-cutaneous junction.
2. Pentagon excision may be suitable for tumors 16 to 20 mm long (ie, 26–30-mm defect), with moderate invasion beyond the vermilion-cutaneous junction. This pattern has considerable vertical extension. It is more applicable to lateral than midline tumors, because more vertical excision is possible in the former, without crossing the mental crease.

Contraindications

1. Lip defects longer than 3 cm
2. Lesions involving the oral commissure
3. Lesions extending deep into the oral cavity
4. Lesions extending deep into the lip musculature

Special Considerations

1. Gross dental infection
2. Nasal sepsis
3. Prior treatment
4. Neck node status

Preoperative Preparation

1. Routine laboratory studies
2. Diagnostic biopsy
3. Panorex if lesion encroaches on the gingivolabial sulcus or the mandible

Special Instruments, Position, and Anesthesia

1. Headlight (optional)
2. Skin hooks, toothed Adson forceps, fine Metzenbaum scissors, measuring caliper
3. Table in neutral position, with the head turned toward the surgeon
4. Local anesthesia by lip infiltration or bilateral mental nerve block if the patient is unfit for general anesthesia

Tips and Pearls

1. Design the W excision to create two inferior angles of 30°
2. Design the pentagon excision to create an inferior angle of 30°
3. Avoid extending excision lines across mental crease, wherever possible
4. Send frozen sections to confirm the adequacy of the excision
5. Close in three layers, with eversion of mucosal and skin edges

Pitfalls and Complications

1. Microstomia occurs if more than one third of the lip diameter is sacrificed.
2. Accurate reapproximation of the vermilion edges is essential to avoid notching.

Postoperative Care Issues

1. Splint the wound to decrease tension and movement.
2. Apply antibiotic ointment during healing phase
3. Counsel to decrease sun exposure and quit tobacco
4. Five-year cancer follow-up

References

Bailey BJ. Wedge and shield excision. In: Bailey BJ, ed. Surgery of the oral cavity. Chicago: Year Book Medical Publishers, 1989:6.

Renner GL, Zitsch RP. Reconstruction of the lip. Otolaryngol Clin North Am 1990;23:975.

Wheeland RG. Reconstruction of the lower lip and chin using local and random-pattern flaps. J Dermatol Surg Oncol 1991;17:605.

Operative Procedure

The patient is placed on the operating table in a prone position. Nasal endotracheal intubation keeps the airway out of the operative field. The proposed excision lines are marked with methylene blue, after carefully estimating the tumor extension by inspection and palpation. For a W excision, design two inferior angles of 30°. The central peak of the W must not return too close to the tumor (Fig. 19-1). If in any doubt, convert to a pentagon. In the case of a pentagonal excision, the inferior angle should also be kept close to 30° but can be a little larger (Fig. 19-2). Try to stay superior to the mental crease.

The surgeon grasps one side of the lip, while the assistant countertracts the other side. This steadies the lip and cuts down on blood loss when the labial artery is transected.

A #15 blade scalpel is used to carry out a through-and-through W or pentagonal excision, starting superiorly at the free edge of the lip and working inferiorly (Figs. 19-3 and 19-4). Complete the surgical excision before attending to hemostasis. Clamp and tie each end of the labial artery with 2.0 silk. Send margins for frozen-section analysis to confirm the adequacy of surgical excision.

The W or pentagonal defect is then closed in three layers. The transected orbicularis oris musculature is carefully reapproximated with 3.0 Dexon or Vicryl to give the wound a strong foundation. Begin at the apex and work superiorly. The subcutaneous layer is reapproximated with 4.0 Dexon or Vicryl, and the skin and mucosa are closed with 5.0 silk, taking care to evert the edges (Figs. 19-5 and 19-6). The vermilion edges must be reapproximated with great accuracy or an unsightly step deformity will result.

Antibiotic ointment is applied to the suture lines during the healing phase. Always splint the wound with an elastic band dressing, as described for the wedge excision (see Procedure 18). This helps to counteract the tendency for these wounds to pull apart, which produces hypertrophic scarring and lip notching.

JOHN B. KINSELLA

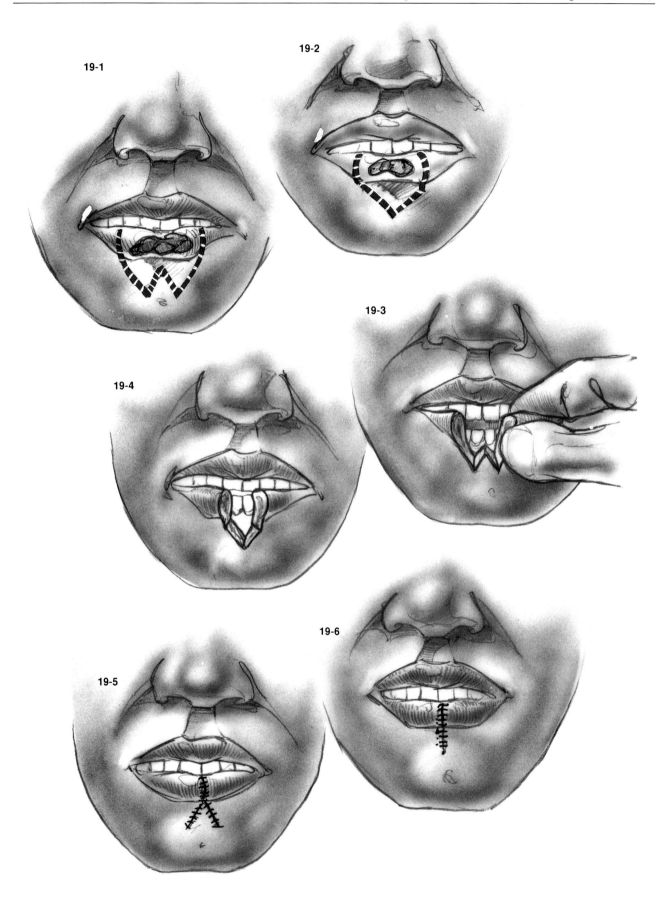

■ 20. ABBE-ESTLANDER RECONSTRUCTION OF THE LIPS (LIP SWITCH FLAP)—Surgical reconstruction of lip defects using tissue from opposite lip

Indications
1. Used to reconstruct lip defects of one half to two thirds of the lip
2. Abbe flap designed to reconstruct medial defects of opposite lip
3. Estlander flap designed to reconstruct lateral defects involving commissure
4. Abbe flap used in secondary reconstruction of the philtral segment of central upper lip, especially in bilateral cleft lip patients

Contraindications
1. Patient unable to tolerate vascular pedicle and keeping lips closed for 2 to 3 weeks because of vascular pedicle

Special Considerations
1. Defects greater than two thirds of the lip should be reconstructed by other methods.
2. The Abbe flap requires a second stage to detach the flap pedicle.

Preoperative Preparation
1. Routine laboratory studies
2. Bleeding, clotting studies (if history warrants)

Special Instruments, Positioning, and Anesthesia
1. Fine, sharp plastic instruments to minimize tissue trauma
2. Patient supine
3. May be performed under local anesthesia, local with sedation anesthesia, or with general anesthesia

Tips and Pearls
1. Best results are achieved when using the lower lip to reconstruct upper lip defects.
2. When using the upper lip as donor site, keep the donor area lateral to avoid distortion of central lip architecture.
3. Match flap height to height of defect.
4. The flap width should be about one half of the width of the defect to maintain appropriate lip proportions.
5. Use same flap width as the defect size when reconstructing central philtral segment.
6. Minimize extension of lower lip vertical donor scar beyond sublabial crease.
7. The upper lip Estlander flap donor site may be matched with the melolabial crease.
8. Small mucosal flaps may be necessary to equalize thinner lateral vermilion with fuller medial vermilion.
9. Pedicles should be placed to allow largest possible oral opening.
10. Match the vermilion on closure.
11. Three-layer closure
12. Preserve the vascular pedicle.
13. Flap division may be performed in approximately 14 days.
14. Commisuroplasty may be required after an Estlander flap reconstruction.

Pitfalls and Complications
1. Vascular compromise
2. Vermilion notching
3. Lip asymmetry
4. Scarring extending beyond sublabial crease

Postoperative Care
1. Minimize oral opening to ease tension on the vascular pedicle. This may be helped with tape around the chin up to the cheeks to minimize jaw opening.

References
Baker SR, Krause CJ. Pedicle flaps in reconstruction of the lip. Facial Plast Surg 1983;1:61.
Becker FF. Facial reconstruction with local and regional flaps. New York: Thieme, 1985:61.

Operative Procedure
With the patient supine and the lips prepped and anesthetized, the height and width of the defect is measured. A donor flap positioned directly opposite the flap with the same height and one half of the width is marked. The donor flap pedicle should be designed to minimize tension on the vascular pedicle during the healing phase. The vermilion edges of the donor and recipient sites are marked with a scalpel to facilitate precise alignment. Local anesthetic with epinephrine may be instilled for hemostasis after the surface markings have been completed. The donor flap is divided in a full-thickness fashion, with the position of the labial artery observed on the side of the division (Fig. 20-1). This is usually easily controlled with electrocautery.

The donor flap is further elevated until it is attached by the vascular pedicle. The flap is then swung into position into the defect (Fig. 20-2) and the donor site is closed in three layers. The donor flap is sewn into the recipient lip with a three layer closure as well. Care is taken to align precisely the vermilion borders (Fig. 20-3). If necessary, the lateral vermilion, which is less full than medial vermilion, may be made fuller by a small vermilion advancement through a small back-cut horizontally on the lip mucosal side to allow advancement of the thinner vermilion. The pedicle is left attached for 2 weeks and transected under straight local anesthesia. Minor trimming may be required to restore normal lip contour.

The same sequence is used in an Estlander flap reconstruction. For an an upper lip donor site, the lateral limb of the incision may be placed along the medial labial crease to help camouflage the donor site incision. The Estlander flap is swung into position, and sutures close the site in three layers, taking care to realign the vermilion borders (Figs. 20-4 and 20-5). Care needs to be taken to preserve the vascular pedicle, which is incorporated within the flap and closed (Fig. 20-6). Occasionally, secondarily commisuroplasties are required in Estlander reconstructions to reestablish the normal commissure.

TOM D. WANG

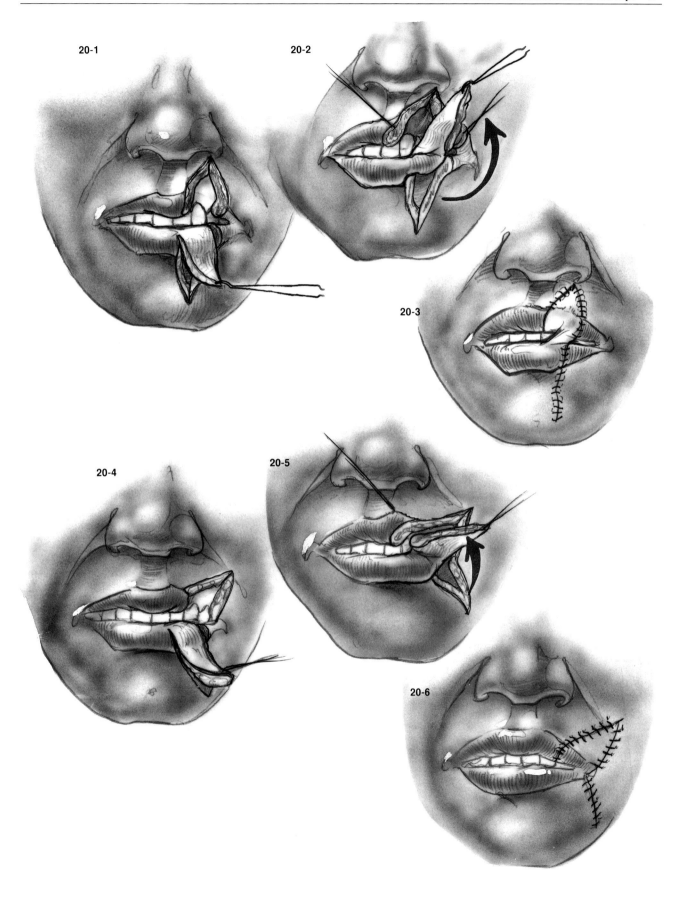

20-1

20-2

20-3

20-4

20-5

20-6

■ 21. GILLIES FAN FLAP

A reconstructive option for upper or lower lip defects

Indications

1. Lateral defects of the upper lip or lower lip that abut the oral commissure
2. Large, central lip defects (using bilateral fan flaps)
3. Defects resulting from trauma, excision of tumors, or infections

Contraindications

1. Lack of a labial arterial pedicle
2. Defects greater than 75% of the lip
3. Patient with tendency to develop hypertrophic scars or keloids

Special Considerations

1. The hematocrit should be ≥30.
2. Surgical margins should be cleared in tumor cases.
3. Further tissue loss may be anticipated in gunshot injuries, and the flap should be delayed to avoid transferring nonviable tissue.

Preoperative Preparation

1. Routine laboratory studies, including complete blood count and clotting profile
2. Photographs
3. Informed consent

Special Instruments, Position, and Anesthesia

1. Plastic surgery instruments
2. Bipolar cautery
3. Supine position
4. General anesthesia preferred

Tips and Pearls

1. The fan flap is rectangular.
2. Dissection is a full-thickness, through-and-through excision of the entire lip into the oral cavity.
3. Flap is based on the superior or inferior labial arteries.
4. Closure is in a continuous line (an advantage).
5. The procedure can be completed in a single stage (an advantage).
6. The commissure is shifted from its natural position, causing it to become rounded (a disadvantage).
7. The lip is denervated; motor and sensory reinnervation may occur in 6 to 18 months, but this still represents a disadvantage.
8. Microstomia can result.

Pitfalls and Complications

1. Flap failure
2. Hypertrophic scar or keloid
3. Tumor recurrence
4. Minor wound separation or infection
5. Hematoma or hemorrhage
6. Anesthetic complications (longer procedure than other reconstructive options)

Postoperative Care Issues

1. Careful monitoring of flap initially for signs of hematoma or venous congestion, which may be managed by removal of one suture
2. The suture line should be cleaned with 1.5% solution of H_2O_2 on a cotton swab, and antibiotic ointment should be applied three or more times daily.
3. Sutures should be removed at 5 to 7 days postoperatively.

References

Calhoun KH. Reconstruction of subtotal and total defects of the lips. In: Calhoun KH. Stiernberg CM, eds. Surgery of the lip. London: Thieme, 1992:42.

Mullin WR, Millard DR. Fan flaps. In: Straugh B, Vasconez LO, Hall-Findlay EJ, eds. Grabb's encyclopedia of flaps, vol 1. Boston: Little, Brown, 1990:686.

Operative Procedure

For upper lip reconstruction, a mark is made with gentian violet at the point of the planned new commissure (Fig. 21-1). The length to be transferred is approximated on the vermilion, and a perpendicular line is marked from the white roll at the mark (Fig. 21-2). The flap is marked with an upward extension of the first line at an angle of approximately 60°. The length of the flap depends on the size of the defect and may involve transecting the nasolabial fold. The vertical height of the defect determines the flap width. The injection of a 1:100,000 epinephrine solution is allowed to work for 5 minutes.

The incision is made by placing the #11 blade through the lip, beginning at the commissure mark to protect the vascular pedicle (Fig. 21-2A). As the flap is rotated, the 60° triangular segment is adapted into position, forming a Z-plasty closure pattern with an appropriate cut, which connects with the defect and parallels the fibers of the orbicularis oris. The flap is full thickness into the oral cavity, and care must be taken to avoid injury to the parotid duct. Mucosa is undermined for vermilion reconstruction (Fig. 21-2B). A back-cut may be required for cosmetic closure. Suturing begins at the vermilion and proceeds laterally (Fig. 21-3). Three layers are closed: 3-0 chromic for the mucosa, 4-0 Vicryl in the muscle, and 6-0 nylon in the skin. A linear closure is achieved by making the back-cut after the remainder of the flap has been transposed. The full-thickness flap in place is shown in Figure 21-4.

For comparison, a partial lower lip reconstruction design is shown in Figure 21-5, and a total lower lip reconstruction, also called the McGregor modification of the fan flap, is shown in Figure 21-6. The same design is used on the other side.

CHRISTOPHER H. RASSEKH

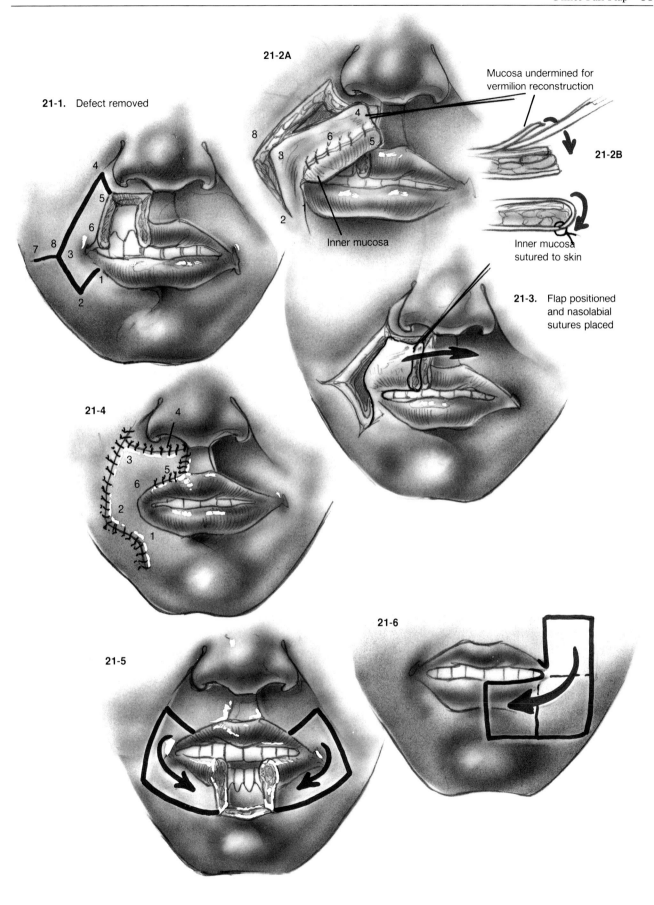

21-1. Defect removed

21-2A

Mucosa undermined for vermilion reconstruction

21-2B

Inner mucosa

Inner mucosa sutured to skin

21-3. Flap positioned and nasolabial sutures placed

21-4

21-5

21-6

■ *22.* KARAPANDZIC FLAP LIP RECON-
STRUCTION—A modification of the Gillies fan flap in which the motor and sensory innervation of the lip is preserved

Indications
1. The Karapandzic flap is recommended to repair defects produced by oncologic surgery or trauma involving 30% to 80% of the lip.

Contraindications
1. Not recommended for the reconstruction of lateral defects of the upper lip
2. Extension to the mandible
3. Involvement of mental skin

Special Considerations
1. Distance from the commissure
2. Anesthesia of the lip or chin may indicate perineural spread.
3. Extent of cancer
4. Neck node status
5. Prior lip resection or facial scars

Special Instruments
1. With or without magnifying loupes
2. Small, delicate plastic surgery instruments
3. Bipolar cautery
4. The patient is placed in a supine position, with the head in neutral position and stabilized within a foam doughnut.
5. Local anesthesia and sedation or general endotracheal anesthesia

Preoperative Preparation
1. Routine laboratory studies
2. Computed tomography scan of the mandible and neck if concerned for occult nodes, mandibular invasion, or perineural spread
3. Fine-needle aspiration biopsy of suspicious lymph nodes

Tips and Pearls
1. The incisions should be placed exactly over the melolabial and mentolabial creases.
2. Mark the skin creases and the vermilion edge lateral to the planned margins of resection before injecting the anesthetic-vasoconstrictor solution.
3. For patients with deep creases, the wound may be sutured, allowing a slight inversion of the edges. This re-creates the crease and hides the scars more effectively.
4. Microstomia can be somewhat corrected by manual or prosthetic dilatation.
5. If dentures cannot be introduced, the problem may be circumvented with the use of split or hinged dentures that may be folded or disassembled.

Pitfalls and Complications
1. Results in microstomia
2. Difficult to introduce full dentures
3. Causes inversion of the vermilion and flattening of the mentolabial junction
4. Persistent pain, dysesthesia, or anesthesia may be a sign of persistence or recurrence.

Postoperative Care
1. Cover the wound with antibiotic ointment.
2. Instruct the patient to use one-half– or one-third–strength hydrogen peroxide for "swish and spit" four times each day for 7 to 10 days.
3. A broad-spectrum oral antibiotic is taken for 24 hours after surgery.
4. Instruct the patient to protect the lips with sunscreen lip balm (eg, 20 SPF).

References
Karapandzic M. Reconstruction of lip defects by local arterial flaps. Br J Plastic Surg 1974;27:93.

Myers EN, Carrau RL. Reconstruction of the oral cavity. In: English G, ed. Otolaryngology. Philadelphia: JB Lippincott, 1993.

Operative Procedure
The patient is positioned supine on the operating table with the head in a neutral position resting over a foam doughnut. The choice between monitored anesthesia control (ie, local anesthesia and conscious sedation) or general anesthesia is based on the patient's or surgeon's preference. Monitored anesthesia control usually is preferred over general anesthesia. The melolabial and mentolabial creases and the estimated margins of resection are marked with methylene blue dye (Fig. 22-1). The patient is given intravenous pentothal immediately before the injections of the anesthetic-vasoconstrictor solution. The mental nerves are blocked using a Marcaine (0.05%) with epinephrine (1:100,000) solution. The margins of resection and the skin over the planned incisions are infiltrated with a solution of lidocaine (1%) with epinephrine (1:100,000). Injections of the latter solution in the deep planes corresponding to the incision lines are not recommended, because they may produce vasoconstriction of the vessels that supply the flap and produce ischemia. The injections of the lidocaine with epinephrine solution provide immediate anesthesia and assist with hemostasis. A mental block offers long-lasting pain control even in patients who prefer general anesthesia. When general anesthesia is chosen, the patient is intubated nasotracheally.

The tumor is resected, including 0.5 cm of normal lip at each side, and the specimen is sent for frozen-section analysis. The flap may be designed while awaiting the pathologic analysis.

The design of the Karapandzic flap involves the separation of two skin–orbicularis oris muscle flaps with intact neurovascular supply from the surrounding muscles of expression. The skin incisions are placed over the melolabial and mentolabial creases (see Fig. 22-1). The extent of the incisions is determined by the size of the defect. The incisions are carried through the skin and subcutaneous tissue but not through the fascia of the orbicularis muscle. A Beaver knife with a #6700 blade is ideal for these incisions. This blade is smaller and sharper than a #15 blade, offering maximum control. The interdigitations of the orbicularis oris muscle with the surrounding muscles of facial expression are carefully separated, using blunt dissection with a fine-tip hemostat or dissecting scissors. This dissection is carried out through the depth of the muscle but not through the buccal mucosa. During this dissection, the neurovascular bundles of the orbicularis oris muscle are identified and preserved (Fig. 22-2). The most medial 1 cm of the buccal mucosa is transected to facilitate the mobilization and suturing of the flap. The dissection is continued until the flaps may be mobilized to achieve a tension-free closure (Fig. 22-3). These maneuvers produce a myocutaneous flap with motor and sensory innervation that can be advanced to close the defect while preserving the vertical height of the lip and the gingivobuccal sulcus.

The mucosa is repaired with interrupted vertical mattress stitches, using an absorbable suture. The muscle is approximated with interrupted Vicryl or Dexon 4-0 stitches. The subcutaneous tissue is approximated with Vicryl or Dexon 5-0 (undyed) stitches. The skin is closed with running mild chromic 6-0 sutures. Steristrips may be used to relieve the tension at the suture line (Fig. 22-4).

RICARDO L. CARRAU

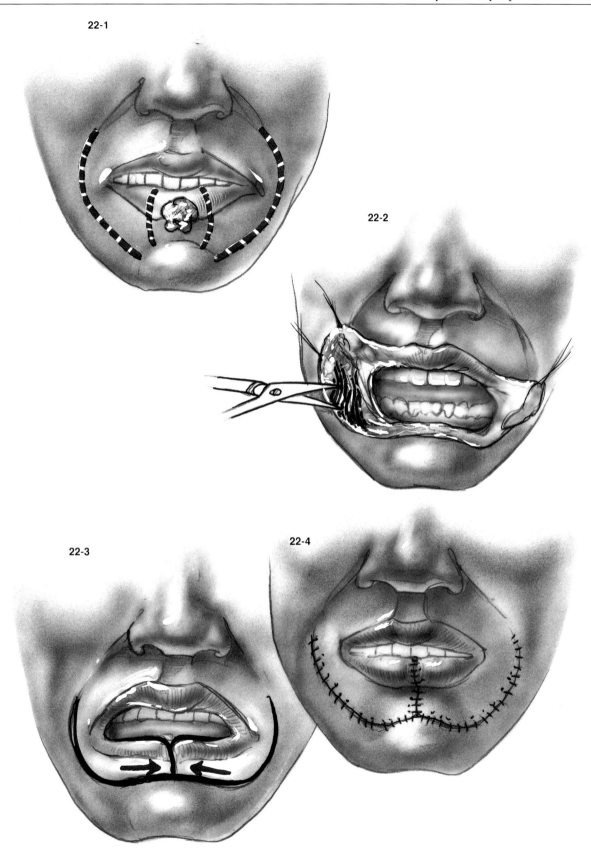

22-1

22-2

22-3

22-4

■ *23.* CHEEK ADVANCEMENT FLAPS FOR LIP RECONSTRUCTION

23a. **Webster Flap**—Modification of the flap originally described by Bernard in which a sliding rectangular flap from the cheek is used to reconstruct the lower lip

Indications
1. Traumatic or surgical defects of the lower lip larger than two thirds of the lip
2. The flap is best used for reconstruction of full-thickness defects of the lower lip that do not extend below the mental crease.

Contraindications
1. Inadequate adjacent cheek tissue
2. Inadequate blood supply; caution in case of loss of the external maxillary artery, as usually occurs in neck dissection
3. Early period after gunshot injuries

Special Considerations
1. Reconstruction of the vermilion
2. Hemostasis
3. Oral commissure involvement
4. Size of defect
5. Prior radiation therapy
6. Adequacy of surgical margins for malignancy

Preoperative Preparation
1. Routine laboratory studies
2. Pathology consultation for tumor cases
3. Consent should include the possibility of staged (multiple) procedures

Special Instruments, Position, and Anesthesia
1. Supine position with general anesthesia preferred
2. Fine plastic surgery instruments
3. Bipolar cautery
4. Nerve stimulator
5. Loupe magnification

Tips and Pearls
1. Burow's triangles are designed preserving muscular layer
2. An inferiorly based mucosal flap is designed to extend above the skin incision and later sutured to the skin edge for vermilion reconstruction.
3. The length of the flap incision should be approximately one-half width of the defect.
4. Preservation of sphincteric function with acceptable cosmesis and usually no microstomia

Pitfalls and Complications
1. Flap necrosis
2. Lower lip may appear tight, with excessive overhang of the upper lip.
3. Vertical scar contracture may occur in the midline region.

Postoperative Care Issues
1. Careful monitoring of the flap
2. If venous congestion or hematoma develop, one or two sutures may be removed
3. Oral musculature exercises after healing
4. Dermabrasion or steroid injection for scarring problems

(continued)

Operative Procedures
Webster Modification of Bernard Technique

The patient is brought to the operating room and placed in the supine position. Sufficient anesthesia is delivered, and the patient's lower face is prepped with Betadine. The size of the defect is measured. A 1:100,000 epinephrine solution is injected into the planned incision lines and allowed to infiltrate for 5 minutes. A full-thickness incision (ie, skin, muscle, and mucosa) is made laterally from the corner of the defect adjacent to the commissure. This incision is approximately one half of the length of the defect and curves slightly upward. A shorter incision is made parallel to the first incision, beginning near the mental crease and curving downward as it is extended laterally (Fig. 23-1).

Mobilization of the flap proceeds laterally to the edge of the masseter muscle, with care to avoid injury to the external facial artery. This creates a rectangular flap that can be sutured to the medial edge of the defect. Adequate gingival mucosa is preserved on the alveolar ridge for suturing to the mucosa of the flap. The resulting closure leaves a standing cone (ie, "dog ear") at the superior lateral corner that is excised as a Burow's triangle, preserving the mucosa that is eventually used as a flap for vermilion reconstruction. The Burow's triangle base should be slanted slightly upward laterally and the medial aspect designed to follow the nasolabial fold (Fig. 23-2). The mucosal flap is rotated and advanced to allow it to be sutured to the superior edge of the cheek flap (Fig. 23-3). Unilateral flaps may be used, or for total lip defects, bilateral flaps can be used. Figure 23-4 shows the completed procedure for bilateral flaps.

(continued)

23-1   Incisions

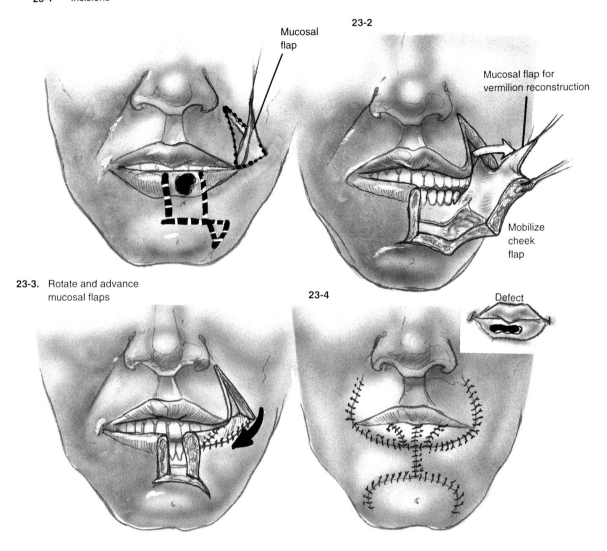

Mucosal
flap

23-2

Mucosal flap for
vermilion reconstruction

Mobilize
cheek
flap

23-3.   Rotate and advance
mucosal flaps

23-4

Defect

23. CHEEK ADVANCEMENT FLAPS FOR LIP RECONSTRUCTION *(continued)*

***23b.* McHugh Flap**—Modification of Dieffenbach's original cheek flap reconstruction of the lower lip in which a neurovascular island is used to reconstruct total or subtotal lower lip defects

Indications
1. Traumatic or surgical defects of the lower lip larger than two thirds of the lip
2. The flap is best used for reconstruction of full-thickness defects of the lower lip that do not extend below the mental crease.

Contraindications
1. Inadequate adjacent cheek tissue
2. Inadequate blood supply; caution in case of loss of the external maxillary artery, as usually occurs in neck dissection
3. Early period after gunshot injuries

Special Considerations
1. Reconstruction of the vermilion
2. Hemostasis
3. Oral commissure involvement
4. Size of defect
5. Prior radiation therapy
6. Adequacy of surgical margins for malignancy

Preoperative Preparation
1. Routine laboratory studies
2. Pathology consultation for tumor cases
3. Consent should include the possibility of staged (multiple) procedures

Special Instruments, Position, and Anesthesia
1. Supine position with general anesthesia preferred
2. Fine plastic surgery instruments
3. Bipolar cautery
4. Nerve stimulator
5. Loupe magnification

Tips and Pearls
1. The flap differs from Bernard type in that it tapers to a triangle laterally, allowing donor site closure without Burow's triangles. This is done in a V-Y fashion.
2. Only skin and mucosa are incised, and muscle, vessels, and nerves must be carefully preserved.
3. Preservation of sphincter function with adequate cosmesis is possible.
4. This flap preserves muscle, vessels, and motor and sensory innervation.

Pitfalls and Complications
1. Damage to facial nerve
2. Flap necrosis or vascular injury
3. Inadequate cosmesis may occur if a horizontal scar is obvious.
4. Parotid duct injury

References
Webster Flap

Calhoun KH. Reconstruction of subtotal and total defects of the lips. In: Calhoun KH, Stiernberg CM eds. Surgery of the lip. London: Thieme, 1992:42.

Webster RC, Coffey RJ, Kelleher RE. Total and partial reconstruction of the lower lip with innervated muscle-bearing flaps. Plast Reconstr Surg 1960;25:360.

McHugh Flap

McHugh M. Reconstruction of the lower lip using a neurovascular island flap. Br J Plast Surg 1977;30:316.

Alternate methods of vermilion reconstruction include using an inferiorly based mucosal flap (see description of McHugh flap), tongue flaps, or a two-stage, bipedicled mucosal flap from the inside of the lip. The mucosal closure usually is accomplished with 4-0 chromic suture, muscle is closed with 4-0 Vicryl suture, and the skin is approximated with 6-0 black nylon. The suture lines are covered with a thin layer of antimicrobial ointment. A small rubber band drain may be used laterally in the inferior incision.

McHugh Sliding Cheek Flap

The patient is brought to the operating room and placed in the supine position. After sufficient anesthesia with nasotracheal intubation, the lower face is prepped with Betadine, and the patient is draped. The injection of a 1:100,000 epinephrine solution is allowed to take effect.

The flap design is a long, narrow triangle oriented horizontally, with the base at the lateral aspect of the defect. The apex is in the inferior pretragal region, and the incisions slope superiorly as they are carried laterally. The flap includes the skin and mucosa; the muscle with its vessels and nerves are preserved by careful blunt dissection. The mucosa is incised for 4 cm superior to the upper skin incision for later use in vermilion reconstruction (Fig. 23-5). The flap is mobilized and sutured in a manner similar to that described for the Bernard technique. The donor site is closed in layers with a V-to-Y advancement technique (Fig. 23-6).

CHRISTOPHER H. RASSEKH

23-5.   McHugh sliding cheek flap   **23-6**   Closure

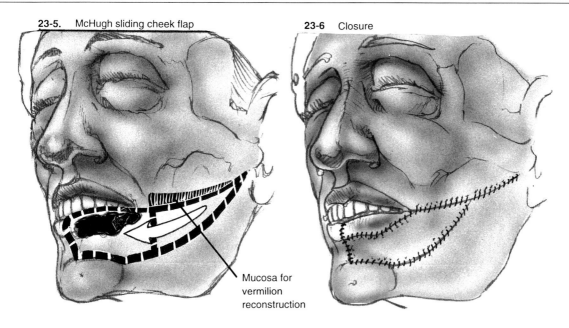

Mucosa for
vermilion
reconstruction

■ 24. PECTORALIS MAJOR FLAP AND DELTOPECTORAL FLAP RECONSTRUCTION OF THE LIPS

Indications
1. Loss of 75% or more of lip secondary to trauma or extirpative surgery
2. Loss of skin or full thickness of lip

Special Considerations
1. Consider a simpler solution.
2. Use a local tissue transfer if available.
3. Not suitable for mandibular replacement if needed
4. Multiple stages are necessary.
5. Rarely necessary

Preoperative Preparation
1. Routine laboratory studies
2. Careful planning of extirpation and defect preparation
3. Appropriate imaging to rule out bony invasion by neoplastic condition

Special Instruments, Position, and Anesthesia
1. Headlight
2. Supine position
3. Consider nasal intubation or tracheostomy.
4. Consider a feeding tube.

Tips and Pearls
1. Reserved for situation in which simpler techniques or local tissue are not available
2. Attempt reconstruction of the lip in units or subunits.
3. Plan to create units and subunits with revision surgery.
4. Preserve as much functional lip tissue as is safely possible.
5. Plan for the eventuality of gravitational pull on tissue.
6. Plan for contraction of tissue, particularly in the commissure area.

Pitfalls and Complications
1. Flap loss
2. Replaces dynamic tissue with static filler
3. Flaps are insensate.

References
Burget GC, Menick FJ. Aesthetic restoration of one-half the upper lip. Plast Reconstr Surg 1986;78:583.
Conley J. Pendulosity in regional flaps about the head and neck. Ann Otolaryngol 1986;16:75.

Operative Procedure

Resection of the tumor or preparation of the donor site is accomplished first. In the former, strict adherence to oncologic principles should be paramount. Compromise of the resection to accommodate a particular reconstructive technique is not appropriate. Proposed resection borders are marked and can often be accomplished by resection of aesthetic lip units (Fig. 24-1). Preservation of small portions of these units does not facilitate repair. Superficial lesions are resected in a supramuscular plane. For deeper lesions, through-and-through, composite resections of the lip are necessary. In extirpative cases, appropriate margins are ensured by frozen-section analysis. Preparation of the recipient site is then accomplished. For defects of skin only, undermining is performed about the periphery of the defect. To facilitate a multilayer closure in through-and-through defects, undermine the subdermal and submucosal planes immediately adjacent to the orbicularis musculature.

For skin-only reconstructions, the deltopectoral flap or a cutaneous extension of the pectoralis musculocutaneous flap can supply large amounts of dermal tissue. The former reconstructive modality is a cutaneous anterior chest wall flap that is medially based on the blood supply from the first through the fourth internal mammary artery perforators (Fig. 24-2). A delay should always be considered and is often necessary in cases of significant systemic disorders or long flap extensions. Consider split-thickness skin grafting of the distal flap during delay.

Flap inset is accomplished with appropriate suture material such as Vicryl or polydioxanone (PDS) in the subcutaneous and subcuticular layers and with nylon, Prolene, or plain gut for skin. Closures should be accomplished from proximal to distal to avoid tension on the distal portions of the flap.

When accomplishing a skin-only repair, using the pectoralis musculocutaneous skin extension, similar principles are maintained in defect closure. Tubing of this flap is unnecessary. The pedicle should be dressed with antibiotic ointment and gauze.

When large, full-thickness, composite resections of the lip are to be reconstructed, the pectoralis musculocutaneous flap offers external skin and underlying muscle. The pectoralis musculocutaneous flap is an anterior chest wall flap supplied by the thoracoacromial artery (Fig. 24-3). Internal lining is obtained with turned-over skin or a skin-mucosal graft on the undersurface of the muscle.

The muscle boundaries are identified on the patient, and appropriate incisions for exposure and flap design are marked. Incisions are opened down to the level of the pectoralis muscle. The lateral border of the muscle is identified, and dissection is carried around its edge into the plane between the pectoralis major and minor. The thoracoacromial artery and its branch to the pectoralis are identified, and adequacy of the blood supply is ensured. The remaining skin incisions are carefully made, isolating the skin paddle. Guard against shearing of the paddle on the muscle.

The flap may then be moved into the recipient's site, which may be superficial or deep to the cervical skin. After the best position for the flap is decided, an internal lining with that position in mind is accomplished by use of split-thickness skin or mucosal grafts secured to the deep surface of the muscle.

A layered closure is accomplished with attempts to overlap orbicularis and pectoralis muscle, using Vicryl, PDS, or similar suture. Careful subcutaneous, subcuticular, and skin approximation are accomplished with respect for anatomic units if possible. Commissure reconstruction necessitates careful splitting of the flap and maturation of the skin-mucosal graft to the cutaneous flap segment. When full-thickness segments of the lateral commissures are reconstructed (Fig. 24-4), overcorrection of commissure placement is necessary to allow contraction of the flap and medial displacement of the final commissure position. The bulky pectoralis flap is subject to constant gravitational pull, which can be helped by suspension stitches or overcorrection in a vertical plane.

After 2 to 3 weeks of flap healing, the deltopectoral or pectoralis pedicle may be divided and second-stage revisions accomplished. After flap viability is ensured and the pedicle divided, the flap is inset with minimal disturbance of the underlying vasculature.

FRANK W. SHAGETS

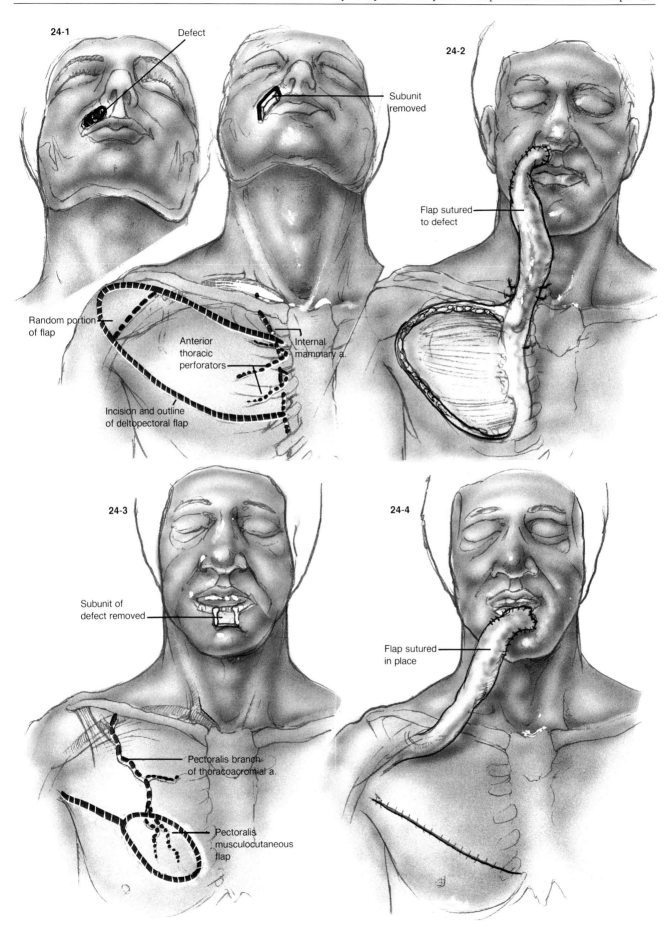

24-1

Defect

Subunit removed

Random portion of flap

Anterior thoracic perforators

Internal mammary a.

Incision and outline of deltopectoral flap

24-2

Flap sutured to defect

24-3

Subunit of defect removed

Pectoralis branch of thoracoacromial a.

Pectoralis musculocutaneous flap

24-4

Flap sutured in place

■ 25. NASOLABIAL FLAP FOR UPPER LIP
A reconstructive local flap

Indications
Defects of the lateral upper lip due to:
1. Trauma
2. Benign neoplasms
3. Malignant neoplasms

Contraindications
1. Positive margins
2. Lack of arterial pedicle
3. Involvement of the vermilion–cutaneous border (relative)
4. Inadequate adjacent cheek tissue

Preoperative Preparation
1. Hematocrit > 30
2. Normal clotting studies
3. No prior trauma or surgery of the facial artery

Special Instruments, Position, and Anesthesia
1. May be done under general or local anesthetic
2. Supine position
3. Routine flap instruments, including fine dissection scissors and tissue handling forceps or hooks

Tips and Pearls
1. The flap is usually of the subcutaneous transposition type, but also can be raised as a musculocutaneous flap based on a branch of the facial artery.
2. The flap is single stage, usually inferiorly based.
3. Donor site closure is achieved in a linear fashion in the nasolabial fold, where it is hidden nicely.
4. This flap provides an excellent color and texture match for the upper lip
5. This flap procedure is generally performed in one stage, but may be performed in two stages.
6. Bilateral flaps may be used to reconstruct near-total upper lip defects.

Pitfalls and Complications
1. Tumor recurrence
2. Dog-ear deformity resulting from inadequate intermediate flap
3. Flap failure due to inadequate thickness, excessive length, infection, or hematoma

Postoperative Care
1. Suture care
2. Suture removal at 5 to 7 days

References
Baaron JN, Saad MN: Subcutaneous pedicle flaps to the lip. In Strauch B, Vasconez LO, Hall-Findlay EJ, eds. Grabb's encyclopedia of flaps, vol. 1. Boston: Little Brown, 1990: 644.

Jackson IT Lip Reconstruction. In: Jackson IT, ed. Local flaps in head and neck reconstruction. St. Louis: Mosby, pp. 352-354.

Operative Procedure
The patient is brought to the operating table and placed in the supine position. Adequate anesthesia is given, including an injection of the margins of the defect and the donor site. The face is painted with Betadine paint (not soap due to the proximity to the eyes) and the patient draped. The length of the flap is determined by the width of the defect; the width of the flap is determined by the height of the defect. The incision is designed as shown in Figure 25-1. An intermediate flap that is thus created at the base of the ala assists in the closure of the donor site (Fig. 25-2). The flap is rotated into position and sutured as shown in Figure 25-3. The intermediate flap is then used to close the donor site after undermining the lateral skin margin (Fig. 25-4). Suturing is done in two layers: 4-0 Vicryl interrupted inverted sutures in the deep dermis followed by 6-0 black nylon in the skin (interrupted). Antimicrobial ointment is applied, and the procedure is terminated. If an intermediate flap cannot be created, it is wise to perform the flap in two stages (Fig. 25-5). The procedure may also be done using a superiorly based flap (Fig. 25-6).

CHRISTOPHER H. RASSEKH

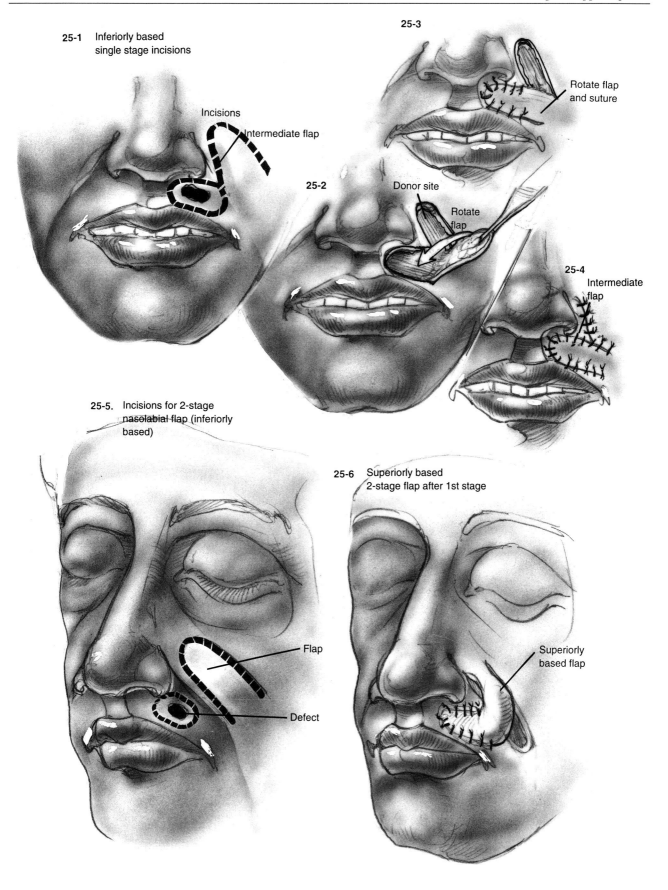

25-1 Inferiorly based single stage incisions

Incisions

Intermediate flap

25-3

Rotate flap and suture

Donor site

Rotate flap

25-2

25-4

Intermediate flap

25-5. Incisions for 2-stage nasolabial flap (inferiorly based)

Flap

Defect

25-6 Superiorly based 2-stage flap after 1st stage

Superiorly based flap

■ 26. RECONSTRUCTION OF THE UPPER LIP: ADVANCEMENT FLAPS WITH MODIFIED BUROW'S TECHNIQUE—Excision of a crescentic area of normal perialar skin to facilitate advancing the remaining two segments of upper lip (ie, Webster's modification of Burow's triangles)

Indications
1. Median or slightly paramedian defects that include less than 30% of the upper lip

Contraindications
1. Lateral lesions, because too much distortion is produced

Special Considerations
1. Involvement of alveolus or gingivobuccal sulcus
2. Involvement of nasal sill or columella
3. Status of parotid and neck nodes
4. Anesthesia of upper lip and incisors
5. Previous scars

Preoperative Preparation
1. Routine laboratory studies
2. Computed tomography scan for positive or negative parotid nodes, suspected perineural spread, or involvement of maxilla
3. Fine-needle aspiration biopsy for suspicious lymph nodes

Special Instruments, Position, and Anesthesia
1. Magnifying loupes (optional)
2. Small, delicate plastic surgery instruments
3. Bipolar cautery
4. Supine position, with head in a neutral position, stabilized in a foam doughnut
5. Local anesthesia and sedation or general endotracheal anesthesia
6. Do not inject epinephrine solution at the base of the flaps (ie, melolabial area).
7. When general anesthesia is preferred, intubate orotracheally and fix tube to midline of lower jaw.

Tips and Pearls
1. Visualize the upper lip as formed by a central subunit (philtrum) and two lateral subunits.
2. The reconstruction should be tension free, and the position and symmetry of the three subunits should be reestablished.
3. Mark the vermilion border lateral to the margins of resection and the crescentic perialar area before injecting the lidocaine with epinephrine solution.
4. Undermine widely to facilitate mobilization of the flaps.

Pitfalls and Complications
1. The upper lip tolerates less loss of tissue than the lower lip.
2. Primary repair of any but the smallest defects results in asymmetry of the Cupid's bow, oral commissures, and nasolabial creases.
3. Any tension obliterates the normal protrusion of the upper lip over the lower lip.
4. Any distortion of these landmarks results in a conspicuous deformity.

Postoperative Care
1. Cover the wound with Bacitracin ointment.
2. Instruct the patient to swish one-half– or one-third–strength hydrogen peroxide mouthwash four times each day for 1 week.
3. Broad-spectrum coverage with an oral antibiotic for 24 hours after surgery
4. The patient should avoid using a spoon for 15 to 21 days.
5. Instruct patient to protect lips with sunscreen lip balm (eg, SPF 20).

References
Burget GC, Menick FJ. Aesthetic restoration of one-half the upper lip. Plast Reconstr Surg 1986;78:583.

Webster JP. Crescentic peri-alar cheek excision for upper lip flap advancement with a short history of upper lip repair. Plast Reconstr Surg 1960;26:40.

Operative Procedure
The patient is positioned supine on the operating table with the head in a neutral position resting on a foam doughnut. The choice between monitored anesthesia control (ie, local anesthesia with conscious sedation) or general anesthesia is based on the patient's or surgeon's preference. Generally, monitored anesthesia control is preferred over general anesthesia. The nasolabial junction, the estimated margins of resection, and the estimated crescentic perialar skin to be resected are marked with methylene blue dye. The margins of resection and the incision lines are infiltrated with lidocaine with epinephrine. The injection of lidocaine with epinephrine provides immediate anesthesia. Marcaine with epinephrine solution may be injected for long-lasting pain control, even in patients who prefer general anesthesia. When general anesthesia is chosen, the patient is intubated orotracheally, and the endotracheal tube is fixed over the midline of the lower jaw.

The cephalic margins for the resection of the tumor are marked at the nasolabial junction or slightly posterior to the visible area of the nostril. Perialar crescentic areas of a width equivalent to the distance that the ipsilateral flap should be advanced are marked and excised (Fig. 26-1). The tumor is resected, including 0.5 cm of normal lip at both sides, and the specimen is sent for frozen-section analysis (Fig. 26-2). The superior labial arteries and other significant bleeders are controlled with a bipolar cautery. The flap may be designed while awaiting the pathologic results. The depth of excision of the perialar crescents extends to the muscles of facial expression. The perialar skin crescents do not need to be symmetric, because more advancement may be required on one side than the other (eg, paramedian tumor). The buccal mucosa is incised at the gingivobuccal sulcus of the upper lip. This incision is usually placed close to the actual sulcus to preserve enough alveolar mucosa to facilitate closure.

The upper lip is widely undermined subperiosteally to allow adequate mobilization of the two flaps to the midline (Fig. 26-3). A Freer or Cottle elevator or electrocautery may be used for subperiosteal dissection. For paramedian defects, the mobilization and advancement of each of the flaps are adjusted in such a manner that the position of the philtrum or lateral subunit is preserved as much as possible. If the closure is not tension free after wide mobilization, other adjunctive techniques may be employed. The philtrum may be reconstructed with an Abbe flap, restoring the anatomical subunits of the upper lip (Fig. 26-4). Alternatively, a Karapandzic flap may be used to provide further mobilization. However, the Karapandzic flap produces distortion and rounding of the oral commissures.

The lip is closed with a meticulous multilayered technique. The mucosa is repaired with Dexon or Vicryl 4-0 (tapered needle) vertical mattress stitches. The orbicularis oris is repaired with Dexon or Vicryl 4-0 (tapered needle) single interrupted stitches. The subcutaneous tissue is approximated with undyed Dexon or Vicryl 5-0 interrupted stitches (Fig. 26-5).

RICARDO L. CARRAU

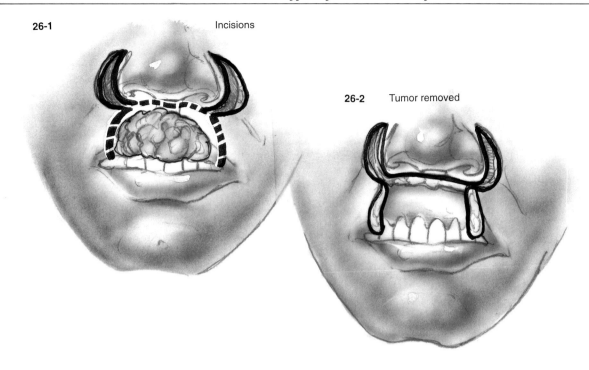

26-1   Incisions

26-2   Tumor removed

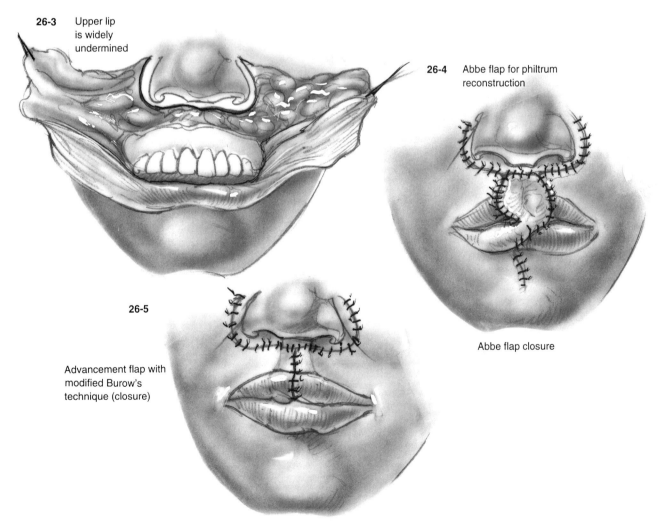

26-3   Upper lip
is widely
undermined

26-4   Abbe flap for philtrum
reconstruction

Abbe flap closure

26-5

Advancement flap with
modified Burow's
technique (closure)

■ *27.* LATERAL COMMISSURE REPAIR

Restoration of the shape and contour of the lateral commissure using the Gillies technique (ie, Lore technique), commissuroplasty for paralytic deformity of the lateral commissure, or stenting techniques for bilateral cicatricial contraction of the corners of the mouth

Indications

1. Traumatic loss or surgical excision of the modiolus
2. Rounded commissure of the lip after pedicled or advancement flap lip reconstruction
3. Paralytic distortion of the lower lip and lateral commissure
4. Electrical burns and thermal injury resulting in cicatricial contraction of the corners of the mouth

Special Instrumentation, Position, and Anesthesia

1. Nasal intubation
2. Oral preparation
3. Local injection with 1% lidocaine with 1:100,000 epinephrine
4. Delicate plastic surgery instruments
5. Bipolar cautery
6. Measuring calipers
7. Methylene blue or a fine skin scribe
8. Nonexothermic prosthetic material
9. Preoperative and postoperative photographs

Tips and Pearls

1. Delicate handling of tissue
2. Meticulous hemostasis
3. Careful preoperative analysis and comparison with undistorted side
4. Careful placement of deep sutures to avoid tension on mucosal flaps
5. Precise approximation of skin and mucosal edges

Pitfalls and Complications

1. The elastic properties of the normal lip make the use of a postoperative splint for unilateral cicatricial contraction of the commissure unsuccessful.
2. Steroid injections (eg, Kenalog) are of potential benefit in patients with tendencies for forming keloids or hypertrophic scars.
3. Minor plastic surgical revisions may be necessary to achieve the most satisfactory result, and the possible need for revision should be discussed with the patient preoperatively.

Postoperative Care Issues

1. Diet considerations according to defect; no oral intake or use of a nasogastric tube is rarely required, but a complete liquid diet through a straw may be required.
2. Commissure splint (consider for highly selected bilateral commissure procedures only)
3. Postoperative care of the incision and oral cavity (ie, peroxide cleaning of incisions and liberal antibiotic ointment application; dilute peroxide oral rinses and dental care)

References

Gillies H, Millard DR. The principles and art of plastic surgery. Boston: Little, Brown and Company, 1957.

Glenn MG, Goode RL. Surgical treatment of the "marginal mandibular lip" deformity. Otolaryngol Head Neck Surg 1987;97:462.

Holt GR, Parel S, Richardson DS, et al. The prosthetic management of oral commissure burns. Laryngoscope 1982;92:407.

Operative Procedures

Treatment of Rounded Commissure After Lip Reconstructive Surgery (Gillies Technique)

After achieving adequate anesthesia, incisions are planned along the lateral corner of the mouth. A small equilateral triangle is designed (Fig. 27-1). The base of this triangle is made of the vermilion border of the rounded portion of the corner of the mouth. The apex of this triangle is placed at or just lateral to the desired location of the commissure. If the contralateral commissure is undistorted, and caliper measurements can be made to determine precisely the location of the new commissure. The small triangle of skin is excised. The incision along the vermilion border of the lower lip is continued medially and angled away from the vermilion border as it is carried more medially. This mucosa is then freed and rotated superiorly. The orbicularis oris muscle within the triangle is divided along the axis of the intercommissure line (Fig. 27-2). This is carried through the buccal layer of mucous membrane, which is also carefully freed from the inner surface of the orbicularis oris muscle. The inner mucosa of the lower lip is advanced and approximated to the skin margin (ie, lower side of excised triangle). The freed vermilion mucosa from the lower lip is rotated to approximate the skin edge (ie, upper side of the triangle; Fig. 27-3). The remaining intraoral mucosal edges are reapproximated using interrupted 4-0 chromic sutures, and 5-0 nylons are used to reapproximate the skin mucosal junctions of the commissure.

Technique for Repair of Paralytic Distortion of the Lip or Marginal Mandibular Lip Deformity (Glenn and Goode Technique)

One of several techniques for restoring symmetry to the corner of mouth and lower lip after entry to the marginal mandibular branch of the facial nerve includes surgical excision of a portion of the paralyzed lower lateral lip. This technique can decrease the size of oral sphincter and can help tighten and depress the lower lip.

The lateral extent of this wedge resection is positioned approximately 5 to 7 mm from the lateral commissure. It can be measured precisely with calipers and marked with methylene blue or a fine skin scribe. The lip is pulled laterally to help determine the width of the wedge resection (2.0–2.5 cm). The orbicularis oris muscle is reapproximated using several interrupted 4-0 Vicryl sutures. Intentional mismatching of the vermilion border by as much as 3 mm can help in reestablishing lost eversion of the lower lip. A horizontal cheiloplasty can be performed to further evert the lower lip. The mucosa is advanced to the skin edge and reapproximated using interrupted 5-0 nylon suture that is carefully placed.

In blunting or foreshortening of the commissure secondary to thermal injuries or avulsion of the modiolus, a two- or three-flap commissuroplasty can be used to restore definition to the commissure. In this technique, the equilateral triangle is designed with its apex at the desired location of the new commissure. Underlying scar and skin within this triangle can be excised. Using mucosal advancement flaps, the length of the intercommissural line can be extended. Occasionally, if the orbicularis muscle has been interrupted, a muscle plication can be performed to help reestablish sphincteric function. In cases of bilateral cicatricial contraction of the corners of the mouth, a prosthetic stent can be used postoperatively. In more severe cases of loss of extrinsic musculature or denervation of the facial nerve, a dynamic or static sling may be necessary to help suspend the lateral commissure to a more desirable position.

DAVID V. WAGNER
HENRY T. HOFFMAN

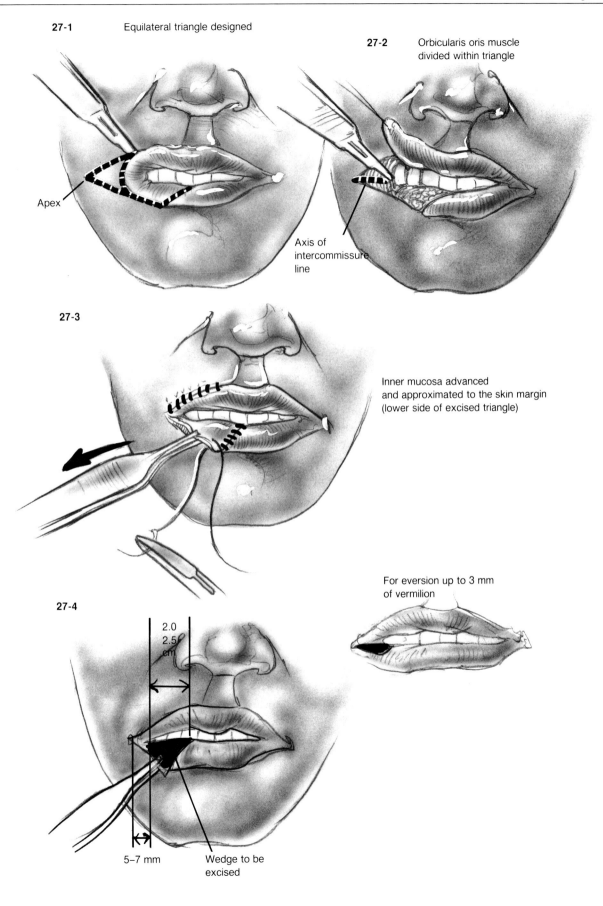

27-1 Equilateral triangle designed

Apex

27-2 Orbicularis oris muscle divided within triangle

Axis of intercommissure line

27-3

Inner mucosa advanced and approximated to the skin margin (lower side of excised triangle)

For eversion up to 3 mm of vermilion

27-4

2.0
2.5
cm

5–7 mm

Wedge to be excised

■ *28.* SURGICAL APPROACHES
Surgical approaches to the oral cavity

Indications
1. Transoral approach for lesions less than 2 cm and for selected lesions up to 4 cm
2. Mandibulotomy approach for posterior oral cavity tumors that do not involve the mandible
3. Visor flap for small lesions of the anterior oral cavity, such as the floor of the mouth, anterior mandibular alveolar ridge, and anterior tongue
4. Transhyoid for small lesions of posterior tongue and posterior wall of hypopharynx; for lesions larger than 2 cm in diameter or cases with cervical adenopathy, another surgical approach is indicated.
5. Median labiomandibular glossotomy for larger lesions of the tongue base, the posterior hypopharynx, tip of epiglottis, and chordoma; palpable cervical adenopathy suggests the need for another surgical approach.

Special Considerations
1. Body habitus
2. Location of tumor
3. Previous irradiation
4. Prior surgical procedures

Preoperative Preparation
1. Informed consent
2. Prophylactic antibiotics
3. Autologous blood if the estimated blood loss is more than 500 mL

Special Instruments, Position, and Anesthesia
1. Fiberoptic headlight
2. Goggles for the surgeon and assistants
3. Soft tissue instruments
4. Yankauer tongue speculum
5. Jennings mouth gag
6. Nasotracheal intubation
7. Laser precautions if the laser is to be used

(continued)

Operative Procedure
The patient is placed in a supine position on the operating room table. The appropriate intravenous catheters and monitoring devices are applied before the institution of anesthesia. Anesthesia may be achieved by means of oral, nasotracheal, or tracheostomy routes; I prefer nasotracheal intubation. A tracheostomy is performed during the procedure if considered to be indicated by the surgeon and the anesthesiologist. By proceeding directly with nasotracheal intubation, the need for performing a tracheostomy under local anesthesia and redraping the patient twice can be avoided. Prophylactic antibiotics, if used, are given before any incision.

For small lesions of the oral cavity or mobile tongue, transoral excision of the lesion can be carried out. Exposure is obtained by means of a Jennings mouth gag or side mouth gag distracting the mandible for a distance of 3 to 4 cm. A small 2-0 silk suture placed through the tip of the tongue and attached to a hemostat works well as a traction suture. The surgical assistant can perform this traction while remaining out of the operative field. Further exposure, if needed, can be achieved by means of a Navy-Army retractor in the lateral oral commissure (Fig. 28-1).

A useful technique for exposure of tumors of the oral cavity is mandibulotomy. A stair-step incision is made in the lip. I generally carry the incision to the lateral aspect of the chin to improve camouflaging the postoperative scar and extend the excision into a natural skin crease on the upper neck. A T-shaped extension from this upper cervical flap can be extended into the neck if a radical neck dissection is required. Alternately, a second horizontal skin incision can be added inferiorly to form a McFee-type incision (Fig. 28-2). The mandible can then be split anteriorly to form a "mandibular swing approach." This can be combined with a paralingual incision to expose tumors of the posterior floor of mouth or tongue base (Fig. 28-3). The mandible can also be split in the region of the angle of

(continued)

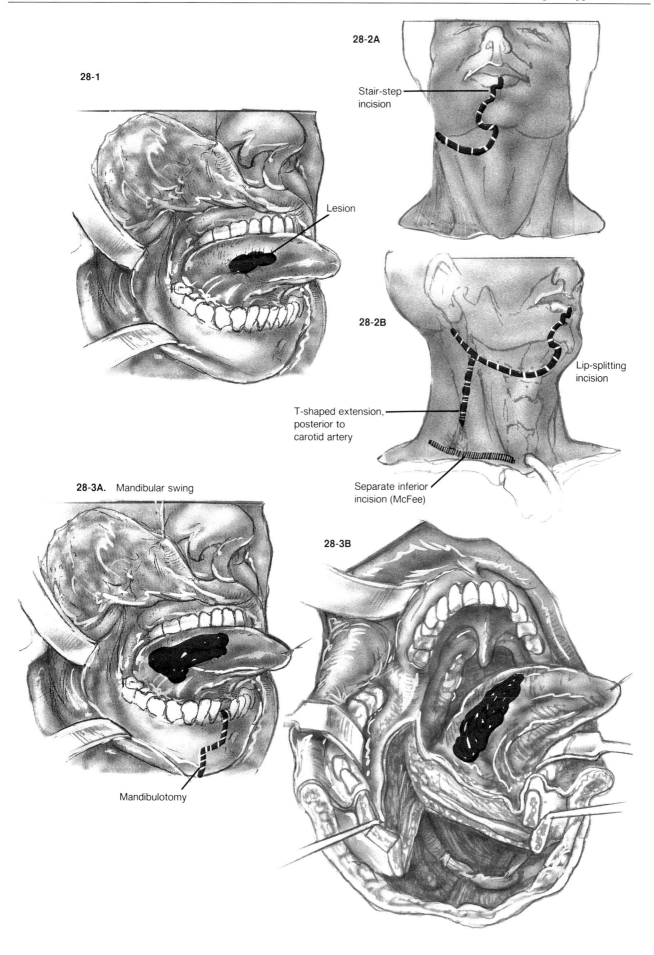

28-1

Lesion

28-2A

Stair-step incision

28-2B

Lip-splitting incision

T-shaped extension, posterior to carotid artery

Separate inferior incision (McFee)

28-3A. Mandibular swing

Mandibulotomy

28-3B

■ *28.* SURGICAL APPROACHES *(continued)*

Tips and Pearls

1. Stepped incisions for the incisions across the lip
2. Careful approximation of the vermilion borders
3. Meticulous hemostasis
4. Staple the drapes on to save time
5. Stair-step or chevron incisions across the mandible
6. Compression plates

Pitfalls and Complications

1. Laser burns or fires if the laser is used
2. Fistula
3. Hemorrhage
4. Dysphagia
5. Cosmetic deformity

Postoperative Care Issues

1. Monitor airway
2. Volume, blood replacement
3. Active (Hemovac) versus passive (Penrose) drains
4. Dedicated nursing unit or intensive care unit
5. Wound care

References

Dichtel WJ, Miller RH, Woodson GE, et al. Lateral mandibulotomy: a technique of exposure for penetrating injuries of the internal carotid at the base of the skull. Laryngoscope 1984;94:1140.

Leipzig B, Cummings CW, Chung CT, et al. Carcinoma of the anterior tongue. Ann Otol Rhinol Laryngol 1982;91:94.

Spiro RH, Gerald FB, Strong EW. Mandibular "swing" approach for oral and oropharyngeal tumors. Head Neck Surg 1981;3:371.

the mandible to provide exposure for the tongue base and hypopharyngeal area. If a mandibular approach is used, it is useful to cut the mandible with a stair-step or chevron-type incision, which increases the surface area of the mandibular wound and aids precise and secure stabilization of the mandible. Another useful technique is to repair the mandible at the mandibulotomy site with a compression plate. The compression plate should be measured and ligated to the mandible before the mandibulotomy is performed, ensuring precise realignment of the mandible (see Fig. 28-3).

A visor flap (Fig. 28-4) is useful for smaller lesions of the oral cavity, including those of the floor of the mouth, alveolar ridge, and anterior tongue. This flap has the advantage of avoiding skin incision; however, both mental nerves must be sacrificed, leaving the patient with cutaneous paresthesia of the chin bilaterally.

A useful approach to the tongue base and posterior hypopharyngeal wall is that of a transhyoid pharyngotomy (Fig. 28-5). A horizontal incision is made over the hyoid bone. The suprahyoid musculature is released with electrocautery. Using blunt dissection, the tongue base is approached by dissecting from anterior to posterior. The central portion of the hyoid bone is removed. Care must be taken to identify and preserve the superior laryngeal nerves and the hypoglossal nerves.

In larger malignant lesions of the posterior hypopharynx or base of the tongue, the median labiomandibular glossotomy is indicated (Fig. 28-6). A midline lip-splitting and chin-splitting incision is employed. The midline mandible is transected in a stair-step fashion. The tongue and suprahyoid musculature are then transected exactly in the midline. The line of the incision inferiorly extends down along the mylohyoid raphe. Using this midline approach, larger tumors of the tongue base can be resected, and the subsequent defect closed in a primary fashion.

C. RON CANNON

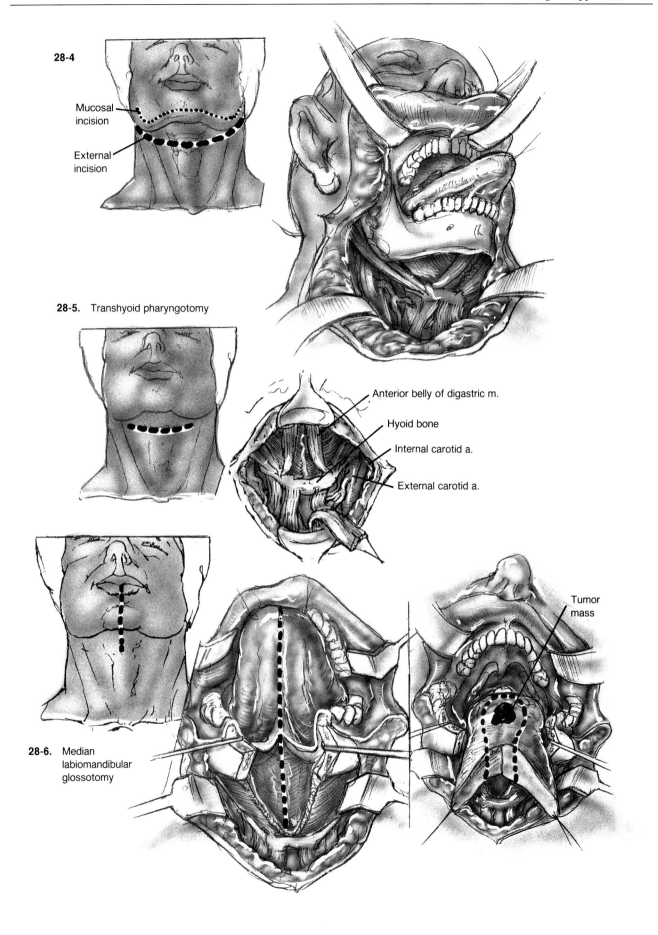

28-4

Mucosal incision

External incision

28-5. Transhyoid pharyngotomy

Anterior belly of digastric m.

Hyoid bone

Internal carotid a.

External carotid a.

28-6. Median labiomandibular glossotomy

Tumor mass

■ 29. PARTIAL ANTERIOR GLOSSECTOMY

Removal of portion of the mobile tongue or portions of the tongue anterior to the circumvallate papilla

Indications

1. Removal of small (<2 cm) or selected, moderate-size (<4 cm) squamous cell carcinoma of tongue
2. Removal of other malignant lesions, such as minor salivary gland carcinoma
3. Removal of benign lesions, such as hemangioma or granular cell myoblastoma
4. No evidence of metastatic disease in neck

Special Considerations

1. Patient's age
2. Status of dentition
3. Presence of regional or distant metastatic disease
4. Other medical problems, such as organic heart disease, diabetes, chronic obstructive pulmonary disease, or anemia
5. Patients with all of their dentition or patients with narrow mandibular arches may require a mandibulotomy approach.

Preoperative Preparation

1. Informed operative consent, including explanations of the diagnosis, purpose of treatment, prognosis with or without treatment, chances of success of treatment, alternative modes of treatment, and potential complications
2. Laboratory evaluation, including clotting studies and x-ray films
3. Panendoscopy to exclude other synchronous tumors of the upper aerodigestive tract can be performed before the definitive procedure or simultaneously with the frozen-section diagnosis. If there is any doubt about the diagnosis, the definitive surgical procedure should be deferred pending the final histologic diagnosis.

Special Instruments, Position, and Anesthesia

1. Headlight
2. Goggles for the surgeons and assistants
3. Jennings mouth gag
4. Nasotracheal intubation
5. Appropriate-size retractors

Tips and Pearls

1. Prophylactic antibiotics
2. Silk suture (2-0) as retraction suture through anterior tongue
3. Block-type resection of lesion
4. Dual suction with Frazier and tonsil suction tips
5. For small lesions, particularly if laser is used, the surgical defect can be left open to heal by secondary intention.
6. A single intraoperative dose of steroids may decrease postoperative tongue edema without adversely affecting healing.

Pitfalls and Complications

1. With larger tongue lesions, the patient may develop airway edema.
2. Dehiscence of tongue closure
3. Bleeding from lingual artery or its branches

Postoperative Care

1. For more posterior and larger lesions of the tongue, the patient must be watched closely for edema and subsequent airway compromise.
2. Excessive tongue movement may lead to wound dehiscence. It is prudent to advise voice rest for 3 to 5 days postoperatively. The use of a "straw" diet (ie, whatever the patient can drink through a straw) is helpful.
3. Bleeding
4. Complications related to other medical problems

References

Johnson JT, Aramany MA, Myers EN. Management of T1 carcinoma of the anterior aspect of the tongue. Arch Otolaryngol 1980;106:249.

Marks JE, Lee F, Freeman RB, et al. Carcinoma of the oral tongue: a study of patient selection and treatment results. Laryngoscope 1981;91:1548.

Operative Procedure

The patient is placed in a supine position. The patient's head is stabilized with a foam doughnut. Anesthesia is generally obtained through a nasotracheal route. Occasionally, for very small lesions of the anterior one third of the tongue, an orotracheal tube may be used, with the tube passed to one side or the other of the oral cavity.

The tongue lesion is exposed by using a Jennings mouth gag or a side mouth gag. A towel clip or single ligature of 2-0 silk placed through the anterior portion of the tongue provides good retraction of the tongue (Fig. 29-1). If further exposure is needed, a Navy-Army or other similar retractor can be placed in the region of the oral commissure.

After adequate visualization of the lesion is obtained, incisions around the lesion itself can be made. Mucosal margins of at least 1 cm should be sought. Incisions can be made with a cold scalpel, electrocautery, or a laser. The carbon dioxide laser has the advantages of cauterizing vessels smaller than 0.5 mm in diameter without bleeding and of sealing some of the lymphatics in the operative field. If the laser is used, however, appropriate laser precautions should be used. For purposes of discussion in this procedure, the use of the electrocautery is described. Using a setting of about 40 watts, an incision is made around the lesion (Figs. 29-2 and 29-3).

The dissection is carried down through the mucosa and tongue musculature. Other silk sutures can be used at this point for further retraction, although they usually are unnecessary. The dissection is carried in an anterior to posterior direction. It is important to remove the tissue as a block and not shave away the lesion. The tumor characteristics are important in this resection. For example, more superficial or exophytic tumors may need a relatively shallow resection. More infiltrative lesions require a larger block resection of the underlying tongue musculature. For deeper resections of the tongue musculature, care must be taken to identify and preserve the lingual and hypoglossal nerves. Branches of the lingual artery may require ligation with silk sutures.

Depending on the location of the lesion on the tongue, various types of excisions may be carried out (Figs. 29-4 and 29-5). After the lesion has been removed, frozen-section–confirmed margins are obtained from the anterior, posterior, medial, lateral, and deep surgical margins. The specimens are marked with ink and given to the pathologist for frozen-section diagnosis. Ideally, the pathologist has seen the lesion before excision and is present in the operating room while the margins for frozen-section analysis are being obtained. While waiting for analysis of the frozen-section margins, further hemostasis is obtained with the electrocautery.

After frozen-section analysis has confirmed that the margins are free of tumor, closure of the wound is begun (Fig. 29-6). The tongue usually is closed in layers, with the deep layers closed with a 3-0 Vicryl suture and the tongue mucosa closed with a ligature of 4-0 Vicryl or 4-0 chromic suture. A single dose of steroids, such as Decadron (8–12 mg), is given as a single dose intraoperatively to decrease postoperative tongue swelling.

C. RON CANNON

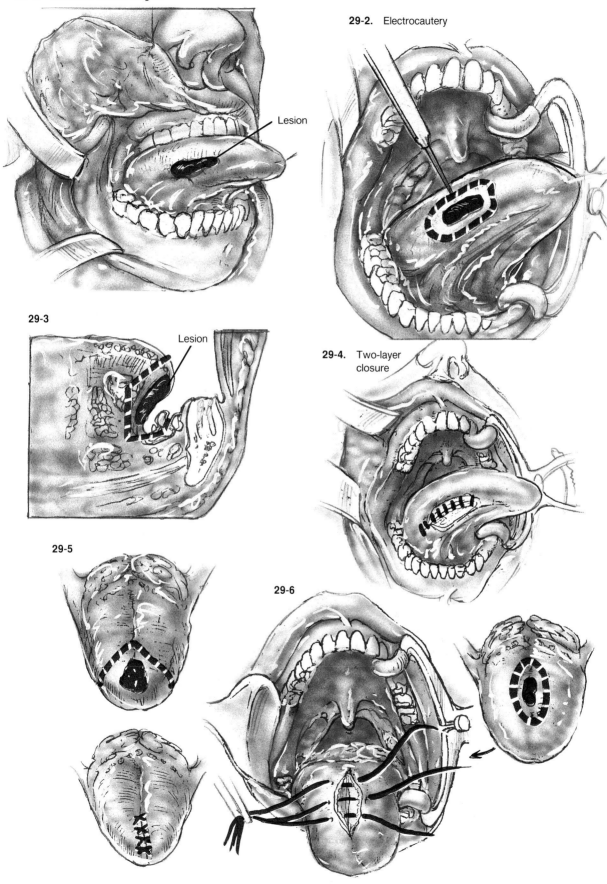

29-1. Lesion on mobile tongue

Lesion

29-2. Electrocautery

29-3

Lesion

29-4. Two-layer closure

29-5

29-6

■ 30. PARTIAL POSTERIOR GLOSSECTOMY OF THE TONGUE BASE— Removal of a portion of the tongue posterior to the circumvallate papilla

Indications

1. Small and medium size carcinomas of tongue base
2. En bloc resection of adjacent soft tissue and bone such as the mandible
3. Neck dissection may be performed in continuity.

Special Considerations

1. Presence of metastatic disease in the neck
2. Use of computed tomography or magnetic resonance imaging to aid in determining tumor extension, particularly inferiorly
3. Confirmation of margins by frozen-section analysis as a guide in adequacy of resection
4. Excision of a cuff of 1 to 2 cm of normal tissue beyond visible or palpable tumor, if possible
5. For smaller, inferior lesions of the tongue, it may be possible to resect a portion of angle of mandible and avoid mandibulotomy.
6. Inferiorly displaced lesions may require a supraglottic laryngectomy to obtain adequate margins.

Preoperative Preparation

1. Informed operative consent, including explanations of the diagnosis, purpose of treatment, prognosis with or without treatment, chances of success of treatment, alternative modes of treatment, and potential complications
2. A first-generation cephalosporin is generally sufficient for prophylactic treatment of normal skin and mucosal contamination. In more extensive dissections, flap reconstruction, or the irradiated patient, an aminoglycoside or clindamycin may be added. For antibiotic prophylaxis to be successful, the antibiotics must be given before surgical incision. The duration of the antibiotic regimen postoperatively (ie, 1, 2, or 7 days) is controversial.
3. The tongue is very vascular. For larger lesions of the tongue base, particularly when a concomitant radical neck dissection is to be performed, the patient donates 1 or 2 units of blood preoperatively.
4. Smaller lesions may be excised without requiring a tracheostomy. If there is any doubt about the adequacy of the airway, a tracheostomy should be performed.
5. Appropriate medical care and consultations of other medical problems such as organic heart disease, diabetes mellitus, or chronic obstructive pulmonary disease
6. Nutritional assessment to ensure prompt healing postoperatively

Special Instruments, Position, and Anesthesia

1. Headlight (fiberoptic)
2. Soft tissue instruments
3. Oscillating saw
4. Goggles
5. Shoulder roll and a foam doughnut used as head rest
6. Compression plate with appropriate instrument (eg, depth gauge, tap instrument, various screws plus plates)
7. Electric drill
8. Use of active drains, such as Hemovac or Jackson-Pratt
9. Appropriate monitoring devices, such as a Foley catheter, arterial line, or central venous pressure line, as determined for each patient's needs

(continued)

Operative Procedure

The patient is placed in a supine position on the operating room table. The appropriate intravenous lines and monitoring devices are applied. After the anesthesiologist institutes general nasotracheal anesthesia, a shoulder roll is placed beneath the patient's shoulders, and the head positioned on a foam doughnut. The operating room table is then turned to the side so that the surgeon and one or two assistants can comfortably work about the patient's head and neck. If the patient does not have severe underlying cardiovascular disease or hypertension, the proposed skin incisions are infiltrated with a solution of 1% Xylocaine with 1:100,000 epinephrine. After the anesthetic has been injected, the patient's facial area, neck, and anterior chest are prepped and draped in sterile fashion. The operative skin incisions are drawn with a marking pen.

The skin incision consists of a stair-step type incision across the lower lip, which is directed inferiorly to the point of soft tissue prominence of the chin (Fig. 30-1). The skin incision is then directed laterally around the soft tissue protuberance and into the neck. The cervical portion of the skin incision is approximately 2 cm beneath the margin of the mandible. If palpable adenopathy is present, a T-shaped extension of the cervical skin incision, inferiorly to facilitate a radical neck dissection, is marked out. This T-shaped incision should be posterior to the region of the carotid artery. An alternate incision for neck dissection is an inferior horizontal incision in the neck (ie, McFee-type incision). After the skin incisions are marked out, the patient's head is turned to the side opposite that with the tumor. The incision begins at the lip area. The surgeon grasps one side of the lip incision and the assistant the other, pinching the labial arteries and decreasing blood loss. The labial arteries can be ligated with 3-0 silk sutures or cauterized with the electrocautery. The skin incision then follows the soft tissue prominence of the chin into the neck. In the neck, the incision extends through the soft subcutaneous tissues and the platysma muscle. The mucosal incision in the lip is directed vertically to the gingivobuccal sulcus and then laterally along the mandible.

After the skin incisions have been made, hemostasis is obtained with the electrocautery or the bipolar cautery. The plane of dissection of the cheek flap is superficial to the periosteum of the mandible. The dissection is carried in an anterior to posterior direction to the region of the angle of the mandible. Some of the fibers of the masseter muscle may have to be divided to give adequate exposure in this area. A mandibulotomy incision is then marked out in a stair-step fashion. The limbs of this incision generally should be 1 to 1.5 cm long, depending on the size of the patient's mandible.

As tongue base lesions have a high propensity for metastasis, a neck dissection is usually included with this procedure. For N0 necks, a modified neck dissection, preserving the spinal accessory nerve, sternocleidomastoid muscle, and internal jugular vein, is usually carried out. For the node-positive neck, a formal radical neck dissection is carried out. The neck dissection contents are shown transected for the sake of clarity in this discussion. The neck dissection is usually carried out before the mandibulotomy.

Before performing the mandibulotomy, a compression plate is placed over the proposed mandibulotomy site (Fig. 30-2). The plate should be large enough so that two screws may be placed through the compression site on each side of the mandibulotomy incision. The compression plate is held in place with a bone forceps. The plate is bent to conform to the vagaries of the mandible. Drill holes are placed through the compression plate in the mandible using an electric drill. A depth gauge is used to select the appropriate length for each screw used for securing the compression plate (Fig. 30-3). A tapping tool, which places the threads in the drill hole for the individual screws, is next used (Fig. 30-4). The compression plate is then secured into place with the screws, ensuring that the screws are the appropriate size and can hold the plate firmly to the mandible. After this has been accomplished, the compression plate and screws are removed and placed on a back table.

A small malleable retractor is placed beneath the mandible to protect the soft tissues and the lingual and hypoglossal nerves from the saw. An oscillating saw is used to perform the mandibulotomy. The mandibulotomy segments can be distracted using small bone

(continued)

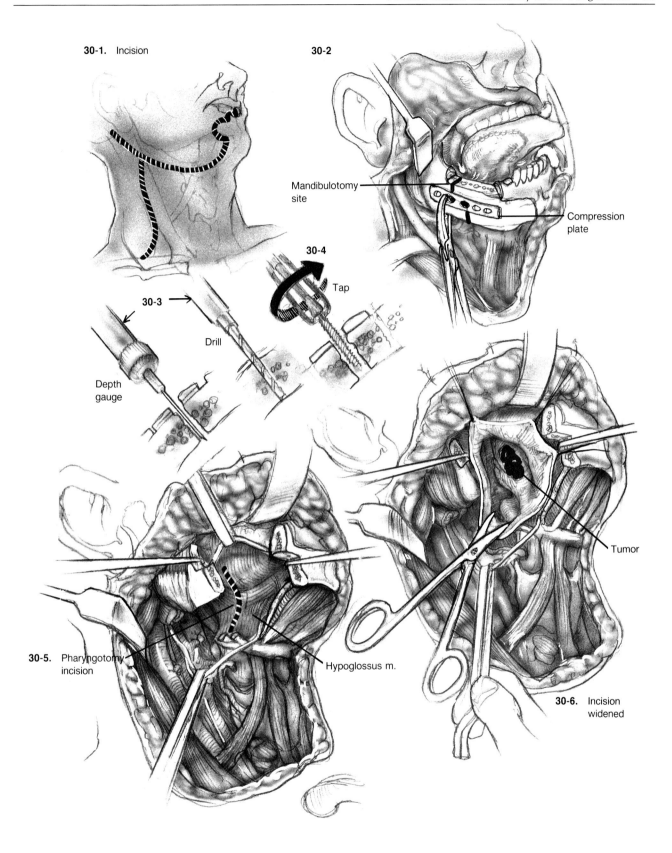

30-1. Incision

30-2

Mandibulotomy
site

Compression
plate

30-3

Drill

Depth
gauge

30-4

Tap

Tumor

30-5. Pharyngotomy
incision

Hypoglossus m.

30-6. Incision
widened

■ *30.* **PARTIAL POSTERIOR GLOSSECTOMY OF THE TONGUE BASE** *(continued)*

Tips and Pearls

1. Preoperative discussion with anesthesiologist regarding tumor size and site and development of plan for airway management
2. For difficult airway, may intubate over a bronchoscope
3. In cases of mandibulotomy, drill holes and apply a compression plate before sectioning the mandible. This enables a better repair of the mandible after mandibulotomy.
4. Use a small feeding tube such as Dobbhoff or Keofeed instead of a regular size nasogastric tube. The smaller tube is more comfortable for the patient and causes less hypopharyngeal irritation and edema.
5. Secure the feeding tube in place with twill tape to prevent accidental loss of the tube.

Pitfalls and Complications

1. Closely observe the airway, particularly for the 48 to 72 postoperative hours. If tracheostomy has been performed, frequent suctioning and adequate tracheostomy care are necessary.
2. For fistula formation in the irradiated patient in whom a radical neck dissection has been performed, consider a dermal graft or muscle flap to cover the carotid artery.
3. Infection or osteomyelitis of the mandibulotomy site
4. Inadequate exposure leading to subtotal tumor excision
5. Closure of the tongue base defect with a running suture in the irradiated patient can lead to necrosis of the mucosal margins. Interrupted sutures are preferred in this situation.

Postoperative Care Issues

1. Use a dedicated nursing unit (ie, nurses familiar with head and neck surgery and with management issues). If not available, employ an overnight intensive care unit stay for monitoring.
2. Empty and recharge suction canister every 8 hours. Drainage tubes may be removed after 2 to 3 days if the drainage is less than 50 mL per 24 hours.
3. Close attention to new wound complications, such as urinary tract infection, phlebitis, atelectasis, or pneumonia
4. Early ambulation
5. Pulmonary toilet (eg, deep breathing, cough, intermittent positive-pressure breathing, incentive spirometry)
6. Tube feedings by bolus (five times daily) or continuous infusion; use of Reglan may prevent gastric stasis
7. Oral feedings usually commence at 1 week postoperatively. If concerned about a fistula, give two or three drops of methylene blue in a glass of water and observe the suture line for a leak.
8. Immediately postoperatively, pain can be controlled with a patient-controlled analgesia infuser. After tube feedings begin, the patient can receive analgesics through the feeding tube.

References

Schechter GL, Sey DE, Roper AL, Jackson RT, Bomstay J. Set-back tongue flap for carcinoma of the tongue base. Arch Otolaryngol 1985;106:668.

Spiro RH, Gerold FP, Shah JP, et al. Mandibulotomy approach to oropharyngeal tumors. Am J Surg 1985;130:466.

hooks (Fig. 30-5). The surgeon's finger is then inserted into the oral cavity and along the lateral pharyngeal wall. An incision is made with a #15 scalpel blade to enter the lateral pharynx. Care is taken to avoid damaging the hypoglossal nerve superiorly and the superior laryngeal nerve inferiorly during this portion of the dissection. After the pharynx is entered, the pharyngotomy is extended superiorly and inferiorly with Metzenbaum scissors (Fig. 30-6).

Under direct vision, the tongue base lesion is inspected and palpated. Using electrocautery, an incision is made around the tumor in a block fashion, obtaining margins of at least 1 cm. Visualization of the tumor can be somewhat difficult, and the surgeon should proceed slowly and patiently to prevent injuring any of the surrounding vital structures or performing a less than total excision of the cancer. After the tumor has been removed, the specimen is marked with a silk ligature and with ink, allowing the pathologist to orient the specimen. Frozen-section analysis is used to confirm the peripheral margins of the wound and the deep surgical margin. Hemostasis of any bleeding vessels is usually obtained with electrocautery (Fig. 30-7).

The surgical defect of the tongue base is not closed until all margins have been examined and found to be free of tumor by frozen-section analysis. For most patients, the wound can be closed in a primary fashion. I prefer a layered closure, using ligatures of 2-0 or 3-0 Vicryl to reapproximate the musculature and the tongue base. The mucosal margins are usually closed with a ligature of 4-0 Vicryl. In a previously irradiated patient, a running suture may cause ischemia of the mucosal margins and subsequent necrosis of the wound margins, leading to wound infection or fistula formation (Fig. 30-8).

The pharyngotomy site is closed in a layered fashion. The first layer uses a 4-0 Vicryl placed in a Connell fashion, everting the mucosa medially. A second reinforcing layered closure is obtained using ligatures of 3-0 silk. I have found it useful to preserve the posterior belly of the digastric muscle during the neck dissection. It can be detached and then used as a third layer of closure over the pharyngotomy site (Fig. 30-9).

After the pharyngotomy site has been closed, the mandible is reapproximated using the compression plates, which had previously been contoured, to approximate the mandible in this area (Fig. 30-10). Before closure of the pharyngotomy site, a small Keofeed or Dobbhoff feeding tube is inserted. Its position in the stomach is verified by applying the suction to the tip of the nasogastric tube, verifying the presence of gastric contents within the suction tip. An alternate method is to use a catheter-tipped syringe and have the anesthesiologist listen to the patient's stomach while a bolus of air is injected into the tube. A final assessment of the patient's airway is then carried out. For small laterally placed tongue base lesions without much operative edema, a tracheostomy may not be indicated. An intravenous dose of Decadron (8 mg) during the procedure may also decrease some of the operative edema. In most cases, however, a tracheostomy is indicated. A vertical incision is made just to the side of the midline on the contralateral side. Care must be taken during the neck dissection to prevent entering the region of the tracheostomy. The tracheostomy tube is usually secured in place with several ligatures of 2-0 silk. Tracheostomy tapes may be placed loosely around the patient's neck. If a flap reconstruction has been carried out, tracheostomy tape is not used.

The gingivobuccal sulcus incision is closed with ligature of 4-0 coated Vicryl in a continuous or interrupted fashion. Careful attention is paid to the region of the vermilion border of the lower lip, which is reapproximated with a ligature of 5-0 Nylon. The chin incision is closed with ligatures of 4-0 coated Vicryl to reapproximate the soft tissues and 5-0 Nylon to reapproximate the skin margins. The platysma muscle and soft tissues of the neck are closed with interrupted ligatures of 3-0 Vicryl. The skin incisions are closed with stainless steel staples. Drainage of the surgical wound is usually carried out by means of a Hemovac drain or other active types of suction, which are brought in through separate stab incisions inferiorly placed over the skin of the anterior chest (Fig. 30-11). The Hemovac drains are secured in place with 2-0 silk.

C. RON CANNON

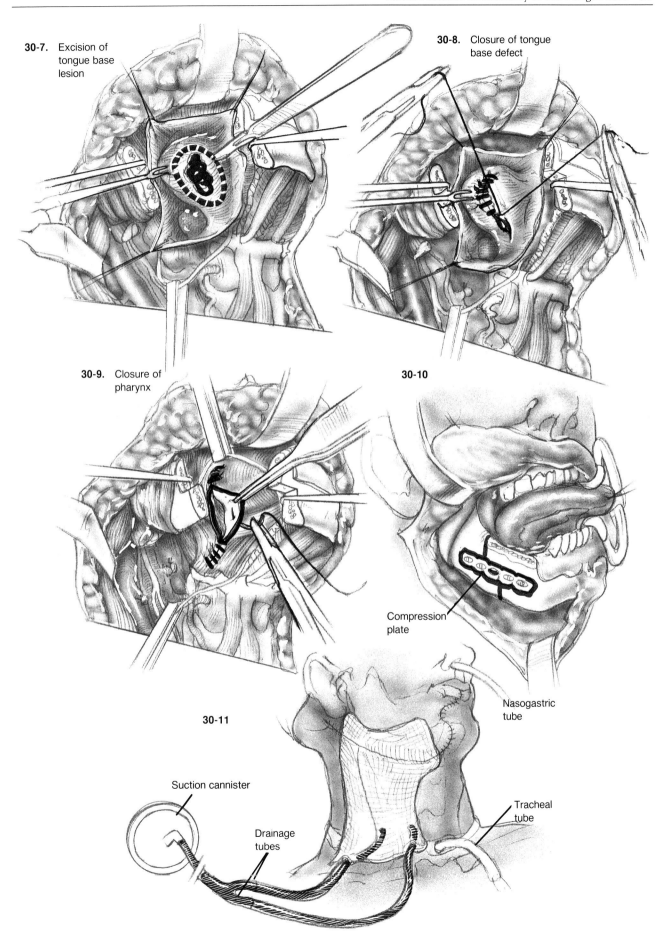

30-7. Excision of tongue base lesion

30-8. Closure of tongue base defect

30-9. Closure of pharynx

30-10

Compression plate

Nasogastric tube

30-11

Suction cannister

Drainage tubes

Tracheal tube

■ *31.* PARTIAL MIDLINE GLOSSECTOMY OF THE TONGUE BASE—Surgical resection of the tongue posterior to the circumvallate papillae

Indications
1. Carcinoma limited to tongue base

Special Considerations
1. Patient must have adequate cardiopulmonary function, and must be active and able to climb stairs.
2. Tumor must not extend to larynx, tonsil, or anterior to circumvallate papillae.

Preoperative Evaluation
1. Magnetic resonance scan
2. Direct laryngoscopy and bimanual palpation

Special Instruments, Position, and Anesthesia
1. Supine on a shoulder roll
2. General anesthesia through a tracheotomy

Tips and Pearls
1. Release suprahyoid musculature along the superior edge of the hyoid.
2. Undertake bilateral neck dissection of zones I, II, and III if the patient is node negative (N0).
3. Identify, dissect out, and preserve the hypoglossal nerve bilaterally.
4. Obtain frozen-section control of all margins.
5. Reapproximate fibroaponeurotic layer of the tongue to the hyoid bone to suspend the larynx.

Pitfalls and Complications
1. Do not underestimate the size of the primary tumor. This procedure is not indicated if the lesion extends to the larynx, anterior tongue, or tonsil.
2. Do not fail to obtain complete hemostasis at the tongue base.
3. Do not fail to visually identify the hypoglossal nerve bilaterally.

Postoperative Care Issues
1. Administer perioperative antibiotics for 24 hours.
2. Nutritional support through a nasogastric tube
3. Maintain suction drains until the output is less than 15 mL in 24 hours.

References
Moore DM, Calcaterra TC. Cancer of the tongue base treated by a transpharyngeal approach. Ann Otol Rhinol Laryngol 1990;99:300.
Weber PC, Johnson JT, Myers EN. The suprahyoid approach for squamous cell carcinoma of the base of the tongue. Laryngoscope 1992;102:637.
Weisberger EC, Lingeman RE. Modified supraglottic laryngectomy and resection of lesions of the base of the tongue. Laryngoscope 1983;93:20.

Operative Procedure
An antibiotic effective against oral flora should be administered before the patient is taken to the operating room or before induction of anesthesia. With the patient in the supine position, the head is extended with a soft roll placed under the shoulders.

A superiorly based apron flap is developed in the subplatysmal plane. This flap can provide adequate exposure for a bilateral, simultaneous, selective (or modified) neck dissection, as appropriate (Fig. 31-1). The tracheotomy is performed through the third tracheal cartilage. The endotracheal tube is withdrawn, an anode tube inserted into the tracheotomy, and anesthesia continued.

Neck dissection should be performed bilaterally for patients with squamous cell carcinoma of the tongue base. Selective dissection of zones I, II, and III is undertaken if there is no demonstrable evidence of metastatic carcinoma. Patients with metastatic cancer should undergo modified radical neck dissection, which preserves the spinal accessory nerve. An effort is made to preserve and maintain the internal jugular vein on the less involved side.

The hypoglossal nerves are identified bilaterally (Fig. 31-2). The nerve is freed from tissue medial and deep to it, which allows gentle retraction superiorly out of the field of surgery.

The suprahyoid musculature is divided along the superior aspect of the hyoid bone (see Fig. 31-1) in the midline to expose the mucosa of the vallecula, which is opened in the midline initially and then extended laterally toward either side to afford a patulous pharyngotomy (Fig. 31-3).

The tongue base is grasped with a tenaculum and delivered into the wound (Fig. 31-4). The tumor is widely resected with 1.5 to 2.0 cm of apparently normal tissue on all sides of the lesion (Fig. 31-5). The specimen is oriented and submitted immediately for frozen-section evaluation of the adequacy of margins. Hemostasis in the residual tongue is obtained with suture ligatures.

Cricopharyngeal myotomy may be performed to facilitate postoperative swallowing. The carotid sheath is separated from the visceral compartment on the left side. The pharynx is rolled away from the surgeon (toward the right), and the cricopharyngeus muscle is incised down to mucosa in the midline posteriorly. This is facilitated if the surgeon's finger is placed into the lumen of the cervical esophagus to distend and fix the fibers of the cricopharyngeal muscle.

The pharyngotomy is then closed by suturing the hyoid bone to the fibrous aponeurotic layer of the tongue base. A 2-0 silk suture or other heavy, nonabsorbable suture is preferred. Sutures should be placed every 7 to 9 mm. The closure is reinforced by approximating suprahyoid musculature to the infrahyoid musculature.

The wound is drained with suction drains bilaterally. The drains are brought out through separate stab incisions in the skin. The skin is subsequently closed in layers, employing a resorbable suture to reapproximate the platysma and staples for the skin.

If the tracheotomy has been placed through the lower border of the apron flap, care must be taken to ensure that tracheal secretions cannot dissect under the flap to contaminate the neck dissection.

JONAS T. JOHNSON

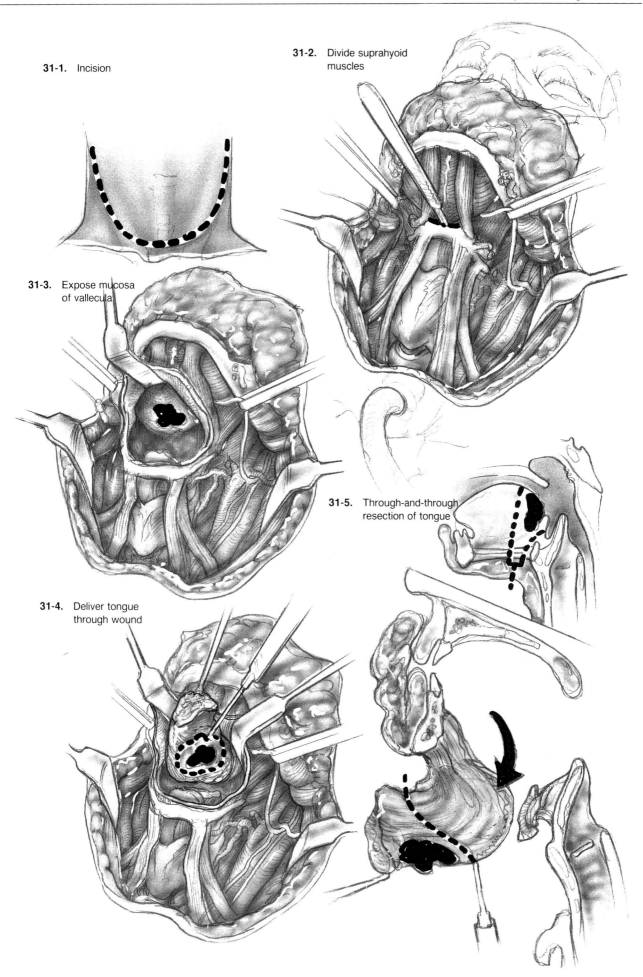

31-1. Incision

31-2. Divide suprahyoid muscles

31-3. Expose mucosa of vallecula

31-5. Through-and-through resection of tongue

31-4. Deliver tongue through wound

■ *32.* NEAR-TOTAL GLOSSECTOMY

Surgical removal of greater than half of tongue, often associated with simultaneous excision of adjacent involved tissues of the floor of the mouth, retromolar trigone, or lateral pharyngeal wall

Indications

1. Stage T3 or T4 carcinoma of the tongue
2. Recurrence after prior radiation therapy for advanced tongue cancer

Special Considerations

1. Floor of mouth involvement
2. Mandibular involvement
3. Retromolar involvement
4. Lateral pharyngeal involvement
5. Functional capacity of patient
6. Nodal status
7. Reconstruction
8. Perioperative antibiotics administered

Preoperative Preparation

1. Magnetic resonance imaging of primary and cervical nodes
2. Assessment of cardiopulmonary status
3. Endoscopic evaluation of tumor and biopsy

Tips and Pearls

1. Use anterior mandibulotomy if the mandible is not involved by tumor.
2. Consider the temporary use of a percutaneous endoscopic gastrostomy tube or gastrostomy tube.
3. Reconstruction with split-thickness skin graft (STSG) is advocated if a mobile, innervated tongue can be preserved.
4. Tracheotomy is always required.
5. Ipsilateral neck dissection is performed concurrently.
6. Margins are controlled with frozen-section evaluation.
7. Mandibular reconstruction is undertaken with free flaps selectively. Skin reconstruction may compromise tongue function.

(continued)

Operative Procedure

The patient is placed on the operating table in the supine position. Intravenous antibiotics should be administered at or just before the initial incision. After the induction of satisfactory general endotracheal anesthesia, a tracheotomy is performed through a horizontal incision in the midline through the second or third tracheal ring. As the endotracheal tube is withdrawn, an anode tube is inserted through the tracheotomy site, and general anesthesia is continued.

If direct laryngoscopy has not been previously performed, formal examination under anesthesia is undertaken at this time. This should include careful inspection and palpation of the extent of the tongue tumor, observing carefully for involvement of adjacent tissues of the floor of the mouth, retromolar trigone, or lateral pharyngeal wall. Observe also fixation or proximity of the tumor to the mandible. If 1 cm or more of normal tissue intervenes between the lingual cortex of the mandible and the tongue, a mandibular-sparing procedure should be undertaken. If the tumor is adherent to or invades the mandible, segmental mandibulectomy is undertaken in continuity with near-total glossectomy. Tumor involvement of the body of the mandible necessitates segmental resection of the entire mental canal. If tumor involves the angle and the ascending ramus of the mandible, segmental mandibulectomy should be undertaken from the mental foramen anteriorly to the condylar neck posteriorly.

A three-quarters H skin incision is employed. The vertical incision begins at the mastoid tip and generally follows the anterior border of the trapezius muscle to the clavicle. The horizontal limb comes off in a naturally occurring skin crease at approximately a midneck level and is brought to the midline (Fig. 32-1). The vertical limb is carried directly through the midline of the lip and mentum down to meet the horizontal limb of the incision in the midline. The lip-splitting incision is vertical and straight. No attempt is made to notch or curve it. Skin flaps are elevated in the subplatysmal plane. Hemostasis is achieved with the use of electrocautery and suture ligatures.

Ipsilateral neck dissection precedes resection of the primary. The neck dissection specimen is left attached to the primary specimen. When segmental mandibulectomy is to be performed, the neck dissection is left attached at the inferior aspect of the mandible in the submandibular region.

Attention is turned to the oral cavity. When a mandibular-sparing operation is deemed feasible, mandibulotomy is performed to improve exposure of the oral cavity. Mandibulotomy is undertaken through an area of mandible with no dentition (Fig. 32-2). If all the teeth are present, the lateral incisor is extracted, and the mandibulotomy is performed in this region. The mandibulotomy should always be performed anterior (mesial) to the mental foramen. A mandibular plate should be placed and the holes drilled before actual performance of the mandibulotomy in anticipation of the reconstruction at the completion of the extirpative portion of the procedure. If segmental mandibulectomy is required, the mandible is divided just anterior to the mental foramen.

Near-total glossectomy, when achieved with mandibulotomy, requires that the ipsilateral floor of the mouth mucosa be divided as the mandible is displaced for improved exposure. The mucosal incision should allow the maximum amount of mucosa to remain on the alveolus to afford a good cuff of tissue for subsequent reconstruction (Fig. 32-3). However, the tumor should be removed with a minimum of 1 cm of normal tissue. In performing near-total glossectomy, resection of the ipsilateral hypoglossal nerve is the rule. Similarly, the lingual nerve is resected with the specimen. Careful inspection and palpation are correlated with preoperative imaging studies to determine the appropriate location of the incision separating the tumor from contralateral structures. A minimum of 1 cm of normal tissue is recommended. All margins should be carefully assessed by the pathologist, and any areas with suspected or close involvement should be subjected to frozen-section analysis.

Absolute hemostasis is critical to the success of the reconstructive procedure. Electrocautery is relatively ineffective in controlling bleeding on the cut surface of the tongue muscle. Hemostatic 3-0 chromic sutures should be placed on an atraumatic needle using a

(continued)

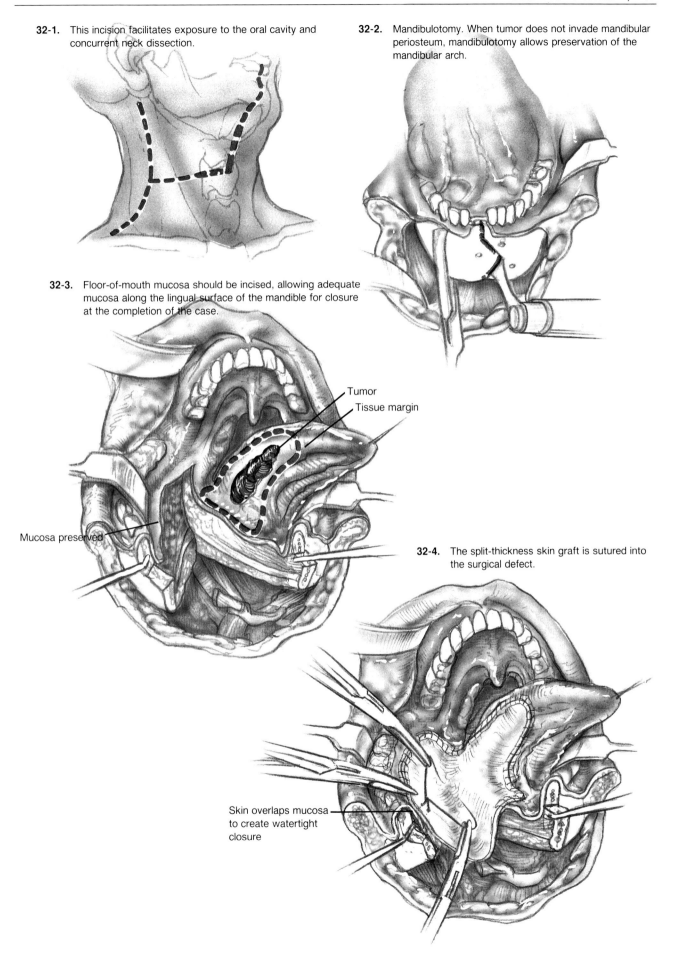

32-1. This incision facilitates exposure to the oral cavity and concurrent neck dissection.

32-2. Mandibulotomy. When tumor does not invade mandibular periosteum, mandibulotomy allows preservation of the mandibular arch.

32-3. Floor-of-mouth mucosa should be incised, allowing adequate mucosa along the lingual surface of the mandible for closure at the completion of the case.

Tumor

Tissue margin

Mucosa preserved

32-4. The split-thickness skin graft is sutured into the surgical defect.

Skin overlaps mucosa to create watertight closure

■ 32. NEAR-TOTAL GLOSSECTOMY (continued)

Pitfalls and Complications
1. Absolute hemostasis before reconstruction
2. STSG must be harvested intact.
3. STSG is immobilized with a bolus and external compressive dressing.
4. The integrity of the contralateral hypoglossal nerve is critical.

Postoperative Care Issues
1. Initiate tube feedings as soon as the bowel functions.
2. Deflate tracheotomy tube cuff to assess the ability to resist aspiration.
3. When the patient no longer aspirates, change to a #4 uncuffed tracheostomy tube, which can also be used to assess adequacy of the airway.
4. Decannulate before institution of oral feeding.
5. Nonpourable pureed diet is often best tolerated.
6. Modified barium swallow may help guide rehabilitation of swallow.

Reference
Stanley RB. Mandibular lingual releasing approach to oral and oropharyngeal carcinomas. Laryngoscope 1984;94:596.

figure-of-eight technique. Bleeding from the cut edge of the mucosa is managed with electrocautery. The lingual artery is identified and tied.

If a "finger" of residual tongue can be maintained on the contralateral side with intact innervation from the hypoglossal nerve, resurfacing the defect with STSG offers the patient the best chance for functional recovery. Reconstruction with bulkier techniques, such as a pectoralis major myocutaneous flap or free full-thickness tissue obtained from a distant site, results in a tethering of the residual tongue with adynamic, insensate tissue. These techniques offer reliable reconstruction at the expense of function.

The STSG is obtained from the ipsilateral thigh employing a dermatome that can provide an adequate amount of skin that is 0.0018 in (0.046 mm) thick. It is generally preferable that the skin graft be free of perforations. This is critical when the STSG is used to separate the oral cavity from the neck wound. The absolute surface area of the STSG is determined by the surface area of the defect to be reconstructed, but the success of the reconstruction requires that the STSG be of ample size to prevent a tight closure; the minimum size is approximately 8 × 12 cm.

The reconstruction is begun by closing the cut edge of the tongue base to the oropharynx and primarily closing the tip of the tongue to itself as indicated. The STSG is then sutured to the cut edge of the tongue mucosa employing a "pie-crusting" technique in which the 2-0 silk suture is driven first through the skin graft then through the cut edge of the mucosa and then back through the skin graft (Fig. 32-4). The suture is tied and left approximately 6 in (15 cm) long to be used to overtie the surgical bolus that is placed at the completion of the reconstruction. The reconstruction is carried posteriorly around the defect, laterally to the residual floor of mouth mucosa, and then anteriorly to the site of the mandibulotomy (Fig. 32-5). As the reconstruction is completed, it becomes apparent that the skin graft needs to be trimmed to fit the shape and size of the defect. Tension on the skin graft is to be avoided, and overtrimming is an error. The mandibulotomy is wired or plated with two screws on either side (Fig. 32-6).

The STSG may be sutured to the underlying tongue musculature in a quilting fashion to help ensure its immobilization. A bolus of antibiotic-impregnated gauze is carefully applied to the STSG to ensure immobilization and to reinforce hemostasis. The bolus is overtied with silks previously left long after insertion of the STSG (Fig. 32-7).

Patients requiring lateral segmental mandibulectomy in whom mandibular reconstruction is not anticipated are reconstructed in a similar fashion using a STSG. In this circumstance, the skin graft separates the oral cavity from the neck dissection defect. The STSG must be free of perforation, and quilting sutures may not be placed in the floor of the mouth.

When simultaneous mandibular reconstruction is deemed appropriate, based on the patient's preoperative good dentition and high performance status, simultaneous reconstruction with a free tissue transfer employing microvascular techniques is the most reliable technique currently available. The impact of this reconstruction on the function of the residual tongue muscle should be considered. Improved cosmesis is rarely a satisfactory trade-off for compromise of tongue function.

The skin flaps are returned to their anatomic position and closed in layers. Positive-pressure drains are placed in dependent portions of the neck dissection and brought out through separate stab wounds. The drain must not touch the STSG. The subcutaneous tissues are reapproximated with a resorbable suture, and the skin is closed with staples. The anode tube is removed and replaced with a cuffed tracheotomy tube, and the patient is returned to the postanesthesia recovery room. A bulky compressive dressing is applied to coapt the skin flap to the deep tissues in the neck. This dressing serves also to further immobilize the STSG.

Continued positive pressure must be maintained on the suction drains during transfer and on arrival in the postanesthesia room.

JONAS T. JOHNSON

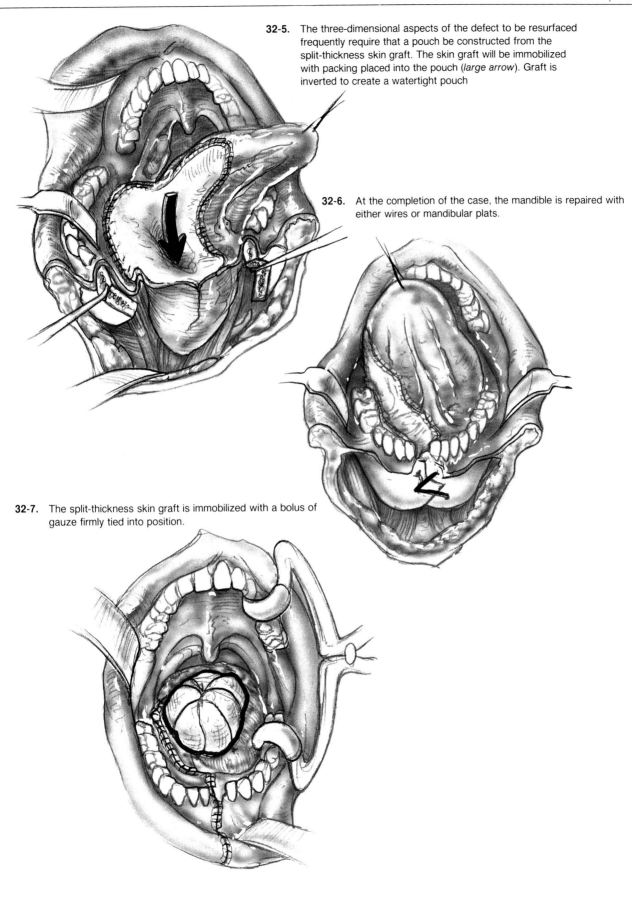

32-5. The three-dimensional aspects of the defect to be resurfaced frequently require that a pouch be constructed from the split-thickness skin graft. The skin graft will be immobilized with packing placed into the pouch (*large arrow*). Graft is inverted to create a watertight pouch

32-6. At the completion of the case, the mandible is repaired with either wires or mandibular plats.

32-7. The split-thickness skin graft is immobilized with a bolus of gauze firmly tied into position.

■ *33.* TOTAL GLOSSECTOMY

Surgical removal of the entire tongue

Indications

1. Extensive carcinoma with involvement of the root of the tongue requiring total glossectomy
2. Tongue base cancer with infiltration anteriorly to involve the mobile tongue

Special Considerations

1. Floor of the mouth involved
2. Mandibular involvement
3. Laryngeal extension
4. Functional capacity of patient
5. Nodal status
6. Reconstruction

Preoperative Studies

1. Magnetic resonance imaging of primary and cervical lymphatics
2. Assessment of cardiopulmonary function
3. Functional status of patient
4. Endoscopy and biopsy

Tips and Pearls

1. Tumors limited to the tongue can be "dropped" through intact mandible, but the reconstruction is technically more demanding.
2. Involvement of the mandible by tumor requires concurrent segmental mandibulectomy. Bone reconstruction of the lateral segmental mandibulectomy is rarely indicated. Anterior segmental defects are best managed with free osteocutaneous tissue transfers.
3. Mandibulotomy may effectively improve exposure in most patients.
4. Concurrent total laryngectomy is advisable in patients with significant cardiopulmonary disease. This is best assessed through evaluation of functional status. The ability to ambulate (minimal two flights of stairs) is critical.
5. Temporary use of a percutaneous endoscopic gastrostomy tube should be considered.
6. Soft tissue reconstruction is satisfactory with pectoralis myocutaneous flaps.
7. Suspension of hyoid-laryngeal complex to mandible
8. Bilateral neck dissection almost always indicated
9. Use of frozen section to ensure tumor-free margin
10. Cricopharyngeal myotomy may aid in rehabilitation.

Pitfalls and Complications

1. Failure to adequately drain wound
2. Closure with tension leads to wound separation and infection.
3. Larynx-sparing procedures in patient with chronic debilitating disease may result in life-threatening pneumonia.

Postoperative Care Issues

1. Deflate tracheotomy tube well to assess ability to defend against aspiration.
2. Change to a small (#4), plugged, uncuffed tube to assess the adequacy of the airway.
3. Decannulate before beginning oral feeding.

References

Gehanno P, Guedon C, Barry B, Depondt J, Kebaili C. Advanced carcinoma of the tongue: total glossectomy without total laryngectomy. Review of 80 cases. Laryngoscope 1992;102:1369.

Myers EN. Tumors of the nose and sinuses. Consultant 1973;13:93.

Tiwari R, Karim AB, Greven AJ, Snow GB. Total glossectomy with laryngeal preservation. Arch Otolaryngol Head Neck Surg 1993;119:945.

Operative Procedure

After induction of general anesthesia, the patient is placed in the supine position, with the head extended over a shoulder roll. The head and neck are prepped and draped in the usual position. Tracheotomy is carried out through the anterior segment of the third tracheal ring. An anode tube is inserted into the tracheostomy and anesthesia maintained.

If the continuity of the mandible is to be preserved, a superiorly based apron flap is elevated in a subplatysmal plane up to the inferior border of the mandible (Fig. 33-1). If tumor considerations require a segmental mandibulectomy to be undertaken, I prefer to use a midline lip-splitting incision to afford appropriate exposure to the mandible (Fig. 33-2). Bilateral selective neck dissection is accomplished (ie, zones I, II, III) in the node-negative (N0) patient, and modified radical neck dissection is performed for patients with palpable adenopathy.

After completion of neck dissection, the superiorly based apron flap is lifted as a visor to afford exposure to the oral cavity. Periosteum should be preserved on the anterior aspect of the mandible. Accordingly, the visor flap should be separated sharply from the mandible. It is appropriate to incise the labial mucosa transorally to ensure that approximately 1 cm of mucosa remains on the mandible to afford adequate mucosa for a water-tight closure at the completion of the case. The neurovascular structures exiting the mental foramen must be divided and ligated. The intraoral incision must be cared all the way to the third molar bilaterally to afford adequate exposure.

In some circumstances, the visor flap may be unnecessary, and the oral component of the procedure can be carried out transorally. This seems most appropriate for thin, edentulous patients. When the extent of tumor requires segmental mandibulectomy, the exposure afforded by visor flap may be inadequate, and a one-half H-type incision may be required with a vertical extension through the midline of the lip, allowing reflection of the cheek flap to afford adequate visibility (see Fig. 33-2).

The mucosa of the floor of the mouth is incised from the retromolar area on one side and around anteriorly to the retromolar area on the opposite side, with care taken to preserve as much floor mouth mucosa as is possible (Figs. 33-3 and 33-4). This approach assists in creating a water-tight closure at the completion of the case. At this point, attention is turned to the mylohyoid, digastric, and genioglossal muscles, which are separated from the mandible anteriorly, allowing the tongue to be dropped through the mandibular arch and brought out into the neck (Figs. 33-5 and 33-6). The lingual artery is divided bilaterally, and the carotid vascular system is separated from the tongue musculature. The hypoglossal nerve and lingual nerve are divided bilaterally.

The posterior margin of resection is dictated by the extent of tumor. Total glossectomy implies that the tongue is separated from the larynx through the vallecula. Under some circumstances, a portion of tongue base may be free of tumor and can be preserved. This is of functional importance and should be undertaken if possible.

In many circumstances, extension of tumor to involve mandible requires a concurrent segmental mandibulectomy. When gross involvement of the mandibular cortex is apparent, it is critical to achieve clear bone margins. From a practical point of view, intraoperative assessment of margins is not practical. Accordingly, patients with involvement of the mandibular body should undergo resection of the entire mental canal. Patients with involvement of the symphysis should have 2 cm bone margins on either side of the area of involvement.

Total glossectomy defects are reconstructed with a pectoralis major myocutaneous flap. The flap is elevated and mobilized such that it reaches the anterior mentum without tension. The skin of the flap is sutured to the recipient mucosa of the floor of mouth and lateral oropharynx. The fascia of the pectoralis muscle is sutured to the mentum anteriorly and to the hyoid bone inferiorly. Wire sutures passed through holes in the lower aspect of the mandible may help suspend the flap and support it against the pull of gravity. The muscle is used to reinforce the wound circumferentially. Suction drains are placed along the region of the construction bilaterally.

JONAS T. JOHNSON

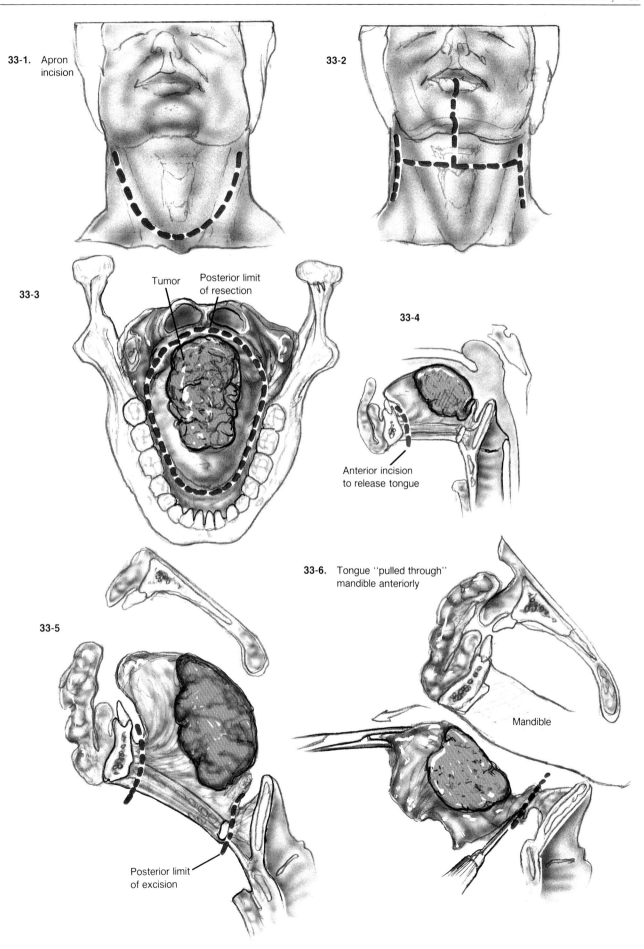

33-1. Apron incision

33-2

33-3 Tumor Posterior limit of resection

33-4

Anterior incision to release tongue

33-5 Posterior limit of excision

33-6. Tongue "pulled through" mandible anteriorly

Mandible

■ *34.* ANTERIOR FLOOR OF MOUTH RESECTION— Transoral excision of the anterior floor of mouth with or without marginal mandibulectomy

Indications
1. Excision of squamous cell carcinoma of the floor of mouth, stage T1 through T3, superficial in nature
2. Removal of other benign or malignant lesions, superficial in nature, arising in the floor of the mouth

Special Considerations
1. Lack of mandibular involvement
2. Status of residual dentition
3. Selective neck dissections, except in patients with T1 very exophytic lesions
4. Marginal mandibulectomy for tumor crossing but not invading the alveolus, tumor adherent to mandibular periosteum, or an inability to achieve anterior margin resection without removing the alveolus
5. Skin graft is used to reconstruct the floor of the mouth in all cases except after failed radiation therapy.
6. Tracheotomy is used in all cases.

Preoperative Preparation
1. Thorough history and physical examination
2. Chest radiograph and barium esophagram to exclude other synchronous tumors of the upper aerodigestive tract
3. Panendoscopy to exclude synchronous tumors of the upper and lower aerodigestive tract
4. Dental consultation about restoration or extraction of residual teeth
5. Confirmation of tissue diagnosis
6. Computed tomography scan of mandible, when necessary to exclude bone invasion

Special Instruments, Position, and Anesthesia
1. General anesthesia delivered through tracheotomy
2. Jennings mouth gag
3. Headlight for the surgeon
4. Stryker saw with right-angled blade if marginal mandibulectomy is necessary

Tips and Pearls
1. The inferior margin of soft tissue dissection is deep to the sublingual glands.
2. Mandibular osteotomies should be carried through completely into the soft tissues to avoid fracture of the mandible.
3. Meticulous hemostasis
4. Appropriate-thickness skin graft
5. Treatment unnecessary for transected Wharton's ducts, even if neck dissections are not carried out

Pitfalls and Complications
1. Postoperative bleeding
2. Loss of skin graft from incomplete hemostasis or inadequate immobilization
3. Fracture of the mandible from inappropriate osteotomies

Postoperative Care
1. Perioperative antibiotics for 24 hours
2. Removal of gauze bolus on the fifth postoperative day
3. Prompt decannulation within 48 to 72 hours after removal of the bolus
4. Maintenance of nutrition with nasogastric tube until decannulation
5. Dental referral for prosthesis after complete healing has occurred

References
McGuirt WF, Johnson JT, Myers EN, Rothfield R, Wagner R. Floor of mouth carcinoma: the management of the clinically negative neck. Arch Otolaryngol Head Neck Surg 1993; : .

Schramm VL, Myers EN, Sigler BA. Surgical management of early epidermoid carcinoma of the anterior floor of the mouth. Laryngoscope 1980;90:207–215.

Operative Procedure
Using the coagulation current or knife, the mucosa is incised, 2-0 silk suture is placed through the anterior margin of resection, and the circulating nurse is notified to mark this on the pathology form. Using small dissecting scissors, the soft tissue is sharply and blunted dissected from anterior to posterior (Fig. 34-1). The deep margin of resection in superficial cancers in this area is the sublingual gland (Fig. 34-2). After the sublingual glands have been identified, dissection is carried deep to the sublingual glands to provide this deep margin (see Fig. 34-2B). Wharton's duct is transected on both sides while dissecting the deep margin of resection. It is unnecessary to reconstruct the ducts. The remainder of the lesion is then excised with sharp and blunt resection.

During the time hemostasis is being obtained, the surgeon and his assistant change into new gowns and gloves and harvest the skin graft. We use a Brown dermatome set at 0.016 to 0.018 in (0.4–0.46 mm). The skin graft should be thick enough to handle easily and not tear but thin enough to be pliable and to have a high possibility of success. Using a "pie-crusting" technique, the skin graft is sewn to the mucosa of the floor of the mouth, leaving every other suture long to tie over. One or two "tacking" stitches are placed in the floor of the mouth with absorbable catgut suture to help adherence of the skin graft to the underlying tissues. One to two Xeroform gauze packs are used as a bolus and tied over with the long ties.

If marginal mandibulectomy is to be done, then the operation is modified somewhat. At the outset of the operation, the soft tissue incisions and osteotomies are outlined with a marking pen. The initial incisions are made in the soft tissue and carried over the alveolar process down to bone and then connected anteriorly. The mucoperiosteum of the mandible is elevated inferiorly to make a precise osteotomy. In patients who are dentulous, the bone cuts for an anterior marginal mandibulectomy usually encompass the central and lateral incisors. In such cases, both canine teeth should be extracted and the osteotomy made in the middle of the socket or medial to it. This preserves bone around the remaining teeth, which allows later application of partial removable dentures with clasps. If the incision is made just next to the remaining teeth, bone resorption eventually destroys the support of the teeth, which become loose and require removal.

Because the alveolar process is not involved with the tumor but rather is a margin of resection around the tumor, it is important to resect only the alveolar process and not go inferiorly into the body of the mandible. The vertical dimension of the mandible is quite substantial, but because it is still possible to fracture the bone, a rim of bone containing only alveolar process should be taken. A Stryker saw with a right-angled blade should be used first in making the vertical bone cuts and then in connecting this with a horizontal bone cut. It is important that the bone be cut completely through. It may be tempting to use an osteotome or a heavy elevator to try to pry the bone and fracture the lingual cortex, but this may fracture the mandible and is contraindicated. After the lingual cortex and mandibular fragment have been cut through, the bone fragment is retracted superiorly and posteriorly along with the soft tissue, and the rest of the resection is then carried out as described previously (Fig. 34-3), again finding the sublingual glands and including them as a margin of resection (Fig. 34-4).

A split-thickness skin graft can be used to resurface the soft tissue and the residual mandibular bone (Fig. 34-5). This is possible because most of the exposed bone of the mandible, after the alveolar process has been removed, is cancellous bone with a thin rim of cortical bone on the buccal and lingual sides. The skin graft heals nicely in this area if care is taken to provide immobilization of the graft over the bone and the soft tissue.

Skin grafts should not be used in patients who are being operated on for recurrent cancer of the floor of the mouth after failed radiation therapy. Skin grafting is contraindicated in such patients because if the skin graft fails, irradiated bone becomes exposed and almost certainly develops osteoradionecrosis. In such cases, my colleagues and I prefer to use a radial forearm free flap with microvascular anastomosis.

EUGENE N. MYERS

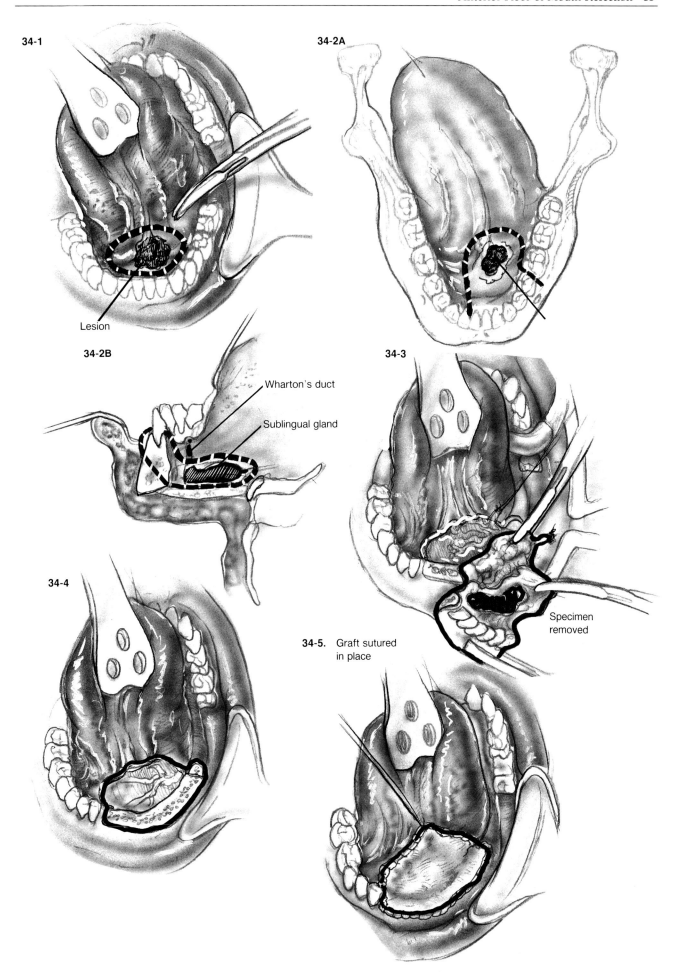

34-1

Lesion

34-2A

34-2B

Wharton's duct

Sublingual gland

34-3

Specimen
removed

34-4

34-5. Graft sutured
in place

■ *35.* LATERAL FLOOR OF MOUTH RESEC-TION—Transoral excision of the lateral floor of the mouth with or without marginal mandibulectomy

Indications

1. Resection of malignant tumors in the lateral floor of the mouth
2. Removal of other benign or malignant lesions, superficial in nature, arising in the floor of the mouth

Special Considerations

1. Lack of mandibular involvement
2. Status of residual dentition
3. Selective neck dissections, except in patients with T1 very exophytic lesions
4. Marginal mandibulectomy for tumor crossing but not invading the alveolus, tumor adherent to mandibular periosteum, or an inability to achieve anterior margin resection without removing the alveolus
5. Skin graft is used to reconstruct the floor of the mouth except after failed radiation therapy.
6. Tracheotomy is used in all cases.
7. In the dentulous patient, if an osteotomy is to be carried out, care must be taken for conservative removal of the alveolus, because the body of the mandible laterally does not have the same high vertical dimension as the anterior mandible.

Preoperative Preparation

1. Chest radiograph and barium esophagram to exclude other synchronous tumors of the upper aerodigestive tract
2. Panendoscopy to exclude other synchronous tumors of the upper and lower aerodigestive tract
3. Dental consultation about restoration or extraction of residual teeth
4. Confirmation of tissue diagnosis
5. Computed tomography scan of mandible, when necessary to exclude bone invasion

Special Instruments, Position, and Anesthesia

1. General anesthesia delivered through tracheotomy
2. Jennings mouth gag
3. Headlight for the surgeon
4. Stryker saw with right-angled blade if marginal mandibulectomy is necessary

Tips and Pearls

1. Superior margin of soft tissue dissection is deep to the sublingual glands.
2. Mandibular osteotomies should be carried through completely into the soft tissues to avoid fracture of the mandible.
3. Meticulous hemostasis
4. Appropriate-thickness skin graft
5. Treatment unnecessary for transected Wharton's ducts, even if neck dissections are not carried out

Pitfalls and Complications

1. Postoperative bleeding
2. Incomplete hemostasis interfering with healing of skin graft
3. Fracture of the mandible from inappropriate osteotomies

Postoperative Care Issues

1. Perioperative antibiotics for 24 hours
2. Removal of skin graft bolus on the fifth postoperative day
3. Maintenance of nutrition with nasogastric tube until decannulation
4. Dental referral for prosthesis after complete healing has occurred

References

McGuirt WF, Johnson JT, Myers EN, Rothfield R, Wagner R. Floor of mouth carcinoma: the management of the clinically negative neck. Arch Otolaryngol Head Neck Surg 1995;121:278.

Schramm VL, Myers EN, Sigler BA. Surgical management of early epidermoid carcinoma of the anterior floor of the mouth. Laryngoscope 1980;90:207.

Operative Procedure

Preoperative evaluation should have revealed whether the plan of management would include a marginal mandibulectomy (Figs. 35-1 and 35-2). Indications for marginal mandibulectomy include:

- Inability to obtain an anterior margin of resection without removing the alveolar process of the mandible
- Attachment of the lesion to the lingual aspect of the mandibular periosteum
- In the edentulous patient, tumor that crosses the mandible and involves the gingival buccal sulcus

Using the coagulation current or knife, the mucosa is incised. After the mucosa is incised, a 2-0 silk suture is placed through the anterior margin of resection, and the operating personnel are notified to mark this on the pathology form. Using small dissecting scissors, the soft tissue is sharply and bluntly dissected from anterior to posterior. The deep margin of resection in superficial cancers in this area is the sublingual gland. Afteglamd. After the sublingual glands have been identified, dissection is carried deep to the sublingual glands to provide this deep margin. Cutting through the margins, particularly in deep-margin resection, transects the Wharton's duct on both sides. No attempt is made to reconstruct the ducts. The remainder of the lesion is then excised with sharp and blunt resection.

During the time that hemostasis is being obtained, the surgeon and his assistant change into new gowns and gloves and harvest the skin graft. We use a Brown dermatome set at 0.016 to 0.018 in (0.4–0.46 mm). The skin graft should be thick enough to handle easily and not tear but thin enough to be pliable and to have a high possibility of good take. Using a "pie-crusting" technique, the skin graft is sewn to the mucosa of the floor of the mouth, leaving every other suture long to tie over. One or two "tacking" stitches are placed in the floor of the mouth with absorbable catgut suture to help adherence of the skin graft to the underlying tissues. One to two Xeroform gauze packs are used as a bolus and tied over with long ties. A nasogastric tube is inserted and this aspect of the procedure is terminated. If neck dissections are to be included, the patient is again prepped and draped, and the appropriate neck dissection is carried out.

Because the alveolar process is not involved with the tumor but rather is a margin of resection around the tumor, it is important to resect only the alveolar process and not go inferiorly into the body of the mandible. Because it is possible to fracture the bone, the vertical dimension of the mandible is quite substantial, even in edentulous patients, and a rim containing only alveolar process should be taken. A Stryker saw with a right-angled blade should be used first in making the vertical bone cuts (Figs. 35-3 and 35-4) and then in connecting this with a horizontal bone cut. It is important that the bones be cut completely through. It may be tempting to use an osteotome or a heavy elevator to try to pry open the bone and fracture the lingual surface. This approach may fracture the mandible and is contraindicated. After the lingual cortex and mandibular fragment have been cut through, the bone fragment is retracted superiorly and medially along with the soft tissue. The remainder of the resection is then carried out as described previously, finding the sublingual glands and including them as a margin of resection.

A split-thickness skin graft can be used to resurface the soft tissue and the residual mandibular bone (Fig. 35-5). This is possible because most of the exposed bone of the mandible, after the alveolar process has been removed, is primarily cancellous bone with a thin rim of cortical bone on the buccal and lingual sides. The skin graft heals nicely in this area if care is taken to provide immobilization of the graft over the bone and the soft tissue.

EUGENE N. MYERS

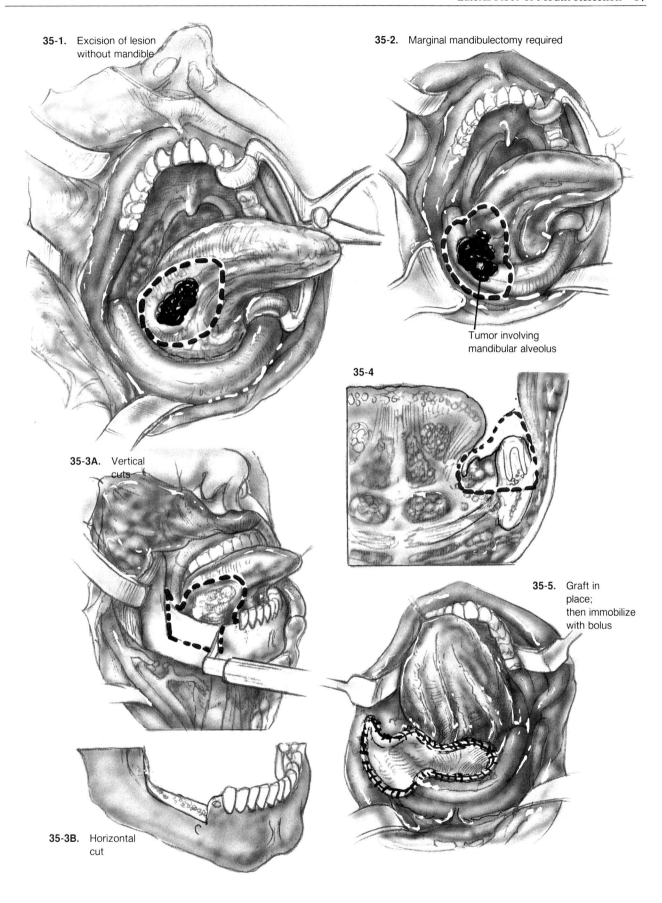

35-1. Excision of lesion without mandible

35-2. Marginal mandibulectomy required

Tumor involving mandibular alveolus

35-4

35-3A. Vertical cuts

35-5. Graft in place; then immobilize with bolus

35-3B. Horizontal cut

■ 36. FLOOR OF MOUTH RESECTION WITH ANTERIOR MANDIBLE INVASION—Resection of the floor of the mouth with anterior involvement of the mandible by carcinoma

Indications

1. Resection of squamous cell carcinoma with clinical or radiographic evidence of invasion of mandible

Special Considerations

1. In massive invasion, the patient may have destruction of the mandible, with cancer infiltrating the skin of the chin.
2. Planning with other surgical colleagues, when necessary, the reconstruction of the mandible and floor of the mouth

Preoperative Preparation

1. Evaluation of the nutritional status, with possible delay of surgery for nutritional replenishment
2. Chest radiograph and barium esophagram to exclude synchronous tumors of the upper aerodigestive tract
3. Computed tomography scan of mandible to determine extent of bone invasion
4. Dental consultation as to restoration or extraction of residual teeth
5. Panendoscopy to exclude synchronous tumors of the upper and lower aerodigestive tract

Special Instruments, Position, and Anesthesia

1. General anesthesia delivered through tracheotomy
2. Headlight for the surgeon
3. Oscillating saw for use in mandibular osteotomy

Tips and Pearls

1. Appropriate neck dissections preliminary to resection of the primary based on the nodal status of both sides of the neck
2. Expose both lingual arteries during preliminary neck dissections to preserve these structures when possible.
3. Dissection through mylohyoid and anterior belly of digastric muscles to provide access to the deep planes of the floor of the mouth and to provide adequate margins

Pitfalls and Complications

1. Inadvertent damage to lingual artery or hypoglossal nerve
2. Postoperative bleeding because of inadequate hemostasis
3. Failure to recognize infiltration of the skin of the chin by tumor, leaving inadequate tumor resection

Postoperative Care Issues

1. Care of bone and skin grafts (discussed elsewhere)
2. Decannulation after grafts have healed
3. Nasogastric feeding after decannulation

References

McGuirt WF, Johnson JT, Myers EN, Rothfield R, Wagner R. Floor of mouth carcinoma: the management of the clinically negative neck. Arch Otolaryngol Head Neck Surg 1995; 121:278.

Schramm VL, Myers EN, Sigler BA. Surgical management of early epidermoid carcinoma of the anterior floor of the mouth. Laryngoscope 1980;90:207.

Operative Procedure

An antibiotic effective against oral flora should be administered when the patient enters the operating room. Patients who have advanced-stage lesions, particularly T4, which deeply involve the substance of the tongue and involve the mandible, require composite resection in conjunction with neck dissection to achieve locoregional control.

Patients with these advanced-stage lesions also are frequently found to be node positive by physical examination on one or both sides of the neck. They require radical or modified radical neck dissection if node positive on one side and selective neck dissection if node negative on the opposite side. Patients who have deep infiltration of the floor of the mouth without bone resection are not candidates for transoral resection and should be approached externally.

The patient is placed in the supine position, and panendoscopy is carried out under general anesthesia. A tracheotomy is performed, and an endotracheal tube is placed in the stoma. The patient is then prepped and draped for the composite resection.

Some patients have deeply infiltrative carcinomas arising in the floor of the mouth and have anterior involvement of the mandible. If any mandible is involved, a segmental resection of the mandible should be carried out, because penetration of the mandible by cancer may involve bone marrow spaces, which mitigates against complete resection by less than segmental resection. The tumor is approached using a lip-splitting incision, although in some patients, particularly in females, a visor flap may be created. This is carried out by incising the lower gingival buccal sulcus from angle of mandible to angle of mandible (Fig. 36-1). The mandibular periosteum is then undermined, and the skin of the face, chin, and lower lip is elevated using Penrose drains to elevate these structures upward off the mandible. Alternatively, a lip-splitting incision with elevation of the periosteum and skin flaps off of the mandible to be resected may be used. Vertical osteotomies are carried out to take the anterior portion of the mandible as a block (Fig. 36-2). The preoperative imaging should be studied to determine how much margin of resection is necessary to gain tumor clearance. When possible, the patient can benefit by preservation of the mental nerves.

After the osteotomies, the bone fragments of the remaining mandible are distracted, leaving the anterior segment of the mandible attached to the soft tissues. The tumor itself is then approached by entering the deep aspect of the floor of the mouth through the mylohyoid muscles and anterior belly of the digastric muscle.

A modification of this approach is necessary when the patient has penetration of cancer through the floor of the mouth and the mandible into the skin of the chin. In this case, the skin of the chin is incised as far peripherally as necessary to gain what appears to be clear margins, and the skin is left on the anterior segment of the mandible to be included in the en bloc resection (Fig. 36-3). If the lower lip is not involved, care must be taken not to interrupt its vascular supply. If it is necessary to take all or part of the lip, this area is included in the appropriate reconstruction.

Reconstruction of the anterior mandible is to be carried out at this time with an osteocutaneous flap reconstruction with microvascular anastomosis (Fig. 36-4). Depending on the size of the bone fragment to be replaced, a radial osteocutaneous free flap, scapular osteocutaneous free flap, or fibular osteocutaneous free flap may be selected. If microvascular surgeons are unavailable, plating of the bone and epithelial coverage with a pectoralis major myocutaneous flap is an option. The regional flap and the free flaps have skin paddles that can be bivalved to provide external coverage in patients requiring excision of the skin of the chin.

EUGENE N. MYERS

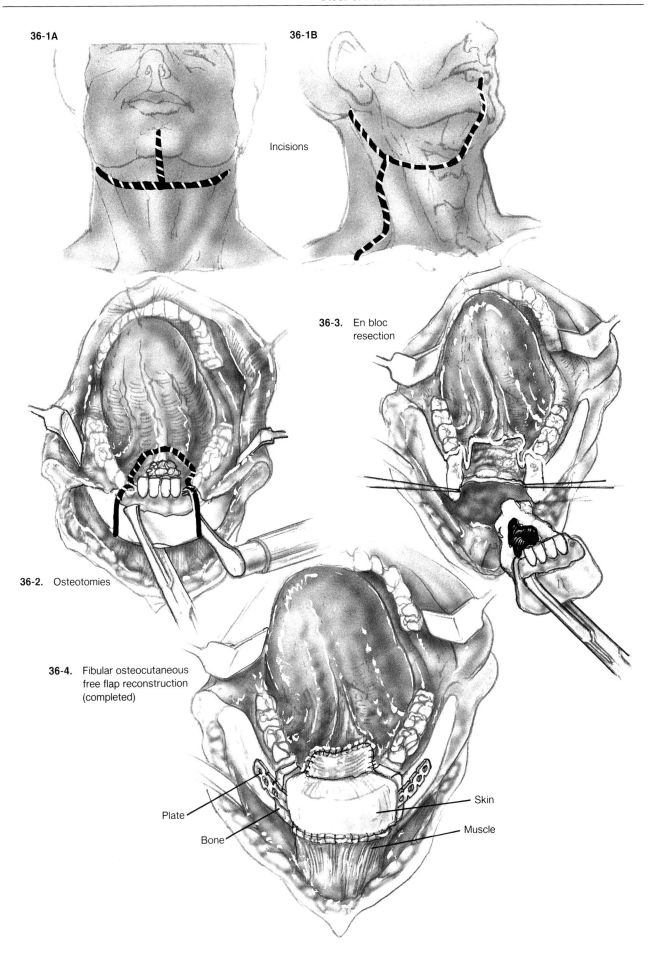

36-1A

36-1B

Incisions

36-3. En bloc resection

36-2. Osteotomies

36-4. Fibular osteocutaneous free flap reconstruction (completed)

Plate

Bone

Skin

Muscle

■ *37.* FLOOR OF MOUTH RESECTION WITH LATERAL MANDIBLE INVASION—When cancer of the floor of the mouth invades the lateral aspect of the mandible. This segment of mandible must be removed. This is done en bloc with soft tissue of the floor of the mouth.

Indications
1. Squamous cell carcinoma of the floor of the mouth with invasion of the mandible
2. Secondary involvement of the floor of the mouth and mandible from malignant tumors of the submandibular gland
3. Other malignant tumors arising in bone

Special Considerations
1. Preoperative consultation with dental colleagues to assess the need for restoration or extraction of teeth
2. Plan the reconstruction of the mandible and floor of the mouth.

Preoperative Preparation
1. Evaluation of nutritional status, with possible delay of surgery for nutritional replenishment
2. Chest radiograph and barium esophagram to exclude other synchronous tumors of the upper aerodigestive tract
3. CT scan of the mandible to evaluate bone destruction
4. Dental consultation about restoration or extraction of residual teeth
5. Panendoscopy to exclude other synchronous tumors of the upper and lower aerodigestive tract
6. Perioperative intravenous antibiotics
7. Confirmation of tissue diagnosis

Special Instruments, Position, and Anesthesia
1. General anesthesia delivered through a tracheotomy
2. Headlight for the surgeon
3. Oscillating saw for osteotomy

Tips and Pearls
1. A visor flap may be used in patients to preserve the cosmetic appearance.
2. Cutting the pterygoid muscles helps in providing good exposure.
3. The neck dissection should be performed first.
4. Elevation of the masseter muscle off the body of the ramus should be done with sharp dissection using a knife or electrocautery.
5. Transection of the mandible anteriorly is determined by the location of the cancer.
6. Wide margins of resection must be taken on the mandible.
7. It is important to obtain access to the deep margin tissues of the floor of the mouth through the mylohyoid muscle. Lingual and hypoglossal nerves and lingual artery are at risk and may need to be taken with the specimen.
8. Each case should be individualized with respect to mandibular reconstruction.

Pitfalls and Complications
1. Inadequate bony resection due to misjudgment of the extent of the tumor
2. The proximal osteotomy must be considerably higher than the angle of the mandible. If a long segment of the ascending ramus is left intact, it will distort the oral cavity by an inward and upward pull of the remaining pterygoid muscles.
3. Bleeding from the large arteries in the upper neck or tongue not adequately dealt with at the time of resection
4. Failure of the skin graft to survive due to inadequate hemostasis or inadequate surgical technique
5. Potential for fluid overload in patients who have long reconstructive procedures

References
Schramm VL, Myers EN. How I do it—head and neck. A targeted problem and its solution. Skin graft reconstruction following composite resection. Laryngoscope 1980;90:1737.

Operative Procedure
An antibiotic effective against oral flora should be administered intravenously. The patient is placed in the supine position with extension of the neck. The head is positioned on a rubber doughnut.

Neck dissection is then carried out. In a node-negative neck, this should be a selective neck dissection of zones I, II, III, and IV. If the patient is node positive, a radical or modified radical neck dissection is carried out.

After neck dissection, the patient's head is returned to the midline. The midline of the lower lip and chin is identified and marked with a pen (Figs. 37-1 and 37-2). No notches or curves around the chin are necessary. The vermilion border and the crease just above chin are marked for later proper realignment. The lip is grasped off the midline with a Lahey clamp. The incision is carried down to the periosteum. The mucoperiosteum is then incised along the body of the ramus of the mandible. A knife or sharp heavy periosteal elevator is then used to undermine the periosteum. The mental nerve is transected. The masseter muscle is incised along the inferior aspect of the mandible, and is dissected off the bone. Retraction with two right-angled retractors is helpful. If necessary, the mandible may be disarticulated or the osteotomy carried up further on the neck of the condyle.

The oscillating saw is then used to transect the mandible anteriorly and posteriorly (Fig. 37-3). The anterior aspect of the segment to be removed is distracted with a bone hook, as is the mandibular arch. This allows access into the oral cavity. An incision is then made along the mylohyoid muscle to get deep into the floor of the mouth.

Having transected the mylohyoid and entering the floor of the mouth, dissection is carried up along the lateral aspect of the tongue. The cheek flap is retracted to gain visualization. Dissection is carried posteriorly along the medial margin of resection.

The bone hook is transferred to the proximal aspect of the mandibular fragment and distracted inferiorly. Using heavy scissors, the pterygoid muscles are sharply dissected. The specimen is then removed. The margins of resection are studied by the pathologist. Closure should be delayed until tumor clearance is assured. After the resection, the exposed ends of the mandible are smoothed with a file and, if possible, covered by a periosteal flap or local soft tissue.

In patients in whom no mandibular reconstruction is to be carried out, a split-thickness skin graft can then be used. The skin graft of 0.016 to 0.018 in (0.4 to 0.46 mm) is harvested from the thigh. The graft is applied by sewing it in an oblique fashion, starting posteriorly and sewing one edge of the skin graft, usually beginning at the posterior aspect of the resection, and progressing anteriorly along the buccal mucosa laterally and on the tongue medially. The success of the skin graft reconstruction depends on a watertight closure. To achieve this, the skin graft is draped over the defect so that it overlaps the mucosa by several millimeters. The graft is then secured by vertically placed 3-0 silk sutures that traverse the skin graft, submucosa, mucosa, and the skin graft a second time (ie, pie-crusting technique). Every second or third suture is left long to be used as ties to hold the bolus dressing.

The skin graft should be left redundant so that a pouch is formed as the open anterior aspect of the graft is closed. This part of the closure is accomplished by sewing the remaining free margin of the graft on itself, beginning at the center and gathering the graft to form the anterior boundary of the pouch. The skin graft lies in an inverted position after the anterior border has been closed and must be everted into the neck. The skin graft pouch is filled with Xeroform gauze to create a bolus of sufficient volume to keep the skin in contact with adjacent soft tissues. The bolus is secured by tying the long sutures to secure the gauze bolus against the skin graft.

Hemovac drains are placed in the neck to help obtain apposition of the cheek and neck flap of the skin graft. A bulky, soft, external compression dressing is also applied to ensure coaptation of the skin graft, soft tissues, and neck skin flaps.

EUGENE N. MYERS

Lip and chin incisions

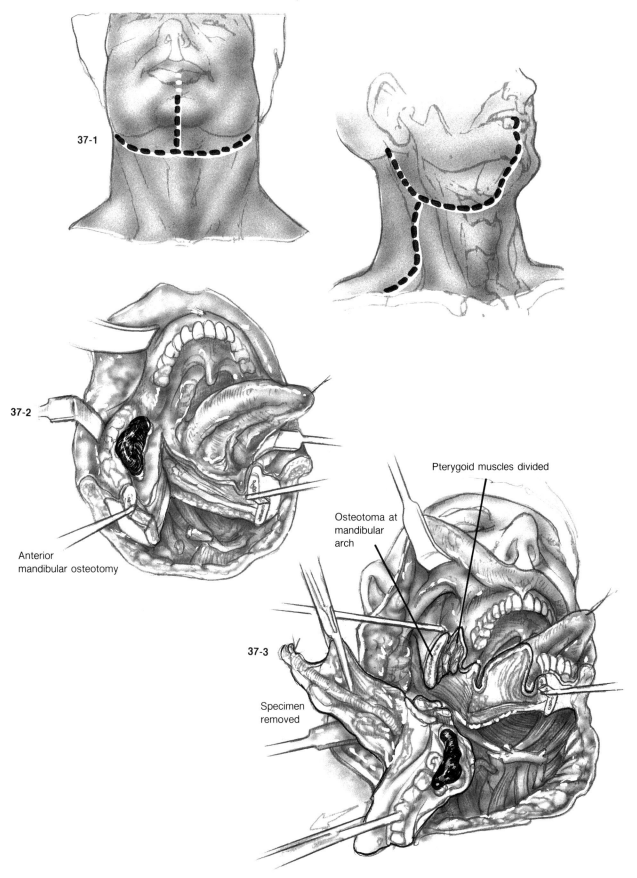

37-1

37-2

Anterior
mandibular osteotomy

Pterygoid muscles divided

Osteotoma at
mandibular
arch

37-3

Specimen
removed

■ *38.* MARGINAL RESECTION OF POSTERIOR FLOOR OF MOUTH WITH MANDIBULAR

INVASION— Marginal resection of the mandible in cases of carcinoma of the posterior floor of the mouth with mandible invasion

Indications

1. Small squamous cell carcinoma with clinical or radiographic evidence of mandibular invasion
2. Tumor mass adherent to the mandible and paresthesia of inferior alveolar nerve
3. Mandibular invasion seen on plain films, Panorex, and computed tomography scan; bone scans show localized activity only.

Special Considerations

1. Block-type resection
2. Patient's age and habitus
3. Status of dentition and size of mandible. For example, in a patient who has worn dentures for many years and has a small atrophic mandible, a segmental mandibulectomy may be necessary.
4. Presence of other medical problems, such as organic heart disease, diabetes mellitus, or chronic obstructive pulmonary disease
5. Presence of exposed bone (ie, mandible), particularly in the irradiated patient, obviates the use of skin grafts. In this group of patients, local or regional flaps are more appropriate.
6. A platysma myocutaneous flap is useful for a one-stage procedure.

Preoperative Evaluation

1. Informed operative consent.
2. Autologous blood transfusion for a large primary tumor or RND anticipated as part of procedure; the patient donates 1 or 2 units of blood preoperatively.
3. Nutritional assessment to ensure proper healing postoperatively

Special Instruments, Position, and Anesthesia

1. Headlight
2. Goggles
3. Oscillating saw
4. Double suction (ie, one using a straight Frazier tip, the other a tonsil suction)
5. Cautery, monopolar and bipolar
6. Shoulder roll, foam doughnut for head
7. Nasotracheal intubation is used to begin the procedure.

Tips and Pearls

1. Outline neck incision and perform neck dissection first.
2. Saline irrigation while using oscillating saw to avoid heat dissipation and soft tissue trauma
3. Use of frozen-section analysis of margins to aid in determining adequate tumor resection
4. Tonsil suction at bedside for patient's comfort

Pitfalls and Complications

1. Inadequate exposure leading to subtotal tumor resection
2. Fistula formation
3. Damage to lingual or hypoglossal nerves
4. Bleeding particularly from lingual artery or its branches

Postoperative Care Issues

1. Use of a dedicated nursing unit or intensive care unit
2. Use of active suction system such as Hemovac or Jackson-Pratt system; may remove drains when drainage is less than 50 mL in 24 hours.
3. Tube feedings by bolus or in continuous fashion
4. Local wound care daily
5. Intubation for 2 to 3 days postoperatively or tracheostomy if there are any questions about the airway

References

Cannon CR, Cantrell RW. Management of carcinoma of the lateral floor of mouth without mandibular invasion. In: Bailey B, ed. Surgery of the oral cavity. Chicago: Year Book Publishers, 1989;97.

Cannon CR, Johns ME, Atkins JP, Keane WM, Cantrell RW. Reconstruction of the oral cavity using the platysma myocutaneous flap. Arch Otolaryngol 1982;108:491.

Operative Procedure

The patient is placed in a supine position on the operating room table. The patient's head is turned to the side opposite the lesion. A shoulder roll is used to extend the neck, and the head is positioned on a foam doughnut. Anesthesia is achieved through a nasotracheal route. The patient's facial area, neck, and anterior chest are draped in the usual sterile fashion. If a skin graft is anticipated, it is wise to prep and drape one of the patient's thighs at the same time.

If the lesion is large and an extensive resection is anticipated, a tracheostomy is performed initially. If the tracheostomy is performed, a wire-woven tube is inserted, and the patient's endotracheal tube is withdrawn. The wire-woven tube is secured in place with ligatures of 2-0 silk. A tracheostomy tube is inserted only at the end of the procedure. The proposed skin incision site is infiltrated with a solution of 1% Xylocaine with 1:100,000 epinephrine unless the patient has history of hypertension or severe organic heart disease.

In this instance, envision a small carcinoma adherent and invading the mandible in the posterior floor of the mouth (Fig. 38-1). Reconstruction is planned with a platysma myocutaneous flap. This flap is outlined and elevated before the tumor ablative surgery. A horizontal skin crease in the middle or lower neck is identified, and a dotted line 10 to 15 cm long is drawn. Using an unfolded 4″ × 4″ gauze is an easy way to measure pedicle length. An ellipse of skin is outlined to match the size of the anticipated surgical defect. The superior skin flap is then elevated, being careful to keep the superior flap as thin as possible (Fig. 38-2). As a general rule, the flap in men should be thin enough to see hair follicles on the underside of the flap. This portion of the dissection is facilitated by the use of a #10 scalpel blade and the use of double skin hooks for retraction. By keeping the dissection superficial in the area, the platysma muscle and its blood supply are left undisturbed. The inferior limb of the flap is then incised and carried down through the subcutaneous tissues and platysma muscle. The platysma muscle and skin paddle are elevated and separated from the underlying deep tissues of the neck.

After the skin flap has been elevated, neck dissection is carried out. This may consist of a supraomohyoid modified or radical neck dissection, depending on the extent of the disease in the patient's neck and the surgeon's training and expertise.

Electrocautery using a cutting current of 40 watts is used for the oral incisions. The resection is begun medially and usually encompasses a small portion of the lateral tongue. Clinically surgical margins of at least 1 cm should be sought. Anterior, posterior, and lateral incisions are then made and the resection carried toward the mandible, leaving the soft tissues attached to the mandible. The resection also extends through the deep musculature and connects the floor of the mouth with the neck dissection. An oscillating saw with an angulated blade is used to perform a marginal mandibulectomy. Use of saline irrigation during the mandibulectomy dissipates the heat generated by the saw and prevents soft tissue injury.

When performing a marginal mandibulectomy, the superior or medial portions of the mandible can be excised, but the mandibular arch is left intact (Fig. 38-3). If the patient is found to have bony invasion of the mandible, it is wise to perform a segmental resection of the mandible (Fig. 38-4).

After the intraoral resection has been completed, the flap is reflected 270° around the mandible to face superiorly into the floor of the mouth (Fig. 38-5). The former inferior edge of the skin paddle lies laterally (adjacent to the mandible), and the superior edge of the skin paddle faces medially. The flap is trimmed to the appropriate size and is sutured into place with interrupted ligatures of 4-0 Vicryl (polyglycolic acid) sutures.

The skin flaps are returned to their original position, and a Jackson-Pratt drain or Hemovac drain is inserted. When using an active drain such as a Hemovac, the drainage system must be observed closely, making sure that oral secretions are not pulled through the suture line, leading to wound infection or fistula formation. A small Penrose drain is an acceptable substitute. The soft tissues in the neck are closed with 3-0 Vicryl sutures and the skin margins reapproximated with stainless steel staples.

C. RON CANNON

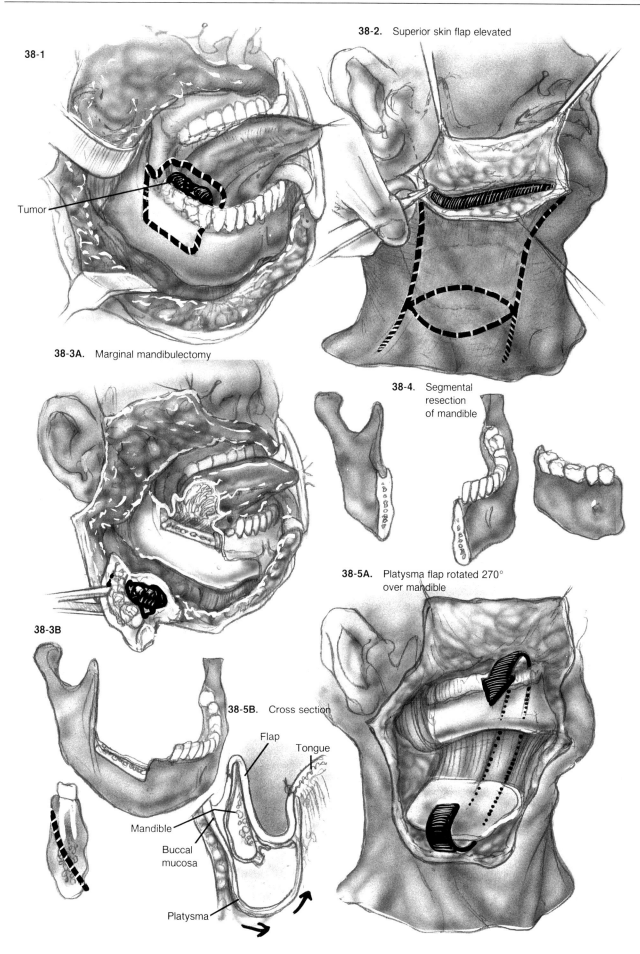

38-1

Tumor

38-2.   Superior skin flap elevated

38-3A.   Marginal mandibulectomy

38-3B

38-4.   Segmental resection of mandible

38-5A.   Platysma flap rotated 270° over mandible

38-5B.   Cross section

Flap

Tongue

Mandible

Buccal mucosa

Platysma

■ 39. ALVEOLAR RIDGE RESECTION
Removal of upper alveolar ridge, teeth, and mucosa en bloc

Indications
1. T1 squamous cell carcinomas of the gingiva may be treated with equal efficacy with surgery or irradiation.
2. T2 squamous cell or salivary gland malignancies are more typically treated with surgical resection.
3. Localized benign tumors of the upper alveolar ridge

Contraindications
1. Lesions such as lymphomas or metastatic tumors more appropriately treated with irradiation or chemotherapy
2. Inability to tolerate general anesthesia
3. Extensive tumor requiring more extensive resection, such as maxillectomy

Special Considerations
1. Rule out inferior extension of maxillary sinus tumor.
2. Upper alveolar ridge carcinoma has a lower incidence of metastasis than lower gingival carcinoma.
3. Tumor may metastasize to buccal or parotid nodes.
4. If dental extraction is performed at the time of the initial biopsy, assume deep invasion into the bone.

Preoperative Preparation
1. Routine laboratory studies and staging
2. Optional computed tomography scan to define the extent of lesion
3. Nasal endoscopy
4. Prosthodontic or dental consultation

Special Instruments, Position, and Anesthesia
1. Headlight, Dingman mouth gag, oscillating bone saw, chisels, and soft tissue instruments
2. Supine position, with head stabilized in a doughnut holder
3. General anesthesia with oral RAE tube
4. Temporary prosthetic device

Tips and Pearls
1. Bone cuts with 1- to 1.5-cm margins
2. Frozen-section control of mucosal margins
3. Neural involvement by tumor should be routinely ruled out.
4. Prophylactic neck dissection is usually not performed.

Pitfalls and Complications
1. Poor oral function
2. Hemorrhage from greater palatine artery
3. Oroantral fistula

Postoperative Care Issues
1. Soft diet is allowed for patients with very small defects. Patients with large defects may require nasogastric feeding until suture lines are well healed.
2. Prosthodontic referral for dental obturator
3. Oral rinse with disinfectant solutions (eg, half-strength hydrogen peroxide) is helpful in keeping the intraoral surgical site clean.

References
Davis RK, Lee CV. Resection of the alveolar ridge. In: Bailey BJ, ed. Surgery of the oral cavity. Chicago: Year Book Medical Publishers, 1989:139.

Strong EW, Spiro RH. Cancer of the oral cavity. In: Myers EN, Suen JY, eds. Cancer of the head and neck. New York: Churchill Livingstone, 1989:417.

Operative Procedure
Prophylactic antibiotics are given during induction of anesthesia. We employ cefazolin and metronidazole for coverage of gram-positive organisms and anaerobes. The antibiotics are routinely employed for 48 hours. The patient is placed in the supine position, and a Dingman mouth gag is inserted if it does not obscure the region to be resected. The buccal retractors help to provide unencumbered exposure of the lesion. If the Dingman mouth gag prevents exposure of the lesion, retraction of the tongue and buccal mucosa may be accomplished with a variety of hand-held retractors. Paralytic agents facilitate such exposure. A local anesthetic with vasoconstrictor (1% solution of Xylocaine with a 1:100,000 dilution of epinephrine) is injected along the lines of resection to enhance hemostasis.

Dental extractions are performed at the sites where osteotomies will be performed. Osteotomies should not be placed between teeth, because there is significant risk for loss of both teeth with this maneuver. Incisions are made in the mucosa with generous margins (approximately 1 cm). The periosteum is elevated proximal and distal, exposing the osteotomy sites (Fig. 39-1). Osteotomies may be performed with a hammer and chisel or with an oscillating saw. After the osteotomies are complete, the segment to be resected can be rocked free and removed. If done carefully, small segments can be removed without disrupting maxillary sinus mucosa. When removal of the mucosa of the floor of the maxillary sinus is desired, a Caldwell-Luc approach to the sinus may provide adequate visualization to ensure tumor extirpation. Surgical margins are sent for frozen-section confirmation. If the maxillary sinus is violated, any diseased mucosa can be removed at that time, and any active sinus disease should be treated with a wide nasoantral window for drainage.

After tumor extirpation, bleeding is controlled with electrocautery or suture ligature, and the wound is irrigated with copious amounts of saline. Very small defects can be reconstructed by placing relaxing incisions and advancing the mucosa for primary closure. Larger defects require placement of a local flap, such as a posteriorly based palatal flap or a buccal flap (Figs. 39-2 and 39-3). Care should be taken not to injure the greater palatine artery. The wound should be closed with minimal or no tension using absorbable sutures. Areas of the donor site for the local flap are left to heal by secondary intention or primary closure, if possible. A dental obturator provides the basis for dental reconstruction (Fig. 39-4).

ROBERT H. MILLER
GERARD J. GIANOLI

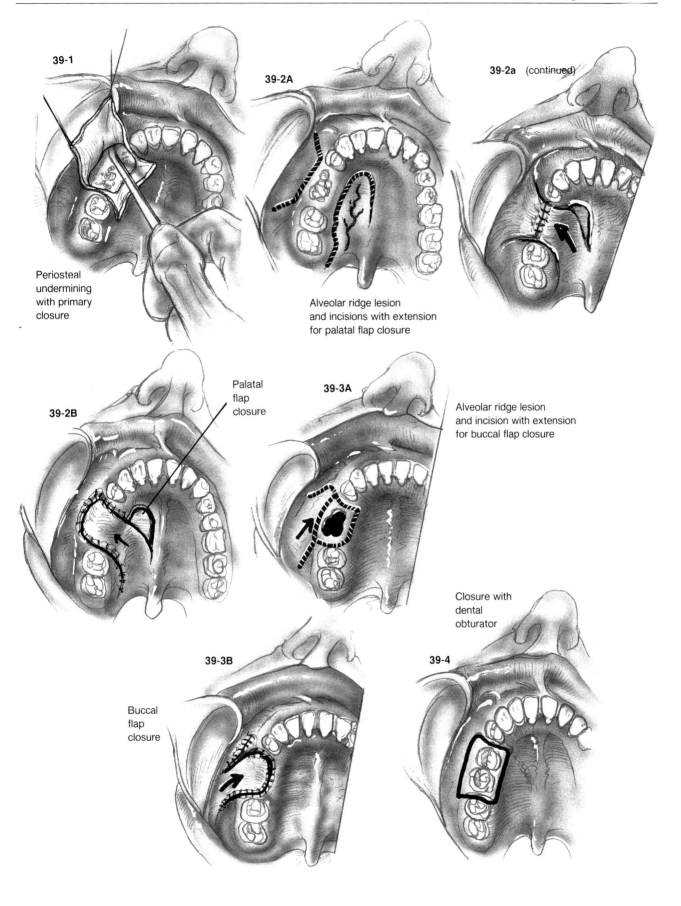

39-1

Periosteal
undermining
with primary
closure

39-2A

Alveolar ridge lesion
and incisions with extension
for palatal flap closure

39-2a (continued)

39-2B

Palatal
flap
closure

39-3A

Alveolar ridge lesion
and incision with extension
for buccal flap closure

39-3B

Buccal
flap
closure

Closure with
dental
obturator

39-4

■ 40. RESECTION OF THE HARD PALATE

Removal of the hard palate bone and overlying mucosa and removal of adjacent tissues, as needed

Indications

1. Malignant and premalignant lesions of the hard palate
2. Benign tumors of the hard palate

Contraindications

1. Contraindications to general anesthesia
2. Extensive lesion that would require a more extensive resection, such as maxillectomy
3. Tumors more appropriately treated with alternative therapies, such as irradiation or chemotherapy

Special Considerations

1. Rule out inferior extension of a maxillary sinus tumor.
2. Bilateral lymphatic drainage and node metastasis within buccal or parotid nodes
3. Because the incidence of occult metastasis is low, prophylactic neck dissection is not generally recommended.
4. Neural invasion may occur with the nasopalatine (incisive foramen) and the greater palatine (greater palatine foramen) nerves, particularly in patients with adenoid cystic carcinoma.

Preoperative Preparation

1. Routine laboratory studies and staging
2. Optional computed tomography scan to define extent of lesion
3. Nasal endoscopy
4. Prosthodontic or dental consultation

Special Instruments, Position, and Anesthesia

1. Headlight, Dingman or Crowe-Davis mouth gag, oscillating bone saw, chisels, and soft tissue instruments
2. Supine position, with head stabilized in a doughnut holder
3. General anesthesia with oral RAE tube
4. Temporary palatal obturator

Tips and Pearls

1. Bone cuts with 1- to 1.5-cm margins
2. Frozen-section control of mucosal margins
3. More variety of histologic tumor types than other sites in the oral cavity

Pitfalls and Complications

1. Poor oral function
2. Hemorrhage from greater palatine artery
3. Oroantral fistula or oronasal fistula

Postoperative Care Issues

1. A soft diet is allowed for patients who are reconstructed immediately with a temporary palatal obturator. Patients who undergo mucosal closure primarily or with a local flap may require nasogastric feeding until the suture lines are well healed.
2. Prosthodontic referral for palatal obturator when appropriate
3. Oral rinse with disinfectant solutions (eg, half-strength hydrogen peroxide) is helpful in keeping the intraoral surgical site clean

References

Evans JF, Shah JP. Epidermoid carcinoma of the palate. Am J Surg 1981;142:451.

Lanier DM. Carcinoma of the hard palate. In: Bailey BJ, ed. Surgery of the oral cavity. Chicago: Year Book Medical Publishers, 1989:163.

Operative Procedure

Prophylactic antibiotics are given during induction of anesthesia. We employ cefazolin and metronidazole for coverage of gram-positive organisms and anaerobes. The antibiotics are routinely employed for 48 hours. The patient is placed in the supine position, with the head extended. A mouth gag is used to retract the tongue and endotracheal tube out of the field while widely opening the mouth. If necessary, various retractors are used to retract the cheeks. Paralytic agents improve oral cavity exposure. A local anesthetic with vasoconstrictor (1% solution of Xylocaine with a 1:100,000 dilution of epinephrine) is injected along the lines of resection to enhance hemostasis.

An incision is made around the periphery of the lesion, allowing for 1- to 1.5-cm tumor-free margins. The incision is carried down through the periosteum (Fig. 40-1). The periosteum is elevated away from the incision site with appropriate periosteal elevators. This allows room to introduce bone-cutting instruments without damaging the overlying soft tissues. An osteotome or oscillating saw is then used to make bone cuts around the area to be resected. After the lesion has been circumscribed by bony cuts, the specimen can often be rocked free and removed. If the specimen is still not freed, additional horizontal bone cuts may be required to release attachments to the maxillary crest or lateral nasal wall. These cuts are made by transnasal placement of the osteotome (Fig. 40-2).

A through-and-through resection generally is employed to allay fears of residual disease on the superior aspect of the specimen, although a bone-sparing procedure may be employed for benign or very superficial lesions (Fig. 40-3). The resected palate is marked before submission for pathologic examination to ensure correlation of anatomic location in case residual tumor is found in the resected margins. Frozen-section control of the margins is routinely employed.

After tumor extirpation, bleeding is controlled with electrocautery or suture ligature, and the wound is irrigated with copious amounts of saline. Very small defects may be closed by lateral placement of relaxing incisions and advancement of mucosa for primary closure (Figs. 40-4 and 40-5). Somewhat larger defects can be closed with local palatal mucosal flaps, with the donor site left to close by secondary intention. Most through-and-through defects require a palatal obturator for reconstruction.

ROBERT H. MILLER
GERARD J. GIANOLI

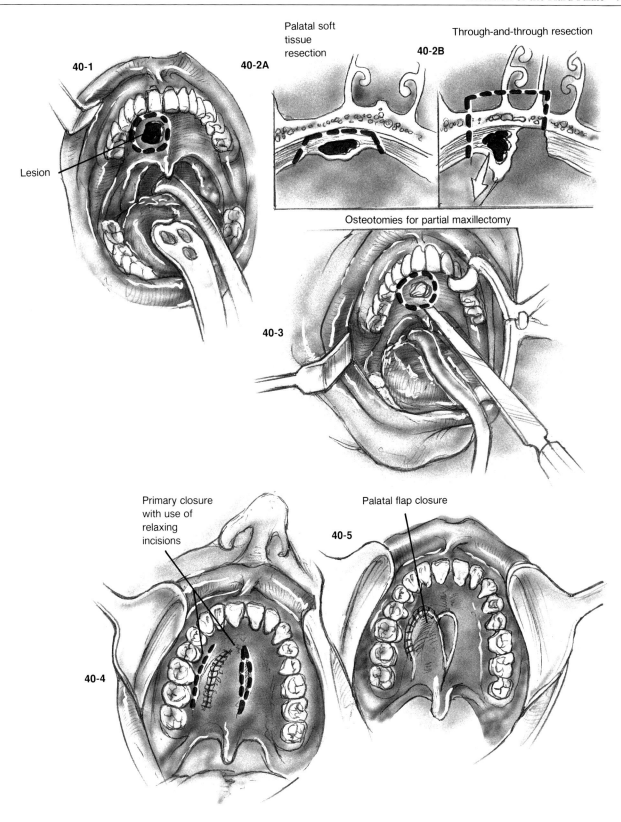

40-1

Lesion

40-2A Palatal soft tissue resection

40-2B Through-and-through resection

Osteotomies for partial maxillectomy

40-3

40-4 Primary closure with use of relaxing incisions

40-5 Palatal flap closure

■ *41.* RESECTION OF THE SOFT PALATE

Surgical resection of part or all of the soft tissues that comprise the soft palate

Indications

1. Malignant and premalignant lesions of the soft palate, especially superficially invasive lesions and small tumors
2. Benign tumors of the soft palate

Contraindications

1. Contraindications to general anesthesia
2. Extensive lesions that extend to the mandibular or maxillary bone are more appropriately treated by composite resection.
3. Lesions, such as lymphomas or metastatic tumors, more appropriately treated by irradiation or chemotherapy

Special Considerations

1. Controversy surrounds the effective treatment of early (T1 or T2) soft palate carcinoma because of the important physiologic role the soft palate plays in speech and deglutition. Some surgeons propose radiation therapy as the initial form of therapy for such lesions.
2. Bilateral lymphatic drainage and metastasis to buccal or parotid nodes
3. The incidence of concurrent second primary tumors (15%–30%) is higher for soft palate carcinomas than most other head and neck malignancies; consequently, aggressive investigation for such lesions is warranted.

Preoperative Preparation

1. Routine laboratory studies and staging
2. Endoscopy of the nasal cavity, nasopharynx, and oropharynx for evaluation of tumor extent
3. Prosthodontic consultation

Special Instruments, Position, and Anesthesia

1. Headlight, Dingman or Crowe-Davis mouth gag, soft tissue instruments, and electrocautery
2. Supine position, with the head stabilized in a doughnut holder
3. General anesthesia with oral RAE tube
4. CO_2 laser and microscope (optional)

Tips and Pearls

1. Surgical resection with 1- to 1.5-cm margins.
2. Frozen-section control of margins
3. Prophylactic neck dissection usually is not performed.

Pitfalls and Complications

1. Dysphagia
2. Hemorrhage from greater palatine artery
3. Velopharyngeal insufficiency

Postoperative Care Issues

1. Nasogastric feeding for patients with very large defects until a palatal obturator is available
2. Patients with smaller defects can be started on a semisolid diet, taking velopharyngeal reflux precautions.
3. Speech therapy for swallowing rehabilitation
4. Oral rinse with disinfectant solutions (eg, half-strength hydrogen peroxide) is helpful in keeping the intraoral surgical site clean.

References

Evans JF, Shah JP. Epidermoid carcinoma of the palate. Am J Surg 1981;142:451.

Netterville JL, Ossoff RH. Carcinoma of the soft palate. In: Bailey BJ, ed. Surgery of the oral cavity. Chicago: Year Book Medical Publishers, 1989:168.

Operative Procedure

Prophylactic antibiotics are given during induction of anesthesia. We employ cefazolin and metronidazole for coverage of gram-positive organisms and anaerobes. The antibiotics are routinely employed for 48 hours. The patient is placed in the supine position, with the head extended. A mouth gag is used to retract the tongue and endotracheal tube out of the field while widely opening the mouth. Buccal retractors are used to retract the cheeks. Paralytic agents are helpful in improving oral cavity exposure. A local anesthetic with vasoconstrictor (1% solution of Xylocaine with a 1:100,000 dilution of epinephrine) is injected along the lines of resection to enhance hemostasis.

The soft palate is placed under tension with retraction from a tenaculum placed at the uvular edge or with sutures placed through the palate and held in position by the suture retainers on the Dingman mouth gag (Fig. 41-1). An incision is made around the periphery of the lesion, allowing for 1- to 1.5-cm tumor-free margins. Resection of the tonsils can be easily combined with the soft palate resection (Fig. 41-2). The incision can be performed with a knife, electrocautery, or the laser. Because the palate is a very vascular structure, attention to hemostasis is important to ensure for accurate lines of resection. If the laser is used, appropriate laser precautions should be instituted. The area to be resected is removed, with careful attention paid to potential submucosal extension. Care is taken to ensure a line of resection that is perpendicular to the plane of the soft palate so that the palatal cut is not beveled. Beveling the palate could result in much narrower margins than anticipated. Superficial lesions may be removed with excision of the mucosa only (without a through-and-through defect). Frozen-section control of the margins is routinely employed.

After tumor extirpation, bleeding is controlled with electrocautery or suture ligature, and the wound is irrigated with copious amounts of saline. The wound can be closed primarily or is left to heal by secondary intention (Fig. 41-3). The patient is counseled about velopharyngeal incompetence. Velopharyngeal insufficiency commonly occurs but is usually temporary for limited resections. For the more extensive resections (eg, total soft palatectomy), nasogastric tube feeding may be required until the patient can be rehabilitated with a palatal prosthesis (Fig. 41-4).

ROBERT H. MILLER
GERARD J. GIANOLI

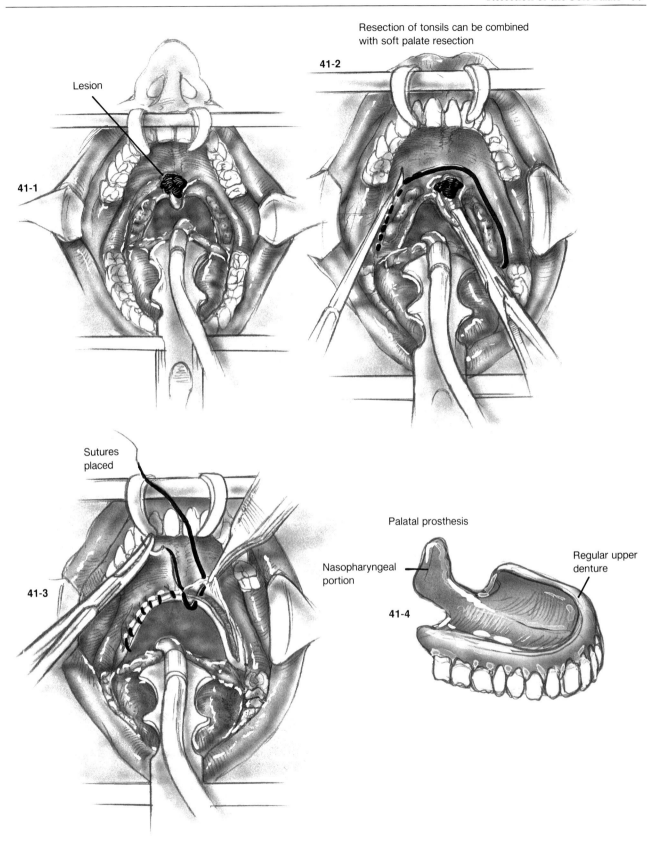

41-1 Lesion

41-2 Resection of tonsils can be combined with soft palate resection

41-3 Sutures placed

41-4 Palatal prosthesis

Nasopharyngeal portion

Regular upper denture

■ *42.* PARTIAL-THICKNESS AND FULL-THICKNESS BUCCAL RESECTION—Surgical resection of the oral mucosa comprising the inner lining of the cheeks, extending from the oral commissure to the retromolar trigone and bounded inferiorly and superiorly by the gingivobuccal sulci

Indications

1. Malignant and premalignant lesions of the buccal mucosa
2. Benign tumors of the buccal mucosa and associated soft tissue

Contraindications

1. Contraindications to general anesthesia do not necessarily contraindicate resection, because most T1 and small T2 lesions are amenable to resection under local anesthesia. More extensive lesions typically require general endotracheal anesthesia.
2. Extensive lesions that extend to the alveolar ridge or retromolar trigone are more appropriately treated by composite resection.
3. Lesions, such as lymphomas or metastatic tumors, more appropriately treated by irradiation or chemotherapy

Special Considerations

1. T1 and small T2 lesions have a less than 20% incidence of nodal metastasis, but most patients present with more advanced lesions that have a higher incidence of nodal metastasis, giving an overall incidence of approximately 50%.
2. Parotid nodes are along the first line of lymphatic drainage for buccal tumors.
3. The prognosis is more ominous for cervical metastasis, more posteriorly located lesions, and larger tumors.

Preoperative Preparation

1. Routine laboratory studies and staging
2. Evaluation of facial nerve function to determine possible neural invasion
3. Palpation of parotid gland and neck for evaluation of possible nodal metastases
4. Bimanual palpation of the tumor to determine the relation of the tumor to Stensen's duct, the alveolar ridges, and the retromolar trigone
5. Determine limitation of mouth opening that may be secondary to masseter or pterygoid muscle invasion.

Special Instruments, Position, and Anesthesia

1. Headlight, Dingman or Crowe-Davis mouth gag, soft tissue instruments, electrocautery, and hand-held nerve stimulator
2. Supine position, with the head stabilized in a doughnut holder
3. General anesthesia with oral RAE tube for large lesions; T1 and small T2 lesions may be comfortably resected under local anesthesia.

Tips and Pearls

1. Surgical resection with 1- to 1.5-cm mucosal margins and an intact fascial layer as the deep margin; some lesions require full-thickness resection for deep-margin control.
2. Frozen-section control of margins
3. These lesions tend to be more advanced than appreciated during the initial examination.

Pitfalls and Complications

1. Bleeding and infection
2. Orocutaneous fistula
3. Total or partial facial paralysis
4. Interference with mastication and speech

Postoperative Care Issues

1. Nasogastric tube feeding until mucosal suture lines are well healed
2. A speech therapy consultation may be helpful.

References

Bloom ND, Spiro RH. Carcinoma of the cheek mucosa. Am J Surg 1980;140:556.

Osguthorpe JD, Putney FJ. Carcinoma of the buccal mucosa. In: Bailey BJ, ed. Surgery of the oral cavity. Chicago: Year Book Medical Publishers, 1989:153.

Operative Procedure

Prophylactic antibiotics are given during induction of anesthesia. We employ cefazolin and metronidazole for coverage of gram-positive organisms and anaerobes. The antibiotics are routinely employed for 48 hours. The patient is placed in the supine position, with the head extended. A mouth gag is used to retract the tongue and endotracheal tube out of the field while widely opening the mouth. Buccal retractors are used to retract the cheeks. Paralytic agents are helpful in improving oral cavity exposure, but if the facial nerve needs to be identified, paralytic agents are relatively contraindicated. A local anesthetic with vasoconstrictor (1% solution of Xylocaine with a 1:100,000 dilution of epinephrine) is injected.

The mucosal incision should include a 1- to 1.5-cm margin around the tumor periphery (Fig. 42-1). The deep margin should be the first unviolated fascial plane that is encountered; a full-thickness resection is performed for deeply invasive tumors (Fig. 42-2). Frozen-section analyses are performed for an additional 2 to 3 mm excised from the periphery of the defect (not from the tumor specimen). We think the use of frozen sections is imperative for enhanced local control and as a practical maneuver to limit the need for additional resections. Tumors that involve the mandibular or maxillary bones should be treated by composite resection.

If Stensen's duct is included in the resection, the remaining duct can be reconstructed or ligated. If sufficient length exists, the duct is sutured to the posterior aspect of the defect. Stenting with 1-mm polyethylene tubing that is sutured in place for 2 weeks helps to prevent stenosis. If the duct has been transected posterior to the masseter muscle or otherwise is of insufficient length, it is ligated.

The facial nerve usually should be preserved during resection of benign lesions and whenever feasible during resection of malignant lesions. For cases of preoperative facial nerve dysfunction, for a tumor in proximity to the facial nerve, or for tumors with a propensity for neural invasion (eg, adenoid cystic carcinoma), tumor invasion of the nerve should be strongly suspected. In such instances, consideration should be given to resection of the involved nerve segment with frozen-section analysis performed to ensure complete resection. Any involved nerve should be excised to a point confirmed to be histologically clear by frozen-section analysis. Neural repair by interposition grafting is performed for any significant neural resection.

Total parotidectomy is indicated for a tumor that invades the gland capsule and for palpable intraparotid nodes. Elective parotidectomy may be useful if facial nerve dissection is required and for larger tumors (eg, large T2, T3, T4). Elective neck dissection or postoperative neck irradiation is performed for T2 or larger lesions, because the incidence of occult metastasis is almost 50%.

Small partial-thickness defects are readily reconstructed by primary closure or split-thickness skin grafting. Primary closure is typically performed in multiple layers with absorbable sutures (Fig. 42-3). Split-thickness skin grafts are fashioned with a pie-crusting technique, and a bolster is sutured into place for 5 to 7 days (Fig. 42-4). Local mucosal flaps from the palate, tongue, or other nearby tissue are also useful.

Larger defects and full-thickness defects require more significant reconstructive efforts. Local or regional flaps may be used in conjunction with a split-thickness skin graft for intraoral lining. Local flaps that have been used to reconstruct such defects include flaps from the tongue, palate, and forehead and the cervical advancement-rotation flap. Myocutaneous flaps have included pectoralis major, trapezius, latissimus dorsi, and sternocleidomastoid flaps. Reconstruction with free tissue transfer from distant sites has proven to be an invaluable means of reconstruction, but it requires expertise in microvascular surgery or a second operative team and often prolongs the operative time significantly (Fig. 42-5).

Postoperatively, the patient is fed through a nasogastric tube until the mucosal suture lines are well sealed, usually 5 to 7 days for partial-thickness reconstructions and 10 to 12 days for full-thickness reconstructions. The patient is then given a full liquid diet, which is advanced as healing progresses. Range of motion exercises are useful to limit scar contracture and restriction of mouth opening.

ROBERT H. MILLER
GERARD J. GIANOLI

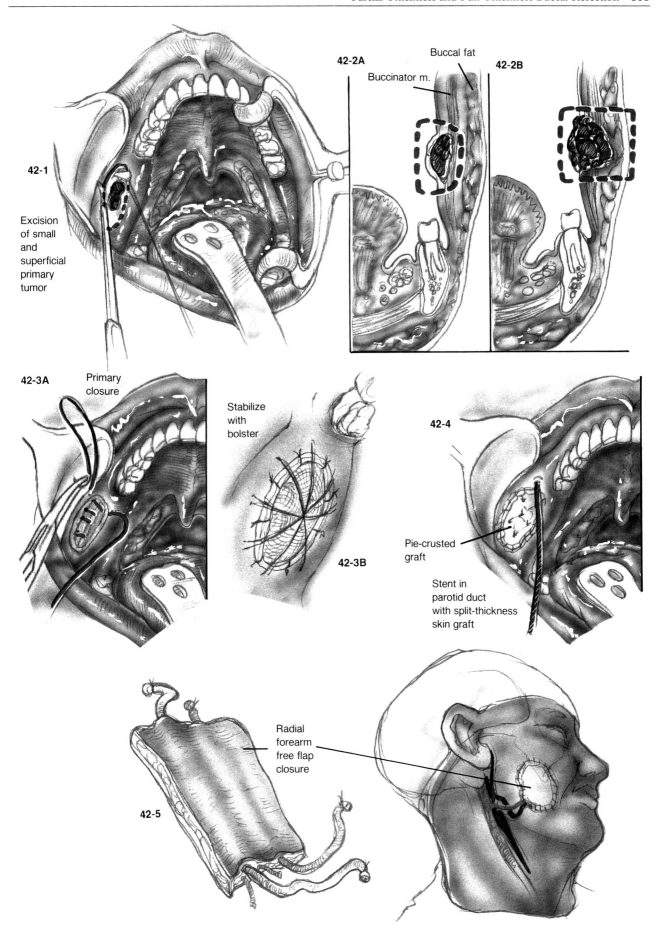

42-1

Excision of small and superficial primary tumor

42-2A

Buccinator m.

Buccal fat

42-2B

42-3A Primary closure

Stabilize with bolster

42-3B

42-4

Pie-crusted graft

Stent in parotid duct with split-thickness skin graft

Radial forearm free flap closure

42-5

■ *43.* MIDLINE, PARAMEDIAN, LATERAL, AND ASCENDING RAMUS MANDIBULAR OSTEOTOMY— Surgical cut through the mandibular bone that is performed as a procedure unto itself.

Indications

1. To provide wide exposure for the resection of benign or malignant neoplasms affecting the oropharynx, posterior oral cavity, pharyngomaxillary space, or skull base
2. As part of a segmental mandibulectomy for benign or malignant neoplasms affecting the mandible
3. As a means to expose the most superior extracranial portion of the internal carotid artery

Contraindications

1. Lesions that are adequately exposed with a less extensive procedure
2. Lesions, such as lymphomas and metastatic tumors, more appropriately treated by irradiation or chemotherapy

Special Considerations

1. Immediate repair of osteotomy with fixation plates or interosseous wiring
2. Tracheotomy for airway management

Preoperative Preparation

1. Preoperative dental consultation may be helpful for patients with poor dentition.
2. Radiographic imaging with computed tomograph or magnetic resonance imaging may be very helpful.

Special Instruments, Position, and Anesthesia

1. Oscillating saw, Gigli saw, bone plate fixation set, osteotomes, periosteal elevators, and soft tissue instruments
2. Supine position, with the head stabilized in doughnut holder

Tips and Pearls

1. Stair-stepped or staggered osteotomy to aid in postoperative stabilization if plates are not used
2. If a fixation plate is used for reconstruction, plate bending or formation and screw hole drilling is done before osteotomy.
3. If segmental resection is required, the initial osteotomy should be placed coincident with the resection site.
4. Dental extraction at the osteotomy site is recommended instead of placement of the osteotomy between two viable teeth.
5. Adequate mucosa is left attached to the mandibular segment to allow easy soft tissue closure at the end of the procedure.

Pitfalls and Complications

1. Hemorrhage, Malocclusion, nerve injury
2. Infection, pharyngocutaneous fistula, orocutaneous fistula, or osteomyelitis
3. Malunion or nonunion
4. Mandibular pain, dysfunction, or trismus
5. Dysphagia and aspiration
6. Airway obstruction

Postoperative Care Issues

1. The tracheotomy is maintained until the airway is adequate.
2. Nasogastric tube feeding is maintained until the mucosal suture lines are well sealed and the patient is able to swallow.
3. Oral rinse with disinfectant solutions.
4. Speech therapy for deglutition rehabilitation may be helpful.
5. Intermaxillary fixation (approximately 6 weeks) is required for the dentulous patient that is repaired with wire fixation.

References

Dichtel WJ, Miller RH, Feliciano DV, Woodson GE, Hurt J. Lateral mandibulotomy: a technique of exposure for penetrating injuries of the internal carotid artery at the skull base. Laryngoscope 1984;94: 1140.

Maves MD, Yessenow RS. Mandibular osteotomy approach to tumors of the tonsil fossa and oropharynx. In: Bailey BJ, ed. Surgery of the oral cavity. Chicago: Year Book Medical Publishers, 1989:183.

Operative Procedure

The mandibular osteotomy may be performed at a variety of sites along the mandible, including the midline, paramedian, lateral body, and ascending ramus (Fig. 43-1).

Midline, Paramedian, and Lateral Body Procedures

A midline lip-splitting incision provides the widest exposure (Fig. 43-2). This incision may be easily incorporated into the incision for a neck dissection. A local anesthetic with a vasoconstrictor (1% solution of Xylocaine with a 1:100,000 dilution of epinephrine) is injected along the lines of resection to enhance hemostasis. The incision is carried intraorally as the lip is transected in the midline and the inferior labial arteries are ligated.

If the midline mandibulotomy is performed, the incision is carried directly to a central incisor. The incisor is then extracted to allow room for the bone cut. Periosteum is elevated on both sides of the mandible where the osteotomy is to be performed. Before the bone cut, a fixation plate is formed to fit in the appropriate position and holes are drilled for the screws. The osteotomy is then performed with an oscillating saw or a Gigli saw. Care is taken to prevent damage to the surrounding soft tissues.

Reconstruction is performed after the resection is complete. The mucosal incision and muscular insertions are reattached with absorbable sutures. The osteotomy site is repaired with the previously formed fixation plate or with interosseous wires. The lip is repaired in three stages: muscle, submucosa, and skin with subcutaneous layers.

If the paramedian mandibulotomy is performed, a similar incision is used, except the midline mucosal incision is carried into the labial-buccal sulcus to the paramedian osteotomy site. The soft tissues lateral to the mandible are elevated as a cheek flap until the osteotomy site is exposed. The paramedian osteotomy site is just anterior to the mental foramen to preserve neural integrity.

Ascending Ramus Procedure

The skin incision for the ascending ramus mandibulotomy extends from the mastoid tip to the submental region. It is made parallel to and approximately 3 cm below the inferior border of the mandible. The inferior aspect of the mandible is exposed, and the periosteum is incised at the inferior border.

The periosteum is elevated on both the medial and lateral surfaces of the mandible at the site where the osteotomy is to be performed (Fig. 43-3). The osteotomy can be performed as a vertical cut through the long axis of the ramus (posterior to the mandibular foramen), as an oblique cut through the angle, or at a more anterior site (eg, lateral, paramedian, midline), as previously described. The advantage of this approach instead of the lip-splitting approach in the previous section is the limitation of intraoral contamination. A bone plate is fashioned to approximate the postosteotomy defect, and screw holes are drilled (Fig. 43-4). The osteotomy is then performed with an oscillating saw or a Gigli saw (Fig. 43-5). Muscular attachments to the medial aspect of the mandible must be severed to allow increased mobility of the posterior mandibular segment. The insertions of the posterior belly of digastric and the medial pterygoid muscles usually require division. After these muscles are divided, the posterior segment of the mandible is rotated laterally and superiorly (Fig. 43-6). Additional muscles that require division for better exposure of the carotid artery and parapharyngeal space include the stylohyoid, stylopharyngeus, and styloglossus muscles. Cranial nerves VII, IX, X, XI, and XII should be carefully identified during any approach to the parapharyngeal space.

Closure begins with reapproximating the previously sectioned muscles with absorbable sutures. Closure of the mandibulotomy defect is performed in a manner similar to that described in the previous section. We prefer the use of fixation plates to increase stability of closure and to eliminate the need for intermaxillary fixation in the postoperative period.

Postoperatively, if no intraoral defect has been created, as as in a vertical ramus mandibulotomy, an angle mandibulotomy, and in some edentulous patients, oral feeding with a soft diet is begun on postoperative day 1.

ROBERT H. MILLER

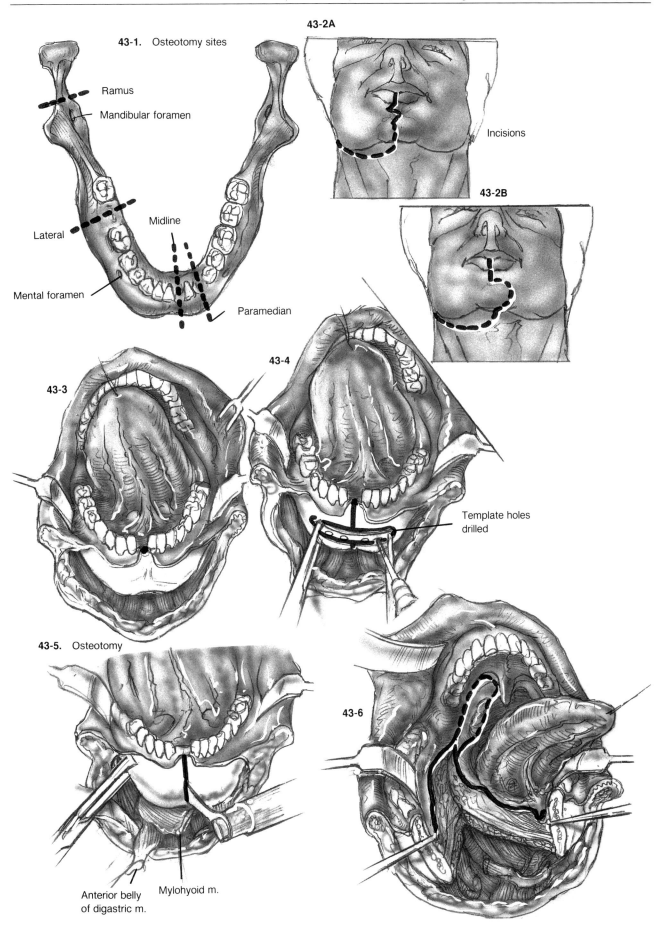

43-1. Osteotomy sites

Ramus

Mandibular foramen

Lateral

Midline

Mental foramen

Paramedian

43-2A

Incisions

43-2B

43-3

43-4

Template holes drilled

43-5. Osteotomy

43-6

Anterior belly of digastric m.

Mylohyoid m.

■ 44. TONGUE FLAPS FOR RECONSTRUC-

TION—The tongue flap is a local flap useful for reconstruction of the posterior oral pharynx defects after resection for cancer. There are two basic flaps with modifications.

Indications

1. Defects of the tonsil area
2. Defects of the tongue base
3. Defects of the soft palate
4. Defects of the buccal mucosa
5. Defects of the floor of the mouth

Contraindications

1. Pharyngeal resection defects that are gigantic and extend inferiorly to the inferior piriform sinus
2. Small defects that can be closed primarily or with a free skin graft
3. Surface defects that can be left to heal by secondary intention

Preoperative Preparation

1. An informed consent from the patient referring to the reconstruction options and the consequence of each option
2. Routine laboratory studies required for a safe anesthetic

Special Instruments, Position, and Anesthesia

1. Only those needed for the primary cancer resection

Tips and Pearls

1. The lingual artery can be ligated on the flap side and still have predictable survival.
2. If the flap side external carotid artery is ligated, another reconstruction option should be selected.

Pitfalls and Complications

1. If the hypoglossal nerve is divided by the cancer resection, the anterior tongue no longer contributes to speech and swallowing. The use of the anterior remaining tongue is ideal for reconstruction.
2. If the tongue used for reconstruction is innervated, it can contribute to swallowing and speech in a different position when used for reconstruction but with some change in speech.
3. Speech and swallowing problems are more often related to tongue restriction, not to tongue size.
4. Swallowing is hardly altered by using a tongue flap. Speech is altered when a posterior tongue flap is rotated into the cheek or floor of mouth. The speech change is obvious early, but with time, speech improves. Tongue size also increases with time, because the tongue is a well exercised muscle. Tongues seem to "grow back."

Postoperative Care Issues

1. Most patients with a major resection have a tracheotomy and a feeding tube placed at the time of resection. A rare exception is the patient with tongue flaps used for buccal mucosa or floor of the mouth reconstruction for whom the airway is safe. A feeding tube is used.
2. Oral feeding starts slowly after 5 to 7 days if there is no sign of infection or a fistula.
3. For the first few days, tongue flaps do not look very healthy. If there is no fistula, it is wise not to inspect the flap too often. The early job of the flap is to prevent a fistula. A later role is to help with tongue mobility. In the early days, if there is no fistula, the flap is a success.
4. After oral feeding starts, any obvious necrotic flap can be trimmed away in the office or treatment room.

References

DeSanto LW, Yarington CT. Tongue flaps: repair of oral and pharyngeal defects after resection of cancer. Otolaryngol Clin North Am 1983;16: 343.

Olsen KD, DeSanto LW. Tongue flaps for reconstruction. In: Bailey BJ, Babin AW, Jafek BW, et al, eds. Surgery of the oral cavity. Chicago: Year Book Medical Publishers, 1989:82-80.

Operative Procedure

The surgical defect determines direction and the arc of rotation, the length of the flap, and the amount of unfurling required. There are two basic flaps: those based posteriorly and those based laterally.

The laterally based flap is used for defects in the posterior oral cavity. The flap is based in the floor of the mouth. The defects that can be repaired are those of the tongue base, tonsil area, soft palate, and lateral hypopharynx. Regardless of the actual designated primary site after resection, the defects look much the same, and the flaps are consistent. Many of these resections are done through a mandibular osteotomy—usually a lateral osteotomy but sometimes an anterior one (Fig. 44-1). These flaps are also used after composite resection if primary closure is not done.

After tumor-free margins are ascertained by frozen-section study, reconstruction begins. The lingual artery and hypoglossal nerve has usually been divided on the flap side. Two sutures are placed in the anterior tongue for traction. With cutting cautery (our preference) or a scalpel, the tongue is incised down the midline back to the surgical defect. Using clamps for traction, the surgeon unrolls the tongue to create a wide flap about 6 to 10 mm thick. The flap is composed of surface epithelium and muscle (Figs. 44-2, 44-3, and 44-4).

The flap is pedicled and shaped as necessary to fill the defect. Shaping often means shortening. The flap can be rotated 180° in either direction, and the arc of rotation is determined by fitting the flap into its destination by trial. The idea is to rotate the flap in the direction that gives the least tension and best fills the defect.

Hemostasis must be meticulous, because a postoperative hematoma can be fatal to the flap. Gentle handling of the flap and hemostasis are axiomatic for reconstruction.

The flap is sutured into place with interrupted 2-0 chromic sutures. Suturing begins at the tongue base and inferolateral pharyngeal wall. Alternating simple and inverting vertical mattress sutures ensures a saliva-tight closure. Sutures are placed 1 cm apart. Closure continues around the soft palate and tonsil area and then to the floor of the mouth. The anterior tongue donor site is closed on itself (Fig. 44-5).

Posteriorly Based Tongue Flap

A posteriorly based tongue flap is used when all or most of the tongue remains intact. The lingual artery and hypoglossal nerve are usually intact. For large defects of the tonsil area, palate, retromolar area, or buccal mucosa, the entire ipsilateral tongue can be used. Traction sutures are placed on each side of the tongue tip, and the tongue is split down the midline back to or into the tongue base. Remember that the arterial supply is lateral and rather far forward. Clamps are placed on the flaps edge, and a flap that measures approximately 6 to 10 mm thick is created. Much of the tongue's intrinsic muscle is left behind. The flap is then filleted to flatten and sculpture it. Hemostasis must be meticulous. The flap is then rotated laterally and sutured as described previously. No bolus is used, and the donor tongue is closed on itself primarily. Any uncovered donor tongue can be felt open (Figs. 44-6, 44-7, and 44-8).

Smaller defects of the floor of mouth can be closed using smaller tongue flaps. It is unnecessary to use the entire hemitongue.

Tongue flaps are not the only flap that is used in oral and oropharyngeal reconstruction. They are a safe, quick, and efficient tool to help in a relatively predictable preconstruction problem. The flap uses tissue that is "at home" in the oral cavity. The marathon reconstruction in terms of time, changing of operative fields, and other inefficiencies that are required with chest, trapezius, pectoralis, and free flaps are avoided. In the anteriorly based flaps, tissue that is redundant (ie, denervated tongue) is given a new role to play in a cost-effective way.

LAWRENCE W. DESANTO
KERRY D. OLSEN

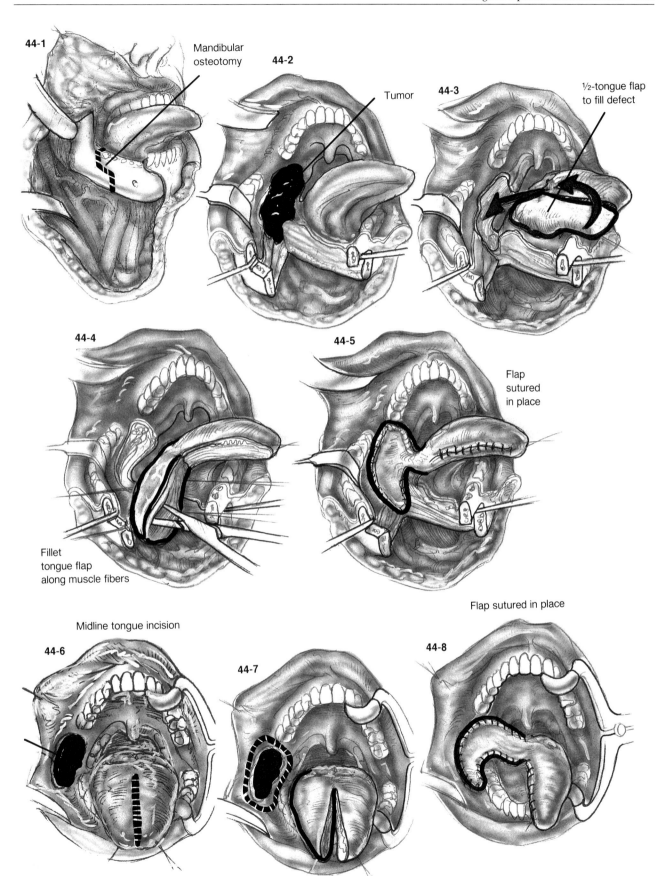

44-1 Mandibular osteotomy

44-2 Tumor

44-3 ½-tongue flap to fill defect

44-4 Fillet tongue flap along muscle fibers

44-5 Flap sutured in place

Midline tongue incision

44-6

44-7

Flap sutured in place

44-8

■ 45. INTRAORAL SKIN GRAFTING

Free skin grafts are used to resurface oral cavity and oropharyngeal defects where there is an underlying recipient bed. The graft provides a biologic dressing that hastens healing without excessive scar formation.

Indications
1. Surface defects of the buccal mucosa
2. Surface defects of the floor of the mouth
3. Surface defects of the hard and soft palate
4. Intranasal surface defects after resection of the hard palate
5. Rarely, a tongue surface defect for which primary closure is not practical

Contraindications
1. Any through-and-through defect where the oral cavity, oropharynx, or pharyngeal defect extends full thickness into the neck

Preoperative Preparation
1. Signed informed consent from the patient should refer to the reconstruction options discussed and the consequence of each option. For a skin graft, the donor site consequences should be included (eg, scar, discoloration, cosmetic liability, donor site options).
2. Routine laboratory studies needed for a safe anesthesia
3. Studies such as endoscopy and imaging that are needed for treatment planning for an operation that requires reconstruction

Special Instruments, Position, and Anesthesia
1. Instruments needed for treatment of the primary problem
2. A variable-depth dermatome
3. Bolus material: dental rolls, parachute silk, polyurethane foam

Tips and Pearls
1. Not every raw surface needs to be covered. Small defects can be left open, and they will heal quickly.
2. Split-thickness skin is not the only biologic dressing that is used. Little known, but remarkable, is the dressing value of human amnion. Amnion, taken from the delivery room, can be used to dress surface defects of the floor of mouth, alveolus, cheek, and most every surface where a split-thickness skin graft is applied. Both function as biologic dressings, and both contract significantly.
3. Skin grafts are not applied like wall paper or even laid like tile. This is one situation in medicine where more is better. Grafts should be big and not tent up.
4. Skin grafts can be put in place in a delayed manner, because skin can be stored for a time and remain viable. The graft is wrapped in sterile gauze soaked in saline and placed in a sterile container, which is refrigerated until needed. A temperature of 4°C is recommended.

Pitfalls and Complications
1. Not much can go wrong except graft failure if the graft option is appropriate. A dead graft can be trimmed off in the office or treatment room and allowed to heal secondarily.

Postoperative Care Issues
1. The bolus needed to hold a skin graft in place in the oral cavity, sinus, nasal cavity, or oropharynx can quickly become soaked with saliva, food, and bacteria. This can be avoided by using a smooth and water-resistant material for the bolus. I like parachute silk, but polyurethane sponge is satisfactory.
2. A feeding tube inserted at the time of surgery buys time and avoids some of the bolus problems, and it ensures nutrition while the bolus and graft are in place.
3. Airway concerns are minimal if the bolus is anterior to the anterior tonsil pillar. For a bolus placed more posteriorly, the airway is better protected by a tracheotomy. Airway protection allows everyone a safer rest, and tracheotomies that are unnecessary are easier to remove than those that are necessary are to insert.

Reference
McGregor, IA. Fundamental techniques of plastic surgery. 7th ed. New York: Churchill Livingstone, 1980.

Operative Procedure
Two prototype operations are presented.

Resection of the Entire Buccal Mucosa for a Verrucous Cancer
The resection involves cheek mucosa and underlying fat down to the overlying skin; the graft base is the undersurface of the cheek skin (Fig. 45-1). The size of the defect is unimportant, except that defects of 2 cm or less can simply be left open. A split-thickness skin graft that is larger by several centimeters is taken from the chosen donor site. The actual thickness is not very important. Some donor sites are the anterior thigh, abdomen, and flank. Posterior donor site are best avoided.

The skin graft is sewn into place with the edges overlapping, and the graft is draped into the concave defect. Every other stitch is left long. After the graft is sutured, the bolus is overlaid and tied in place using the ends of the sutures (Fig. 45-2).

I usually make a bolus by wrapping dental sponges in a wrap of parachute silk, sewing the silk around the bolus. Just as effective is a piece of polyurethane sponge that is cut to fit in place. There may be other bolus materials that are as effective.

Bolus grafting is most useful where the is minimal motion and the underlying surface can provide some stability. Concave defects are ideal. Tenting across the defect is denied by an oversized graft and a suitable bolus. Bolus grafting does not work well on mobile structures such as the anterior tongue.

The bolus can be removed in 4 or 5 days, after which any redundant skin can be trimmed away.

Quilted grafts can eliminate the bolus in some instances. If the defect is reasonably stable, a quilted graft can be used without a bolus. The technique is the same; an oversized graft is placed in the defect and sewn to its edge. Absorbable anchoring sutures are placed around the graft mesh to fix it to the bed. Multiple sutures are needed in the bed to provide an immobile graft.

With either method, meticulous hemostasis to the graft bed is essential. I use cautery before placing a graft. In the bolus graft, I place multiple scalpel "pie cuts" to accommodate any blood that may otherwise accumulate under the graft. In the meshed graft, these cuts are already made. I prefer the meshed grafts.

Dental Appliance Method
Skin grafts to the upper alveolus, hard palate, and maxillectomy defects are not comfortably immobilized with a bolus. A denture or a dental splint are nicely adapted to hold a graft in place.

In the edentulous patient, the denture can be used or a fabricated dental splint made before surgery and then modified in the operating room to adapt to the defect. The dental plate or the splint fits as before the procedure on the unresected part of the palate but must to be adapted to the resection area. This is done by molding soft dental compound to the denture and modeling it to the defect and skin graft. The dental compound then cools and hardens, welded to the denture and molded to the graft site. To ensure a good weld to the denture, holes are drilled into the appliance or denture. After the dental material is fixed to the denture, it is rewarmed in hot water and contoured to the graft site. The skin graft is then placed and sutured where possible, and the modified stent is placed over the graft to immobilize it.

To maintain a stable denture and stent, the appliance can be wired to the remaining alveolus or fixed by wire suspension suture from the zygoma. I prefer the later method.

If there is enough alveolus, holes can be drilled and the appliance or denture wired in place directly.

If the patient has teeth, the problem is more complicated and dental help is appreciated. Cap splints can be made to attach to the teeth outside of the resection to provide a point of fixation for a metal bar that bridges the defect. This is inserted in the operating room. The graft is set in place, and the dental compound is molded around the metal bar to hold the graft in place. Skin grafting a partial mucosal defect in a dentulous patient is a rare exercise. Usually, the patient has a full-thickness defect, and no graft (Figs. 45-3 and 45-4) is needed. The defect is managed later with a partial dental prosthesis.

LAWRENCE W. DESANTO

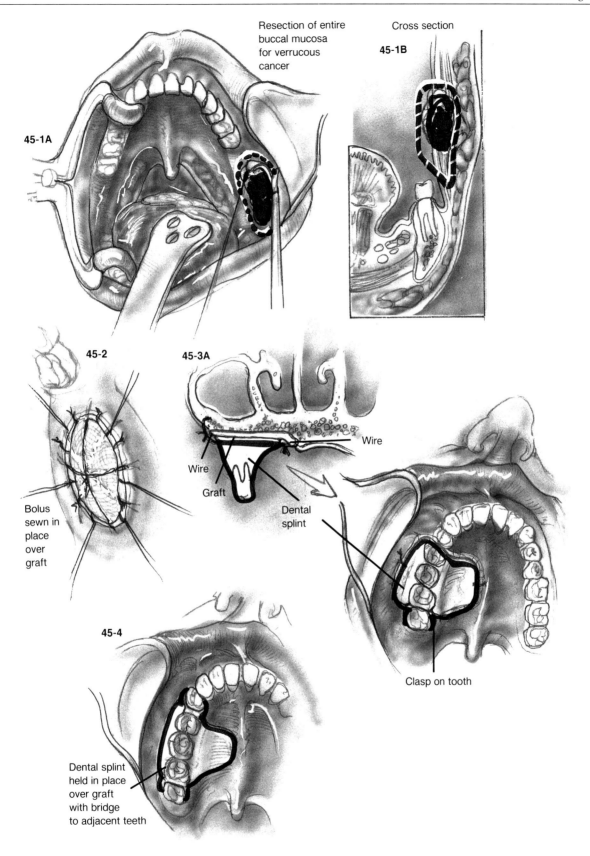

Resection of entire buccal mucosa for verrucous cancer

45-1A

Cross section
45-1B

45-2

Bolus sewn in place over graft

45-3A

Wire

Wire

Graft

Dental splint

Clasp on tooth

45-4

Dental splint held in place over graft with bridge to adjacent teeth

■ 46. SEGMENTAL RESECTION FOR MANDIBULAR CYSTS AND TUMORS—Resection of a full-thickness segment of the mandible with or without surrounding soft tissue for the treatment of benign and malignant processes of the mandible

Indications
1. Malignant neoplasms affecting the mandible primarily or by virtue of invasion from adjacent tissue
2. Benign neoplasms of the mandibular bone

Contraindications
1. Lesions adequately treated by a marginal mandibulectomy
2. Lesions, such as lymphomas or metastatic tumors, more appropriately treated by irradiation or chemotherapy

Special Considerations
1. Immediate reconstruction is preferred, especially for resections that extend anteriorly to the mental foramen.
2. Tracheotomy for airway management
3. The skin incision can easily be extended for neck dissection.
4. Anterior floor of the mouth lesions typically cross the midline and place the patient at risk for bilateral cervical metastases.

Preoperative Preparation
1. Routine laboratory studies and staging
2. Preoperative dental consultation may be helpful for patients with poor dentition and especially for those who will ultimately require postoperative radiation therapy.
3. Mental nerve integrity is routinely checked to assess possible neural invasion of the inferior alveolar nerve.
4. Assess the extent of mandibular involvement and be prepared for required appropriate reconstructive techniques.

Special Instruments, Position, and Anesthesia
1. Oscillating saw, Gigli saw, bone plate reconstruction and fixation set, osteotomes, periosteal elevators, and soft tissue instruments
2. Supine position, with the head stabilized in a doughnut holder
3. General endotracheal anesthesia, with a tracheotomy done at the outset of the procedure

Tips and Pearls
1. If a fixation plate is used for reconstruction, plate bending or formation and screw hole drilling are done before the osteotomies to ensure exact relocation of the mandibular segments.
2. Dental extraction at the osteotomy site is recommended instead of placing the osteotomy between two viable teeth that are closely approximated.

Pitfalls and Complications
1. Hemorrhage
2. Infection, pharyngocutaneous fistula, orocutaneous fistula, or osteomyelitis
3. Mandibular pain and dysfunction
4. Dysphagia and aspiration
5. Airway obstruction
6. Extrusion of reconstruction plate (if used)
7. Mandibular nerve injury

Postoperative Care Issues
1. The tracheotomy is maintained until the airway is adequate. The patient should also be able to keep an adequate airway while sleeping, because surgical resection and reconstruction of the upper airway may precipitate obstructive sleep apnea.
2. Nasogastric tube feeding is maintained until the mucosal suture lines are well sealed and the patient is able to swallow without aspiration.
3. Speech therapy for deglutition rehabilitation may be helpful.

References
Johnson JT. Large lateral posterior floor-of-mouth lesion with mandibular invasion. In: Bailey BJ, ed. Surgery of the oral cavity. Chicago: Year Book Medical Publishers, 1989:116.

Wald RM, Calcaterra TC. Lower alveolar carcinoma. Segmental v. marginal resection. Arch Otolaryngol 1983;109:578.

Operative Procedure
Prophylactic antibiotics are given during induction of anesthesia. We employ cefazolin and metronidazole for coverage of gram-positive organisms and anaerobes. The antibiotics are routinely employed for 48 hours. The patient is placed in the supine position, with the head extended. If a distant graft site (eg, fibular or scapular grafts) is anticipated, it should be properly positioned and readied for surgery. Paralytic agents can improve oral cavity exposure, but if the facial nerve needs to be identified, paralytic agents are relatively contraindicated. A tracheotomy is performed at the outset of the procedure to ensure a stable airway and enhance intraoral exposure. A reinforced endotracheal tube is placed into the tracheotomy site.

A lip-splitting incision or a visor flap incision is used. The skin flap is elevated, carefully ensuring the integrity of the marginal mandibular nerve (Fig. 46-1). If the resection is performed for a benign mandibular tumor, and then the periosteum is elevated off of the entire segment to be resected (Fig. 46-2). If the resection is for malignant disease, the mandibular bone is resected en bloc with surrounding soft tissue (Fig. 46-3). Generally, surgical margins of 1 to 1.5 cm are appropriate. If there is any question of mental nerve anesthesia preoperatively, biopsies of the inferior alveolar nerve are sent for frozen-section examination. The nerve should be traced superiorly until a clear neural margin can be attained.

Reconstruction of a segmental defect of the mandible is a somewhat controversial subject. We suggest a tailored approach for each individual patient. Generally, all defects that extend anterior to the mental foramen should undergo some type of immediate reconstruction. Defects that are posterior to the angle of the mandible frequently do well with soft tissue closure or closure with a pedicled myocutaneous flap. However, we tend to recommend reconstruction for most patients.

The microvascular osteomyocutaneous free flap provides excellent reconstruction of the bony mandible and associated soft tissues (Fig. 46-4). However, this requires expertise in microvascular surgery or the use of a second surgical team. The operative time is significantly increased. For patients who have significantly impaired cardiovascular status and if there is concern about prolonging the surgical procedure, a mandibular reconstructive plate with a pectoralis major pedicled flap can be used for a relatively expedient reconstruction (Fig. 46-5). A second-stage reconstruction can be performed for these patients.

An alternative to segmental mandibulotomy for a select group of patients is marginal mandibulectomy or a mandibular shave. For patients who have tumor that approximates but does not invade the mandibular bone, this technique offers a means of obtaining a healthy margin while maintaining mandibular continuity. A marginal mandibulectomy can be performed in a vertical, horizontal, or oblique plane (Fig. 46-6).

ROBERT H. MILLER
GERARD J. GIANOLI

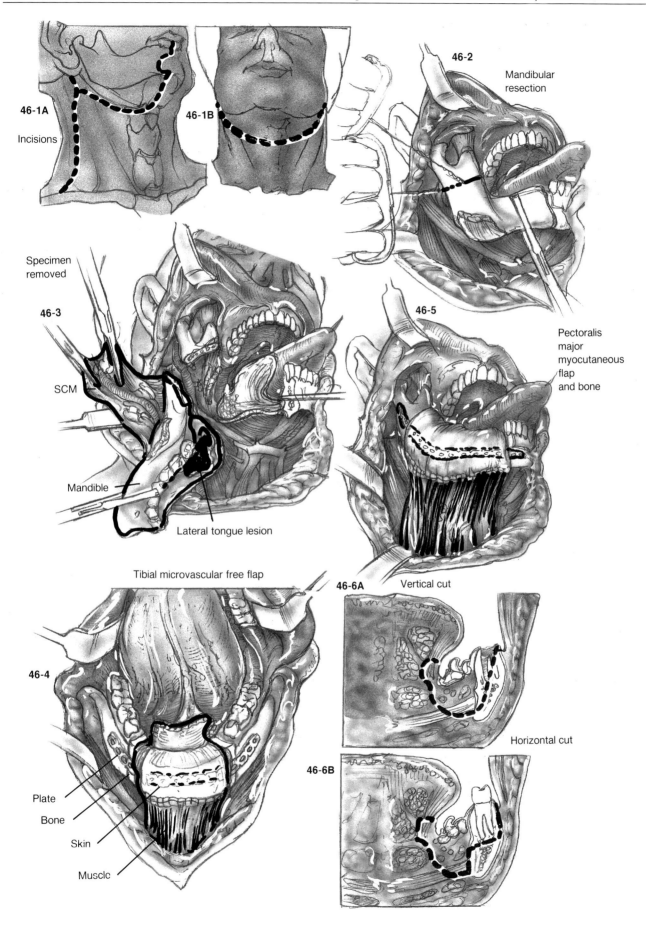

46-1A
Incisions

46-1B

46-2
Mandibular resection

Specimen removed

46-3

SCM

Mandible

Lateral tongue lesion

46-5

Pectoralis major myocutaneous flap and bone

Tibial microvascular free flap

46-4

Plate

Bone

Skin

Musclc

46-6A Vertical cut

Horizontal cut

46-6B

■ 47. SUPERFICIAL AND PLUNGING RANULA

EXCISION—Surgical removal of a mucocele or pseudocyst of the floor of mouth with or without cervical extension

Indications
1. Small ranulas, for which marsupialization may be effective treatment
2. Excision is preferred for recurrent ranulas, plunging ranulas, ranulas associated with prior oral trauma or surgery, and ranulas associated with submandibular duct relocation procedures

Special Considerations
1. Ranulas occur as cystic-appearing swellings in the floor of mouth and are usually lateralized.
2. They may be true mucus-filled cysts (ie, mucoceles) or pseudocysts (ie, extravasation of saliva).
3. Ranulas with extension into the neck (ie, plunging ranulas) may be confused with branchial cleft cyst, thyroglossal duct cyst, dermoid or epidermoid cyst, teratoid cyst, cystic hygroma, laryngocele, arteriovenous malformation, or lymphadenopathy.

Preoperative Preparation
1. Routine laboratory studies
2. Sialography not indicated

Special Instruments, Position, and Anesthesia
1. Oral RAE endotracheal tube
2. Foam doughnut for head, shoulder roll
3. Headlight
4. Molt retractor and tongue retractor
5. Iodoform gauze packing

Tips and Pearls
1. Sublingual gland excised with plunging ranula and recurrent ranulas
2. Cervical exploration unnecessary, because neck component resolves spontaneously with removal of ipsilateral sublingual gland
3. Complete excision of pseudocyst unnecessary
4. Results of marsupialization improved with gauze packing

Pitfalls and Complications
1. High recurrence rates with simple marsupialization or incision and drainage
2. Injury to lingual nerve with subsequent anesthesia of ipsilateral tongue
3. Injury to Wharton's duct leading to stenosis or salivary leakage

Postoperative Care Issues
1. Good oral hygiene
2. Oral rinses after meals
3. If used, gauze packing should be removed by postoperative day 10.
4. Oral antibiotics for 1 week or until gauze packing removed

References
Crysdale WS, Mendelsohn JD, Conley S. Ranulas—mucoceles of the oral cavity: experience in 26 children. Laryngoscope 1988;98:296.
Galloway RH, Gross PD, Thompson SH, Patterson AL. Pathogenesis and treatment of ranula: report of three cases. J Oral Maxillofac Surg 1989;47:299.

Operative Procedure

The patient is positioned supine and intubated with an oral RAE endotracheal tube taped to the contralateral corner of the mouth. A shoulder roll may be placed as needed. Betadine prep includes the lower face and upper neck. An oral prep should also be done with a throat pack temporarily placed. A Molt retractor is placed in the mouth opposite the ranula. A tongue retractor facilitates access to the floor of mouth. Local anesthetic consisting of a solution of 1% lidocaine with 1:100,000 epinephrine is injected in the area of the intraoral incision for hemostasis.

Two surgical approaches may be used at this point, depending on the history and presentation of the ranula. For small lesions confined to the floor of mouth, simple marsupialization with gauze packing may be an appropriate initial procedure. For larger cysts, recurrent ranula, or a history of oral trauma, marsupialization has a high rate of failure. These presentations along with plunging ranula require excision of the ipsilateral sublingual gland for successful management. Treatment of plunging ranula does not require cervical exploration. Excision of the offending mucus-secreting gland results in spontaneous resolution of the cervical component.

Marsupialization for smaller, nonrecurrent ranulas is performed under local or general anesthesia. The cystic mass is unroofed, and the mucus is evacuated (Fig. 47-1). The margins of the cyst are sutured to the mucosa with absorbable suture such as Vicryl. The exposed cavity is packed with iodoform gauze (Fig. 47-2). After 10 days, the gauze is removed. Extrusion of the gauze may begin before 10 days as the cavity heals from inside out.

Classically, larger or recurrent ranulas have been treated with complete surgical removal, including the cystic mass and the associated sublingual gland. The initial incision is made directly over the ranula on its superior aspect. Dissection removes the ranula and the sublingual gland from the neighboring structures (Fig. 47-3). Bipolar cautery is useful for hemostasis and to minimize electrical stimulation of adjacent nerves. Careful dissection technique is necessary to avoid injury to the lingual nerve, submandibular duct, and terminal branches of the hypoglossal nerve. Cannulation of the duct helps to prevent inadvertent transection of the structure. If it occurs, it can be directly sutured to the adjacent floor of mouth mucosa (ie, sialodochoplasty).

Some surgeons have advocated a more conservative approach for large, recurrent, or plunging ranulas. The description that follows is related from their experience. Plunging or recurrent ranulas should be managed with transoral excision of the sublingual gland and evacuation of the pseudocyst. Complete extirpation of the cyst is difficult and unnecessary. With appropriate retractors in place and the floor of mouth adequately exposed, an incision is made with a #15 blade in the lingual gingival sulcus, extending from the ipsilateral first molar anteriorly to the midline as necessary for access (Fig. 47-4). A submucoperiosteal plane is developed using an elevator along the medial aspect of the mandible to the level of the floor of the mouth. With the soft tissue flap retracted medially and posteriorly, the sublingual gland is identified bulging against the opposite side of the periosteum. An incision is made along the periosteum over the gland. Separation of the gland from the surrounding tissues is accomplished using blunt and sharp dissection (Fig. 47-5). The lingual nerve and submandibular duct are located medial to the initial dissection. Blunt techniques are used when approaching these structures. The vascular pedicle is located medially and posteriorly and is ligated before complete removal (Fig. 47-6). The contents of the pseudocyst, including that extravasating below the mylohyoid muscle, may be evacuated through this intraoral approach before closure of the incisions.

WILLIAM W. SHOCKLEY
C. GAELYN GARRETT

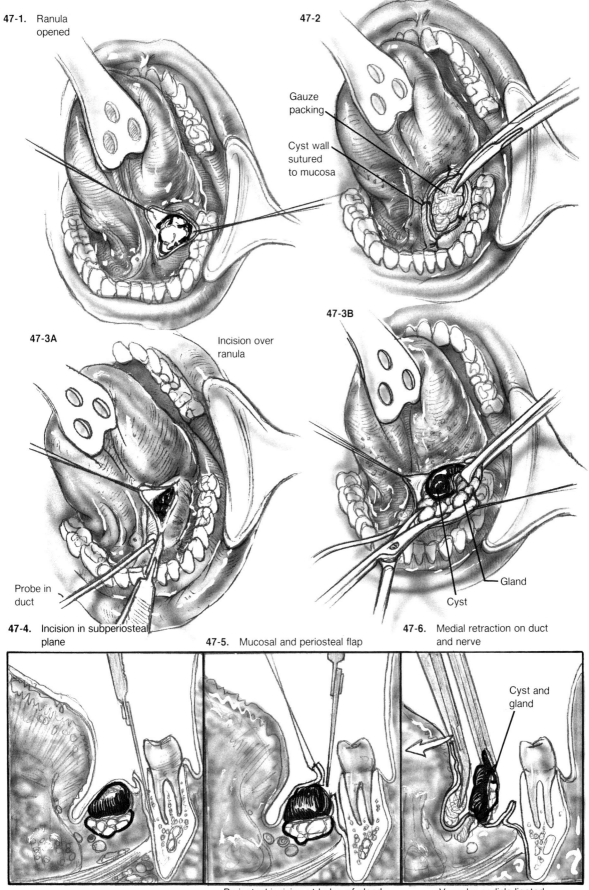

47-1. Ranula opened

47-2

Gauze packing

Cyst wall sutured to mucosa

47-3A

Incision over ranula

47-3B

Probe in duct

Gland

Cyst

47-4. Incision in subperiosteal plane

47-5. Mucosal and periosteal flap

47-6. Medial retraction on duct and nerve

Cyst and gland

Periosteal incision at bulge of gland

Vascular pedicle ligated

■ 48. RESECTION OF TONSIL AND RETRO-MOLAR TRIGONE WITH AND WITHOUT MANDIBULAR INVOLVEMENT

— Removal of involved tissues in the tonsillar and retromolar trigone region because of neoplasms with no or minimal mandibular invasion

Indications

1. Cancer of the retromolar trigone and tonsillar region
2. Other unusual neoplasms involving this anatomic region
3. Transoral approach is reserved for early, superficial, well-circumscribed tumors and usually is reserved for selected T1 or T2 lesions.
4. Lip-splitting approach allows additional exposure without violation of mandibular continuity.
5. Lip-splitting with midline mandibulectomy allows further access posteriorly for enhanced visualization of the tumor and adjacent tissues.
6. Transcervical approach provides access to selected lesions, avoiding inherent cosmetic deformity with lip-splitting procedure.
7. Marginal mandibulectomy is appropriate for early lesions affixed to mandible but without evidence of bony invasion.
8. Segmental mandibulectomy generally is reserved for advanced-stage disease or definite mandibular invasion.

Contraindications

1. Gross bony erosion on clinical examination (if mandibular sparing anticipated)
2. Radiographic evidence of significant bony involvement (if mandibular sparing anticipated)
3. Skull base invasion
4. Unresectable neck disease: cervical metastasis or direct tumor extension
5. Intracranial extension, as in tumor extension through the foramen ovale
6. Involvement of nasopharynx or paravertebral musculature

Special Considerations

1. Trismus must be investigated fully to assess cause; usually 2° to pterygoid invasion
2. Assessment of potential mandibular invasion
3. Tongue base or root of tongue involvement
4. Submucosal extension into nasopharynx or hypopharynx
5. Infiltration into muscles of mastication (ie, pterygoid and masseter muscles)
6. Radiographic evidence of enlargement of foramen ovale, indicative of intracranial extension through cranial nerve V, mandibular branch
7. Selected early lesions better treated with primary radiation therapy
8. Reconstructive maneuvers must be tailored to resulting defect and should be anticipated.
9. Consideration of combined therapy (irradiation with or without chemotherapy) for advanced lesions
10. Cervical node status

Preoperative Preparation

1. Routine laboratory studies including radiographs and liver function tests
2. Panorex of mandible for lesions encroaching on the bone
3. Computed tomography (CT) scans from skull base to clavicles for assessing tumor extent, skull base foramina, mandibular invasion (bone windows), and cervical nodes
4. Fiberoptic endoscopy and complete panendoscopy, including examination of nasopharynx
5. Evaluation of tumor extent at endoscopy, including careful palpation

(continued)

Operative Procedure

Resection of Tonsil and Retromolar Trigone: Mandibular Sparing

The surgical resection is tailored to removal of the tumor with a 1.5-m cuff of normal tissue. The following description assumes a T3N0M0 squamous cell carcinoma of the right tonsil, involving the anterior and posterior pillars, soft palate, retromolar trigone, and a small portion of the tongue base. A lip-splitting approach (without mandibulotomy) has been deemed the optimal method of exposure.

The incision is marked with a marking pen, indicating a curvilinear transverse incision with extension into midpoint of the lip, preserving the mentum as a cosmetic unit (Fig. 48-1). Before preparation, the proposed incision is injected with a solution of 1% lidocaine with 1:100,000 epinephrine.

Neck incision is made up to the chin and subplatysmal flaps are elevated. The nerve is identified, dissected free, and swept superiorly. Neck dissection is completed, including removal of submandibular gland.

The periosteum is incised along entire inferior border of mandible (Fig. 48-2). Subperiosteal elevation is undertaken up to superior border of mandibular body, with exposure of the ramus up to the mandibular notch.

A lip-splitting incision is accomplished and continued into the oral cavity with the scissors, as a through-and-through incision is made in the gingivobuccal sulcus (Fig. 48-3). The labiofacial soft tissues are reflected, and the entire tumor can be readily visualized.

The tumor is again inspected and palpated, and the proposed resection is marked with the tip of the cautery in a dotted-line fashion (Fig. 48-4). The optimal resection margin is 1.5 to 2.0 cm. A small resection of mandibular rim is planned to provide a cuff of tissue in the region of the retromolar trigone (Fig. 48-5). The osteotomy is accomplished with a reciprocating saw, and the resection is accomplished using the cutting cautery, using the coagulation mode when necessary for bleeding.

In this case, the defect was amenable to a split-thickness skin graft. The graft (0.015 in [0.38 mm]) is obtained and "pie crusted." It is sutured into position using the quilting technique, although the use of a bolster may be necessary as well (Fig. 48-6).

The lip is closed in four layers: muscle, dermis, skin with vermilion, and mucosa. Jackson-Pratt drains are inserted and brought out through stab incisions. The remaining soft tissues are closed using a platysma-dermal layered closure, followed by skin closure.

Resection of Tonsil and Retromolar Trigone: Segmental Mandibular Resection

The patient has a T4N0M0 squamous cell carcinoma of the right retromolar trigone with clinical and radiographic invasion of mandible, minimal tongue involvement, and invasion of the tonsil, pillars, and pharyngeal wall. The plan is for a lip-splitting approach, segmental mandibulectomy, and reconstruction using a pectoralis myocutaneous flap. A supraomohyoid neck dissection is planned to evaluate nodal status and to improve access for the surgical resection.

The cervical portion of the incision is made, and subplatysmal flaps are elevated. Neck dissection is completed after identification of the marginal mandibular nerve.

The resection begins by making a transoral incision in the gingivobuccal sulcus, 1.5 cm away from the visible and palpable tumor. This incision is carried down to bone on the lateral aspect of the mandible (Fig. 48-7).

The periosteum at the inferior border of the mandible is incised and elevated *up to but not beyond* the buccal cut. This avoids elevating into the region of mandibular invasion (Fig. 48-8). At this point, the lip-splitting incision is made and connected with the gingivobuccal resection margin.

The tumor is in full view, as is the entire body and ramus of the mandible. The lateral margin of resection is already completed. A 1.5-cm resection margin is marked out in dotted-line fashion with the cautery, and the proposed incision is injected with a vasoconstrictor (Fig. 48-9).

The mandibular resection margins are determined based on

(continued)

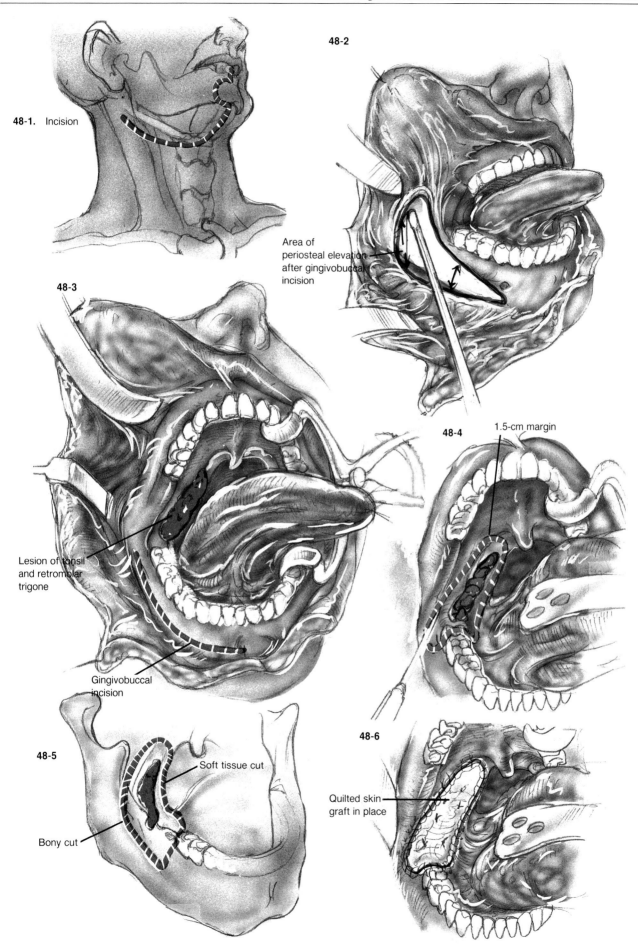

48-1. Incision

48-2

Area of
periosteal elevation
after gingivobuccal
incision

48-3

Lesion of tonsil
and retromolar
trigone

Gingivobuccal
incision

48-4

1.5-cm margin

48-5

Soft tissue cut

Bony cut

48-6

Quilted skin
graft in place

■ **48.** RESECTION OF TONSIL AND RETRO-MOLAR TRIGONE WITH AND WITHOUT MANDIBULAR INVOLVEMENT *(continued)*

Special Instrumentation, Position, and Anesthesia

1. Headlight and bipolar cautery
2. Nerve stimulator and periosteal elevators
3. Oscillating or reciprocating saw and cutting bur
4. Dermatome (if skin graft anticipated)
5. Shoulders on roll, head in circular foam doughnut
6. Anesthesia through the nasotracheal tube or tracheostomy tube, depending on extent of surgery; use of paralyzing agents limited to initiation of procedure

Tips and Pearls

1. Beware of submucosal extension, usually manifested as mucosal edema.
2. Be sure CT cuts with bone windows encompass the area of concern. Both axial and coronal planes are recommended, with 2-mm cuts through the region at highest risk for mandibular invasion.
3. Always palpate tumor and adjacent structures, especially the tongue base and root of tongue.
4. Selected lesions of the tonsil and retromolar trigone are better treated with irradiation.
5. Decisions regarding approach (eg, transoral, transcervical, lip-splitting, midline mandibulotomy) are tied to the necessary exposure and the need for mandibular resection.
6. The vermilion border is carefully marked before incision in the lip to allow a precise reapproximation at the time of closure.
7. Look for perineural invasion along inferior alveolar nerve preoperatively and intraoperatively.
8. Reconstructive options include healing by secondary intention, prosthetic rehabilitation (for palatal defects), primary closure, skin graft, and flap reconstruction.

Pitfalls and Complications

1. Inadequate or inaccurate tumor assessment, compromising resection
2. Orocutaneous or pharyngocutaneous fistula
3. Poor healing leading to exposed bone
4. Malunion or nonunion at mandibular osteotomy site
5. Tethering of tongue or velopharyngeal insufficiency compromises speech, mastication, and swallowing.

Postoperative Care Issues

1. Full liquid diet resumed at 7 days and advanced as tolerated; feeding tube removed at this point
2. Decannulation (if tracheostomy is performed) is accomplished as soon as secretions are manageable and the airway is stable (usually 7–10 days).
3. Speech pathologist is essential for speech and swallowing rehabilitation.
4. Postoperative irradiation should begin 3 to 6 weeks postoperatively, if indicated by tumor stage, nodal disease, or positive margins.
5. Early lesions removed with resultant positive margins should be reexcised, avoiding radiation therapy.

References

Spiro RH, Gerold FP, Strong EW. Mandibular "swing" approach for oral and oropharyngeal tumors. Head Neck 1981;3:371.

Stiernberg CM, Shockley WW, Pillsbury HC. Surgical approaches to tumors of the oropharynx. In: Johnson JJ, Derkay CS, Mandell-Brown MK, Newman RK, eds. Instructional courses, vol 6. St. Louis: Mosby-Year Book, 1993;241.

surgical philosophy and radiographic evidence of involvement (Fig. 48-10). Typically, this involves resection from the mental nerve foramen to the mandibular notch, leaving the coronoid and condylar neck in situ. If mandibular continuity is to be restored with a reconstruction plate or osseous free flap, appropriate holes are drilled before resection with the oscillating saw. Soft tissue resection is performed with the cutting current, using cautery when needed. From the anterior osteotomy, the mandible is retracted laterally and hinged posteriorly. In this fashion, tumor resection advances posteriorly and medially (Fig. 48-11).

The resected tissue is marked and oriented for the pathologist. Tissue for frozen section is obtained from the adjacent tissue. The surgeon has decided not to reconstruct the mandible and to use a pectoralis myocutaneous flap for soft tissue reconstruction (Fig. 48-12). This is sutured into place using a two-layer closure, taking robust bites of flap and recipient tissue in an interrupted fashion.

Surgical Variations

Transoral Resection

For minimally invasive localized lesions, transoral resection may be a viable therapeutic option. For the N0 neck, elective neck dissection or elective radiation therapy may be appropriate, depending on the individual case. Tumors approached transorally should have no clinical or radiographic evidence of bony invasion. Tumor infiltration of periosteum (even microscopic involvement) mandates resection of at least the adjacent cortical bone. As with other approaches, a 1.5-cm margin around the visible and palpable tumor is recommended. Closure is usually accomplished by primary closure, skin graft, or healing by secondary intention.

Midline Mandibulotomy

The decision to use a midline mandibulotomy is based on the need for posterolateral exposure. Typically, this approach is reserved for large tonsillar or tongue base cancers without mandibular invasion. For tumors "stuck to" the mandibular ramus but without mandibular evidence of invasion on CT scan, resection of the involved segment is still advisable.

Through a lip-splitting incision, the symphysis is exposed, the proposed osteotomy down the midline is marked out, a mandibular fracture plate is applied, and holes are drilled and tapped. The plate is removed, and the osteotomy accomplished with a reciprocating or an oscillating saw. For the dentulous patient, a small saw can be used to create the osteotomy between the central incisors. Alternatively, a tooth can be removed with the bony cut being made through the tooth socket. An incision is made in the floor of the mouth in the gingivolingual sulcus as the mandible is swung out laterally for exposure. With careful dissection, the lingual nerve usually can be spared.

After resection, frozen sections, and reconstruction, the mandibular segments are reopposed, and the fracture plate applied. In the dentulous patient, a compression plate changes the occlusion and should be avoided. Problems with stiffness and pain in the TMJ are common after mandibular swing procedures.

In a variation of the midline mandibulotomy, a paramedian osteotomy is performed just in front of the mental nerve and behind the attachment of the mylohyoid muscle. The exposure seems to be equivalent but provides less disruption of the tongue musculature.

Lateral Mandibulotomy

Many surgeons prefer a lateral mandibulotomy site for the osteotomy. Although in this situation, ipsilateral anesthesia of the lip and chin are expected sequelae, the advantage of this technique is that a lip-splitting incision can generally be avoided. The other advantage of a lateral mandibulotomy is that this segment may be resected if intraoperatively it appears that tumor invasion precludes sparing of the mandible. If it is unclear whether the body or ramus of the mandible is free of tumor, lateral mandibulotomy provides flexibility, with sparing this segment when feasible and resection when it appears necessary.

WILLIAM W. SHOCKLEY

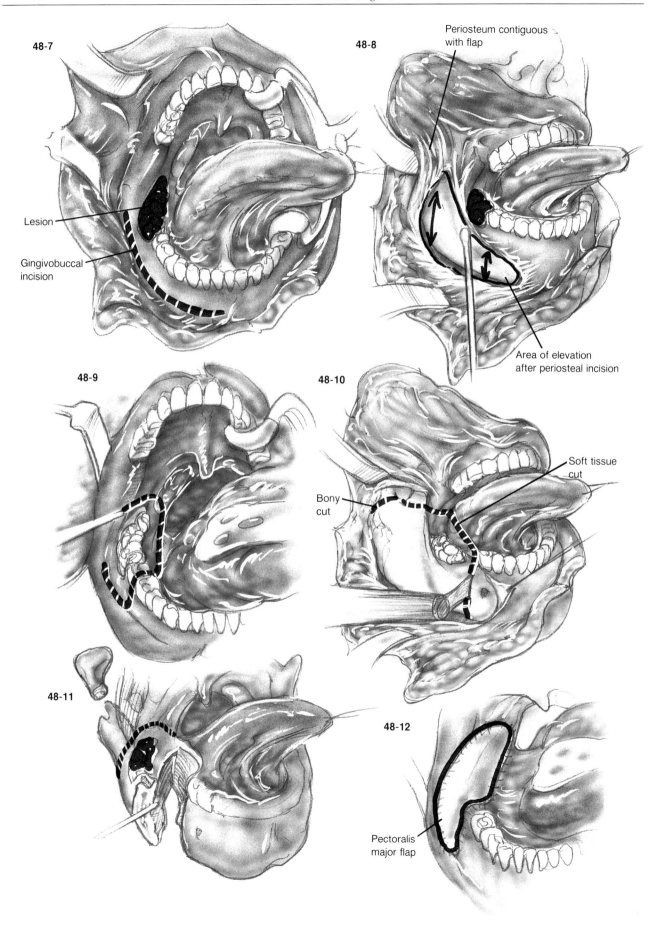

48-7

Lesion

Gingivobuccal
incision

48-8

Periosteum contiguous
with flap

Area of elevation
after periosteal incision

48-9

48-10

Bony
cut

Soft tissue
cut

48-11

48-12

Pectoralis
major flap

■ 49. VESTIBULOPLASTY

Surgical extension of the oral vestibule for the purpose of improving and enlarging the denture bearing area of the mandible

Indications

1. Significant resorption of the alveolar bone of the edentulous mandible or maxilla
2. A shallow vestibular sulcus
3. Inadequate denture bearing area with dislodgment of dental prostheses by local muscle attachments

Special Considerations

1. Adequate alveolar bone (15 mm of vertical height) for support of dental prosthetics or implants
2. Need for additional procedures, including alveolar ridge augmentation or osseointegrated implants

Preoperative Preparation

1. Preoperative evaluation and recommendations by the patient's dentist or prosthodontist
2. Panorex and cephalometric x-ray films of the mandible
3. Routine laboratory studies and physical examination
4. Splint preparation

Special Instruments, Position, and Anesthesia

1. Supine position
2. General anesthesia through nasotracheal tube
3. Injection with solution of 1% lidocaine with 1:100,000 epinephrine
4. Dermatome

Tips and Pearls

1. Elevation of mucosal flaps is facilitated by generous submucous injection of local anesthetic
2. The patient's existing denture can be modified for use as a postoperative splint in some cases

Pitfalls and Complications

1. Final result of vestibular extension may be smaller after healing.
2. Scarring in the depth of the vestibule can cause poor denture fit.
3. Nonkeratinized tissue over alveolar bone may become mobile.
4. Possibility of injury to mental or lingual nerves
5. Accelerated resorption of alveolar crest bone after vestibuloplasty
6. Facial soft tissue profile changes

Postoperative Care Issues

1. Splint is left in place for 7 to 10 days
2. Antibiotics are continued until the splint is removed
3. Impressions for new dentures can be made in 4 to 6 weeks

References

Davis WH, Davis CL. Surgical management of soft tissue problems. In: Fonseca RJ, Davis WH, eds. Reconstructive maxillofacial surgery. Philadelphia: WB Saunders, 1986:69.

Harle F. Mandibular vestibuloplasty using skin. In: Stoelinga PJ ed. Proceedings of the Consensus Conference: the relative roles of vestibuloplasty and ridge augmentation in the management of the atrophic mandible. Chicago: Quintessence Publishing, 1984:25.

Operative Procedure

The patient is placed supine with his or her head slightly elevated and extended. General anesthesia is administered.

The split-thickness skin graft is harvested first. The most common donor sites are the anterior thigh or parallel and slightly inferior to the iliac crest. The width of the skin graft is dictated by the height of the alveolar bone that is to be covered. A 5- to 6-cm-wide graft is usually sufficient for adequate coverage. The graft should be thin (0.012–0.015 in [0.3–0.38 mm]) and 15 to 18 cm long. The donor site is sprayed with thrombin, and a moist dressing is applied.

Attention is turned to the oral cavity. The pharynx should be loosely packed with a gauze sponge to prevent aspiration of blood. The alveolar and labiobuccal mucosa is injected with local anesthetic with epinephrine. This submucous injection facilitates elevation of mucosal flaps and aids hemostasis. Using a #15 blade, an incision is made along the crest of the alveolar ridge at the junction of the free and attached mucosa (Fig. 49-1). The labiobuccal incision begins at the lateral margin of one retromolar pad and continues to the opposite side (see Fig. 49-1). Sharp dissection should be carried through the submucosa only, leaving the periosteum intact. A 1-cm transverse incision is made at the posterior end of the crest incision, extending to the inferior margin of the mandible (see Fig. 49-1). A supraperiosteal mucosal flap is raised, ensuring that the underlying periosteum is cleared of soft tissue.

The external oblique ridge marks the posterior extent of the dissection (Fig. 49-2), which should be carried to the inferior border of the mandible in most areas except the most posterior extent of the dissection, the mental neurovascular bundle region, and the midline of the mandible. In these areas, dissection should be less extensive to preserve important functional and cosmetic structures.

Generous local anesthesia is injected on the lingual side of the alveolar crest in the same fashion as before. The tongue is retracted medially to facilitate exposure and flap elevation. Using a #15 blade, an incision is made in the lingual alveolar mucosa at the junction of the free and attached mucosa. The incision begins at the level of one retromolar pad and extends to the opposite side (see Fig. 49-1). Care must be taken in the most posterior region to avoid injury to the lingual nerves. A supraperiosteal plane of dissection is achieved as before. The mylohyoid muscle is divided with a scalpel or tissue scissors as part of the lingual dissection. Bipolar cauterization before lysis of the muscle aids in hemostasis. Division of the mylohyoid continues anteriorly to the point where its mandibular attachment is covered by the genial muscles. Using blunt dissection, the flap is elevated to the inferior border of the mandible.

Any loose crest tissue must be excised, leaving only firmly attached keratinized mucosa along the alveolar crest. Sharp bony angles and ridges are smoothed, removing mucosa as necessary for exposure. The labiobuccal and lingual flaps are sutured in place at the depth of the newly enlarged vestibule using eight to ten submandibular sutures. Sutures of 3-0 chromic are first placed through the lingual flap. A surgical awl is passed through the cervical skin, along the posterior border of the mandible, and anterior to the lingual flap. The sutures are threaded through the awl and passed under and anterior to the mandible. Next, the suture is passed through the buccolabial flap and tied at the depth of the vestibule. The free ends of the respective flaps are connected to each other and to the periosteal junction (Fig. 49-3).

The splint is made. Preoperatively, an impression is made of the existing alveolar ridge. A cast is made from this impression using dental stone. A heat-polymerizing clear acrylic resin splint is fabricated on the stone cast. After reflection and stabilization of the flaps, this splint is relined with impression compound to adapt it to the enlarged alveolar ridge. After the splint has dried, the skin graft is applied to it using dermatome glue. The epithelial surface is applied to the splint, leaving the dermal surface to contact the mandibular periosteum. The splint and graft are placed over the mandible (Fig. 49-4) and secured with 1-0 nylon circummandibular ligatures.

WILLIAM W. SHOCKLEY
WILLIAM R. BLYTHE

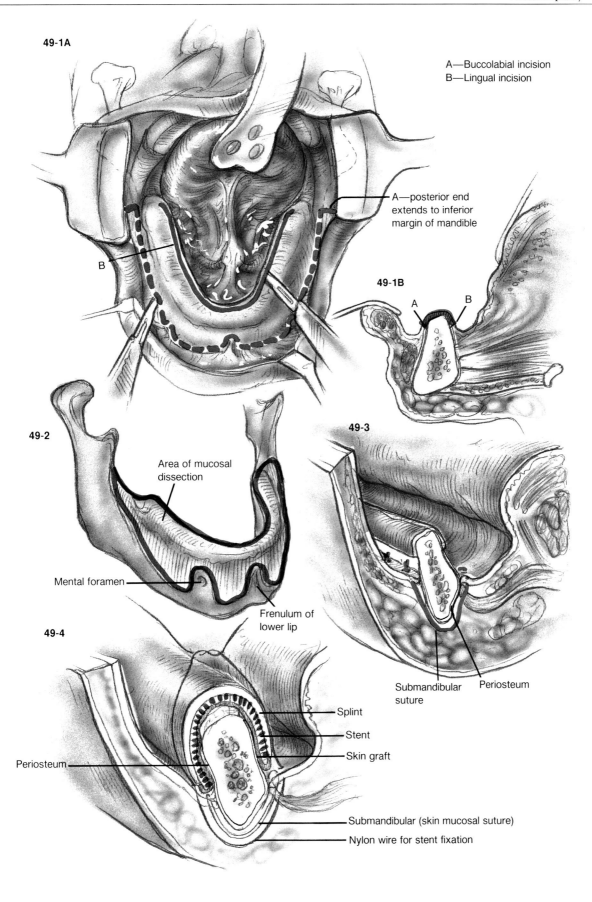

49-1A

A—Buccolabial incision
B—Lingual incision

A—posterior end
extends to inferior
margin of mandible

B

49-1B

A   B

49-2

Area of mucosal
dissection

Mental foramen

Frenulum of
lower lip

49-3

Submandibular
suture   Periosteum

49-4

Periosteum

Splint

Stent

Skin graft

Submandibular (skin mucosal suture)

Nylon wire for stent fixation

■ 50. MANDIBULAR RECONSTRUCTION

Reconstruction of mandibular defects with cortical "block" bone grafts, particulate cancellous bone grafts, a mandibular reconstruction plate, or vascularized free bone grafts

Indications
1. Traumatic defects
2. Defects related to bone loss from infection
3. Segmental defects following cancer resection
4. Congenital mandibular deficiency or asymmetry

Contraindications
1. Poor anesthetic risk
2. Damaged, poorly vascularized recipient tissues
3. Prior therapeutic radiation (relative risk)

Special Considerations
1. Primary versus secondary reconstruction
2. Prior radiation therapy
3. Insufficient soft tissue envelope
4. Anticipated donor site deformity, disability, or risks
5. Timing of reconstruction

(continued)

Operative Procedure: Secondary Mandibular Reconstruction

Titanium Tray With Particulate Bone and Cancellous Marrow (PBCM)

Numerous options are available in secondary reconstruction of mandibular defects. In a nonirradiated field, virtually any of the aforementioned techniques and many others may be appropriate. In the irradiated patient, hyperbaric oxygen treatments before and after surgery have been beneficial. However, this may not be necessary if vascularized tissue is being used in the reconstruction.

For purposes of this discussion, we describe the reconstruction of a segmental defect of the body of the mandible related to trauma in an otherwise healthy patient. A nasotracheal intubation is preferred. If not already in maxillary-mandibular fixation, this should be accomplished to establish proper occlusion, usually employing Erich arch bars. The ipsilateral face, neck, and hip are prepared and draped.

An iliac crest bone graft is obtained and additional marrow harvested (Fig. 50-1). The donor site is closed after obtaining hemostasis, and a suction drain is inserted. The proposed horizontal cervical incision is marked and injected with a solution of 1% lidocaine with 1:100,000 epinephrine.

The incision is made down through platysma, and subplatysmal flaps are elevated. The marginal mandibular nerve is identified and reflected superiorly. In the posttraumatic patient, the nerve may be difficult to identify, in which case, the inferior border of the mandible is approached with cautious blunt and sharp dissection, using the nerve stimulator liberally. In the region of the intact mandible, soft tissues are elevated in a subperiosteal plane.

After the intact segments have been identified, the soft tissues can be separated from the edges of the mandibular stumps. Debridement may be necessary. The edges of the bone are then "freshened" using a cutting bur or saw (Fig. 50-2). The wound is copiously irrigated with saline, and hemostasis is obtained using the bipolar cautery. Careful inspection should confirm no communication with the oral cavity.

The titanium tray is then fashioned to fit the defect, dissecting soft tissues as necessary for a proper fit. Holes are drilled and screws applied to maintain stable fixation of the tray. The PBCM is then placed in the tray and packed to fill the defect (Fig. 50-3). After further hemostasis and irrigation, a Jackson-Pratt drain is inserted through a small stab incision. Meticulous closure is accomplished.

Variations
- Alloplastic trays (eg, Dacron, Vitallium, Teflon)
- Use of cancellous bone chips only
- Use of allogeneic bone chips
- Biodegradable cribs, such as the rib, ilium, or cadaver mandible (Fig. 50-4)
- Solitary iliac crest block, secured with reconstruction plate (Fig. 50-5)
- Vascularized free bone flaps from the iliac crest, scapula, fibula, or radius (Fig. 50-6)

(continued)

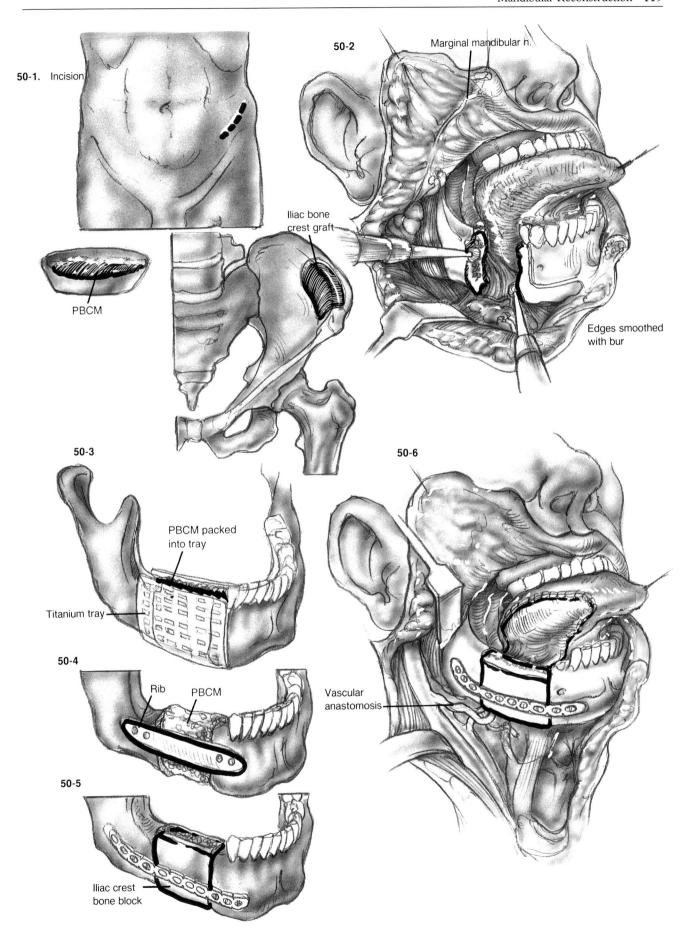

50-1. Incision

PBCM

Iliac bone
crest graft

50-2

Marginal mandibular n.

Edges smoothed
with bur

50-3

PBCM packed
into tray

Titanium tray

50-4

Rib   PBCM

50-5

Iliac crest
bone block

50-6

Vascular
anastomosis

■ **50.** MANDIBULAR RECONSTRUCTION
(continued)

Preoperative Preparation
1. Panorex of mandible
2. Computed tomography (CT) or three-dimensional CT scans in selected patients
3. Consideration of hyperbaric oxygen therapy for poorly vascularized or irradiated tissues
4. Routine laboratory tests and coagulation profile
5. Preoperative prophylactic antibiotics

Special Instruments, Position, and Anesthesia
1. Supine position, shoulder roll, and head support
2. Nasotracheal intubation and no muscle relaxants
3. Drills, burs, plating sets, and reciprocating or oscillating saw
4. Microvascular instruments if free flap planned
5. Nerve stimulator and bipolar cautery

Tips and Pearls
1. Identification or avoidance of marginal mandibular nerve
2. In secondary reconstruction, avoid entry into oral cavity (ie, contamination).
3. Establish proper occlusion before reconstruction of defect with arch bars, splints, or other methods.
4. Avoid dead space and hematoma formation.
5. Proper fixation of graft or flap in position

(continued)

Operative Procedure: Primary Mandibular Reconstruction
In the setting of primary reconstruction, the implication is that there is continuity between the defect and the oral cavity. In most situations, this occurs after resection of an oral or oropharyngeal tumor with composite resection of a mandibular segment.

Although not emphasized in this discussion, the associated soft tissue deficit must be addressed simultaneously. Assuming soft tissue reconstruction is also needed, the most common methods include using a myocutaneous flap with a mandibular reconstruction plate or a vascularized osseous free flap. Pedicled osteomyocutaneous flaps have been used successfully but are less popular at this time.

Pectoralis Flap With Mandibular Reconstruction Plate
Depending on the anticipated defect, a nasotracheal tube or tracheostomy is used. After preparation and draping, the appropriate incision is made to access the tumor for resection. The inferior border of the mandible is exposed after identifying and reflecting the marginal mandibular nerve. Unless contraindicated by tumor extent, subperiosteal dissection exposes the body, angle, and ramus of the mandible.

Based on the extent of the tumor, mandibular invasion, and the proposed margins of resection, the osteotomy sites are marked. Before making these cuts, the mandibular reconstruction plate is applied to the lateral surface of the mandible and contoured appropriately. Holes are drilled and tapped. Screws are loosely applied to ensure proper alignment and contour of the plate (Fig. 50-7). The screws are then removed and the resection undertaken.

After confirming tumor-free margins with frozen-section analysis, the wound is irrigated, and reconstructive plans are formulated. If primary closure can be accomplished without distortion of the tongue, it is preferable. For major defects, a flap is necessary. The mandibular plate is affixed and a pectoralis myocutaneous flap is harvested and sutured into position (Fig. 50-8). The subcutaneous tissue of the flap should overlap the plate. Cervicofacial and chest incisions are closed over suction drains.

Oromandibular Reconstruction With Vascularized Free Bone Flaps
The greatest advances in oral cavity and mandibular reconstruction are associated with refinements in free-flap reconstructive techniques. The flaps enjoying the greatest popularity are composite flaps from the scapula, fibula, and ilium. Although alternative donor sites for vascularized bone–containing flaps include the radius, rib, ulna, humerus, and metatarsus, these have not been found to be particularly effective for mandibular reconstruction.

The defect is approached as outlined previously. The mandible should be marked accordingly to maintain the appropriate contour. The mandibular reconstructive plate technique described may be applicable to stabilize the free bone flaps between the mandibular stumps (Fig. 50-9). After the flap is obtained, it is cut to fit the defect, and osteotomies may be necessary to create curvature, especially with fibular flaps (Fig. 50-10).

After the osseous portion of the flap is stabilized with plates, the microvascular anastomosis is accomplished. The soft tissue component of the flap is tailored to the defect and sutured into position. A small paddle of skin may be placed externally to serve as a monitor of flap viability. The donor sites are closed, and the cervical facial incision is closed over suction drains.

(continued)

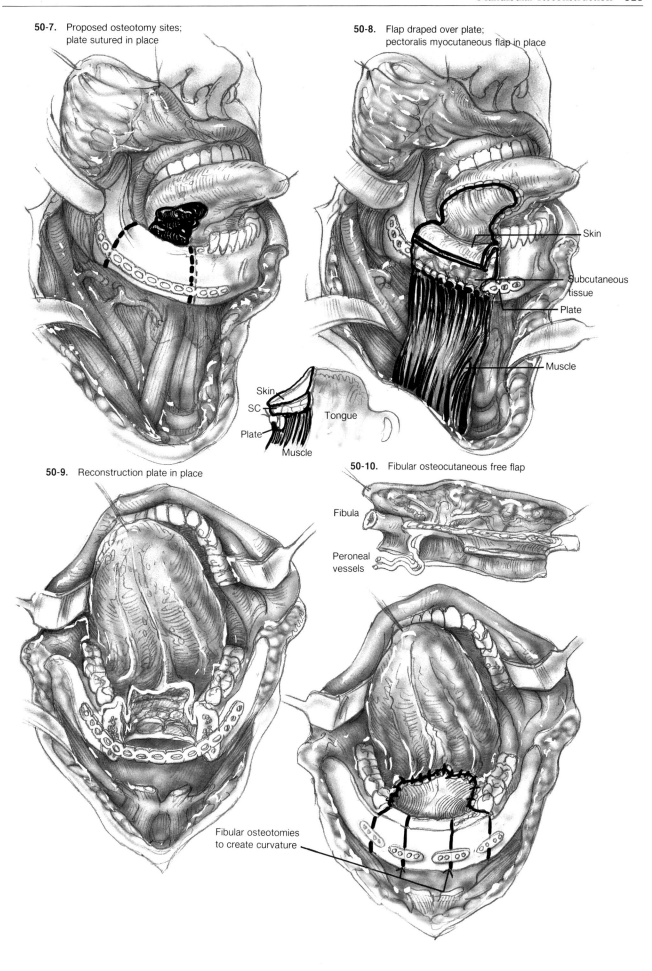

50-7. Proposed osteotomy sites; plate sutured in place

50-8. Flap draped over plate; pectoralis myocutaneous flap in place

Skin

Subcutaneous tissue

Plate

Muscle

Skin

SC

Plate

Muscle

Tongue

50-9. Reconstruction plate in place

50-10. Fibular osteocutaneous free flap

Fibula

Peroneal vessels

Fibular osteotomies to create curvature

■ 50. MANDIBULAR RECONSTRUCTION

(continued)

Pitfalls and Complications

1. Infection and graft failure
2. Exposure (externally or orally) of plate, graft, or tray
3. Absorption of graft
4. Nonunion at graft site or instability
5. Acute loss of flap in microvascular cases

Postoperative Care Issues

1. Closed suction drainage
2. Perioperative antibiotics
3. Full liquid diet; avoid chewing
4. For mucosal suture lines, no oral intake for 7 days and then resume full liquid diet.
5. For microvascular cases, monitor flap viability (use of skin paddle intraorally or extraorally).

References

Shockley WW, Weissler MC. Reconstructive alternatives following segmental mandibulectomy. Am J Otolaryngol 1992;13:156.

Urken ML, Weinburg H, Vickery C, et al. The internal oblique iliac crest osteomyocutaneous flap in reconstruction of composite defects of oral cavity involving bone, mucosa, and skin. Laryngoscope 1991;101:257.

Urken has been a proponent of the internal oblique iliac crest osseomyocutaneous flap. This tripartite flap is ideal for posterolateral defects and is harvested from the ipsilateral hip (Fig. 50-11). The shape may be designed to recreate the mandibular body-angle-ramus segment. A skin graft is used over the iliac crest muscle to resurface to oral cavity and oropharyngeal defect (Fig. 50-12).

WILLIAM W. SHOCKLEY

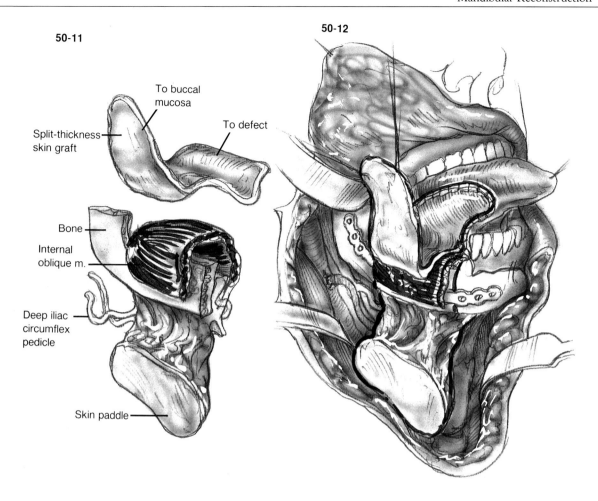

50-11

To buccal mucosa

To defect

Split-thickness skin graft

Bone

Internal oblique m.

Deep iliac circumflex pedicle

Skin paddle

50-12

■ 51. AURICULECTOMY
Surgical removal of the external ear

Indications
1. Carcinoma involving the entire auricle
2. Infection or avascular necrosis consuming the external ear (unlikely, because all efforts should be made to preserve some remnant of the auricle for later reconstruction)

Special Considerations
1. Total auriculectomy is seldom performed; partial preservation of the external ear improves the likelihood of subsequent reconstruction.
2. Patients requiring auriculectomy for carcinoma should also be considered for en bloc superficial parotidectomy because of the potential extension of tumor along fascial planes. Neck dissection is indicated for cervical or parotid adenopathy.
3. Carcinomas involving the medial half of the external auditory canal should be managed by temporal bone resection.

Preoperative Preparation
1. Routine laboratory studies
2. Chest x-ray and liver function tests to rule out metastatic disease in patients with extensive tumors
3. Computed tomography scan of temporal bone for extensive disease

Special Instruments, Position, and Anesthesia
1. Neck dissection set
2. Dermatome
3. Head rest

Tips and Pearls
1. A margin of at least 1 cm of normal tissue should be taken in patients with squamous cell carcinomas of the external ear.
2. Careful orientation of the specimen for the pathologists is necessary to avoid tumor-involved margins. This possibility can be minimized by sending margins for frozen-section examination from the patient after removing the tumor and adjacent normal appearing tissue.

Postoperative Care Issues
1. Radiation therapy should be strongly considered in the postoperative period for the patient with extensive local or regional disease.
2. Careful cleaning of the external auditory canal is necessary to maintain patency.

References
Conley JJ, Novak AJ. The surgical treatment of tumors of the ear and temporal bone. Arch Otolaryngol 1960;71:635.
Lewis JS, Page R. Radical surgery for tumors of the ear. Arch Otolaryngol 1966;83:114.

Operative Procedure
The patient is placed in the supine position, with the involved ear, adjacent scalp, and neck in the surgical field. The incisions should be planned to incorporate possible neck dissection or parotidectomy. In such patients, my colleagues and I prefer to perform the regional lymphadenectomy or parotid surgery as the first phase of the procedure (Figs. 51-1 and 51-2). The skin of the external canal is incised, and the canal skin elevated from medial to lateral positions. The auricle is widely resected en bloc, including the periosteum of the lateral temporal bone. Margin specimens are obtained from the patient and sent for histopathologic examination.

After confirming the surgical margins are free of disease, reconstruction should focus on three areas: soft tissue coverage of the lateral skull, preservation of the external auditory canal, and preparation for prosthetic or surgical restoration of the auricle. The choice of soft tissue coverage of the lateral skull depends on the availability of adjacent skin, which can be advanced or rotated to cover the surgical defect. One of the simpler techniques is to widely undermine the adjacent scalp and to undercut the galea. This procedure allows for increased elasticity of the galea. Local advancement flaps are relatively simple, but they are cosmetically less than desirable.

A more complicated repair includes mobilization of adjacent cervical skin, using the neck incision. An alternative and increasingly employed approach is to use myocutaneous or free flaps (Fig. 51-3). Both flaps have the advantage of providing large amounts of soft tissue for wound coverage and a high likelihood of success. The disadvantage is that they are significantly longer procedures. However, I prefer these flaps in wounds larger than 6 cm in the greatest diameter and recommend some rather than extensive mobilization of the scalp.

Preservation of the external auditory canal requires careful approximation of the soft tissue used for coverage of the lateral skull to the external canal and the lining of the canal with skin. The latter is best accomplished using a split-thickness skin graft (0.012 in [0.3 mm]). The graft should be sutured to the adjacent soft tissue and held within the canal with packing (Fig. 51-4). The suture line should be irregular or a variation of Z-plasty to minimize stenosis of the ear canal. I recommend the canal packing placed against the restored canal skin should be absorbable to avoid disturbing the skin at the time of packing removal.

Prosthetic reconstruction of the auricle is practical and much simplified with the advent of osteointegrated implants. These implants are placed directly into the lateral temporal bone at the time of the initial surgery. Success of the implant requires detailed preoperative planning, proper placement within the bone, and satisfactory soft tissue coverage (Figs. 51-5 and 51-6). The implants are available as one- or two-stage devices. The two-stage device requires a minor second procedure to expose the implant. The implant is placed approximately 4 mm into the temporal bone, and the lateral or exposed portion of the device is 1 to 3 mm superficial to the skin. The prosthetic ear can be prepared during the postoperative period and used several months after completion of all treatment modalities.

STEVEN D. SCHAEFER

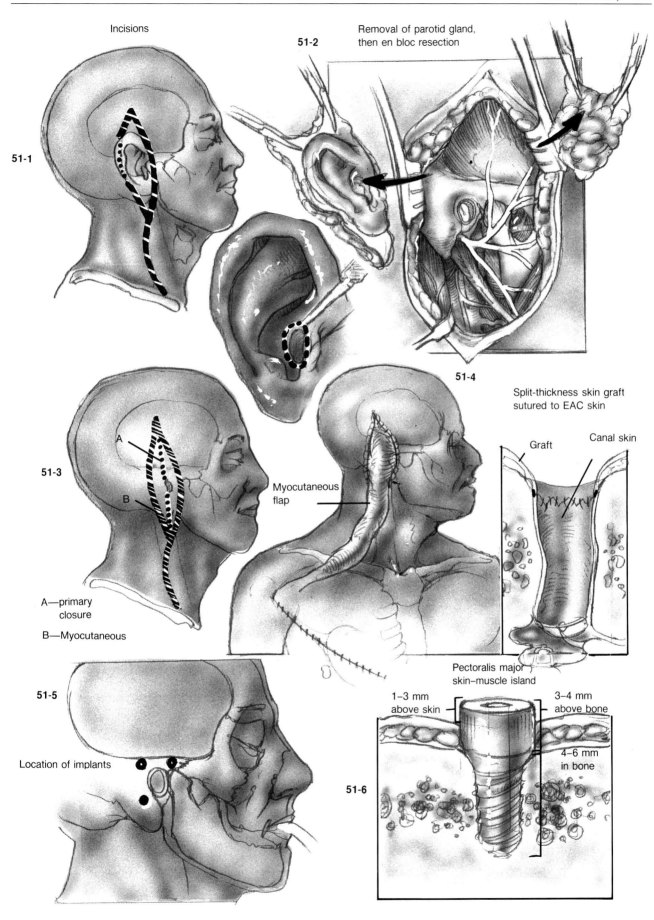

51-1   Incisions

51-2   Removal of parotid gland,
then en bloc resection

51-4

51-3

A—primary
closure

B—Myocutaneous

Myocutaneous
flap

Split-thickness skin graft
sutured to EAC skin

Graft   Canal skin

Pectoralis major
skin–muscle island

51-5   Location of implants

1–3 mm
above skin

3–4 mm
above bone

4–6 mm
in bone

51-6

■ *52.* PINNA RECONSTRUCTION: REGIONAL, WEDGE, AND STELLATE EXCISION—Reconstruction of the pinna after tumor excision or trauma

Indications

1. Primary closure for small lesions along the helical rim or antihelix without perichondrial invasion
2. Skin graft or local skin flap for larger, superficial defects of the helix or antihelix not involving cartilage
3. Composite graft or stellate-wedge excision for defects of the helical skin and cartilage requiring reconstruction of the cartilaginous framework

Contraindications

1. Any closure under tension heals poorly and distorts the shape of the pinna.
2. Grossly contaminated wounds more than 5 hours old and complex wounds from human bites should undergo delayed closure.
3. Uncertain status of margins of resection

Special Considerations

1. For high-risk patients (eg, recurrent carcinoma, invasive melanoma, tumors of the concha or postauricular sulcus), consider Mohs resection or 9- to 12-month delay before reconstruction.

Preoperative Preparation

1. Routine laboratory studies

Special Instruments, Position, and Anesthesia

1. General anesthesia or local infiltration and sedation
2. Expose and prepare both pinnae.

(continued)

Operative Procedure

Small, superficial defects along the helix and antihelix can be closed primarily after undermining (mostly posteriorly). The wound is closed with 6-0 nylon (Figs. 52-1 and 52-2).

The proposed area of wedge excision is outlined in Figure 52-3. Notice the inner, normal tissue, which is sacrificed to reestablish symmetry between peripheral and central areas. The wedge is excised, and the upper portion of pinna is rotated downward (Fig. 52-4). The perichondrium is closed with 5-0 Vicryl, and the skin is reapproximated with 6-0 nylon. An alternative method would be to use a composite graft approximately half the size of the surgical defect from the contralateral external ear (Fig 52-5). This would result in both ears appearing similar in size.

The wedge and stellate excisions are planned for identical lesions (Figs. 52-6 and 52-7). Notice that the stellate incision produces a break at conchoantihelical junction and that the wedge excision is

(continued)

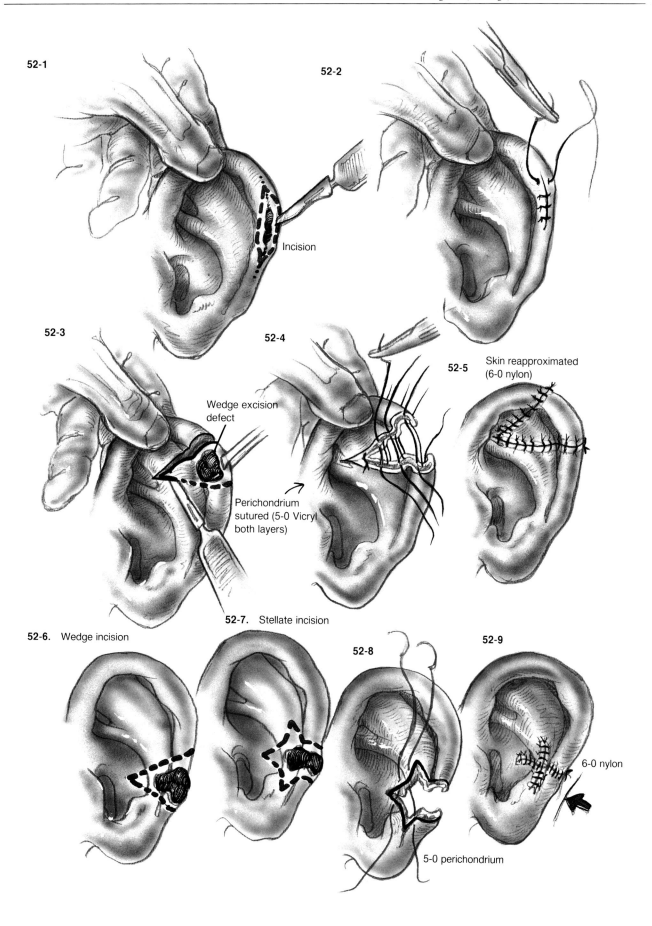

52-1

52-2

Incision

52-3

Wedge excision defect

Perichondrium sutured (5-0 Vicryl both layers)

52-4

52-5   Skin reapproximated (6-0 nylon)

52-6.   Wedge incision

52-7.   Stellate incision

52-8

52-9

6-0 nylon

5-0 perichondrium

■ *52.* PINNA RECONSTRUCTION: REGIONAL, WEDGE, AND STELLATE EXCISION (continued)

Tips and Pearls

1. Cartilage must be present at the helical margin to prevent late postoperative collapse.
2. Primary closure of defects of the helix and antihelix should be oriented parallel to the long axis to minimize reduction in pinna height.
3. Branches of the external carotid artery, the posterior auricular Artery (PAA) and superficial temporal artery extensively collateralize, forming two networks, one in the concha and one along the triangular and scaphoid fossae. The lobule is supplied by PAA.
4. Venous drainage parallels the arterial pattern. Posterior veins drain into the external jugular vein, occasionally connecting with the mastoid emissary vein. Anterior veins empty into the superficial temporal and retromandibular veins.
5. The lower half of the pinna is innervated by branches of the great auricular nerve. Branches of the auriculotemporal nerve innervate the superior lateral portion, and the superior medial surface is supplied by the lesser occipital nerve.

Pitfalls and Complications

1. Distortion and dehiscence due to closure under tension
2. Chondritis

Postoperative Considerations

1. Sterile cotton and mineral oil dressing to immobilize pinna
2. Skin sutures removed on postoperative day 7

References

Allison GR. Anatomy of the auricle. Clin Plast Surg 1990;17:209.

Antia NH, Buch VI. Chondrocutaneous advancement flap for the marginal defect of the ear. Plast Reconstr Surg 1967;39:472.

Converse JM, Brent B. Acquired deformities of the auricle. In: Converse JM, ed. Reconstructive plastic surgery. Philadelphia: WB Saunders, 1977:1724.

Menick FJ. Reconstruction of the ear after tumor excision. Clin Plast Surg 1990;17:405.

a straight line with a 90° angulation. Corresponding limbs of the excision should be of equal length. A composite excision is performed (Fig. 52-8). The flaps formed are then closed; 5-0 Vicryl closes both layers of the perichondrium, and 6-0 nylon is used to close the skin (Fig. 52-9).

For larger defects of the helical rim, a chondrocutaneous advancement flap can be performed. The lateral skin and cartilage of the helical root and superior pole, as well as inferiorly, are sharply incised (Fig. 52-10, *dashed lines*). The medial skin should be carefully preserved, because it serves as the pedicle of the flap. The flaps are then rotated into place. The helical root is closed in a V-to-Y fashion. The perichondrium is closed with 5-0 Vicryl, and the skin is closed with 6-0 nylon (Fig. 52-11).

STEVEN D. SCHAEFER
THOMAS ROMO III

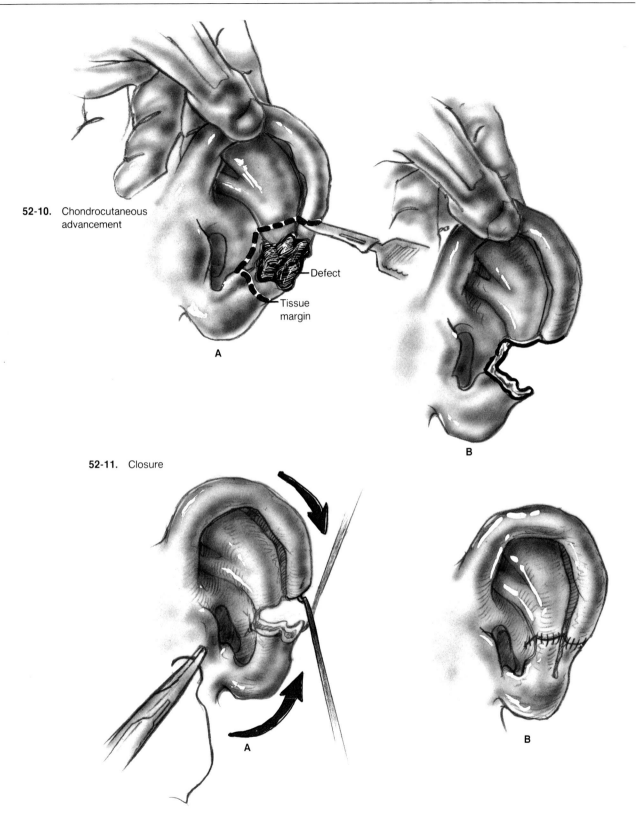

52-10. Chondrocutaneous advancement

Defect

Tissue margin

A

B

52-11. Closure

A

B

■ *53.* PINNA AND CONCHAL RECONSTRUCTION WITH COMPOSITE GRAFTS—Reconstruction of the pinna after tumor excision or trauma

Indications
1. Composite grafts and flaps for large defects of the pinna
2. Tunnel technique for cases of partial avulsions of the pinna more than 1.5 cm wide

Contraindications
1. Any closure under tension will heal poorly and distort the shape of the pinna.
2. Grossly contaminated wounds more than 5 hours old and complex wounds from human bites should undergo delayed closure.
3. Uncertain status of margins of resection

Special Considerations
1. For high-risk patients (eg, recurrent carcinoma, invasive melanoma, tumors of the concha or postauricular sulcus), consider Mohs resection or a 9- to 12-month delay before reconstruction.

Preoperative Preparation
1. Routine laboratory studies

Special Instruments, Position, and Anesthesia
1. General anesthesia or local infiltration and sedation.
2. Expose and prep both pinnae.

Tips and Pearls
1. Cartilage must exist at the helical margin to prevent late postoperative collapse.

Pitfalls and Complications
1. Distortion and dehiscence due to closure under tension
2. Chondritis

Postoperative Considerations
1. Sterile cotton or mineral oil dressing to immobilize the pinna
2. Skin sutures removed on the seventh postoperative day

References
Allison GR. Anatomy of the auricle. Clin Plast Surg 1990;17:209.

Converse JM, Brent B. Acquired deformities of the auricle. In: Converse JM, ed. Reconstructive plastic surgery. Philadelphia: WB Saunders, 1977:1724.

Menick FJ. Reconstruction of the ear after tumor excision. Clin Plast Surg 1990;17:405.

Pitanguy I, Flemming I. Plastic operations on the auricle. In: Neumann HH, ed. Head and neck surgery, vol 3. Philadelphia: WB Saunders, 1982:20.

Operative Procedure

Defects of the conchal skin, with or without cartilage, may be reconstructed with a full-thickness skin graft applied directly to perichondrium or periosteum (Fig. 53-1). Composite wedge grafts may be taken from the contralateral ear to replace large helical defects. The wedge removed should be exactly one-half the size of the defect to achieve maximal symmetry (Fig. 53-2). Larger defects of the helix can be reconstructed with the tunnel technique of Converse or with an anteriorly based postauricular skin flap (Fig. 53-3).

The Converse technique is useful in trauma cases if the avulsed portion of pinna is available; alternatively, cartilage may be harvested from the contralateral concha or scaphoid fossa. The pinna is folded back and the outline of the defect is drawn on the post-auricular skin (Fig. 53-4). The outlined incision is made with a #15 blade down to mastoid periosteum. The wound edges are undermined (mostly posteriorly). The posterior skin edge of the pinna defect is also incised with a #15 blade, and medial and lateral flaps are developed to expose the remaining cartilage. The medial pinna skin flap is then sutured to the anterior postauricular skin flap with interrupted 4-0 chromic sutures. The avulsed cartilage can be dermabraded to yield a cartilage-dermal graft, or the skin can be completely removed and only the cartilage used. Alternatively, cartilage can be harvested contralaterally from the concha or scapha. The cartilage is attached by suturing both layers of perichondrium with 5-0 Vicryl. The posterior flap of the postauricular incision is then sutured to the lateral flap of the pinna with interrupted 6-0 nylon.

Three to four weeks later, the suture lines can be released and the pinna lateralized. If dermis was left on the cartilage, it is allowed to epithelialize; if a free cartilage graft was used, the raw areas on the medial surface of the pinna and the postauricular region are skin grafted.

The postauricular skin flap of Dieffenbach has been modified to include cartilage for contour. A skin flap is developed that extends from the lateral helical surface, along the medial pinna, across the postauricular sulcus and onto the mastoid (see Fig. 53-4). Previously harvested cartilage is then sutured to the edge of the helical cartilage by approximating perichondrium with interrupted 5-0 Vicryl. The skin flap is then reflected back over the reconstructed cartilage framework and sutured in place with 6-0 nylon. A small area posterior to the end of the flap may be grafted with full-thickness skin.

A composite chondrocutaneous rotational flap can be harvested from the concha (based at the helical root) for reconstruction of the superior pole of the pinna (Fig. 53-5). Conchal skin and cartilage are raised and rotated superiorly to fill the defect. Perichondrium is sutured with interrupted 5-0 Vicryl, and the skin is closed with 6-0 nylon. The conchal bowl and medial surface of the flap are skin grafted.

STEVEN SCHAEFER
THOMAS ROMO III

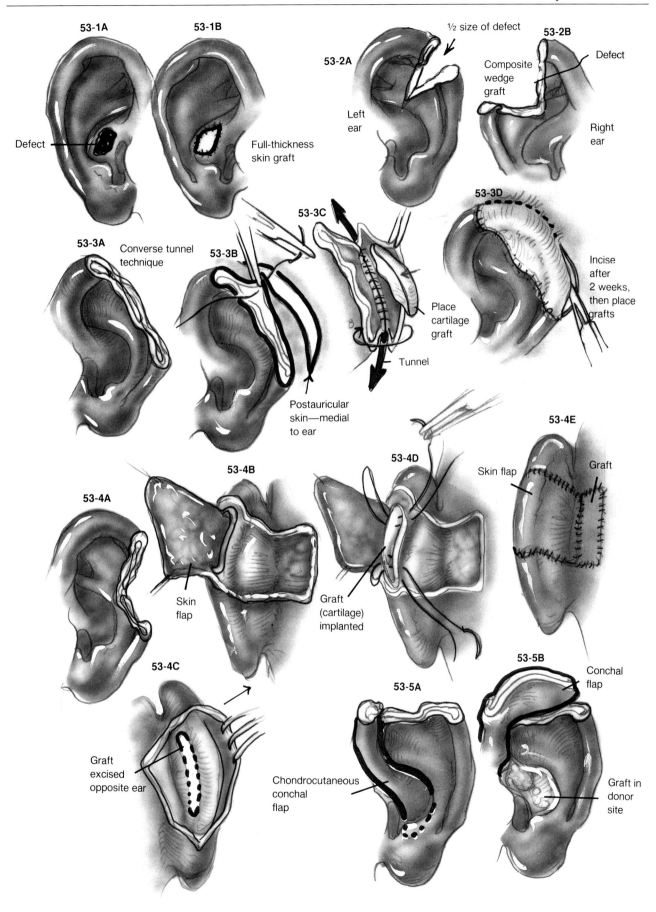

53-1A Defect

53-1B Full-thickness skin graft

53-2A Left ear ½ size of defect

53-2B Composite wedge graft Defect Right ear

53-3A Converse tunnel technique

53-3B Postauricular skin—medial to ear

53-3C Place cartilage graft Tunnel

53-3D Incise after 2 weeks, then place grafts

53-4A

53-4B Skin flap

53-4C Graft excised opposite ear

53-4D Graft (cartilage) implanted

53-4E Skin flap Graft

53-5A Chondrocutaneous conchal flap

53-5B Conchal flap Graft in donor site

■ *54.* LOCAL EXCISION AND SKIN GRAFT

Surgical removal of an auricular lesion with adequate margins and coverage with a split-thickness skin graft

Indications

1. Benign and malignant neoplastic processes within the confines of the auricle
2. Chronic suppurative processes unresponsive to medical management and local wound care

Special Considerations

1. Careful preoperative history and physical examination with attention to adnexal structures and the neck so that the extent of the disease is not underestimated
2. Plan to do a larger resection than indicated by visual margins.
3. Consider a composite graft of cartilage and skin if underlying cartilage must be taken.
4. Preoperative planning and coordination with a pathologist experienced in microsurgical marginal control (ie, Mohs chemosurgery)

Preoperative Preparation

1. Routine laboratory studies
2. Clotting studies, if applicable
3. Clearance for general anesthesia
4. Consider contralateral audition before surgery. The operated ear must be temporarily packed, which may cause a conductive hearing loss.

Special Instruments, Position, and Anesthesia

1. Adequate illumination
2. Prepare the ear and the donor site; consider local, regional, and distant sites.
3. Dermatome
4. General anesthesia is preferable if more than a pinch graft is required.

Tips and Pearls

1. Mark the boundaries of the lesion under magnification (loupes or microscope) before the injection of local anesthetic.
2. Ensure sufficient negative surgical margins before grafting.
3. Exposed cartilage must be covered.
4. Consider several methods of grafting and closure before surgery.
5. The skin graft must be thin enough to reveal an early recurrence.
6. "Pie crust" the graft, and compress it with a bolster.

Pitfalls and Complications

1. Underestimation of disease—be prepared to do a larger operation, including regional lymphadenectomy.
2. Lack of adequate coverage. Chondritis or perichondritis (rare) may result from infection of exposed cartilage.
3. Recurrence of disease is less likely with chemosurgical control.
4. Graft failure may require secondary grafting.

Postoperative Care Issues

1. Infection (especially perichondritis or chondritis) is best prevented with complete coverage. Superficial infection is managed with local wound care.
2. Graft failure may result from infection, hematoma or seroma formation, or inadequate recipient blood supply.
3. Careful follow-up for recurrence of disease
4. A hearing aid may be worn after the graft has completely taken.

References

Larson PO, Ragi B, Mohs FE, Snow SN. Excision of exposed cartilage for management of Mohs surgery defects of the ear. J Dermatol Surg Oncol 1991;9:749.

Niparko JK, Swanson NA, Baker SR, Telian SA, Sullivan MJ, Kemink JL. Local control of auricular, preauricular and external canal cutaneous malignancies with Mohs surgery. Laryngoscope 1990;100L:1047.

Stone JL. Mohs micrographic surgery: a synopsis. Hawaii Med J 1993;5:134.

Operative Procedure

The ear is sterilely prepped and draped, and the lesion to be excised is outlined. A margin of approximately 0.5 to 1.0 cm is usually added to allow for complete removal. This should be marked before infiltration of local anesthetic (Fig. 54-1). A graft site providing sufficient non–hair-bearing skin with a good match for color and texture is selected. Choices include the postauricular area, the medial surface of the upper arm, the suprapubic area, and the buttock.

The lesion is next infiltrated with a solution of 1% lidocaine with 1:100,000 epinephrine. A stronger solution of 1% lidocaine with 1:30,000 epinephrine may be used if desired. The lesion in excised en toto, with a margin of normal tissue included (Fig. 54-2). The microscope or loupes may be used to facilitate resection. The lesion is oriented with a sketch and sent en bloc to the pathologist for Mohs chemosurgical control (Fig. 54-3). It is helpful to break scrub at this time and personally take the specimen to the pathologist.

If margins are positive, additional tissue is taken until tumor-negative margins have been obtained. The bed is then inspected for any questionable areas, and hemostasis is obtained. It is important not to overly cauterize the recipient site.

Most surgical defects are quite small and require minimal grafting. Lesions smaller than 0.5 cm may be allowed to granulate and close by secondary intention if cartilage has not been exposed. Exposed cartilage must be covered to prevent infection.

A split-thickness skin graft is obtained with a hand-held dermatome or a sharp blade. The area to be grafted may be approximated by placing a sterile piece of paper or the foil wrapper from a suture over the site and marking it accordingly (Fig. 54-4). This pattern is then transferred to the skin graft. The graft is "pie crusted" to allow for drainage of blood and serum and placed on the bed of the defect. Any final sizing is done as it is sutured in place (Fig. 54-5). Sewing from the graft to the surrounding tissue (ie, "from ship to shore") helps prevent distortion.

The graft should be stabilized by packing the ear with strips of lubricated gauze (eg, Xeroderm) or tied under a bolster of cotton wool or gauze to prevent shearing during the healing period (Fig. 54-6). The donor site is dressed with Xeroderm or a clear plastic dressing, such as Tegaderm.

STEVEN D. SCHAEFER
CHRISTOPHER J. LINSTROM

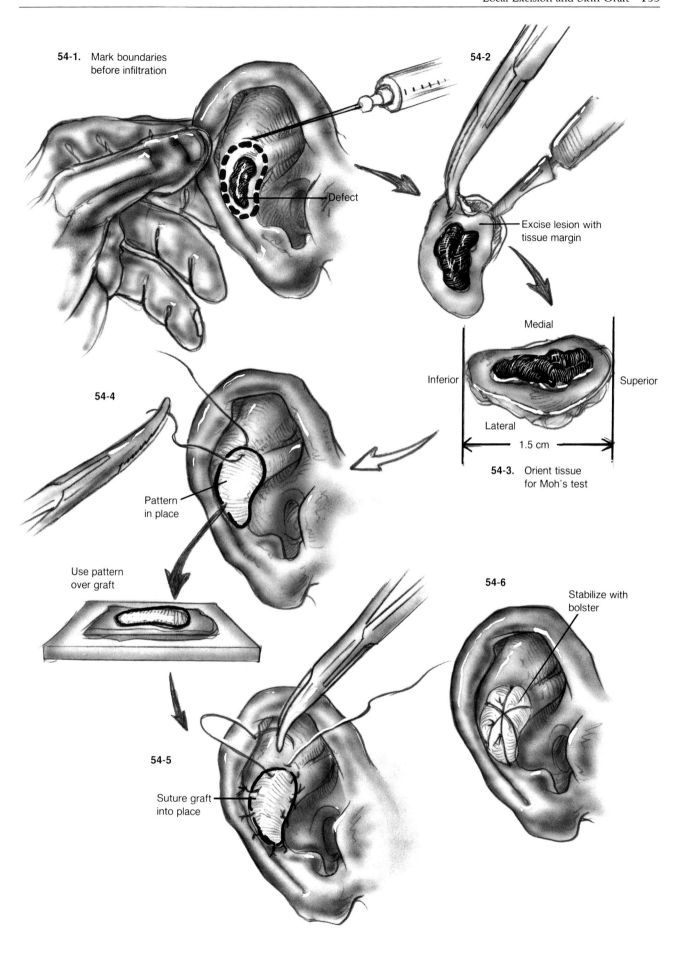

54-1. Mark boundaries before infiltration

Defect

54-2 Excise lesion with tissue margin

Medial

Inferior

Lateral

Superior

1.5 cm

54-3. Orient tissue for Moh's test

54-4 Pattern in place

Use pattern over graft

54-6 Stabilize with bolster

54-5 Suture graft into place

■ *55.* SUPERFICIAL, INTERMEDIATE, AND RADICAL TEMPORAL BONE RESECTION—Partial or nearly complete en bloc resection of the temporal bone

Indications
1. Cancer originating on the auricle
2. Cancers originating within the middle ear or mastoid
3. Skin cancers extending to the auditory canal
4. Neoplasms adjacent to the stylomastoid foramen

Contraindications
1. Malignant tumor extension medial to the carotid
2. Malignant tumor extension beyond the dura

Special Considerations
1. Attempts to save all or a portion of the helix
2. Attempts to resect less than all of the external auditory canal
3. Tumor at or posterior to the postauricular sulcus
4. Tumor extending into the glenoid fossa
5. Tumors with limited encroachment on the temporal bone
6. Prosthetics

Preoperative Preparation
1. Computed tomography (CT) scans of the temporal bone, parotid, and neck
2. Careful review of the pathology, clinical characteristics, CT scans, and plans for intraoperative resection and closure and postoperative treatment, including radiotherapy and prostheses

Special Instruments, Position, and Anesthesia
1. The patient is supine on one side of the table, with the head at the foot of the table to allow the surgeon to sit when necessary
2. Special head holders, such as a Mayfield, are usually unnecessary.
3. Tape or belt the patient to the table across the shoulders, hips, and thighs so the table may be rotated about its longitudinal axis.
4. Otologic operating microscope and otologic drill
5. Microvascular operating microscope
6. Anesthesiologist at the patient's feet

Tips and Pearls
1. Mark resection lines carefully, leaving adequate margins.
2. When the skin incisions about the tumor have been made, staple or suture plastic or gauze to the tumor side of the skin margins.
3. Never dissect such that the tumor is seen. Resection should be performed with adequate soft tissue and bone margins.
4. Plan deep intraosseous bone cuts and landmarks available to be seen and followed from that perspective; the standard landmarks used in other temporal bone work may not be available.
5. Extend transcortical and transmastoid epitympanic cuts through the anterior attic compartment to enter the glenoid fossa.
6. Extend the fascial recess approach, working through the wide expanse of the tympanic bone inferiorly, to the glenoid fossa.
7. The tympanic bone inferiorly gives an intraosseous route about 1 cm wide for dissection between the landmarks of the preserved osseous lumen of the external auditory canal and the neck muscle attachments to the skull base.
8. Under direct vision, a connecting cut between the superior and inferior glenoid fossa entries may be made with the otologic drill medial to the anterior tympanic annulus by lowering the medial facial recess margin to the nerve and horizontal canal and retracting the manubrium and tympanic membrane laterally to the plane of the fibrous annulus.
9. The facial nerve occupies the anterior-most aspect of the stylomastoid foramen–digastric periosteal sheath and must be exposed to allow precise dissection through the foramen.
10. If the middle ear or any pneumatized space is invaded by tumor, a near-total temporal bone resection is necessary for en bloc resection of all pneumatized spaces without entry.
11. The otic capsule, internal auditory canal, internal carotid canal, and jugular foramen are key intraosseous pathways for near-

(continued)

Operative Procedures
Intermediate or Lateral Temporal Bone Resection

The ear incisions are marked, being careful to give at least 1 cm or more margin around a malignant tumor and being careful to remember the three-dimensional nature of the temporal bone, tumor, and necessary resection. If some of the helix and antihelix are to be saved, extending the pretragal parotid–neck flap incision superiorly into a partial coronal flap allows the remaining pinna and postauricular tissues to be displaced posteriorly (Fig. 55-1). If all of the auricle is to be resected circumferentially, this superior extension may not be necessary (Fig. 55-2). The tragus, concha, all soft tissue medial to these structures, and the adjacent medial bone is taken en bloc with the specimen; this bone includes the pericanal mastoid cortex and complete circumference of the cartilaginous and osseous external auditory canal. A superficial parotidectomy and upper neck dissection are included in the en bloc dissection (Fig. 55-3). A total parotidectomy, full neck dissection, condylectomy, and resection of the complete glenoid fossa may be necessary if other structures are involved with tumor.

The mastoid cortex, posterior and superior to the cortex to be taken with the specimen, is exposed, and a transcortical mastoidectomy is performed, undercutting the cortex to be maintained in continuity with the intact external auditory canal specimen. The middle fossa dura that is seen through the thinned bone and a thinned osseous canal are the landmarks to be followed to enter the glenoid fossa superiorly and cut through the root of the zygoma (Fig. 55-4). Periosteum over the neck muscles attaching to the skull base, the thinned osseous canal, fibrous annulus, the fallopian canal, and the lateral circumference of the stylomastoid foramen are the landmarks to be followed while extending the fascial recess through the tympanic bone to enter the glenoid fossa inferiorly (Fig. 55-5).

The mastoid tip lateral to the posterior belly of the digastric muscles is removed or separated to be taken with the specimen, and the facial nerve is dissected through the stylomastoid foramen to begin the parotidectomy and neck dissection, beginning posterosuperiorly (Fig. 55-6).

After the specimen has been removed, the mastoid defect is closed by obliteration with a viable anteroinferiorly based temporalis muscle flap and skin graft or radial forearm microvascular skin and subcutaneous tissue free flap.

Radical Temporal Bone Resection

Radical temporal bone resection is necessary if the middle ear or any pneumatized space is invaded with malignant tumor.

The patient is positioned in a Mayfield head holder with tongs and prepared for middle and posterior fossa craniectomy.

The incision is a postauricular-suboccipital incision, with gentle curves anterosuperiorly into a coronal incision and anteroinferiorly into a neck incision, cutting across the pinna-canal area. Circumferential removal of all the pinna en bloc with the specimen removes the tip of this broad, bipedicled flap. If some of the pinna is to be spared, it remains attached to the anteriorly reflected flap (Fig. 55-7).

Middle and posterior fossa craniectomies are performed extradurally. The dura and the dural sinuses are dissected from the posterior and middle fossa attachments to the temporal bone as far as possible. At this point, the neck and the parotid may be dissected or await most of the osseous cuts to be made.

The osseous cuts begin in the middle fossa by skeletonizing and entering the carotid canal, cochlea, vestibule, and bone medial to the semicircular canals and perilabyrinthine cells, taking care not to enter air cells and to preserve the lateral osseous walls of these structures. The soft tissue and osseous incisions transect the seventh and eighth cranial nerves. The dura and dural sinuses continue to be exposed and dissected from the specimen. Dissection through the cochlea, internal auditory canal, vestibule, and dissection of the

(continued)

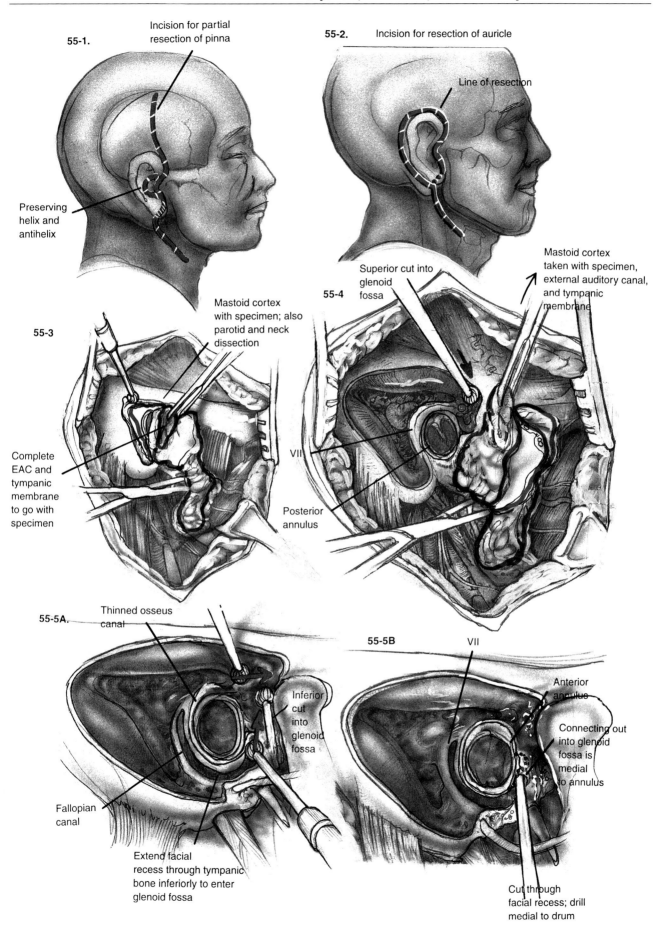

55-1.   Incision for partial resection of pinna

Preserving helix and antihelix

55-2.   Incision for resection of auricle

Line of resection

55-3

Mastoid cortex with specimen; also parotid and neck dissection

Complete EAC and tympanic membrane to go with specimen

55-4   Superior cut into glenoid fossa

Mastoid cortex taken with specimen, external auditory canal, and tympanic membrane

VII

Posterior annulus

55-5A.   Thinned osseus canal

Inferior cut into glenoid fossa

Fallopian canal

Extend facial recess through tympanic bone inferiorly to enter glenoid fossa

55-5B   VII

Anterior annulus

Connecting out into glenoid fossa is medial to annulus

Cut through facial recess; drill medial to drum

■ 55. SUPERFICIAL, INTERMEDIATE, AND RADICAL TEMPORAL BONE RESECTION

(continued)

total temporal bone resection. Dissections through these sites must maintain osseous barrier between dissection and tumor.

12. Near-total temporal bone resection requires large middle fossa and posterior fossa craniectomies, necessitating the assistance of a neurosurgeon.

13. In the near-total temporal bone resection, the surgeon approaches the internal carotid canal from the middle fossa superomedially and dissects the carotid from the canal, leaving intact the lateral wall of the carotid canal to go with the tumor.

14. In the near-total resection, the surgeon enters the jugular foramen medially and maintains the superior bony foramen wall intact to be excised with the tumor.

15. Although the sigmoid and internal jugular vein are ligated, severe bleeding still comes from the inferior petrosal sinus; this must be occluded immediately from the jugular bulb lumen when opened.

16. Watertight closure of dural defects must be accomplished.

17. Viable soft tissue flaps or microvascular free grafts are usually required for closure, especially if cerebrospinal fluid leaks occur or postoperative radiotherapy is planned.

18. The skin of the external canal medial to the resection margins must be biopsied if attempting to save some of the canal.

19. Circumferential section of the glenoid fossa and condyle is required if tumor invades the glenoid fossa.

20. After a superficial or intermediate resection, it is possible to let the modified or radical mastoid cavity obliterate, healing by secondary intention; however, healing is much more rapid and controlled if the defect is primarily repaired.

Pitfalls and Complications

1. Stenosis of a partially saved external auditory canal
2. Late osteoradionecrosis with infection may occasionally occur in cases not obliterated with viable tissue.
3. Intraoperative tumor exposure and subsequent tumor recurrence may result if postauricular tumor elevated off mastoid cortex.
4. If invaded by tumor, attempts at less than en bloc resection of the glenoid fossa may result in recurrence.
5. Resections of invaded petrous apex marrow medial to the carotid may be futile if done for cure.
6. Resections of invading tumor deep to the dura may be futile.
7. Attempts to resect malignant tumors at the mastoid tip or stylomastoid foramen without including limited temporal bone resections as part of the en bloc approach may lead to tumor recurrence.
8. Attempts to make blind chisel cuts may result in fractures that expose the tumor or cause excessive bleeding.
9. "Sleeve" resections of the external auditory canal skin alone have no place in the resection of these malignancies.
10. When dissecting through the tympanic bone, care must be taken to avoid injury to the jugular bulb and internal carotid artery.
11. When dissecting medial to the anterior annulus, care must be taken to avoid injury to the internal carotid artery.
12. If malignant tumor invades any pneumatized space and all pneumatized spaces are not resected en bloc, tumor recurrence is expected.
13. Cerebrospinal fluid leaks are probable if a watertight closure and viable soft tissue obliterative closure have not been achieved.

Postoperative Care Issues

1. If a cerebrospinal fluid leak occurs, lumbar spinal fluid drainage may help the defect heal spontaneously.
2. Perioperative antibiotics may be useful.
3. If required, an auricular prosthesis should be used for cosmesis.

References

Neely JG, Forrester M. Anatomic considerations of the medial cuts in the subtotal temporal bone resection. Otolaryngol Head Neck Surg 1982;90:641.

internal carotid artery from its canal are completed through the temporal bone to the neck, removing bone medially to the dura and maintaining the integrity of the osseous barrier between the dissection plane and the tumor (Fig. 55-8).

The dissection is carried anterolaterally through the glenoid fossa and posterolaterally along the sigmoid and jugular bulb to the neck, carotid, and internal jugular vein, avoiding entering these vascular structures. Care must be taken to completely detach the intact carotid artery from the temporal bone. At this point, the parotid, neck dissection area, and temporal bone are attached only at the jugular foramen and inferior petrosal sinus; care must be taken not to fracture through the jugular bulb.

The sigmoid sinus and internal jugular vein are ligated. The jugular bulb is entered from posterolaterally, and the inferior petrosal sinus is occluded immediately (Fig. 55-9). The specimen is delivered.

The only cerebrospinal fluid leak is usually at the porus acusticus, which is repaired with fascia in a watertight closure. The facial nerve is repaired with cable grafts and the defect obliterated with viable soft tissue and skin.

Superficial Temporal Bone Resection

Superficial temporal bone resections are reserved for special cases of minimal involvement of the temporal bone. If a tumor involves only the tragus or the concha and is benign or malignant with very superficial involvement of the skin and does not involve cartilage or external canal, it may be locally excised down to but not into bone, taking full-thickness cartilage. If a very small and limited malignant tumor superficially involves the lateral-most cartilaginous canal and clearly does not approach to within 1 cm of the osseous canal, this same operation may be done. All margins must be checked histologically during surgery; beware of underestimating these cases.

If a similarly limited malignant tumor enters the external auditory canal or penetrates cartilage, lateral mastoid cortex medial to the concha and circumferential osseous canal are taken with the specimen. The party wall of the anterior external canal and posterior glenoid fossa are removed en bloc with the specimen; "sleeve" resection of the skin alone should never be done. The osseous canal may be transected lateral to the tympanic membrane if the skin margins that remain with the patient are histologically free of tumor (Fig. 55-10).

If tumor is fixed to the mastoid tip laterally and does not involve the pinna or canal, the tip lateral to the posterior belly of digastric muscle is resected en bloc with the specimen. This begins by performing a mastoidectomy, following the facial nerve through the stylomastoid foramen and detaching the tip anteriorly with a drill bone cut laterally from the foramen, posteriorly, with a cut through the cortex along the digastric, and medially, with exposure of the digastric (Fig. 55-11).

If malignant tumor from the parotid or neck involves the stylomastoid foramen, the foramen, with that segment of the facial nerve, may be resected en bloc with the tumor. This procedure begins with a mastoidectomy and exposure of the proximal mastoid segment of the facial nerve. The fallopian canal and nerve are transected just inferior to the posterior semicircular canal. The dissection is carried along the digastric posteriorly, as previously described, but it then proceeds medially deep to the stylomastoid foramen, into and through the medial tip cells to the neck and jugular foramen (without entering the bulb). The dissection is carried through the facial nerve and through the substance of the inferior portion of the tympanic bone, maintaining the intact osseous lumen of the external auditory canal, along a plane just lateral to the lateral wall of the jugular foramen and internal carotid artery to the glenoid fossa and neck medial to the tumor and stylomastoid foramen (Fig. 55-12).

J. GAIL NEELY
HAROLD C. PILLSBURY

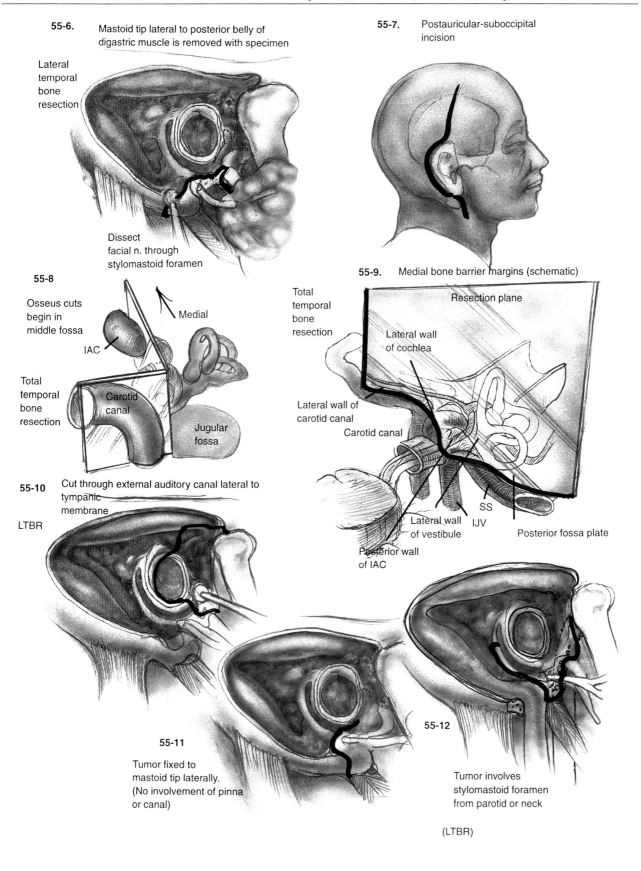

55-6. Mastoid tip lateral to posterior belly of digastric muscle is removed with specimen

Lateral temporal bone resection

Dissect facial n. through stylomastoid foramen

55-7. Postauricular-suboccipital incision

55-8

Osseus cuts begin in middle fossa

IAC

Medial

Total temporal bone resection

Carotid canal

Jugular fossa

55-9. Medial bone barrier margins (schematic)

Total temporal bone resection

Resection plane

Lateral wall of cochlea

Lateral wall of carotid canal

Carotid canal

Lateral wall of vestibule

Posterior wall of IAC

SS

IJV

Posterior fossa plate

55-10 Cut through external auditory canal lateral to tympanic membrane

LTBR

55-11 Tumor fixed to mastoid tip laterally. (No involvement of pinna or canal)

55-12 Tumor involves stylomastoid foramen from parotid or neck

(LTBR)

■ 56. VARIOUS INCISIONS FOR NECK SURGERY

—Incisions for neck surgery may require exposure for a limited area of dissection (eg, lymph node biopsy) or for complete exposure of the neck (eg, radical neck dissection).

Indications

1. Providing adequate exposure of the cervical lymph node groups targeted for removal
2. Permitting extension of the incision for removal of additional lymph node groups (eg, ipsilateral, contralateral)
3. Providing proper surgical exposure when the primary cancer is concomitantly excised

Special Considerations

1. The incision should be placed over the area to be exposed. If wider exposure is subsequently required, the initial incision should be placed to permit extending it in a manner that optimally meets the goals outlined earlier.

Preoperative Preparation

1. Neck skin and upper chest should be shaved and prepped.
2. Maintain important surface landmarks in the draped field (eg, chin, ear lobe, clavicle).
3. A folded sterile towel provides support for the drapes along the posterolateral neck.

Tips and Pearls

1. Place incisions along natural crease lines to camouflage the scar.
2. Use deeper sutures to relieve tension on the skin closure.

Pitfalls and Complications

1. Avoid the use of trifurcating incisions, particularly in radiated tissue.
2. Incisions and flaps should be designed to maintain optimal blood supply to the flap, to minimize the risk for flap necrosis and wound dehiscence, and to provide the best cosmetic result possible.

Postoperative Care Issues

1. Maintain neck drains on constant suction until fluid accumulation ceases, which is usually in 3 to 5 days, depending on the nature and extent of the surgery.

Reference

Robbins KT. Neck dissection: classification and incisions. In: Shockley W, Pillsbury H, eds. The neck: diagnosis and treatment. St. Louis: Mosby, 1993.

Operative Procedure

Three types of neck incisions are recommended: modified apron, hockey stick, and inverted hockey stick.

Modified Apron Incision

The modified apron incision (Fig. 56-1) is used for exposure of level I, II, and III lymph node groups (ie, selective neck dissection of the supraomohyoid type). The lateral vertical limb extends from the mastoid tip superiorly to where the omohyoid muscle crosses the carotid sheath inferiorly. The medial vertical limb starts in the submental triangle and extends inferiorly in a smooth, gradual curve to meet the lateral limb. The incision line curves around the thyroid prominence to minimize its visibility. The medial limb can be readily extended superiorly for access to the oral cavity (ie, lip-splitting incision). The blood supply to this flap is from cutaneous branches of the facial artery.

For bilateral procedures, the incision is extended across the midline to create a symmetric apron flap. When raised, this flap provides exposure of the corresponding contralateral lymph node groups of levels I through III.

Hockey Stick Incision

The hockey stick incision (Fig. 56-2) is used for exposure of level II through V lymph node groups associated with cancers arising in the pharynx, larynx, or other midline visceral structures. The vertical limb starts at the mastoid process superiorly and extends inferiorly across the posterior triangle toward the clavicle. The superior part of this vertical limb extends across the upper part of the sternocleidomastoid muscle, and the lower part lies behind the sternal head of this muscle, paralleling its posterior border. The hockey stick incision then curves sharply toward the midline in the midregion of the posterior triangle, paralleling the clavicle about 3 cm above it.

If necessary, the incision can be extended across the midline to create a symmetric, broadly based apron flap for bilateral dissections. If tracheostomy is required, the incision can be incorporated into the horizontal component of the neck incision. Blood is supplied by the cutaneous branches of the facial artery.

Inverted Hockey Stick Incision

The inverted hockey stick incision (Fig. 56-3) is used as an alternative to the modified apron incision for unilateral neck dissections associated with cancers arising in the oral cavity and oropharynx. It provides excellent exposure of level I, II, and III lymph nodes (ie, in supraomohyoid neck dissection). Its vertical limb extends inferiorly, providing adequate exposure for the additional removal of levels IV and V (ie, in modified radical or radical neck dissection). The horizontal component of the incision extends across the upper neck from the submental triangle medially, paralleling the body of the mandible, toward the mastoid tip laterally. The vertical component extends inferiorly across the posterior triangle toward the junction of the clavicle with the anterior border of the trapezius.

The horizontal component of the incision can be extended across the midline for bilateral neck dissections. The blood supply of the resulting inferiorly based flap is from the cutaneous branches of the transverse cervical and supraclavicular arteries extending superiorly in a vertical direction. Care is taken to place the vertical limb of the incision over the lateral part of the lower posterior triangle to encompass the arterial branches from the transverse cervical artery entering laterally. The angle of the junction between the horizontal and vertical limbs is 90° or greater.

Variations

Incisions for most other neck procedures can be incorporated into part or all of one of the recommended patterns. For example, exposure of the midline anterior compartment for thyroidectomy is provided through the horizontal component of the bilateral hockey stick incision. Exposure of the submandibular triangle for removal of the gland is provided through the horizontal component of the unilateral inverted hockey stick incision. Exposure for parotidectomy in conjunction with neck dissection is provided by extending the vertical component of the unilateral modified apron incision superiorly in the preauricular crease.

K. THOMAS ROBBINS

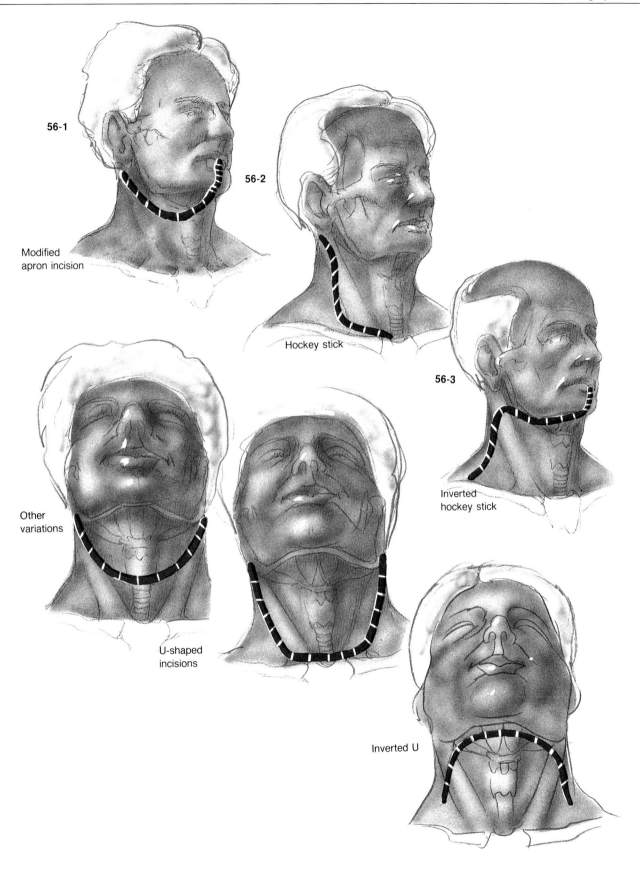

56-1

Modified
apron incision

56-2

Hockey stick

56-3

Inverted
hockey stick

Other
variations

U-shaped
incisions

Inverted U

■ *57*. RADICAL NECK DISSECTION

A comprehensive neck dissection that removes lymph node groups I through V, the sternocleidomastoid muscle, the internal jugular vein, and XI nerve.

Indications

1. Cancer involving multiple cervical lymph node metastases, particularly if they are located in the posterior triangle of the neck near the spinal accessory nerve
2. A large metastatic tumor mass or multiple matted nodes in the upper portion of the neck
3. After ill-advised open incisional biopsy of a neck node, when extensive undermining and postoperative inflammation obscure the relation of the tumor to the sternocleidomastoid muscle, spinal accessory nerve, and internal jugular vein

Contraindications

1. No palpable cervical metastases, as in the treatment of the node-negative neck

Special Considerations

1. The site and extent of the primary tumor
2. Bilateral palpable metastases make it desirable to preserve the internal or the external jugular vein on the side of the neck less involved.
3. Encroachment or involvement of the skin of the neck
4. Encroachment or involvement of the carotid artery
5. Previous radiation treatment
6. Previous neck surgery

Preoperative Preparation

1. Appropriate laboratory studies
2. A computed tomography scan may be necessary to assess the relation of the tumor to the carotid artery, paraspinal muscles, and cervical vertebrae.
3. Four-vessel angiogram, with balloon occlusion test, if carotid resection is considered

Special Instruments, Position, and Anesthesia

1. Vascular instruments if carotid resection or a graft is anticipated.
2. Neck extended with roll under shoulders, with the head turned to opposite side and stabilized in a foam doughnut
3. Alert the anesthesia department to the possibility of resecting both internal jugular veins. Fluid administration should be reduced to about 50 mL/hour after ligation of the second internal jugular vein to avoid cerebral edema.

(continued)

Operative Procedure

The incisions most commonly used to perform a neck dissection are discussed in Procedure 56. Skin flaps are elevated in a subplatysmal plane. However, for a large tumor mass, the platysma is left attached to it as the skin flaps are elevated.

Dissection of the Submandibular Triangle

As the superior neck flap is elevated, the ramus mandibularis is exposed by incising the superficial layer of the deep cervical fascia that envelopes the submandibular gland, immediately above the gland and about 1 cm in front and below the angle of the mandible. The incised fascia is gently pushed superiorly, exposing the nerve that lies deep to it but superficial to the adventitia of the anterior facial vein. The submandibular prevascular and retrovascular lymph nodes, which are usually close to the nerve, are carefully dissected away from it. In doing so, the facial vessels are exposed and divided (Fig. 57-1).

The fibrous fatty tissue of the submental triangle is dissected off of the anterior bellies of the digastric muscles and the mylohyoid. The fascia is then dissected off of the anterior belly of the digastric muscle, and the specimen is retracted posteriorly, removing the fibrous fatty tissue containing lymph nodes lateral to the mylohyoid muscle. When the dissection reaches the posterior border of the mylohyoid, the muscle is retracted anteriorly, exposing the lingual nerve and the submandibular gland duct, which are divided (Fig. 57-2). The hypoglossal nerve and the veins that usually accompany it are left undisturbed as the dissection continues in a posterior direction. The facial artery is ligated as it crosses forward, under the posterior belly of the digastric, completing the dissection of the submandibular gland (Fig. 57-3).

Upper Dissection

The tail of the parotid gland is transected, and the posterior facial vein and the greater auricular nerve are divided. The sternocleidomastoid muscle is then incised close to its insertion in the mastoid process. The fibrofatty tissue medial to the muscle is incised, exposing the splenius capitis and the levator scapulae muscles. Depending on the location and the extent of the tumor in the neck, it may be necessary to include the posterior belly of the digastric in the dissected specimen. Otherwise, incising the fascia below the digastric and gentle inferior traction of the specimen allows identification of the hypoglossal nerve, the upper end of the internal jugular vein, and the spinal accessory nerve. At this point in the dissection, the internal jugular vein and the spinal accessory nerve are divided if the location and extent of the tumor permit it (Fig. 57-4).

Posterior Dissection

The dissection is continued posteriorly and inferiorly along the anterior border of the trapezius muscle. The fibrofatty tissue of the posterior triangle of the neck is then dissected forward and downward in a plane immediately lateral to the fascia of the splenius and the levator scapulae muscles. The spinal accessory nerve and the transverse cervical vessels are divided as they cross the anterior border of the trapezius muscle (Fig. 57-5). During this portion of the operation, it is important to preserve the branches of the cervical plexus that innervate the levator scapulae muscle, unless the extent of the disease in the neck precludes it.

(continued)

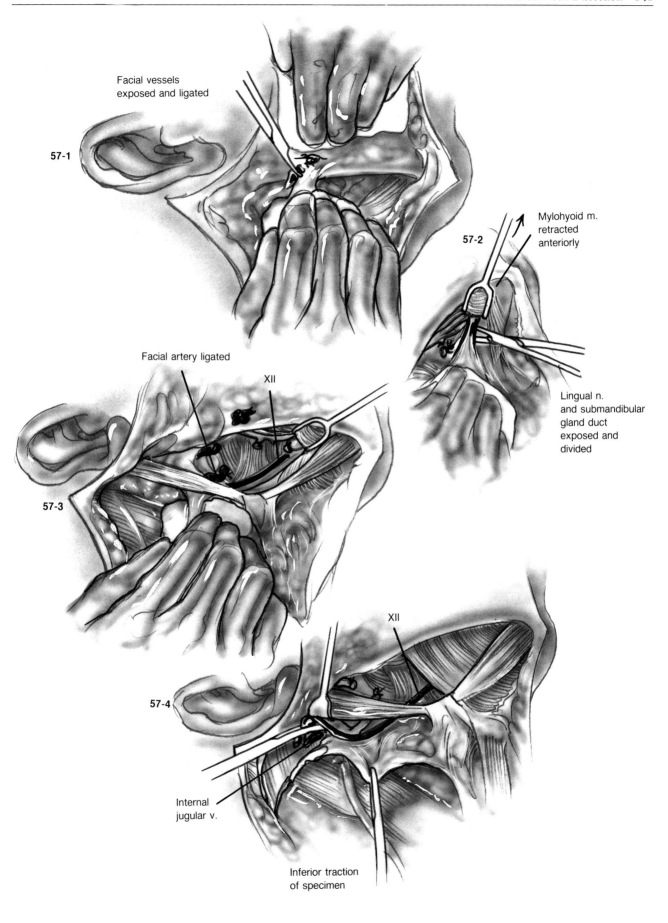

Facial vessels
exposed and ligated

57-1

57-2

Mylohyoid m.
retracted
anteriorly

Lingual n.
and submandibular
gland duct
exposed and
divided

Facial artery ligated

XII

57-3

XII

57-4

Internal
jugular v.

Inferior traction
of specimen

■ *57.* RADICAL NECK DISSECTION *(continued)*

Tips and Pearls

1. Avoid trifurcate incisions.
2. Identification of the marginal mandibular nerve ensures adequate removal of the submandibular nodes.
3. To avoid a chyle leak, meticulously dissect the fat adjacent to the lower end of the internal jugular vein. Use clips liberally before dividing the fatty tissue that may contain lymphatics.
4. Attempt to preserve the nerves to the levator scapula.
5. Ligate the cutaneous branches of the cervical plexus to prevent formation of neuromas.
6. Avoid dissecting behind the carotid artery.
7. Avoid continuous suturing in the wound closure.
8. Always orient the surgical specimen for the pathologist.

Pitfalls and Complications

1. Postoperative hematoma usually occurs within the first few hours. Evacuation of clots and control of the bleeding vessel are best accomplished in the operating room, using sterile technique.
2. Postoperative seromas are common. If small, aspirate; if large or difficult to control with aspiration, insert a suction drain in a sterile fashion.
3. A chyle leak of more than 400 mL/day or any chyle leak that can not be adequately evacuated with the drains should be explored immediately. Otherwise, a low-fat diet and suction drainage suffice in most cases.

Postoperative Care Issues

1. In patients undergoing bilateral radical neck dissection, monitor serum and urine osmolality to guide postoperative fluid replacement.
2. Institute shoulder rehabilitation exercises as soon as possible.

References

McQuarrie DG, Mayberg M, Ferguson M, et al. A physiologic approach to the problem of simultaneous bilateral neck dissection. Am J Neurosurg 1977;134:455.

Strong EW, Sheman LJ. Radical neck dissection for squamous cell carcinoma of the head and neck. In: Larson DL, Ballantyne AJ, Guillamondegui OM, eds. Cancer in the neck. New York: Macmillan Publishing, 1986:121.

Inferior Dissection

The sternocleidomastoid muscle and the superficial layer of the deep cervical fascia are incised above the superior border of the clavicle. The external jugular vein and the omohyoid muscle are divided (Fig. 57-6). The fibrofatty tissue in this region is then gently pushed in upward, exposing the brachial plexus, the scalenus anticus muscle, and the phrenic nerve.

Medial Dissection

The dissection is carried forward as the specimen is dissected off of the scalenus medius, the brachial plexus, and the scalenus anticus. Care must be taken not to injure the phrenic nerve inferiorly. In this area of the neck, the thoracic duct on the left side or an accessory duct on the right may need to be ligated. The duct is anterior or superficial to the anterior scalene muscle and the phrenic nerve and posterior to the carotid and the vagus nerve. To avoid a chyle leak through contributing lymphatic channels, the fat in this region is clipped and then cut.

As the dissection continues superiorly, the cutaneous branches of the cervical plexus are divided. After this is done, only a relatively thin layer of tissue remains to be incised before the vagus nerve, the common carotid artery, and the internal jugular vein are exposed.

The internal jugular vein can be divided superiorly or inferiorly, depending on the location of the disease in the neck. If the tumor mass is located low in the jugulodigastric region or in the midjugular region, the internal jugular vein is first ligated and divided superiorly. The dissection then continues in an inferior direction, separating the specimen from the vagus nerve, the carotid, and the superior thyroid vessels. The medial limit of the dissection is marked by the strap muscles. If, however, the disease is located high in the jugulodigastric region, especially if the tumor is extensive and may require removal of the external carotid artery or the hypoglossal nerve, the internal jugular vein is divided inferiorly, and the dissection is carried in a superior direction along the common carotid artery (Fig. 57-7). By doing so, mobilization of the surgical specimen allows easier dissection of it from the internal carotid artery and, if possible, the external carotid and the hypoglossal nerve. The completed dissection is shown in Figure 57-8.

The incision is usually closed in two layers; the first one approximates the platysma anteriorly and the subcutaneous tissue laterally, and the second one approximates the skin. One or two suction drains are left in place; they should not rest immediately over the carotid artery or in the area of the thoracic duct. Bulky or pressure dressings are unnecessary.

JESUS E. MEDINA

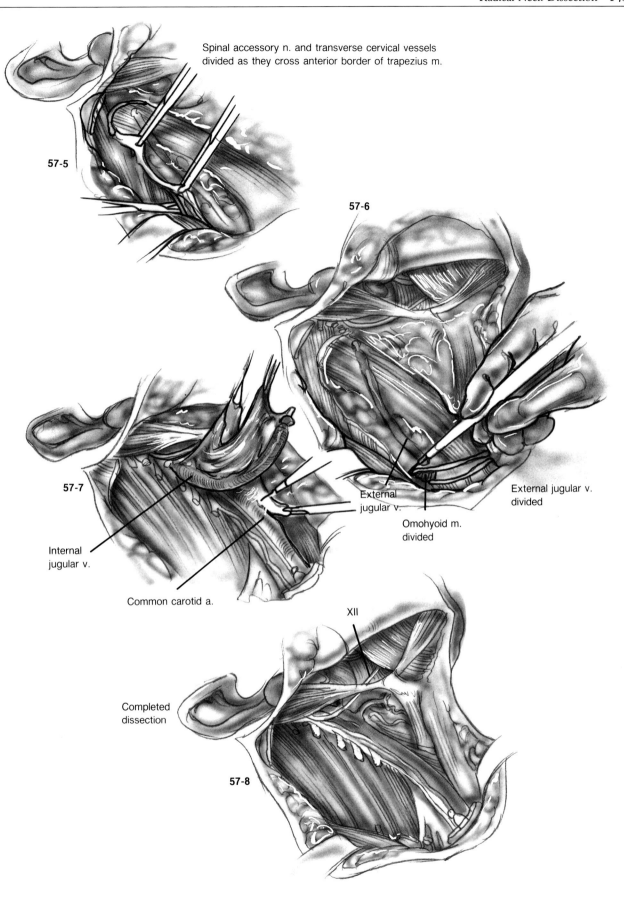

Spinal accessory n. and transverse cervical vessels
divided as they cross anterior border of trapezius m.

57-5

57-6

External
jugular v.

External jugular v.
divided

Omohyoid m.
divided

57-7

Internal
jugular v.

Common carotid a.

XII

Completed
dissection

57-8

■ *58.* SUPRAOMOHYOID NECK DISSECTION

A selective neck dissection that consists of the en bloc removal of nodal regions I, II, and III[1]

Indications

1. Surgical treatment of the neck of patients with squamous cell carcinoma of the oral cavity staged T2–T4N0 or TxN1 if the palpable node was less than 3 cm, clearly mobile, and located in level I or II. The operation must be done on both sides of the neck in patients with cancers of the anterior tongue and floor of the mouth.
2. Elective treatment of the neck in patients with squamous cell carcinoma of the lip or skin of the midportion of the face and when these lesions are associated with clinically discrete, single metastases to the submental or submandibular nodes. A bilateral dissection is performed if the lesion is located at or near the midline.

Contraindications

1. Metastases larger than 3 cm in the upper or midjugular regions
2. "Matted" nodes anywhere along the jugular vein that may require removal of the sternocleidomastoid muscle or the internal jugular vein
3. Metastases in the nodes of the posterior triangle of the neck

Special Considerations

1. Site and extent of the primary tumor
2. Metastases in both sides of the neck
3. Previous radiation treatment
4. Previous neck surgery

Preoperative Preparation

1. Appropriate laboratory studies
2. Obtaining a computed tomography scan, magnetic resonance image, or ultrasound scan of patients' necks without clinically palpable nodes is questionable.

Special Instruments, Position, and Anesthesia

1. Special instruments are usually unnecessary. However, immediate availability of vascular instruments and sutures is desirable in case the need arises to repair a tear of the internal jugular vein.
2. The neck is extended with roll under shoulders, and the head is turned to the opposite side and stabilized in a foam doughnut.
3. Unlike the case in which a bilateral radical neck dissection is performed, there is no need for the anesthesiologist to curtail fluid administration when a bilateral supraomohyoid neck dissection is performed, particularly if the external jugular vein is preserved in one or both sides.

(continued)

Operative Procedure

The incision preferred to perform a unilateral supraomohyoid neck dissection extends in an apron-like fashion from the mastoid tip to the mandibular symphysis. The lowest point of this incision is usually placed at the level of the thyrohyoid membrane. This incision can be extended into a lip-splitting incision, and if a more extensive dissection of the neck is indicated by the surgical findings, a descending limb can easily be added for exposure. If bilateral dissection is necessary, an apron-like incision is made from mastoid to mastoid overlying the thyrohyoid membrane.[2]

A superior flap is elevated in a subplatysmal plane up to the inferior border of the mandible. The marginal mandibular branch of the facial nerve is identified and preserved, unless it is grossly involved by tumor in a submandibular node. The greater auricular nerve and the external jugular vein are also preserved during the elevation of the flap. An inferior flap is elevated, usually to about 1 in (0.5 cm) above the clavicles. However, elevation of the flap can be carried down to the level of the clavicles, if necessary.

The dissection of the submental and submandibular triangles is carried out in the same manner described for the radical neck dissection. The dissection continues below the digastric and posterior to the omohyoid, removing sharply all the fibroadipose tissue in this area, exposing and preserving the hypoglossal nerve and the superior thyroid vessels. The fascia of the omohyoid muscle is included with the specimen, outlining the anteroinferior limit of the dissection (Fig. 58-1). It usually is possible to continue the dissection posteriorly, exposing the internal jugular vein and the upper end of the spinal accessory nerve.

The fascia along the anterior border of the sternocleidomastoid muscle is incised. The fascia is then dissected off of the anterior border and medial aspect of the upper two thirds of the muscle (Fig. 58-2). Superiorly, the dissection is carried around the muscle up to the point where the spinal accessory nerve enters it. The spinal accessory nerve is carefully dissected free from the surrounding tissues (Fig. 58-3).

(continued)

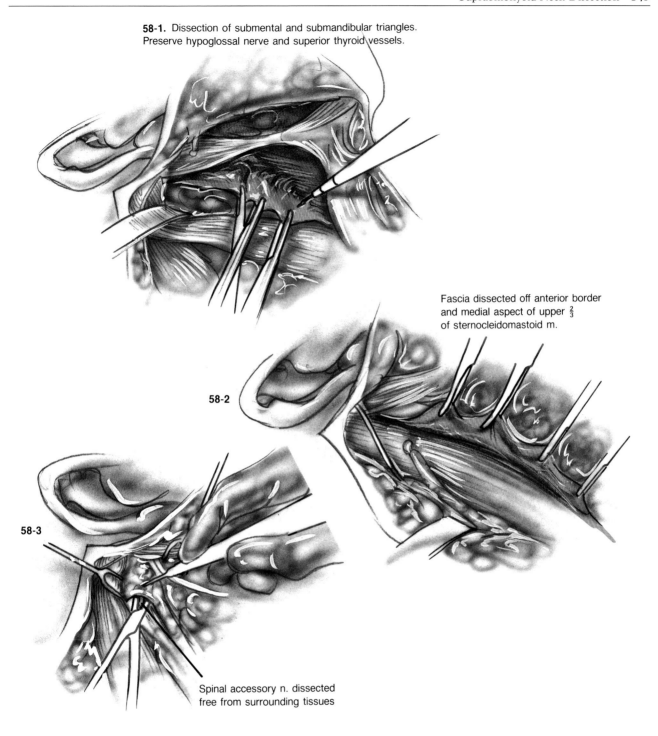

58-1. Dissection of submental and submandibular triangles. Preserve hypoglossal nerve and superior thyroid vessels.

Fascia dissected off anterior border and medial aspect of upper $\frac{2}{3}$ of sternocleidomastoid m.

58-2

58-3

Spinal accessory n. dissected free from surrounding tissues

■ *58.* SUPRAOMOHYOID NECK DISSECTION
(continued)

Tips and Pearls
1. It is seldom necessary to use a trifurcate incision.
2. Identification of the marginal mandibular nerve is essential to ensure adequate removal of the submandibular nodes.
3. Avoid undue retraction of the spinal accessory nerve during the dissection medial to the upper third of the sternocleidomastoid muscle.
4. Routine frozen-section examination of the nodes in the specimen is unnecessary. If an enlarged node, suspected of containing metastasis, is found in the jugulo-omohyoid region, the dissection is extended to include the nodes in region IV.
5. An enlarged node, clearly positive for metastasis, is more commonly found in the course of the dissection of the jugulodigastric region. Depending on the characteristics of the node, it may be necessary to remove the internal jugular vein to resect it adequately. It is unnecessary to convert the operation to a radical or modified radical neck dissection.
6. Avoid dissecting behind the carotid artery.
7. Avoid continuous suturing in the wound closure.
8. Orient the surgical specimen for the pathologist.

Pitfalls and Complications
1. Postoperative hematoma usually occurs within the first few hours. Evacuation of clots and control of the bleeding vessel are best accomplished in the operating room, using sterile technique.
2. Postoperative seromas and chyle leaks are rare.

Postoperative Care Issues
1. Preserving the spinal accessory nerve does not ensure adequate postoperative function of the trapezius. Mild to moderate electromyographic abnormalities and temporary dysfunction of the trapezius have been observed in patients undergoing this operation. Shoulder rehabilitation exercises should be instituted as soon as possible to prevent additional shoulder dysfunction while the nerve recovers.

References
1. Shah JP. Patterns of cervical lymph node metastasis from squamous carcinomas of the upper aerodigestive tract. Am J Surg 1990;160: 405.
2. Medina JE, Byers RM. Supraomohyoid neck dissection: rationale, indications and surgical technique. Head Neck Surg 1989;11:111.

Above the level of the nerve, the splenius capitis and the levator scapula muscles are dissected clean. The fibroadipose tissue containing lymph nodes from this area is brought forward, underneath the spinal accessory nerve (Fig. 58-4). Below this level, the posterior limit of the dissection is marked by the cutaneous branches of the cervical plexus, which are preserved. A block of nodal and adipose tissue is formed and is reflected anteriorly (Fig. 58-5). The dissection is then carried along the vagus nerve, the common and internal carotid arteries, and the internal jugular vein. The inferior limit of the dissection is usually the omohyoid muscle as it crosses forward, lateral to the internal jugular vein (Fig. 58-6). However, if a node is found in this area that appears to be involved by tumor, the omohyoid is divided and the lymph nodes and adipose tissue anterior to the scalene muscles and the brachial plexus (ie, lymph node group IV) are included in the specimen.

The common facial vein is divided, and the surgical specimen is removed, or it is reflected toward the midline, beginning the dissection on the opposite side (Fig. 58-7).

JESUS E. MEDINA

Fibroadipose tissue brought forward
under the spinal accessory n.

58-4

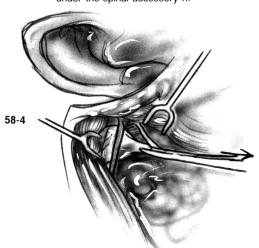

58-5. Block of nodal and adipose tissue reflected anteriorly.
Dissection carried along internal carotid artery
and internal jugular vein.

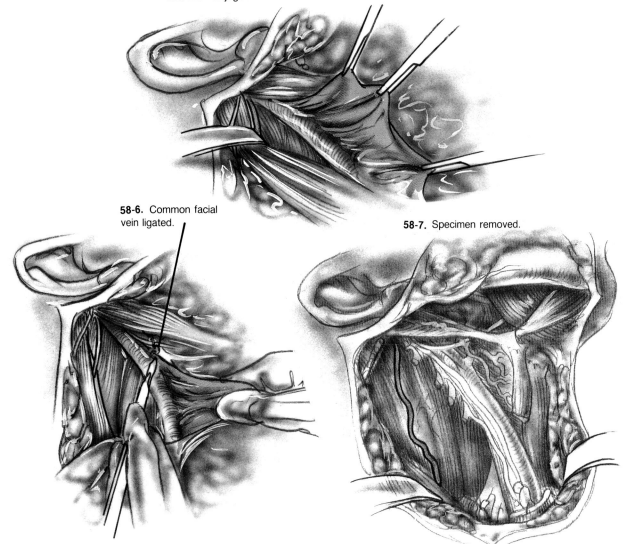

58-6. Common facial
vein ligated.

58-7. Specimen removed.

■ 59. MODIFIED RADICAL NECK DISSECTION PRESERVING THE SPINAL ACCESSORY NERVE

This operation has an important role in the surgical treatment of patients with palpable nodal metastases.

Indications

1. Clinically obvious lymph node metastases; preservation of the spinal accessory nerve is possible and indicated whenever it is not directly involved by tumor, regardless of the number, size, and location of the involved lymph nodes.

Contraindications

1. Although some surgeons advocate performing this operation in patients with node-negative neck disease, the removal of the internal jugular vein and the sternocleidomastoid muscle is no longer warranted in such cases.

Special Considerations

1. Site and extent of the primary tumor
2. Metastases in both sides of the neck
3. Previous radiation treatment
4. Previous neck surgery

Preoperative Preparation

1. Appropriate laboratory studies
2. A computed tomography scan may be necessary to assess the relation of the tumor to the carotid artery, paraspinal muscles, and cervical vertebrae.

Special Instruments, Position, and Anesthesia

1. Vascular instruments if carotid resection or a graft is anticipated.
2. Neck extended with a roll under shoulders, with the head turned to the opposite side and stabilized in a foam doughnut
3. Alert the anesthesia department of the possibility of resecting both internal jugular veins. Fluid administration should be reduced to about 50 mL/hour after ligation of the second internal jugular vein to avoid cerebral edema.

Tips and Pearls

1. Avoid trifurcate incisions.
2. Remember that the cranial nerve XI is superficially located in the midposterior triangle of the neck and can be injured during the elevation of the flaps.
3. To avoid a chyle leak, meticulously dissect the fat adjacent to the lower end of the internal jugular vein. Use clips liberally before dividing the fatty tissue that may contain lymphatics.
4. Attempt to preserve the nerves to the levator scapula.
5. Ligate the cutaneous branches of the cervical plexus to prevent formation of neuromas.
6. Avoid dissecting behind the carotid artery.
7. Avoid continuous suturing in the wound closure.

Pitfalls and Complications

1. Postoperative hematoma usually occurs within the first few hours.
2. Postoperative seromas are common. If small, aspirate; if large or difficult to control with aspiration, insert a suction drain in a sterile fashion.
3. A chyle leak of more than 400 mL/day or any chyle leak that cannot be adequately evacuated should be explored.

Postoperative Care Issues

1. Preserving the spinal accessory nerve does not ensure adequate postoperative function of the trapezius.
2. It is critical to handle the nerve carefully during surgery, avoiding undue traction and stretching.

References

Pearlman NW, Meyers AD, Sullivan WG. Modified radical neck dissection for squamous cell carcinoma of the head and neck. Surg Gynecol Obstet 1982;154:214.

Remmler D, Byers RM, Scheetz J, et al. A prospective study of shoulder disability resulting from radical and modified neck dissections. Head Neck Surg 1986;8:280.

Operative Procedure

The incision is selected from among those described in Procedure 56. The incision used must allow easy exposure of the entire side of the neck from the clavicle to the mandible and from the midline anteriorly to the anterior border of the trapezius posteriorly. The spinal accessory nerve can be located superficially as it courses through the posterior triangle of the neck; the skin flaps elevated over this region must be kept relatively thin to avoid injuring the nerve.

After the skin flaps have been raised, the submandibular triangle is dissected in the same manner as that described for the radical neck dissection (see Procedure 56).

Attention is then focused on the initial exposure and dissection of the spinal accessory nerve, which can be accomplished in three ways. First, after the posterior belly of the digastric muscle is exposed, blunt and careful sharp dissection of the fibroadipose tissue below it expose the hypoglossal nerve, the internal jugular vein, and the upper end of the spinal accessory nerve. The nerve is usually found immediately posterior to the jugular vein, but it may lay obliquely across the anterolateral surface of the vein or, less commonly, be several millimeters posterior to it. Downward exposure and isolation of the nerve requires incising the upper one third of the sternocleidomastoid muscle, obliquely, over the course of the nerve (Fig. 59-1).

A second approach is to incise the fascia along the lower one third of the anterior border of the trapezius muscle. The underlying fibroadipose tissue is then incised, one layer at a time, until the nerve is visualized (see Fig. 59-2).

A third approach is to incise the fascia and underlying tissue immediately behind the posterior border of the trapezius muscle, in the vicinity of Erb's point, where the greater auricular nerve curves forward, around the posterior border of the sternocleidomastoid muscle. In doing this, the surgeon should keep in mind that the relation of the spinal accessory nerve to Erb's point is not as consistent as some anatomy texts proclaim; that in this area, the location of the spinal accessory nerve is the deepest in its course through the posterior triangle of the neck; and that the nerve can be easily confused with the cutaneous branches of the cervical plexus.

After the nerve has been exposed and isolated through its entire course in the neck, the upper and posterior dissection of the neck can proceed in the same manner as in the radical neck dissection. The specimen is then passed forward, under the nerve (Fig. 59-3), and the inferior and medial portions of the neck dissection are completed as described for the radical neck dissection (see Procedure 56). The completed dissection is shown in Figure 59-4.

JESUS E. MEDINA

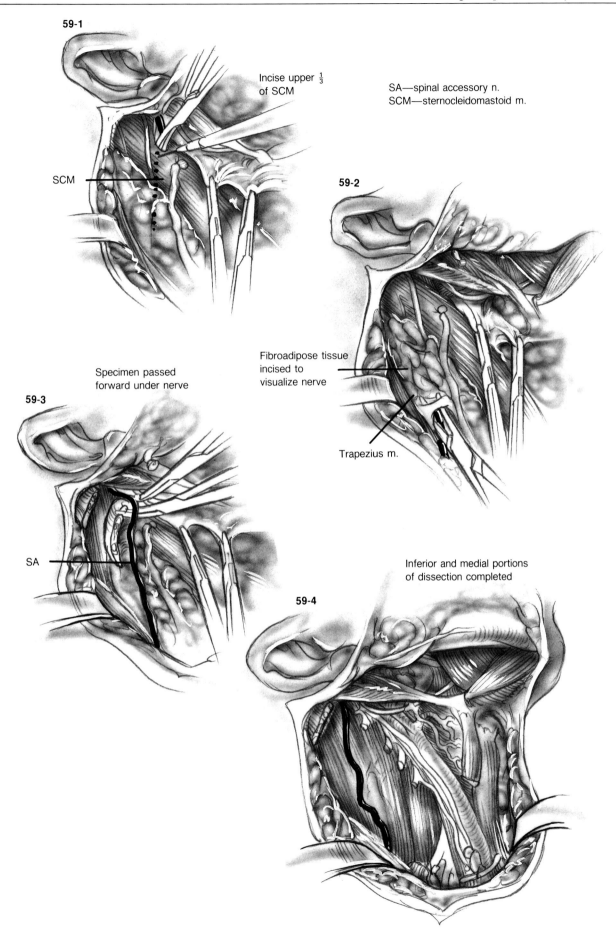

59-1

Incise upper ⅓ of SCM

SA—spinal accessory n.
SCM—sternocleidomastoid m.

SCM

59-2

Fibroadipose tissue incised to visualize nerve

Trapezius m.

Specimen passed forward under nerve

59-3

SA

Inferior and medial portions of dissection completed

59-4

■ 60. MODIFIED RADICAL NECK DISSECTION PRESERVING THE SPINAL ACCESSORY NERVE, THE INTERNAL JUGULAR VEIN, AND THE STERNOCLEIDOMASTOID

MUSCLE—En bloc removal of the lymph node–bearing tissues of one side of the neck, including lymph nodes in levels I through V, preserving the spinal accessory nerve, the internal jugular vein, and the sternocleidomastoid muscle. The submandibular gland may or may not be removed.

Indications

1. Treatment of the node-negative (N0) neck in patients with squamous cell carcinoma of the upper aerodigestive tract, especially when the primary tumor is located in the larynx and hypopharynx. In that case, the nodes in the submandibular triangle are at low risk of containing metastases and do not need to be removed.
2. Treatment of the nodal stage N1 neck if the metastatic nodes are mobile and no greater than 2.5 to 3 cm[1]
3. According to Bocca, this type of neck dissection is indicated for the treatment of metastases in the neck at any stage, except if the metastasis is "fixed."[2]
4. Treatment of the neck in patients with differentiated carcinoma of the thyroid who have palpable lymph node metastases in the lateral or posterior compartments of the neck

Contraindications

1. Although some surgeons advocate performing this operation in patients with N0 neck disease, routine dissection of the posterior triangle of the neck in these cases is not justified.

Special Considerations

1. Site and extent of the primary tumor
2. Metastases in both sides of the neck
3. Previous radiation treatment
4. Previous neck surgery

Preoperative Preparation

1. Appropriate laboratory studies
2. A computed tomography scan may be necessary to assess the relation of the tumor to the carotid artery, paraspinal muscles, and cervical vertebrae.

Special Instruments, Position, and Anesthesia

1. Vascular instruments if carotid resection or a graft is anticipated.
2. Neck extended with roll under shoulders, with the head turned to the opposite side and stabilized in foam doughnut

(continued)

Operative Procedure

The incisions, the elevation of the cervical flaps, and the dissection of the submental and submandibular triangles are performed in the manner described for the radical neck dissection. After the dissection of the submandibular triangle has been completed, the dissection continues in a posterior direction, identifying and preserving the hypoglossal nerve and the superior thyroid vessels (Fig. 60-1). As this is done, the upper end of the internal jugular vein and the spinal accessory nerve are exposed below the posterior belly of the digastric muscle. The fascia of the sternocleidomastoid muscle is incised along the posterior border of the muscle. It is then dissected off the lateral aspect of the muscle in an anterior direction. The greater auricular nerve and, occasionally, the external jugular vein are preserved during this part of the procedure. The dissection of the fascia continues around the anterior border of the muscle and onto its medial surface. Retracting the muscle laterally, the spinal accessory nerve is identified as it enters the muscle, at about the level of the junction of its upper and middle thirds. The fibrofatty tissue overlying the spinal accessory nerve is carefully divided, exposing the nerve between its exit at the jugular foramen and its entrance into the sternocleidomastoid muscle (Fig. 60-2).

The dissection proceeds above and behind the spinal accessory nerve, where the fibrofatty tissues containing lymph nodes are dissected from the splenius capitis and the levator scapulae muscles (Fig. 60-3). The dissected tissue from this area of the neck is then brought forward under the spinal accessory nerve (Fig. 60-4). Below the level of the nerve, the cutaneous branches of the cervical plexus are divided as they cross the posterior border of the sternocleidomastoid muscle.

At this point, the dissection of the posterior triangle begins by identifying the spinal accessory nerve at the point where it exits from under the sternocleidomastoid muscle or, more easily, as it crosses

(continued)

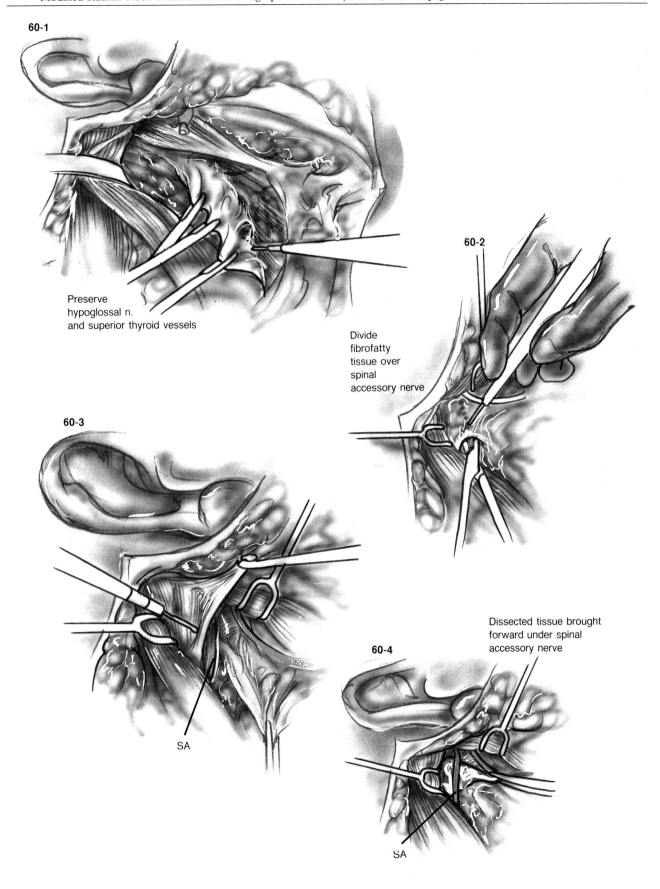

60-1

Preserve
hypoglossal n.
and superior thyroid vessels

60-2

Divide
fibrofatty
tissue over
spinal
accessory nerve

60-3

SA

Dissected tissue brought
forward under spinal
accessory nerve

60-4

SA

■ 60. MODIFIED RADICAL NECK DISSECTION PRESERVING THE SPINAL ACCESSORY NERVE, THE INTERNAL JUGULAR VEIN, AND THE STERNOCLEIDOMASTOID MUSCLE *(continued)*

Tips and Pearls

1. Cranial nerve XI is superficially located in the midposterior triangle of the neck and can be injured during elevation of the skin flaps.
2. To avoid a chyle leak, meticulously dissect the fat adjacent to the lower end of the internal jugular vein. Use clips liberally before dividing the fatty tissue that may contain lymphatics.
3. Attempt to preserve the greater auricular nerve.
4. Attempt to preserve the nerves to the levator scapula.
5. Ligate the cutaneous branches of the cervical plexus to prevent formation of neuromas.
6. Avoid dissecting behind the carotid artery.
7. Avoid continuous suturing in the wound closure.
8. Orient the surgical specimen for the pathologist.

Pitfalls and Complications

1. Postoperative hematoma usually occurs within the first few hours. Evacuation of clots and control of the bleeding vessel are best accomplished in the operating room, using sterile technique.
2. Postoperative seromas are particularly common after this type of neck dissection because of the large "dead space" created between the sternocleidomastoid and the trapezius muscles. Do not hesitate to leave the drains in for 6 to 8 days to ensure adherence of the skin flaps to the "floor" of the posterior triangle.
3. A chyle leak of more than 400 mL/day or any chyle leak that can not be adequately evacuated with the drains should be explored immediately. Otherwise, a low-fat diet and suction drainage suffice in most cases.
4. There is no good way to apply a pressure dressing to the neck.

Postoperative Care Issues

1. Preserving the spinal accessory nerve does not ensure adequate postoperative function of the trapezius. Moderate to severe electromyographic abnormalities and temporary dysfunction of the trapezius have been observed after this operation. Institute shoulder rehabilitation exercises as soon as possible.

References

1. Molinari R, Chiesa F, Cantu G, Grandi C. Retrospective comparison of conservative and radical neck dissection in laryngeal cancer. Ann Otolaryngol 1980;89:578.
2. Bocca E, Pignataro O, Oldini C. Functional neck dissection: an evaluation and review of 843 cases. Laryngoscope 1984;94:942.

the anterior border of the trapezius muscle (Fig. 60-5). Using very gentle traction on the nerve, the spinal accessory nerve is freed from the surrounding tissues using a scalpel. With the nerve isolated, the fascia and fibroadipose tissues are incised along the anterior border of the trapezius muscle. The tissue that contains lymph nodes is then dissected in an anterior direction off the splenius capitis, the levator scapulae, and the scalenus medius muscles. These tissue are then brought forward under the spinal accessory nerve (Fig. 60-6).

The fascia of the sternocleidomastoid muscle is dissected off the medial aspect of the muscle until the anterior border of the muscle is reached (Fig. 60-7). The superficial layer of the deep cervical fascia is then incised along the superior border of the clavicle, between the posterior border of the sternocleidomastoid muscle and the anterior border of the trapezius. The external jugular vein is divided between clamps, and the omohyoid muscle is transected. The fibrofatty tissue in this area is gently pushed in a superior direction, identifying the proper plane of dissection superficial to the fascia of the scalenus medius, the brachial plexus, the scalenus anticus, and the phrenic nerve (see Fig. 60-7). The contents of the posterior triangle of the neck, completely freed, can be brought forward, under the sternocleidomastoid muscle (Fig. 60-8).

The dissection continues in an anterior direction by dividing the inferior cutaneous branches of the cervical plexus. The specimen is dissected sharply from the vagus nerve, the carotid artery, and the internal jugular vein. To avoid injury to the thoracic duct, the dissection in the anteroinferior area of the neck, lateral to the internal jugular vein and the common carotid artery, is carried out carefully as described for radical neck dissection (see Chap. 56). The dissection of the specimen from the internal jugular vein continues superiorly toward the upper portion of the neck that was previously dissected, completing the operation (Fig. 60-9).

JESUS E. MEDINA

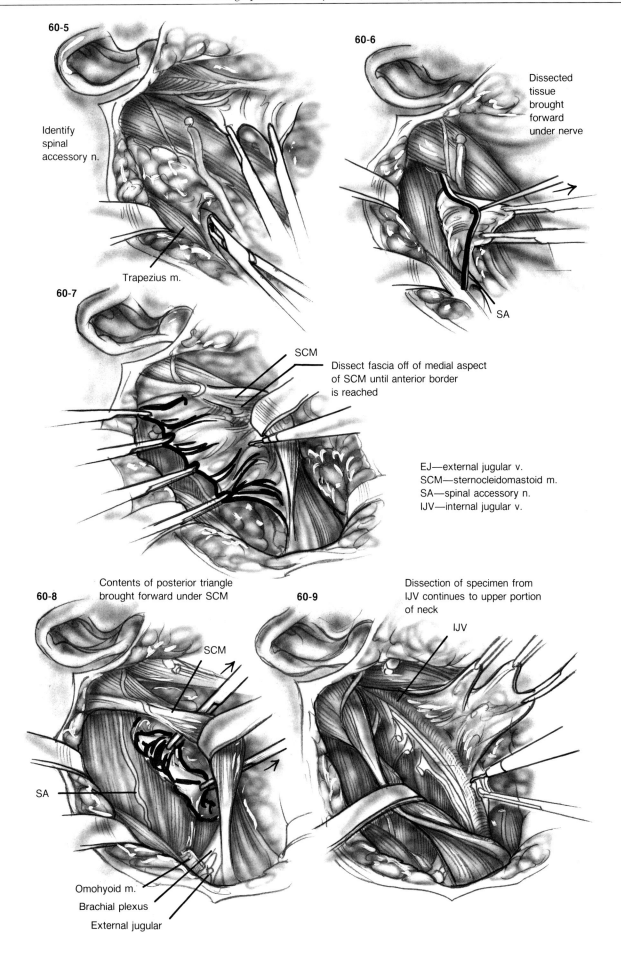

60-5

Identify
spinal
accessory n.

Trapezius m.

60-6

Dissected
tissue
brought
forward
under nerve

SA

60-7

SCM

Dissect fascia off of medial aspect
of SCM until anterior border
is reached

EJ—external jugular v.
SCM—sternocleidomastoid m.
SA—spinal accessory n.
IJV—internal jugular v.

Contents of posterior triangle
brought forward under SCM

60-8

SCM

SA

Omohyoid m.
Brachial plexus
External jugular

Dissection of specimen from
IJV continues to upper portion
of neck

60-9

IJV

■ 61. TRANSSTERNAL MEDIASTINAL NODE
DISSECTION— A procedure designed to remove lymphatic tissue from the superior mediastinum and a route of access to the distal trachea and esophagus in cases of recurrent carcinoma or stomal recurrences after total laryngectomy

Indications
1. Stomal recurrence
2. Carcinoma extending into the superior mediastinum

Contraindications
1. Involvement of the great vessels of the mediastinum (Fig. 61-1)
2. Distant metastatic disease
3. Medically unsuitable patients

Special Considerations
1. This approach is challenging from an anatomic standpoint. The extension of neck surgery into the chest poses a major physiologic challenge to the patient.

Preoperative Preparation
1. Computed tomography scans of the chest with contrast
2. The operation should be performed only if there is a realistic expectation of a successful outcome.

Special Instruments, Position, and Anesthesia
1. Sternal saw
2. Heavy instruments to resect the ribs and clavicles
3. Provision for the placement of chest tubes

(continued)

Operative Procedure
Stomal recurrence commonly develops in patients whose wound-healing capabilities have been compromised by previous surgery and irradiation. Advanced age and associated medical problems make the situation even more tenuous. If the pharynx or esophagus are not entered, the complication rate is low, and the postoperative course is relatively predictable. However, the need to resect the esophagus or pharynx increases the risk to the patient because of the risk of fistula formation.

The patient is placed on the operating room table in a supine position. The entire chest is prepped so that it is available for a pectoralis flap and chest tube placement. The anesthesiologist must understand that the tracheotomy tube or endotracheal tube should be removed periodically throughout the procedure. Several large-bore intravenous catheters need to be placed along with central venous monitoring with a central venous pressure or Swan-Ganz catheter. A Foley catheter is required. Appropriate perioperative antibiotics are indicated in this procedure.

The specific incision depends on the clinical situation (Fig. 61-2). In most instances, the operation is being done for a stomal recurrence, and a wide circular excision of skin around the prior tracheostomy site needs to be resected. If a neck dissection or additional head and neck procedure is required in conjunction with the transsternal mediastinal dissection, a separate cervical incision must be incorporated into the plan. The surgeon must draw all anticipated incisions at the outset of the operation, including the anticipated reconstruction, so that the viability of all skin flaps is ensured.

The operation is begun by incising around the stomal recurrence using an inferior semicircular incision. The entire incision is not incised in case an unanticipated unresectable feature of the operation is discovered early in the operation; this approach allows the wound to be closed and the operation aborted. If the skin paddle around the stomal recurrence is incised in its entirety, this option may not be possible.

The sternum and proximal heads of the clavicles are exposed first. Care should be taken to avoid unnecessary dissection laterally along the distal extent of the clavicle, where interruption of the pectoral branch of the thyroacromial artery may occur. This technical point is important to preserve the potential vascular supply to the pectoralis major myocutaneous flap if this is the method of choice.

The clavicles may be divided proximally by using an oscillating saw or a Gigli saw (Fig. 61-3). The manubrium is divided near the sternal angle with an oscillating saw or sternal saw (Fig. 61-4). The second rib may be divided at this point as well, depending on the level of sectioning of the manubrium and the location of the second rib insertion into the sternum. The bony specimen is retracted, and the underlying soft tissues are dissected free. If the tumor is associated with infiltration of the sternum or clavicle, the bony specimen should remain in continuity with the main specimen; otherwise, it may be removed as a separate specimen.

(continued)

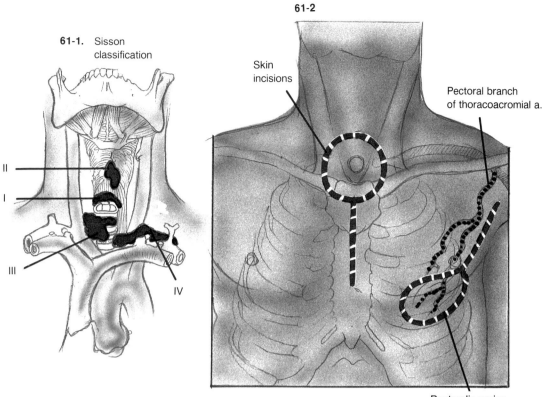

61-1. Sisson classification

II

I

III

IV

61-2

Skin incisions

Pectoral branch of thoracoacromial a.

Pectoralis major skin island

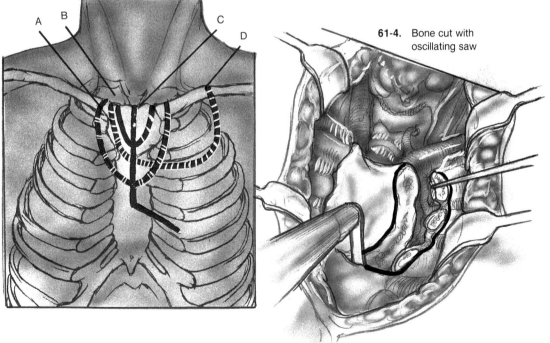

61-3. Types of bony sternal incisions

A B   C

D

61-4. Bone cut with oscillating saw

■ 61. TRANSSTERNAL MEDIASTINAL NODE DISSECTION *(continued)*

Tips and Pearls

1. It is not always necessary to resect the entire manubrium or first ribs. If the stomal recurrence is small or the need to gain entrance to the mediastinum limited, the surgeon may gain access to the chest by piecemeal resection of the manubrium with a rongeur.
2. In larger dissections, the surgeon should resect the entire manubrium, proximal heads of the clavicles, and the proximal head of the first ribs.

Pitfalls and Complications

1. The main problem is providing adequate postoperative coverage of the tissues. The pectoralis myocutaneous flap provides excellent coverage of the chest wound.
2. Preventing accumulation of a seroma

Postoperative Care Issues

1. Individuals undergoing transsternal mediastinal dissection have thoracic splinting.
2. The patient may require vigorous chest physiotherapy and assisted ventilation.

References

Sisson GA, Bytell DE, Becker SP. Mediastinal dissection—1976: indications and newer techniques. Laryngoscope 1976;87:751.

Sisson GA, Straehley CJ, Johnson NE. Mediastinal dissection for recurrent cancer after laryngectomy. Laryngoscope 1962;73:1069.

Mobilization of the specimen is performed in a lateral to medial direction, following the great vessels of the neck into the mediastinum. One or, occasionally, both of the internal jugular veins have been sectioned in the radical neck dissection. The surgeon should avoid disruption of the subclavian vein as the internal jugular vein is ligated. If one side of the neck requires operation at the time of the mediastinal dissection, I generally approach the chest beginning on that side because of the improved visualization of the anatomic landmarks. The subclavian veins (or brachiocephalic vein on the right) are followed inferiorly first because they are superficially located in the upper mediastinum. This is best done with a fine hemostat along the vein and an assistant cutting along the dissected tissues (Fig. 61-5). Instruments should be available for vascular repairs if inadvertent injuries occur.

The carotid arteries are also followed at a deeper plane into the mediastinum in a similar fashion to the dissection along the subclavian veins. This course follows the carotid on the left and the brachiocephalic artery on the right. This dissection involves the removal of the thymic remnant along with the thyroid gland unless this structure can be preserved. An attempt should be made to identify the parathyroid glands and to preserve the blood supply to them if possible. In many cases, this is not an option, but if removed from the specimen or tissues, the parathyroids may be reimplanted into the forearm or sternocleidomastoid muscle.

Simultaneous with the mediastinal dissection, the trachea and esophagus are mobilized to allow resection of the stomal recurrence (Fig. 61-6). The trachea is sectioned distal to the stomal recurrence to obtain 1- to 2-cm tumor-negative margins that are confirmed by frozen-section analysis. The pharynx and esophagus are dissected free of tumor using frozen-section confirmation.

The reconstruction is begun by rounding the ends of the clavicles, ribs, and sternum so that they are smooth and will not impinge on soft tissues. A pectoralis major myocutaneous flap is harvested and rotated into position to close the wound and obliterate the dead space (Fig. 61-7). Other reconstructive techniques may be required to close the pharynx, such as an opposite pectoralis or trapezius myocutaneous flap, gastric pull-up, free tissue transfer, or free jejunal flap. Suction drains are positioned to remove serum and blood but are positioned so as not to impinge on the exposed great vessels. If entry has been made into the pleura, chest tubes are placed and secured to an underwater seal.

A portion of the pectoralis flap should be placed within the depths of the wound to approximate the trachea. This may require making a hole in the center of the flap or fashioning the skin paddle into a cone with the apex the site of the new tracheostoma. The wound is closed in layers, using 2-0 or 3-0 chromic for the subcutaneous tissues and staples on the skin (Fig. 61-8).

The patient is admitted to the intensive care unit for careful monitoring of vital signs, fluid balance, urine output, respiratory status, serum calcium, and Hemovac output.

MICHAEL D. MAVES

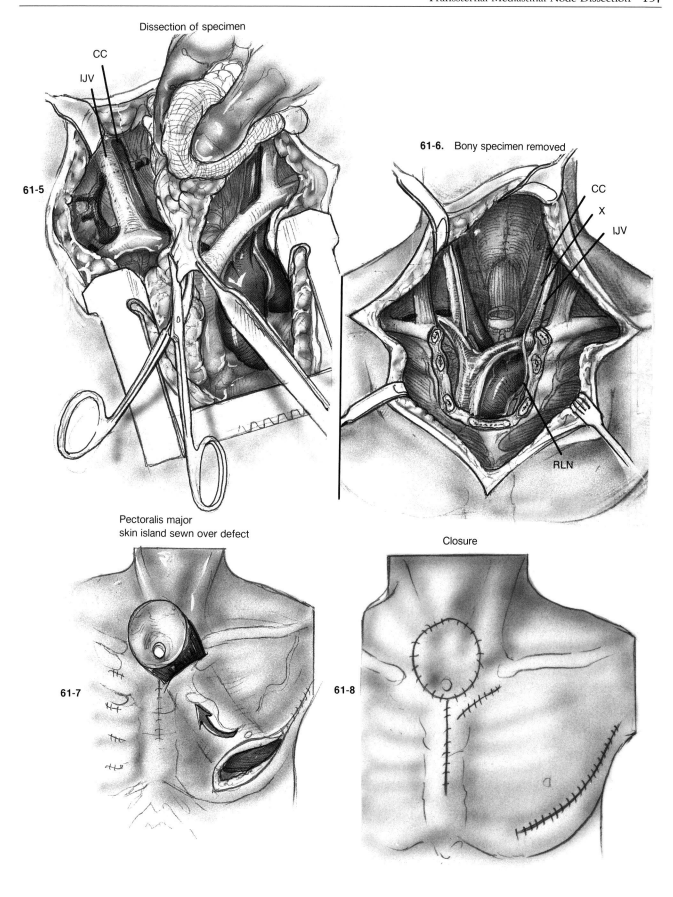

Dissection of specimen

CC

IJV

61-5

61-6. Bony specimen removed

CC

X

IJV

RLN

Pectoralis major
skin island sewn over defect

61-7

Closure

61-8

■ 62. CERVICAL NODE BIOPSY—Cervical lymph node biopsy is one of the most frequently performed diagnostic surgical procedures, although it has been supplanted somewhat by the use of fine-needle aspiration for evaluating cervical masses.

Indications
1. Histologic confirmation of the nature of cervical masses of undetermined cause
2. Suspicion of malignancy
3. Establishment of diagnosis and staging of lymphoma
4. Confirmation of fine-needle aspiration results
5. Removal of suspected tuberculous nodes

Contraindications
1. For suspected metastatic squamous cell carcinoma if a full preparatory diagnostic workup has not been completed
2. If general medical condition of the patient is unacceptable
3. If it will not add to the evaluation of the patient

Special Considerations
1. Incisions for lymph node biopsies should be planned with cosmesis in mind and should consider the possibility of conversion to a more extensive operation, such as a neck dissection.

Preoperative Preparation
1. Consideration of the information to be obtained
2. Review of the pertinent radiographs
3. Consultation with a pathologist to determine the amount and type of tissue to be obtained and how it will be processed to obtain the maximum amount of information

Special Instruments, Position, and Anesthesia
1. The patient is be positioned with the head extended as appropriate, using a shoulder roll.
2. The mass is marked preoperatively if it is small or extremely mobile.
3. I prefer the use of general anesthesia in the biopsy of lateral cervical triangle for lymph nodes located along the spinal accessory chain to avoid inadvertent damage to the spinal accessory nerve.

Tips and Pearls
1. Avoid the temptation to place an Allis clamp on the nodes to be removed. This causes a crush artifact and makes interpretation of the tissue by the pathologists more difficult.
2. I prefer to use a 2-0 silk suture through the node if necessary or to dissect the tissues away from the node and remove it in a "clean" fashion.
3. Do not try to "sneak" a node out from near the anticipated course of the facial nerve! Do it correctly by identifying and preserving the appropriate branches of the facial nerve.

Pitfalls and Complications
1. Avoid rupturing cancerous nodes with central necrosis if possible. The necrotic material may increase seeding of the wound bed.
2. Remember that lymph nodes in the carotid sheath lie anterior or posterior to the internal jugular, vein which should be left uninjured.

Postoperative Care Issues
1. A small Penrose or rubber-dam drain with a pressure dressing is an excellent method of managing such wounds. The patient can return the following day for removal.
2. Always suture drains to prevent their loss.

References
Gianoli GJ, Miller RH. Cervical lymph node biopsy. J La State Med Soc 1992;144:91.

Jones AS, Cook JA, Phillips DE, Roland NR. Squamous carcinoma presenting as an enlarged cervical lymph node. Cancer 1993;72:1756. [Comment in Cancer 1994;73:2008.]

Operative Procedure
The patient is positioned with the head extended to facilitate identification and localization of the targeted lymph node. The node selected should be one thought to be involved in the primary process and located in a position that makes its removal as straightforward as possible. Avoid nodes that may represent secondary reactive lymphadenopathy, and those associated with the facial nerve should be avoided. Similarly, be careful to avoid damage to the spinal accessory nerve in the lateral cervical triangle. I prefer to biopsy nodes near the facial or spinal accessory nerves of a patient under general anesthesia, which avoids the use of Xylocaine and allows the use of a nerve stimulator for their identification and preservation.

The incision is marked, and local anesthetic (1% solution of Xylocaine with a 1:100,000 dilution of epinephrine) is injected before prepping the patient (Fig. 62-1). This allows the incision to be considered in terms of its cosmetic significance and of subsequent procedures. When draping the patient under local anesthesia, avoid covering the patient's face, which causes a sensation of claustrophobia for some individuals and almost certainly induces apprehension for all patients.

The wound is opened in layers: skin with subcutaneous tissue, platysma, and deeper tissues (Fig. 62-2). I prefer to make small superior and inferior flaps in a subplatysmal plane. A self-retaining retractor may be placed or the wound opened by individual retraction (Fig. 62-3).

The node is located by palpation and direct visualization. The tissues are released from the surrounding tissues. The surgeon should notice the relative vascularity of the surrounding tissues and infiltration of any structures. A 2-0 silk suture provides excellent retraction of the node, while limiting the damage to the tissue for the pathologist (Fig. 62-4). Cultures are performed for any purulent drainage encountered. Hemostasis is provided by bipolar or Bovie electrocautery.

The node should be placed in a saline-moistened sponge and kept in the sterile field until tissue for pathology has been sent. I prefer to take the node directly to the frozen-section room for analysis before it is placed in formalin. The quality of information received from the pathologist is directly related to the quality of information given to the pathologist by the surgeon.

The wound is gently irrigated. Final hemostasis is obtained, and a small Penrose or rubber-dam drain is placed (Fig. 62-5). A compressive dressing is applied, and the patient is taken to the recovery room or observation area.

MICHAEL D. MAVES

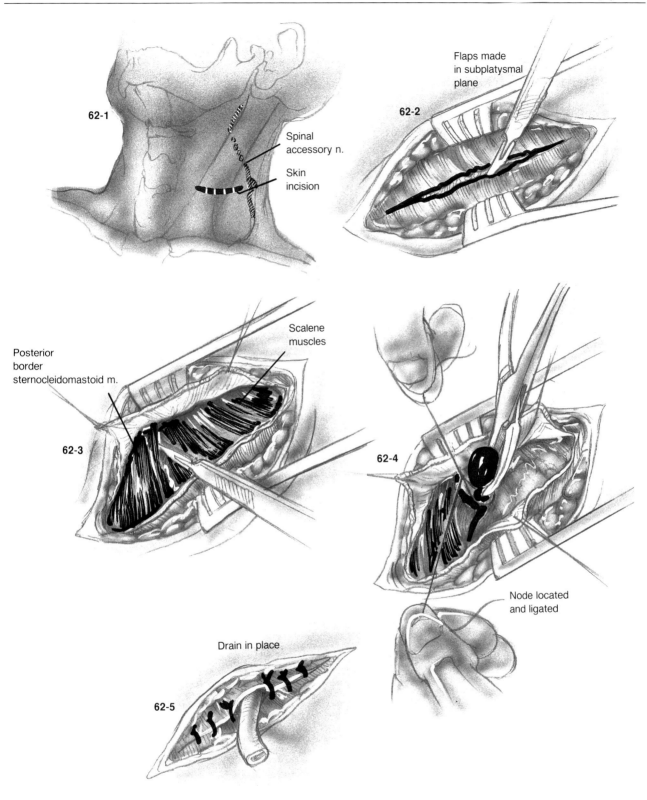

62-1
Spinal accessory n.

Skin incision

62-2
Flaps made in subplatysmal plane

62-3
Posterior border sternocleidomastoid m.

Scalene muscles

62-4
Node located and ligated

62-5
Drain in place

■ 63. SCALENE NODE BIOPSY—Scalene node biopsy is
a diagnostic tool used to examine the scalene fat pad in the supraclavicular fossa. The diagnostic modality is used for investigation
of head and neck primary lesions, but it is more commonly employed
to rule out metastatic spread of abdominal or thoracic disease to the
neck.

Indications
1. To obtain histologic confirmation of the status of the supraclavicular node pad in patients suspected of having metastatic spread
of abdominal or thoracic malignancies to the neck

Contraindications
1. Patients who are medically unstable or otherwise could not undergo the procedure
2. When the desired information could be obtained in a less invasive
fashion or will not add to the clinical situation

Special Considerations
1. The left thoracic duct drains the body below the diaphragm and
the left chest. The right thoracic duct drains only the right chest.
These structures are at risk in scalene lymph node biopsy and
should be kept in mind in any dissection in this area.

Preoperative Preparation
1. Evaluation of the status of the neck and presence of any observable
lymphadenopathy, thyromegaly, or other anatomic abnormality
that would make execution of the operation difficult

Special Instruments, Position, and Anesthesia
1. Usually, general anesthesia, which can be done with local anesthesia and intravenous sedation (if required)
2. Provision for inadvertent entry into or injury to the pleural space,
internal jugular vein, and thoracic duct

Tips and Pearls
1. This operation may be conceptualized as a small part of the traditional dissection of the lateral cervical triangle in neck dissection.
The same approach and precautions are necessary as in neck
dissection, which is an excellent preparatory procedure.

Pitfalls and Complications
1. Pneumothorax
2. Chyle fistula
3. Injury to the internal jugular vein, phrenic nerve, vagus nerve,
brachial plexus, musculocutaneous nerve, and common carotid
artery

Postoperative Care Issues
1. A suction drain system reduces the incidence of seroma formation
and promotes apposition of tissues. Use of a Penrose drain is
also allowable.
2. Early shoulder rehabilitation aids in reducing the postoperative
discomfort.

References
Bigsby R, Greengrass R, Unruh H. Diagnostic algorithm for acute superior
vena caval obstruction (SVCO). J Cardiovasc Surg 1993;34:347.
Petru E, Pickel H, Tamussino K, Lahousen M, et al. Pretherapeutic
scalene lymph node biopsy in ovarian cancer. Gynecol Oncol 1991;43:
262.

Operative Procedure
The patient is placed on the operating room table in a supine position.
The neck is extended on a shoulder roll. The operation is conducted
on the left side of the neck if the procedure is being done to investigate
the potential spread of malignancy from distant sites to the neck.
The procedure may be performed on the right side of the neck if a
mass is present or there is suspected spread of disease from the distribution of the right thoracic duct.

A transverse incision approximately 6 to 8 cm long is placed 2
to 4 cm above the clavicle (Fig. 63-1). This allows excellent exposure
and conversion of the wound to a McFee or apron incision if necessary. The wound is opened in a layered fashion: skin and subcutaneous tissue followed by platysma. Superior and inferior flaps are
developed in a subplatysmal plane. A self-retaining retractor is placed
for exposure (Fig. 63-2).

The superficial layer of the deep investing cervical fascia is incised
1 cm above the clavicle to expose the fascia of the supraclavicular
fascia. The supraclavicular fat is swept cephalad in a method similar
to a neck dissection (Fig. 63-3). The aim of the dissection is to remove
a sample of supraclavicular fat with contained nodes for pathologic
analysis. There is no need to remove the omohyoid muscle. The
surgeon should avoid needless sectioning of the transverse cervical
artery or the suprascapular artery. These vessels lie close to the floor
of the lateral cervical triangle and may be displaced inferiorly in
most instances (Fig. 63-4). The dissection remains centrally in the
lateral triangle of the neck, away from the trapezius muscle and
spinal accessory nerve laterally. The brachial plexus can be identified
at the level of the floor of the lateral triangle of the neck. The deep
layer of fascia overlying the scalene muscles and the brachial plexus
should be preserved. The phrenic nerve is identified medially. The
dissection should not require further extension medially unless disease extension dictates.

After the supraclavicular fat pad is dissected from the floor of
the lateral cervical triangle, it may be sectioned across the superior
aspect of the wound and taken to the pathologist in a fresh state for
immediate processing. The wound is inspected for any evidence of
a chyle leak, which requires ligation with 4-0 or 5-0 silk before wound
closure.

A suction drain is placed, and the wound is closed in layers with
absorbable 3-0 or 4-0 chromic sutures to approximate the platysma
and the subcutaneous tissue. The skin may be closed with staples,
interrupted nonabsorbable suture (5-0 nylon), or tape skin closures.

MICHAEL D. MAVES

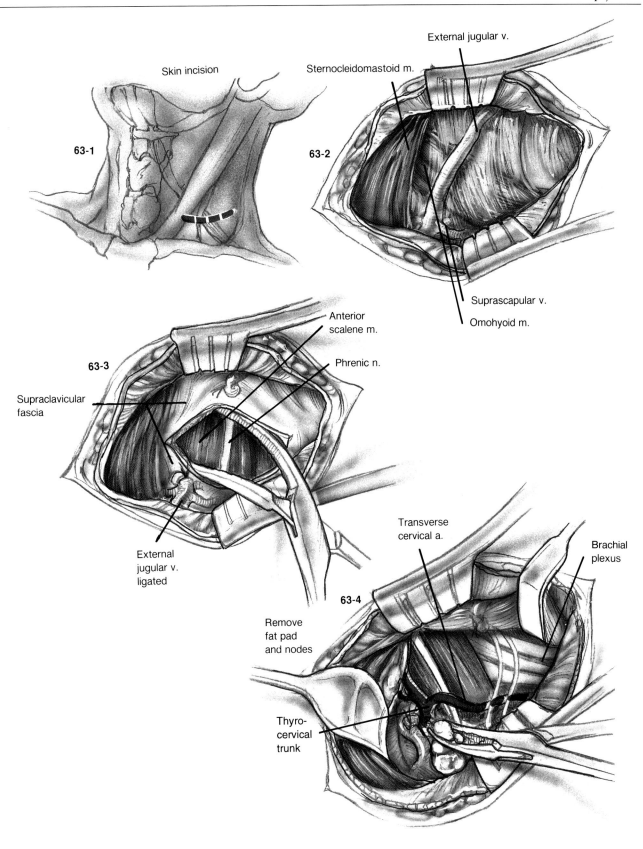

63-1   Skin incision

63-2   External jugular v.
Sternocleidomastoid m.
Suprascapular v.
Omohyoid m.

63-3   Anterior scalene m.
Phrenic n.
Supraclavicular fascia
External jugular v. ligated

63-4   Transverse cervical a.
Brachial plexus
Remove fat pad and nodes
Thyro-cervical trunk

■ *64.* POSTEROLATERAL NECK DISSECTION

Removal of the suboccipital and retroauricular lymph node groups and nodal regions II, III, IV, and V

Indications

1. Treatment of melanomas, squamous cell carcinomas, or other skin tumors with metastatic potential, such as the Merkel cell carcinomas, that originate in the posterior and posterolateral aspects of the neck and the occipital scalp

Special Considerations

1. Site and extent of the primary tumor
2. Metastases in one or both sides of the neck
3. Previous radiation treatment
4. Previous neck surgery

Preoperative Preparation

1. Appropriate laboratory studies

Special Instruments, Position, and Anesthesia

1. When a unilateral dissection is to be performed, the patient is placed in a near-lateral decubitus position with the help of a "bean bag." The neck is extended, and the head is turned toward the opposite side. A foam doughnut or a horseshoe head rest is used to stabilize the head. When a bilateral dissection is to be performed, the patient is placed on the operating table in the prone position, and the neck is slightly flexed.

Tips and Pearls

1. Cranial nerve XI is superficially located in the midposterior triangle of the neck and can be injured during the elevation of the flaps.
2. The thickness of the posterior skin flaps is paramount in this operation. A flap that is too thick can include the superficial suboccipital lymph nodes and defeat the purpose of the operation. A flap that is too thin is likely to necrose.
3. Avoid continuous suturing in the wound closure.
4. Orient the surgical specimen for the pathologist.

Pitfalls and Complications

1. Postoperative hematoma usually occurs within the first few hours. Evacuation of clots and control of the bleeding vessel are best accomplished in the operating room, using sterile technique.
2. Postoperative seromas are common. If small, aspirate; if large or difficult to control with aspiration, insert a suction drain in a sterile fashion.

Postoperative Care Issues

1. Preserving the spinal accessory nerve does not ensure adequate postoperative function of the trapezius. Careful handling of the nerve during surgery, avoiding undue traction and stretching of it, is essential to minimize postoperative dysfunction. This is twice as important when the operation is done on both sides simultaneously. Postoperative shoulder rehabilitation exercises should be instituted as soon as any dysfunction becomes apparent.

References

Goepfert H, Jesse RH, Ballantyne AJ. Posterolateral neck dissection. Arch Otolaryngol 1980;106:618.

Medina JE. Modified neck dissection. In: Shockley WW, Pillsbury HC, eds. The neck—diagnosis and surgery. St.Louis: CV Mosby, 1994: 551.

Operative Procedure

The hockey stick incision extends from the nuchal line to about 1 inch above the clavicle; the vertical portion of the incision is placed about halfway between the posterior border of the sternocleidomastoid muscle and the anterior border of the trapezius.

A thin posterior skin flap is elevated up to the posterior midline of the neck. If the flap is too thick, the superficial suboccipital nodes may be elevated with it. An anterior flap is elevated to the level of the anterior border of the sternocleidomastoid muscle.

The spinal accessory nerve should be preserved if the location of the primary tumor in the skin or the location and extent of the nodal metastases do not preclude it. If the nerve is to be preserved, it is identified early in the dissection and exposed throughout its course in the neck (Fig. 64-1). The different ways to accomplish this are described in Procedure 59.

The dissection begins posteriorly. The fibroadipose tissue that contains the suboccipital lymph nodes is located superficially and deep to the upper one third of the trapezius muscle. Some surgeons describe lymph nodes deep to the splenius capitis muscle, along the deep portion of the occipital artery, and advocate resecting the upper portion of the splenius to ensure their removal. Most surgeons, however, do not include the splenius in the resection and carry the dissection in a plane immediately superficial to this muscle. Identification of this plane is easily accomplished "from below" by incising the trapezius muscle obliquely, starting from a point in the anterior border of the muscle (located approximately at the junction of the upper and middle thirds of it) and continuing upward and backward, toward the posterior midline of the neck at the nuchal line (Fig. 64-2).

The specimen is then dissected forward, off the splenius capitis. In doing so, the superior insertion of the trapezius is incised.

As the dissection is continued forward, the retroauricular lymph node is included in the specimen, and the superior insertion of the sternocleidomastoid muscle is incised near the mastoid process (Fig. 64-3). In the depth, the plane of dissection changes from the splenius capitis to the levator scapulae. When the specimen is freed enough, it is brought forward under the spinal accessory nerve, if it is being preserved (Fig. 64-4).

The remainder of the operation is carried out in a manner similar to the radical and modified radical neck dissections (see Procedures 57 and 59; Fig. 64-5). Depending on the characteristics of the tumor in the neck, it is often possible to preserve the internal jugular vein. The completed dissection is shown in Figure 64-6.

JESUS E. MEDINA

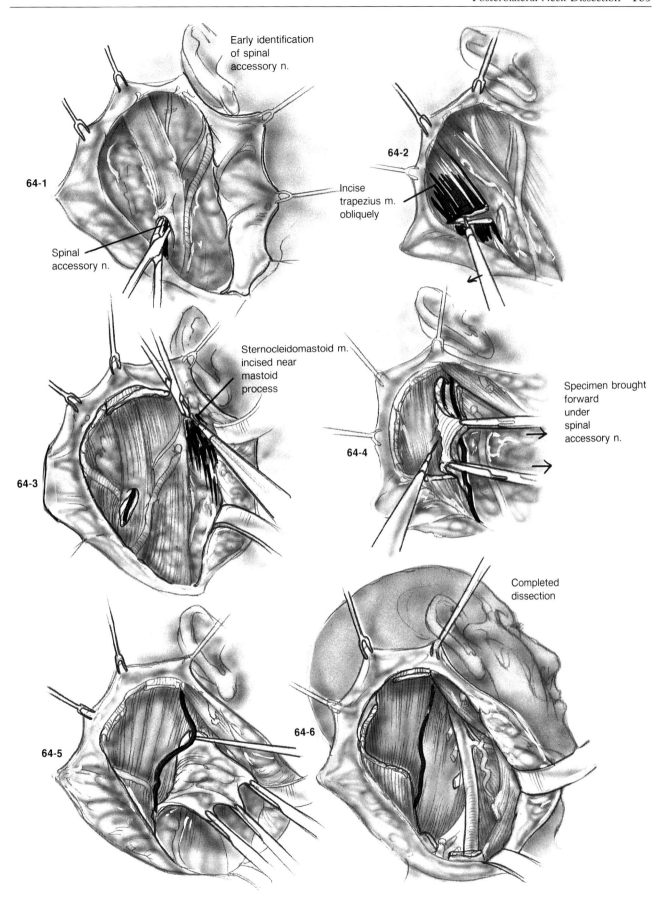

Early identification
of spinal
accessory n.

64-1

Spinal
accessory n.

64-2

Incise
trapezius m.
obliquely

Sternocleidomastoid m.
incised near
mastoid
process

64-3

64-4

Specimen brought
forward
under
spinal
accessory n.

Completed
dissection

64-5

64-6

■ 65. EXCISION OF SUPRACLAVICULAR

SPACE MASSES—Supraclavicular space masses are a heterogeneous group of tumors requiring surgical excision. Most commonly, these are metastatic malignant tumors, but lesions such as lipomas, neurilemomas, angiomas, cystic hygromas, lymphangiomas, or aneurysms of supraclavicular vessels are found.

Indications
1. Lesions presenting in the supraclavicular fossa that require excision because of the potential for malignancy
2. Functional problems related to interference of normal function of the shoulder or low neck
3. Masses that present a cosmetic deformity

Contraindications
1. There is no real contraindication, but the surgeon must ascertain the limits of such a lesion to avoid injury to the great vessels, brachial plexus, and pleura.

Special Considerations
1. Lipomas may be easily dissected through a relatively small incision.
2. Consider the possibility of a brachial plexus tumor for any supraclavicular mass.

Preoperative Preparation
1. Computed tomography and magnetic resonance scans should be reviewed carefully.
2. Cystic hygromas may extend well beyond their apparent clinical boundaries.

Special Instruments, Position, and Anesthesia
1. The patient is supine, with the head extended.
2. A nerve stimulator should be available.

Tips and Pearls
1. Lipomas are easy to remove.
2. Neuromas of the brachial plexus can masquerade as neoplastic lesions.
3. Cystic hygromas and lymphangiomas should be dissected in a systematic fashion to ensure complete excision.

Pitfalls and Complications
1. Attempting to excise a neurogenous tumor of the brachial plexus without necessary preparation, coordination with additional specialists, or an informed patient can lead to a flail limb due to inadvertent injury to the brachial plexus.

Postoperative Care Issues
1. Similar to neck dissection
2. Suction drainage system

References
Livermore GH, Kryzer TC, Patow CA. Aneurysm of the thoracic duct presenting as an asymptomatic left supraclavicular neck mass. Otolaryngol Head Neck Surg 1993;109:530.

Wax MK, Treloar ME. Thoracic duct cyst: an unusual supraclavicular mass. Head Neck 1992;14:502.

Operative Procedure
The patient is placed on the operating room table in a supine position. The head is extended and rotated away from the supraclavicular fossa in question. The 4- to 10-cm incision is placed 2 cm superior and parallel to the clavicle (Fig. 65-1). This incision may be injected with a 1% solution of Xylocaine with a 1:100,000 concentration of epinephrine for hemostasis. I prefer the use of the Shaw scalpel and bipolar electrocautery for hemostasis and clear definition of the dissected tissue planes.

The wound is opened in layers: skin with subcutaneous tissue and platysma. Superior and inferior flaps are developed in a subplatysmal plane (Fig. 65-2). A self-retaining retractor is placed.

Usually, the mass can be exposed by direct dissection (Fig. 65-3). Care should be taken to identify the suprascapular sensory nerves and to preserve these nerves, if feasible. I do not hesitate to section these sensory nerves if necessary for exposure (Fig. 65-4). However, the musculocutaneous nerve is frequently at risk in such a dissection, and its sacrifice may lead to loss of deltoid muscle and shoulder function.

The essence of the operation is the systematic identification and preservation of (medial to lateral) the carotid sheath with contained common carotid artery, internal jugular vein and vagus nerve, the cervical sympathetic chain, the several channels of the thoracic duct, phrenic nerve, transverse cervical artery and vein, omohyoid muscle, and brachial plexus with the musculocutaneous nerve (ie, reference anatomy). The underlying muscles of the floor of the lateral triangle of the neck are observed: anterior, middle, and lateral scalene and the trapezius muscle laterally.

Masses may arise from any of these structures, and it is only through a meticulous and thorough dissection of the supraclavicular fossa that the surgeon can conclusively establish the disease process. If the process is a lipoma, it may be dissected free of the surrounding tissues. If the problem is related to the nerves of the brachial plexus, consultation with a neurosurgeon, orthopedic surgeon, or hand surgeon is prudent to enable an orderly dissection and repair of the problem. Alternatively, the wound may be closed and the patients approached on another day to allow full discussion with the patient and family.

Cystic hygromas are approached in a systematic fashion, similar to the approach of a modified neck dissection, to preserve and protect vital structures and to dissect and remove of all of the lymphangioma.

On completion of the procedure, hemostasis is obtained, and a suction drain is placed. The wound is closed in layers with absorbable 3-0 or 4-0 chromic sutures to approximate the platysma and the subcutaneous tissue. The skin may be closed with staples, interrupted nonabsorbable suture (5-0 nylon), or tape skin closures.

MICHAEL D. MAVES

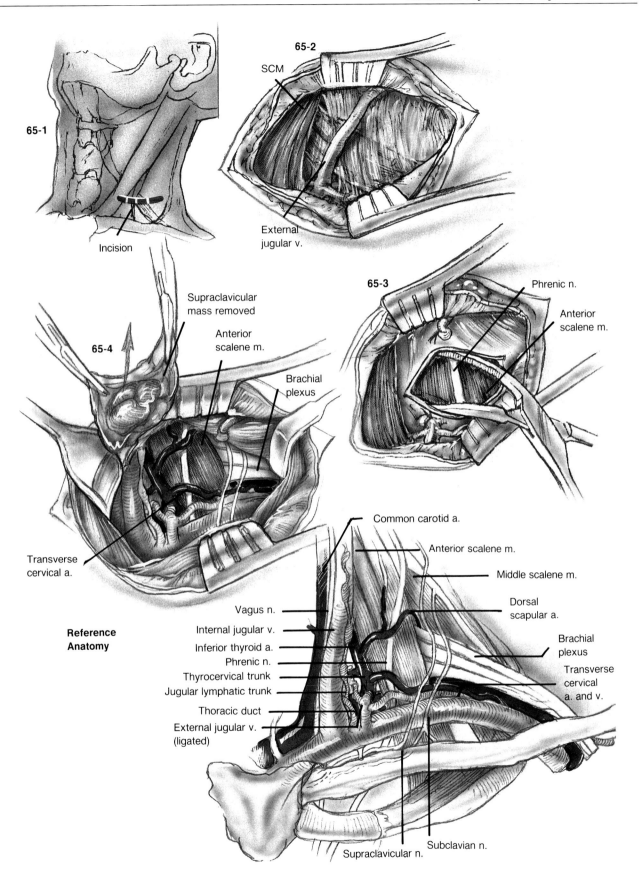

65-1

Incision

65-2

SCM

External
jugular v.

65-3

Phrenic n.

Anterior
scalene m.

65-4

Supraclavicular
mass removed

Anterior
scalene m.

Brachial
plexus

Transverse
cervical a.

**Reference
Anatomy**

Common carotid a.

Anterior scalene m.

Middle scalene m.

Dorsal
scapular a.

Brachial
plexus

Transverse
cervical
a. and v.

Vagus n.

Internal jugular v.

Inferior thyroid a.

Phrenic n.

Thyrocervical trunk

Jugular lymphatic trunk

Thoracic duct

External jugular v.
(ligated)

Supraclavicular n.

Subclavian n.

■ 66. DRAINAGE OF DEEP NECK SPACE AB-
SCESSES—Drainage of collections of purulent material from within the deeper fascial spaces of the neck. Superficial abscesses may be drained with a simple stab wound.

Indications
1. Drainage of deep space neck infections; rarely is actual fluctuance of the neck apparent, and when it does occur, it is very late in the disease process.

Contraindications
1. There are no absolute contraindications to the drainage of a deep neck space abscess.
2. Relative contraindications include clotting abnormalities or a medically unstable patient. In extreme cases, drainage may be necessary at the bedside, using local anesthesia supplemented with intravenous sedation.

Special Considerations
1. Computed tomography and magnetic resonance imaging may be helpful, but reliance on imaging techniques should not substitute for clinical evaluation of patients with suspected deep cervical space abscesses. Rarely is actual fluctuance of the neck seen.

Preoperative Preparation
1. Direct laryngoscopy or esophagoscopy allows inspection and identification of the site of infection.
2. A tracheotomy should be considered if there is concern about the patient's airway.
3. If the patient is not already on antibiotics, perioperative antibiotics are indicated.

Special Instruments, Position, and Anesthesia
1. The patient is placed in a supine position.
2. The anesthesiologist should be aware that the patient may have distorted upper airway anatomy due to the abscess.

Tips and Pearls
1. Try to correct the abscess on the initial cervical exploration. There may not be another opportunity to return the patient to the operating room again, or the patient may not be medically stable.

Pitfalls and Complications
1. Inspect all areas of the neck for collections of purulent material. The abscess may be phlegmonous instead of purulent. Such a process requires drainage but does not yield much frankly purulent material.

Postoperative Care Issues
1. Be patient in removing the cervical drains during the postoperative period. Label the drains with a suture or safety pin so that they may be removed in a logical sequence (eg, distal to proximal) after the patient is stable and cervical drainage has ceased.

References
Har-El G, Aroesty JH, Shaha A, Lucente FE. Changing trends in deep neck abscess. A retrospective study of 110 patients. Oral Surg Oral Med Oral Pathol 1994;77:446.
Johnson JT. Abscesses and deep space infections of the head and neck. Infect Dis Clin North Am 1992;6:705.

Operative Procedure
The ideal approach to a deep neck abscess is one that affords an excellent exposure of the entire neck so that the infectious process can be followed and drained completely. The incision should be able to be converted into a more extensive procedure easily, and it should be somewhat cosmetic, realizing the potentially life-threatening, but benign nature of such problems. I have found a high apron incision to be the ideal route of access for such operations.

The patient is placed on the operating room table in a supine position. An apron incision is marked from the mastoid tip, descending inferiorly and extending toward the midline at the level of the thyroid ala (Fig. 66-1). This incision allows exposure of the critical areas of the neck and may be extended with a vertical limb if required.

The wound is opened in layers: skin with subcutaneous tissue and then platysma. Because of the infected tissues, the surgeon should anticipate more bleeding than usual. This can be managed with Bovie electrocautery. Superior and inferior flaps are developed in the subplatysmal plane. A self-retaining retractor is placed.

I begin the exploration of the neck by identifying the anterior border of the sternocleidomastoid muscle and retracting it posteriorly to expose the carotid sheath. The carotid sheath is opened and drained if necessary. I observe the condition of the internal jugular vein to ensure that there is no thrombosis. The great vessels are retracted posteriorly, and the retrovisceral space of the neck is exposed and entered (Fig. 66-2). The fascia overlying the cervical vertebrae can be seen, and wide exposure of this space is afforded by digital dissection (Fig. 66-3). The surgeon's index finger opens the retroesophageal space superiorly to the base of the skull and inferiorly to the thoracic inlet. Any purulent material encountered should be cultured for aerobic and anaerobic bacteria. In many instances, frank purulent material may not exist; instead, a phlegmonous "dishwater" discharge is discovered.

If required by the clinical condition, the pterygoid space, masseteric space, and parotid space can be inspected and opened by extension of the previously described procedure. The pterygoid and masseteric space may be reached through the superior portion of the wound at the margin of the mandible (Fig. 66-4). The parotid space requires an extension of the incision in the preauricular area similar to a parotidectomy. Multiple stab incisions in the periparotid fascia provide drainage of the abscess.

After all required areas of the neck have been drained, the wound is copiously irrigated with saline, and several large, 2-cm-wide Penrose drains are inserted in the neck. One drain is placed superiorly to the level of the base of the skull. Another drain is placed inferiorly in the retropharynx toward the mediastinum. Additional drains are placed in specific areas of loculation (Fig. 66-5).

The wound is closed loosely in layers. The skin is closed loosely, and a large cervical wrap is placed. The patient is monitored closely during the postoperative period, with particular attention to the patient's temperature and leukocyte count. Drains are slowly advanced after the patient has defervesced and the leukocyte count has become normal. The most distal drains are advanced first, followed by the more proximal ones, to allow the wound to close from the depths.

MICHAEL D. MAVES

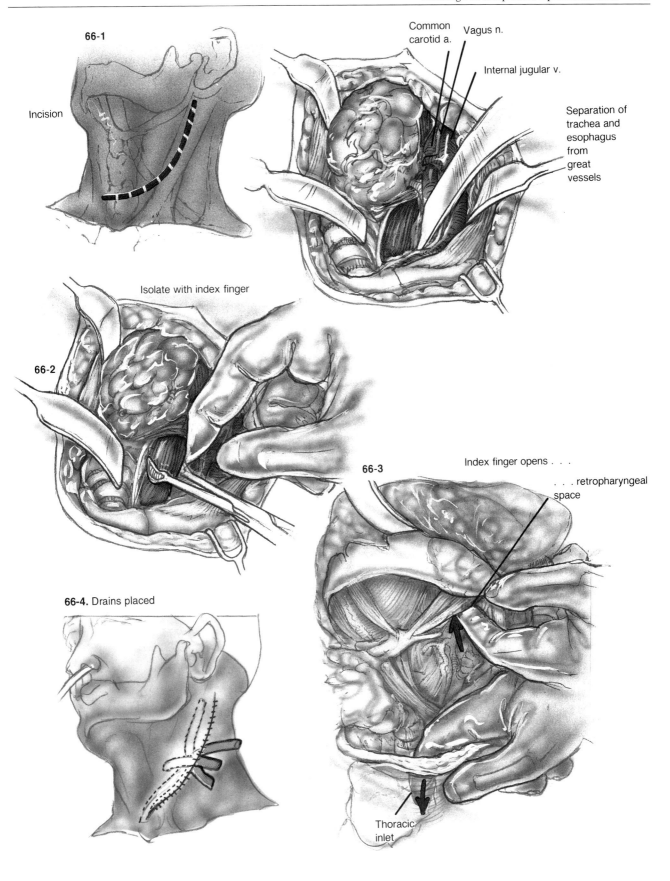

66-1

Incision

Common carotid a.

Vagus n.

Internal jugular v.

Separation of trachea and esophagus from great vessels

Isolate with index finger

66-2

66-3

Index finger opens . . .

. . . retropharyngeal space

66-4. Drains placed

Thoracic inlet

■ 67. MANAGEMENT OF PENETRATING IN-JURIES TO THE NECK— Exploration and repair of injuries to the neck caused by external high-velocity instruments (eg, bullets), external low-velocity instruments (eg, knives, icepicks), iatrogenic trauma due to endoscopic instrumentation, or internal injuries due to foreign bodies

Indications

1. Neck exploration should be considered for every patient with neck trauma. The decision depends on the results of the physical examination, fiberoptic endoscopy, computed tomography (CT) scans, arteriography, diagnostic endoscopy, and the level of injury (ie, neck trauma levels).

Contraindications

1. There are no contraindications to exploration of the neck in cervical trauma. Delay or not performing an exploration of the neck when indicated may jeopardize the patient's life.

Special Considerations

1. If the patient is stable hemodynamically, without evidence of an expanding hematoma or a level II injury, an orderly evaluation of the problem should be made. Initial fiberoptic examination of the upper aerodigestive tract is completed in the emergency room.
2. If indicated, the patient should have a CT examination of the neck and arteriography to rule out significant trauma to the vascular tree. If there is no evidence of transgression of the vascular axis, penetration of the aerodigestive tract, or compromise of the airway, the patient may be observed without undertaking exploration.
3. If there is apparent or suspected injury to the vascular system or pharynx with airway compromise or an expanding hematoma, urgent exploration of the neck is required.

Preoperative Preparation

1. Complete head and neck examination
2. A comprehensive examination of the rest of the body to rule out other trauma
3. Establishment of an airway
4. Initiation of fluid resuscitation
5. Tetanus prophylaxis is imperative.
6. Perioperative antibiotics are indicated.

Special Instruments, Position, and Anesthesia

1. An experienced anesthesiologist is required for this type of surgery.
2. Sufficient blood (≥6 units)
3. Vascular instruments
4. The ability or another surgeon to repair major vascular injuries is imperative.

Tips and Pearls

1. The planes of dissection in emergent surgery are not as clean as in an elective case.
2. Hematoma can distort, discolor, and make quite difficult identification of even major landmarks in the neck.

Pitfalls and Complications

1. Obtain proximal and distal control of the vascular system as the initial step in any exploration.
2. Leave the area of maximum injury relatively undisturbed until vital structures can be identified.
3. Be prepared for the unexpected in neck exploration. Anticipate!

Postoperative Care Issues

1. Penrose drains are superior to suction drains in most instances.

References

Clark GC, Lim RC Jr, Rosenburg JM. Cervicothoracic vascular injuries. Presentation, management, and outcome. Am Surg 1991;57:582.

Kelly P, Sanson T, Strange G, Orsay E. A prospective study of the impact of helmet usage on motorcycle trauma. Ann Emerg Med 1991;20:852.

Operative Procedure

The patient is brought to the operating room and placed supine on the table. The patient should have several large-bore intravenous lines, a central venous pressure or Swan-Ganz catheter, and a Foley catheter in place. If the airway was not secured in the emergency room, the patient should be intubated by an experienced anesthesiologist or undergo tracheotomy. Sufficient blood and colloid or crystalloid solutions should be on hand, along with personnel to conduct a resuscitation if the patient's condition deteriorates.

Preparatory direct laryngoscopy, esophagoscopy, and bronchoscopy are performed to examine the upper aerodigestive tract for injury. This can confirm impressions made on the initial examination and discover occult injuries.

An apron or hockey stick incision with the long limb parallel to the anterior border of the sternocleidomastoid muscle provides exposure to all areas of the neck and complete linear exposure of the vascular tree for proximal and distal control (Fig. 67-1). The wound is opened in layers: skin with subcutaneous tissue and then platysma. Because of the trauma, the surgeon should anticipate more discoloration of the tissues, distortion of even major structures, and more bleeding than usually encountered in a nontraumatic case.

Proximal and distal control of the common, internal, and external carotid arteries is provided by retraction of the anterior border of the sternomastoid muscle (Fig. 67-2). The jugular vein is encountered with the vagus and hypoglossal nerves, which should be protected. Considerable bleeding may occur from the internal jugular vein, which may seem like arterial bleeding in a patient who is well oxygenated by the anesthesiologist. This can be controlled with digital pressure while proximal and distal control is achieved. The patient should be brought quickly into the Trendelenburg position to prevent air embolization.

Injuries to the carotid arterial system are handled by repair, replacement, or ligation, depending on the location and size of the injury. A mandibulotomy may be necessary for exposure to the superior aspects of the neck (Fig. 67-3). The significance of the vessel makes a difference; internal carotid artery integrity is paramount. Close cooperation with the general surgery, vascular surgery, or trauma surgery team is indicated if the head and neck surgeon is not comfortable or capable of performing vascular surgery of the head and neck.

After the arterial injuries are addressed, the neural structures of the neck in the area of the injury should be inventoried (Fig. 67-4). The vagus, facial, phrenic, hypoglossal, spinal accessory, brachial plexus, and cervical sympathetic chain are major neural structures that should be preserved or repaired.

The "organs" of the neck are examined for injury as the next phase of the exploration. The tongue, pharynx, larynx, thyroid, and esophagus are inspected for injury and repaired. Large Penrose drains are placed in proximity to the areas of disruption to afford drainage postoperatively. It may not be possible to repair some visceral injuries, and these injuries must be drained and allowed to heal secondarily. A nasogastric tube is placed and secured for postoperative feeding.

The neck is closed in layers with passive Penrose drains in place. A large cervical wrap is placed, and the patient is placed in an area of the hospital where close observation may be conducted. The hemodynamic status of the patient requires continued monitoring and frequent inspection of the wounds. The patient's temperature curve is monitored, but I find serial assessment of the white blood cell count to be an early, reliable indicator of a fistula.

MICHAEL D. MAVES

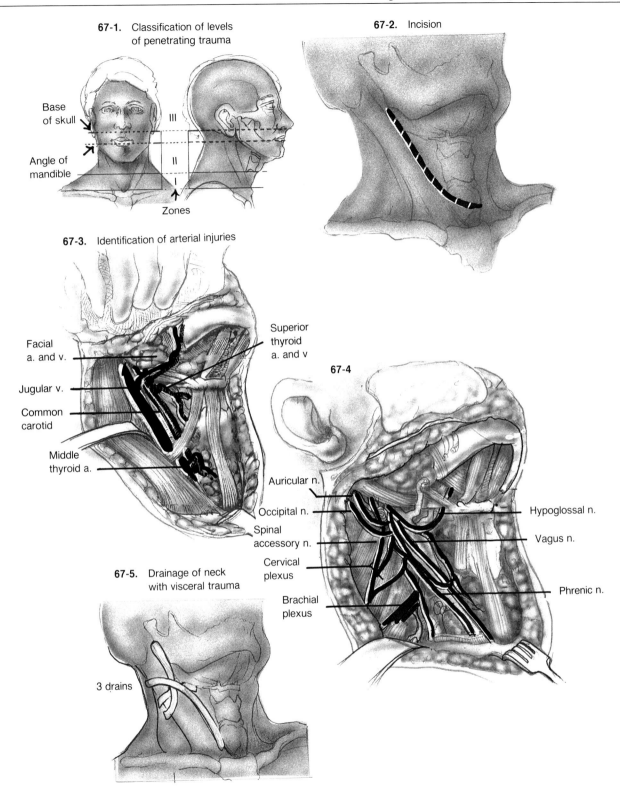

67-1. Classification of levels of penetrating trauma

Base of skull

Angle of mandible

III

II

I

Zones

67-2. Incision

67-3. Identification of arterial injuries

Facial a. and v.

Jugular v.

Common carotid

Middle thyroid a.

Superior thyroid a. and v

67-4

Auricular n.

Occipital n.

Spinal accessory n.

Cervical plexus

Brachial plexus

Hypoglossal n.

Vagus n.

Phrenic n.

67-5. Drainage of neck with visceral trauma

3 drains

■ 68. ENDOSCOPIC PARTIAL LARYNGEC-TOMY FOR SUPRAGLOTTIC DISEASE—Endoscopic excision of a portion or all of the supraglottic larynx

Indications

1. Selected early cancers (T1, T2) of the suprahyoid epiglottis (eg, suprahyoepiglottic ligament) epiglottis, aryepiglottic fold, or the vestibular fold
2. Selected larger supraglottic cancers (T2, T3) that are confined to the supraglottis in patients who are not suitable for an open supraglottic laryngectomy. These patients should receive full-course radiation therapy after the excisional biopsy of the supraglottic cancer.
3. Selected benign neoplasms of the supraglottic larynx
4. Selected inflammation-induced supraglottic swelling (eg, radiation edema, sarcoid) resulting in airway obstruction that is refractory to medical management

Contraindications

1. Inability to obtain adequate endoscopic exposure of the surgical site
2. Inability for the patient to undergo general anesthesia
3. Cancer invasion of the laryngeal framework, except if the surgical goal is airway palliation

Special Considerations

1. Patients with a history of swallowing impairment secondary to a neurologic deficit or previous head and neck surgery
2. Management of cervical metastases
3. Patients with cervical spine disorders

Preoperative Preparation

1. Routine laboratory studies
2. Careful office examination, including flexible fiberoptic or telescopic laryngoscopy
3. Optional radiographic imaging to assist in determining the extent of the primary or regional metastatic disease
4. Careful discussion with the patient about all treatment options and the goals of the endoscopic excision: treatment, excisional biopsy before irradiation, or airway palliation
5. After the intravenous line is placed, 10 to 16 mg of Decadron is administered
6. Optional perioperative antibiotics

Special Instruments, Position, and Anesthesia

1. Adjustable supraglottiscope with a wide malleable retractor (Richard Wolf Co., Rosemont, IL)
2. Carbon dioxide laser preferably with a microspot
3. Surgical microscope
4. Boston University gallows (Pilling Co., Fort Washington, PA) to maintain Boyce-Jackson position (elevated-vector suspension)
5. Large (Jackson) alligator laryngeal forceps (Pilling Co.)
6. Electrocautery
7. Laser-protected endotracheal tube for general anesthesia

Tips and Pearls

1. Obtain ideal exposure before beginning the resection.
2. Meticulous hemostasis

Pitfalls and Complications

1. Aspiration after resection of larger lesions
2. Slow wound healing if there is significant gastroesophageal reflux

Postoperative Care Issues

1. Nasogastric enteral nutrition, depending on the extent of the resection
2. Swallowing therapy, depending on the extent of resection
3. Optional antireflux management

References

Shapiro J, Zeitels SM, Fried MF. Laser surgery for laryngeal cancer. Operative techniques. Otolaryngol Head Neck Surg 1992;3:84.

Zeitels SM, Koufman JA, Davis RK, Vaughan CW. Endoscopic treatment of supraglottic and hypopharynx cancer. Laryngoscope, 1994;104:71.

Operative Procedure

Endoscopic Exposure

The patient is intubated with a laser-protected endotracheal tube. Direct laryngoscopy is performed with a standard-tube laryngoscope (eg, Dedo, Jako) to assess the lesion for possible transoral resection. If the lesion is thought to be a cancer, it is staged and mapped. A small biopsy with frozen-section analysis can be performed to confirm the cancer diagnosis before proceeding with the excisional biopsy.

The adjustable supraglottiscope is placed with the blades closed. The laryngoscope blades are first separated in a parallel fashion, and then the inferior blade is distracted posteriorly to allow the widest possible surgical exposure (Fig. 68-1 and 68-2). A wide malleable retractor is placed alongside the laryngoscope to prevent the tongue from insinuating between the laryngoscope blades, which would obscure laryngeal visualization (Fig. 68-3). During the laryngoscopy, the patient is placed in the Boyce-Jackson position (ie, flexion of the neck on the chest and extension of the head on the neck) and maintained in that position with the Boston University gallows. This position is called elevated-vector suspension (see Fig. 68-1). The endotracheal tube is maintained out of the surgical field by the inferior laryngoscope blade.

The microscope and the carbon dioxide laser are then brought into position. A wet cottonoid is placed over the cuff of the endotracheal tube. The laser is typically programmed for a repeated pulse mode with a spot size of 0.3 to 0.8 mm. The power is set at 3 to 5 watts, with a 0.1-second pulse duration and 0.1-second interval between pulses. As necessary, bleeding may be controlled with the electrocautery by applying the current to an insulated suction or to an alligator forceps that has grasped the offending vessel.

Epiglottic Resection

The superior laryngoscope blade is placed in the vallecula glossoepiglottica. The suprahyoid epiglottis is grasped with a large alligator-type Jackson laryngeal forceps and retracted posteriorly. The vallecula mucosa is incised to expose the white fibers of the hyoepiglottic ligament. This ligament is incised to expose the preepiglottic fat (Fig. 68-3). The dissection continues caudad toward the petiole on the anterior aspect of the epiglottis. As necessary, the epiglottis is retracted laterally to incise the mucosa and lateral epiglottic attachments of the quadrangular membrane. This lateral epiglottic dissection is performed cephalad to caudad until the epiglottic petiole is reached and the epiglottis is excised (Fig. 68-4).

Aryepiglottic Fold Resection

The superior laryngoscope blade is placed under the epiglottis, and the mucosal incisions anterior to the arytenoid, posterior to the epiglottis, and along the vestibular fold are made to outline the lesion. The superior laryngoscope blade can be replaced in the vallecula glossoepiglottica if it is necessary to resect a portion of the epiglottis for an adequate tumor-free margin (Fig. 68-5). There are no significant healing problems from leaving exposed epiglottic cartilage if the patient is not immunocompromised. The exposed cartilage of the residual epiglottis will mucosalize without consequence.

Vestibular Fold Resection

The adjustable supraglottiscope or a large-tube laryngoscope are placed to expose the lesion. A flat, wet cottonoid is placed over the ipsilateral true vocal fold into the ventricle and under the vestibular fold. This protects the true vocal fold from unintended trauma from the laser during the vestibular fold resection. The vestibular fold and the lesion are retracted medially, and the lesion is excised.

Combined Resection

Any combination of these procedures can be employed, but larger resections require greater skill and experience. Exposure of larger lesions may be problematic, and maintaining an adequate deep cancer-free margin can be difficult (Fig. 68-6). Bleeding from branches of the superior laryngeal vasculature obscures visualization and requires electrocautery. The laryngoscope typically needs to be repositioned during the procedure.

STEVEN M. ZEITELS

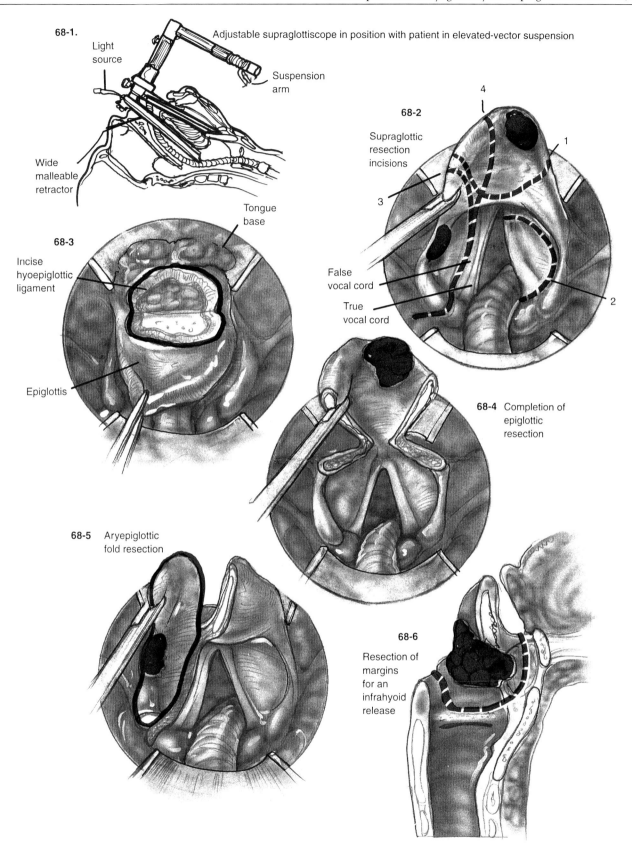

68-1.   Adjustable supraglottiscope in position with patient in elevated-vector suspension

Light source

Suspension arm

Wide malleable retractor

Tongue base

68-2

Supraglottic resection incisions

4

1

3

False vocal cord

True vocal cord

2

68-3

Incise hyoepiglottic ligament

Epiglottis

68-4   Completion of epiglottic resection

68-5   Aryepiglottic fold resection

68-6

Resection of margins for an infrahyoid release

■ 69. ENDOSCOPIC PARTIAL LARYNGEC-TOMY AT THE GLOTTIC LEVEL—Transoral excision of neoplasms located on the true vocal folds

Indications
1. Squamous cell carcinoma, limited to the midportion of a mobile vocal fold
2. Verrucous carcinoma

Special Considerations
1. Adequate surgical margins for histologic inspection
2. Extensive resection produces an inadequate postoperative voice
3. Vocal fold anatomy and histology
4. Laser safety for patient and operating room staff

Preoperative Evaluation
1. Routine laboratory studies
2. Electrocardiogram
3. Photographic documentation
4. Endostroboscopic evaluation

Special Instrumentation, Position, and Anesthesia
1. Binocular microlaryngoscope
2. Suspension device
3. Microsurgical instrumentation
4. Laser-safe endotracheal tube
5. Patient eye and skin protection
6. Neck flexion, with head extension
7. Total patient paralysis and relaxation
8. Decreased fraction of inspired oxygen (FIO_2) with helium, nitrogen, or room air

Tips and Pearls
1. Exposure with a suitable laryngoscope and suspension device
2. Define the extent of resection before surgical retraction, which distorts the field.

Pitfalls and Complications
1. Extension to the anterior commissure
2. Extension to the vocal process
3. Lateral extension into the ventricle
4. Subglottic extension
5. Overaggressive resection leading to loss of postoperative voicing
6. Intraoperative and postoperative bleeding

Postoperative Care Issues
1. Airway observation
2. Humidification after large resection

References
Ossoff RH, Sisson GA, Shapshay SM. Endoscopic management of selected early vocal cord carcinoma. Ann Otol Rhinol Laryngol 1985;94: 560.

Shapshay SM, Hybels RL, Bohigian RK. Laser excision of early vocal cord carcinoma: indications, limitations, and precautions. Ann Otol Rhinol Laryngol 1990;99:46.

Operative Procedure

Endoscopic partial laryngectomy at the glottic level begins with exposure. The largest-caliber laryngoscope possible is placed, and a suspension device is used. We prefer a modification of the Dedo laryngoscope. The Dedo laryngoscopes with an upward flair at the distal tip provide improved exposure of the anterior commissure over the standard Jako microlaryngoscope. The Dedo laryngoscopes also permit ample proximal space for binocular vision and work with microlaryngeal instruments. Alternatively, if a modification of the Dedo laryngoscope cannot be placed because of anatomic limitations, a modified Holinger laryngoscope, which permits binocular vision, can be inserted. This Ossoff-Pilling laryngoscope is extremely useful for obtaining exposure of the anterior commissure in retrognathic patients. Characteristics of useful microlaryngoscopes for endoscopic procedures include adequate lighting and a smoke evacuation port to facilitate use with the carbon dioxide laser.

Exposure is achieved with a suitable laryngoscope and suspension device applied. The glottis is inspected with a 0° telescope. This provides excellent monocular visualization and can be coupled with a video or still camera for teaching or documentation purposes. The operating microscope is then aligned with the visual field. The 400-mm focal length lens provides an acceptable working distance. Precision is enhanced by using the microscope on 16× magnification.

The lesion is visualized and palpated to determine if it can be separated from the vocal ligament. Neoplasms arise within the mucosa. By incising the vocal fold membrane lateral to the lesion (Fig. 69-1), a blunt elevator may be inserted into Reinke's space (Fig. 69-2) and used to separate the vocal fold cover, consisting of the mucosa and superficial lamina propria, from the underlying ligament (Fig. 69-3). Specially designed microlaryngeal scissors are then used to excise the mucosal flap (Fig. 69-4). These steps can be tedious. If successful, this serves as adequate therapy for severe dysplasia or carcinoma in situ (CIS). If it is not possible to separate the lesion from the vocal ligament, a superficial biopsy is taken. Frozen-section analysis is employed to determine the extent of invasion. If carcinoma with invasion is found, additional margins are required.

The carbon dioxide laser is attached to the operating microscope with the micromanipulator. The newer-generation microspot micromanipulators provide a laser spot size of 250 to 300 μm at a 400-mm focal length working distance. The enhanced precision afforded by the smaller spot size is significantly preferable to the older-generation micromanipulators, which provided an 800-μm spot size at the same working distance. The laser is then used in a focused single pulse mode to outline the area of additional resection (Fig. 69-5). The portion to be excised is retracted with cup forceps or a microlaryngeal suction while the laser in a repeat pulse mode of approximately 2000 watts/cm^2 is used to excise the portion of vocal fold previously outlined (Fig. 69-6).

It is possible to excise the entire membranous vocal fold in this manner. However, voice results may worsen as more aggressive resection is pursued. Resection limited to mobile middle-third vocal fold lesions usually result in the formation of a scar band during healing. Although this scar band does not develop normal vibratory characteristics, it usually provides a surface for the normal vocal fold to vibrate against during phonation. Voice results are comparable to those obtained after radiation therapy.

Endoscopic partial laryngectomy at the glottic level should be reserved for lesions limited to the midportion of a mobile true vocal fold. With this restriction, endoscopic excision provides cure rates equal to other, more radical procedures such as radiation therapy or open cordectomy. Endoscopic partial laryngectomy at the glottic level is also appropriate for lesions that are not radiosensitive, such as verrucous carcinoma, in which good endoscopic exposure can be obtained and adequate surgical margins are not limited by cartilaginous encroachment. Inappropriate use of endoscopic partial laryngectomy at the glottic level for lesions that encroach on the anterior commissure or the vocal process of the arytenoid leads to failure because of early cartilaginous extension and enhanced lymphatic lateral (paraglottic space) extension.

ROBERT H. OSSOFF
MARK S. COUREY

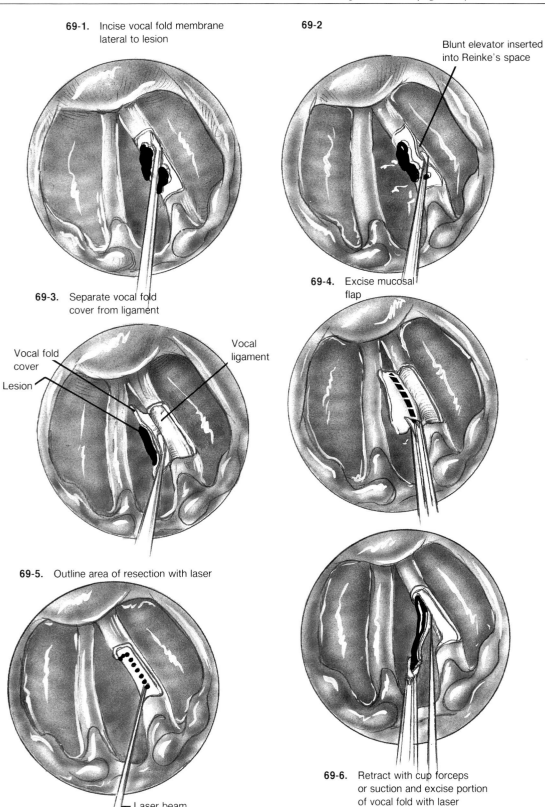

69-1. Incise vocal fold membrane lateral to lesion

69-2

Blunt elevator inserted into Reinke's space

69-3. Separate vocal fold cover from ligament

Vocal fold cover

Lesion

Vocal ligament

69-4. Excise mucosal flap

69-5. Outline area of resection with laser

Laser beam

69-6. Retract with cup forceps or suction and excise portion of vocal fold with laser

■ 70. LARYNGOFISSURE AND CORDECTOMY

The simplest form of vertical partial laryngectomy. It is the least invasive and the most limited of the open procedures because only the vocal cord and its adjacent internal perichondrium are removed.

Indications

1. Stage T1 invasive carcinoma of the true vocal fold limited to the middle one third of the cord and localized to the free margin of the cord; these lesions may also be appropriate for endoscopic resection or radiation therapy.
2. T1 verrucous or papillary carcinoma may be the most appropriate indication.

Contraindications

1. Stage T2, T3, or T4 lesions
2. Bulky lesions obscuring mucosal margins
3. Arytenoid involvement
4. Deep anterior commissure involvement
5. Recurrence after radiation therapy

Special Considerations

1. Functional results of the procedure may not be optimal with this procedure, because the missing cord is not reconstructed.
2. A modification of this procedure is cordectomy, including the adjacent thyroid ala and imbrication laryngoplasty, forming a "neocord" with the patients own false vocal cord. This procedure is not necessarily contraindicated for radiation therapy failures or deep anterior commissure involvement, but cordectomy alone is contraindicated in these situations. This imbrication procedure is also safer for lesions larger than 2 mm.

Preoperative Preparation

1. Staging, including imaging and endoscopy
2. Routine laboratory tests

Tips and Pearls

1. Do not select this procedure for any lesion for which there is a question about the adequacy of this approach.
2. Temporary tracheotomy may be advisable in some patients for airway management during the postoperative period.

Pitfalls and Complications

1. Hoarseness
2. Aspiration
3. Incomplete tumor excision
4. Airway obstruction and postoperative edema

Special Instruments, Position, and Anesthesia

1. Headlight
2. Laryngectomy tray
3. Oscillating saw

Postoperative Care Issues

1. Remove drain on the first postoperative day.
2. Begin trials of cuff deflation on the first postoperative day.
3. Examine the airway with flexible laryngoscopy.
4. Decannulate late in the first postoperative week.
5. Begin feeding as tolerated, even before decannulation.
6. Speech therapy

References

Bailey BJ. Early glottic carcinoma. In: Bailey BJ, Johnson JT, Pillsbury HC, et al, eds. Head and neck surgery—otolaryngology. Philadelphia: JB Lippincott, 1993;1313.

Liu C, Ward PH, Pleet L. Imbrication reconstruction following partial laryngectomy. Ann Otol Rhinol Laryngol 1986;95:567.

Olsen KD, Thomas JV, DeSanto LW, Suman VJ. Indications and results of cordectomy for early glottic carcinoma. Otolaryngol Head Neck Surg 1993;108:277.

Operative Procedure

Laryngofissure and Cordectomy

The patient is positioned supine on the operating table. The tracheotomy should be performed under local anesthesia or under general anesthesia after oral intubation, depending on the ease of airway management. A transverse skin incision is made in the region of the lower thyroid ala, and an attempt is made to keep the dissection separate from the tracheotomy. Cervical flaps are elevated in a subplatysmal plane until the hyoid is exposed superiorly and the cricoid exposed inferiorly. The strap muscles are incised in the midline, and the external thyroid perichondrium is incised in the midline and at the superior and inferior ala. The oscillating saw is used to perform a midline thyrotomy (Fig. 70-1), and the cricothyroid membrane is incised at the lower border of the thyroid, but only in the midline. The incision is carried superiorly through the thyrotomy upward, dividing the anterior commissure or the ipsilateral vocal cord just proximal to the anterior commissure and taking care to avoid cutting into the tumor.

The tumor is resected, including the entire true vocal cord, vocal process of the arytenoid, and all adjacent tissue, complete with the internal perichondrium of the thyroid cartilage (Fig. 70-2). Margins are checked with frozen sections. The free edges of the mucosa are approximated using interrupted 4-0 chromic suture (Fig. 70-3). The laryngofissure is closed using 2-0 Vicryl sutures placed through drill holes if the thyroid cartilage is calcified. The perichondrium is closed with 3-0 Vicryl sutures, and the skin closed in two layers with 3-0 Vicryl inverted interrupted sutures in the deep dermis and 5-0 fast-absorbing gut in the skin. A Penrose drain is used with a dressing consisting of a sterile gauze wrap. The cuffed tracheotomy tube is secured with sutures and ties.

Imbrication Laryngoplasty After Cordectomy

In this procedure, the steps are the same except that the resection includes the adjacent horizontal strip of thyroid cartilage (Fig. 70-4). The superior cartilaginous segment is then imbricated medial to the inferior strut and secured with an imbricating suture of 2-0 Prolene (Figs. 70-5 and 70-6). The false vocal cord is brought down and sutured to the subglottic mucosa, allowing a predictable tension-free mucosal closure and a neocord consisting of vascularized, innervated tissue. The closure is the same as for the laryngofissure and cordectomy.

CHRISTOPHER H. RASSEKH

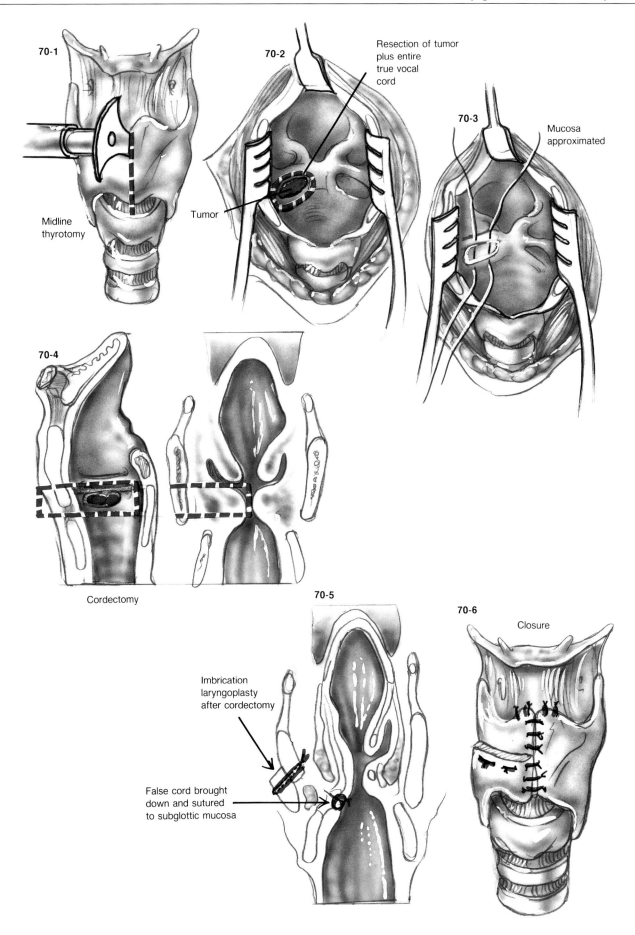

70-1

Midline
thyrotomy

70-2

Tumor

Resection of tumor
plus entire
true vocal
cord

70-3

Mucosa
approximated

70-4

Cordectomy

70-5

Imbrication
laryngoplasty
after cordectomy

False cord brought
down and sutured
to subglottic mucosa

70-6

Closure

■ 71. VERTICAL PARTIAL LARYNGECTOMY, INCLUDING THE THYROID CARTILAGE— Removal of one vocal cord and a portion of the overlying thyroid cartilage through an external approach

Indications

1. Carcinoma of the glottis with extension to the vocal process of the arytenoid or involvement of the floor of the ventricle
2. Transglottic tumor without cord fixation
3. Recurrent glottic carcinoma after radiation therapy

Contraindications

1. Cord fixation (not an absolute contraindication, although surgery may be feasible only for a few selected cases)
2. Subglottic extension of more than 10 mm anteriorly or 5 to 6 mm posteriorly
3. Invasion of the cricoarytenoid joint
4. Involvement of the interarytenoid area
5. Involvement of the anterior commissure or the contralateral vocal cord
6. Fair to poor pulmonary status
7. Thyroid cartilage invasion
8. Involvement of both arytenoids

Special Considerations

1. For anterior commissure or contralateral cord involvement, an anterior commissure or frontolateral laryngectomy should be performed.
2. Involvement of the arytenoid cartilage
3. Impaired cord mobility
4. Deep ventricular involvement
5. Transglottic tumor
6. Subglottic extension
7. Submucosal spread
8. Prior radiation therapy
9. Patient's medical condition, especially the pulmonary status
10. Reliability of follow-up
11. Neck node status
12. Informed consent must be obtained for total laryngectomy or partial procedures in case the tumor extends beyond the involved vocal cord.

Preoperative Evaluation

1. Routine laboratory studies
2. Pulmonary function tests
3. Computed tomography or magnetic resonance scan if occult tumor-positive nodes and cartilaginous invasion are considerations.
4. Upper endoscopy, laryngoscopy
5. Strobovideolaryngoscopy (optional)
6. Preoperative evaluation of speech and swallowing

Special Instruments, Position, and Anesthesia

1. Headlight
2. Delicate instruments
3. Sagittal saw to enter larynx
4. Supine position, with the head extended
5. Bipolar cautery
6. General anesthesia
7. Tracheotomy is necessary.
8. Nasogastric or gastrostomy tubes are necessary.

Tips and Pearls

1. Palpate or dissect the jugular nodal chains to identify adenopathy that may have been missed preoperatively.
2. For more than 5 mm of subglottic tumor extension, consider ipsilateral thyroidectomy and resection of the superior one half of the ipsilateral cricoid cartilage.

(continued)

Operative Procedure

The patient is placed in the supine position on the operating table, using a transverse shoulder roll and head extension. General anesthesia is induced, and an endotracheal tube is inserted, or a tracheostomy is performed under local anesthesia, and general anesthesia is then induced. A nasogastric feeding tube is placed.

A laryngoscopy is performed to reevaluate the extent of the tumor (Fig. 71-2). A transverse incision is made, curving superiorly as it goes laterally over the sternocleidomastoid muscles, enabling an apron flap to be raised (Fig. 71-1). The inferior portion of the incision (overlying the larynx) is one fingerbreadth below the cricoid cartilage. A superior subplatysmal flap is raised to the level of the hyoid bone. If a tracheotomy has not been performed, a separate transverse incision can be made inferior and parallel to the other incision. The skin island between the two incisions must be at least 2 cm wide. Laterally, exposure can include the anterior sternocleidomastoid muscle, allowing the jugular lymph node chains to be examined for metastatic adenopathy. Any suspicious nodes are sent for frozen-section analysis.

The strap muscles and the sternocleidomastoid muscles should be clearly visible. The strap muscles are bluntly dissected in the midline to expose the thyroid perichondrium. Gently elevating the strap muscles laterally exposes the thyroid cartilage. The thyroid perichondrium is incised along its superior and inferior borders directly in the midline. The perichondrium is elevated laterally to within 3 mm of the posterior border of the thyroid cartilage on the involved side and halfway posteriorly on the uninvolved side. The thyroid perichondrium is sutured to the adjacent strap muscle to protect it from trauma. It is important to maintain the integrity of the perichondrium and strap muscles, because they are necessary for reconstruction of the defect after resection. If thyroid or cricoid cartilage invasion is seen at this time, a total laryngectomy should be performed.

The thyroid cartilage is divided vertically in the midline with a sagittal saw (Fig. 71-3). The internal thyroid perichondrium is not violated. The internal perichondrium is elevated gently with a blunt elevator 2 to 3 mm laterally on the tumor side. The thyroid cartilage is also divided vertically on the involved side 4 mm anterior to its posterior border. The external thyroid perichondrium should not be damaged.

The larynx is entered in the midline through a small horizontal incision in the cricothyroid membrane. The cricoid and the thyroid cartilage are separated with hooks to expose the tumor on the involved side. The surgeon must wear a headlight for this portion of the procedure. As exposure of the tumor is gained, the laryngeal soft tissue in the midline of the anterior portion of the involved cord (if it is uninvolved), is incised in an inferior to superior direction. A good way to do this is to place a scissors with one blade inside and one blade outside the lumen. The internal branches of the superior laryngeal neurovascular bundle on the involved side can be divided at this time. The incision is carried horizontally and laterally within the thyrohyoid membrane at the superior end of the thyroid cartilage. The tumor is well visualized (Fig. 71-4). The mobilized portion of the larynx is retracted laterally. The tumor is resected, including the ipsilateral mobilized thyroid cartilage. The ipsilateral arytenoid is removed by separating the cricoarytenoid joint if the vocal process is involved. It is not necessary to remove the arytenoid if the vocal process is uninvolved; in fact, its preservation enhances postoperative vocal rehabilitation. The inferior border of the resection is usually the superior surface of the cricoid cartilage, but the superior half of the ipsilateral cricoid can be resected if necessary.

Frozen sections are performed on all margins to determine the adequacy of the resection. Once free of tumor, closure and reconstruction can begin. After resection, a raw surface remains in the endolarynx. It can be resurfaced with a rotated flap of piriform sinus

(continued)

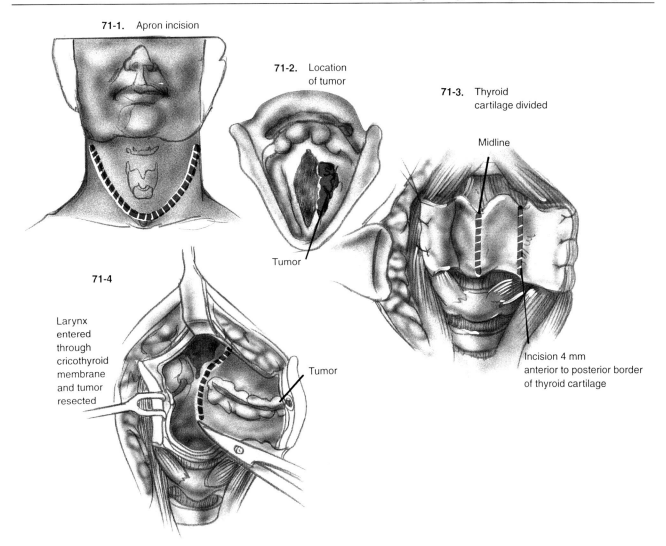

71-1.   Apron incision

71-2.   Location of tumor

Tumor

71-3.   Thyroid cartilage divided

Midline

Incision 4 mm anterior to posterior border of thyroid cartilage

71-4

Larynx entered through cricothyroid membrane and tumor resected

Tumor

■ *71.* VERTICAL PARTIAL LARYNGECTOMY, INCLUDING THE THYROID CARTILAGE

(continued)

3. For T3 lesions and for T2 lesions with impaired vocal cord mobility, an ipsilateral neck dissection—preferably with preservation of the internal jugular vein, sternocleidomastoid muscle, and XIth cranial nerve—is usually indicated.
4. Enter the larynx on the side opposite the tumor.
5. Because the lymphatics at the glottic level are scarce, margins may be close. However, complete excision of the tumor must be confirmed by frozen-section analysis.
6. The entire epiglottis should be preserved to prevent aspiration.
7. Preservation of at least the posterior portion of one arytenoid eases postoperative recovery of voice and deglutition.
8. Laryngoplasty and construction of a neocord improves vocal rehabilitation, but it may increase the risk of airway compromise if the muscle flap is too bulky.
9. Mucosal coverage of raw surfaces hastens postoperative recovery.
10. For most T1 and T2 tumors, radiation therapy, laser cordectomy, or laryngofissure with cordectomy are the primary treatment options.
11. The vertical thyroid cartilage cuts can be adjusted such that less thyroid ala is removed. This is especially true for a unilateral posterior lesion, in which case as much as one half of the ipsilateral anterior thyroid cartilage can be preserved.

Pitfalls and Complications

1. In patients with significant obstructive pulmonary disease preoperatively, postoperative rehabilitation is extremely difficult and often impossible.
2. Aspiration is common in the initial postoperative period, but it should stop by the sixth week postoperatively.
3. Laryngeal stenosis is possible, especially if more than one third of the opposite vocal cord is removed. Placement of a laryngeal keel can prevent anterior webbing, but it can also create local irritation and stimulate the formation of granulation tissue.
4. Frequent follow-up examinations are essential, especially for patients who have dysplasia of the opposite vocal cord.
5. Patients must stop smoking.
6. Tumor recurrence is heralded by a voice change or laryngeal stenosis.

Postoperative Care Issues

1. If a Silastic keel is placed, it is removed in 3 to 4 weeks.
2. Although decannulation is usually preferable before initiating swallowing, we prefer to leave the tracheotomy tube in for 1 month and to initiate swallowing late in the second week.
3. A speech pathologist is essential to aid in the patient's postoperative recovery.

References

Bailey BJ. Glottic carcinoma. In: Bailey BJ, Biller HF, eds. Surgery of the larynx, eds. Philadelphia: WB Saunders, 1985:263.

Biller HF, Ogura JH, Pratt CG. Hemilaryngectomy for T2 glottic cancers. Arch Otolaryngol 1971;93:238.

Kleinsasser O. Tumors of the larynx and hypopharynx. New York: Thieme Medical Publishers, 1988:161.

mucosa or the area can be left to granulate. If the piriform sinus mucosa is available, it is preferable to cover the raw area (Fig. 71-5). Absorbable suture is used to attach this mucosa.

Reconstruction can be achieved by simple closure of the perichondrium and strap muscles over the defect. Without thyroid cartilage, these collapse into the defect and create a serviceable neocord. However, many surgeons prefer to perform a "laryngoplasty" in which a portion of strap muscle or omohyoid muscle is tunnelled laterally through a small perichondral incision into the area of resection. A neocord is constructed to act as a fixed surface against which the opposite vocal cord can vibrate (Fig. 71-6).

The muscle flap is sutured to both the anterior commissure (or the remaining ipsilateral vocal cord) and the arytenoid (or the raw bed overlying the cricoid lamina) (see Fig. 71-6). The remaining true vocal cord is also sutured to the anterior thyroid ala. At this time a Silastic keel can be placed between the remaining vocal cord and the neocord to prevent webbing. The keel is secured in place with permanent monofilament sutures and is removed 3 weeks postoperatively. We prefer not to use a keel, because it necessitates a second surgical procedure and again leads to the risks of wound infection and fistulization.

The thyroid perichondrium and the strap muscles are closed across the midline with long-lasting absorbable suture. A suction or Penrose drain is placed in this layer. The wound is thoroughly irrigated, and then is closed in two layers.

HARSHA V. GOPAL
MARVIN P. FRIED

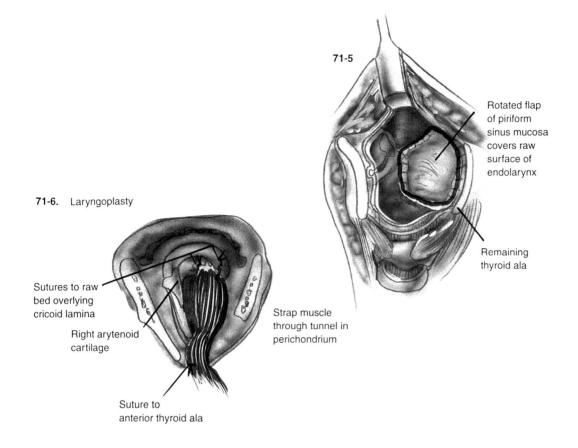

71-5

Rotated flap
of piriform
sinus mucosa
covers raw
surface of
endolarynx

Remaining
thyroid ala

71-6.   Laryngoplasty

Sutures to raw
bed overlying
cricoid lamina

Right arytenoid
cartilage

Strap muscle
through tunnel in
perichondrium

Suture to
anterior thyroid ala

■ *72.* ANTERIOR COMMISSURE AND ANTEROLATERAL VERTICAL PARTIAL LARYNGECTOMY— Removal of one vocal cord, a portion of the other vocal cord, and a portion of the thyroid cartilage

Indications
1. Carcinoma of the glottis, with extension to the vocal process of the arytenoid, involvement of the floor of the ventricle, or involvement of the anterior commissure
2. Involvement of as much as one third of the anterior portion of the contralateral vocal cord
3. Transglottic tumor without cord fixation
4. Recurrent glottic carcinoma after radiation therapy

Contraindications
1. Cord fixation (not an absolute contraindication, although surgery may be feasible only for a few selected cases)
2. Subglottic extension of more than 10 mm anteriorly or 5 to 6 mm posteriorly
3. Invasion of the cricoarytenoid joint
4. Involvement of the interarytenoid area
5. Involvement of more than the anterior one third of the contralateral vocal cord; if more is removed, near-total laryngectomy should be performed.
6. Fair to poor pulmonary status
7. Thyroid cartilage invasion
8. Involvement of both arytenoids

Special Considerations
1. Anterior commissure or contralateral cord involvement
2. Involvement of the arytenoid
3. Impaired cord mobility
4. Deep ventricular involvement
5. Transglottic tumor
6. Subglottic extension
7. Submucosal spread
8. Prior radiation therapy
9. Patient's medical condition, especially the pulmonary status
10. Reliability of follow-up
11. Neck node status
12. Informed consent must be obtained for total or near-total laryngectomy, in case the tumor is found to extend beyond the involved vocal cord.

Preoperative Evaluation
1. Routine laboratory studies
2. Pulmonary function tests
3. Computed tomography or magnetic resonance scans if occult nodes and cartilaginous invasion are considerations.
4. Upper endoscopy, laryngoscopy
5. Strobovideolaryngoscopy (optional)
6. Preoperative evaluation of speech and swallowing

Special Instruments, Position, and Anesthesia
1. Headlight
2. Delicate instruments
3. Sagittal saw to enter the larynx
4. Supine position, with the head extended
5. Bipolar cautery
6. General anesthesia
7. Tracheotomy is necessary.
8. Nasogastric or gastrostomy tube is necessary.

Tips and Pearls
1. Palpate or dissect the jugular nodal chains to identify adenopathy that may have been missed preoperatively.
2. For more than 5 mm of extension, the surgeon should consider ipsilateral thyroidectomy and resection of the superior one half of the ipsilateral cricoid cartilage.

(continued)

Operative Procedure
The patient is placed in the supine position on the operating table, using a transverse shoulder roll and head extension. General anesthesia is induced, and an endotracheal tube is inserted, or a tracheotomy is performed under local anesthesia, and general anesthesia is then induced. A nasogastric feeding tube is placed.

Laryngoscopy is performed to reevaluate the extent of the tumor (Fig. 72-2). A transverse incision is made, curving superiorly as it goes laterally over the sternocleidomastoid muscles, enabling an apron flap to be raised (Fig. 72-1). The inferior portion of the incision (overlying the larynx) is one fingerbreadth below the cricoid cartilage. A superior subplatysmal flap is raised to the level of the hyoid bone. If a tracheotomy has not been performed, a separate transverse incision can be made inferior and parallel to the other incision. The skin island between the two incisions must be at least 2 cm wide. Laterally, exposure can include the anterior sternocleidomastoid muscle, allowing the jugular lymph node chains to be examined for metastatic adenopathy. Any suspicious nodes are sent for frozen-section analysis. A node dissection is necessary if any nodes contain metastatic cancer.

The strap muscles and the sternocleidomastoid muscles should be clearly visible. The strap muscles are bluntly dissected in the midline to expose the thyroid perichondrium. Gently elevating the strap muscles laterally exposes the thyroid cartilage. The thyroid perichondrium is incised along its superior and inferior borders, directly in the midline. The perichondrium is elevated laterally to within 3 mm of the posterior border of the thyroid cartilage on the more involved side and halfway posteriorly on the less uninvolved side. The thyroid perichondrium is sutured to the adjacent strap muscle to protect it from trauma. It is important to maintain the integrity of the perichondrium and strap muscles, because they are necessary for reconstruction of the defect after resection. If thyroid or cricoid cartilage invasion is seen at this time, a total laryngectomy should be performed.

In this case, the anterior commissure is involved. The thyroid cartilage is divided 2 to 3 mm lateral to the midline on the less involved side (Fig. 72-3). If there is involvement of the anterior contralateral vocal cord, the cartilage incision can be placed posteriorly, allowing more of the anterior vocal cord to be resected vertically with a sagittal saw in the midline. The internal thyroid perichondrium is not violated. The internal perichondrium is elevated gently with a blunt elevator 2 to 3 mm laterally on the tumor side. The thyroid cartilage is also divided vertically on the more involved side 4 mm anterior to its posterior border. The external thyroid perichondrium should not be damaged.

The larynx is entered on the less involved side through the cricothyroid membrane. The cricoid and the thyroid cartilages are separated with hooks to expose the tumor on the opposite side. The surgeon must wear a headlight for this portion of the procedure. As exposure of the tumor is gained, the laryngeal soft tissue on the less involved side is incised in an inferior to superior direction. A good way to do this is to place a scissors with one tine inside and one tine outside the lumen. The cut on the less involved side should be anterior to the posterior half of the vocal cord. The internal branches of the superior laryngeal neurovascular bundle on the involved side can be divided at this time. The incision is carried horizontally and past the midline of the superior end of the thyroid cartilage. The mobilized portion of the larynx is retracted laterally, such that the tumor can be well visualized (Fig. 72-4). The tumor is resected, including the ipsilateral thyroid cartilage. The ipsilateral arytenoid is removed by separating the cricoarytenoid joint if the vocal process is involved. It is not necessary to remove the arytenoid if the vocal process is uninvolved; its preservation enhances postoperative vocal rehabilitation. The inferior border of the resection is usually the superior surface of the cricoid cartilage, but the superior half of the ipsilateral cricoid can be resected if necessary. Frozen-section analyses

(continued)

72-1.   Incision

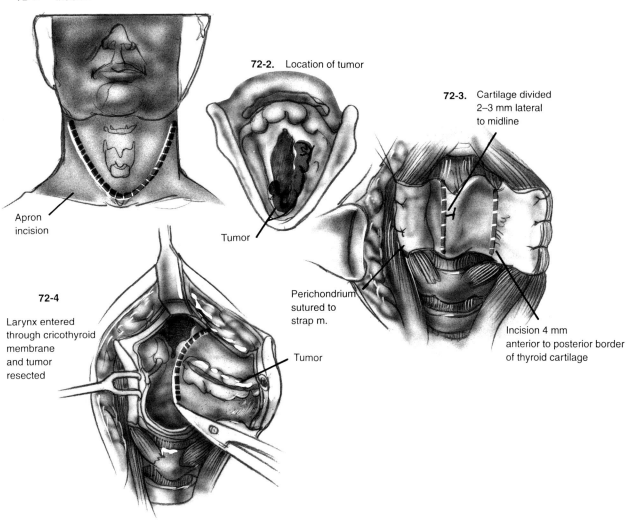

Apron
incision

72-2.   Location of tumor

Tumor

72-3.   Cartilage divided
2–3 mm lateral
to midline

Perichondrium
sutured to
strap m.

Incision 4 mm
anterior to posterior border
of thyroid cartilage

72-4

Larynx entered
through cricothyroid
membrane
and tumor
resected

Tumor

■ 72. ANTERIOR COMMISSURE AND ANTEROLATERAL VERTICAL PARTIAL LARYNGECTOMY (continued)

3. For T3 lesions and for T2 lesions with impaired vocal cord mobility, an ipsilateral neck dissection—preferably with preservation of the internal jugular vein, sternocleidomastoid muscle, and XIth cranial nerve—is usually indicated.
4. Enter the larynx on the side opposite the tumor.
5. Because lymphatics at the glottic level are scarce, margins may be close. However, complete excision of the tumor must be confirmed by frozen-section analysis.
6. The entire epiglottis should be preserved to prevent aspiration.
7. Preservation of at least the posterior portion of one arytenoid eases postoperative recovery of the voice and deglutition.
8. Laryngoplasty and construction of a neocord improve vocal rehabilitation but may increase the risk of airway compromise if the muscle flap is too bulky.
9. Mucosal coverage of raw surfaces hastens postoperative recovery.
10. For most T1 and some T2 tumors, radiation therapy, laser cordectomy, or laryngofissure with cordectomy are the primary treatment options.
11. The vertical thyroid cartilage cuts can be adjusted such that less thyroid ala is removed. This is especially true for a unilateral posterior lesion in which case as much as one half of the ipsilateral anterior thyroid cartilage can be preserved.

Pitfalls and Complications

1. In patients with significant obstructive pulmonary disease preoperatively, postoperative rehabilitation is extremely difficult and often impossible.
2. Aspiration is common in the initial postoperative period, but it should stop by the sixth week postoperatively.
3. Laryngeal stenosis is possible, especially if more than one third of the opposite vocal cord is removed. Placement of a laryngeal keel can prevent anterior webbing, but it can also create local irritation and stimulate the formation of granulation tissue.
4. Frequent follow-up examinations are essential, especially for patients who have dysplasia of the opposite vocal cord.
5. Patients must stop smoking.
6. Tumor recurrence is heralded by a voice change or laryngeal stenosis.

Postoperative Care Issues

1. If a Silastic keel is placed, it is removed in 3 to 4 weeks.
2. Although decannulation is usually preferable before initiating swallowing, we prefer to leave the tracheotomy tube in for 1 month and to initiate swallowing late in the second week.
3. A speech pathologist is essential to aid in the patient's postoperative recovery.

References

Bailey BJ. Glottic carcinoma. In: Bailey BJ, Biller HF, eds. Surgery of the larynx. Philadelphia: WB Saunders 1985:263.

Biller HF, Ogura JH, Pratt CG. Hemilaryngectomy for T2 glottic cancers. Arch Otolaryngol 1971;93:238.

Kleinsasser O. Tumors of the larynx and hypopharynx. New York: Thieme Medical Publishers, 1988:161.

are performed on all margins to determine the adequacy of the resection. After all margins are determined to be free of tumor, closure and reconstruction can begin.

After resection, a raw surface remains in the endolarynx (Fig. 72-5). It can be resurfaced with a rotated flap of piriform sinus mucosa, or the area can be left to granulate. Covering the raw area with the the piriform sinus mucosa is preferable. Absorbable stitches are used to attach the mucosa.

Reconstruction can be achieved by simple closure of the perichondrium and strap muscles over the defect. However, many surgeons prefer to perform a laryngoplasty in which a portion of strap muscle or omohyoid is tunneled laterally through a small perichondral incision into the area of resection. A neocord is constructed to act as a fixed surface against which the opposite vocal cord can vibrate. The muscle flap is sutured to the anterior thyroid ala remnant and to the arytenoid or the raw bed overlying the cricoid lamina (Fig. 72-6). The remaining true vocal cord is also sutured to the anterior thyroid ala. At this time, a Silastic keel can be placed between the remaining vocal cord and the neocord to prevent webbing. The keel is secured in place with permanent monofilament sutures and is removed 3 weeks postoperatively. We prefer not to use a keel, because it necessitates a second surgical procedure and increases the risks of wound infection and fistulization.

The thyroid perichondrium and the strap muscles are closed across the midline with long-lasting absorbable suture. A suction or Penrose drain is placed in this layer. The wound is thoroughly irrigated and is closed in two layers.

HARSHA V. GOPAL
MARVIN P. FRIED

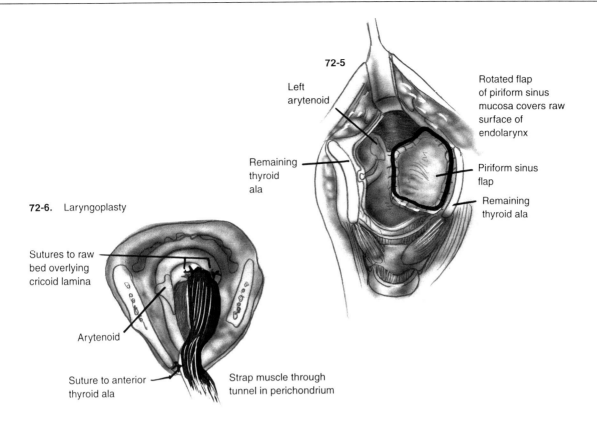

72-5

Left
arytenoid

Remaining
thyroid
ala

Rotated flap
of piriform sinus
mucosa covers raw
surface of
endolarynx

Piriform sinus
flap

Remaining
thyroid ala

72-6.   Laryngoplasty

Sutures to raw
bed overlying
cricoid lamina

Arytenoid

Suture to anterior
thyroid ala

Strap muscle through
tunnel in perichondrium

■ *73.* VERTICAL PARTIAL LARYNGECTOMY

Partial removal of laryngeal tissue in the vertical dimension by employing a family of conservation surgical procedures

1. Hemilaryngectomy—standardized excision of lateral laryngeal contents, including most or all of true cord, false cord, ventricle, and overlying thyroid cartilage
2. Vertical partial laryngectomy (VPL) with sparing of thyroid cartilage—may be for cordectomy only or may include true cord, ventricle, and portion of false cord
3. VPL and laryngoplasty—excision followed by repair of the surgical defect by various techniques
4. Extended (frontolateral) bilateral VPL—excision of more than half of the endolaryngeal soft tissue for treating bilateral glottic tumors

Indications

1. Cancer involving the anterior commissure
2. Cancer involving the vocal process of the arytenoid cartilage
3. Bilateral glottic cancer
4. Early, "superficial" transglottic cancer
5. Recurrent glottic cancer after radiation therapy

Contraindications

1. Cord fixation
2. Posterior commissure involvement
3. Involvement of both arytenoids
4. Bulky transglottic cancer
5. Thyroid cartilage invasion

Special Considerations

1. Encroachment or involvement of anterior commissure
2. Encroachment or involvement of vocal process arytenoid cartilage
3. Assessment of cord mobility
4. Extension to ventricle or false cord
5. Status of mucosa adjacent to obvious tumors
6. Prior treatment
7. Pulmonary status; general medical problems
8. Communication needs in work and other activities
9. Reliability for follow-up
10. Neck node status

Preoperative Preparation

1. Routine laboratory studies
2. Computed tomography scan, if concerned about occult nodes or cartilage invasion
3. Careful mapping DL
4. Fiberoptic endoscopy with or without videostroboscopy

Special Instruments, Position, and Anesthesia

1. Headlight
2. Small, delicate plastic surgery instruments
3. Senn retractor, bipolar cautery
4. Shoulders on roll, neck extender, head stabilized in foam doughnut
5. Deepen anesthesia when entering larynx

(continued)

Operative Procedure

For unilateral partial laryngectomy and laryngoplasty, the patient is positioned on the operating table in a prone position with the head extended. Oral endotracheal intubation or tracheotomy under local anesthesia may be performed to allow the induction of anesthesia. A transverse incision is made, passing one fingerbreadth below the inferior margin of the cricoid cartilage and curving outward and superiorly in the natural skin folds of the neck. As the incision passes lateral to the anterior jugular veins, it is curved superiorly toward the mastoid tip and carried up to a level just inferior to the greater cornua of the hyoid bone. A vertical midline incision is dropped from the midpoint of the transverse incision and extends about 2 cm inferiorly, and through this incision, a tracheotomy can be performed if it was not accomplished initially.

The anterior cervical flap of skin and platysma muscle is elevated superiorly until the entire hyoid bone is exposed. Care is taken to avoid injury to the superior laryngeal neurovascular bundle, because this innervation is important for postoperative function. The inferior skin flap is elevated laterally for a distance of several centimeters to allow access to the tissue of the neck for direct palpation along the jugular lymphatic chains bilaterally. These chains of lymph nodes are palpated to identify any suspicious nodes to confirm the absence of metastatic carcinoma. Any suspect nodes are sent for frozen-section evaluation. The sternohyoid, sternothyroid, and thyrohyoid muscles (ie, strap muscles) and the larynx from the level of the hyoid bone down to the cricoid cartilage are clearly visible. The external thyroid perichondrium is incised in the midline and along the superior and inferior margins of the thyroid alae bilaterally. The external thyroid perichondrium is then elevated, being careful to avoid tearing the perichondrium. The perichondrium is sutured to the overlying strap muscles to prevent shrinkage of the injury.

The plane between the external thyroid perichondrium and the overlying strap muscles is not entered, because these tissues will be repositioned to lie deep to the thyroid ala to provide bulk and to stabilize the thyroid cartilage. The external thyroid perichondrium and muscle flap are the essential ingredients for the laryngeal reconstruction (ie, laryngoplasty) phase of the procedure. The external thyroid perichondrium is elevated back to the posterior margin of the thyroid ala (Fig. 73-1). The thyroid cartilage is divided in the midline using an oscillating surgical saw, being careful to avoid injury to the underlying soft tissue. As the internal thyroid perichondrium is reached, it is elevated carefully from the thyroid cartilage, and the dissection is carried three quarters of the way back in the direction of the superior and inferior thyroid cornua.

The airway is entered below the level of the glottis by employing a transverse incision through the cricothyroid membrane. This incision is extended on both sides approximately 1 cm from the midline. At this point, the surgeon employs a headlight to permit visualization in a superior direction and progressively enlarges the opening into the airway by extending the incision superiorly so that it passes through the anterior commissure and up to the superior thyroid notch.

With the tumor directly in the vision of the surgeon, the incision is then extended laterally across the midportion of the false vocal fold (ie, ventricular band). The inferior line of resection is then extended along the superior margin of the cricoid cartilage as it begins to curve superiorly and posteriorly (Fig. 73-2). The surgeon then arbitrarily selects the posterior resection line, often at about the point where the vocal process of the arytenoid cartilage joins the body of the arytenoid cartilage. My colleagues and I make a strong effort to preserve the body of the arytenoid cartilage to have dynamic glottic tissue involved in the rehabilitation of larynx postoperatively.

Typically for the unilateral lesion, the specimen comprises all of the tissue from the midline of that side back to the body of the arytenoid cartilage posteriorly. In the vertical dimension, it extends from the level of the cricoid cartilage up to a point superiorly that includes one half to one third of the false vocal fold. The internal perichondrium of the thyroid cartilage forms the deep margin of the tumor specimen.

We routinely use frozen-section analysis to evaluate surgical

(continued)

73-1. Elevation of external perichondrium and midline thyrotomy

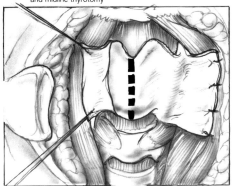

73-2. Resection of tumor

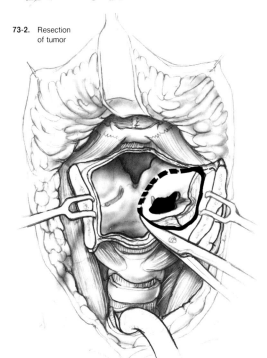

73-3

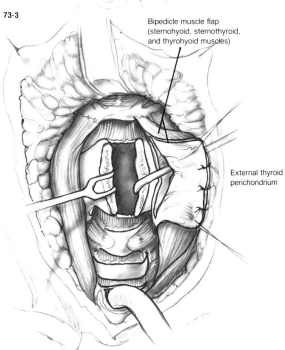

Bipedicle muscle flap (sternohyoid, sternothyroid, and thyrohyoid muscles)

External thyroid perichondrium

73-4 Bipedicle muscle flap used for reconstruction

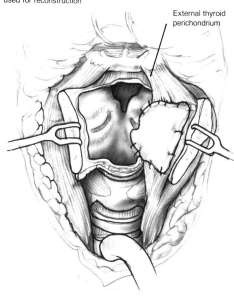

External thyroid perichondrium

73-5. Unilateral reconstruction (axial view)

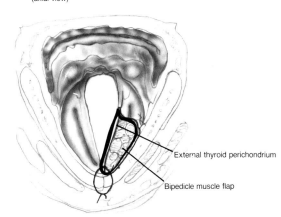

External thyroid perichondrium

Bipedicle muscle flap

73-6. Partial laryngectomy—cordectomy via midline thyrotomy (excision true vocal fold)

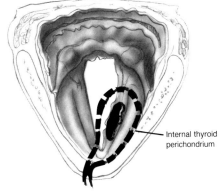

Internal thyroid perichondrium

■ 73. VERTICAL PARTIAL LARYNGECTOMY
(continued)

Tips and Pearls

1. Explore the neck to detect occult metastatic nodes that were missed preoperatively.
2. Enter the larynx at a safe distance from the tumor.
3. Resect the tumor with close margins, and then send margin strips for frozen-section confirmation of the adequacy of the excision.
4. Attempt to spare the posterior segment of the arytenoid cartilage, because it will enhance postoperative glottic function.
5. Avoid extending the resection into the epiglottis; otherwise, postoperative problems with aspiration are likely.
6. "Severe dysplasia" has almost the same long-term prognosis as carcinoma in situ.
7. Preserve a central strip of midline thyroid cartilage if the cancer involves the anterior commissure.
8. Techniques that limit granulation tissue formation yield more predictable outcomes.
9. The safety and efficacy of partial laryngeal surgery for cancer has been documented.

Pitfalls and Complications

1. Aspiration may occur during the first 2 weeks after surgery, but it should not persist beyond the fifth week.
2. Granulation tissue may develop in the surgical field and should be excised endoscopically.
3. Laryngeal stenosis is a rare complication and should raise the suspicion of recurrence.
4. Recurrence usually is associated with voice changes as an early sign.
5. Regular follow-up examinations are important during the first 3 to 5 years after surgery.

Postoperative Care Issues

1. When a Silastic keel is used to separate raw surfaces, my colleagues and I prefer to remove the keel at 3 weeks.
2. Liquids may be swallowed 5 to 7 days after surgery, and a soft diet may be initiated 10 to 14 days postoperatively.
3. Decannulation is usually accomplished about 3 weeks postoperatively, after it has been possible to plug the tracheostomy tube for extended periods.
4. The speech pathologist is a key individual in assisting the patient to regain maximum voice quality.

References

Bailey BJ. Early glottic carcinoma. In: Bailey BJ, et al, eds. Head and Neck Surgery—Otolaryngology. Philadelphia: JB Lippincott, 1993: 1313.

Nichols RD, Mickelson SA. Partial laryngectomy after irradiation failure. Ann Otol Rhinol Laryngol 1991;100:176.

margins to ensure that the resection has been adequate. After the specimen has been excised, we then remove mucosal strips from all four epithelial margins.

Care is taken to avoid resection of substantial portions of the epiglottic cartilage, because experience has shown that this invites postoperative aspiration. On some occasions, we have employed the surgical operating microscope to visualize epithelial changes under higher-powered magnification, especially in patients with patchy dysplasia or carcinoma in situ.

Having ensured the adequacy of the tumor resection, we begin the laryngoplasty or reconstructive phase of the operation. We employ a bipedicle muscle flap consisting of most of the sternohyoid, sternothyroid, and thyrohyoid muscles. This strap muscle bundle is separated from its posterolateral tissue attachment by a vertical incision made arbitrarily so as to develop a pedicle muscle flap about the size of the small finger or index finger, depending on the size of the surgical defect. The flap appears excessively large initially, but experience has shown that there will be muscular atrophy of about 30%.

The incision that isolates the bipedicle muscle flap is made from a point about 1 cm above the superior margin of the thyroid cartilage to a similar point about 1 cm below the inferior margin of the thyroid cartilage. The bipedicle muscle flap preserves its attachment to the external thyroid perichondrium on its deep or under surface and is also intact superiorly and inferiorly. This tissue complex is then repositioned so that it comes to lie deep to the thyroid ala, which is still attached posteriorly to its muscular insertion by the inferior pharyngeal constrictor (Fig. 73-3). The muscle flap tends to flatten out along the inner surface of the thyroid ala, and the external perichondrium forms the lining of the laryngeal lumen. The perichondrium is sutured to the adjacent mucosa with a few loose tacking sutures (Fig. 73-4). The thyroid alae are then sutured together, and the wound is drained using a 0.5-in (1-cm) Penrose rubber drain or a small flap drain (Fig. 73-5). A #5 or #6 tracheotomy tube replaces the endotracheal tube, and a light compression dressing is applied over the skin.

Surgical Variations

Laryngofissure

The laryngofissure procedure represents the earliest form of vertical partial laryngectomy and consists of either a midline or paramedian vertical incision in the thyroid cartilage to afford access to the anterior of the larynx. Through this incision, a limited resection (ie, cordectomy) of one true vocal cord can be performed for a small, early-stage glottic carcinoma involving the mobile portion of the true cord (Fig. 73-6). An upward extension of the operative field allows the laryngeal ventricle and the lower half of the false vocal cord to be included with the specimen (Fig. 73-7). The resection stops short of the arytenoid cartilage, and its deepest layer is the internal perichondrium of the thyroid ala (Fig. 73-8).

Hemilaryngectomy

The hemilaryngectomy procedure is indicated for the management of T1 or T2 glottic carcinoma, and it is appropriate for lesions that arise on the true cord and extend to the false cord. The technique involves a full-thickness incision from the laryngeal epithelium through the entire soft tissue depth, including most of the thyroid ala on the same side as an en bloc resection of one half of the larynx (Fig. 73-9). The posterior resection line can be extended to the midline of the posterior commissure (Fig. 73-10).

Anterior Commissure Partial Laryngectomy

Anterior commissure partial laryngectomy is used for lesions involving the anterior commissure and extending a significant distance posteriorly along both true vocal cords. There may also be superior extension toward the petiole of the epiglottis. The anterior one third to two thirds of the true vocal cord is excised en bloc with a smaller amount of the midline portion of the thyroid cartilage (Fig. 73-11). The defect can be reconstructed by advancing a triangular segment of the epiglottis superiorly to inferiorly into the defect, or it can be allowed to fill in with granulation tissue if a keel is left in place for 4 to 6 weeks postoperatively (Fig. 73-12).

BYRON J. BAILEY

73-7. Extended cordectomy via midline thyrotomy
(true and false vocal folds)

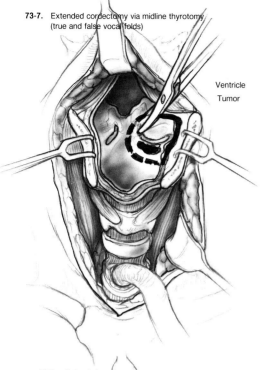

Ventricle

Tumor

73-10. Hemilaryngectomy with arytenoid
included with specimen

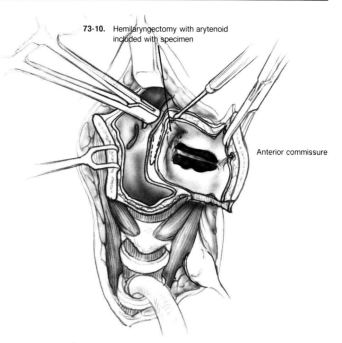

Anterior commissure

73-8. Extended cordectomy—specimen removed
(no reconstruction)

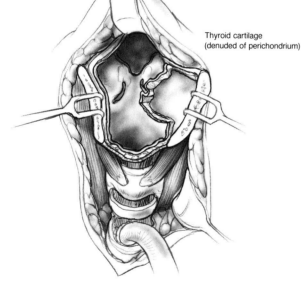

Thyroid cartilage
(denuded of perichondrium)

73-11. Vertical partial laryngectomy
for anterior commissure/bilateral tumor involvement

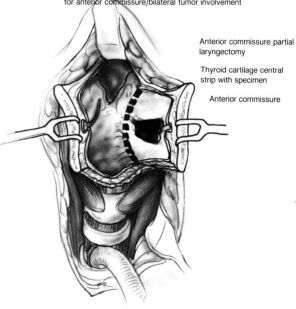

Anterior commissure partial
laryngectomy

Thyroid cartilage central
strip with specimen

Anterior commissure

73-9. Hemilaryngectomy with arytenoid cartilage
also resected (axial view)

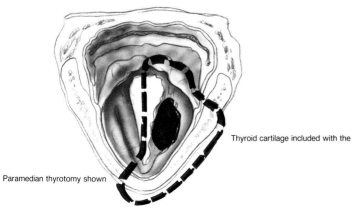

Thyroid cartilage included with the

Paramedian thyrotomy shown

73-12. Frontolateral vertical partial laryngectomy
with bilateral flap reconstruction

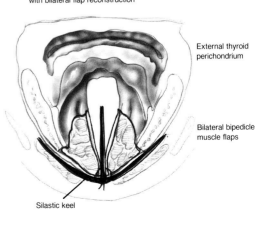

External thyroid
perichondrium

Bilateral bipedicle
muscle flaps

Silastic keel

■ 74. VERTICAL PARTIAL LARYNGECTOMY WITH EXTENSION (SUBTOTAL OR THREE-QUARTER LARYNGECTOMY—Resection of supraglottic larynx with ipsilateral vocal cord and overlying thyroid cartilage.

Indications

1. Supraglottic carcinoma with ipsilateral extension to vocal cord (no fixation) (small transglottic)
2. Most favorable—lateral angle tumors of epiglottis and vestibular fold
3. Vestibular fold carcinoma
4. Marginal carcinoma of aryepiglottic fold and arytenoid

Contraindications

1. Vocal cord fixation (? relative contraindication)
2. Subglottic extension (>10mm anterior, >5mm posterior)
3. Cartilage or cricoarytenoid joint invasion
4. Prior XRT (? relative contraindication)
5. Involvement of interarytenoid region
6. Involvement of both arytenoids
7. Fair to poor pulmonary status
8. Involvement of > $\frac{1}{3}$ contralateral cord
9. Inability to preserve- (a) contralateral; vestibular fold, A-E fold, mobile arytenoid; (b) ipsilateral inferior cricoid strut
10. Extensive supraglottic/tongue base involvement
11. Pyriform apex involvement

Special Considerations/Tips and Pearls

1. One half of glottis and all of supraglottis are removed
2. Neck dissections performed—high risk of nodal metastases
3. Informed consent for near-total or total laryngectomy
4. Accurate frozen section margins
5. Preserve contralateral recurrent laryngeal nerve and, if possible, external laryngeal nerve
6. Reconstruction requires preservation of one mobile arytenoid, restoration of posterior glottic bulk to prevent aspiration, and maintenance of sufficient anteroposterior diameter of glottic remnant to preserve adequate airway and phonation.
7. With > 5mm subglottic extension, ipsilateral thyroid lobectomy is performed
8. Initial pharyngotomy—contralateral to tumor and along vallecula or piriform, depending on involvement of lingual epiglottis.

Preoperative Evaluation

1. PFT's and CT/MRI scans
2. Panendoscopy
3. Preop speech/swallow therapy evaluation

Pitfalls and Complications

1. Patients with severe COPD may be difficult or impossible to rehabilitate.
2. Aspiration is common initially but subsides in most patients.
3. Failure to reconstruct resected cord results in severe aspiration/poor phonation. Airway narrowing from reconstruction can later be debulked (eg, CO_2 laser).
4. Voice or airway changes, pain, dysphagia may signal recurrence.

Postoperative Care Issues

1. NGT or G-tube to suction until bowel function returns.
2. H_2 blockers
3. Decannulation is preferable before initiating deglutition. Supraglottic swallow may prevent aspiration. If decannulation is not possible by 2 weeks postoperatively, begin swallowing therapy.

References

Lore JM Jr (ed.) An atlas of head and neck surgery. Philadelphia: WB Saunders, 1988;912.

Friedman WH. Katsantonis GP. Subtotal laryngectomy with contralateral laryngoplasty. In Silver CE (ed). Laryngeal cancer, New York: Thieme, 1991;183.

Operative Procedure

Patient is supine under general anesthesia. Perform direct laryngoscopy, place NGT (or G-tube), and tracheotomy if not already present.

Raise apron flap, anterior portion 2 cm below cricoid. Subplatysmal flap raised above hyoid bone. Exposure allows evaluation of adenopathy.

Strap muscles are transected from hyoid and retracted inferiorly. Perichondrium is incised along superior aspect of thyroid lamina, contralateral to tumor and vertically in the midline. Perichondrial flap is elevated inferiorly just below the midpoint of the thyroid cartilage. The perichondrium on the ipsilateral thyroid cartilage is removed with the specimen. The thyroid cartilage incision is a horizontal line across the contralateral thyroid lamina at the level of the laryngeal ventricle, midway between the thyroid notch and the inferior thyroid cartilage border. The incision is carried to the midline, then directed vertically and inferiorly. Posteriorly, the horizontal incision is carried within several millimeters of the posterior margin of this thyroid lamina and then carried superiorly (vertically). A posterior strut of contralateral thyroid lamina, superior cornu, and attached constrictor muscles is thus preserved for reconstruction. Suprahyoid muscles are transected at the hyoid and the pharynx is entered contralateral to the tumor. If tumor involves lingual epiglottis, pharyngotomy proceeds inferiorly through the thyrohyoid membrane to the prior thyroid cartilage cut, transecting the internal but preserving the external laryngeal nerve. If the lingual epiglottis is uninvolved, the pharyngotomy traverses the vallecula first.

The dissection proceeds under direct visualization of the tumor along the contralateral thyroid cartilage cut as well as through the vallecula. The hyoid is grasped with Allis clamps and the thyroid lamina retracted forward with skin hooks. Soft tissue at the level of the contralateral thyroid cartilage out is divided with curved Mayo scissors, passing through the ventricle, avoiding the contralateral arytenoid. At the midline, dissection is vertical in an inferior direction through anterior commissure and cricothyroid membrane to the superior cricoid.

Ipsilateral cricoid is incised (sagittal saw) several mm below the superior margin, preserving an inferior strut. Proceeding posteriorly, the cut ends medial to the cricoarytenoid joint. Soft tissue of the subglottis is incised with Mayo scissors, anterior to posterior, resecting ipsilateral arytenoid and underlying cricoid at the level of the cricoarytenoid joint.

Inferior constrictors are dissected from the ipsilateral thyroid lamina and the pyriform sinus mucosa divided up to the level of the prior vallecula cut. The ipsilateral hyoid is transected lateral to the lesser cornu and the specimen removed. The ipsilateral paraglottic space has been removed with the tumor.

Cricopharyngeal myotomy is performed. Frozen section analysis of all margins is obtained.

The glottis is reconstructed using the preserved posterior strut of contralateral thyroid cartilage. A medial vertical mucosal cut is performed to expose the superior cornu. A scissors is used to greenstick fracture the posterior thyroid strut in a medial direction. An additional fracture of the distal strut is performed to allow the superior cornu to be sutured to the anterior midline. The strut is anchored anteriorly and posteriorly with 2-0 nylon sutures. Pyriform sinus and hypopharyngeal mucosa is advanced to cover the cartilage-muscle pedicle, securing mucosa to the cut edge of thyroid cartilage. The contralateral vocal cord is sutured anteriorly to the outer thyroid perichondrium.

The remaining larynx is sutured to bare tongue base musculature, placing the larynx anteriorly to reduce aspiration. Closure is performed with 3-0 Vicryl sutures, approximating perichondrium and strap muscles to the tongue base. Lateral pharyngeal defects are closed and reinforced with strap and digastric muscles, and routine skin closure and wound drainage are performed. A tracheostomy tube is sutured in place.

ARTHUR M. LAURETANO
MARVIN P. FRIED

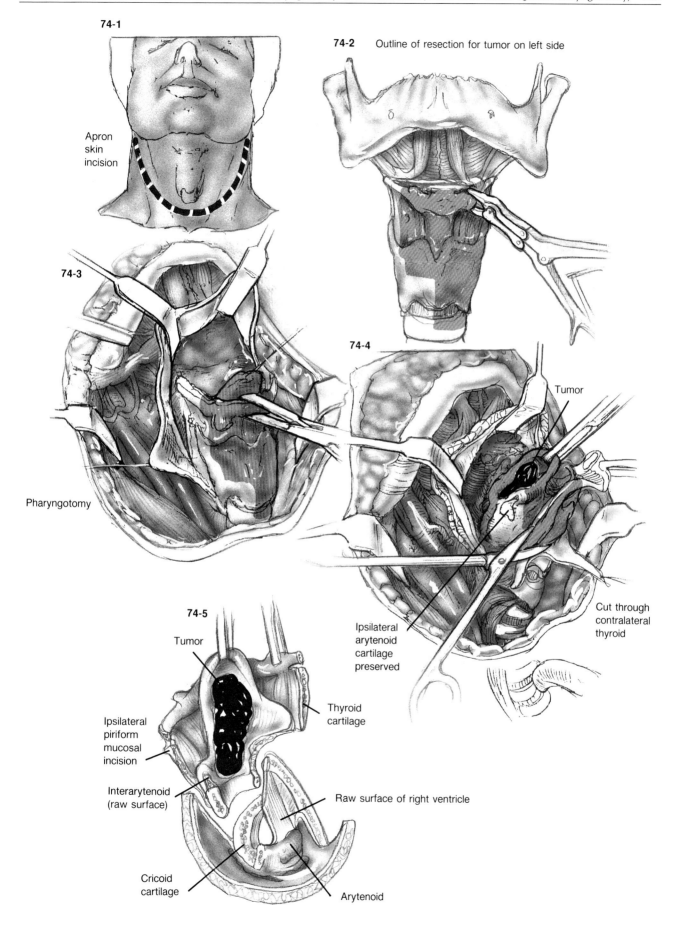

74-1

Apron
skin
incision

74-2 Outline of resection for tumor on left side

74-3

Pharyngotomy

74-4

Tumor

Ipsilateral
arytenoid
cartilage
preserved

Cut through
contralateral
thyroid

74-5

Tumor

Ipsilateral
piriform
mucosal
incision

Thyroid
cartilage

Interarytenoid
(raw surface)

Raw surface of right ventricle

Cricoid
cartilage

Arytenoid

■ 75. SUPRAGLOTTIC LARYNGECTOMY (HORIZONTAL HEMILARYNGECTOMY)—Removal of laryngeal structures above the floor of the ventricle (true vocal fold)

Indications

1. T1, T2 supraglottic carcinomas, eg, cancers involving laryngeal surface of the epiglottis, infrahyoid and suprahyoid epiglottis, ventricular folds, and aryepiglottic folds
2. Supraglottic carcinomas that are T3 by virtue of pre-epiglottic space involvement

Contraindications

1. Fixation or impaired motion of vocal fold
2. Poor medical condition, especially extreme age, poor pulmonary reserve, or both
3. Tumor within 5 mm of anterior commissure
4. Thyroid cartilage involvement
5. Prior radiation therapy is a relative contraindication

Special Considerations

1. The Jackson "anterior commissure" laryngoscope is a useful tool in the detection of vocal fold involvement
2. A bulky supraglottic tumor makes it difficult to assess by endoscopy inferior extension toward the ventricle and the vocal fold. Preoperative CT may help
3. Bilateral selective neck disection should be done concomitantly
4. Enter the airway as far away from the tumor as possible

Preoperative Preparation

1. Preoperative barium esophagogram and upper GI series are helpful in detecting esophageal motility disorders and reflux, which may delay or interfere with postoperative swallowing rehabilitation
2. Consent must always be obtained for total laryngectomy

(continued)

Operative Procedure

An apron type incision from mastoid tip to mastoid tip is preferred (Fig. 75-1). Bilateral selective neck dissection is carried out in the usual fashion. The neck specimen can be left attached to the thyrohyoid membrane or be totally removed.

The hyoid bone is skeletonized from the greater horn of the involved side to the lesser horn of the uninvolved side. The infrahyoid muscles are divided just inferior to the hyoid bone, and the suprahyoid muscles are also detached from the hyoid bone. The neurovascular bundle of the involved side is identified near the superior horn of the thyroid cartilage and ligated. On the uninvolved side, the hyoid bone is transected just lateral to the lesser horn (Fig. 75-2). The superior laryngeal nerve on this side is preserved if possible. Incision of the perichondrium is carried out along the superior border of the thyroid cartilage and the perichondrium is carefully elevated inferiorly to just below the middle of the thyroid cartilage (Fig. 75-3). On the involved side, the cartilage is cut horizontally with the oscillating saw at the middle of the thyroid cartilage in male patients, and at the junction of the upper and middle third in females. This level should be above the level of the vocal folds. On the uninvolved side, the cartilage cut sweeps upward to the the superior edge of the thyroid cartilage, intersecting at a point midway between the thyroid notch and the superior horn (Fig. 75-4).

The pharynx is now entered, either through the piriform sinus of the uninvolved side or through the valleculae just above the hyoid bone. Once the pharynx is entered, the epiglottis is grasped with an Allis clamp (the patient should be fully paralyzed at this point) so the full extent of the tumor can be determined. After ensuring no involvement of the lingual surface of the epiglottis, the incision is continued across the valleculae (Fig. 75-5). The arytenoid prominence and the laryngeal ventricle should be clearly identified. The mucosal cut is carried along the aryepiglottic fold toward the anterior end of the arytenoid into the laryngeal ventricle. The mucosa over-

(continued)

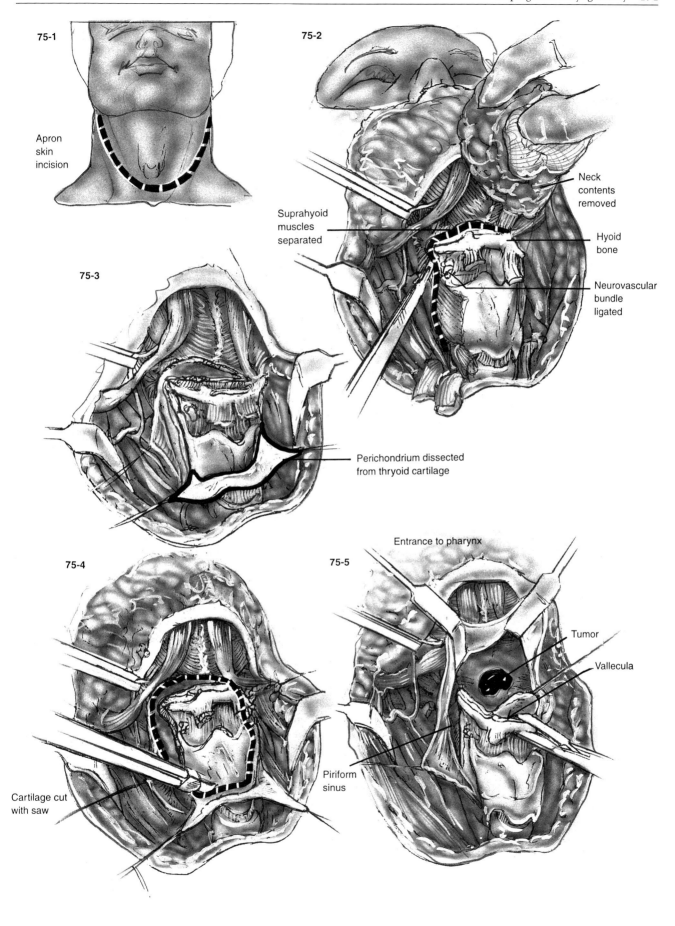

75-1

Apron
skin
incision

75-2

Suprahyoid
muscles
separated

Neck
contents
removed

Hyoid
bone

Neurovascular
bundle
ligated

75-3

Perichondrium dissected
from thryoid cartilage

75-4

Cartilage cut
with saw

75-5

Entrance to pharynx

Tumor

Vallecula

Piriform
sinus

■ 75. SUPRAGLOTTIC LARYNGECTOMY (HORIZONTAL HEMILARYNGECTOMY)

(continued)

Special Instruments, Position, and Anesthesia

1. Headlight
2. Skin hooks
3. Oscillating saws
4. Shoulder roll with neck extended
5. If there is no danger of airway compromise, anesthesia may be initiated by endotracheal intubation, with a tracheotomy performed after general anesthesia induction
6. Local tracheostomy followed by induction of general anesthesia is required in cases of bulky tumor
7. Deepen anesthesia and make certain the patient is paralyzed when the larynx is entered

Tips and Pearls

1. The line of transection in supraglottic laryngectomy is the valleculae superiorly and both ventricles inferiorly
2. The inferior margin must be free of tumor for at least 2 to 3 mm

Pitfalls and Complications

1. Aspiration and pneumonia are the most common complications of supraglottic laryngectomy
2. Fistula
3. Postoperative edema, particularly if the field has been radiated
4. Airway obstruction

Postoperative Care Issues

1. If the nasogastric tube is dislodged during the early postoperative period, it should be replaced with extreme care to avoid disrupting the suture line
2. Bedside evaluation by the swallowing team prior to oral feeding is helpful. Diet should start with semi-solids.
3. Be sure the airway is adequate prior to the removal of the tracheotomy tube.

References

Coates HL, DeSanto LW, Devine KN, Elveback LA. Carcinoma of the supraglottic larynx. A review of 221 cases. Arch Otol 1976;102:686.
Som ML. Conservation surgery for carcinoma of the supraglottis. J Laryngol Otol 1970;84:655.

lying the arytenoid may be removed, but the cartilage should not be exposed (Fig. 75-6). If tumor extent requires removal of the arytenoid, the vocal fold should be sutured to the cricoid (see Procedure 76). Using the scissors, one blade is engaged in the ventricle and the other blade cuts along the cartilage incision on the uninvolved side. Care must be taken to avoid injury to the thyroid perichondrium. Once the uninvolved side has been incised, then the remnant of the larynx with the tumor can be exposed like an open book. The incision on the involved side is carried along the aryepiglottic fold through the posterior part of the false cord into the ventricle continuing anteriorly to the midline of the thyroid cartilage (Fig. 75-7). The rest of the supraglottic structures should be removed with at least a 2- to 3-mm margin (inset). Frozen section is mandatory to determine the adequacy of the margin.

A generous cricopharyngeal myotomy is carried out by inserting the index finger into the lumen of the esophagus and then dividing the inferior constrictors (Fig. 75-8).

Before beginning closure, a nasogastric tube is inserted through the nose into the stomach. The shoulder roll should be removed and the neck flexed to facilitate closure. Mucosa-to-mucosa closure is not achievable and should not be attempted. Some mucosa approximation from tongue base to piriform sinus is achievable with 3-0 atraumatic absorbable sutures (Fig. 75-9). The rest of the closure is achieved by suturing the base of the tongue to the perichondrium of the thyroid cartilage. Interrupted sutures are first placed without tying (Fig. 75-10). Later all are tied at the same time after placement of a suspension suture of 0-nylon from the remnant of the thyroid cartilage midline to the soft tissue adjacent to the genial area of the periosteum of the mandible. The wound is thoroughly irrigated, and a closed suction drainage device is placed. The skin is closed in two layers. A cuffed size 8 tracheostomy tube replaces the endotracheal tube. A retention suture with 0-Prolene is placed from the chin to the chest wall to prevent extension of the neck.

FRANK WONG

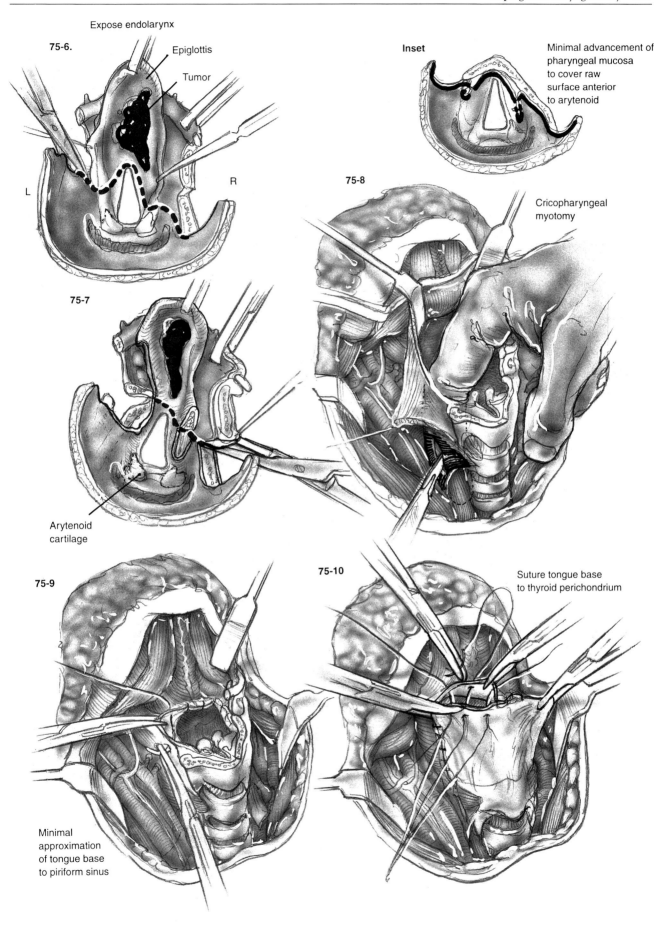

Expose endolarynx

75-6.

Epiglottis

Tumor

L

R

Inset

Minimal advancement of
pharyngeal mucosa
to cover raw
surface anterior
to arytenoid

75-8

Cricopharyngeal
myotomy

75-7

Arytenoid
cartilage

75-9

Minimal
approximation
of tongue base
to piriform sinus

75-10

Suture tongue base
to thyroid perichondrium

■ 76. EXTENDED SUPRAGLOTTIC PARTIAL LARYNGECTOMY

LARYNGECTOMY—Removal of the supraglottic larynx in combination with the removal of part or almost all of the tongue base, the piriform sinus, or one vocal fold

Indications

1. Cancer involving the lingual surface of the epiglottis
2. Cancer involving tongue base
3. Cancer involving aryepiglottic fold and one arytenoid
4. T1 cancer of the piriform sinus

Contraindications

1. Impaired vocal fold mobility
2. Involvement of circumvallate papillae
3. Involvement of the posterior glottis
4. Poor pulmonary reserve
5. Extension of tumor to within 1.5 cm of the apex of the piriform sinus

Special Considerations

1. Do not suture tongue mucosa directly to larynx.
2. Resection of the tongue anterior to the circumvallate papillae may severely compromise swallowing so that supraglottic laryngectomy is not feasible, and a total laryngectomy is required.

Special Instruments, Position, and Anesthesia

1. Same as for supraglottic laryngectomy

Tips and Pearls

1. When the procedure is performed for piriform sinus cancer, arytenoidectomy is often necessary.
2. When arytenoidectomy is required to eradicate carcinoma, the posterior end of the ipsilateral vocal ligament must to be surgically fixed in the midline to the cricoid cartilage.

Complications

1. Aspiration and pneumonia are more common than in standard supraglottic laryngectomy.
2. Inclusion of an arytenoid cartilage in the resection significantly compromises vocal and swallowing functions.
3. Fistula formation

Postoperative Care Issues

1. Same as for standard supraglottic laryngectomy

References

Ogura JH, Dedo H. Glottic reconstruction following subtotal supraglottic laryngectomy. Laryngoscope 1965;75:865.

Ogura JH, Marks JE, Freeman RB. Results of conservation surgery for cancers of the supraglottis and piriform sinus. Laryngoscope 1980;90:591.

Operative Procedure

The initial exposure and cartilage cuts are the same as for standard supraglottic laryngectomy.

For tongue base cancer, entrance to the pharynx is through the piriform sinus of the uninvolved side. Laryngeal resection is carried out by first cutting through the ventricles of both sides of the larynx under direct vision (Fig. 76-2). Resection is then carried upward toward the tongue base. A full thickness of the tongue base is resected with adequate margins as determined by frozen-section examination. Closure is similar to standard supraglottic laryngectomy, achieved by suturing the remnant of the tongue to the perichondrium of the thyroid cartilage. In a total tongue base resection, a flap reconstruction may be required to close the defect between the remnant of the tongue and the remnant of the larynx. The remnant of the larynx is suspended toward the mandible as in standard supraglottic laryngectomy.

When the procedure is performed for piriform sinus cancer, the pharynx is entered through the vallecula. The mucosal incision is carried down inferiorly on the contralateral side of the tumor. The incision is extended through the aryepiglottic fold, just anterior to the arytenoid and then through the ventricle, as in standard supraglottic laryngectomy. The larynx is then rotated to expose the tumor. Resection is carried horizontally through the ventricle and the involved piriform sinus at the same plane, under direct vision and with adequate margins, as confirmed by frozen-section examination (Fig. 76-1). The piriform sinus incision should be well below the tumor. Closure is the same as for supraglottic laryngectomy, achieved by approximating the tongue base to the thyroid perichondrium.

Suction drainage is used and skin flap closed in two layers. The neck is kept flexed by retention sutures. The endotracheal tube is replaced by a regular cuffed tracheostomy tube.

When cancer involves the arytenoid mucosa without vocal fold fixation, the resection must include the arytenoid cartilage. After entering the pharynx through the vallecula, the mucosa of the posterior glottis is incised posterior to the arytenoid cartilage. Arytenoidectomy is carried out by disarticulating the cricoarytenoid joint, amputating the vocal process, and removing the body of the cartilage along with its covering mucosa (Fig. 76-3). The supraglottic structure and piriform sinus are removed en bloc with adequate margins (Fig. 76-4). Margins of the surgical resection are examined by frozen section. After removal of the specimen, the vocal ligament is transfixed to the midline of the cricoid cartilage with 3-0 Vicryl suture (Fig. 76-5). Anesthesia should then be lightened to ensure adequate vocal fold approximation. The remainder of the pharyngeal closure is carried out as in standard supraglottic laryngectomy.

If the supraglottic tumor extends to the mucosa of the vocal fold without fixation, the procedure may also include excision of the involved vocal fold. This resection approximates near-total laryngectomy.

FRANK WONG

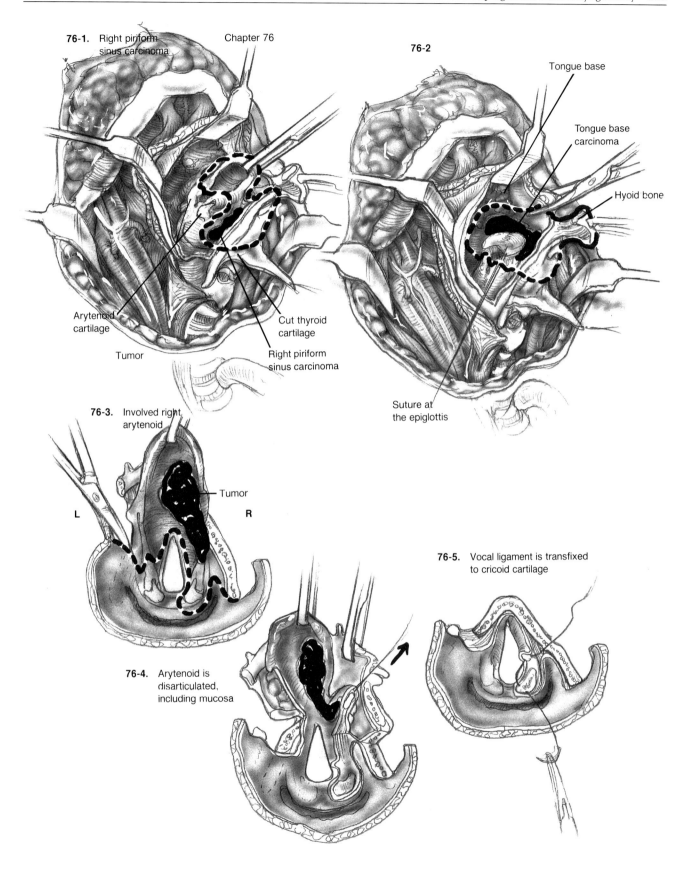

76-1. Right piriform sinus carcinoma

Chapter 76

Arytenoid cartilage

Tumor

Cut thyroid cartilage

Right piriform sinus carcinoma

76-2

Tongue base

Tongue base carcinoma

Hyoid bone

Suture at the epiglottis

76-3. Involved right arytenoid

Tumor

L   R

76-4. Arytenoid is disarticulated, including mucosa

76-5. Vocal ligament is transfixed to cricoid cartilage

■ 77. NEAR-TOTAL LARYNGECTOMY

A family of surgical procedures for lateralized squamous cancers of the larynx and piriform fossa with limitations of vocal fold movement. The entire larynx is removed, from tongue to trachea, except for the narrow posterolateral column of uninvolved subglottic, arytenoid, and piriform tissue, which can be preserved safely on the uninvolved side. A dynamic tracheopharyngeal myomucosal shunt is used for generating a voice using pulmonary air. The procedure is determined by the extent of disease:

- Near-total laryngectomy is a standardized en bloc excision of one cancerous paraglottic space plus all of its contiguous neighbors.
- A composite shunt is a dynamic tracheopharyngeal myomucosal shunt for the generation of a voice by pulmonary air. It is built from two sources the column of innervated soft tissues remaining from the larynx and from a small, local rotation flap from the ipsilateral pharynx.
- Near-total laryngopharyngectomy includes a wider margin of the pharynx, beyond the piriform, because the cancer involvement is primarily piriform.
- Extended near-total laryngopharyngectomy is a near-total laryngopharyngectomy in which so much pharyngeal wall is resected for hypopharyngeal cancer that primary closure of the pharyngeal defect is impractical. Flap reconstruction of the hypopharynx and perhaps the oropharynx is required.

Indications

1. Near-total laryngectomy
   a. Lateralized glottic or transglottic cancers with impaired movement, fixation, or subglottic extension, for which conventional vertical partial laryngectomies or supracricoid partial laryngectomy would be unsafe
   b. Lateralized supraglottic or aryepiglottic fold cancers with impaired movement, fixation, or glottic extension, for which conventional supraglottic partial laryngectomy, partial laryngopharyngectomy, or supracricoid laryngectomy would be unsafe
   c. Most supraglottic cancers in patients physiologically unfit for supraglottic or supracricoid partial laryngectomies, obviating escalation to a total laryngectomy
2. Near-total laryngopharyngectomy
   a. Piriform cancers with impaired movement (indicating paraglottic space invasion) or supraglottic and aryepiglottic cancers with pharyngeal wall spread or tongue base extension such that partial laryngopharyngectomy or extended supraglottic partial laryngectomy would be unsafe
3. Extended near-total laryngopharyngectomy
   a. All that remains of the hypopharynx after adequate resection of large piriform and hypopharyngeal wall cancers is the contralateral piriform fossa and the postcricoid region. The piriform can serve as the usual recipient of the voice shunt, but the rest of the swallowing tube depends on reconstruction with extrapharyngeal tissues.

Contraindications

1. Previous irradiation failure or partial laryngectomy failure is a relative contraindication.
2. Bilateral anterior "horseshoe" glottic/transglottic cancers infiltrating both ventricles
3. Primary subglottic cancers
4. Posterior cancer, such as postcricoid cancer

Special Considerations

1. The concept of continuing diagnosis
2. Neck dissections are often indicated.
3. Postoperative irradiation is tolerable.

(continued)

Operative Procedures

Direct Laryngoscopy and Biopsy

Carefully examine the column of laryngeal tissue slated for preservation. The ventricle to be entered should be free of tumor. The surgeon should not overlook submucosal extension or satellitosis, especially in pharyngeal cases. The center of the lesion should be biopsied, taking care not to obscure the lesion's borders. The surgeon must communicate her or his exact suspicions, the specimen site and orientation, and the history of previous treatment directly to the histopathologist performing the frozen-section analysis. Conclude by inserting the nasogastric feeding tube.

Tracheotomy

The trachea is approached through the transverse segment of the future apron flap incision. The surgeon separates the straps, and divides and ligates the inferior thyroid veins. The trachea is exposed below the thyroid isthmus. The operator again checks the transoperative tube's cuff and the sterile anesthetic hose. An aliquot of local anesthetic is instilled into the trachea without puncturing the balloon. After stabilizing the trachea with a hook, an opening incision is made. The band retractors are placed into the tracheal lumen, and the new tube is inserted as the anesthetist pulls out the old one. Careful placement prevents excessive advancement and ventilation of one lung. After the new tube is connected, it should be anchored to the skin.

Neck Dissection

After elevating the flaps in the subplatysmal prevenous plane, all the fat, fascia, and lymph nodes of the submental, submandibular, carotid, muscular, and posterior triangles of the neck are removed. The accessory, phrenic, vagus, hypoglossal, and marginal mandibular nerves, as well as the brachial plexus and the carotid arterial system, are preserved. In the neck of a high-risk patient, the internal jugular vein, the omohyoid and digastric muscles, and the submandibular gland and cervical plexus should be included in the resection. For elective surgery on a node-negative neck, these components are often preserved.

Near-Total Laryngectomy

The neck dissection exposes the strap muscles over the larynx on the principal side of the tumor. These are transected low, exposing the thyroid lobe to be included in the resection. The fascia is incised along the anterior border of the contralateral straps so the midline prelaryngeal soft tissues stay with the specimen. The contralateral straps are preserved. The surgeon divides and oversews the union between the contralateral thyroid lobe and the isthmus. The isthmus will accompany the specimen.

The surgeon next rolls away the larynx and the "specimen side" lobe of the thyroid. The superior, middle, and inferior thyroid veins are visualized and divided. (They may have already been released by a neck dissection.) The superior and inferior neural and arterial pedicles are identified as they cross to the specimen. The surgeon divides and ligates the superior thyroid artery and laryngeal nerve and similarly transects the inferior thyroid artery and recurrent nerve. The posterior border of the thyroid ala and the hyoid are skeletonized and freed from the inferior constrictor muscle (Fig. 77-1). The suprahyoid muscles are cut free to release the hyoid to be removed with the specimen. The operator shadows the upper border of the hyoid across the midline to the opposite lesser horn, taking care to evade the nearby hypoglossal nerve and the loop of the lingual artery.

The surgeon identified the column of the larynx to be preserved for the shunt on the side of least tumor involvement. It was previously confirmed during laryngoscopy that the ventricle on that side was tumor free. It is safe to enter there to begin the separation between the laryngeal elements of the composite shunt and the anterolateral margin of the resection specimen.

(continued)

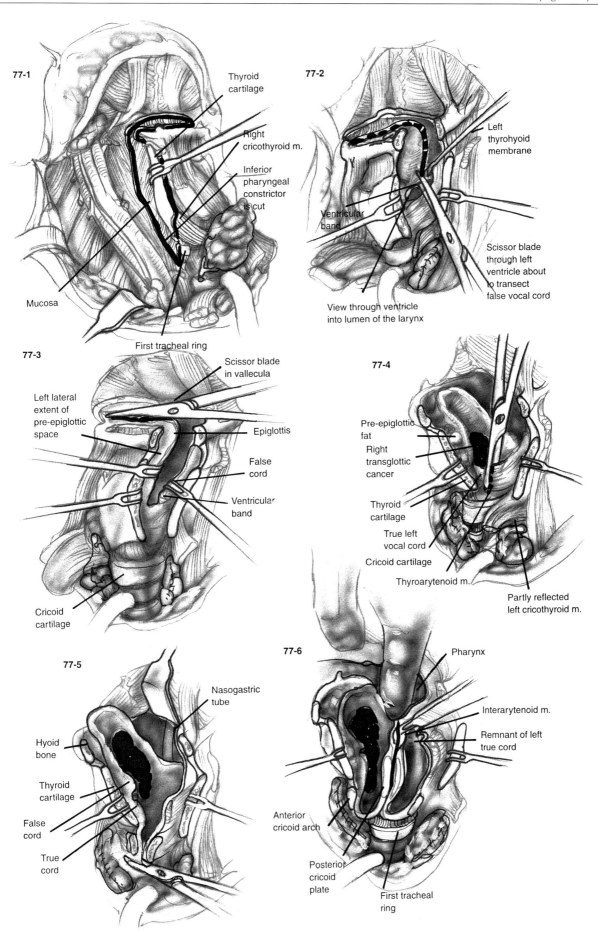

77-1
Thyroid cartilage
Right cricothyroid m.
Inferior pharyngeal constrictor is cut
Mucosa
First tracheal ring

77-2
Left thyrohyoid membrane
Ventricular band
Scissor blade through left ventricle about to transect false vocal cord
View through ventricle into lumen of the larynx

77-3
Scissor blade in vallecula
Left lateral extent of pre-epiglottic space
Epiglottis
False cord
Ventricular band
Cricoid cartilage

77-4
Pre-epiglottic fat
Right transglottic cancer
Thyroid cartilage
True left vocal cord
Cricoid cartilage
Thyroarytenoid m.
Partly reflected left cricothyroid m.

77-5
Nasogastric tube
Hyoid bone
Thyroid cartilage
False cord
True cord

77-6
Pharynx
Interarytenoid m.
Remnant of left true cord
Anterior cricoid arch
Posterior cricoid plate
First tracheal ring

■ 77. NEAR-TOTAL LARYNGECTOMY (continued)

Preoperative Preparation
1. Suspicion of the likely diagnosis of cancer before biopsy
2. Mapping the surface extent of the tumor
3. Use videolaryngoscopy, and document the tumor extent with prints.
4. Imaging studies, if they help demonstrate the depth of invasion
5. Speech pathology consultation
6. Tracheotomy demonstration by a nurse
7. Appropriate educational materials for the patient and family

Special Instruments, Position, and Anesthesia
1. A small (5.5 or 6), cuffed initial endotracheal anesthesia tube
2. Lindholm vallecular laryngoscope and 0° and 70° telescopes (Storz)
3. The neck is extended. The anesthesia tube is accessible and can be removed when the tracheotomy is made.
4. A fiberoptic headlight, preferably xenon
5. Light bone shears; nasal perichondral elevators; bipolar cautery
6. A 14-Fr catheter to size the voice shunt

Tips and Pearls
1. The more subglottic mucosa is preserved, the more favorable to voice production is the internal taper of the eventual tracheo-pharyngeal shunt.
2. A chalice-shaped configuration of the upper (pharyngeal) opening of the shunt is undesirable; it catches food and favors aspiration.
3. Sometimes, supraglottic cancer is found beyond the supraglottis, and a supraglottic laryngectomy may need to be extended beyond the expected pulmonary tolerance of the patient. In these situations, a near-total laryngectomy should be considered before a total procedure.

Pitfalls and Complications
1. Regional and distant metastases, second primaries, and local recurrences (rare)
2. Near-total laryngectomy was primarily designed for untreated, well-defined, relatively predictable cancers centered in the paraglottic space. Beware of radiation treatment failure.
3. Delayed acquisition of voice is probably the most common complication of near-total laryngectomy.
4. Aspiration will ensue if the recurrent laryngeal nerve to the shunt is destroyed or if the muscle in the laryngeal remnant is overcauterized.
5. The anterior tracheal wall stoma is slower to stabilize than the usual end-on stoma that follows a total laryngectomy.

Postoperative Care Issues
1. The dressing is removed on postoperative day 1.
2. Closed wound suction for approximately 3 days.
3. Feed through a nasogastric tube for about 10 days.
4. Speech pathology plays an integral role.

References

Keith RL. Looking forward . . . a guidebook for the laryngectomee. 2nd ed. New York: Thieme Medical Publishers, 1991.

Pearson BW, DeSanto LW. Near-total laryngectomy. Operative techniques. Otolaryngol Head Neck Surg 1990;1:28.

Pearson BW. Management of the primary site: larynx and hypopharynx. In: Pillsbury HC, Goldsmith MM, eds. Operative challenges in otolaryngology. Chicago: Year Book Medical Publishers, 1990:346.

A middle "column" or wedge is removed from the ala of the thyroid cartilage on the conserved side after releasing the hyoid origin of the sternohyoid covering it and dividing the hyoid. The hyoid body stays with the specimen. A periosteal elevator is insinuated under the deep surface of the middle third of the thyroid ala, starting at the superior margin to prepare the overlying wedge of cartilage or bone (alotomy) for removal between saw cuts. The operator must be careful not to traumatize the outer fibers of the underlying thyroarytenoid muscle or to enter yet into the ventricle just above it. The laryngeal lumen is entered through the fibroglandular tissue that caps the ventricle on the noninvolved side (Fig. 77-2).

The mucosal edges of the ventriculotomy are retracted with hooks, and the larynx is entered with the outstretched blade of a scissors. An upward cut is made across the false cord. Turning toward the tumor side, the vallecula is transected (Fig. 77-3). The specimen is folded forward as the headlight shines into the open larynx, enabling a good look at the cancer. The surgeon determines where to safely transect the "good" true cord and cuts down from above through this point (Fig. 77-4) and on into the anterior subglottis. The posterior cricoid plate is cut in the midline and broken to open the cricoid ring, and then the anterior and posterior cuts are joined at a safe distance under the tumor (Fig. 77-5). The surgeon continues cutting up through the break in the posterior cricoid plate and divides the interarytenoid (Fig. 77-6). The specimen, attached only by pharyngeal mucosa, is lifted and removed completely (Fig. 77-7).

Samples of the surgical margins are sent with the specimen for histopathologic review (Fig. 77-8). While waiting for the pathologist's report, the surgeon carries out a submucosal resection of the residual cricoid cartilage (Fig. 77-9). The remaining recurrent laryngeal nerve is essential to aspiration prevention and must be preserved, but the surgeon should ensure that the shunt becomes flaccid. After a report of tumor-free surgical margins, the reconstruction commences.

Reconstruction With the Composite Shunt

The surgeon stretches out the hypopharyngeal mucosa remaining on the newly cleared tumor side (Fig. 77-10A) and makes a simple backcut to develop an inferiorly based pennant-shaped flap from the margin (Fig. 77-10B). The base is level with the residual corniculate. The tip is high enough on the pharynx to give a flap that can rotate down and lie alongside the entire length of the shunt (Fig. 77-11). The width is whatever size is needed to form an appropriate shunt diameter after it is combined with the laryngeal component. In cases with much residual larynx, a flap may be minimal or unnecessary.

The surgeon next forms the tubular shunt. The flap and the laryngeal remnant are united in parallel to create the posterior wall (Fig. 77-12A). The composite is tubed, and the anterior wall is completed by sewing the vertical anterior seam that completes the tubular configuration (Fig. 77-12B). A 14-Fr catheter is a useful temporary gauge for the diameter.

The remaining pharyngotomy is closed (Fig. 77-12C,D), and the permanent stoma in the anterior tracheal wall is completed (Fig. 77-12E). Suction drains are placed in the neck, and the skin flaps are closed with an airtight deep layer of running chromic suture and a well-aligned skin closure of staples. To complete the operation, the surgeon dresses the stoma and the neck as necessary (eg, Xeroform around the tracheal tube and bulky gauze around the neck). The physician makes sure the bladder is not distended, and the patient is transported to the recovery room.

BRUCE W. PEARSON

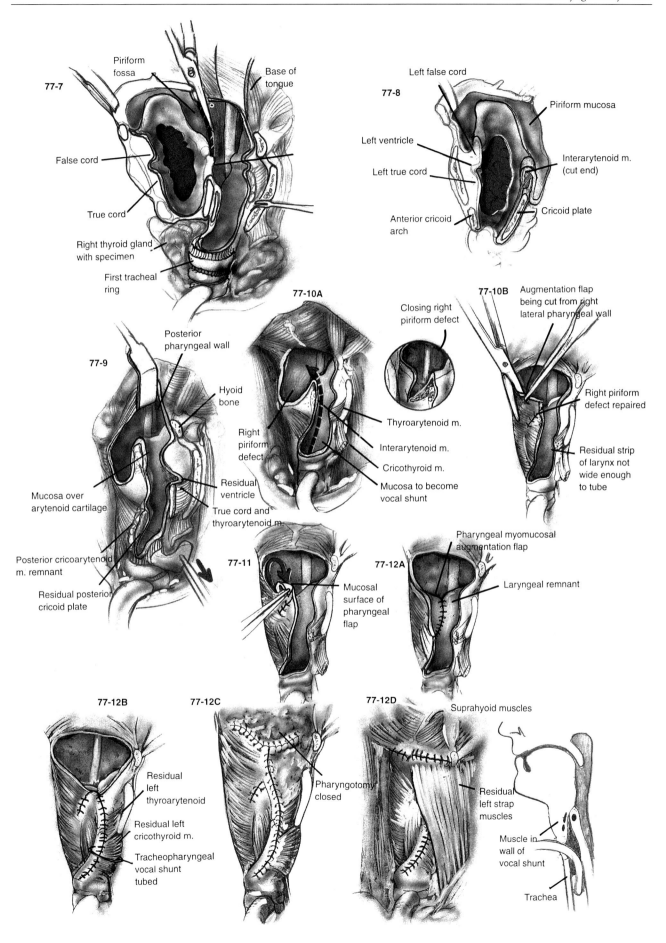

77-7
Piriform fossa
Base of tongue
False cord
True cord
Right thyroid gland with specimen
First tracheal ring

77-8
Left false cord
Piriform mucosa
Left ventricle
Left true cord
Interarytenoid m. (cut end)
Anterior cricoid arch
Cricoid plate

77-9
Posterior pharyngeal wall
Hyoid bone
Mucosa over arytenoid cartilage
Posterior cricoarytenoid m. remnant
Residual posterior cricoid plate
Residual ventricle
True cord and thyroarytenoid m.

77-10A
Right piriform defect
Closing right piriform defect
Thyroarytenoid m.
Interarytenoid m.
Cricothyroid m.
Mucosa to become vocal shunt

77-10B
Augmentation flap being cut from right lateral pharyngeal wall
Right piriform defect repaired
Residual strip of larynx not wide enough to tube

77-11
Mucosal surface of pharyngeal flap

77-12A
Pharyngeal myomucosal augmentation flap
Laryngeal remnant

77-12B
Residual left thyroarytenoid
Residual left cricothyroid m.
Tracheopharyngeal vocal shunt tubed

77-12C
Pharyngotomy closed

77-12D
Suprahyoid muscles
Residual left strap muscles
Muscle in wall of vocal shunt
Trachea

■ 78. TOTAL LARYNGECTOMY

Removal of entire larynx, including thyroid and cricoid cartilages and the hyoid bone

Indications

1. Stage T3 and T4 carcinoma of the larynx
2. Stage T2 carcinoma unsuitable for partial laryngectomy
3. Subglottic carcinoma or glottic carcinoma with subglottic extension of more than 1.5 cm
4. Carcinoma of the base of the tongue extending beyond the circumvallate papillae
5. Failed radiotherapy for laryngeal carcinoma

Contraindications

1. Distant metastasis
2. Extreme age or poor medical status

Special Considerations

1. Social work consultation regarding home care or disposition
2. Meticulous reconstruction of the tracheostoma, avoiding tension in the approximation of skin to tracheal mucosa and avoiding exposure of the tracheal cartilage
3. Meticulous mucosal closure of the pharynx using inverting Connell stitch
4. Tracheostomy for obstructive lesion as a separate procedure and if total laryngectomy is delayed for more than 48 hours, the incidence of stomal recurrence may increase. Emergent total laryngectomy should be considered after tracheostomy under local anesthesia.

Preoperative Preparation

1. Speech consultation with counseling regarding postoperative voice restoration. Meeting with a laryngectomee or support group is highly desirable.
2. Routine laboratory studies
3. Computed tomography scan to delineate the extent of the disease and neck node status
4. Preoperative and perioperative antibiotics

Special Instruments, Position, and Anesthesia

1. Anesthesia may be administered initially by orotracheal intubation, if the lesion is not large.
2. Tracheostomy under local anesthesia is advisable before induction of anesthesia for bulky obstructive lesions.
3. Supine position with a shoulder roll to keep the neck extended

(continued)

Operative Procedure

A transverse collar incision is carried out about two fingerbreadths (3 cm) above the sternal notch, extending superiorly and laterally on both sides (Fig. 78-1). Skin flaps are elevated in the subplatysmal plane. Bilateral selective neck dissection may be carried out as indicated, with the contents left attached to the thyrohyoid area. Total laryngectomy commences by skeletonizing the larynx. The strap muscles are transected inferiorly low in the neck, and the thyroid gland is exposed. One lobe of the thyroid can be removed if extralaryngeal spread is suspected; otherwise, the thyroid gland can be dissected free from the trachea and larynx after dividing the thyroid isthmus (Figs. 78-2 and 78-3).

This procedure is carried out on both sides of the larynx. The posterior border of the thyroid cartilage is identified, and the larynx is rotated to expose the attachment of the inferior constrictor muscle. This muscle is incised along the posterior border of the thyroid ala (Fig. 78-4). The thyrohyoid membrane is then exposed. The superior laryngeal neurovascular bundle is easily identified medial to the superior horn of the thyroid cartilage, and it is ligated and divided. If there is no extension into the piriform sinus, the superior horn of the thyroid cartilage should be isolated and the piriform sinus mucosa dissected from the thyroid cartilage without entering the pharynx.

The hyoid bone is grasped in the midline with an Allis forceps, and the attachments of the suprahyoid muscles are transected. These muscles are thick and must be divided completely with Bovie electrocautery until the external aspect of the vallecular mucosa is reached. Care must be taken to avoid damage to the hypoglossal nerve. The larynx is mobilized from surrounding structures.

(continued)

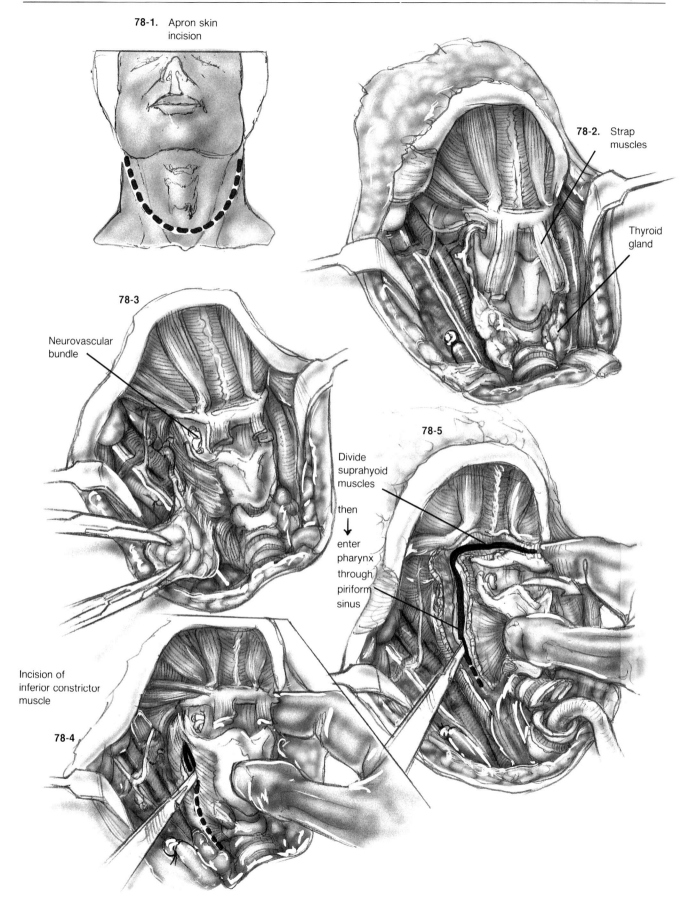

78-1. Apron skin incision

78-2. Strap muscles

Thyroid gland

78-3

Neurovascular bundle

78-5

Divide suprahyoid muscles

then

↓

enter pharynx through piriform sinus

Incision of inferior constrictor muscle

78-4

78. TOTAL LARYNGECTOMY *(continued)*

Tips and Pearls

1. Enter the pharynx on the side opposite the tumor.
2. An oropharyngeal suction inserted through the mouth into the vallecula can facilitate location of that mucosa.
3. Save as much mucosa as possible without compromising complete tumor resection margins.
4. After pharyngeal closure, water (plain or with methylene blue) may be instilled to test the suture line.
5. Some surgeons perform incomplete closure of the muscle layer to facilitate esophageal speech or prosthetic voice rehabilitation. Alternatively, a cricopharyngeal myotomy may be performed.

Pitfalls and Complications

1. Pharyngocutaneous fistula usually results from inadequate pharyngeal closure, insufficient mucosa, or previous radiation damage.
2. Stomal stenosis may result from infection, wound tension, or inadequate size of initial construction.
3. Subcutaneous hematoma may result in infection and flap loss. Meticulous hemostasis before closure is mandatory, and functional suction drainage is essential to prevent wound infection.
4. Airway obstruction from slight oozing and crust formation can be prevented by inserting a #12 laryngectomy tube into the newly created permanent tracheostoma.
5. Postoperative swallowing difficulty may be caused by cricopharyngeal muscle hypertrophy.
6. Stomal recurrence
7. Hypothyroidism or hypoparathyroidism

Postoperative Care Issues

1. The patient is fed through a nasogastric tube as soon as bowel function returns.
2. Oral intake usually starts between the 7th and 10th postoperative day if there are no signs of infection.
3. Speech therapy is usually started after swallowing is established.

References

Alberti PW. The historical development of laryngectomy. II. The evolution of laryngology and laryngectomy in the mid-nineteenth century. Laryngoscope 1975;85:288.

Lore JM. An atlas of head an neck surgery. 3rd ed. Philadelphia: WB Saunders, 1988:892.

The trachea is transected at the level of the intended resection around the fourth tracheal ring. If subglottic extension is suspected, at least four rings should be included. The posterior wall of the trachea is incised, avoiding entering the esophagus. The posterior tracheal wall and cricoid cartilage are separated from the esophagus. The anterior tracheal wall is secured to the neck skin with a heavy nylon suture. An armored tube is placed into the distal trachea (Fig. 78-5).

The pharynx is entered either through the vallecula or from the piriform sinus in an area that is free of tumor. The mucosal incision is enlarged with Metzenbaum scissors transversely along the valleculae superiorly or from the piriform sinus toward the tongue base under direct vision. The epiglottis is grasped with an Allis or Babcock clamp. The mucosal cut is continued along both medial walls of the piriform sinuses. After the incision reaches the cricoid level, the superior dissection can be joined with the inferior dissection from the trachea. The mucosa is transected and the larynx is removed (Fig. 78-6).

Before pharyngeal closure, a nasogastric feeding tube is passed and fixed to the nose (Figs. 78-7 and 78-8). The pharyngeal mucosal defect is closed meticulously with Connell inverting stitch using 3-0 Vicryl atraumatic absorbable sutures. A T-shaped closure is preferable to a straight-line closure (Fig. 78-9). Second-layer closure may be achieved by approximating the constrictor muscles. After the pharynx is closed, the wound is thoroughly irrigated.

A permanent tracheostoma is constructed by bringing the skin of the neck to cover the tracheal edge mucosa without exposing the cartilage. The tracheostoma can be enlarged by beveling the tracheal cut. Construction of the tracheostoma should be free of tension. The skin flap is closed in two layers after placement of suction drainage (Fig. 78-10).

FRANK WONG

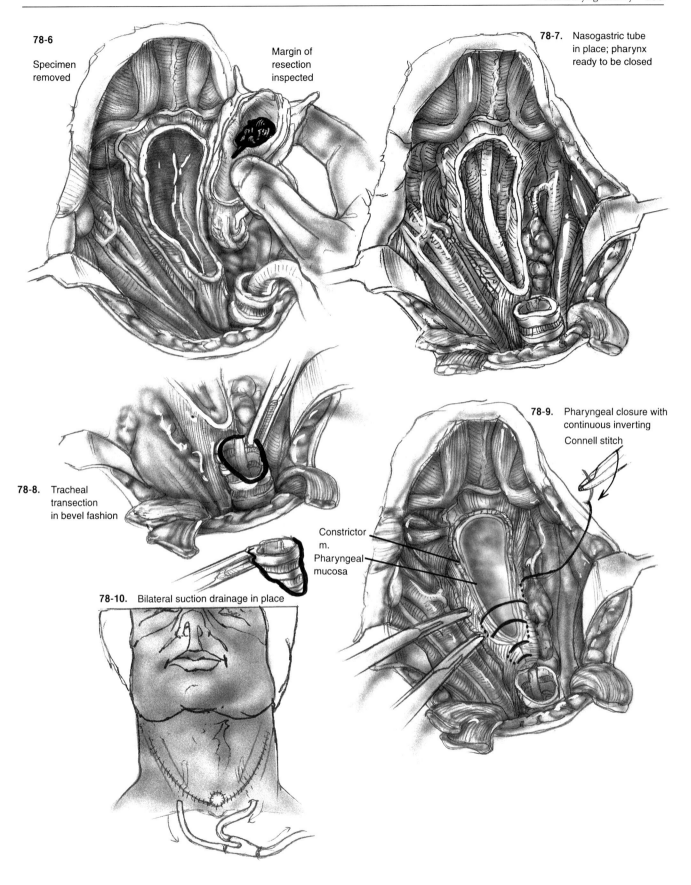

78-6

Specimen
removed

Margin of
resection
inspected

78-7. Nasogastric tube
in place; pharynx
ready to be closed

78-8. Tracheal
transection
in bevel fashion

78-9. Pharyngeal closure with
continuous inverting

Connell stitch

Constrictor
m.
Pharyngeal
mucosa

78-10. Bilateral suction drainage in place

■ 79. TOTAL LARYNGECTOMY WITH EXTENSION—Excision of the larynx with up to one half the circumference of the pharynx or a portion of the posterior tongue

Indications

1. Piriform sinus carcinoma involving the medial wall or apex, or laryngeal cancer extending to the piriform sinus
2. Larynx carcinoma extending into the base of the tongue or base of tongue cancer extending to or beyond the circumvallate papillae

Contraindications

1. Cervical esophageal or postcricoid extension
2. Extension of tumor to or across the midline of the posterior pharyngeal wall
3. Inability to preserve one lingual artery and one hypoglossal nerve

Special Considerations

1. Intraoperative frozen-section analysis is essential to assess margins.
2. Inspection and palpation during resection to rule out submucosal spread and multicentricity of the tumor
3. Flap reconstruction frequently required
4. Bilateral selective neck dissection is often indicated.

Preoperative Preparation

1. Routine laboratory studies
2. Barium swallow and esophagoscopy to delineate the extent of tumor
3. Consent for flap reconstruction should be incorporated in consent for surgery.

Pitfalls and Complications

1. Possible submucosal spread of tumor
2. Fistula formation
3. Stricture

Postoperative Care

1. Same as for laryngectomy

References

Eisbach KJ, Krause CJ. Carcinoma of the pyriform sinus. A comparison of treatment modalities. Laryngoscope 1977;87:1904.

El Badawi SA, Goepfert H, Fletcher GH, Herson J, Oswald MJ. Squamous cell carcinoma of the pyriform sinus. Laryngoscope 1982;92: 357.

Surgical Procedure

An apron-type skin incision, from mastoid tip to mastoid tip, is performed to accommodate bilateral neck dissection. Inferiorly, this incision is at the level of the planned tracheotomy. The larynx is mobilized by transecting the strap muscles inferiorly, freeing the hyoid bone from its muscle attachments and freeing the larynx from the carotid sheath.

If the piriform sinus is involved, the next step is careful inspection to rule out extrapharyngeal extension. The constrictor muscle of the involved side remains untouched until the total extent of the tumor can be evaluated under direct vision of the mucosal surface. On the uninvolved side, the inferior constrictor is transected near its attachment to the thyroid cartilage, and the neurovascular bundle is divided as in standard total laryngectomy. The piriform mucosa on the uninvolved side is dissected from the posterior surface of the thyroid cartilage and the posterior cricoarytenoid muscle. The pharynx is entered through the vallecula, and the tumor is inspected. This incision is carried around the larynx, saving as much mucosa as possible on the uninvolved side. On the side of the tumor, a full thickness of pharyngeal mucosa and constrictor muscle is removed along with the larynx (Fig. 79-1).

Closure of the pharynx proceeds as for total laryngectomy if adequate residual pharyngeal mucosa is available. To assess for adequate mucosa, a #36 Maloney bougie is inserted through the mouth to the esophagus. If the pharynx mucosa can be closed without tension around this bougie, the mucosa is adequate. If the mucosa is inadequate, a flap is interposed to ensure an adequate lumen for swallowing and to decrease the risk of salivary fistula formation (Figs. 79-2 and 79-3).

For tongue base cancer, entry into the pharynx is through the piriform sinus of the least involved side. The larynx is removed as in total laryngectomy, proceeding cephalic from the trachea. After the tumor is adequately exposed, the tongue is transected anteriorly. At least a 2-cm margin should be allowed, determined by inspection and by digital palpation. Margins should be confirmed by frozen-section analysis (Figs. 79-4 and 79-5).Closure proceeds as in total laryngectomy. If the tongue excision is extensive, pedicle myocutaneous flap reconstruction may be required.

FRANK WONG

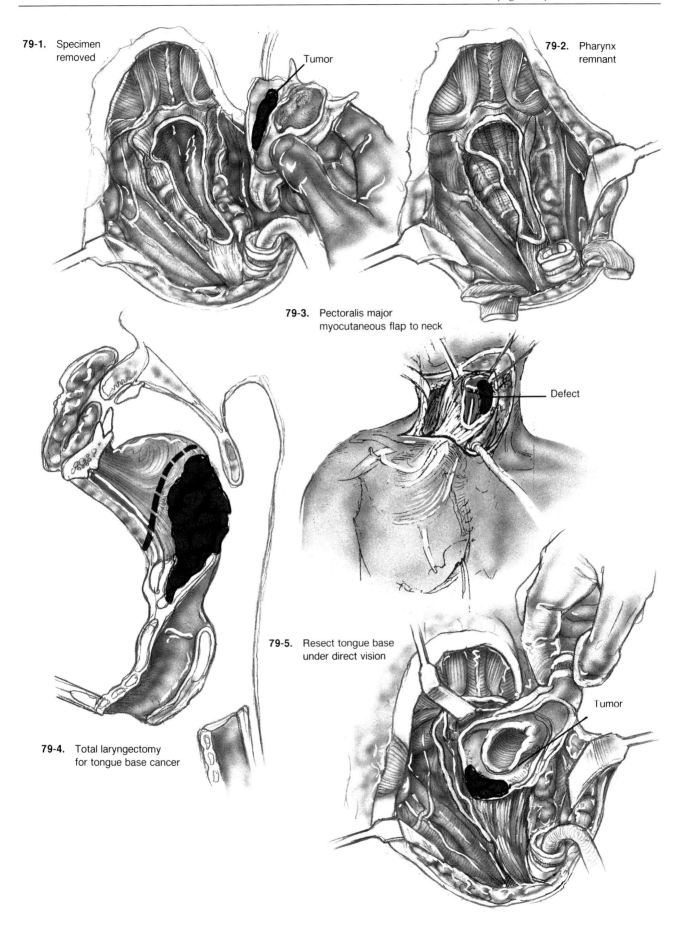

79-1. Specimen removed

Tumor

79-2. Pharynx remnant

79-3. Pectoralis major myocutaneous flap to neck

Defect

79-4. Total laryngectomy for tongue base cancer

79-5. Resect tongue base under direct vision

Tumor

■ 80. TOTAL PHARYNGOLARYNGECTOMY

Excision of the larynx, hypopharynx, and upper cervical esophagus

Indications

1. Hypopharyngeal carcinoma or larynx cancer extending to involve two thirds of the circumference of the hypopharynx
2. Extensive tumor involvement of the posterior pharyngeal wall
3. Pharyngeal carcinoma with minimal cervical esophagus extension
4. Postcricoid cancer

Contraindications

1. Distant metastasis
2. Mediastinal involvement
3. Prevertebral fascial involvement

Special Considerations

1. History of previous abdominal surgery (ie, gastric or esophageal surgery)
2. Chest condition
3. Malnutrition
4. Reconstructive planning

Preoperative Preparation

1. Barium esophagogram and upper gastrointestinal series with follow-through to determine extent of disease and for reconstruction options
2. Computed tomography scan of neck and chest
3. Cinefluoroscopy may be needed to determine prevertebral fascia involvement
4. Consultations with thoracic surgeon, gastrointestinal surgeon, or microvascular surgeon to plan reconstruction
5. Make sure the patient is in positive nitrogen balance. Preoperative nasogastric tube or intravenous hyperalimentation as needed before definite surgery
6. Routine laboratory studies
7. Group and crossmatch at least 2 units of packed cells
8. Prophylactic antibiotics
9. Intensive care unit arrangement for immediate postoperative care

(continued)

Operative Procedure

The patient is placed in a supine position, with the neck extended and shoulders on rolls. General anesthesia is induced through endotracheal intubation or a local tracheotomy if the patient cannot be intubated.

A large, apron-type incision, from mastoid tip to mastoid tip, is made. The lower transverse limb of the incision is placed about two fingerbreadths (3 cm) below the cricoid cartilage (Fig. 80-1). The skin flap is elevated at the subplatysmal plane. Bilateral neck dissection is performed at the outset. Meanwhile, the retropharyngeal and retroesophageal spaces are explored to determine resectability. Exploration of the prevertebral space can be done by retracting the sternocleidomastoid muscle laterally and rotating the larynx medially. The retropharyngeal and retroesophageal space can be entered with sharp and blunt dissection (Fig. 80-2), allowing examination under direct vision.

Any suspicious lesion should be biopsied and sent for frozen-section analysis. If the tumor invades the prevertebral fascia and carotid artery, the procedure should be terminated, or the procedure should be considered only palliative. After completion of the neck dissection, the contents can be removed or left attached to the thyrohyoid area.

The pharyngolaryngectomy can proceed as planned. The larynx is skeletonized as in total laryngectomy, and the pharynx and larynx are mobilized as one unit (Fig. 80-3). The larynx and pharynx are separated from the base of tongue area superiorly to the trachea inferiorly and dissected away from one carotid sheath to the other. Blunt dissection of the retropharynx and retroesophagus is carried out. The contralateral thyroid lobe should be preserved and dissected

(continued)

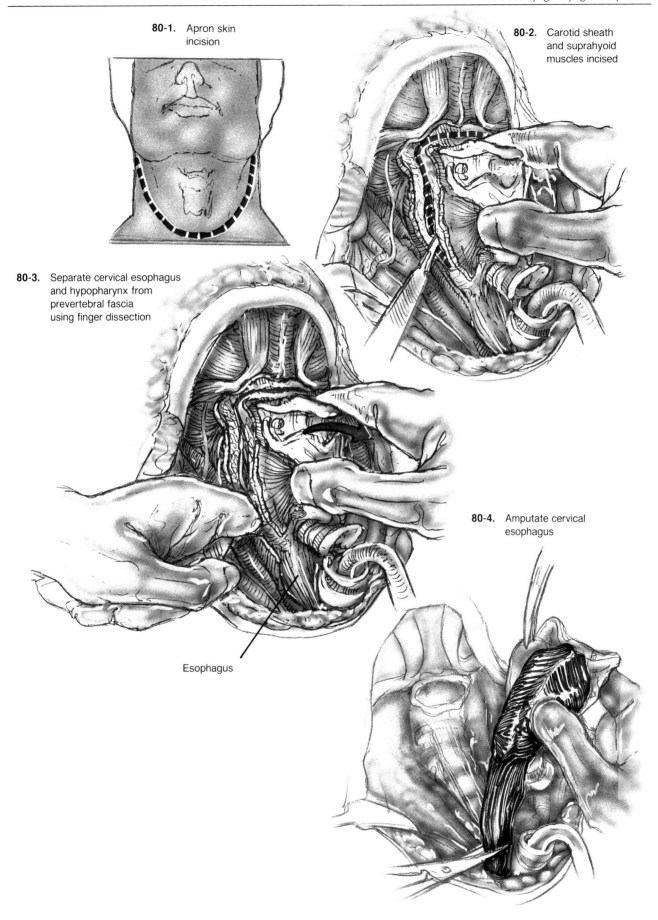

80-1. Apron skin incision

80-2. Carotid sheath and suprahyoid muscles incised

80-3. Separate cervical esophagus and hypopharynx from prevertebral fascia using finger dissection

Esophagus

80-4. Amputate cervical esophagus

■ 80. TOTAL PHARYNGOLARYNGECTOMY
(continued)

Special Instruments, Position, and Anesthesia
1. Headlight
2. Microvascular and abdominal surgical instruments
3. Dermatome for possible skin graft
4. Shoulders on roll and neck extended; patient prepped from lower face to lower abdomen

Tips and Pearls
1. Microvascular reconstruction with radial forearm skin flap or jejunum visceral free flap provides the best functional result.
2. If the cervical esophagus is involved, total esophagectomy is necessary to achieve cure. Gastric pull-up is a good choice for reconstruction.

Pitfalls and Complications
1. Submucosal tumor spread
2. Fistula
3. Stricture at the distal anastomosis site may require dilation.
4. Pneumonia
5. Pleural Effusion
6. Third space fluid deficit after mediastinal and abdominal dissection

Postoperative Care Issues
1. Intensive care unit
2. Monitor fluids carefully
3. Free flaps require special care.
4. Parenteral alimentation is advisable.

References

Harrison DFN, Thompson AE. Pharyngoesophagectomy with pharyngogastric anastomosis for cancer of the hypopharynx. Review of 101 operations. Head Neck Surg 1986;8:418.

Schecter GL, Balor JW, Gilbert DA. Functional evaluation of pharyngoesophageal reconstructive techniques. Arch Otolaryngol Head Neck Surg 1987;113:40.

Schuller DE. Reconstruction options for pharyngeal and/or cervical esophageal defects. Arch Otolaryngol Head Neck Surg 1985; 111: 193.

away from the trachea and larynx. If the thyroid gland is infiltrated with tumor, total thyroidectomy should be carried out. The bilateral superior laryngeal neurovascular bundle is identified, tied, and divided. All strap muscles are detached from the hyoid bone superiorly and inferiorly low in the neck. The trachea is transected at the fourth tracheal ring, and anesthesia is continued through tracheal intubation through an armored tube, which is secured to the chest skin with silk sutures. The anterior tracheal wall is secured to the neck skin. The pharynx is entered through the vallecula as in total laryngectomy. Under direct vision, the circumferential incision is carried out superiorly with adequate margins (Fig. 80-4). The lower circumferential cut is at the cervical esophagus level, separating the esophagus from the trachea with adequate margins (Fig. 80-4). It is imperative to have the lower margin assessed by frozen-section examination. If the lower margin is not clear of carcinoma or the tumor exhibits submucosal extension, total esophagectomy should be carried out. Reconstruction of the defect, from the tongue base to the cervical esophagus, can be achieved with the following options:

1. Skin flap: Bakamjain flap (ie, deltopectoral flap), a two-stage procedure (Figs. 80-5 and 80-6).
2. Myocutaneous flap: pectoralis major or trapezius myocutaneous flap (Figs. 80-7 and 80-8)
3. Microvascular flap: radial forearm skin flap or jejunum vicera-free flap (Fig. 80-9)

After the reconstruction of the pharyngeal defect, the wound is thoroughly irrigated. A permanent tracheostomy is constructed as in total laryngectomy. Bilateral closed suction drainage is placed, and the skin is closed in the usual two layers. The patient is transferred to the intensive care unit.

FRANK WONG

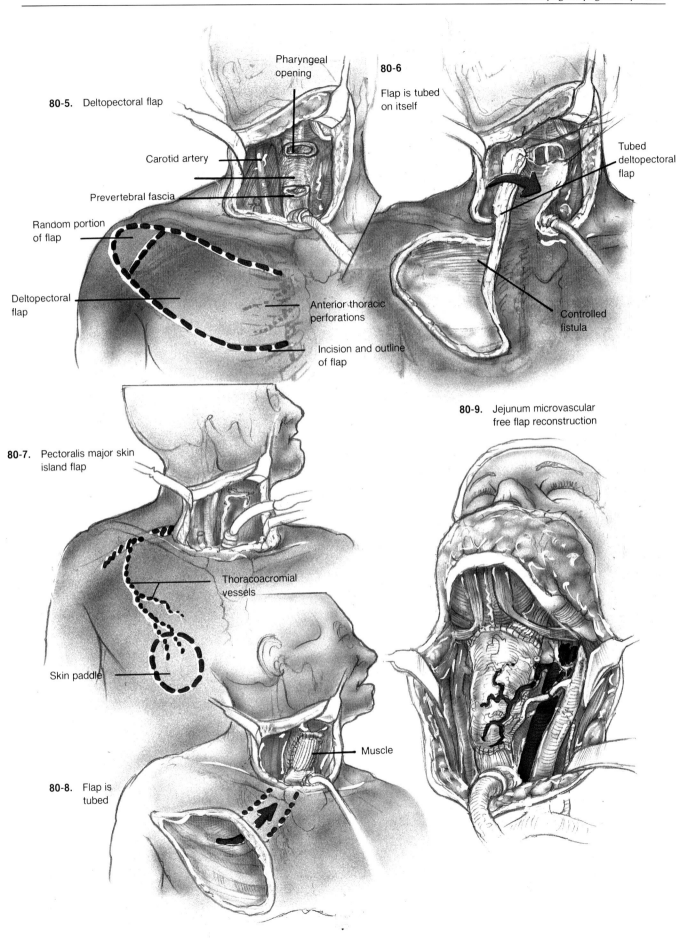

80-5. Deltopectoral flap

Pharyngeal opening

80-6

Flap is tubed on itself

Carotid artery

Tubed deltopectoral flap

Prevertebral fascia

Random portion of flap

Deltopectoral flap

Anterior thoracic perforations

Controlled fistula

Incision and outline of flap

80-9. Jejunum microvascular free flap reconstruction

80-7. Pectoralis major skin island flap

Thoracoacromial vessels

Skin paddle

Muscle

80-8. Flap is tubed

■ 81. TRACHEOESOPHAGEAL SHUNT (VOICE REHABILITATION)—Creation of a functional tracheoesophageal fistula for placement of a prosthesis used for alaryngeal speech after total laryngectomy

Indication
1. Aphonia after total laryngectomy

Contraindications
1. Inability to manage tracheoesophageal prosthesis (eg, severe tremor or poor manual dexterity, blindness, dementia, morbid obesity)
2. Tracheostoma stenosis (<1 cm)
3. Poor patient motivation
4. Severe hearing loss
5. Severe gastroesophageal reflux
6. Severe chronic obstructive pulmonary disease
7. Active alcoholism
8. Poor wound healing potential (eg, diabetes, malnutrition, previous radiation therapy) is a relative contraindication.

Special Considerations
1. Pharyngeal or upper esophageal stricture
2. Constrictor muscle spasm (consider myotomy and pharyngeal plexus neurectomy)

Preoperative Preparation
1. Speech therapy consultation
2. Insufflation test
3. Routine laboratory studies

Special Instruments, Position, and Anesthesia
1. One 29-cm (10 × 14 mm) rigid esophagoscope
2. Two 14-gauge rubber catheters
3. Shoulder roll; neck and head extended
4. General endotracheal anesthesia through the stoma

Tips and Pearls
1. Protect posterior esophageal wall with beveled mouth of the esophagoscope

Pitfalls and Complications
1. Incorrect placement of tracheoesophageal puncture or poor prostheses fit
2. Injury to the posterior or lateral esophageal wall
3. Wound infection or breakdown
4. Leakage and aspiration
5. Stoma stenosis or granulation buildup
6. Stenosis or closure of fistula
7. Poor sound generation or voice quality

Postoperative Care
1. Remove rubber catheter and place tracheoesophageal fistula prostheses between postoperative days 2 and 5.
2. Diet may be rapidly advanced if there is no leakage or aspiration.
3. Consider tube feeding in heavily irradiated patients.
4. Local wound care with H_2O_2 and cotton-tip applicators
5. Antibiotics if indicated

References
Robbins KT, Oppenheimer RW. Reverse catheter placement: a modification of the Blom-Singer technique. J Otolaryngol 1993;22:204.
Singer MI, Blom ED. An endoscopic technique for restoration of voice after total laryngectomy. Ann Otol Rhinol Laryngol 1980;89:529.
Singer MI. Tracheoesophageal speech: vocal rehabilitation after total laryngectomy. Laryngoscope 1983;93:1454.

Operative Procedure
General anesthesia is induced with the patient in the supine position. A shoulder roll is placed, and the head and neck are extended. A 29-cm (10 × 14 mm) rigid esophagoscope is introduced and advanced to the stoma site; the neopharynx and upper esophagus are inspected for strictures and mucosal abnormalities. The esophagoscope is then gently rotated 180° such that the longer side of the bevel is oriented posteriorly. With the room lights dimmed, the party wall can be transilluminated using the esophagoscope light.

A puncture site is identified 5 to 10 mm below the superior mucocutaneous junction of the tracheostoma at midline. The opening of the esophagoscope is oriented beneath the identified puncture site and a stab incision is made under direct vision with a #11 scalpel blade oriented into the opening of the esophagoscope (Fig. 81-1). The knife tip should scrape against the posterior (long) lip of the esophagoscope to ensure complete division of the esophageal mucosa. A hemostat is then placed through the puncture such that the tips are visualized through the scope, and the hemostat is opened. A #14 rubber catheter is fed through the esophagoscope to the open hemostat, and the catheter is grasped with the hemostat (Fig. 81-2). The catheter is then pulled externally through the puncture, and a clamp is placed on the end of the catheter so that it is not accidentally pulled back into the esophagoscope. The esophagoscope is withdrawn, leaving the proximal end of the catheter protruding from the mouth.

A second 14-gauge rubber catheter is placed through the nose and brought out the mouth. The funnel (proximal) end of the lower catheter is cut off, and the two catheter ends are sutured together with 2-0 silk suture. The proximal end of the lower catheter is brought out through the nose by pulling the upper catheter out of the nose (Fig. 81-3). The suture connecting the upper and lower catheters is cut, and the upper catheter is discarded. The proximal and distal ends of the remaining catheter are sutured together using an 0 silk suture (Fig. 81-4). The catheter is further secured with tape to the nasal ala. In 2 to 5 days, the catheter is removed, and a tracheoesophageal voice prosthesis (eg, Blom-Singer) is placed.

Many other methods for creation of a tracheoesophageal shunt that work well have been described. However, the advantages of this method include limited specialized equipment requirements, elimination of problems with postoperative tracheoesophageal fistula stent (ie, catheter) displacement, and technical ease.

AARON J. PRUSSIN

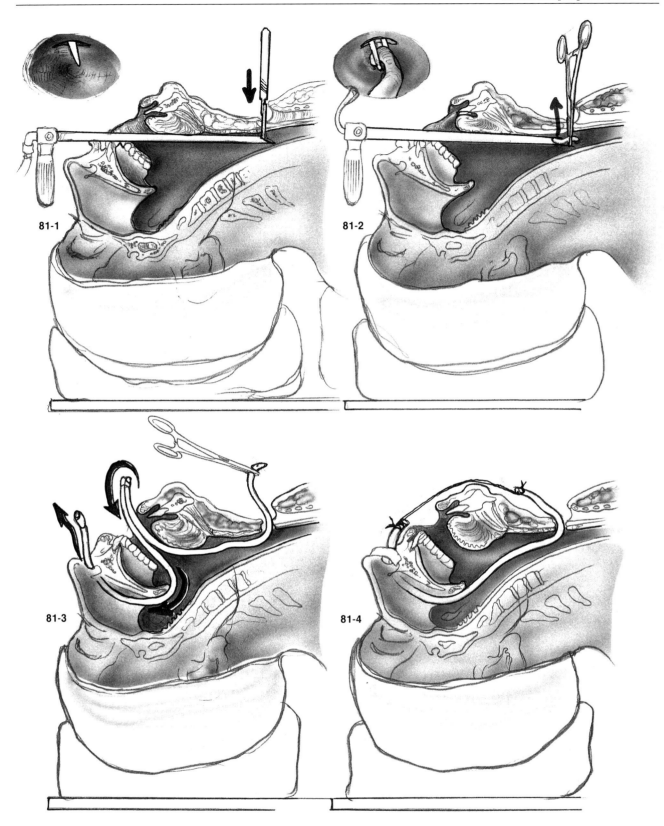

81-1

81-2

81-3

81-4

82. RECURRENT LARYNGEAL NERVE SECTION AND AVULSION—Procedure to sever or remove a segment of a unilateral recurrent laryngeal nerve to produce ipsilateral paralysis

Indications

1. Severe spasmodic dysphonia unresponsive to botulinum toxin
2. Severe spasmodic dysphonia in patient unable to receive botulinum toxin

Special Considerations

1. Previous surgery in the region
2. Normal movement of the contralateral vocal cord
3. Rule out other conditions that may endanger the normal function of the contralateral true vocal cord
4. Absolute accuracy of the diagnosis

Preoperative Preparation

1. Routine laboratory studies
2. Inspection of cervical region for previous surgery or traumatic injury
3. Lidocaine block of recurrent laryngeal nerve to test for effect
4. Extensive, documented discussion with the patient and family about the irreversibility of the procedure
5. Warn the patient that a few patients develop a breathy, weak voice that may require later minimal thyroplasty for the voice to become audible again.

Special Instruments, Position, and Anesthesia

1. Routine major surgical tray
2. Position the patient on a shoulder roll, with the head extended.
3. Usually, section the left nerve because of a greater risk over time of injury to the left nerve from common pulmonary tumors or thoracic surgery.
4. Have direct laryngoscopy equipment available.

Tips and Pearls

1. Perform neural avulsion of the entire cervical segment of the nerve.
2. Nerve section of several centimeters of nerve often results in neural regrowth with recurrent spasmodic dysphonia.

Pitfalls and Complications

1. The recurrent laryngeal nerve may be difficult to locate because of previous thyroid surgery.
2. Nerve crush, division, or removal of a short segment (1 to 4 cm) may lead to recurrence of dysphonia.

Postoperative Care Issues

1. Monitor for cervical hematoma.
2. Monitor patient for moderate aspiration.
3. Speech therapy consultation for swallowing, as needed
4. Follow-up speech therapy consultation for voice

References

Aronson AE, Desanto LW. Adducto spastic dysphonia: three years after recurrent laryngeal nerve section. Laryngoscope 1983;93:1.

Dedo HH, Izdebski K. Intermediate results of 306 recurrent laryngeal nerve sections for spastic dysphonia. Laryngoscope 1983;93:9.

Netterville JL, Stone RE, Rainey C, Zealear DL, Ossoff RH. Recurrent laryngeal nerve avulsion for treatment of spastic dysphonia. Ann Otol Rhinol Laryngol. 1991;100:10.

Operative Procedure

The patient is positioned with the neck in the extended position, with a shoulder roll placed under the back if needed. An incision is outlined several centimeters inferior to the cricoid cartilage, placed in a skin crease if possible (Fig. 82-1). This incision is usually 4 to 5 cm long. The skin and subcutaneous tissue is infiltrated with a solution of lidocaine and epinephrine.

After the incision is completed down through the platysma, skin flaps are raised in all directions, with emphasis on the elevation in the superior and inferior direction. We prefer to remove the left recurrent laryngeal nerve, because the left nerve with its longer course through the chest is at greater risk of injury over time than the right. The sternohyoid is elevated away from the sternothyroid and with further mobilization of the sternothyroid, the paratracheal fat can be seen. Large inferior thyroid veins are divided to gain entry into this space. Dissection down through this fat pad inferior to the thyroid gland leads to identification of the recurrent laryngeal nerve near the level of the tracheoesophageal groove (Fig. 82-2).

The nerve is isolated and followed superiorly deep to the inferior pole of the thyroid gland until it is seen passing deep to the cricopharyngeus muscle. Several branches of the nerve that are seen passing into the lateral wall of the esophagus are avulsed or pulled out of their insertion into the muscle by grasping the nerve with a clamp and gently pulling until the distal end of the branch pulls put of the muscle.

The recurrent laryngeal nerve is dissected away from the inferior thyroid vascular pedicle. The surgeon can often see several branches of the nerve as it passes deep to the cricopharyngeus. Each branch of the nerve is independently avulsed from its insertion into the laryngeal muscles (Fig. 82-3). This is performed by placing traction on the nerve by grasping it with a forceps. As the nerve stretches, another forceps is used to grasp the nerve at a more distal point as the nerve is withdrawn from under the cricopharyngeus. The two forceps are marched over each other, slowly avulsing the nerve branch from its insertion into the laryngeal muscles. This process is repeated for the one or two other branches of the nerve passing deep to the cricopharyngeus muscle. If Galen's anastomosis (ie, sensory branch communicating between the recurrent laryngeal nerve and the superior laryngeal nerve) is identified, it is followed to be sure it does not pass deep to the cricopharyngeus and then is sectioned. If this nerve were avulsed by traction, it could damage the superior laryngeal nerve.

With the distal laryngeal attachments of the nerve completely detached, the the recurrent laryngeal nerve is traced proximally under the clavicle. Several small branches that pass into the muscular wall of the esophagus must be divided or avulsed as the nerve is isolated. The nerve is traced as far proximally into the chest as possible, with good visualization of the surrounding structures. At this point, the nerve is cauterized and divided (Fig. 82-4). The length of the nerve segment excised usually is 8 to 11 cm (Fig. 82-5).

When the easily identified recurrent laryngeal nerve is followed and it passes deep to the cricopharyngeus, I do not perform laryngoscopy with stimulation of the exposed nerve to confirm its identity.

The major reason for using neural avulsion instead of sectioning is that nerves have an amazing ability to regenerate. The regeneration is not complete enough for normal cord motion, but it commonly results in the return of motor tone in the paralyzed cord, which results in the return of spasmodic dysphonia. The neural ingrowth into the distal cut end of the recurrent laryngeal nerve may be from other, smaller motor nerves in the region rather than the proximal cut end of the recurrent laryngeal nerve. For this theoretical reason, we begin performing neural avulsion of the distal nerve end so there will be no distal stump to allow neural regeneration to occur. This method has decreased the likelihood of a return of spasmodic dysphonia with no increased morbidity.

The wound is closed with 4-0 Vicryl in the platysma and the subcuticular layer. A 3-mm closed suction drain is usually left for 12 to 24 hours. The cutaneous layer is leveled with a fine layer of 6-0 fast-absorbing plain gut. With this method of closure, the patients do not need to return for suture removal.

JAMES L. NETTERVILLE

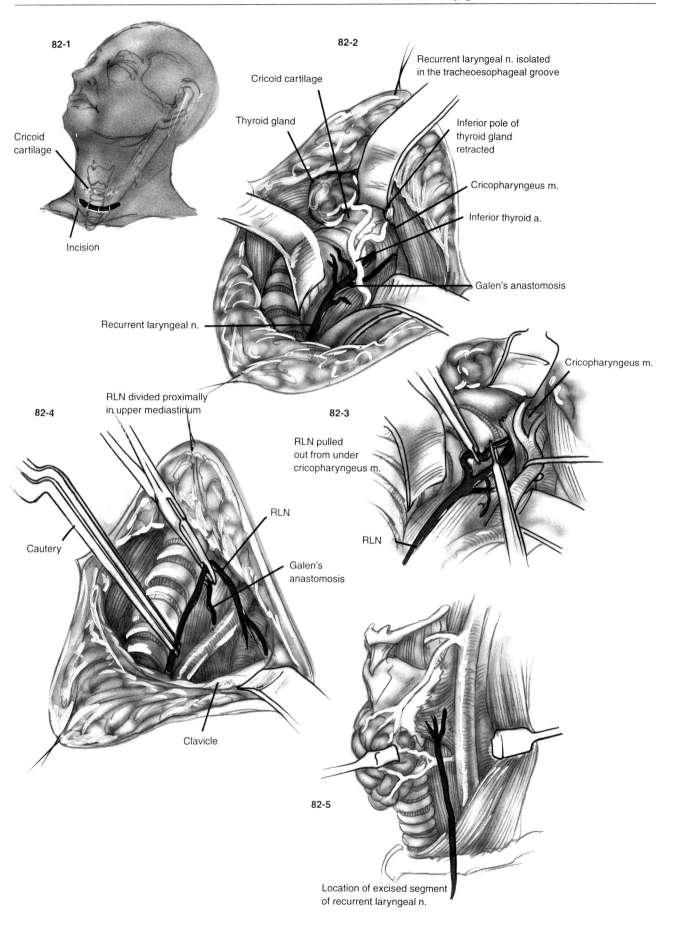

82-1

Cricoid cartilage

Incision

82-2

Cricoid cartilage

Thyroid gland

Recurrent laryngeal n. isolated in the tracheoesophageal groove

Inferior pole of thyroid gland retracted

Cricopharyngeus m.

Inferior thyroid a.

Galen's anastomosis

Recurrent laryngeal n.

Cricopharyngeus m.

82-3

RLN pulled out from under cricopharyngeus m.

RLN

82-4

RLN divided proximally in upper mediastinum

RLN

Cautery

Galen's anastomosis

Clavicle

82-5

Location of excised segment of recurrent laryngeal n.

■ *83.* LARYNGEAL DIVERSION
Separation of the trachea from the larynx and pharynx

Indications
1. Chronic severe aspiration, but potential for reversal of the disease process

Contraindications
1. Preexisting pathology of the upper cervical trachea

Special Instruments, Position, and Anesthesia
1. If a tracheotomy is in place, it should be intubated with an armored tube at the beginning of the procedure.
2. If there is no preexisting tracheotomy, orotracheal intubation should be used, switching to an armored tube when the trachea is entered.

Tips and Pearls
1. Submucosal resection of the last tracheal ring of the rostral stump provides more mucosa for closure.

Pitfalls and Complications
1. Much more difficult in children
2. Preexisting tracheotomy complicates the procedure.
3. Adequate exposure may be impossible in a kyphotic patient with a low-lying larynx.
4. Injury to carotid or embolic showering from carotid retraction
5. Failure at suture line can result in fistula
6. Recurrent laryngeal nerve injury

Postoperative Care Issues
1. Stoma care as for a laryngectomy
2. Feeding is usually withheld for several days, requiring tube feedings.

References
Blitzer A, Krepsi YP, Oppenheimer RW, et al. Surgical management of aspiration. Otolaryngolol Clin North Am 1988;21:743.

Eibling DE, Bacon G, Snyderman CH. Surgical management of chronic aspiration. In: Advances in otolaryngology—head and neck surgery. St. Louis: Mosby-Year Book, 1992.

Operative Procedure
A horizontal skin incision is made at the level of the second tracheal ring and superior and inferior subplatysmal flaps are elevated (Fig. 83-1). The strap muscles are separated in the midline to expose the trachea and thyroid isthmus. The isthmus is divided and suture ligated in the midline. Taking care to preserve the recurrent laryngeal nerves, both halves of the thyroid are reflected laterally along with soft tissue to expose the cricoid cartilage and the upper four or five tracheal rings (Fig. 83-2).

If there is no preexisting tracheotomy, the trachea is incised horizontally in the third or fourth interspace (see Fig. 83-2). The endotracheal tube is retracted until the tip is just above the tracheal opening, and an armored endotracheal tube is placed in the distal trachea. The tracheal incision is then completed circumferentially, and the posterior wall of the distal trachea is separated from the esophagus for about 1 to 2 cm, a sufficient distance to allow mobilization for formation of a stoma.

Most patients have a tracheotomy before the diversion procedure. In these cases, the peritracheal dissection is similar, but the trachea is transected at the level of the tracheotomy. The distal trachea is mobilized from the esophagus for 1 to 2 cm.

To close the proximal tracheal stump, the terminal ring is incised vertically in the anterior midline to allow the sides to be collapsed inward, creating a closure oriented in the anterior to posterior plane (Fig. 83-3). Some surgeons recommend submucosal resection of the terminal ring to provide more soft tissue for closure and collapse the next ring. If proximal trachea is deficient, the inferior portion of the cricoid may be removed. The tracheal mucosa is closed using an inverting running 4-0 absorbable suture (Fig. 83-4). The stump is the oversewn with a second layer or 3-0 suture through the tracheal cartilage (see Fig. 83-4). A sternohyoid muscle pedicle may be used to reinforce the closure.

The distal tracheal stump is then sutured to the skin, as in a laryngectomy (Fig. 83-5), and the residual skin incision is closed over a drain.

GAYLE E. WOODSON

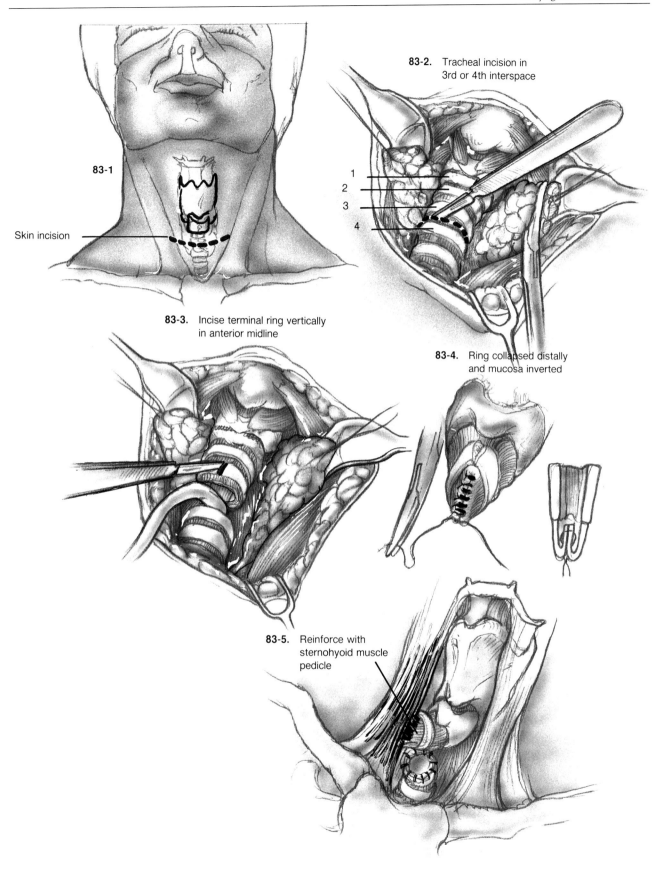

83-1.

Skin incision

83-2. Tracheal incision in 3rd or 4th interspace

1
2
3
4

83-3. Incise terminal ring vertically in anterior midline

83-4. Ring collapsed distally and mucosa inverted

83-5. Reinforce with sternohyoid muscle pedicle

■ 84. ARYTENOIDECTOMY

Removal of arytenoid cartilage

Indications

1. Airway obstruction due to vocal fold immobility
2. Patient dissatisfaction with tracheotomy

Contraindications

1. Potential for recovery of vocal fold motion

Preoperative Preparation

1. Tracheotomy is essential for external arytenoidectomy and usually required for endoscopic arytenoidectomy.

Special Instruments, Position, and Anesthesia

1. Cricoid or other sturdy hook to rotate larynx
2. Fine hook to retract arytenoid

Tips and Pearls

1. The orientation of muscle fibers in the posterior cricoarytenoid muscle indicates locations of the muscular process of the arytenoid.

Pitfalls and Complications

1. The vocal fold returns to the medial position during healing. This is a more common occurrence after endoscopic arytenoidectomy because of contracture of the open wound in the larynx.
2. Submucosal scar tissue can tether the vocal fold, preventing lateralization of the fold by either technique.
3. Fistula

Postoperative Care Issues

1. Voice rest, with avoidance of cough or Valsalva for 10 days

References

Osoff FH, Duncavage JA, Krepsi YP, Shapshay SM, Sisson GA. Endoscopic laser arytenoidectomy revisited. Ann Otol Rhinol Laryngol 1990;99:764.

Woodman D. A modification of the extralaryngeal approach to arytenoidectomy for bilateral abductor paralysis. Arch Otolaryngol 1946;43:63.

Operative Procedure

External Arytenoidectomy

The patient is placed on the operating table in the supine position, with the head turned to the opposite side. A horizontal skin incision is made at about the level of the cricothyroid membrane on the paralyzed side and extends slightly across the midline. Subplatysmal flaps are elevated superiorly to the level of the hyoid bone and inferiorly below the cricoid cartilage. Dissection is carried out anterior to the sternocleidomastoid muscle and lateral to the strap muscles to identify the posterior edge of the thyroid cartilage (Fig. 84-1).

The larynx is rotated by a hook placed on the superior cornu of the cartilage (see Fig. 84-1). The constrictor muscles are incised along the posterior edge of the thyroid (see Fig. 84-1), and the pyriform sinus mucosa is carefully elevated from the undersurface of the cartilage and the surface of the posterior cricoarytenoid muscle and reflected superiorly. The muscular process of the arytenoid is identified (Fig. 84-2) by the convergence of the posterior cricoarytenoid muscle fibers and used as a guide to locate and open the cricoarytenoid joint. A hook on the muscular process is used to retract the arytenoid laterally as it is dissected from the surrounding tissues, until the vocal process is reached (Fig. 84-3). A suture is then placed through the vocal process and tied securely, leaving two long ends (Fig. 84-4). The body of the arytenoid is resected lateral to this suture. One end of the suture is then passed through the posterior edge of the ipsilateral thyroid cartilage and then tied to the other end of the suture to lateralize the vocal fold (Figs. 84-5 and 84-6). The constrictor muscles are reapproximated to the thyroid cartilage, and the wound is drained and closed.

Endoscopic Arytenoidectomy

For endoscopic arytenoidectomy (not illustrated), an operative posterior commissure laryngoscope is introduced and suspended to expose the arytenoid of interest, the posterior portion of the ipsilateral aryepiglottic fold, and the medial portion of the contralateral arytenoid. This procedure is most commonly performed with a laser, but it can also be accomplished with microsurgical instruments. An incision is made in the aryepiglottic fold overlying the arytenoid cartilage. The soft tissues are dissected to expose the superior aspect of the arytenoid cartilage. The cartilage is dissected free from its surrounding tissue and muscle attachments and removed, taking care to preserve the mucosa over the medial surface of the arytenoid.

Another approach is to vaporize the entire arytenoid cartilage and an adjacent segment of the membranous vocal fold. This latter procedure is especially indicated when vocal fold immobility is the result of mechanical fixation rather than nerve injury.

GAYLE E. WOODSON

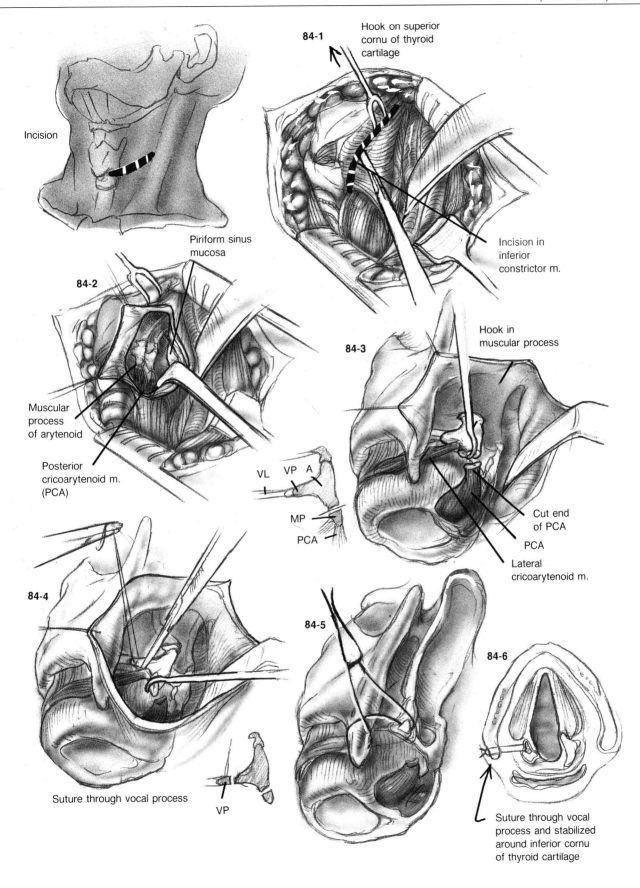

Incision

84-1

Hook on superior cornu of thyroid cartilage

Incision in inferior constrictor m.

Piriform sinus mucosa

84-2

Muscular process of arytenoid

Posterior cricoarytenoid m. (PCA)

84-3

Hook in muscular process

Cut end of PCA

PCA

Lateral cricoarytenoid m.

VL VP A

MP

PCA

84-4

Suture through vocal process

VP

84-5

84-6

Suture through vocal process and stabilized around inferior cornu of thyroid cartilage

■ 85. THYROID LOBECTOMY AND ISTHMUS-
ECTOMY—Surgical removal of one half of the thyroid gland with the thyroid isthmus

Indications
1. Adenomatous disease
   a. Microfollicular adenoma
   b. Follicular adenoma
   c. Hürthle cell adenoma smaller than 2cm in diameter
2. Recurrent thyroid cyst
3. Unilateral thyroid enlargement
4. Suspicious results on fine-needle aspiration

Special Considerations
1. Recurrent laryngeal nerve
2. Superior laryngeal nerve
3. Parathyroid gland preservation

Preoperative Evaluation
1. Routine laboratory work
2. Thyroid function tests
3. Documentation of vocal fold function
4. Thyroid scanning
5. Fine-needle aspiration

Special Instruments, Position, and Anesthesia
1. Fine-tipped hemostats for dissecting the recurrent laryngeal nerve
2. Tracheal retractors
3. Langenbeck retractors
4. Bipolar cautery
5. Shoulder roll, with the patient's neck extended

(continued)

Operative Procedure
A horizontal skin incision is made two fingerbreadths (4 cm) above the clavicles. This is centered in the midline and slightly curved upward (Fig. 85-1). The position can be adjusted slightly superiorly or inferiorly to conform to a natural-appearing skin crease. The incision is carried through the subcutaneous tissue and platysma. Flaps are elevated in the subplatysmal plane, with care taken not to injure the anterior jugular veins. These anterior jugular veins should remain unelevated on the strap muscles. If bleeding from one of these veins occurs, the vein should be ligated with silk or Vicryl ligatures. The superior flap is elevated to the hyoid bone. The inferior flap is elevated to the clavicles and sternum (Fig. 85-2).

The midline of the strap muscles is identified and incised with sharp dissection (Fig. 85-3). The strap muscles can usually be retracted laterally to provide sufficient exposure, without the need for division. If it is necessary to divide the strap muscles, they should be divided above the level of the cricoid ring to prevent injury to the branches of the ansa cervicalis that innervate the muscles. The sternohyoid is separated by blunt dissection from the sternothyroid. This is done bilaterally, and both thyroid lobes are palpated to identify nodules. The thyroid capsule is identified, and the gland is bluntly and sharply dissected from the sternothyroid muscle (Fig. 85-4).

Dissection next occurs at the thoracic inlet. Lateral retraction is placed on the trachea, and superior and lateral retraction is placed on the lower pole of the thyroid gland. This spreads the tissue in the tracheoesophageal groove. Blunt curved hemostats are used with the spreading motion to identify the recurrent laryngeal nerve as it enters the neck. Spreading should be done in the direction parallel to the course of the nerve, because perpendicular dissection may result in nerve avulsion (Fig. 85-5). Only the most superficial inferior thyroid veins should be ligated before identifying the full course of the recurrent laryngeal nerve. Identification of the recurrent laryngeal nerve in this manner allows visualization of the entire course of the cervical portion (Fig. 85-6). All branches can be safely preserved. If the nerve is not identified at the thoracic inlet, suspicion of a nonrecurrent recurrent laryngeal nerve must arise. In this instance, the laryngeal nerve arises laterally from the vagus and courses directly into the larynx.

After identification and preservation of the recurrent laryngeal nerve, the inferior thyroid veins superficial to the nerve are doubly ligated with silk suture (Fig. 85-7). The inferior pole of the thyroid gland is retracted superiorly, and the inferior parathyroid gland is visualized. The gland is caramel colored and located in a more superficial plane than the recurrent laryngeal nerve. The blood supply is usually from the inferior thyroid artery. All arterial branches to the thyroid are ligated as close to the gland as possible to facilitate preservation of the native blood supply to the parathyroid gland. If the parathyroid gland turns black while dissection occurs, it can be excised, minced, and reimplanted as previously described (Loré). If doubt exists about the identification of the gland, a small portion can be sent for frozen-section analysis, while the remainder of the gland is held within the sterile field in saline.

The middle thyroid vein is identified and doubly ligated at it arises from the internal jugular vein (Fig. 85-8).

The thyroid isthmus is dissected from the anterior tracheal wall, clamped, and transected on the contralateral side. Total isthmusectomy enlarges the surgical margin, and the remaining thyroid lobe is adequate to maintain thyroid function if replacement hormone therapy is not used postoperatively. The isthmus may be divided between the clamps and then ligated with Vicryl or silk suture. It is not usually necessary to cauterize the isthmus before ligation (Fig. 85-9).

(continued)

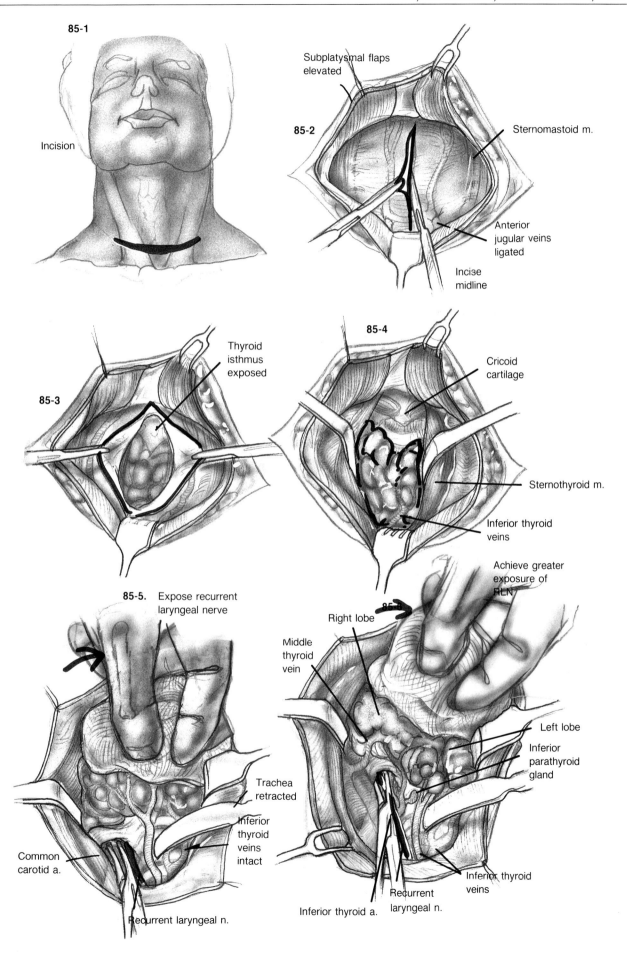

85-1

Incision

85-2

Subplatysmal flaps elevated

Sternomastoid m.

Anterior jugular veins ligated

Incise midline

85-3

Thyroid isthmus exposed

85-4

Cricoid cartilage

Sternothyroid m.

Inferior thyroid veins

85-5. Expose recurrent laryngeal nerve

Trachea retracted

Inferior thyroid veins intact

Common carotid a.

Recurrent laryngeal n.

Achieve greater exposure of RLN

Right lobe

Middle thyroid vein

Left lobe

Inferior parathyroid gland

Inferior thyroid veins

Inferior thyroid a.

Recurrent laryngeal n.

■ *85.* THYROID LOBECTOMY AND ISTHMUS-ECTOMY *(continued)*

Tips and Pearls

1. Identify the recurrent laryngeal nerve at the thoracic inlet as the initial step in the procedure.
2. Follow the nerve from the mediastinum to its insertion into the larynx.
3. Do not transect any structures at or near the inferior pole of the thyroid until the identity and position of the nerve is secure.
4. Reflect the gland from the lateral to medial aspects.
5. Identify and preserve the parathyroids with the blood supply intact, if possible.
6. If the blood supply of the parathyroids is questionable, reimplant them in the strap muscles.
7. Frozen-section analysis is necessary to determine the need for total thyroid lobectomy.
8. Palpate the opposite lobe for nodules.

Pitfalls and Complications

1. Recurrent laryngeal nerve injury from failure to identify or over aggressive retraction
2. Superior laryngeal nerve injury from failure to identify or over aggressive retraction
3. Sacrifice of parathyroid glands
4. Intraoperative and postoperative bleeding

Postoperative Care Issues

1. Observation for hematoma
2. Observation for airway obstruction
3. Observation for hypocalcemia

References

Harvey HK. Diagnosis and management of the thyroid nodule: an overview. In: Harvey HK, ed. Disorders of the thyroid and parathyroid, II. Otolaryngol Clin North Am 1990;23:2.

Loré JM. An atlas of head and neck surgery. 3rd ed. Philadelphia: WB Saunders, 1988:741.

The pyramidal thyroid lobe may be encountered during dissection of the thyroid isthmus. This embryologic remnant may persist from development and contain functioning thyroid tissue. Because only a small portion of thyroid is necessary to maintain normal function, it is usually best to resect the pyramidal lobe during the initial procedure, when surgical scarring is at a minimum. The thyroid gland develops from a medial primordium arising from two lateral primordia that are divided by the fourth and fifth bronchial pouch complexes. By the fifth week of embryonic development, the gland is bilobed and joined by the thyroglossal duct. This duct is attached to the ventral surface of the pharynx. As development continues, the thyroid gland becomes situated lower in the neck, and the isthmus develops from each lobe as functioning thyroid tissue. The pyramidal lobe develops from the distal end of the thyroglossal duct and may contain functioning tissue. The thyroglossal duct may persist to the base of the tongue, and normal functioning thyroid tissue may be found anywhere along its course.

When encountered, the pyramidal lobe is skeletonized with blunt and sharp dissection. Crossing anterior jugular veins are ligated as necessary, and the pyramidal lobe is delivered with the specimen (Fig. 85-10). Occasionally, the thyroglossal duct tract or cyst may continue as the superior aspect of the pyramidal lobe. If a thyroglossal duct cyst is suspected, a Sistrunk procedure may be required for complete excision (see Procedure 84).

The thyroid lobe is reflected medially and dissected from the trachea. Branches of the inferior thyroid artery are ligated as they enter the gland. The posterior suspensory ligament of Berry is identified and incised. The recurrent laryngeal nerve and its branches are kept under constant visualization and should be seen in their entirety as they pierce the inferior constrictor and enter the larynx. The relation of the recurrent laryngeal nerve to the inferior thyroid artery and posterior suspensory ligament is not constant (Fig. 85-11). When performing total thyroid lobectomy, it is imperative to identify the nerve and follow its branches for preservation. Thirty-nine percent of all recurrent laryngeal nerves branch before entering the larynx.

The superior parathyroid gland is identified at this time. It usually exists in a plane deep to the recurrent laryngeal nerve. Its blood supply is most often from the inferior thyroid artery (Fig. 85-12).

The thyroid lobe is pedicled by the superior pole vessels. It can be freely retracted inferiorly while the vessels are skeletonized and doubly ligated, with or without a no-clamp technique (see Fig. 85-12). An attempt is made to ligate arteries and veins separately as close to the gland as possible. This lessens the likelihood of injury to the superior laryngeal nerve, particularly the external branch that supplies the cricothyroid muscles and is important in vocal fold function.

The gland is then inspected within the operative field for parathyroid tissue. Any suspicious tissue is sent for frozen-section analysis. The parathyroid glands, if identified on the specimen, are then reimplanted as previously described. The thyroid lobe is sent for frozen-section analysis and the need for total thyroidectomy determined.

If the operation is complete at this point, the wound is vigorously irrigated, and hemostasis is achieved. Care should be exercised in closing; excessive clamping or cautery near the entrance of the recurrent laryngeal nerve into the larynx may result in injury. Instead, hemostatic substances, such as Surgicel, may be used. A small, fully perforated suction drain is placed under the strap muscles laterally to the recurrent laryngeal nerve and brought out through a separate stab wound. This drain is connected only to bulb suction. Overzealous suction by wall units may lead to recurrent laryngeal nerve injury. The strap muscles are reapproximated in the midline, and the platysma is closed separately from the subcutaneous tissue and skin.

ROBERT H. OSSOFF
MARK S. COUREY

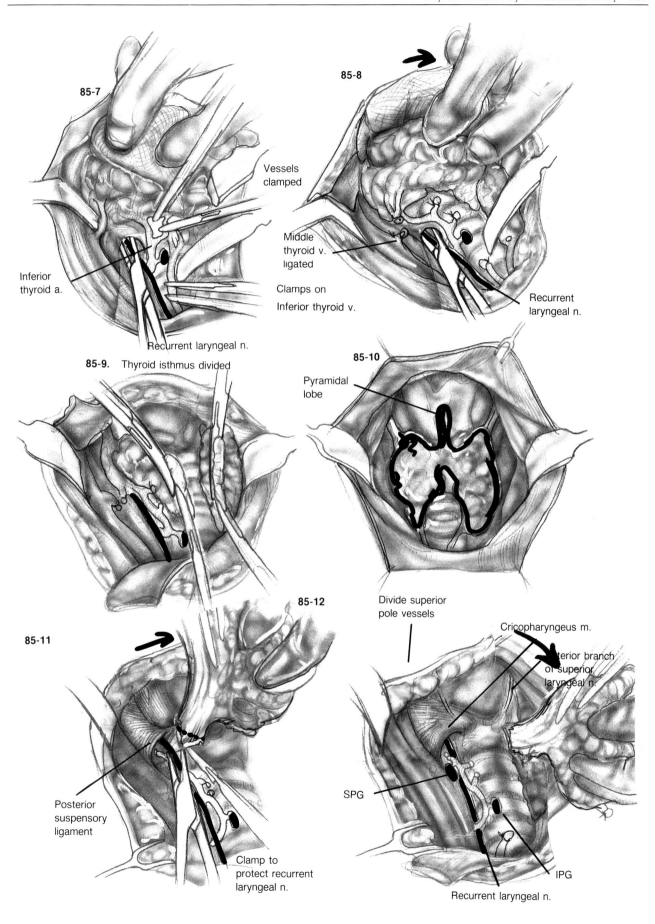

85-7

Inferior thyroid a.

Recurrent laryngeal n.

Vessels clamped

Middle thyroid v. ligated

Clamps on Inferior thyroid v.

85-8

Recurrent laryngeal n.

85-9. Thyroid isthmus divided

85-10

Pyramidal lobe

85-11

Posterior suspensory ligament

85-12

Clamp to protect recurrent laryngeal n.

Divide superior pole vessels

Cricopharyngeus m.

terior branch of superior laryngeal n.

SPG

IPG

Recurrent laryngeal n.

■ 86. SUBTOTAL THYROIDECTOMY

Surgical removal of the thyroid gland while preserving the portion of the gland nearest the suspensory ligament and tracheoesophageal groove

Indications

1. Graves' disease
2. Hashimoto's thyroiditis
3. Multinodular goiter

Special Considerations

1. Identification of recurrent laryngeal nerve
2. Parathyroid gland preservation

Preoperative Evaluation

1. Routine laboratory studies
2. Thyroid function tests
3. Thyroid autoantibodies
4. Documentation of vocal fold function
5. Thyroid scanning
6. Fine-needle aspiration

Special Instruments, Position, and Anesthesia

1. Fine-tipped hemostats for dissecting recurrent laryngeal nerve
2. Tracheal retractors
3. Langenbeck retractors
4. Bipolar cautery
5. Shoulder roll or thyroid pillow; neck extended

Tips and Pearls

1. Identify the recurrent laryngeal nerve at the thoracic inlet as the initial step in the procedure.
2. Follow the nerve from the mediastinum to its insertion into the larynx.
3. Do not transect any structures at or near the inferior pole of the thyroid until the identity and position of the nerve is secure.
4. Reflect the gland from lateral to medial positions.
5. Identify and preserve parathyroids with the blood supply intact, if possible.
6. If the blood supply of the parathyroids is questionable, reimplant them in strap muscles.
7. Frozen-section analysis is necessary to determine the need for total thyroid lobectomy.
8. Palpate the opposite lobe for nodules.

Pitfalls and Complications

1. Recurrent laryngeal nerve injury from failure to identify or overaggressive retraction
2. Sacrifice of parathyroid glands
3. Intraoperative and postoperative bleeding
4. Recurrence of the thyroid disease, with enlargement of the thyroid remnant, necessitating revision thyroidectomy and placing the recurrent laryngeal nerve and parathyroid glands at extreme risk

Postoperative Care Issues

1. Observation for hematoma
2. Observation for airway obstruction
3. Observation for hypocalcemia

References

Block MA. Surgical therapy of thyroid tumors. In: Thawley SE, Panje WR, Batsakis JG, eds. Comprehensive management of head and neck tumors, Vol 2. Philadelphia, WB Saunders, 1987;1616.

Friedman M, Pacella BL. Total versus subtotal thyroidectomy. Disorders of the thyroid and parathyroid. Otolaryngol Clin North Am 1990; 23:413.

Operative Procedure

Initially, the operation proceeds the same as thyroid lobectomy. A horizontal skin incision is used in a cervical skin crease, subplatysmal flaps are elevated to hyoid bone and clavicles, and strap muscles are separated in the midline and divided at a level superior to the cricoid ring if division is deemed necessary for adequate exposure. Both thyroid lobes are palpated. The trachea is then retracted medially while the inferior pole of the thyroid gland is retracted superiorly. This exposes the thoracic inlet and permits identification of the recurrent laryngeal nerve as it enters the neck.

Identification of the nerve is imperative. A blunt hemostat is used in the spreading motion parallel to the direction of the nerve. The nerve is then followed with fine hemostats until it disappears under the posterior suspensory ligament of Berry (see Figs. 85-1 through 85-6).

The inferior pole veins are then doubly ligated (see Fig. 85-7). The gland is reflected medially as the middle thyroid vein is ligated at the insertion into the internal jugular vein (see Fig. 85-9). The thyroid isthmus is dissected from the anterior tracheal wall and ligated between clamps. It is then tied with Vicryl or silk sutures (see Fig. 85-10).

The operation departs from the previously described total thyroid lobectomy as attention is turned to the superior pole of the thyroid gland. The superior pole vessels are skeletonized and doubly ligated. Preferably, a no clamp technique is employed (Fig. 86-1). These vessels are taken close to the gland capsule to prevent inadvertent injury to the superior laryngeal nerve.

The gland remains pedicled to the inferior thyroid artery and posterior and anterior suspensory ligaments. While reflecting the gland medially, the recurrent laryngeal nerve is kept in constant view (Fig. 86-2). The inferior thyroid artery is identified up on the thyroid gland. Its branches are ligated with fine hemostats as they enter the gland (Fig. 86-3). Care is taken not to penetrate the thyroid lobe deeply, because this causes bleeding and may injure the recurrent laryngeal nerve. The gland is transected, leaving a posterior wedge of tissue in the tracheoesophageal groove (Fig. 86-4). This tissue is approximately 1.5 cm wide and 2 to 3 cm long. Hemostasis is achieved with superficial sutures and ligatures in the thyroid tissue. Care is taken not to penetrate the lobe deeply, because this would cause injury to the recurrent laryngeal nerve.

Thyroid lobectomy or subtotal tyroid lobectomy is then performed on the remaining lobe.

The wound is vigorously irrigated and hemostasis inspected. Care is exercised not to employ excessive clamping or cautery near the remaining thyroid remnant, because this may injure the recurrent laryngeal nerve. Hemostatic substances may be placed over the lobe remnants. A small, fully perforated suction drain is then placed under the strap muscles lateral to the recurrent laryngeal nerve and brought through a separate stab wound. This drain is placed only to bulb suction, because overzealous suctioning with wall units may lead to nerve injury. The strap muscles are reapproximated in the midline, and the platysma is closed in separate layers from the subcutaneous tissue and skin.

We want to stress the importance of recurrent laryngeal nerve identification and parathyroid preservation in subtotal thyroidectomy. To achieve adequate preservation, the nerve must be identified in its entire cervical course from the thoracic inlet to its penetration into the larynx. Subtotal thyroid lobectomy offers no advantage to total thyroid lobectomy. We have seen cases of recurrent laryngeal nerve injury resulting after subtotal thyroid lobectomy, and we have witnessed regrowth of the thyroid remnant, necessitating revision thyroid lobectomy and placing the recurrent laryngeal nerve at extreme risk. With the availability of thyroid replacement, the indications for this operation are limited to only noncompliant patients who would be placed at significant risk because of their lack of ability to adequately use thyroid supplementation.

ROBERT H. OSSOFF
MARK S. COUREY

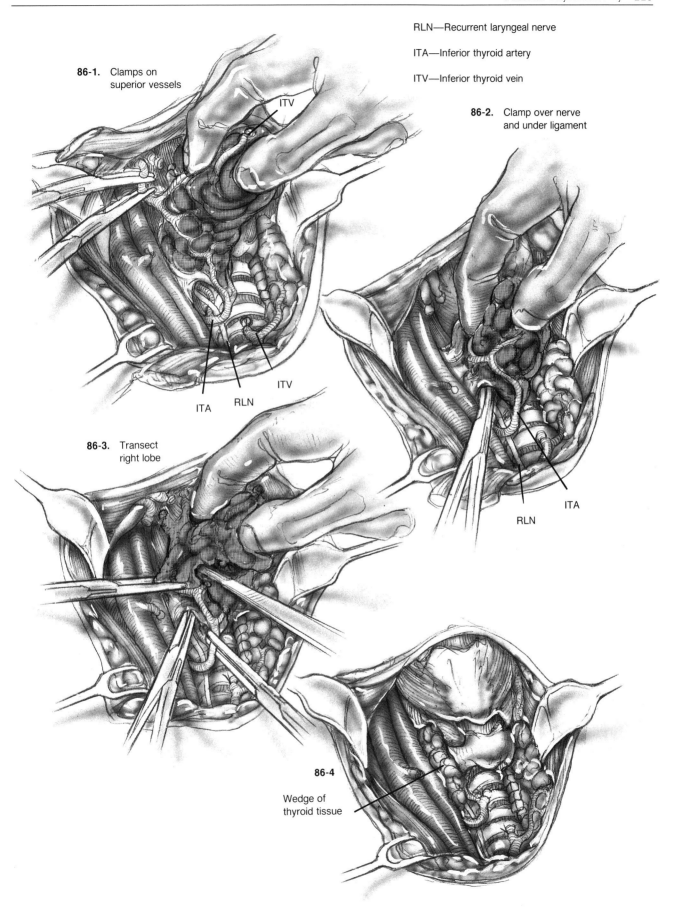

RLN—Recurrent laryngeal nerve

ITA—Inferior thyroid artery

ITV—Inferior thyroid vein

86-1. Clamps on superior vessels

ITV

ITV

ITA RLN

86-2. Clamp over nerve and under ligament

ITA

RLN

86-3. Transect right lobe

86-4

Wedge of thyroid tissue

■ *87.* MEDIASTINAL (RETROSTERNAL) GOITER EXCISION—Surgical extirpation of thyroid tissue located in the superior, anterior mediastinum

Indications
1. Substernal extension of cervical goiter, which cannot be elevated into the neck with cervical extension
2. Substernal cervical component

Special Considerations
1. Identification of the recurrent laryngeal nerve
2. Identification of the inferior thyroid vein and artery
3. Preservation of the parathyroid gland
4. Preservation of the great vessels

Preoperative Evaluation
1. Routine laboratory studies
2. Thyroid function test
3. Documentation of vocal fold function
4. Evaluation of pre-existing tracheal compression
5. Thyroid scanning with iodine[131] to evaluate the substernal component
6. CT scanning to evaluate the position of the thyroid gland with respect to the great vessels and trachea
7. Fine needle aspiration

Special Instruments, Position, and Anesthesia
1. Sternal splitting saw
2. Flexible ribbon retractors
3. Langenbeck retractors
4. Bipolar cautery
5. Shoulder roll with neck extended

(continued)

Operative Procedure
There are two forms of mediastinal goiter. The first and most common is from the thoracic extension of cervical disease (Fig. 87-1). The second, relatively rare, condition occurs as a separate mass of goitrous tissue, which may be either connected to an uninvolved thyroid lobe and fibrous stalk, or without cervical connections.

In the first form, excision of the substernal goiter is often most easily achieved by extending the neck and placing gentle superior retraction on the thyroid lobe. The majority of substernal goiters can be removed via low collar excisions. This technique delivers the thyroid gland into the neck and, because the inferior thyroid vessels still retain their native cervical origin, is a relatively safe maneuver.

Delivery of the substernal portion can usually be facilitated by first dividing the strap muscles. The superior pole vessels are then taken (Fig. 87-2) and the thyroid isthmus transected (Fig. 87-3). The medial thyroid vein is ligated laterally (Fig. 87-4). This provides lateral exposure. Superficial veins arising over the trachea and connecting to the thyroid lobe medially can also be ligated (Fig. 87-5). The lobe is then reflected from lateral to medial and delivered into the cervical region. Dissection of the inferior pole vessels and posterior suspensory ligament is then undertaken as previously described. It is inadvisable to transect the posterior suspensory ligament and inferior thyroid artery until the position of the recurrent laryngeal nerve is secure. Again, attempt at premature ligation of the inferior thyroid artery may result in recurrent laryngeal nerve injury.

If these maneuvers fail to deliver the retrosternal component, improved exposure may be achieved by either superior median sternotomy or resection of the medial third of the clavicle. Although both procedures provide adequate exposure, superior median sternotomy is associated with less postoperative morbidity.

(continued)

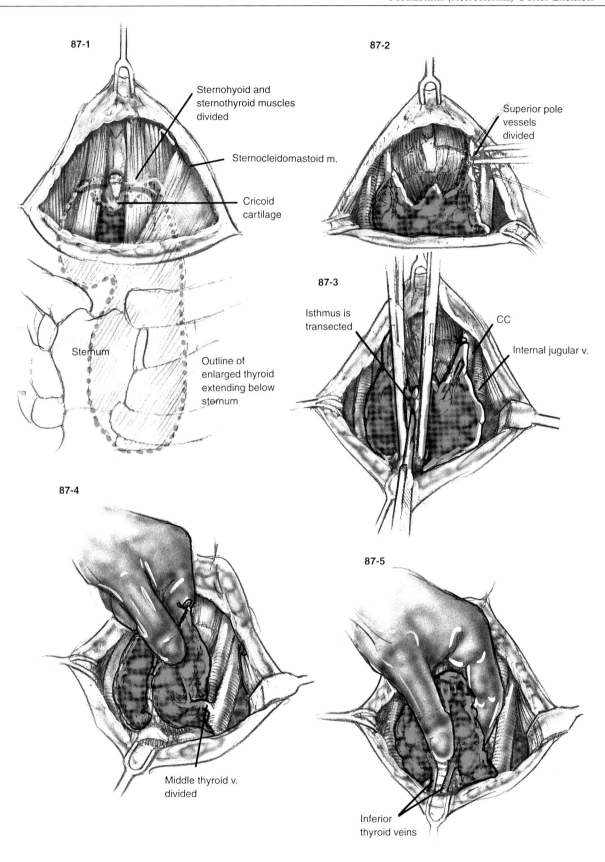

87-1

Sternohyoid and sternothyroid muscles divided

Sternocleidomastoid m.

Cricoid cartilage

Sternum

Outline of enlarged thyroid extending below sternum

87-2

Superior pole vessels divided

87-3

Isthmus is transected

CC

Internal jugular v.

87-4

Middle thyroid v. divided

87-5

Inferior thyroid veins

■ *87.* MEDIASTINAL (RETROSTERNAL) GOITER EXCISION *(continued)*

Tips and Pearls

1. It is imperative to identify the recurrent laryngeal nerve.
2. Release of the superior whole vessels and isthmus may permit delivery of the thyroid tissue into the cervical area.

Pitfalls and Complications

1. Overzealous attempts to deliver the substernal component into the cervical area, which result in:
   a. Great vessel injury
   b. Injury to recurrent laryngeal nerve
   c. Avulsion of an inferior thyroid vessel
2. Sacrifice of the parathyroid glands
3. Intraoperative and postoperative bleeding

Postoperative Care Issues

1. Postobstructive pulmonary edema if the substernal component was causing significant preoperative tracheal compression
2. Pneumothorax
3. Airway hematoma, obstruction, or both
4. Postoperative hypocalcemia

References

Loré JM. An atlas of head and neck surgery, 3rd ed. Philadelphia: WB Saunders, 1988:842.

Shaha AR. Surgery for benign thyroid disease causing tracheoesophageal obstruction. In Harvey HK (ed). Disorders of the thyroid and parathyroid. II. Otolaryngol Clin North Am 1990;23:391.

Median sternotomy begins with a horizontal cervical skin incision in a low neck crease, approximately 4 cm above the clavicles. Superior and inferior subplatysmal flaps are elevated to the hyoid bone and clavicles, respectively. A vertical incision is then made in the inferior skin flap from the midline of the horizontal incision to the third intercostal space. The inferior flaps are reflected laterally, and wide exposure of the thoracic inlet and sternum is provided. Additional exposure on the involved side may be obtained by resecting the sternal and clavicular heads of the sternocleidomastoid muscle (Fig. 87-6). As previously stated, the sternohyoid and sternothyroid muscles have been transected at a level superior to the cricoid ring to prevent injury to their nerve supply.

Blunt retrosternal dissection with the surgeon's finger provides a safe place for the posterior portion of the sternal saw (Fig. 87-7). A ribbon retractor is placed in the superior mediastinun to further protect the great vessels while the saw is in use. The sternal saw is then used to incise the midline of the sternum to the manubrium or third intercostal space. The incision is brought out bilaterally at the manubrium. Fibrous attachments on the posterior surface of the manubrium, potentially connecting to the pleura, are incised. The curved Mayo scissors and a Finochietto rib spreader are inserted to retract the thorax (Fig. 87-8). As the dissection proceeds, the superior vena cava is exposed along with its tributaries, the right and left innominate veins. Vessels from the thymus gland are ligated. The recurrent laryngeal nerve can then be identified as it loops around the arch of the aorta or subclavian artery. This is seen following under the innominate vein. The thyroid lobe is then retracted superiorly, while the inferior thyroid veins are ligated. The inferior thyroid artery can be identified arising from the thyrocervical trunk and ligated as it inserts onto the thyroid gland (Fig. 87-9).

With the thyroid lobe thus excised, closure begins by placing sternal wires in a figure-of-eight fashion, to reapproximate the portion of the split sternum. The divided heads of the sternocleidomastoid muscle and strap muscles can then be reapproximated using heavy silk suture. A fully perforated suction drain is placed into the cavity created by excision of the gland in the superior mediastinum. A second fully perforated suction drain is placed under the strap muscles laterally and brought out through a separate stab incision in the wound. The strap muscles are then reapproximated in the midline, and the platysma, subcutaneous tissue, and skin are closed in separate layers. The previously placed drains are maintained to bulb suction, as oversuction may result in injury to the recurrent laryngeal nerve or great vessel.

ROBERT H. OSSOFF
MARK S. COUREY

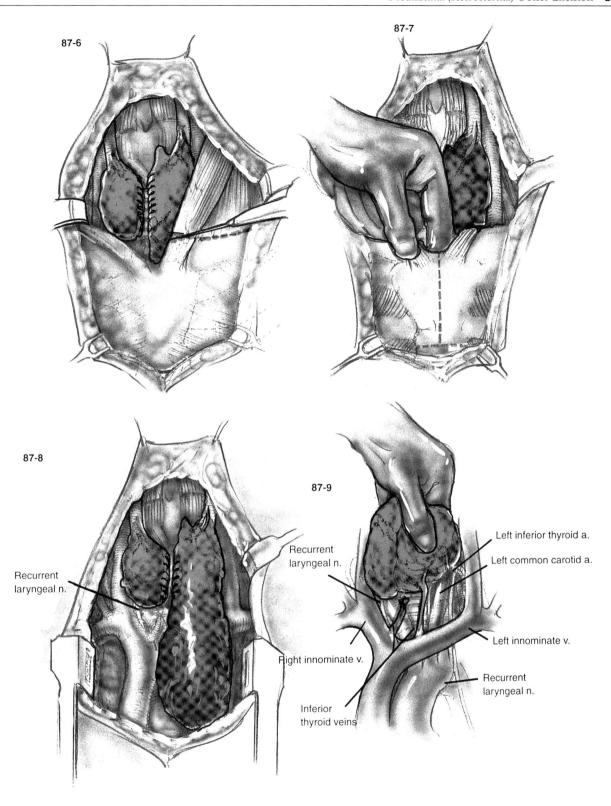

87-6

87-7

87-8

Recurrent
laryngeal n.

87-9

Recurrent
laryngeal n.

Right innominate v.

Inferior
thyroid veins

Left inferior thyroid a.

Left common carotid a.

Left innominate v.

Recurrent
laryngeal n.

■ 88. TOTAL THYROIDECTOMY

Surgical removal of the entire thyroid gland, including both lobes, the isthmus, and pyramidal lobe

Indications

1. Carcinoma of the thyroid
2. Graves' disease
3. Multinodular goiter refractory to thyroid suppression and causing pressure symptoms, cosmetic deformity, or the fear of malignancy

Special Considerations

1. Concern regarding regional or distant metastases
2. Concern regarding retrosternal extension or involvement of the laryngotracheal skeleton

Preoperative Preparation

1. Routine laboratory studies
2. Thyroid function tests
3. Thyroglobulin and calcitonin levels, if indicated
4. Documentation of vocal cord function
5. Computed tomography, ultrasound, or magnetic resonance studies if infiltration of surrounding structures, retrosternal extension, or metastases are suspected.

Special Instruments, Position, and Anesthesia

1. Shoulder roll, with the neck extended
2. Fine-tipped hemostats for dissecting nerve
3. Bipolar cautery

Tips and Pearls

1. Attempt to identify all four parathyroids and preserve at least two of them
2. Use the inferior thyroid artery to identify the recurrent laryngeal nerve
3. Sharp dissection of Berry's ligament off the trachea to avoid nerve damage

Pitfalls and Complications

1. Recurrent laryngeal nerve injury because of failure to identify the nerve along its course into the larynx
2. Hypoparathyroidism because of failure to identify and preserve at least two of the four glands
3. Thyroid storm in Graves' disease because of inadequate preoperative control

Postoperative Care Issues

1. Careful observation for hematoma with airway obstruction
2. Careful observation for transient or permanent hypocalcemia

References

Gluckman JL. Practical approach to thyroid tumors. In: Pillsbury H, Shockley W, eds. The neck: diagnosis and surgery. St. Louis: Mosby-Year Book, 1993.

Sedgwick C. Surgery of the thyroid gland. In: Sedgwick C, Cady B, eds. Surgery of the thyroid and parathyroid glands. Philadelphia: WB Saunders, 1980.

Operative Procedure

A low collar incision is made two fingerbreadths above the clavicles, preferably in a natural skin crease. The incision must be symmetric, extending equidistant from the midline and being slightly curved (Fig. 88-1). If there is a large, unilateral thyroid mass, the incision should be slightly higher on that side, because postoperatively, it will settle symmetrically.

The technique we advocate necessitates dividing the sternohyoid and sternothyroid muscles to facilitate exposure. This has no adverse effect on function or cosmesis. The first step is to divide the deep cervical fascia between the sternohyoid and the sternocleidomastoid muscles. The middle thyroid vein is identified, divided, and ligated. The jugular vein and carotid artery are identified by incising the carotid sheath and retracted laterally. The strap muscles are then separated in the midline, bluntly dissected from the underlying thyroid capsule, and individually isolated. To preserve their innervation from the ansa hypoglossi nerve, they are divided high between clamps and retracted superiorly and inferiorly to expose the underlying gland. Be sure to divide and ligate the anterior jugular veins first at the same level as the divided strap muscles (Fig. 88-2).

The carotid artery is retracted laterally, and the inferior thyroid artery is identified arising deep to the carotid artery. This is traced medially until the recurrent laryngeal nerve is located in the tracheoesophageal groove. With the thyroid gland retracted medially, the nerve is surprisingly superficial. The relation of the inferior thyroid artery to the recurrent nerve is so varied that careful identification of both structures is the key to safe dissection. The nerve is then traced superiorly to its insertion (Fig. 88-3). The nerve may branch, and because it is impossible to know which branch contains the motor fibers, all branches should be preserved.

A decision must be made about where to transect the inferior thyroid artery. If the inferior parathyroid is to be sacrificed with the specimen, the inferior thyroid artery is doubly ligated laterally and divided. If the parathyroid is to be preserved, the branches of the artery are divided distal to the parathyroid, preserving its blood supply. The inferior pole of the thyroid gland is then mobilized superiorly by dividing and ligating the inferior thyroid veins, staying in the plane on the trachea.

Attention is then directed to the superior pole. The thyroid lobe is retracted inferiorly and medially, exposing the superior thyroid vessels, which are carefully isolated and divided. The external branch of the superior laryngeal nerve may be intertwined with these vessels, and to avoid injury to this nerve, the vessels are divided as close as possible to the thyroid capsule (Fig. 88-4).

The superior parathyroid gland is usually easily identified along the posterolateral border of the thyroid gland just deep to the superior lobe. This is dissected off the gland and pedicle laterally and preserved. As the dissected lobe is retracted medially, the recurrent nerve is traced superiorly, dividing the thin lateral portion of the posterior suspensory ligament of Berry that overlies the distal portion of the nerve. With the entire nerve in full view, the remaining portion of the suspensory ligament is divided by sharp dissection, freeing the dissected lobe from the trachea (Fig. 88-5).

The contralateral lobe of the thyroid is resected in an identical manner, paying attention to preservation of the parathyroids, particularly if they have not been well identified on the first side or if the vascular supply might have been compromised. A pyramidal lobe should be actively sought and removed in its entirety up to the hyoid.

After performing the total thyroidectomy, the wound is irrigated, and meticulous hemostasis achieved. Bleeding adjacent to the nerve is controlled with gentle pressure, bipolar cautery, or careful, selective clamping. If necessary, a hemostatic material may be packed over any troublesome bleeding that cannot safely be controlled by the above methods. A Penrose drain is placed instead of a suction drain because of concern for the suction traumatizing the recurrent nerve. The strap muscles are then reapproximated with mattress sutures (Fig. 88-6). The closure is completed in layers with absorbable sutures for the subcutaneous layer and staples for the skin.

JACK L. GLUCKMAN
LOUIS G. PORTUGAL

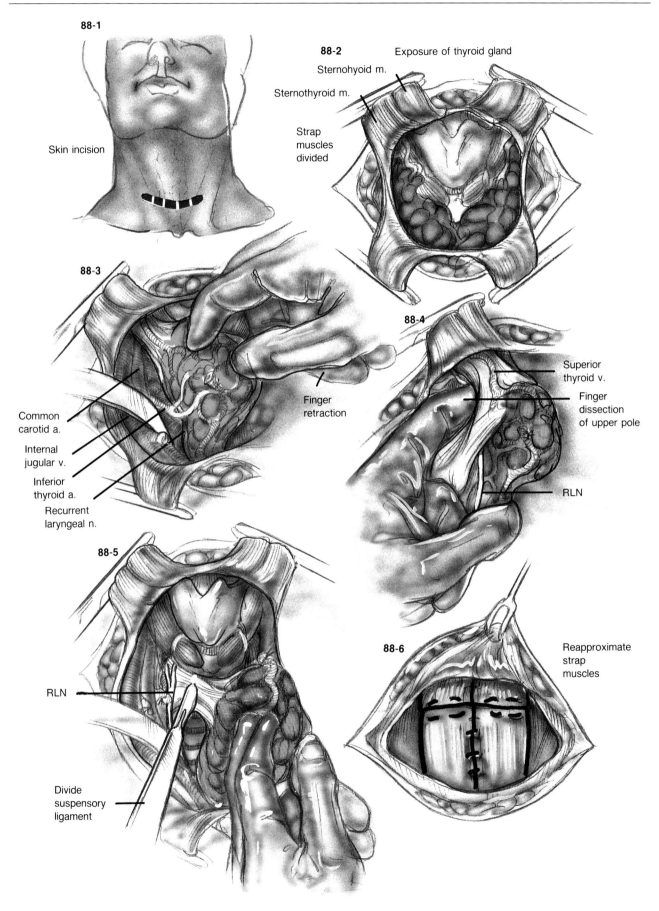

88-1

Skin incision

88-2 Exposure of thyroid gland

Sternohyoid m.

Sternothyroid m.

Strap muscles divided

88-3

Common carotid a.

Internal jugular v.

Inferior thyroid a.

Recurrent laryngeal n.

Finger retraction

88-4

Superior thyroid v.

Finger dissection of upper pole

RLN

88-5

RLN

Divide suspensory ligament

88-6

Reapproximate strap muscles

■ 89. TOTAL THYROIDECTOMY WITH PARA-TRACHEAL AND SUPERIOR MEDIASTINAL NODE DISSECTION—Removal of node-bearing tissue within the paratracheal area and superior mediastinum

Indications
1. Overt or high index of suspicion for metastatic disease from thyroid carcinoma

Special Considerations
1. As for total thyroidectomy
2. Rarely necessary to perform sternotomy

Preoperative Preparation
1. As for total thyroidectomy
2. Computed tomography or magnetic resonance scans to evaluate presence and extent of metastatic cancer

Special Instruments, Position, and Anesthesia
1. Shoulder roll; neck extended
2. Always have sternotomy instruments in operating room.

Tips and Pearls
1. Before paratracheal and mediastinal dissection, attempt to identify and isolate the inferior parathyroids and avoid inadvertently removing them in the dissection.
2. Blunt finger dissection of the superior mediastinum after the planes have been established is the most effective method of dissection.

Pitfalls and Complications
1. Recurrent nerve injury
2. Inadvertent removal of inferior parathyroids
3. Hemorrhage from inferior thyroid veins coursing through mediastinum
4. Pneumothorax

Postoperative Care Issues
1. As for total thyroidectomy
2. Postoperative chest X-ray to rule out pneumothorax

Reference
Gluckman JL. Practical approach to thyroid tumors. In: Pillsbury H, Shockley W, eds. The neck: diagnosis and surgery. St. Louis: Mosby-Year Book, 1993.

Operative Procedure

The paratracheal, superior mediastinal, and lateral neck nodal groups all need to be addressed in patients undergoing thyroidectomy for malignancy. A sequence usually is followed in surgically managing patients with thyroid cancer if there is a suspicion or evidence of regional metastases. After the total thyroidectomy, the paratracheal nodes are routinely dissected. If there is overt nodal metastases in these groups, the superior mediastinum is explored and superior mediastinal dissection performed. If the paratracheal nodes are involved, it is our inclination to perform a lateral neck exploration, and the appropriate nodal dissection performed depends on the operative findings, type of cancer, and philosophy of the surgeon. For a well-differentiated cancer, the dissection may vary from node plucking to a formal functional neck dissection. For medullary cancer, because of the potential for extracapsular spread, a more complete modified radical neck dissection is advised, sparing the accessory nerve or jugular vein if possible. Details of these lateral neck dissection techniques are available elsewhere in this atlas and are therefore not discussed here.

The paratracheal lymph nodes characteristically lie in the tracheoesophageal groove, surrounding the recurrent laryngeal nerves and anterior to the trachea (Fig. 89-1). Nodes in the superior mediastinum lie within the fibrofatty tissue located between the trachea and upper sternum superior to the innominate vessels. Inferior thyroid veins course through this fibrofatty tissue and may hemorrhage if they are not properly controlled as low as possible before commencing this dissection.

After the total thyroidectomy has been performed, the paratracheal and superior mediastinal nodes are resected in continuity. The paratracheal node dissection commences at approximately the level of the cricoid cartilage, with the node-bearing tissue dissected off the recurrent laryngeal nerves superiorly to inferiorly. Care must be taken not to inadvertently remove the inferior parathyroid glands during the dissection. These nodes generally dissect off easily. It is rarely necessary to sacrifice the recurrent laryngeal nerves unless they are overtly involved with cancer (Fig. 89-2).

After this has been performed bilaterally, the superior mediastinal and pretracheal nodes are removed by dividing the fascia above the innominate vessels and by gentle finger dissection, sweeping the node-bearing tissue superiorly into the neck to communicate with the paratracheal and pretracheal nodal dissection. Great care is taken not to injure the recurrent nerves and not to avulse the inferior thyroid veins (Fig. 89-3).

At this stage, the lateral sides of the neck are addressed according to the described philosophy and the appropriate neck dissections performed. The wound is closed as already described for total thyroidectomy.

JACK L. GLUCKMAN
LOUIS G. PORTUGAL

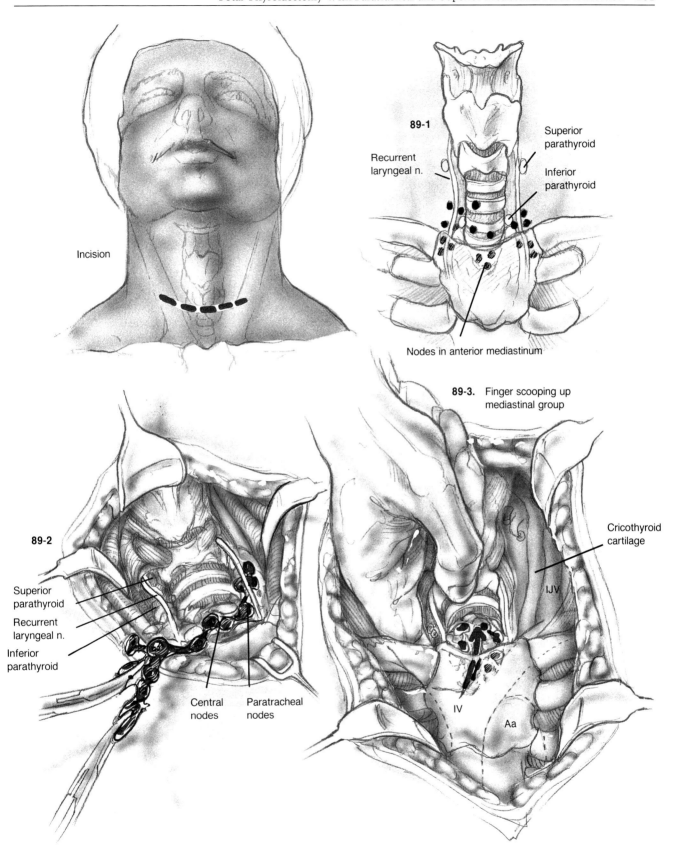

Incision

89-1

Recurrent
laryngeal n.

Superior
parathyroid

Inferior
parathyroid

Nodes in anterior mediastinum

89-3. Finger scooping up
mediastinal group

89-2

Superior
parathyroid

Recurrent
laryngeal n.

Inferior
parathyroid

Central
nodes

Paratracheal
nodes

Cricothyroid
cartilage

IJV

IV

Aa

■ 90. TOTAL THYROIDECTOMY WITH TRACHEAL RESECTION FOR MALIGNANT INVASION—Surgical removal of a segment of the trachea in continuity with the thyroid and reconstruction

Indications
1. Carcinoma of thyroid invading the underlying trachea

Special Considerations
1. Important to determine preoperatively the extent of tracheal involvement using imaging and bronchoscopy

Preoperative Preparation
1. Same as for total thyroidectomy (see Procedure 88)
2. Computed tomography scan with fine axial cuts
3. Magnetic resonance imaging
4. Bronchoscopy
5. Consent for various reconstructive techniques, depending on the pathology encountered

Special Instruments, Position, and Anesthesia
1. As for total thyroidectomy (see Procedure 88)
2. Neck extended during thyroidectomy and then flexed to permit end-to-end anastomosis if a sleeve resection is performed
3. Planned extubation in the operating room or in the recovery room the following day

Tips and Pearls
1. For resection: intraoperative determination of whether a shave, sleeve resection, wedge resection, or resection of an extended portion of anterior wall should be performed
2. For end-to-end anastomosis: mobilization procedures, including suprahyoid release, are essential to provide tension-free anastomosis.
3. For myoperiosteal flap: preservation of the blood supply to sternocleidomastoid muscle by mobilizing as minimally as possible

(continued)

Operative Procedure
The therapeutic approach depends on the type of thyroid cancer and the degree of tracheal involvement. If the patient has advanced anaplastic cancer, radical resection should not be attempted unless the tumor is extremely localized and in its earliest stages. Well-differentiated and medullary cancers with extrathyroidal extension can be effectively treated with surgery, followed by radioactive iodine or external irradiation, as appropriate. Despite sophisticated preoperative evaluation, the ultimate determination of how best to treat the involved trachea is made intraoperatively.

The total thyroidectomy is performed using the technique already described (see Procedure 88), with the gland dissected up to the area of tracheal infiltration. Unless there is evidence of intratracheal extension, an initial attempt is made to shave the tumor from the anterior face of the trachea. This may be accomplished by shaving the cartilage without entering the airway (Fig. 90-1). Deeper infiltration, particularly with intraluminal extension, necessitates a wider excision, possibly requiring a sleeve or wedge resection.

If a *sleeve resection* is indicated, four to five rings can be resected and the defect reconstructed using an end-to-end anastomosis if a suprahyoid release is performed. The skin incision should be extended up to the angle of mandible bilaterally to permit exposure to the suprahyoid area (Fig. 90-2). After the area to be resected has been delineated, the plane between the trachea and esophagus is identified, the already identified nerves protected, and the esophagus freed from the posterior wall of the trachea by a combination of sharp and blunt dissection (Fig. 90-3). After this dissection is completed, the trachea is transected superiorly and inferiorly, and the resected trachea is removed (Fig. 90-4). The endotracheal tube, which had been partially withdrawn to permit the resection, is then advanced into the distal trachea.

To provide a tension-free closure at the anastomotic site, the head is flexed by removing the shoulder roll. Mobilization of the upper tracheal stump is achieved using a suprahyoid release. The suprahyoid musculature is freed from its attachment to the body and lesser horn of the hyoid using cautery. Care is taken not to damage the superior laryngeal or hypoglossal nerves. The body of the hyoid is divided from the greater horn using a scissors or saw, and the body is mobilized inferiorly (Fig. 90-5). The lower trachea is mobilized by circumferential freeing of its fibrous attachments by blunt dissection.

(continued)

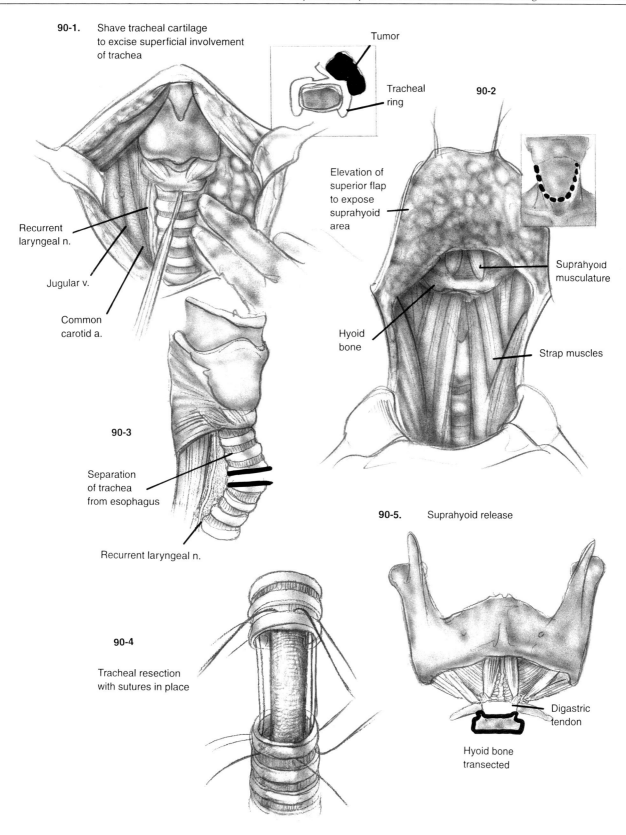

90-1. Shave tracheal cartilage to excise superficial involvement of trachea

Tumor

Tracheal ring

Recurrent laryngeal n.

Jugular v.

Common carotid a.

90-2

Elevation of superior flap to expose suprahyoid area

Suprahyoid musculature

Hyoid bone

Strap muscles

90-3

Separation of trachea from esophagus

Recurrent laryngeal n.

90-5. Suprahyoid release

90-4

Tracheal resection with sutures in place

Digastric tendon

Hyoid bone transected

■ 90. TOTAL THYROIDECTOMY WITH TRACHEAL RESECTION FOR MALIGNANT INVASION *(continued)*

Pitfalls and Complications

1. Injury to the recurrent laryngeal nerves
2. Avulsion of anastomotic suture line due to inadvertent hyperextension of neck
3. Stenosis at anastomotic suture line

Postoperative Care Issues

1. Maintenance of neck flexion by placing suture from mentum to sternum
2. Same as for total thyroidectomy, particularly regarding airway obstruction and bilateral vocal cord paralysis
3. Chest x-ray film for detecting pneumothorax
4. After end-to-end anastomosis, allow no oral intake of food, using instead nasogastric tube feedings for 5 days.

References

Friedman M, Toriumi DM, Owens R, Grybauskas VT. Experience with the sternocleidomastoid myoperiosteal flap for reconstruction of subglottic and tracheal defects: modification of technique and report of long-term results. Laryngoscope 1988;98:1003.

Gluckman JL. Practical approach to thyroid tumors. In: Pillsbury H, Shockley W, eds. The neck: diagnosis and surgery. Chicago: Mosby-Year Book, 1993.

An end-to-end anastomosis is performed using 2-0 nylon suture, commencing with the posterior tracheal wall. Each suture is placed submucosally around the upper and lower tracheal rings, with the knots placed outside the lumen (Fig. 90-6). A tracheostomy should *not* be placed after completion of the anastomosis. A 0-nylon suture is placed between the mentum and the skin of the sternum to prevent inadvertent extension of the neck, and the patient is awakened and extubated in the operating room or in the recovery room the next day.

If only the anterior half of one or two rings are involved, a *wedge resection* of these rings, maintaining the posterior tracheal wall intact, can be performed. The closure is exactly as for a sleeve resection (Fig. 90-7).

If an anterior tracheal wall defect involving a number of rings is present after resection, a sternocleidomastoid myoperiosteal flap can be used (Fig. 90-8). After the resection, the sternal and clavicular attachments of the sternocleidomastoid muscle are isolated and a flap elevated that includes the periosteum at the site of attachment. The amount of periosteum harvested may be as large as 4×4 cm if necessary (Fig. 90-8).

The sternocleidomastoid mobilization should permit the flap to reach the defect without tension while simultaneously attempting to preserve the blood supply of the transverse cervical, superior thyroid, and occipital vessels. The mobilized flap is positioned, and the periosteum is sutured to the cartilage along the margins of the tracheal defect (Fig. 90-9). If the defect is greater than 30% of the circumference of the trachea, this technique is not satisfactory, and tracheal resection and end-to-end anastomosis should be used.

JACK L. GLUCKMAN
L. G. PORTUGAL

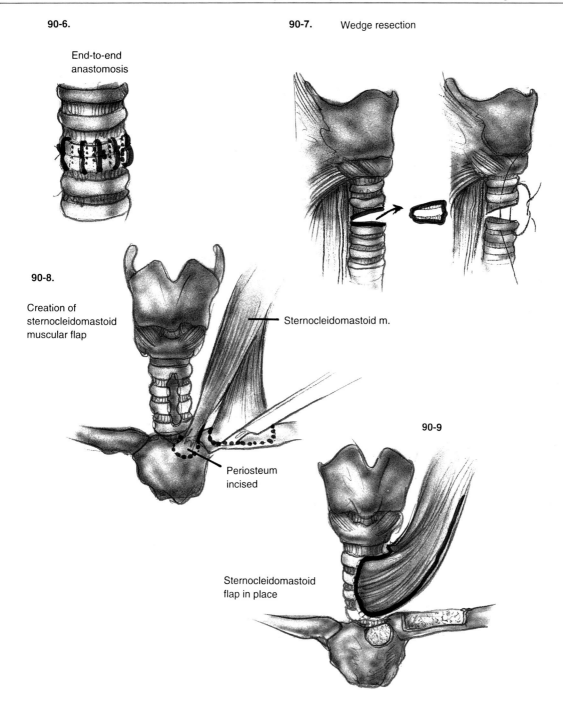

90-6.

End-to-end
anastomosis

90-7.   Wedge resection

90-8.

Creation of
sternocleidomastoid
muscular flap

Sternocleidomastoid m.

Periosteum
incised

90-9

Sternocleidomastoid
flap in place

■ 91. PARATHYROIDECTOMY

Various approaches are employed for removing hyperplastic or neoplastic parathyroids:

1. For adenomas
   a. A unilateral approach is used if, after a localizing preoperative test and exploration of that side, one enlarged pathologic gland is found that on frozen section is compatible with the diagnosis of adenoma and if further exploration of that side identifies a grossly normal parathyroid gland that on histologic examination of a frozen-section sample is found to be normal.
   b. A bilateral approach is used when the preceding criteria are not met; all four glands are identified and biopsied.
2. Parathyroidectomy for hyperplasia
   a. A subtotal parathyroidectomy is done when hyperplasia is found in the absence of renal failure and multiple endocrine neoplasia (MEN) syndrome; a 3- or 3.5-gland excision is completed.
   b. Total parathyroidectomy with autotransplantation of 0.5 gland (ie, 20 to 30 mg of tissue) is completed when there is associated renal failure and hyperplasia with a MEN syndrome.

Indications

1. Symptomatic patients with joint pains, muscle weakness, renal stones, or other features of hyperparathyroidism
2. High serum calcium levels on three occasions
3. An elevated parathyroid hormone level determined by immunoradiometric assay (IRMA)
4. When associated with renal failure

Contraindications

1. Poor metabolic state, with limited life expectancy

Special Considerations

1. Double adenomas
2. Hyperplastic glands with or without renal disease or in the presence of an MEN syndrome
3. Prior surgery; obtain prior records and pathology slides
4. Cancer, when the parathyroid gland that is enlarged is matted to the surrounding tissue

Preoperative Preparation

1. Laboratory tests: serum calcium, IRMA parathyroid hormone, serum proteins, blood urea nitrogen, creatinine, and alkaline phosphatase levels
2. Localization tests at the discretion of the physician
3. Invasive tests: angiography or venography with sampling for parathyroid hormone (usually reserved for recurrent or persistent hyperparathyroidism)
4. Laryngeal examination

Special Instruments, Position, and Anesthesia

Same as for thyroidectomy

(continued)

Operative Procedure

The patient is placed on the operating table with the head extended (caution: in elderly patients, extend with care), and surgical preparation goes from the mandible to the xiphoid. The lower extension allows complete median sternotomy by the thoracic surgeon, if necessary.

The incision and elevation of the flaps is similar to the steps outlined for thyroid surgery. In most cases of parathyroid exploration, the strap muscles are sectioned with a high incision to avoid injury to their nerve supply from the ansa hypoglossi. To safely perform this section, the strap muscles are bluntly dissected away from the underlying thyroid gland (Fig. 91-1). With this exposure, the thyroid gland is palpated to determine if any nodules or enlarged lymph nodes are present that would mandate thyroidectomy. The tissues between the carotid artery and the trachea are palpated for four enlarged parathyroid glands or an enlarged gland (Fig. 91-2).

The dissection is begun inferiorly, freeing the lower pole of the thyroid gland, identifying the recurrent laryngeal nerve, and preserving the inferior thyroid artery with its terminal branches, ligating only those that enter the thyroid gland. This is an attempt to preserve the blood supply to normal parathyroid glands (Fig. 91-3). As the thyroid gland is freed, the parathyroid glands are sought close to the thyroid, and then exploration continues from medial to lateral in the adipose tissue between the carotid artery and the trachea. Sometimes, in the lower neck, posterior or in the same plane as the carotid artery where the common carotid and subclavian arise, the parathyroid glands are found. If the lower dissection is not productive, the dissection is carried superiorly along the course of the recurrent laryngeal nerve as the upper pole of the thyroid is mobilized from a lateral to medial plane. If necessary, the superior thyroid artery can be ligated for greater exposure. The superior parathyroid is often found anterior or posterior to where the recurrent laryngeal nerve penetrates the inferior border of the cricothyroid muscle.

(continued)

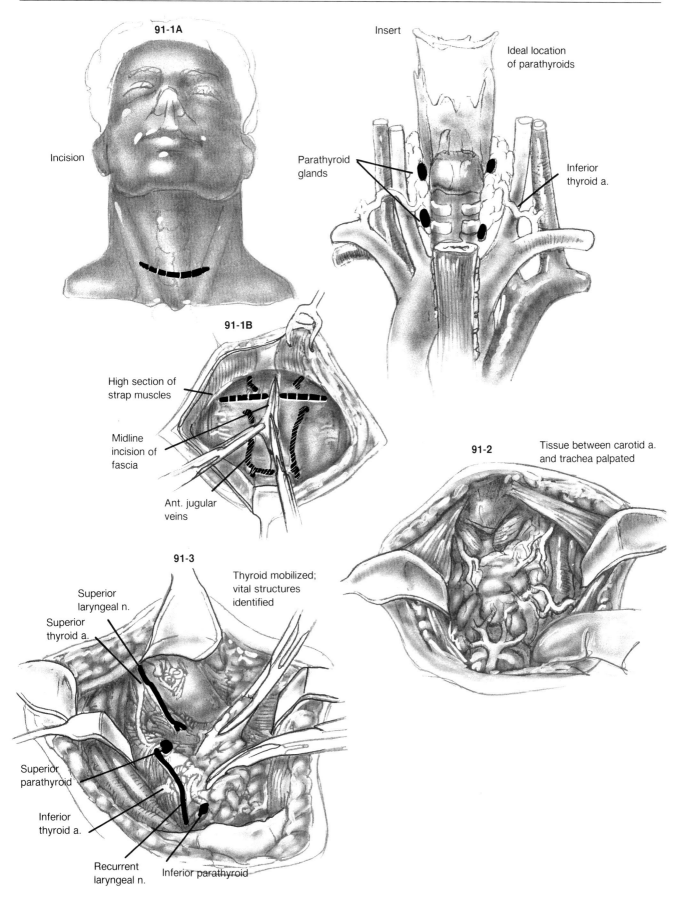

91-1A

Incision

Insert

Ideal location
of parathyroids

Parathyroid
glands

Inferior
thyroid a.

91-1B

High section of
strap muscles

Midline
incision of
fascia

Ant. jugular
veins

91-2

Tissue between carotid a.
and trachea palpated

91-3

Thyroid mobilized;
vital structures
identified

Superior
laryngeal n.

Superior
thyroid a.

Superior
parathyroid

Inferior
thyroid a.

Recurrent
laryngeal n.

Inferior parathyroid

■ 91. PARATHYROIDECTOMY *(continued)*

Tips and Pearls

1. Identify and preserve the inferior thyroid artery.
2. Identify and preserve recurrent laryngeal nerves.
3. The lower parathyroids usually are within 2 cm of the inferior pole of the thyroid and can be in the superior mediastinum with thymic tissue.
4. The upper parathyroids usually are within 1 to 2 cm of the penetration of the recurrent laryngeal nerve at the cricothyroid muscle.
5. Most upper and lower parathyroid glands receive their blood supply from the inferior thyroid artery.
6. For the hard to find parathyroid, check the thyroid gland, retrotracheal area, retroesophageal area, carotid sheath, up to the carotid bifurcation, anterior and posterior superior mediastinum.
7. Be careful not to damage the blood supply to the normal parathyroids. If the gland turns bluish black, consider autotransplantation of the gland to a muscle bed.
8. The biopsy of normal glands is done with the smallest middle ear cup forceps and a Beaver knife blade.
9. Reexplorations are dissected from lateral to medial, rather than medial to lateral, as a surgeon does with primary cases to avoid injury to the recurrent laryngeal nerve and inferior thyroid artery in a scarred tissue bed.
10. In approximately 25% of patients, associated thyroid disease is found, necessitating concomitant thyroidectomy.
11. Use medium suction-type drains during the postoperative period.

Pitfalls and Complications

1. Hematoma or seroma
2. Hypoparathyroidism
3. Recurrent laryngeal or superior laryngeal nerve injury
4. Persistent or recurrent hyperparathyroidism

Postoperative Care Issues

1. Drains are removed when drainage is less than 20 to 25 mL per day.
2. Daily serum calcium determinations are made for 5 days. The ionized calcium reflects the true level of calcium; it does not depend on serum proteins, but it is more expensive to obtain.
3. If patient has symptoms of muscular irritability (ie, Trousseau or Chvostek's signs) and the serum calcium level is normal, check magnesium levels.
4. Institute calcium supplements if the serum calcium level is low, if the patient is symptomatic, and if the patient is elderly with a history of cardiac disease.
5. When starting intravenous supplements, also start supplementation by mouth so the intravenous form can be gradually diminished as serum calcium levels return to normal.

References

Petti GH. Hyperparathyroidism. Otolaryngol Clin North Am 1990;2: 339.

Scholz DA. Asymptomatic primary hyperparathyroidism. Mayo Clinic Proc 1981;56:473.

If no abnormal parathyroid has been identified after the preceding exploration, the prevertebral and retroesophageal space is dissected and inspected inferiorly into the anterior and posterior mediastinum. Thymic tissue may be removed, because a parathyroid from the third arch can be associated with it (Fig. 4).

If no abnormal parathyroid has been identified, a similar exploration is completed on the opposite side.

Thyroidectomy may be done if a discrete hyperactive parathyroid is not confirmed after the dissection is finished, because intrathyroidal parathyroid tissue occurs in 2% to 5% of patients; the surgeon usually can feel a nodular density in the thyroid.

Parathyroid glands that appear bluish black at the conclusion of the operation can be considered devascularized, and at the surgeon's discretion, they may be removed and placed in a sterile iced saline bath in preparation for autotransplantation (Fig. 5). The wound is copiously irrigated, strap muscles closed, superficial and deep drains placed, and the midline fascia closed (Fig. 6). The skin is closed with interrupted #3 or #4 chromic subcuticular sutures and then a running subcuticular Prolene suture that can be pulled out 1 week later. Wound edges are covered with Steri-Strips, and at the surgeon's discretion, a dressing may be applied.

On awakening the patient, a direct laryngoscopy is performed as the endotracheal tube is removed, documenting motion or the lack of it of the vocal cords (Fig. 91-7).

GEORGE H. PETTI

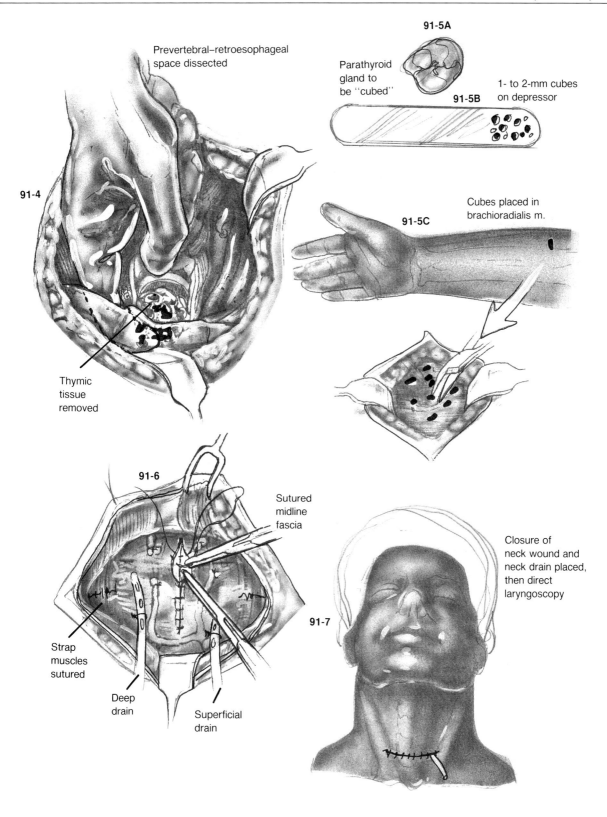

91-5A

Parathyroid gland to be "cubed"

1- to 2-mm cubes on depressor

91-5B

Prevertebral–retroesophageal space dissected

91-4

Thymic tissue removed

91-5C

Cubes placed in brachioradialis m.

91-6

Sutured midline fascia

Strap muscles sutured

Deep drain

Superficial drain

91-7

Closure of neck wound and neck drain placed, then direct laryngoscopy

■ 92. TOTAL PARATHYROIDECTOMY AND
AUTOTRANSPLANTATION—Removal of the parathyroids and transplant of some parathyroid tissue to retain hormonal function

Indications

1. Symptoms of joint pains, muscle weakness, and renal stones
2. High serum calcium results on three samples
3. An elevated parathyroid hormone by immunoradiometric assay
4. Associated renal failure
5. For adenomas
   A unilateral approach is indicated if a preoperative localizing test and exploration of one side detect one enlarged, pathologic gland, which is confirmed by frozen-section analysis to contain an adenoma and a bilateral approach is indicated otherwise.
6. For hyperplasia a subtotal parathyroidectomy is indicated when hyperplasia is found in the absence of renal failure and multiple endocrine neoplasia (MEN) syndrome and a total parathyroidectomy with autotransplantation of one-half gland (20 to 30 mg of tissue) is indicated if there is associated renal failure and hyperplasia with a MEN syndrome.

Contraindications

1. Poor metabolic state with limited life expectancy

Special Considerations

1. Double adenomas
2. Hyperplastic glands with or without renal disease or in the presence of a MEN syndrome
3. If the parathyroid gland that is enlarged is matted to the surrounding tissue and cancer is suspected

Preoperative Preparation

1. Laboratory tests for serum calcium, parathyroid hormone (ie, IRMA), serum proteins, blood urea nitrogen, creatinine, and alkaline phosphatase
2. Localization tests at the discretion of the physician
3. Invasive tests include angiography, venography with sampling for parathyroid hormone (usually reserved for recurrent or persistent hyperparathyroidism)
4. Laryngeal examination

Special Instruments, Position, and Anesthesia

1. Same as for thyroidectomy (see Procedure 88)

Tips and Pearls

1. Lower parathyroids usually are within 2 cm of the inferior pole of the thyroid or in the superior mediastinum.
2. Upper parathyroids usually are within 1 to 2 cm of penetration of the recurrent laryngeal nerve at the cricothyroid muscle.
3. Most upper and lower parathyroid glands receive their blood supply from the inferior thyroid artery.
4. Do not damage blood supply to the normal parathyroids.
5. Reexplorations are dissected from lateral to medial aspects, instead of the medial to lateral approach used in primary cases.
6. In approximately 25% of patients, associated thyroid disease is found, necessitating concomitant thyroidectomy.

Pitfalls and Complications

1. Hypoparathyroidism
2. Recurrent laryngeal or superior laryngeal nerve injury

Postoperative Care Issues

1. Daily serum calcium levels are determined for 5 days.
2. If the patient has symptoms of muscular irritability (eg, Trousseau's or Chvostek's sign) and the serum calcium level is normal, check the magnesium level.
3. Institute calcium supplements when serum calcium is low, the patient is symptomatic, and if the patient is elderly with history of cardiac disease.
4. When starting intravenous supplements, also start oral supplementation so the intravenous form can be gradually diminished.

References

Wells SA. The successful transplantation of frozen parathyroid tissue in man. Surgery 1980;81:86.

Operative Procedure

Total Parathyroidectomy

Total parathyroidectomy is indicated for secondary hyperparathyroidism due to renal failure and for hyperplasia of parathyroids associated with the MEN syndrome; it may be indicated in primary hyperparathyroidism due to diffuse hyperplasia. However, in this condition, a 3.5-gland excision usually suffices.

The surgical technique is similar to the technique as outlined for parathyroid adenoma (see Procedure 91). The surgical technique explores the midneck from carotid artery to carotid artery, from the carotid bifurcation into the superior mediastinum, seeking all abnormal parathyroid glands (Figs. 92-1 and 92-2).

All parathyroid tissue found is excised, and approximately 20 to 30 mg of parathyroid tissue is placed on a side table in a sterile, iced saline bath to be used for autotransplantation.

If the hyperplastic parathyroid tissue is nodular, it is best to not use the nodular areas for autotransplantation because these areas tend to be more active and proliferative and are more likely to cause persistent hyperparathyroidism, necessitating removal of the autograft (Figs. 92-3 and 92-4).

Autotransplantation

After a parathyroid gland is identified for autotransplantation, it is placed in a sterile, iced saline bath until the surgery is completed (Fig. 92-5).. It is then removed from the saline bath, placed on a moistened, sterile wood tongue depressor, and with a #11 scalpel, it is diced into 1- to 2-mm cubes. The average gland produces 10 to 15 cubes, and these are used for autotransplantation.

An incision is made over the brachioradialis muscle; any muscle could be used, but it is easier to remove parathyroid tissue from this region if it becomes hyperplastic than it can be removed from the neck muscle (Fig. 92-6).

After an incision is made and the brachioradialis muscle is identified, individual muscle pockets are created and a cube of parathyroid tissue is placed in each pocket. The pocket is closed with a small surgical clip or may be sutured with nonabsorbent monofilament suture material.

Bleeding must be controlled, and postoperatively, no blood is drawn from that arm, nor are blood pressure readings taken from that arm to ensure that the transplanted parathyroid tissue is not damaged.

GEORGE PETTI

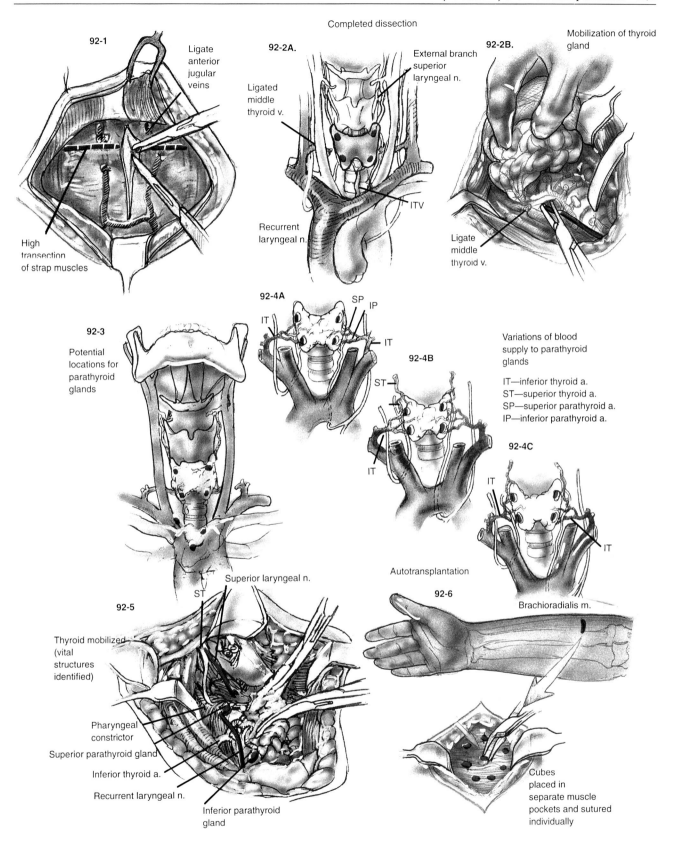

92-1

Ligate anterior jugular veins

High transection of strap muscles

Completed dissection

92-2A.

Ligated middle thyroid v.

External branch superior laryngeal n.

ITV

Recurrent laryngeal n.

92-2B.

Mobilization of thyroid gland

Ligate middle thyroid v.

92-3

Potential locations for parathyroid glands

92-4A

IT

SP IP

IT

92-4B

ST

IT

Variations of blood supply to parathyroid glands

IT—inferior thyroid a.
ST—superior thyroid a.
SP—superior parathyroid a.
IP—inferior parathyroid a.

92-4C

IT

IT

Autotransplantation

92-6

Brachioradialis m.

Superior laryngeal n.

ST

92-5

Thyroid mobilized (vital structures identified)

Pharyngeal constrictor

Superior parathyroid gland

Inferior thyroid a.

Recurrent laryngeal n.

Inferior parathyroid gland

Cubes placed in separate muscle pockets and sutured individually

■ 93. RECURRENT HYPERPARATHYROIDISM AND CANCER OF THE PARATHYROID—Various approaches are employed for removing hyperplastic or neoplastic parathyroids:

1. For adenomas
   a. A unilateral approach is used if, after a localizing preoperative test and exploration of that side, one enlarged pathologic gland is found that on frozen section is compatible with the diagnosis of adenoma and if further exploration of that side identifies a grossly normal parathyroid gland that on histologic examination of a frozen-section sample is found to be normal.
   b. A bilateral approach is used when the preceding criteria are not met; all four glands are identified and biopsied.
2. Parathyroidectomy for hyperplasia
   a. A subtotal parathyroidectomy is done when hyperplasia is found in the absence of renal failure and multiple endocrine neoplasia (MEN) syndrome; a 3- or 3.5-gland excision is completed.
   b. Total parathyroidectomy with autotransplantation of 0.5 gland (ie, 20 to 30 mg of tissue) is completed when there is associated renal failure and hyperplasia with a MEN syndrome.
3. For cancer of the parathyroid, suspected when the parathyroid gland is matted to the surrounding tissue, wide excision with a cuff of normal tissue usually includes thyroidectomy on that side and peritracheal fat and lymph node dissection in the adjacent region. Modified neck dissection is done only if nodes are palpable.
4. For recurrent or persistent hyperparathyroidism, the dissection is started laterally from the carotid and carried medial to avoid initiating the procedure in a scarred previously operated wound.

Indications
1. Symptomatic patients, with joint pains, muscle weakness, renal stones, and other features of hyperparathyroidism
2. High serum calcium levels on three occasions
3. An elevated parathyroid hormone level determined by immunoradiometric assay (IRMA)
4. When associated with renal failure

Contraindications
1. Poor metabolic state, with limited life expectancy

Special Considerations
1. Double adenomas
2. Hyperplastic glands with or without renal disease or in the presence of a multiple endocrine neoplasia (MEN) syndrome
3. Prior surgery; obtain prior records and pathology slides
4. Cancer, when the parathyroid gland that is enlarged is matted to the surrounding tissue

Preoperative Preparation
1. Laboratory tests: serum calcium, IRMA parathyroid hormone, serum proteins, blood urea nitrogen, creatinine, and alkaline phosphatase levels
2. Localization tests at the discretion of the physician
3. Invasive tests: angiography or venography with sampling for parathyroid hormone (usually reserved for recurrent or persistent hyperparathyroidism)
4. Laryngeal examination

(continued)

Operative Procedure
For recurrent or persistent hyperparathyroidism, surgery is started in a lateral position from the carotid artery medial to the trachea (Fig. 93-1) This allows identification of the recurrent laryngeal nerve coming from a position where prior surgery has probably not taken place, making the initial identification of the nerve perhaps easier.

Dissection is completed from the carotid artery to the trachea. The strap muscles have been sectioned as demonstrated in Figure 93-2. The thyroid gland is examined carefully and removed if no parathyroid is located in another position, because in approximately 5% of cases, there may be an intrathyroidal parathyroid. The thymus gland and the superior mediastinum are explored, and the thymus gland is removed along with the fat of the superior mediastinum in an attempt to find parathyroid tissue (Fig. 93-3). The opposite side is then managed in a similar fashion, taking care on both sides to examine the space inferior and posterior to the common carotid subclavian artery take off on the right and the common carotid to the prevertebral fascia on the left side (Fig. 93-4)

(continued)

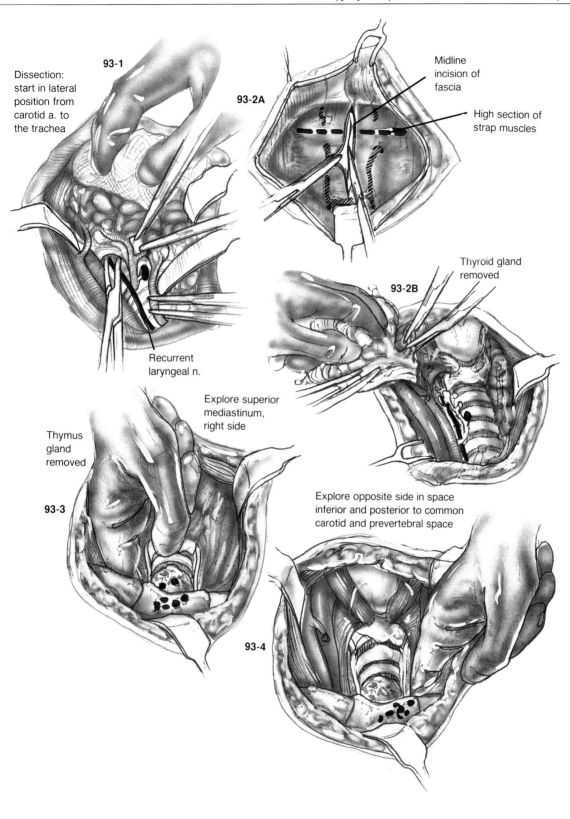

93-1

Dissection: start in lateral position from carotid a. to the trachea

Recurrent laryngeal n.

93-2A

Midline incision of fascia

High section of strap muscles

93-2B

Thyroid gland removed

Thymus gland removed

93-3

Explore superior mediastinum, right side

Explore opposite side in space inferior and posterior to common carotid and prevertebral space

93-4

■ 93. RECURRENT HYPERPARATHYROIDISM AND CANCER OF THE PARATHYROID

(continued)

Special Instruments, Position, and Anesthesia

Same as for thyroidectomy

Tips and Pearls

1. Identify and preserve the inferior thyroid artery.
2. Identify and preserve recurrent laryngeal nerves.
3. The lower parathyroids usually are within 2 cm of the inferior pole of the thyroid and can be in the superior mediastinum with thymic tissue.
4. The upper parathyroids usually are within 1 to 2 cm of the penetration of the recurrent laryngeal nerve at the cricothyroid muscle.
5. Most upper and lower parathyroid glands receive their blood supply from the inferior thyroid artery.
6. For the hard to find parathyroid, check thyroid gland, retrotracheal area, retroesophageal area, carotid sheath, and up and beyond the carotid bifurcation anterior and posterior superior mediastinum.
7. Be careful not to damage blood supply to normal parathyroids. If the gland turns bluish black, consider autotransplantation of the gland to a muscle bed.
8. The biopsy of normal glands is done with the smallest middle ear cup forceps and a Beaver knife blade.
9. Reexplorations are dissected from lateral to medial, rather than medial to lateral, as a surgeon does with primary cases to avoid injury to the recurrent laryngeal nerve and inferior thyroid artery in a scarred tissue bed.
10. In approximately 25% of patients, associated thyroid disease is found, necessitating concomitant thyroidectomy.
11. Use medium suction-type drains during the postoperative period.

Pitfalls and Complications

1. Hematoma or seroma
2. Hypoparathyroidism
3. Recurrent laryngeal or superior laryngeal nerve injury
4. Persistent or recurrent hyperparathyroidism

Postoperative Care Issues

1. Drains are removed when drainage is less than 20 to 25 mL per day.
2. Daily serum calcium determinations are made for 5 days. The ionized calcium reflects the true level of calcium; it does not depend on serum proteins, but it is more expensive to obtain.
3. If patient has symptoms of muscular irritability (ie, Trousseau or Chvostek's' signs) and the serum calcium level is normal, check magnesium levels.
4. Institute calcium supplements if the serum calcium level is low, if the patient is symptomatic, and if the patient is elderly with a history of cardiac disease.
5. When starting intravenous supplements, also start supplementation by mouth so the intravenous form can be gradually diminished as serum calcium levels return to normal.

References

Castleman B. Parathyroid carcinoma: a study of 70 cases. Cancer 1973;31:600.

Clark O. The reasons for failure in parathyroid operations. Arch Surg 1989;124:911.

If a diseased parathyroid is located and there is questionable damage to a normal parathyroid, the normal parathyroid that is damaged has a bluish black devascularized color, and a small portion of this gland is sent for histologic identification. If normal parathyroid is the returned diagnosis, this tissue can be prepared for autotransplantation (Fig. 93-5).

Carcinoma of the Parathyroid

A patient with carcinoma of the parathyroid usually presents with higher serum calcium levels than the average patient with hyperparathyroidism. During the surgical procedure, the parathyroid and its surrounding tissue has a matted and a tacky adherence to the muscle or to the trachea or to the thyroid gland (Fig. 93-6) This matting usually indicates that the surgeon is dealing with carcinoma (Fig. 93-7). The parathyroid with surrounding fat muscle and thyroid gland tissue is removed (Fig. 93-8A). The tissue removed consists of the thyroid lobe on that side, the isthmus of the thyroid gland, the parathyroid carcinoma with surrounding fat and muscle if it is adherent to the strap muscle, and adjacent lymph nodes and paratracheal fat (Fig. 93-8B).

GEORGE H. PETTI

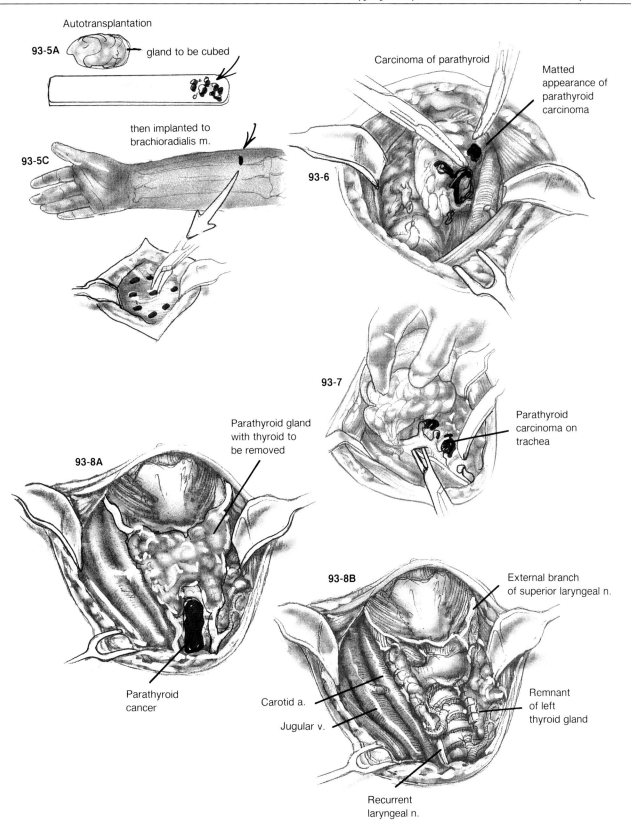

Autotransplantation

93-5A   gland to be cubed

then implanted to
brachioradialis m.

93-5C

Carcinoma of parathyroid

Matted
appearance of
parathyroid
carcinoma

93-6

93-7

Parathyroid
carcinoma on
trachea

Parathyroid gland
with thyroid to
be removed

93-8A

Parathyroid
cancer

93-8B

External branch
of superior laryngeal n.

Carotid a.

Jugular v.

Remnant
of left
thyroid gland

Recurrent
laryngeal n.

■ 94. TRACHEOSTOMY

Surgical creation of an opening into the trachea through the neck, bringing the tracheal mucosa into continuity with the skin

Indications

1. Airway obstruction due to
    a. Inflammatory disease
    b. Benign laryngeal pathology (eg, webs, cysts, papilloma)
    c. Malignant laryngeal tumors
    d. Benign and malignant tracheal tumors
    e. Laryngeal trauma or stenosis
    f. Tracheal stenosis
2. Pulmonary toilet
3. Obstructive sleep apnea

Special Considerations

1. Emergent versus elective surgery
2. Intubation versus operation

Preoperative Preparation

1. Routine laboratory studies
2. Arterial blood gases (optional)

Special Instrumentation, Position, and Anesthesia

1. Headlight
2. Laryngoscope and bronchoscope available
3. Flat or semi-Fowler position
4. Local anesthetic if emergent surgery
5. Trousseau dilator

Tips and Pearls

1. Horizontal incision if elective surgery
2. Vertical incision if emergent surgery
3. Stay in the midline.
4. Divide the thyroid isthmus.

Pitfalls and Complications

1. Airway obstruction
2. Apnea
3. Bleeding (eg, innominate artery)
4. Injury to recurrent nerve
5. Tracheoesophageal fistula
6. Pneumothorax (in children)
7. Subcutaneous emphysema
8. Tracheal malacia
9. Tracheal stenosis
10. Subglottic stenosis
11. Dislodgement of the tracheostomy tube

Postoperative Care Issues

1. Monitor to prevent dislodgement of the tracheostomy tube.
2. Use nebulizer to deliver 40% O_2.
3. Deflate the balloon once each 15 minutes every hour for the first 24 hours; then leave deflated.
4. Do not change the tracheostomy tube for the first 48 hours unless absolutely necessary.
5. Clean the inner cannula at least once every 8 hours.
6. Suction the trachea as needed.
7. A sentinel bleed may indicate innominate artery erosion.

References

Loré JM. An atlas of head and neck surgery. 3rd ed. Philadelphia: WB Saunders, 1988:811.

Montgomery WW. Surgery of the upper respiratory system, vol 2. Philadelphia: Lea & Febiger, 1973:324.

Operative Procedure

If the procedure is performed under general anesthesia, the patient is placed supine, with the head extended by using a shoulder roll. Some patients, because of some degree of airway distress, are unable to lie flat and require local anesthesia for the procedure. These patients are placed in a semi-Fowler position, and the incision is made in the midline of the neck, approximately 2 cm above the sternal notch. The incision is horizontal if the tracheostomy is elective and vertical if urgent or emergent (Fig. 94-1). The strap muscles are separated in the midline until the thyroid isthmus is encountered. If the thyroid isthmus is over the area where the opening into the trachea is to be made, the isthmus is divided by elevating the isthmus with clamps. Clamp and suture ligating each side with 3-0 silk (Fig. 94-2). In most cases, the thyroid can be retracted out of the way after releasing the fascial attachments to the anterior trachea. The fascia overlying the trachea is then identified by using two KD sponges, spreading vertically along the trachea. At this point, if the procedure is under local anesthetic, 1 mL of 4% Xylocaine is injected directly into the trachea to suppress the cough reflex. This procedure is unnecessary if the procedure is being performed under general anesthesia.

A tracheal hook is placed between the second and third tracheal rings, and a horizontal incision is made between the third and fourth tracheal rings. A small segment of the tracheal cartilage is removed, creating a window in the trachea (Fig. 94-3). Some surgeons prefer not to remove cartilage for fear of tracheal malacia and prefer making a cruciate incision between the third and fourth tracheal rings, spreading with a Trousseau dilator and inserting the tracheostomy tube through the opening with the dilator still in place. The tracheostomy tube is then placed through the opening into the trachea (Fig. 94-4). The tracheostomy tube is sutured to the skin using 3-0 silk as an added precaution to avoid accidental dislodgement of the tracheostomy tube. The tracheal tapes are then placed on each side of the tracheostomy tube and secured around the neck, allowing at least one finger to slide easily under the tape. In children, a suture is placed on each side of the tracheal opening and taped to the skin in case the tracheostomy tube should accidentally become dislodged within the first 48 hours. A 4 × 4 inch gauze sponge is cut to allow placement under the tracheostomy tube. Antibiotics are not routinely used.

NICHOLAS J. CASSISI

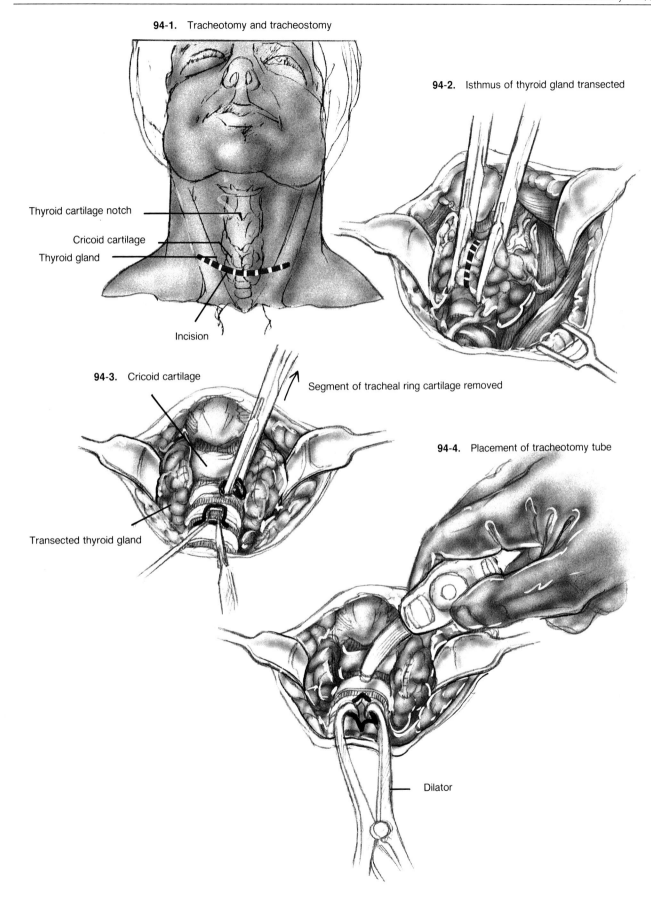

94-1. Tracheotomy and tracheostomy

Thyroid cartilage notch

Cricoid cartilage

Thyroid gland

Incision

94-2. Isthmus of thyroid gland transected

94-3. Cricoid cartilage

Segment of tracheal ring cartilage removed

Transected thyroid gland

94-4. Placement of tracheotomy tube

Dilator

■ 95. TRACHEAL RECONSTRUCTION

Surgical procedure to repair the trachea using grafts and stents

Indications

1. Moderate tracheal stenosis
2. Long tracheal stenosis
3. Tracheomalacia
4. Benign tracheal tumors

Contraindications

1. Patient on a ventilator
2. Patient with a nonfunctioning glottis

Special Considerations

1. Harvesting of rib, septal, or auricular cartilage graft
2. Perichondrium of graft is sutured to the tracheal mucosa.

Preoperative Preparation

1. Routine laboratory studies
2. Indirect examination of the larynx to determine vocal cord mobility

Special Instruments, Position, and Anesthesia

1. Headlight
2. Nasal instruments if septal cartilage is used
3. Chest instruments if rib cartilage is used
4. Abacour stent
5. T-tube
6. Shoulder roll, head holder, and head hyperextended
7. General anesthesia

Tips and Pearls

1. Suture is placed submucosally around tracheal cartilage and sutured to an adjacent strap muscle.
2. Perichondrium should extend beyond the cartilage graft.
3. If a tracheostomy tube is required, place it below the cartilage graft.

Pitfalls and Complications

1. Infection
2. Loss of cartilage graft
3. Blockage of stents with secretions

Postoperative Care Issues

1. Antibiotics
2. If a T-tube stent is used, daily installation of saline to keep secretions from inspissating within the tube
3. Change T-tubes every 6 months.
4. Leave the stent in place for 3 weeks.
5. Bronchoscopy before tracheostomy removal

References

Lusk RP, Kang DR, Muntz HR. Auricular cartilage grafts in laryngotracheal reconstruction. Ann Otol Rhinol Laryngol 1993;102:247.

Streitz JM, Shapshay SM. Airway injury after tracheotomy and endotracheal intubation. Surg Clin North Am 1991;71:1211.

Operative Procedure

Most adult tracheal reconstructions are inferior, involving the cricoid and anterior tracheal walls. If laryngotracheal reconstruction is necessary, the techniques are the same as used for children, which are covered in the chapter on laryngoplasty and tracheoplasty.

The operative procedure begins with the patient supine on a shoulder roll, with the head secured on a foam head holder. General anesthesia is administered, through the tracheostomy if one is present. A collar incision extending from the anterior borders of the sternocleidomastoid muscles is made, and the cervical flap is elevated in the subplatysmal plane to the level of the hyoid bone (Fig. 95-1). The strap muscles are separated in the midline, and the entire trachea is exposed. If the thyroid isthmus is impinging on the area, it is divided and suture ligated (Fig. 95-2). The tracheal defect is then identified, and a vertical incision is made along the anterior wall of the trachea in the area of the defect. The incision should extend slightly above and below the defect (Fig. 95-3). A 4-0 Vicryl suture is placed just lateral to the incision and tied through the strap muscles on each side. This allows the tracheal incision to be held open as wide as possible (Fig. 95-4).

The length and width of the cartilaginous support graft is then determined. A cartilage graft is obtained from the nasal septum, the ear, or the rib. Generally, the auricular or septal cartilage suffices. Procedure 256 describes the methods of obtaining septal cartilage grafts. At least 1 mm of perichondrium should extend beyond the support graft on all sides so that it may be sutured to the tracheal mucosa. If auricular cartilage is to be used, a postauricular incision is made, and cartilage from the conchal bowl, including the perichondrium on both sides, is included. The 4-0 Vicryl sutures are then placed through the perichondrium and tracheal mucosa, if possible; these are not tied until all the sutures have been placed. The sutures are tied, and the cartilage is wedged between the two sides of the trachea (Fig. 95-5). If needed, additional sutures are placed through the cartilage graft and the tracheal cartilages.

Some type of stent is then placed into the trachea to support the cartilage graft. Two types of stent are commonly used. An Abacour stent, which is made of Teflon, or a fingercot filled with foam rubber, sutured closed to prevent spillage of the foam rubber, is placed under the cords. The stents are secured by placing 28-gauge wire through the superior and inferior edges of the stent passed through the trachea, brought out at the tracheostomy site, wrapped around a dental roll, and taped to the stent wall.

Three weeks later, the patient is returned to the operating room, one end of the wire is cut at the skin edge, and the wires and stent are removed (Fig. 95-6). The patient is placed on antibiotics for 5 days postoperatively.

Alternative Treatment

For short, web-like stenosis, the CO_2 laser may be used. It is important that the microspot laser be used so that less power density is used, decreasing the tissue injury beyond the scar. Microflaps fashioned with the laser may be used to minimize scar reformation. Radial incisions in the area of the stenosis can be made and the area dilated with a rigid bronchoscope. However, it is important not to denude the epithelium circumferentially, because the area will restenose in 6 to 8 weeks. If a short tracheal stenosis recurs, sleeve resection with anastomosis may be indicated, but if the stenosis should again recur, a permanent T-tube stent may be the only alternative for the patient. The T-tube should be replaced about every 6 months.

NICHOLAS J. CASSISI

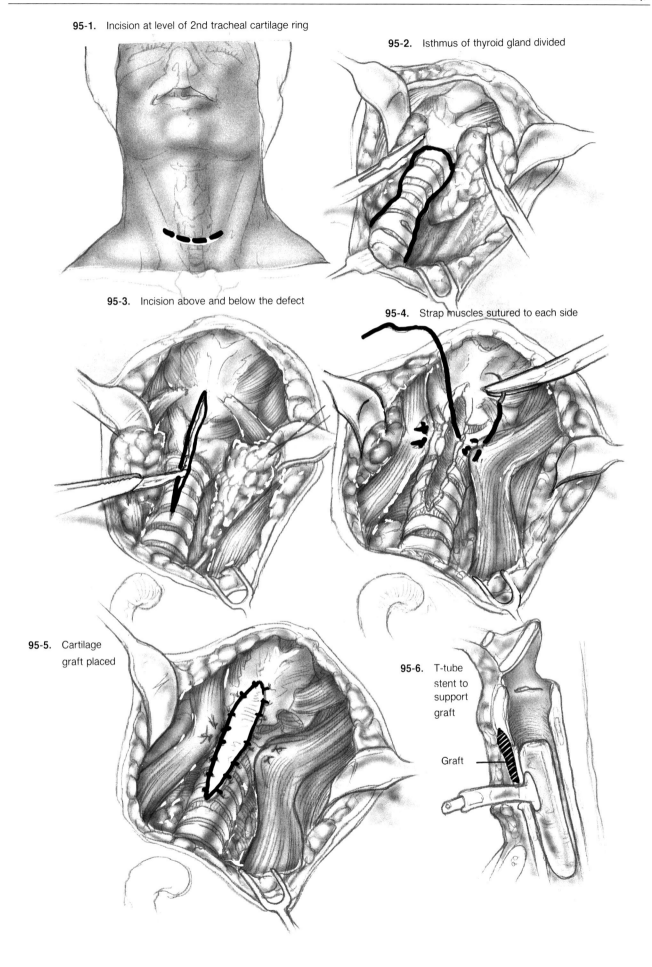

95-1. Incision at level of 2nd tracheal cartilage ring

95-2. Isthmus of thyroid gland divided

95-3. Incision above and below the defect

95-4. Strap muscles sutured to each side

95-5. Cartilage graft placed

95-6. T-tube stent to support graft

Graft

■ 96. TRACHEAL RESECTION AND REANAS-TOMOSIS—Partial removal of the trachea in the vertical dimension and primary reanastomosis of the resected ends

Indications

1. Tracheal stenosis
2. Tracheal tumors

Contraindications

1. Stenosis greater than 50% of the tracheal length
2. Severe subglottic stenosis involving the vocal cords
3. Patients on ventilators

Special Considerations

1. Patients with glottic injuries should have the glottic injury repaired before tracheal resection.
2. The tracheostomy tube must be removed at the time of tracheal resection.
3. Minimal tension on the suture line
4. Cervical flexion
5. Suprahyoid laryngeal release
6. Division of the right inferior pulmonary ligament

Preoperative Preparation

1. Computed tomography scan to evaluate the nature, vertical length, distal extent, and relative narrowing of the stenosis
2. Evaluation of the larynx by mirror or fiberoptic examination to determine vocal cord mobility

(continued)

Operative Procedure

An endotracheal tube is placed transorally to the level of the stenosis, and general anesthesia is administered through the tracheostomy. The patient is placed in the supine position on a shoulder roll, with the neck fully extended. A collar incision, extending from the anterior borders of the sternocleidomastoid muscles, is made, and the cervical flap is elevated in the subplatysmal plane to a level above the hyoid bone. The strap muscles are separated in the midline, and the entire trachea is exposed (Fig. 96-1). The trachea from cricoid to carina is mobilized along the anterior surface to preserve the blood supply to the trachea, which enters laterally. This is accomplished by sharp dissection along the cervical portion of the trachea and by blunt finger dissection in the thoracic portion. Circumferential dissection of the trachea should be limited to the area of the stenosis and just slightly above and below the stenosis. The recurrent laryngeal nerves need not be exposed (Fig. 96-2).

After the stenotic portion of the trachea is exposed, if a tracheostomy stoma exists in the area of the stenosis, the anterior tracheal wall is divided in the midline superiorly and inferiorly from the stoma until normal lumen is encountered. If no stoma exists, resection of the stenosis proximally and distally is performed in stages to avoid resecting excessive length (Fig. 96-3). It is important to resect all of the abnormal trachea to minimize the risk of restenosis. After the resection is complete, an infrahyoid or suprahyoid laryngeal release is performed, unless the stenotic segment is short enough to allow reanastomosis of the trachea with minimal tension on the suture line.

The technique of infrahyoid laryngeal release involves dividing the sternohyoid and omohyoid at the level of the thyrohyoid membrane. The superior cornua of the thyroid cartilage are divided, and the thyrohyoid membrane is divided with sharp dissection, using care to stay against the upper edge of the thyroid cartilage to prevent damage to the superior laryngeal nerve (Fig. 96-4). This infrahyoid release allows about a 2.5-cm "drop" of the larynx (Fig. 96-5). The

(continued)

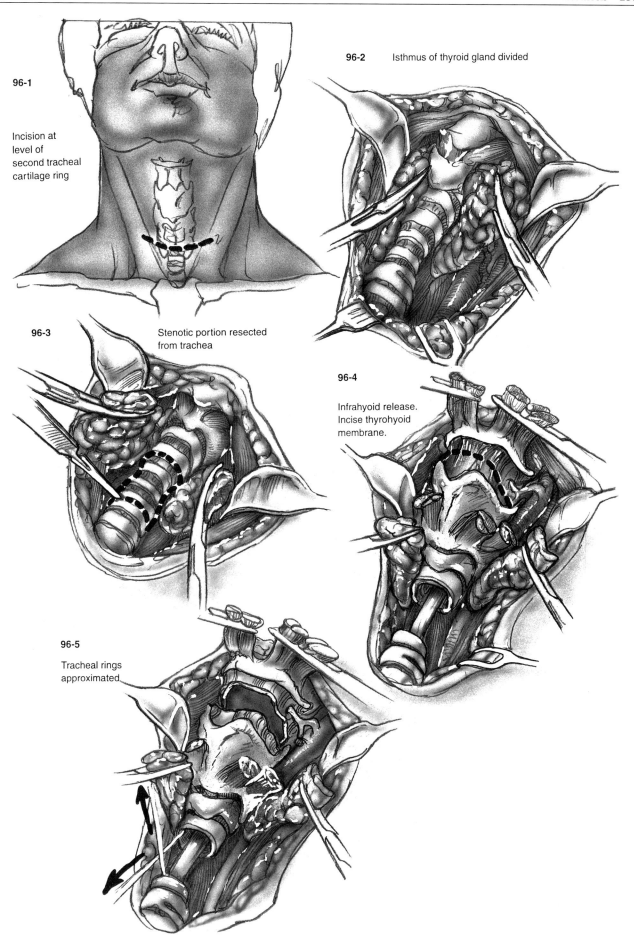

96-1

Incision at
level of
second tracheal
cartilage ring

96-2   Isthmus of thyroid gland divided

96-3   Stenotic portion resected
from trachea

96-4

Infrahyoid release.
Incise thyrohyoid
membrane.

96-5

Tracheal rings
approximated

■ **96.** TRACHEAL RESECTION AND REANAS-
TOMOSIS *(continued)*

Special Instruments, Position, and Anesthesia
1. Headlight
2. Supine position, with head hyperextended
3. General anesthesia
4. Endotracheal tube placed through the vocal cords to the level of the stenosis

Tips and Pearls
1. Heavy suture from the chin to anterior chest to keep the head in flexion for 7 to 10 days

Postoperative Care Issues
1. The patient is extubated when fully awake in the intensive care unit.
2. Nasogastric tube not routinely placed
3. Liquids on second postoperative day

References
Montgomery WW. Suprahyoid release for tracheal anastomosis. Arch Otolaryngol 1974;99:255.
Ross JA. Techniques in the surgical repair of tracheal stenosis. Otolaryngol Clin North Am 1979;12:4:893.

suprahyoid release involves dividing the muscle attachments from the superior surface of the hyoid bone (Fig. 96-6). The hyoid is then transected at the level of the lesser cornu using rongeurs (Fig. 96-7). The body of the hyoid, the thyroid and cricoid cartilages, and the proximal tracheal segment drop inferiorly (Fig. 96-8). If, despite using these techniques, adequate release is not possible and there is continued tension on the suture line, bronchial repositioning and pulmonary ligament release can be done, but this must be done in cooperation with the thoracic surgeon. The tracheal anastomosis is then begun using 2-0 silk or Vicryl sutures, which are passed submucosally from the outside in through the lateral walls of the trachea, one to two rings above and below the level of transection. These sutures are used for traction to pull the segments as far superiorly as possible to minimize tension at the suture line.

The 4-0 Vicryl sutures are first placed across the posterior wall approximately 3 mm apart and left untied until all the posterior sutures have been satisfactorily positioned (Fig. 96-9). The previously placed endotracheal tube is then advanced into the distal trachea; the posterior sutures are then tied, and the 4-0 Vicryl sutures are placed 3 mm apart and 3 mm from the tracheal edge and left untied until all of the lateral and anterior sutures are placed. The neck is then flexed, and the 2-0 Vicryl sutures are tied before tying the 4-0 sutures (Fig. 96-10). Some surgeons recommend removing the 2-0 traction sutures, but they may be left in place to reduce tension on the suture line. Suction drains are placed and brought out laterally through the neck. A heavy suture is placed from the chin to the chest to keep the neck in maximum flexion. A specially made posterior cervical collar can be helpful in maintaining maximum cervical flexion.

Antibiotics are not routinely used. I administer antibiotics only if considerable granulation tissue or infection develops around the previous tracheostomy site. The patient is extubated in the operating room or the intensive care unit the following day when he or she is fully awake. The patient is cared for in the intensive care unit, and liquids are begun orally on the second postoperative day. Oral intake is increased as tolerated. Occasionally, the patient may encounter some swallowing difficulties if the laryngeal release procedure has been done, but this is not permanent.

NICHOLAS J. CASSISI

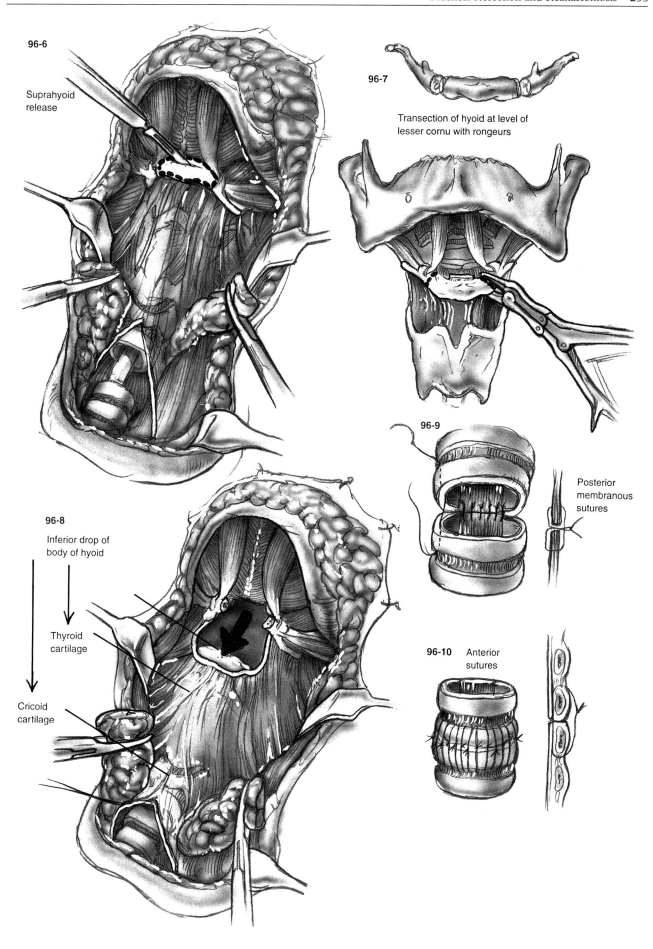

96-6

Suprahyoid release

96-7

Transection of hyoid at level of lesser cornu with rongeurs

96-8

Inferior drop of body of hyoid

Thyroid cartilage

Cricoid cartilage

96-9

Posterior membranous sutures

96-10   Anterior sutures

■ 97. CERVICAL ESOPHAGOSTOMY

Establishing an opening into the cervical esophagus in which a tube is placed for long-term enteral feedings

Indications

1. If more than 2 weeks of enteral feeding is expected after major head and neck resection, during recovery from a cerebrovascular accident, or after major laryngopharyngeal trauma

Contraindications

1. Severe gastroesophageal reflux with esophagitis
2. Open neck wound near esophagostomy site
3. Inadequate muscle for great vessel protection

Preoperative Preparations

1. Barium swallow
2. Esophagoscopy, which may be performed with esophagostomy

Special Instruments, Position, and Anesthesia

1. General or local anesthesia (with intravenous sedation)
2. Esophagoscopes and Maloney dilators
3. An 18-Fr sump feeding tube

Pitfalls and Complications

1. Injury to recurrent laryngeal or cervical sympathetic nerves
2. Erosion of the carotid artery
3. Gastroesophageal reflux

Postoperative Care Issues

1. If patient is taking minimal oral feedings, they may resume on the second postoperative day.
2. Administer broad-spectrum systemic antibiotics for 5 days.
3. Change to a nonsump 18-Fr feeding tube after 5 days.
4. The skin entry point requires cleaning with hydrogen peroxide and application of bacitracin ointment twice daily.

References

Fitz-Hugh GS, Sly DS. Elective cervical esophagostomy. Ann Otol Rhinol Laryngol 1967;76:804.

Schechter GL, Sly DS. Cervical esophagostomy. Am Coll Surg Film Library, Chicago.

Operative Procedure

A shoulder roll is used to extend the neck, and a 18-Fr nasogastric feeding tube is placed. Whether the patient is under general or local anesthesia, an appropriate concentration of Xylocaine with epinephrine is infiltrated along the anterior border of the lower one third of the left sternomastoid muscle, deep into the region of the medial aspect of the carotid sheath. The left side is preferred, because the cervical esophagus is located in a left paramedian position in the lower part of the neck. Entry through the right side is possible and often indicated to provide protection for the great vessels, but this approach is more difficult.

A 4- to 5-cm incision is made along the sternomastoid in the location described, and dissection is carried down to the omohyoid muscle, which is usually maintained in the lower part of the dissection field. The middle thyroid vein should be ligated if it is in the way. Two "Army-Navy" retractors are used to retract the carotid sheath and its contents laterally and the tracheoesophageal complex medially (Fig. 97-1). Dissection is then directed posteriorly and inferiorly toward the esophagus, cervical spine, and longus coli muscle. The cervical sympathetic nerves should be protected as the loose fascia overlying the longus coli is incised. Digital dissection is used for entry into the retroesophageal space and for palpation of the feeding tube within the cervical esophagus. The objective is to grasp the posterolateral aspect of the cervical esophagus and the contained feeding tube with a Babcock clamp. It is helpful to isolate the esophagus and its contained tube with the index finger against the cervical spine and then apply the Babcock clamp (Fig. 97-2). Once accomplished, the clamp and esophagus are carefully drawn anteriorly into the wound. Blunt dissection of the periesophageal fascia helps to identify the esophageal musculature.

A 5-mm longitudinal incision (ie, esophagotomy) is made through the esophageal muscles and mucosa down to the feeding tube that is held with the esophagus by the Babcock clamp (Fig. 97-3). The esophageal mucosal edges are grasped with fine-pointed hemostats, the Babcock clamp is released, and a fresh 18-Fr sump feeding tube is placed through the esophagotomy down into the stomach (Fig. 97-4). In most patients, tube entry into the stomach is indicated by the first mark on the feeding tube at skin level. The original nasogastric tube is then withdrawn carefully by the anesthetist to avoid displacing the tube just placed through the esophagotomy. A pursestring suture of 3-0 Vicryl is then placed around the esophagotomy site. If the sternomastoid muscle is intact, its medial border may be sewn to the posterior edge of the esophagotomy site with several similar Vicryl sutures to provide a muscle barrier between the feeding tube and the great vessels (Fig. 97-5). If the sternomastoid muscle is absent, this may be accomplished using the strap muscles. The strap muscles are dissected from the thyroid gland, retracted laterally, and the feeding tube is drawn up from the esophagotomy medial to them. The tube is then led out at the lower end of the skin incision and sewn in place with two separate 2-0 silk sutures. The tube functions as a drain for the wound, which may then be closed in layers.

GARY L. SCHECHTER

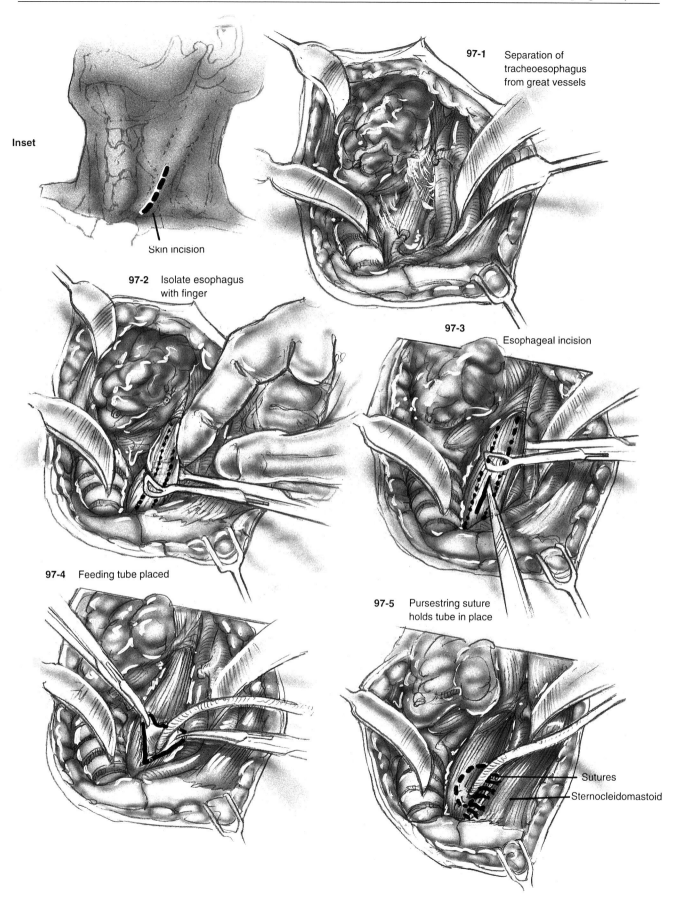

Inset

Skin incision

97-1   Separation of tracheoesophagus from great vessels

97-2   Isolate esophagus with finger

97-3   Esophageal incision

97-4   Feeding tube placed

97-5   Pursestring suture holds tube in place

Sutures

Sternocleidomastoid

■ 98. PHARYNGEAL POUCHES (ZENKER'S DIVERTICULUM)—Posterior herniation of the hypopharyngeal mucosa between the transverse fibers of the cricopharyngeal muscle and the oblique fibers of the inferior constrictor muscles

Indications

1. Oropharyngeal dysphagia secondary to a hypopharyngeal (Zenker's) diverticulum

Special Considerations

1. Size of diverticulum
2. Respiratory complications, such as aspiration
3. Nutritional complications, such as weight loss

Preoperative Preparation

1. Cine and video radiologic studies

Special Instruments, Position, and Anesthesia

1. TA-15 to TA-30 stapling device
2. Headlight
3. Esophageal bougie
4. Esophagoscope
5. General anesthesia

Tips and Pearls

1. Pack the diverticulum with Vaseline gauze placed through the esophagoscope.
2. Place an esophageal bougie after packing the diverticulum to prevent constricting the esophagus after removal of the diverticulum.
3. Stapling device for moderate or large sacs

Pitfalls and Complications

1. Injury to recurrent laryngeal nerve
2. Leakage and subsequent infection
3. Mediastinitis
4. Esophageal stenosis
5. Recurrence of the diverticulum

Postoperative Care Issues

1. Hypaque swallow 24 hours postoperatively
2. Clear liquids if no leakage

References

Morton RP, Bartley RF. Inversion of Zenker's diverticulum: the preferred option. Head Neck 1993;15:253.

Payne SW. The treatment of pharyngoesophageal diverticulum: the simple and complex. Hepatogastroenterology 1992;39:109.

Operative Procedure

General anesthesia is preferred. Before preparation of the skin of the neck, a cervical esophagoscope is placed to the level of the diverticulum, and the diverticulum is packed with Vaseline gauze to allow easier identification of the diverticulum in the neck. The end of the gauze packing is brought out the mouth and taped to the side of the face. An esophageal bougie is then placed into the esophagus to minimize the possibility of esophageal stenosis during the closure of the esophagus.

Some surgeons prefer an oblique incision along the left anterior border of the sternocleidomastoid muscle, but a horizontal incision also allows easy access to the diverticulum (Fig. 98-1). The flap is elevated, and the dissection is carried between the sternocleidomastoid and the strap muscles. The carotid sheath with its contents is retracted laterally, and the omohyoid muscle is identified. The diverticulum is identified, the distal end of the sac is dissected free and then retracted cephalad, and the diverticulum is dissected along its neck to the entrance into the esophagus between the fibers of the inferior constrictor muscle and the cricopharyngeus muscle (Fig. 98-2).

The gauze packing is then removed from the sac, and the diverticulum is then excised using the TA-15 gastrointestinal stapler (Fig. 98-3). If the stapler cannot be used, a suture is placed extramucosally in the esophagus above and below the neck of the diverticulum, and the sac is excised (Fig. 98-4). Interrupted 3-0 Vicryl sutures are used in a Connell fashion to invert the mucosa (Fig. 98-5). A cricopharyngeal myotomy is then performed, being careful not to injure the recurrent laryngeal nerve. This can be achieved by staying posteriorly when doing the myotomy (Fig. 98-6).

The neck wound is closed after placement of a Jackson-Pratt suction drain. Antibiotics are used for the first 24 hours. No nasogastric tube is used. Twenty-four hours postoperatively, a Hypaque swallow is obtained, and if there is no leak, the patient is started on liquids and discharged after the drain has been removed. The patient is kept on a completely liquid diet until the first postoperative visit and then told to resume a normal diet.

Surgical Variations

Some surgeons advocate cricopharyngeal myotomy alone for small diverticula. The technique is the same for cricopharyngeal myotomy for any reason.

In the inversion technique, after identification of the sac, a cricopharyngeal myotomy is performed, a pursestring 3-0 Vicryl suture is passed extramucosally around the neck of the sac, and the esophageal bougie is removed. The sac is then inverted, and the pursestring suture is pulled tight. No feeding tube is needed, and the patient can be fed on the first or second postoperative day. This technique should not be used for very large sacs or if the pouch has been present for many years.

The diverticulopexy and myotomy technique is similar to the inversion technique with cricopharyngeal myotomy, except that the distal end of the sac is inverted and suspended to the prevertebral fascia using 3-0 Prolene suture, which changes the angle of the diverticulum to the esophagus.

NICHOLAS J. CASSISI

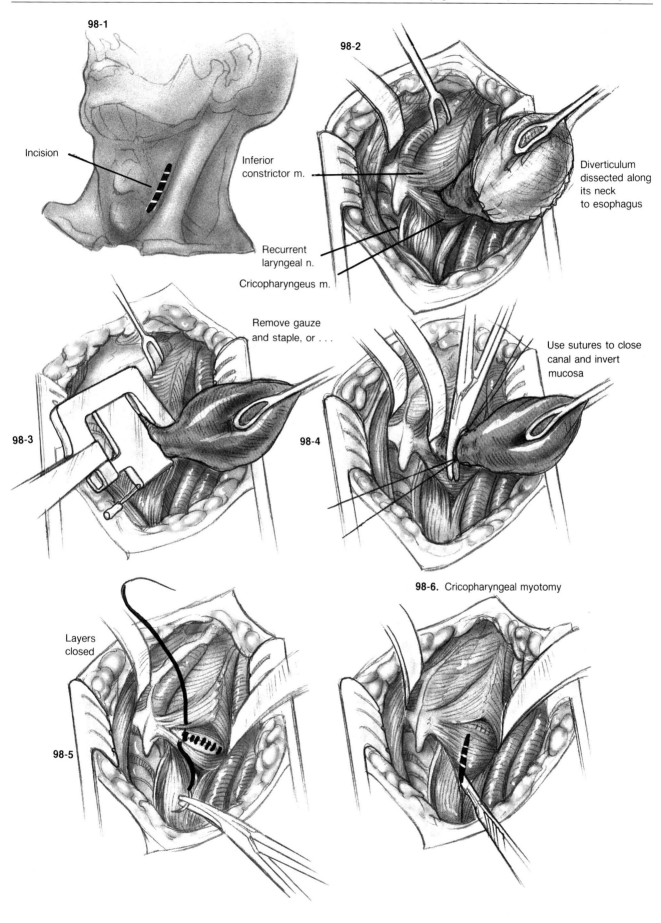

98-1

Incision

Inferior
constrictor m.

Recurrent
laryngeal n.

Cricopharyngeus m.

98-2

Diverticulum
dissected along
its neck
to esophagus

Remove gauze
and staple, or . . .

98-3

Use sutures to close
canal and invert
mucosa

98-4

98-6. Cricopharyngeal myotomy

Layers
closed

98-5

■ 99. MEDIASTINAL EXPLORATION AND DISSECTION—Technique for opening the superior mediastinum through the upper sternum for evaluation of and access to the thymus and superior mediastinal lymphatics, tracheobronchial tree, vascular structures, and the esophagus. The mediastinal dissection is used for resection of head and neck cancers that have extended into the superior mediastinum.

Indications

1. Exploration of the parathyroid glands or parathyroid adenomas, substernal thyroid gland extension, or hemorrhage associated with neck surgery
2. Evaluation of adenopathy
3. Exposure of the trachea for reconstruction
4. Mediastinal dissection associated with stomal recurrence after laryngectomy, thyroid or parathyroid malignancies, or laryngopharyngoesophagectomy

Contraindications

1. Previous coronary vascularization using the internal mammary vessels
2. Presence of aortic or superior vena caval vascular abnormalities

Special Considerations

1. Work closely with cardiothoracic and general thoracic surgeons, taking a team approach to these problems.
2. Determine preoperatively if the problem requires thoracic inlet exploration using the suprasternal approach (eg, substernal thyroid) or formal superior mediastinal exploration (eg, stomal recurrence).

Preoperative Preparation

1. Computed tomography scan of the mediastinum
2. Barium swallow
3. Bronchoscopy and esophagoscopy
4. Type and hold blood for thoracic inlet exploration.
5. Type and crossmatch blood for superior mediastinal exploration or dissection.

(continued)

Operative Procedure

Thoracic Inlet Exploration

Exploration of the thoracic inlet may be performed as a single procedure or as the preliminary step to mediastinal exploration and dissection. The exploration is begun at the midline with identification of the cervical trachea. In patients with short necks, the thyroid isthmus may have to be elevated. This is accomplished by releasing the soft tissue bands attached to its inferior edge, each side of which contains a single vein that extends inferiorly toward the chest. After these are ligated, the isthmus is elevated superiorly, and the anterior tracheal wall may be traced inferiorly into the mediastinum. The soft tissue mass anterior to the trachea in the thoracic inlet contains the innominate artery and vein crossing from right to left. These are encased in a mass of connective tissue that also contains mediastinal lymph nodes and remnants of the thymus (Fig. 99-1).

After the trachea is cleared of soft tissue on its anterior surface, the exploration is extended laterally to the carotid sheaths. The inferior thyroid arteries are encountered extending superiorly along the medial aspects of the sheaths and usually extending to the thyroid gland anterior to the recurrent laryngeal nerves. This anatomic association must be explored carefully, because there may be a small branch of the nerve anterior to the artery as well. On the right side, the recurrent laryngeal nerve may travel toward the tracheoesophageal groove in a lateral to medial direction from the subclavian artery, and care must be taken to avoid injury to it in its lateral position. On the left side, the nerve assumes a position in the tracheoesophageal groove in the mediastinum, but this side has its own perils. The thoracic duct extends superiorly through the left side of the thoracic inlet posterior and lateral to the jugular vein. It enters the junction of the jugular and subclavian veins at a point where there may be numerous thin lymphatic channels (Fig. 99-2). Care must be taken to avoid tearing these vessels to prevent a chyle leak. If chyle appears in the wound during exploration, a careful search for its source should be carried out under magnification, and meticulous ligation is required.

The final part of the thoracic inlet exploration is identification of the vagus nerves in the posterior aspects of the carotid sheaths and tracing the great vessels inferiorly to their junction with their parent vessels behind the manubrium and clavicular heads. Whether removing a substernal thyroid or searching for mediastinal parathyroids or lymph nodes, it is important to identify the major structures described to maintain control of the exploration.

Mediastinal Exploration

More definitive exploration and dissection of the mediastinum above the level of the heart requires sternotomy at a minimum and may require manubrial resection for maximal exposure. Median sternotomy down to the junction of the manubrium and body of the sternum with lateral extensions may be used for limited extension of the thoracic inlet exploration. This is accomplished after incising the periosteum on the posterior aspect of the manubrium and bluntly dissecting a midline plane inferiorly toward the junction with the sternal body (Fig. 99-3). The sternal saw is then inserted, and a midline cut is made inferiorly. The lateral cuts are made in short segments while alternately dissecting the soft tissues from the posterior aspects of the sternum. At the lateral aspects of the sternum, this soft tissue contains the internal mammary vessels. If lymphatic dissection or exposure of the trachea or vasculature is necessary, the manubrium may be resected piecemeal from medial to lateral aspects. In many patients, this approach coupled with a sternal retractor allows adequate exposure of the superior mediastinum (Fig. 99-4).

(continued)

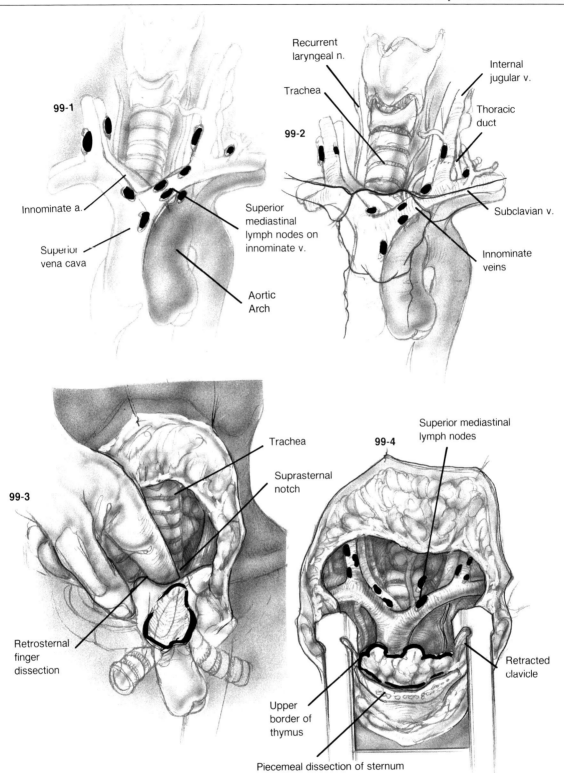

99-1

Innominate a.

Superior
vena cava

Superior
mediastinal
lymph nodes on
innominate v.

Aortic
Arch

Recurrent
laryngeal n.

Trachea

99-2

Internal
jugular v.

Thoracic
duct

Subclavian v.

Innominate
veins

99-3

Trachea

Suprasternal
notch

Retrosternal
finger
dissection

Superior mediastinal
lymph nodes

99-4

Retracted
clavicle

Upper
border of
thymus

Piecemeal dissection of sternum

■ 99. MEDIASTINAL EXPLORATION AND DISSECTION *(continued)*

Special Instruments, Position, and Anesthesia
1. Complete muscle paralysis and controlled ventilation
2. Shoulder roll and neck extension
3. Thoracotomy instruments on standby
4. Vascular instruments

Tips and Pearls
1. Veins can resemble anthracotic lymph nodes.
2. Large veins have thin walls and require special suture technique for repair of holes and tears.
3. The membranous trachea (posterior wall) tears easily during dissection from the esophagus.
4. Pleural reflections are easily penetrated.
5. The right recurrent laryngeal nerve divides from the vagus in the operative field and may be in a lateral position.

Pitfalls and Complications
1. Major venous hemorrhage
2. Pneumomediastinum from tracheal tear
3. Standard or tension pneumothorax
4. Recurrent laryngeal nerve paralysis

Postoperative Care Issues
1. Monitor for mediastinal widening and shifts and for pneumothorax.
2. Check for endotracheal erosion from the tracheotomy tube.

References

Ginsberg RJ. Evaluation of the mediastinum by invasive techniques. Surg Clin North Am 1987;67:1025.

Niederle B, Roka R, Fritsch A. Transsternal operation in thyroid cancer. Surgery 1985;98:1154.

Sisson GA, Bytell DE, Becker SP. Mediastinal dissection, 1976: indications and newer techniques. Laryngoscope 1977;87:751.

Complete superior mediastinal dissection and procedures requiring manipulations of the great vessels for tracheal resections or reconstructions demand removal of the superior sternal plate along with the costochondral and clavicular articulations. This is accomplished after methodically incising the clavicular heads and sternal heads of the first three ribs just lateral to their articulations using a strong oscillating saw. Before making each vertical saw cut, the soft tissues and neurovascular bundles are dissected away from the posterior surface of the bone to prevent hemorrhage (Fig. 99-5). After all vertical cuts are made and a horizontal saw cut is completed at the juncture of the manubrium and sternal body, the sternal plate is removed in one piece. In cases requiring major tracheal resection, such as primary tracheal carcinomas or tracheal stomal recurrence, the bone is not replaced, and a pectoralis myocutaneous flap is rotated in to protect the great vessels from the mediastinal tracheostoma. The bone plate may be preserved and wired back into position where the exposure was used for removal of benign disease or for tracheal reconstruction.

Mediastinal dissection is best begun by defining the inferior limits of the dissection at the aortic arch, superior vena cava, and carina. The lymph nodes and thymic remnants are contained in a fascial envelope that is readily dissected off the structures previously mentioned, and the dissection is extended laterally to the hilar regions (Fig. 99-6). The soft tissues are then elevated superiorly as each vessel and the trachea are traced upward toward the root of the neck. The dissection is complete when the tissue planes are joined with those established at the onset when the thoracic inlet was explored and entered (Fig. 99-7).

The operative site is irrigated profusely with saline and an antibiotic solution of the surgeon's choice. The anesthesiologist is asked to hyperinflate the lungs while a pool of irrigating solution is maintained in the mediastinum. The appearance of air bubbles requires a careful search for pleural tears or tracheobronchial disruption. These should be repaired when found. A chest tube may be necessary. Continuous suction drains are then placed in the mediastinum and under the skin flaps. The wounds are closed in an appropriate manner.

The patient must be observed in an intensive care unit where the personnel are familiar with thoracic surgery patients. Correction of problems that may develop from tension pneumothorax or mediastinal hemorrhage is most effective if the complication is detected early.

GARY L. SCHECHTER

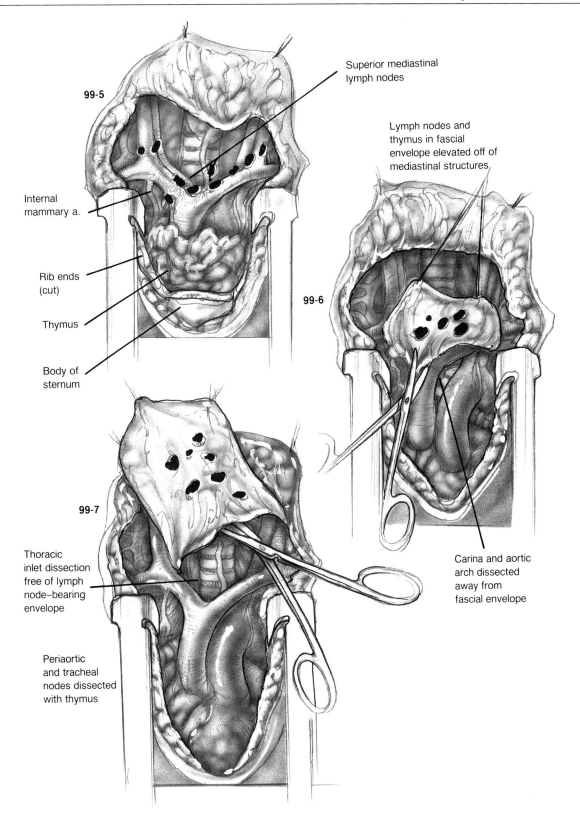

99-5

Superior mediastinal
lymph nodes

Internal
mammary a.

Rib ends
(cut)

Thymus

Body of
sternum

Lymph nodes and
thymus in fascial
envelope elevated off of
mediastinal structures

99-6

99-7

Thoracic
inlet dissection
free of lymph
node–bearing
envelope

Periaortic
and tracheal
nodes dissected
with thymus

Carina and aortic
arch dissected
away from
fascial envelope

■ 100. CRICOPHARYNGEAL MYOTOMY AND MYECTOMY

—Incision or excision of a portion of the cricopharyngeus muscle performed to eliminate the constant tension or spasm of the cricopharyngeus muscle in patients who have had conservation surgery of the larynx or pharyngeal reconstructions and in those with cricopharyngeal achalasia

Indications

1. Isolated cricopharyngeal spasm unresponsive to pharmacologic or dilation therapy
2. Multiple cranial neuropathy associated with central nervous system disease resulting in dysphagia or aspiration
3. Cricopharyngeal stenosis unresponsive to dilation
4. Tracheoesophageal fistula candidates who have cricopharyngeal spasm from retrograde air pressure
5. In association with Zenker's diverticulum resection or suspension and in conservation laryngeal surgery

Contraindications

1. Lack of elevated pressures on manometric studies in patients with suspected primary spasm
2. Multiple cranial neuropathy, usually bilateral, with glottic incompetence and severe aspiration
3. Stricture with transmural fibrosis

Special Considerations

1. A complete neurologic and upper gastrointestinal workup is needed to understand cricopharyngeal dysfunction.

Preoperative Preparation

1. Barium swallow and esophagoscopy
2. Manometric and motility studies

Special Instruments, Position, and Anesthesia

1. Esophagoscopes (rigid and flexible)
2. Maloney mercury-weighted dilators
3. Magnification (microscope or loupes)
4. Bipolar cautery

Tips and Pearls

1. Avoid mucosal penetration to prevent fistula formation.
2. Cricopharyngeus muscle extends into adjacent constrictor and esophageal muscles.
3. Protect the recurrent laryngeal nerve.

Postoperative Care Issues

1. Observe continuous suction for salivary drainage.
2. Wait for edema to subside before feeding patient.

References

Bosma JF, Donner MW, Tanaka E, Robertson D. Anatomy of the pharynx pertinent to swallowing. Dysphagia 1986;1:51.
Esophageal spasm and diverticulum. In: Skinner DB, Belsey RHR, eds. Management of esophageal disease. Philadelphia: WB Saunders, 1988;29:431.

Operative Procedure

Cricopharyngeal myotomy may be performed under local anesthesia, including topical anesthesia of the pharyngoesophagus with intravenous sedation, or under general anesthesia. Slight extension of the neck is desirable. Either side may be approached, unless there is a preexisting unilateral neurologic deficit; the side of the deficit should be used. When myotomy is performed with other operative procedures, the primary operation dictates the approach.

The procedure begins with placement of a 40- to 44-Fr Maloney esophageal dilator and taping it to the patient's cheek for easy access. The anterior border of the sternomastoid muscle and the medial border of the carotid sheath are identified. Venous connections between the internal jugular vein and the thyroid and larynx and those of the the superior thyroid artery are individually ligated (Fig. 100-1). The superior laryngeal nerve is then identified, coursing inferiorly and medially toward the thyrohyoid membrane, and is dissected and retracted carefully to prevent damage to the external motor branch to the cricothyroid muscle.

The posterior border of the thyroid cartilage is palpated and elevated with a double-hook retractor. This exposes the inferior constrictor and, inferior to this, the cricopharyngeus muscle. The Maloney dilator is palpated in the esophageal lumen, and the dissection is continued into the retropharyngeal and retroesophageal spaces. This allows further medial rotation of the laryngotracheal complex and exposes the posterolateral aspect of the cricopharyngeus muscle (Fig. 100-2). It also rotates the entry point of the recurrent laryngeal nerve into the larynx, the Killian-Jameson area, away from the operative site.

The fibers of the cricopharyngeus muscle run perpendicular to those of the pharyngoesophagus, are easily identified in the main portion of the muscle, and interdigitate with the inferior constrictor muscle superiorly and the esophageal muscle inferiorly. The myotomy or myectomy therefore must extend into these adjacent muscles to be complete. I subscribe to the concept that myectomy is necessary to have a permanent disruption of the cricopharyngeus muscle, because I have experienced several cases in which the muscle regained its integrity after myotomy alone.

A microscope or operating loupes are helpful in performing the myotomy and myectomy, because they enable identification of the mucosa with its underlying orange-red Maloney dilator. Bipolar cautery is used to coagulate the muscle and any obvious blood vessels before incision. This allows better hemostasis and easier separation of the muscle fibers. The incision should extend approximately 1.5 to 2.0 cm into the inferior constrictor superiorly and esophageal muscles inferiorly (Fig. 100-3). After the mucosa is identified, a submucosal plane is dissected posteriorly, approximately 1.5 cm along the length of the muscle incision, using blunt-tipped scissors. A 1.0-cm strip of muscle is resected using the bipolar cautery technique mentioned previously (Fig. 100-4).

After the muscle incision and resection are completed, the dilator is removed, and the mucosa is inspected for tears, which should be repaired with an absorbable suture. The wound is then irrigated with an antibiotic-containing solution, and a continuous suction drain is placed close to the muscle incision. The wound is closed in layers. Intraoperative and postoperative antibiotics are recommended because of the possibility of pharyngeal contamination.

The patient is fed according to his overall medical condition. If the myotomy is performed in conjunction with other laryngopharyngeal surgery, the major procedure determines the time of feeding. If the myotomy is performed as a primary procedure, clear liquids may be started on the third postoperative day. The suction drains are removed if there is no increase in wound drainage, and the diet is advanced according to the patient's tolerance.

GARY L. SCHECHTER

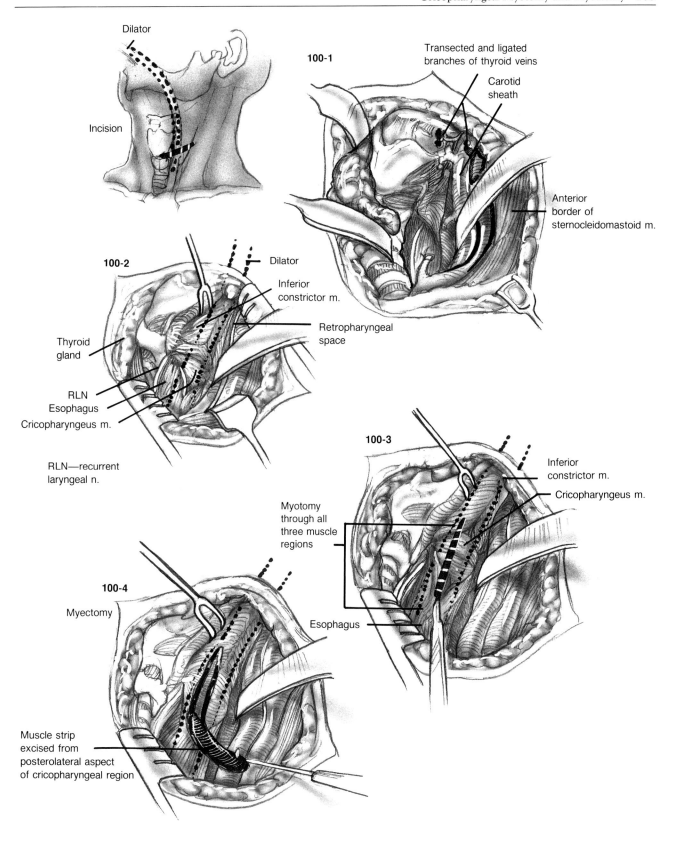

Dilator

Incision

100-1

Transected and ligated branches of thyroid veins

Carotid sheath

Anterior border of sternocleidomastoid m.

100-2

Dilator

Inferior constrictor m.

Retropharyngeal space

Thyroid gland

RLN
Esophagus
Cricopharyngeus m.

RLN—recurrent laryngeal n.

100-3

Inferior constrictor m.

Cricopharyngeus m.

Myotomy through all three muscle regions

Esophagus

100-4

Myectomy

Muscle strip excised from posterolateral aspect of cricopharyngeal region

■ *101.* REVISION OF STENOTIC TRACHEOS-TOMY— Surgical procedure to enlarge a tracheostomy using Z-plasty

Indications
1. Respiratory difficulty
2. Difficulty changing voice prosthesis

Special Considerations
1. Previous radiation therapy
2. Presence of tracheoesophageal puncture

Preoperative Preparation
1. Routine laboratory studies

Special Instruments, Position, and Anesthetic
1. Headlight
2. Shoulder roll and foam head rest
3. Local anesthesia

Tips and Pearls
1. Modify if voice prosthesis is present using only three flaps
2. Trim flaps
3. Meticulous skin to mucosal closure
4. No tension on suture line

Pitfalls and Complications
1. Separation of suture line
2. Restenosis
3. Infection

Postoperative Care Issues
1. Do not use voice prosthesis during healing.
2. Polysporin ointment on suture line

Reference
Berstein L. Transposed and interposed flaps in head and neck surgery. Otolaryngol Clin North Am 1972;5:3:531.

Operative Procedure
Stomal stenosis often can be corrected by incising the skin and dissecting between the scar and the trachea. The scar is then removed, and it is important that the trachea is mobilized enough so that two stay sutures using 3-0 Prolene can be placed from the trachea to the clavicles. The sutures are placed submucosally in the trachea. This allows the tracheostoma to be sutured to the skin with minimal tension on the suture line. Meticulous closure of the skin to the mucosa is mandatory so that no cartilage is exposed, reducing the incidence of chondritis and further scar formation.

Alternate Technique

With the patient supine, the area of the stoma is injected with a solution of 1% Xylocaine with a 1:100,000 dilution of epinephrine. Incisions are made through the skin only at 12, 3, 6, and 9 o'clock (Fig. 101-1). If a tracheoesophageal puncture exists, incisions are made only at 3, 6, and 9 o'clock. The skin flaps are undermined, elevated, and folded outward in all four quadrants (Fig. 101-2). Inner incisions at a 45° axis to the skin incisions are made, and scar tissue is excised (Fig. 101-3). The mucosal flaps formed by these incisions are then elevated and everted (Fig. 101-4). All flaps are then trimmed to form triangles, and the skin flaps are advanced between the mucosal flaps and carefully sutured with 4-0 Vicryl (Fig. 101-5). Care must be taken not to leave any cartilage exposed. The suture line is then covered with an antibiotic ointment such as Polysporin.

NICHOLAS J. CASSISI

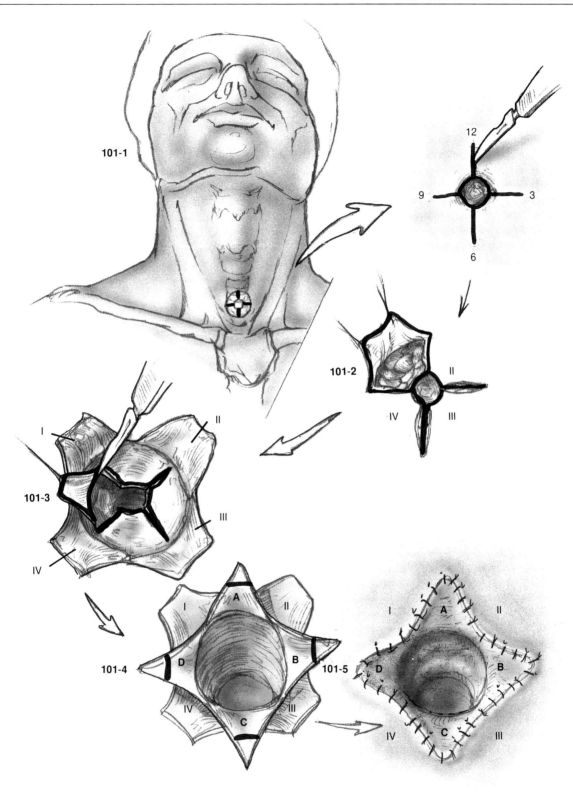

101-1

12
9   3
6

101-2
I
II
IV   III

101-3
I
II
III
IV

101-4
I   A   II
D   B
IV   III
C

101-5
I   A   II
D   B
IV   C   III

■ 102. PARTIAL AND TOTAL PHARYNGEC-
TOMY—The techniques for partial or total excision of the oropharynx or hypopharynx used in the treatment of benign or malignant tumors. These procedures may be performed individually or in conjunction with partial laryngectomy (ie, partial laryngopharyngectomy), laryngectomy (ie, laryngopharyngectomy), or esophagectomy (ie, laryngopharyngoesophagectomy).

Indications
1. Benign or malignant tumors
2. Stricture

Contraindications
1. In patients with severe chronic lung disease, pharyngectomy without laryngectomy is contraindicated.

Special Considerations
1. Cancers in this region have extensive submucosal spread and produce skip metastases.
2. Neck dissection is indicated in virtually all cases of epidermoid carcinoma of the pharynx.
3. Bilateral neck dissection should be considered in midline epidermoid carcinomas larger than 2 cm.
4. Provide for the widest margin of resection necessary, and prepare the patient for the consequences, such as laryngectomy or cervical esophagectomy.

Preoperative Preparation
1. Barium swallow and esophagoscopy
2. Pulmonary function evaluation when the larynx is spared

Special Instruments, Position, an Anesthesia
1. Appropriate saws, plates, and screws for mandibulotomy
2. Headlight

(continued)

Operative Procedure
Because most hypopharyngeal tumors are squamous carcinomas at a stage that requires associated neck dissection, it is important to plan the neck dissection incisions that best complement the approach to the pharynx for pharyngectomy. In general, I prefer the half-H or T-on-side incision (Fig. 102-1). This consists of a vertical limb that extends along the anterior border of the trapezius muscle, from the mastoid tip down to within 3 to 4 cm of the clavicle and a horizontal limb approximately 4 cm below the angle of the mandible, from a contralateral paramedian point meeting the vertical limb at a right angle. This incision gives excellent exposure for neck dissection and allows additional modification for approaches to the pharynx and larynx.

Tracheotomy is essential temporarily in all cases of pharyngeal resection. In addition, I prefer a cervical esophagostomy (see Procedure 97) or a percutaneous esophagogastrostomy for alimentation. These patients usually undergo prolonged oral rehabilitation, and many require postoperative radiotherapy. Eliminating the constraints of a nasogastric tube is helpful for the patient's physical and psychologic comfort. A feeding jejunostomy should be considered if a gastric pull-up reconstruction is being considered.

Posterior and Limited Lateral Wall Resections
Resection of lesions of the superior hypopharynx limited to the piriform fossa are discussed in Procedure 76. Lesions limited to less than 3 to 4 cm on the posterior pharyngeal wall and those less than 3 cm on the lateral wall of the oropharynx are approached preferably through the midline to avoid unnecessary damage to cranial nerves IX, X, and XII. A horizontal incision at the level of the thyrohyoid membrane is used to perform a suprahyoid or median pharyngotomy. Through this approach, the suprahyoid muscles are separated from the body of the hyoid as far laterally as possible without injuring the superior laryngeal nerve branches. After the valleculae are entered, the larynx is retracted inferiorly while the tongue base is retracted superiorly (Fig. 102-2). The resulting exposure allows resection of most small to medium-sized midline oropharyngeal or superior hypopharyngeal tumors down to the prevertebral muscles. Small lateral oropharyngeal wall lesions or extensions of posterior pharyngeal wall lesions, including the underlying constrictor muscles, may also be resected using this approach (Fig. 102-3). The ipsilateral glossopharyngeal nerve must be resected in the latter cases. Although some lateral pharyngeal wall defects smaller than 3 cm may be closed primarily and equivalent-sized posterior pharyngeal wall defects can be sutured open to the prevertebral fascia, most cases require flaps or skin grafts for reconstructions (see Procedure 103).

(continued)

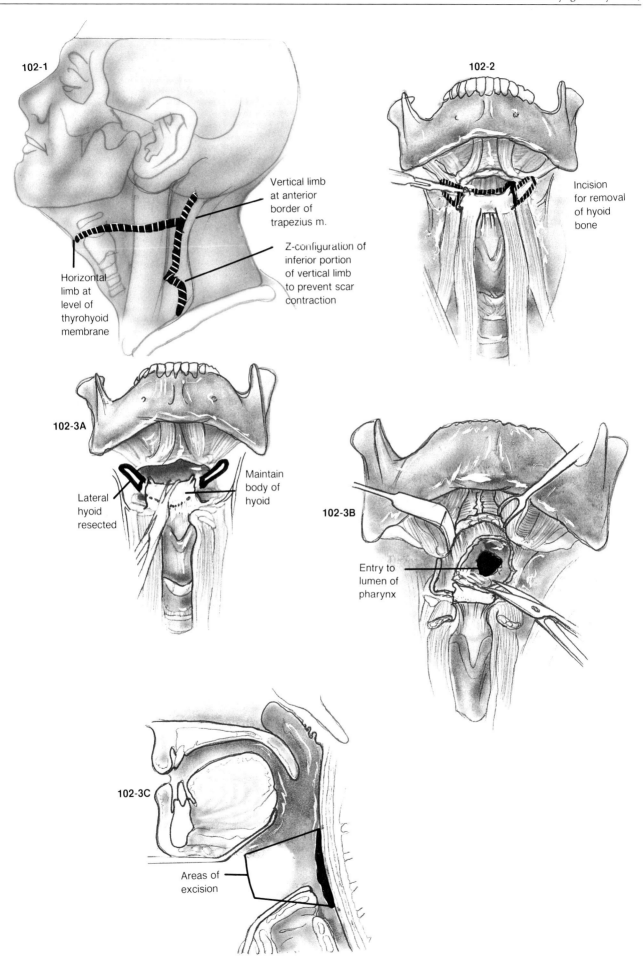

102-1

Vertical limb at anterior border of trapezius m.

Z-configuration of inferior portion of vertical limb to prevent scar contraction

Horizontal limb at level of thyrohyoid membrane

102-2

Incision for removal of hyoid bone

102-3A

Lateral hyoid resected

Maintain body of hyoid

102-3B

Entry to lumen of pharynx

102-3C

Areas of excision

■ *102.* PARTIAL AND TOTAL PHARYNGEC-TOMY *(continued)*

Tips and Pearls

1. At least a 3- to 4-cm tumor-free margin from the cricopharyngeus is required, or laryngectomy and cervical esophagectomy is necessary.
2. Resection of posterior pharyngeal wall lesions may be carried out using a midline suprahyoid approach.
3. In selected patients, tumors of the superior half of the piriform fossa may be resected using the larynx-sparing partial laryngo-pharyngectomy procedure (see Chap. 76).
4. Remove teeth with significant caries or periodontal disease that are in the anticipated mandibulotomy incision to prevent post-operative bone infection.

Pitfalls and Complications

1. Injury to branches of cranial nerves V, IX, X, and XII during mandibular swing or pharyngotomy approaches
2. Resection and reconstruction of more than 35% to 40% of the oropharyngeal and hypopharyngeal walls severely disables deglutition in most patients. If this amount of surgery or more is necessary, particularly if the patient has moderate to severe pulmonary dysfunction, laryngectomy should accompany the resection.
3. Diagnose and treat aggressively gastroesophageal reflux to prevent increased postoperative complications with the reconstruction site and interference with swallowing rehabilitation.

Postoperative Care Issues

1. The type of reconstruction used determines the kind of postoperative issues that arise.

References

Harrison DF. Surgical management of hypopharyngeal cancer. Arch Otolaryngol 1979;105:149.

Marks JE, Smith PG, Sessions DG. Pharyngeal wall cancer: a reappraisal after comparison of treatment methods. Arch Otolaryngol 1985;111:79.

Pingree TF, Davis RK, Reichman O, Derrick L, et al. Treatment of hypopharyngeal cancer: a 10 year review of 1362 cases. Laryngoscope 1987;97:901.

The median pharyngotomy is closed with careful attention to reconstituting the attachments of the suprahyoid muscles. I prefer 2-0 silk or Vicryl and place several sutures deep into the midline and paramedian tongue base musculature and bring them around the body of the hyoid bone (Fig. 102-4). The tongue base mucosa is not reapproximated to the mucosa of the valleculae, but the lateral pharyngeal mucosa must be approximated precisely in primary and flap closures. Constant suction drainage is required in all cases.

Subtotal and Total Pharyngectomy

Large lesions of the pharynx, with or without extension to the tonsil, tongue base, or larynx, usually require more exposure than can be obtained using the median pharyngotomy. I prefer using a mandibulotomy and mandibular swing in these cases. In many patients, a lip-splitting incision does not have to accompany the mandibulotomy to obtain the required exposure.

The mandibulotomy is performed anterior to the mental foramen, using an angle that favors good bone healing (Fig. 102-5). Bone plates of the surgeon's choice are fitted and screwed in place and then removed before completing the bone cuts. Any teeth in the line of the mandibulotomy are removed. The mandibulotomy is performed using a reciprocating saw with a thin blade. In most patients, the ipsilateral submandibular gland and lingual nerve are sacrificed to bring the incision through the floor of the mouth and into the pharynx. With the mandible retracted laterally and the patient paralyzed appropriately, excellent exposure of the pharynx is obtained (Fig. 102-6). If the lateral pharyngeal wall must be incised vertically down into the piriform fossa, the lingual vessels should be ligated. The hypoglossal and superior laryngeal nerves, however, should be individually dissected free and retracted with great care if they are grossly free of tumor or out of the field of resection (Fig. 102-7).

The pharyngeal lesion may be resected under direct vision without injury to the internal carotid artery. Dissection of the retropharyngeal nodes should accompany the resection (Fig. 102-8). If laryngectomy (see Chap. 80) is necessary, the resection may be extended inferiorly. If the inferior margin of resection must involve part or all of the cervical esophagus, this should be anticipated and the patient prepared for more extensive reconstruction techniques (see Chap. 103).

Although the closure depends on the type of reconstruction used, the basic principles remain the same. The reconstruction material should be sutured to the remaining mucosa in a manner that creates a watertight closure. I prefer 3-0 Vicryl sutures and place them using individual mattress stitches at key locations for positioning of the flaps or grafts and then oversew these with a Connell stitch of the same suture material. Continuous suction drains are placed near to, but not against, the suture lines, and the wounds are closed in layers after the mandibulotomy is secured with the bone plate.

GARY L. SCHECHTER

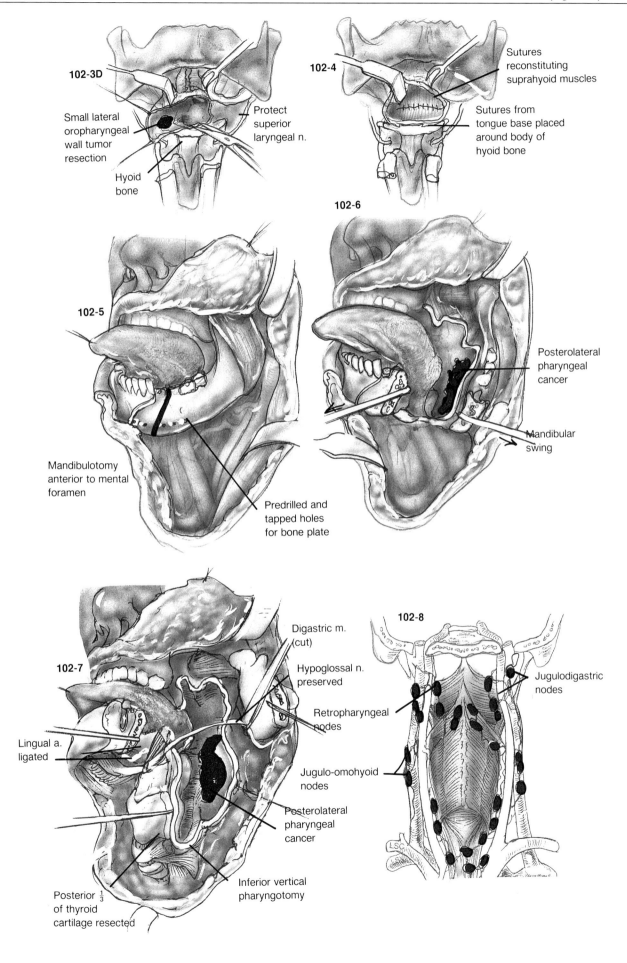

102-3D

Small lateral oropharyngeal wall tumor resection

Protect superior laryngeal n.

Hyoid bone

102-4

Sutures reconstituting suprahyoid muscles

Sutures from tongue base placed around body of hyoid bone

102-6

102-5

Mandibulotomy anterior to mental foramen

Predrilled and tapped holes for bone plate

Posterolateral pharyngeal cancer

Mandibular swing

102-7

Digastric m. (cut)

Hypoglossal n. preserved

Retropharyngeal nodes

Lingual a. ligated

Posterolateral pharyngeal cancer

Posterior ⅓ of thyroid cartilage resected

Inferior vertical pharyngotomy

102-8

Jugulodigastric nodes

Jugulo-omohyoid nodes

■ *103.* PHARYNGEAL RECONSTRUCTION

Procedures used to replace the pharyngeal tissues removed during resection. The donor tissues used in these procedures include skin grafts, skin flaps, stomach, and free flaps of skin, muscle, or jejunum.

Indications

1. Local and regional defects produced by resection of benign and malignant lesions

Special Considerations

1. Reconstruction materials should emulate local tissues.
2. The pharynx is a dynamic structure that must remain pliable after reconstruction.

Preoperative Preparation

1. Donor sites require preoperative preparation such as Phisohex washes for skin sites and small bowel preparation for jejunal autografts.
2. Prepare for two teams working simultaneously, if possible.

Special Instruments, Position, and Anesthesia

1. Microvascular instruments and microscope
2. Stapler for intestinal anastomoses
3. Dermatome for skin grafts
4. Separate scrub team for abdominal and microvascular work

Tips and Pearls

1. Use primary closure for T1 lesions only.
2. Reconstruction should provide abundant donor tissue that allows adequate pharyngeal, laryngeal, and tongue movement during deglutition.
3. Use meticulous suturing technique for watertight closure.
4. Provide additional support for all flaps and grafts to prevent shearing forces and pulling at recipient sites.
5. Protect microvascular anastomoses and prevent kinking of vessels.

(continued)

Operative Procedure

The choice of reconstruction technique after pharyngectomy is determined primarily by the amount and location of resection and secondarily by the overall status of the patient. Small lateral oropharyngeal and superior pyriform fossa defects may be closed primarily. Small posterior pharyngeal wall defects may be closed by suturing the edges of the mucosal defect to the prevertebral fascia. Larger defects in the posterior pharynx, but still limited to the posterior wall, may be assisted with closure by using split-thickness skin grafts on the prevertebral muscles. Larger defects must be closed with composite tissues.

Regional Skin Flaps

The pectoralis myocutaneous or myofascial flap (see Procedure 250) is the choice for single-staged skin flap reconstruction of the pharynx or pharyngoesophagus. I prefer to use the myofascial flap for lateral wall reconstruction, because it results in less bulk than the myocutaneous flap. This flap in any of its forms is adequate in patients who are not candidates for intraabdominal or free flap surgery. With or without the skin paddle, the flap must be elevated from the chest wall and passed through an abundant tunnel under the neck skin that does not compress the vascular pedicle. The skin of the upper chest should be protected for use as a deltopectoral flap if later coverage or backup is required. This necessitates protecting the internal mammary perforating vessels medially and using a horizontal chest incision instead of the traditional vertical or oblique incision, which would transect the potential deltopectoral flap (Fig. 103-1).

At the recipient site, the mucosal edges of the remaining pharyngeal mucosa are stitched directly to the muscle using a 3-0 Vicryl suture. The trailing bulk of the flap is supported in the neck, to prevent tension on the pharyngeal suture line, with multiple sutures placed in the strap muscles medially and the scalene muscles laterally (Fig. 103-2).

Free Composite Skin Flaps

The radial forearm free flap (see Procedure 265) provides the most useful skin for pharyngeal reconstruction because it is pliable and thin. It is excellent for defects involving the lateral and posterior pharyngeal walls. Other donor sites to be considered include the lower abdominal wall and the lateral thigh region. Following the concept of the myofascial flap, any free muscle flap, including the gracilis or rectus abdominis (see Procedure 268) muscles, may be used. All free flaps mentioned in this section require that the microvascular team begin harvesting the flap when the primary resection is begun to have it ready for transfer at the appropriate time.

The free flap vasculature is anastomosed to the recipient vessels first, and the anastomotic site is stabilized. The flap itself is then sutured into position as any other flap. The only difference is that provision must be made for protection of the vascular pedicle to prevent compression or kinking (Fig. 103-3).

Free Jejunal Autograft

I think that the jejunum provides the best material for pharyngeal reconstruction available (see Procedure 269). The general and microvascular surgeons together harvest the flap as the primary resection is taking place. It may be used as a large patch for replacement of one or more of the pharyngeal walls, or it may be maintained in part as a tubular structure for replacement of part or all of the pharynx and the cervical esophagus. The same principles and technique apply after the microvascular anastomoses are completed as for other free flaps, except for the preparation of the jejunum. I place the jejunum in a kidney basin and resect the stapled tissues at each end that are used in the jejunal resection. A bulb syringe is then used to irrigate the lumen with antibiotic-containing saline. If the jejunum is to be used as a patch, it is incised along its antimesenteric border and opened completely. After it is trimmed to size, it is sutured in place as with the other flaps (Fig. 103-4). If it is used for combined pharyngeal and cervical esophageal replacement, only its upper portion is opened, and the lower portion is maintained as a tubular structure. The lower anastomosis must be located above the thoracic inlet (Fig. 103-5).

(continued)

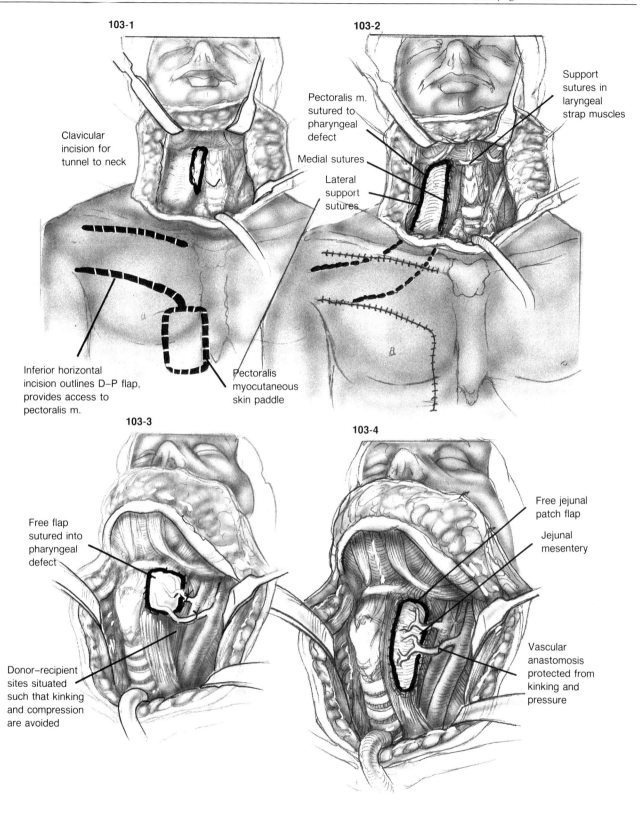

103-1

Clavicular incision for tunnel to neck

Inferior horizontal incision outlines D–P flap, provides access to pectoralis m.

Pectoralis myocutaneous skin paddle

103-2

Pectoralis m. sutured to pharyngeal defect

Medial sutures

Lateral support sutures

Support sutures in laryngeal strap muscles

103-3

Free flap sutured into pharyngeal defect

Donor–recipient sites situated such that kinking and compression are avoided

103-4

Free jejunal patch flap

Jejunal mesentery

Vascular anastomosis protected from kinking and pressure

■ *103.* PHARYNGEAL RECONSTRUCTION
(continued)

Pitfalls and Complications
1. Salivary fistulas
2. Anastomotic stenoses
3. Rigidity and tethering of adjacent structures
4. Donor site complications

Postoperative Care Issues
1. Provide excellent enteral nutrition and hydration over a prolonged period.
2. Rest the reconstruction site until healed, usually 2 to 3 weeks, before orally feeding the patient.
3. Deal with special issues concerning the donor site.

References

Coleman JJ, Searles JMJ, Hester TR, et al. Ten years' experience with the free jejunal autograft. Am J Surg 1987;154:394.

Schechter GL, Baker J, El Mahdi A, Bumatay J. Gastric pullup. Combined treatment for advanced cancer of the laryngopharynx and cervical esophagus. Laryngoscope 1982;92:11.

Takato T, Kiyonori I. Oral and pharyngeal reconstruction using the free forearm flap. Arch Otolaryngol 1987;113:873.

Gastric Pullup

The gastric pullup is only used when laryngopharyngoesophagectomy is performed and the inferior line of resection is below the thoracic inlet. The general thoracic surgeon must begin to mobilize the stomach during the primary tumor resection. The initial steps involve releasing the duodenum with a Kocher maneuver, ligating the vasculature along the greater curvature and at the superior aspect of the lesser curve, and starting the blunt dissection of the esophagus in the posterior mediastinum. The final phase of the primary resection in the neck involves beginning the blunt esophageal dissection from above. Eventually, the blunt esophageal dissection is carried out from above and below simultaneously by one surgeon.

The esophagus is transected at the gastroesophageal junction using a stapling device, and it is removed, leaving a long heavy silk tracer suture that is used to pull the stomach through the mediastinum after it has been manually stretched and placed in a plastic pouch to ease the friction. Once up into the neck, the gastric pouch is slowly pulled toward the pharyngeal defect, and traction sutures are placed at each leading corner (Fig. 103-6). A "smile incision" is then made in its anterior surface, creating a longer posterior flap for extension into the pharynx (Fig. 103-7). If there is need to bring the posterior pharyngeal mucosa down to meet this posterior gastric flap, a deep transverse relaxing incision may be made at the nasooropharyngeal juncture (see Fig. 103-7). The posterior suture line is completed first using interrupted 3-0 Vicryl sutures. As the suturing continues laterally and anteriorly, the tongue base is drawn down to the anterior wall of the stomach pouch for final closure (Fig. 103-8). A nasogastric tube is placed into the stomach pouch for drainage, and continuous suction catheters are placed near, but not against, the anastomosis before closing the skin flaps.

GARY L. SCHECHTER

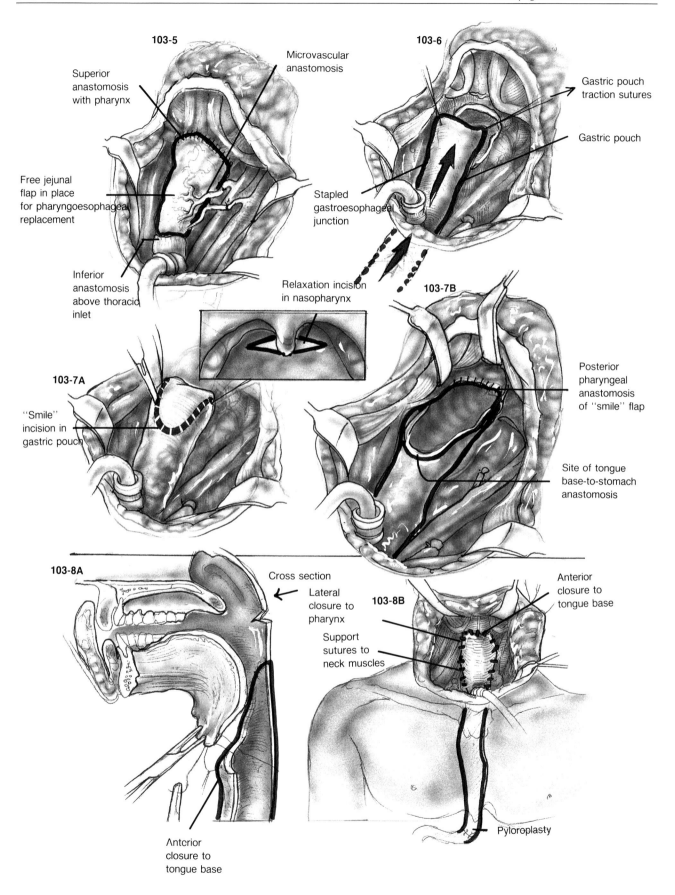

103-5

Superior
anastomosis
with pharynx

Microvascular
anastomosis

Free jejunal
flap in place
for pharyngoesophageal
replacement

Inferior
anastomosis
above thoracic
inlet

Stapled
gastroesophageal
junction

103-6

Gastric pouch
traction sutures

Gastric pouch

Relaxation incision
in nasopharynx

103-7A

"Smile"
incision in
gastric pouch

103-7B

Posterior
pharyngeal
anastomosis
of "smile" flap

Site of tongue
base-to-stomach
anastomosis

103-8A

Cross section

Lateral
closure to
pharynx

Support
sutures to
neck muscles

103-8B

Anterior
closure to
tongue base

Anterior
closure to
tongue base

Pyloroplasty

■ *104.* THYROGLOSSAL DUCT CYST

Excision of a thyroglossal duct cyst, excising remnants of tissue along the thyroid gland's migration from the foramen cecum to the lower neck and commonly involving the hyoid bone

Indications

1. Infection that may lead to abscess formation or septicemia
2. Mass effects, including pain, dysphagia, and dyspnea
3. Cosmetic efects of a mass

Contraindications

1. A relative contraindication is a cyst representing the only functioning thyroid tissue.
2. Acute infection, which should be treated before surgical excision
3. Bleeding disorder
4. Medical contraindications to general anesthesia

Special Considerations

1. A cyst with a sinus tract requires excision of the entire tract, including an ellipse around its opening.
2. Previous attempts at excision require wider and deeper surgical margins, including the center section of the hyoid bone.

Preoperative Preparation

1. Examine the area midline or just lateral to the midline. A pathognomonic sign is vertical motion of the mass with swallowing or tongue protrusion.
2. Imaging studies that may be helpful include ultrasound (ie, shows cystic nature), computed tomography scan, or magnetic resonance scan. A radioactive thyroid scan may be indicated only for children without a palpable thyroid gland to determine if the cyst contains the patient's only functional thyroid tissue.
3. Fine-needle aspiration biopsy can be considered.
4. Antibiotics to resolve acute infections before excision

Special Instrumentation, Position, and Anesthesia

1. Bone-cutting forceps or heavy scissors to cut hyoid bone

Tips and Pearls

1. Always examine the patient for a thyroglossal duct opening on the lingual wall of the vallecula in the region of the foramen cecum.
2. Use two horizontal incisions for fistulas or tracts.
3. Incise along the superior border of the hyoid bone with the duct visualized to prevent transecting it and losing its identity.
4. Always remove the midportion of the hyoid bone, and never reapproximate the ends.
5. Send a frozen-section specimen from all solid masses for histologic analysis.

Pitfalls and Complications

1. Injury to the superior laryngeal and hypoglossal nerves is possible but rare.
2. Incomplete excision leads to a complicated repeat operation.
3. Infection
4. Hematoma

Postoperative Care Issues

1. Send the pathology specimen to detect concomitant neoplastic disease, especially if the patient has a history of neck irradiation.
2. Drain the surgical site at the corner of the wound.
3. Continue intravenous fluids and give nothing orally for 48 hours if the pharynx was entered.
4. Check the patient for an adequate airway, because hematoma may compromise it.
5. Assess the voice quality.
6. Prophylactic antibiotics, especially if the indication for removal was infection

References

Lee KJ, Klein TR. Surgery of cysts and tumors of the neck. 2nd ed. In: Paparella MM, Shumrick DA, eds. Otolaryngology. Philadelphia: W B Saunders, 1980;2991.

Pincus RL. Congenital neck masses and cysts. In: Bailey B, ed. Head and Neck Surgery—Otolaryngology. Philadelphia: JB Lippincott, 1993;755.

Operative Procedure

The patient is positioned on the operating table in the prone position, with the head extended. General anesthesia rather than local anesthesia is advisable, because the excision may extend deeply into the tongue's base. Nasotracheal intubation is unnecessary; an oral tube is quite satisfactory. The surgical field is scrubbed from the clavicles to the lips. Sterile drapes are placed to provide easy identification and palpation of neck landmarks, such as the thyroid notch. The skin incision is placed in accordance with the location of the cyst (Fig. 104-1).

In the typical case, a single transverse incision is made at or just below the level of the hyoid bone and is carried down through the subcutaneous tissue and platysma muscle (Fig. 104-2). A short, superiorly based flap can be developed to provide better exposure. Occasionally, a cyst has a long duct that may require a second incision lower in the neck. This is usually not recognized until the dissection has begun.

Sharp and blunt dissection are used to identify the cyst, which may be found adherent to the hyoid bone, completely surrounding it, or deep in the tongue musculature beneath the bone. Care should be taken to avoid entering the cyst or cutting across the tract, which would make the lesion much more difficult to dissect from the surrounding soft tissues. Before proceeding too far into the depths of the tongue's base, bone-cutting forceps should be used to release the center section of the hyoid bone (Fig. 104-3). This can facilitate the remainder of the excision by allowing the surgeon to grasp the bone and pull the specimen upward and outward as the dissection proceeds (Fig. 104-4). Using a combination of blunt and sharp dissection, the surgeon can get around the entire cyst or follow its tract down to the foramen cecum, where entry into the vallecula and excision of a small area of mucosa can be accomplished if necessary.

The tongue's vascularity makes postoperative bleeding or hematoma one of the more common complications. Electrocautery can be used on small bleeders and silk ties on the larger ones. In this area of the neck, surgery in the midline is relatively safe from injury to important nerves, although the superior laryngeal nerves could be inadvertently injured while cutting the hyoid bone. Injury or lysis of a hypoglossal nerve is unlikely, except in cases of very large cysts or a second operation.

Closure is done from inside out. Absorbable sutures are used to close the dead space in the tongue musculature. Specific closure of the vallecula mucosa is not necessary if the hole is small and the tongue musculature is reapproximated. However, some type of drain should be used. I prefer a 0.25- to 0.5-in (6- to 13-mm) Penrose drain, but a suction-type drain may be acceptable, but it can have an air leak if the vallecula was entered. The platysma and subcutaneous tissues are closed with absorbable 3-0 or 4-0 interrupted sutures and the skin with a running subcuticular Prolene suture. After the drain is secured and the dressing applied, the patient is awakened in the operating room, extubated, and taken to the recovery room.

CHARLES M. STIERNBERG

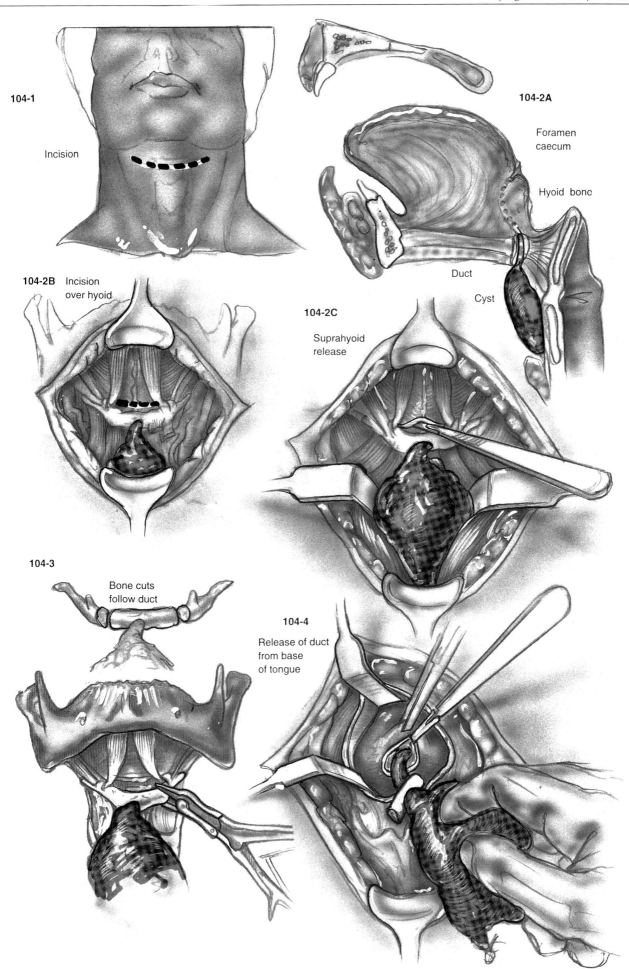

104-1

Incision

104-2A

Foramen
caecum

Hyoid bone

Duct

Cyst

104-2B Incision
over hyoid

104-2C

Suprahyoid
release

104-3

Bone cuts
follow duct

104-4

Release of duct
from base
of tongue

■ 105. BRANCHIAL CLEFT CYSTS

Excision of a branchial cleft cyst, excising remnants of the embryologic branchial clefts, most commonly of the second cleft and less commonly the first, third, or fourth

Indications

1. Infection that may lead to septicemia or abscess formation
2. Mass effects, including pain, dysphagia, stridor, and dyspnea
3. Cosmetic effects of a mass or draining fistula
4. Rule out the possibility of neoplastic disease

Special Considerations

1. Cervical cysts that are infected at presentation can be misdiagnosed as a simple neck abscess.
2. Incision and drainage alone are not adequate treatment. The entire cyst and its tract must be removed to prevent recurrence.
3. Cysts can enlarge rapidly after an upper respiratory tract infection, or they can develop slowly over several weeks or months and be unrelated to an infection. Otorrhea and otalgia are sometimes associated with a first cleft cyst.
4. Location of the cyst depends on the cleft from which it is derived. First cleft cysts may appear on the lateral side of the face anterior to the ear, or they may arise just below the angle of the mandible. Second and third cleft cysts occur in the neck anterior to the anterior edge of the sternocleidomastoid muscle. Fistula openings in the skin can also be present for any of these clefts.

Preoperative Preparation

1. The extent of disease can be delineated by ultrasound (ie, shows cystic nature), computed tomography, magnetic resonance imaging, and radiopaque dyes injected into the fistula tracts.
2. Preoperative antibiotics to resolve acute infection, if possible, before resecting the cysts

Special Instrumentation, Position, and Anesthesia

1. No special surgical instruments are required.

Tips and Pearls

1. When a cyst is infected, intravenous antibiotics should be administered and a drainage procedure avoided if possible. Incision and drainage make removal of the cyst at a later date much more difficult.
2. A preauricular pit may signal the presence of a first branchial cleft cyst. Excise the entire tract through cartilage to the external auditory canal, and be prepared to perform total parotidectomy with facial nerve dissection.
3. For second, third, and fourth branchial cleft cysts, use horizontal incisions in the neck creases for best cosmetic results. "Step ladder" parallel incisions may be necessary for resecting a tract that cannot be reached through one incision.
4. Avoid rupturing the cyst during excision. Do not use forceps with teeth.

Pitfalls and Complications

1. Cranial nerves IX, X, XI, and XII are at risk for injury during surgical excision of second and third cleft cysts. The seventh cranial nerve is exposed to possible injury during excision of a first cleft cyst. Care must also be taken in dissections around the superior laryngeal nerve. A third branchial cleft cyst can have a fistulous tract that penetrates the thyrohyoid membrane near this nerve.
2. Recurrence is certain if the entire tract is not excised.

Postoperative Care

1. The wound should be drained with a Penrose or suction drain.
2. Check the airway and cranial nerves postoperatively.
3. Perioperative antibiotics may be necessary if the cyst has been infected or the aerodigestive tract is entered during the resection.

References

Pincus RL. Congenital neck masses and cysts. In: Bailey BJ, ed. Head and neck surgery—otolaryngology. Philadelphia: JB Lippincott, 1993;1:482.

Operative Procedure

The patient is positioned on the operating table in a supine position, with the head extended and turned to provide best exposure of the cyst. General anesthesia rather than local anesthesia is required, because dissection can be extensive. The surgical field should include the entire ipsilateral neck, the auricle, and the lateral side of the face if a first branchial cleft cyst is suspected. Sterile drapes are placed to provide easy identification and palpation of landmarks, such as the mandibular angle. The skin incision is placed in accordance with the location of the cyst, preferably in a natural skin crease. It should also be designed to remove any skin opening to a fistula. This can sometimes require a second parallel incision lower in the neck (Fig. 105-1). Such fistulas are often seen as punctate openings in the skin and can be draining or dry. For a first branchial cleft cyst, the incision's design should allow the surgeon to perform parotidectomy.

The cyst, which is deep to the superficial fascia, is usually easily identified after the dissection is carried down through the subcutaneous tissue and platysma muscle (Fig. 105-2). If infection has occurred, the cyst can be quite adherent to adjacent structures. Care should be taken to avoid entering the cyst or cutting across its tract, because this makes the lesion much more difficult to trace and dissect. After the cyst has been mobilized from the surrounding soft tissues, the surgeon can usually identify a tract, which should be followed as far as possible (Fig. 105-3). Here is where a second "step ladder" incision can be beneficial. The tract for a second branchial cleft cyst typically arches over the ninth cranial nerve and enters the tonsillar fossa. A third branchial cleft cyst has a tract that pierces the thyrohyoid membrane or piriform sinus (Fig. 105-4). For a first branchial cleft cyst, however, the tract can course through the parotid gland and open into the ear canal. Knowledge of embryologic development of these cysts and their tracts facilitates dissection.

The primary intraoperative complication to avoid is injuring cranial nerves. This can be achieved by having good exposure during dissection. Meticulous hemostasis using electrocautery and ties helps prevent postoperative hematoma or seroma, but a drain should also be used. Closure of the wound begins with absorbable sutures for closing any dead space left in the soft tissues of the neck. I prefer a 0.25- to 0.5-in (6- to 13-mm) Penrose drain, but a suction-type drain is acceptable. The platysma and subcutaneous tissues are closed with absorbable 3-0 or 4-0 interrupted sutures, and the skin is closed with a running subcuticular Prolene suture. After the drain is secured and the dressing applied, the patient is awakened in the operating room, extubated, and taken to the recovery room.

CHARLES M. STIERNBERG

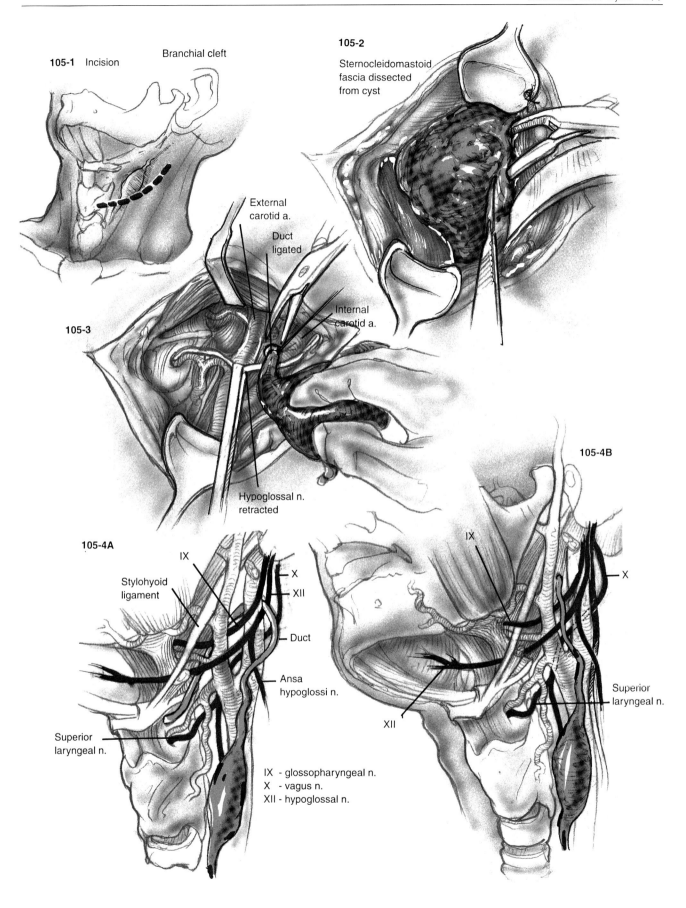

105-1   Incision

Branchial cleft

105-2
Sternocleidomastoid
fascia dissected
from cyst

105-3

External
carotid a.

Duct
ligated

Internal
carotid a.

Hypoglossal n.
retracted

105-4B

105-4A

IX

X

XII

Stylohyoid
ligament

Duct

Ansa
hypoglossi n.

Superior
laryngeal n.

IX

X

XII

Superior
laryngeal n.

IX - glossopharyngeal n.
X - vagus n.
XII - hypoglossal n.

■ 106. LYMPHANGIOMA

Removal of a lymphangioma is achieved by the excision of the congenital cystic lymphatic structures formed by aberrant development or obstruction of the normal lymphatic system. Also known as cystic hygromas, these cystic structures may occur anywhere in the lymphatic system but are usually found in the neck.

Indications

1. Infection can progress to abscess formation. Excision should be performed after appropriate antibiotic treatment.
2. Mass effects can distort and obstruct the jugular vein, carotid arteries, and vagus nerve. They may also cause pain, dysphagia, dyspnea, or stridor.
3. Hemorrhage into these cystic structures can cause rapid enlargement.
4. Cosmesis

Contraindications

1. Bleeding disorder
2. Other medical contraindications to general anesthesia

Special Considerations

1. Lymphangiomas are commonly far more extensive than is initially appreciated on physical examination.
2. An important surgical principal is preservation of normal structures of the neck.
3. Recurrence is common.

Preoperative Preparation

1. The most common chief complaint is a neck mass, which can fluctuate in size, especially enlarging during upper respiratory tract infections.
2. Physical examination reveals a soft, cystic, multiloculated mass that can be transilluminated.
3. Helpful studies include ultrasound (ie, shows cystic nature), computed tomography, and magnetic resonance imaging.
4. Preoperative antibiotics can resolve acute infections before excision.

Special Instrumentation, Position, and Anesthesia

1. No special surgical instruments are required.

Tips and Pearls

1. Use two horizontal step incisions if necessary for adequate exposure.
2. Avoid rupturing the cysts during resection.

Pitfalls and Complications

1. Cranial nerves VII, X, XI, and XII and the superior laryngeal nerve are particularly susceptible to injury.
2. Incomplete excision or recurrence may lead to a more complicated repeat operation.
3. Wound infection
4. Hematoma or seroma

Postoperative Care Issues

1. Drain the wound.
2. Check patient's airway and voice postoperatively.

References

Kennedy TL. Cystic hygroma—lymphangioma: a rare and still unclear entity. Laryngoscope 1989;99(Suppl 49):1.

Lee KJ, Klein TR. Surgery of cysts and tumors of the neck. In: Paparella MM, Shumrick DA, eds. Otolaryngology. 2nd ed, vol 3. Philadelphia: WB Saunders, 1980;2988.

Operative Procedure

The patient is positioned on the operating table in the prone position, with the head extended and turned to get the best exposure of the lesion. General anesthesia rather than local anesthesia is essential unless the lymphangioma is very small and the patient is an adult. The surgeon should be aware, however, that these lesions are frequently much larger and more extensive than they appear on the surface. They often wrap around structures in the neck and can penetrate deeply into muscles. The surgical field is scrubbed and draped in a manner that allows easy palpation of landmarks and an additional incision if it becomes necessary. The skin incision is horizontal, but its exact design and placement depends on the location of the lymphangioma (Fig. 106-1). The lesions may be in the posterior or anterior triangles and extend to the midline or deeply into the tongue musculature. The initial incision is carried down through the subcutaneous tissue and platysma muscle. A short superiorly based flap can be helpful in obtaining exposure and may avoid a second parallel incision.

Lymphangiomas are usually obvious after the neck is opened. They are multiloculated, fluid filled, and envelop nerves, vessels, and muscles (Fig. 106-2). By necessity, dissection is most often slow and tedious, because the lymphangioma walls tear easily. Sharp and blunt dissection are used to expose and dissect the cyst, which may be found wrapping around various structures in the neck. Despite this difficulty, an important principle is preservation of normal structures (Figs. 106-3 and 106-4).

Potential complications are mostly those that are common to any procedure in the neck. Postoperative hematoma is possible and can be avoided by meticulous attention to hemostasis. Electrocautery can be used on small bleeding vessels and silk ties used on the larger ones. Unfortunately, recurrence is a common complication and probably reflects the difficulty in resecting these lesions.

Absorbable sutures are used to close any dead space left by the resection. Some type of drain should be used. I prefer a 0.25- to 0.5-in (6- to 13-mm) Penrose drain, but a suction-type drain is acceptable. The platysma and subcutaneous tissues are closed with absorbable 3-0 or 4-0 interrupted sutures, and the skin is closed with a running subcuticular Prolene suture. After the drain is secured and the dressing applied, the patient is awakened in the operating room, extubated, and taken to the recovery room.

CHARLES M. STIERNBERG

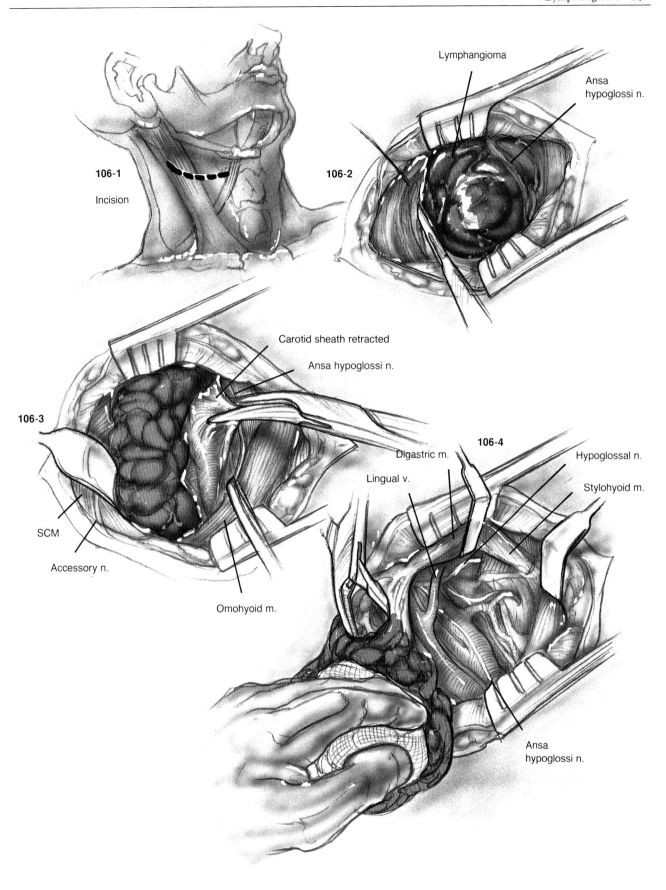

106-1

Incision

106-2

Lymphangioma

Ansa hypoglossi n.

106-3

Carotid sheath retracted

Ansa hypoglossi n.

SCM

Accessory n.

Omohyoid m.

106-4

Digastric m.

Lingual v.

Hypoglossal n.

Stylohyoid m.

Ansa hypoglossi n.

■ *107.* DERMOID CYST OF THE NECK

Excision of a benign cystic mass that has differentiated from pluri-potential embryonal cells of at least two of the three germinal layers. These aberrant cysts can occur anywhere in the body, but more than 10% arise in the head and neck.

Indications

1. Infection
2. Mass effects causing dysphagia
3. Cosmesis

Special Considerations

1. Differential diagnoses include thyroglossal duct cyst, epidermal inclusion cyst, and sebaceous cyst

Preoperative Preparation

1. A painless, slow-growing mass, usually in the midline of the sub-mental triangle when occurring in the neck.
2. The usually firm mass can have a fistulous tract with an opening to the skin. It does not elevate when the patient swallows.
3. X-ray studies can show calcifications or tooth-like structures. A computed tomography scan may be used to delineate its extent.

Special Instrumentation, Position, and Anesthesia

1. No special surgical instruments are needed.

Tips and Pearls

1. Cysts lie deep to the cervical fascia and contain sebaceous material on biopsy.
2. Keep the curved incision well below the edge of the mandible to avoid cranial nerve VII.
3. Use sharp dissection to remove the cyst.

Pitfalls and Complications

1. Recurrence
2. Infection
3. Hematoma or seroma

Postoperative Care Issues

1. Pathologic examination of the specimen to rule out a neoplasm
2. A small surgical drain to avoid hematoma or seroma is removed in 24 hours.

References

McGuirt WF. Differential diagnosis of neck masses. 2nd ed. In: Cummings CW, Schuller DE, eds. Otolaryngology—head and neck surgery. St. Louis: Mosby-Year Book, 1993:1551.

Maran AGD. Benign diseases of the neck. In: Kerr AG, Evans JNG, eds. Scott-Brown's otolaryngology. 5th ed. Boston: Butterworth, 1987: 295.

Operative Procedure

The patient is positioned on the operating table in the supine position, with the head extended for best exposure of the cyst. General or local anesthesia can be used, although general anesthesia is best for children. The surgical field is scrubbed from the clavicles to the lips. Sterile drapes are placed to provide easy identification and palpation of neck landmarks, such as the thyroid notch. The skin incision is placed in accordance with the location of the cyst, which can vary but is usually in the midline of the submental triangle (Fig. 107-1).

In the typical case, a single transverse incision is made and is carried down through the subcutaneous tissue and platysma muscle. If the dermoid cyst is large, a short superiorly based flap can be developed to provide better exposure. If a fistula exists, it should be excised en bloc with the cyst and an elliptical area of skin around its opening.

Sharp and blunt dissection are used to identify the cyst, which may be adherent to the hyoid bone (Fig. 107-2). Care should be taken to avoid entering the cyst, which would make the lesion much more difficult to dissect from the surrounding soft tissues (Fig. 107-3). Postoperative bleeding or hematoma can be avoided by meticulous hemostasis using electrocautery and ties. In this area of the neck, surgery in the midline is relatively safe from injury to important nerves. If the cyst is off center, however, a superior laryngeal or hypoglossal nerve could be injured inadvertently (Fig. 107-4).

Closure is begun with absorbable sutures for closure of the dead space that is left after removal of the cyst. A drain should be placed to help prevent a postoperative hematoma or seroma. I prefer a 0.25- to 0.5-in (6- to 13-mm) Penrose drain, but a suction-type drain is acceptable (Fig. 107-5). The platysma and subcutaneous tissues are closed with absorbable 3-0 or 4-0 interrupted sutures, and the skin is closed with a running subcuticular Prolene suture (see Fig. 107-3). After the drain is secured and the dressing applied, the patient is awakened in the operating room, extubated, and taken to the recovery room.

CHARLES M. STIERNBERG

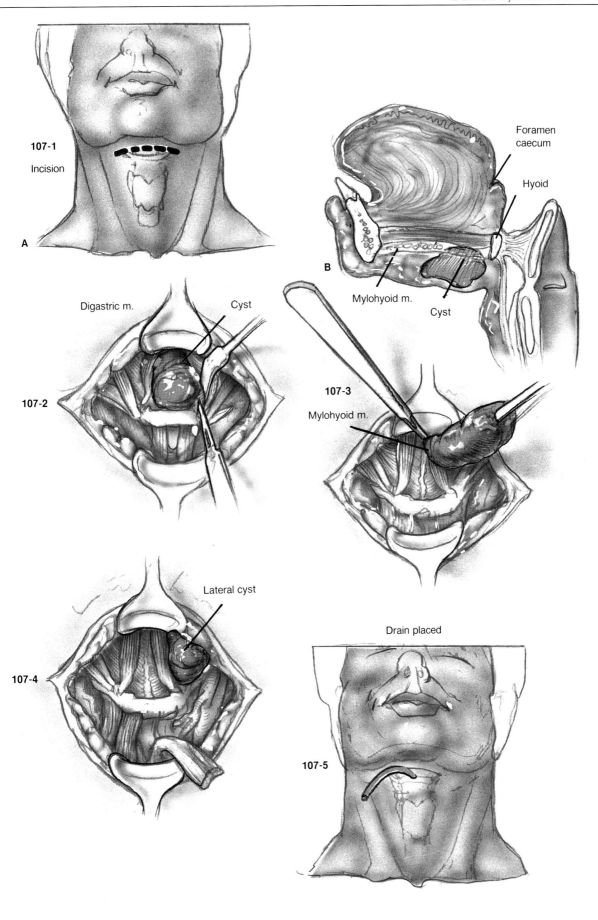

107-1

Incision

A

Foramen
caecum

Hyoid

B

Mylohyoid m.

Cyst

Digastric m.   Cyst

107-2

107-3

Mylohyoid m.

Lateral cyst

107-4

Drain placed

107-5

■ 108. EXCISION OF LARYNGOCELE

Removal of laryngocele, an air-filled dilatation of the saccule of the laryngeal ventricle. An internal laryngocele is a cystic dilatation confined within larynx, and an external laryngocele is a cyst that perforates through the thyrohyoid membrane and occurs primarily in the soft tissues of the neck. A combined laryngocele is a dumbbell cyst, with significant internal and external components and its connection "neck" at the thyrohyoid membrane.

Indications
1. Symptoms
2. Infections, such as laryngopyocele
3. Suspicion of malignancy

Special Considerations
1. Internal or external laryngocele
2. Entire cyst to be excised
3. Avoiding superior laryngeal nerve injury
4. Tracheotomy unnecessary
5. Laryngoscopy to be certain no partially obstructing ventricular mass

Preoperative Preparation
1. Laryngoscopy, fiberoptic and rigid
2. Routine laboratory studies
3. Imaging studies
4. Oscillating saw for a large internal component
5. Shoulders on roll, neck extended, and head stabilized on a doughnut

Tips and Pearls
1. Sac dissection facilitated by cotton-tipped applicator sticks
2. Lateral thyrotomy eases internal dissection and avoids potential blunting of the anterior commissure.

Pitfalls and Complications
1. Failure to recognize cause of lesion
2. Unroofing or partial resection frequently causes a recurrence.
3. Penetration of laryngeal lumen may necessitate a tracheotomy.
4. Lateral dissection may injure the superior laryngeal nerve pedicle.

Postoperative Care Issues
1. Penrose drain left overnight
2. Observe for postoperative bleeding, airway compromise, or subcutaneous emphysema.

References
Holinger LD. Laryngocele and saccular cysts. Ann Otol Rhinol Laryngol 1970;87:675.
Komisar A. Laser laryngoscopic management of internal laryngocele. Laryngoscope 1987;97:368.
Yarington CT, Frazer JP. An approach to the internal laryngocele and other submucosal lesions of the larynx. Ann Otol Rhinol Laryngol 1966;75(4):956.

Operative Procedure

For the removal of an external laryngocele, the patient first undergoes direct laryngoscopy and biopsy of any suspicious ventricular lesion. Carcinoma is found in 2% to 18% of patients with laryngoceles. On the operating room table, the patient is then positioned supine, with the neck extended and turned to the side. An incision is outlined and crosshatched over the cystic lesion, in a skin crease, at or below the level of the hyoid bone (Fig. 108-1).

The incision is made and brought down through the platysma. Subplatysmal flaps are elevated and sewn to the drapes for retraction. The cyst is encountered anterior to the carotid sheath, which should be identified and protected from the dissection (Fig. 108-2). The strap muscles are retracted anteriorly. The soft tissues over the cyst are dissected until the cyst is completely identified (Fig. 108-3). The cyst is then traced to its neck at the thyrohyoid membrane. Care is taken to stay on the cyst wall. An applicator stick may facilitate this dissection. The cyst may perforate where the superior laryngeal nerve enters the larynx. The nerve should be identified and carefully preserved. The cyst is next traced through the thyrohyoid membrane. If there is no significant internal component, the larynx need not be entered. The stump is ligated (Fig. 108-4).

Small, isolated internal laryngoceles have been treated successfully with laser laryngoscopic excision. However, if there is a large, combined internal-external laryngocele or an isolated, large internal laryngocele, a lateral thyrotomy can facilitate the dissection. The sternohyoid muscle is incised at the upper border of the thyroid cartilage. The thyrohyoid muscle is retracted or similarly divided. The perichondrium along the upper border of the cartilage is incised to the thyroid notch. The perichondrium is reflected inferiorly with a peanut forceps and Freer elevator. The superior laryngeal nerve is identified and exposed. The elevated periosteum is sewn to the strap muscle with chromic suture as a stay to aid in later identification. The height of the larynx is measured. A point just above the midpoint is marked and connected to a point on the upper border of the thyroid cartilage just medial to the superior laryngeal nerve's entrance. A limited lateral thyrotomy is then made with an oscillating saw (Fig. 108-5). In children and some adults, a knife may suffice for these cuts. Care is taken to avoid entering the laryngeal lumen. Perforation may necessitate tracheotomy. The cartilage is then elevated. The internal laryngocele is identified (or the internal part of the combined laryngocele identified) in the paraglottic space. The tract is traced submucosally to its origin.

The perichondrium and strap muscles are closed in layers. A drain is placed.

ROBERT PINCUS

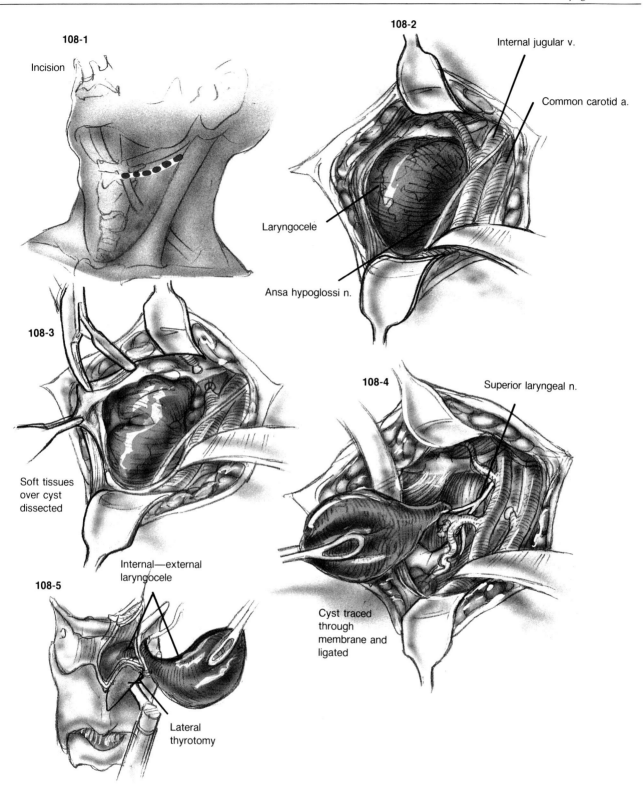

108-1

Incision

108-2

Internal jugular v.

Common carotid a.

Laryngocele

Ansa hypoglossi n.

108-3

Soft tissues
over cyst
dissected

108-4

Superior laryngeal n.

Cyst traced
through
membrane and
ligated

Internal—external
laryngocele

108-5

Lateral
thyrotomy

■ 109. CAROTID BODY TUMOR RESECTION

Surgical removal of the paraganglioma, which arises in the carotid bifurcation

Indications

1. A radiologically proven mass arising in the bifurcation of the carotid artery in any healthy patient younger than 60 years of age and in selected older patients
2. Deficits in ipsilateral cranial nerves IX, X, XI, and XII
3. Chronic pain

Special Considerations

1. Determination if the mass is a secreting tumor
2. For elderly, asymptomatic patients, observation alone may be adequate.
3. Angiographic evidence of adequate profusion across the circle of Willis
4. Greater likelihood of malignancy or multiple tumors in patients with positive family histories
5. Consideration of preoperative embolization of large tumors immediately before surgery

Preoperative Preparation

1. Routine laboratory studies
2. Urine catecholamine levels in hypertensive patients
3. Coagulation studies
4. Ipsilateral and contralateral arteriography with balloon occlusion of the ipsilateral carotid artery, if indicated
5. Immediate preoperative embolization in selected patients with large tumors

Special Instruments, Position, and Anesthesia

1. Headlight
2. Vascular clamps
3. Javid shunt

Tips and Pearls

1. Resection of the ipsilateral submandibular gland with large tumors to open the parapharyngeal space and increase visualization
2. Ligation of the external carotid system for large tumors
3. Identification of the hypoglossal nerve in the submandibular triangle
4. Identification of the spinal accessory nerve where it enters the sternocleidomastoid muscle
5. Dissection of the tumor in a subadventitial plane, starting superiorly at the site of cranial control of the carotid artery
6. Posterior to anterior dissection
7. Resection of all overlying lymphoid tissue (area 2 and perhaps area 3) before tumor resection

Pitfalls and Complications

1. Intense fibrosis and possible carotid artery injury from embolization earlier than immediately before surgery
2. Cranial nerve injury, especially cranial nerves X and XII

Postoperative Care Issues

1. Monitoring of neurologic status
2. Assessment of cranial nerve function
3. Early assessment of swallowing ability, with therapy as needed
4. Evaluation of the arteriography (groin) site if immediate preoperative embolization was done

References

LaMuraglia GM, et al. The current surgical management of carotid body paragangliomas. J Vasc Surg.

Wax MK, Briant TDR. Carotid body tumors: a review. J Otolaryngol 1992;21:277.

Williams MD, et al. Carotid body tumor. Arch Surg 1992;127:963.

Operative Procedure

The patient is prepped, draped, and positioned in standard fashion.

The incision extends from an area 2 cm below the mastoid tip in a curvilinear fashion anteriorly to the submental area (Fig. 109-1). It can be extended to a lip-splitting incision if needed. After dividing skin, subcutaneous tissue, and the platysma muscle, the fascia overlying the lower edge of the submandibular gland is identified and the dissection carried in a plane immediately over the submandibular gland, with attention directed toward visualization and preservation of the marginal mandibular branch of the facial nerve. Posteriorly, the incision is extended superiorly to the inferior aspect of the parotid gland, with the sternocleidomastoid muscle exposed all the way to the mastoid tip.

In large tumors, the submandibular gland is first removed. After the gland is removed, the hypoglossal nerve is found in the bed of the submandibular gland. Dissection is carried posteriorly along this nerve toward the carotid system. In small tumors, cranial nerve XII nerve is rarely adherent to the paraganglioma, but in larger tumors, the nerve must be carefully dissected from the neoplasm. In all cases, the sternocleidomastoid branch of the occipital artery is divided and ligated to allow the XIIth nerve to be displaced superiorly, facilitating dissection of the nerve away from the paraganglioma.

The next step in the surgery is to accomplish a Bocca-type functional neck dissection, removing all lymphoid tissue that overlies the tumor (Fig. 109-2). Proximal and distal control of the carotid artery is gained by carefully exposing the artery and placing vascular loops (Fig. 109-3).

If the tumor is especially large and abuts the skull base, the carotid is best exposed by first following the vagus nerve toward the skull base. With the vagus nerve freed from the tumor, attention is directed to the posterior aspect of the internal carotid near the skull base. After this artery is fully identified, a vascular loop is placed.

The paraganglioma is carefully dissected from adjacent vital structures. Superiorly and medially, branches of the external carotid artery are followed back toward the carotid body tumor and ligated where necessary to gain appropriate access to the paraganglioma. Posterosuperiorly, the previously identified internal carotid artery is carefully dissected free from the tumor. Typically, the posterior aspect of the artery can be identified, and by careful dissection of the adventitia of the artery, the internal carotid can be freed in almost its entire extent from the paraganglioma. The posterior dissection plane most typically is used, because carotid body tumors tend to be less adherent to the deep structures in this area. Injury to the sympathetic trunk or the already identified vagus nerve must be avoided.

Dissection is continued from posterosuperiorly toward the carotid bulb. Typically, branches of the external carotid system are encountered and can be divided. These vessels are controlled by 3-0 silk suture ligatures on the small branches and 2-0 silk suture ligatures on the larger branches.

As the dissection approaches the carotid bulb, care must be taken to gain control of several tiny branches coming from the deep area of the carotid bifurcation and extending directly into the paraganglioma. These vessels are identified by dissection in a subadventitial plain carried very cautiously forward with Lincoln scissors. Hemostasis is ensured with 3-0 silk suture ligatures.

The dissection of the paraganglioma off the carotid system depends on carefully following the subadventitial plane of the arteries (Fig. 109-4). In most cases, tumor vascularity extends beyond the bifurcation along the posterior aspect of the internal carotid artery. These small vessels can either be controlled with careful bipolar cautery or suture ligature.

After the paraganglioma is fully removed, the excisional bed is carefully irrigated with saline, hemostasis meticulously ensured, and an active drain (eg, 10-mm fully perforated Jackson-Pratt) is placed through a separate stab incision. Standard closure is then accomplished.

R. KIM DAVIS

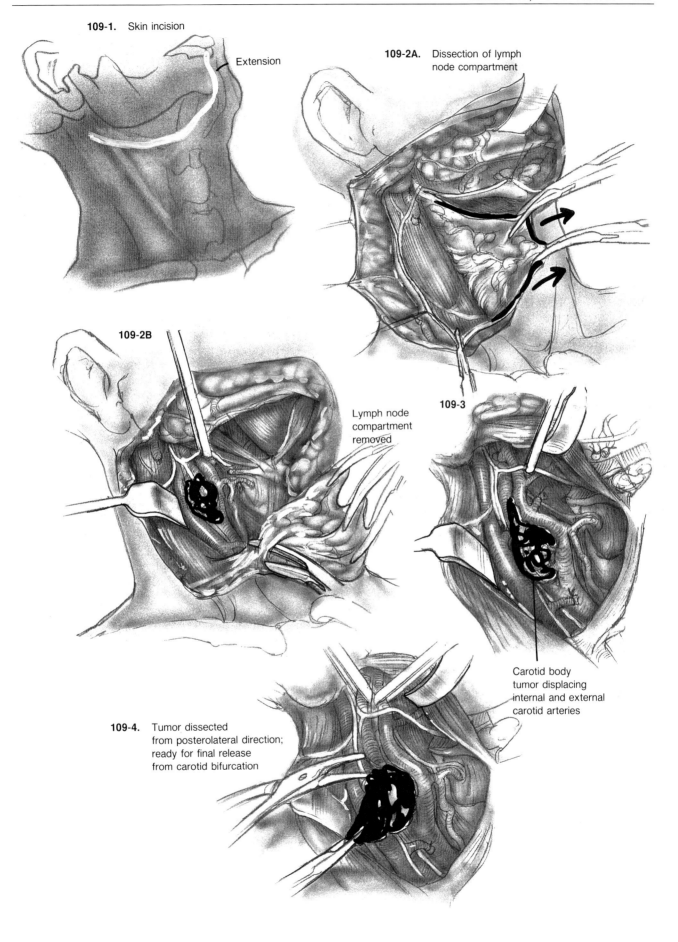

109-1. Skin incision

Extension

109-2A. Dissection of lymph node compartment

109-2B

Lymph node compartment removed

109-3

Carotid body tumor displacing internal and external carotid arteries

109-4. Tumor dissected from posterolateral direction; ready for final release from carotid bifurcation

■ *110.* EXTERNAL CAROTID ARTERY LIGATION—Obliteration of artery supplying main vasculature to head and neck, excluding the brain

Indications

1. Control of bleeding from branches of the external carotid artery distal to the site of ligation
2. Diminishment of blood supply to the area of the tumor bed as adjunctive procedure prior to tumor resection
3. Involvement of vessel or major branches in tumor

Special Considerations

1. Internal carotid artery does not branch in neck, except for rare exceptions
2. Patency of internal carotid artery should be assured prior to external carotid artery ligation to avoid interruption of collateral flow through ophthalmic artery
3. May fail for control of posterior epistaxis due to distance from bleeding site and possible vascular contributions from other vessels

Preoperative Preparation

1. Routine laboratory studies
2. Blood products to be available in patient with hemorrhage
3. If arteriogram contemplated, should be done prior to surgery
4. Vascular imaging may be helpful.

Special Instruments, Position, and Anesthesia

1. Headlight
2. Vascular loops and sutures
3. Vascular clamps
4. 1% lidocaine without epinephrine for infiltration of carotid bulb, if necessary
5. Shoulder on roll, neck extended, head on doughnut
6. General anesthesia (local when necessary)

Tips and Pearls

1. Obtain control of the common carotid artery below bifurcation.
2. Follow the external carotid artery to its second branch, at least.
3. The external carotid artery is usually anterior and more superficial, but not always.
4. Bradycardia is common with carotid bulb manipulation; hypotension may be suggestive of a vascular event.
5. Be certain the vagus nerve, internal jugular vein, hypoglossal nerve, and superior laryngeal nerve are identified and not violated.

Pitfalls and Complications

1. Persistence of bleeding due to collateral flow
2. Damage to other structures in head and neck
3. Propagation of thrombus due to manipulation of sclerotic vessels
4. Retrograde thrombus formation

Postoperative Care Issues

1. Primarily related to problem necessitating ligation

References

Hyde FT. Ligation of the external carotid artery for control of ideopathic nasal hemorrhage. Laryngoscope 1925;35:899.
Konno A, Togawa K, Iizuka K. Analysis of factors affecting complications of carotid artery ligation. Ann Otol Rhinol Laryngol 1981;90:222.

Operative Procedure

A horizontal skin incision is outlined and cross-hatched at the level of the hyoid bone and submandibular gland, 2 to 3 fingerbreadths below the angle of the mandible. The incision is placed in a skin crease (Fig. 110-1). The posterior third of the incision is over the sternocleidomastoid muscle (SCM). The incision is then carried down through skin and platysma, until the anterior border of the SCM is identified. The dissection is carried along the anterior border of the SCM. The anterior border of the SCM is retracted posteriorly and a clamp is used to dissect anterior the muscle, spreading parallel to the great vessels, being careful not to injure them. The carotid sheath is identified first inferiorly, by palpation.

Dissection is continued, spreading in the direction of the carotid artery until the carotid sheath is well identified. The common carotid artery is carefully separated from the other contents of the sheath. The internal jugular vein, ansa hypoglossi, and vagus nerve are retracted posteriorly. At this point I usually place a vascular loop loosely around the common carotid artery in case later control is essential. The dissection is carried up along the common carotid artery past the carotid bulb. If bradycardia ensues, 1% lidocaine without epinephrine may be injected into the areolar tissue around the bulb with a small-gauge needle.

At this point, the hypoglossal nerve is identified crossing the branches, and carefully preserved (Figs. 110-2 and 110-3). The external branch of the carotid artery is *usually* anterior and superficial to the internal branch. The internal carotid artery does not branch in the neck. The dissector must be certain that he or she has identified at least two branches of the vessel to be certain that it is the external carotid artery. If uncertain, dissection can be continued further superiorly. A 2-0 silk tie is placed between the first (superior thyroid artery) and second anterior branch (lingual artery) (Fig. 110-4). In cases of vascular resection for tumor, the vessel is double tied inferiorly, prior to transection. Resection may also be done at more superior branches but is not recommended inferior to the first branch because of the risk of thrombus extending proximally.

The wound is then closed in layers after the vascular loop is removed from the common carotid artery. No drain is necessary.

ROBERT PINCUS

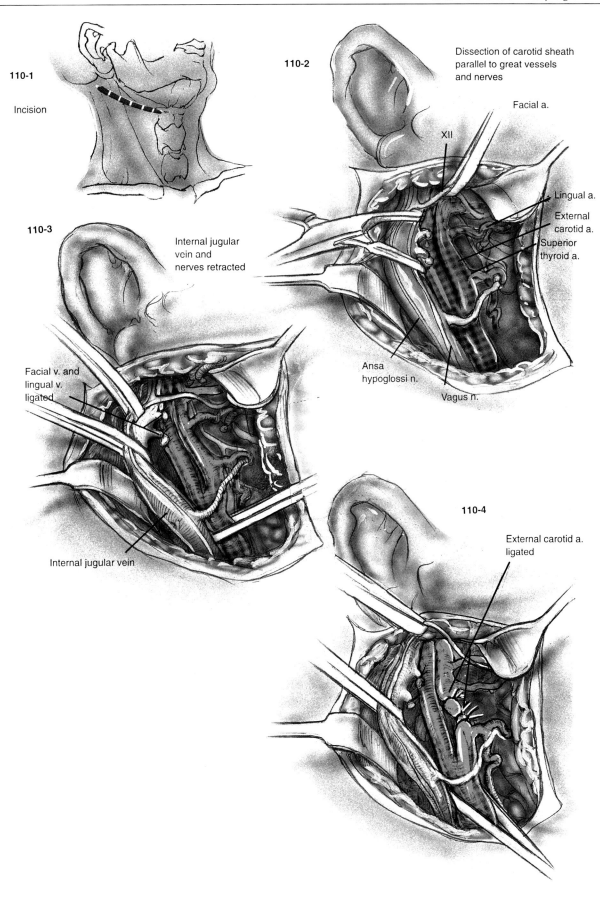

110-1

Incision

110-2

Dissection of carotid sheath
parallel to great vessels
and nerves

Facial a.

XII

Lingual a.

External
carotid a.

Superior
thyroid a.

Ansa
hypoglossi n.

Vagus n.

110-3

Internal jugular
vein and
nerves retracted

Facial v. and
lingual v.
ligated

Internal jugular vein

110-4

External carotid a.
ligated

■ *111.* LIPOMA EXCISION OR LIPOSUCTION

Removal of a benign adipose tissue mass in the neck. Although these benign neoplasms can occur anywhere in the head and neck region, they are usually in the posterior triangle, the supraclavicular triangle, or the occipital area.

Indications

1. Cosmesis (most common indication)
2. Mass effect, occasionally causing decreased mobility
3. Rule out possible malignancy

Preoperative Preparation

1. The patient's history indicates a painless, slow-growing mass.
2. The physical examination reveals a mass that is usually soft and mobile when palpated.
3. Plain radiographs are of limited use. Magnetic resonance imaging reveals a mass with the signal density of fat. A computed tomography scan shows a homogeneous mass.
4. Fine-needle aspiration results are consistent with normal adipose tissue.

Special Considerations

1. The differential diagnosis may include epidermal inclusion cyst and sebaceous cyst.
2. During excision of a posterior triangle lipoma, care should be taken to avoid injury to the spinal accessory nerve.
3. If the lipoma is larger than about 5 cm, liposuction can be performed instead of surgical excision.

Special Instrumentation, Position, and Anesthesia

1. Liposuction instruments are necessary if this procedure is performed. Otherwise, no special instruments are necessary for surgical excision.

Tips and Pearls

1. Lipomas can often be excised under local anesthesia.
2. For small lipomas, the cosmetic results of surgical excision can be equal to liposuction.
3. During liposuction, direct the cannula's opening away from the skin surface.
4. It is usually not the intent of liposuction to remove all adipose tissue.

Pitfalls and Complications

1. Postoperative hematoma, seroma, or infection
2. Injury to the spinal accessory nerve in the posterior triangle of the neck
3. Injury to the thoracic duct during excision of a lipoma in the supraclavicular triangle

Postoperative Care Issues

1. The pathology specimen should be examined to rule out a neoplasm.
2. The small surgical drain used to avoid a hematoma or seroma is removed in 24 hours.

References

Pinski KS, Roenigk HH. Liposuction of lipomas. Dermatol Clin 1990;8: 483.

Spinowitz AL. The treatment of multiple lipomas by liposuction. J Dermatol Surg Oncol 1989;15:538.

Operative Procedure

The patient is positioned on the operating table in the supine position for a lipoma in the anterior neck. If the lipoma is located in the posterior neck, the patient may need to lie on one side or be completely prone. Although most cases can be performed under local anesthesia, a general anesthetic is better for children or if the lipoma is near the spinal accessory nerve. After the surgical field is scrubbed, sterile drapes are placed to provide easy identification and palpation of neck landmarks. The skin is incised in accordance with the location of the lipoma and in relaxed skin tension lines (Fig. 111-1). In the typical case, a single transverse incision is made and is carried down through the skin and subcutaneous tissue to the level of the lipoma.

If the lipoma does not have any identifiable capsule around it, it may not "shell out." Sharp dissection is used for its removal (Fig. 111-2). The surgical principle is removal that results in a cosmetic improvement. Overly aggressive excision could result in a depressed area.

Except for the smallest lipomas, a drain should be placed in the wound before closure. This usually can be removed within 24 hours. Closure is accomplished in a routine fashion. The platysma and subcutaneous tissues are closed with absorbable 3-0 or 4-0 interrupted sutures, and the skin is closed with a running subcuticular Prolene suture. After the drain is secured and the dressing applied, the patient is awakened in the operating room, extubated, and taken to the recovery room.

An alternative to surgical excision is liposuction, but it should be employed only if the surgeon is sure the lesion is a lipoma and not a malignancy. The principle of cosmetic liposuction is not total fat removal but rather contouring of fat in an area where it is in excess, and liposuction of a lipoma may not remove all of the adipose tissue. The procedure can be performed under local or general anesthetic. It begins with a small stab incision at the border of the lipoma in a relaxed skin tension line and preferably in a well hidden spot (Fig. 111-3). The 4- to 6-mm cannulas are passed through the lipoma numerous times in a crisscross fashion, creating a Swiss cheese or honey comb effect in the tissue and allowing the area to flatten, but without surface irregularities (Fig. 111-4). The smaller cannulas require more passes but have a less chance for surface irregularity. Between 0.5 and 1 atm of suction is used, and the cannula is passed 8 to 12 times through each tunnel. It is important to direct the aperture of cannula away from the skin surface. Disconnecting the suction and passing the cannula around the periphery several times enhances a smooth transition to the normal surrounding skin. Closure is performed with simple, interrupted 5-0 or 6-0 Prolene. Elastic tape over the liposuctioned area helps to provide support and prevent hematoma. The patient is instructed to rest for 1 week.

CHARLES M. STIERNBERG

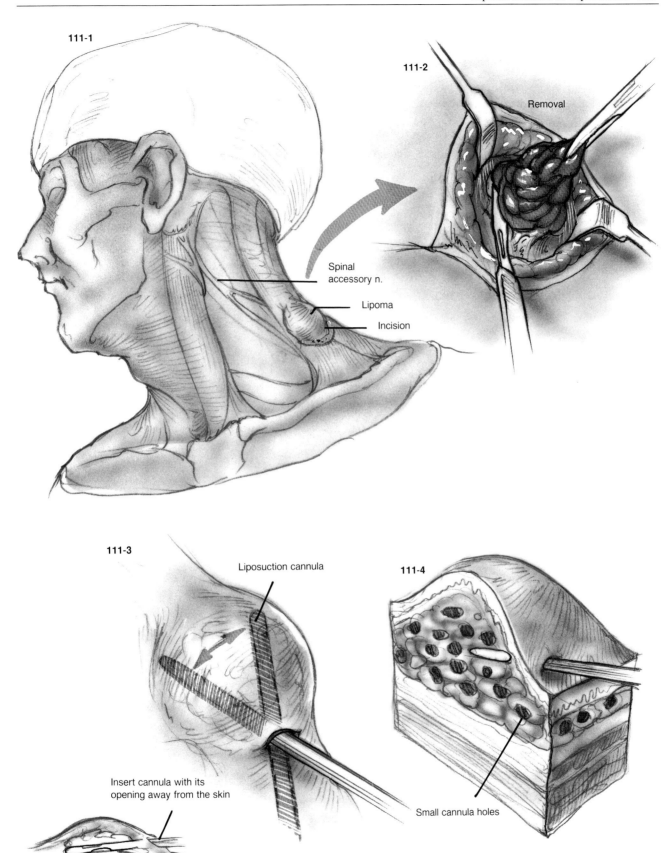

111-1

Spinal
accessory n.

Lipoma

Incision

111-2

Removal

111-3

Liposuction cannula

Insert cannula with its
opening away from the skin

111-4

Small cannula holes

■ *112.* DRAINAGE OF NECK ABSCESSES
Surgical opening of a collection of purulent debris in the neck

Indications
1. Neural, vascular, airway, or septic complications
2. Risk of complication
3. Persistence or worsening despite appropriate antibiotic therapy

Special Considerations
1. Knowledge of fascial spaces of head and neck and symptoms of each space involved
2. Appropriate antibiotic therapy
3. Treatment of underlying cause (eg, dental extraction)

Preoperative Preparation
1. Appropriate antibiotic therapy
2. Imaging if warranted and if clinical considerations allow
3. Airway management

Special Instruments, Position, and Anesthesia
1. Headlight
2. Shoulder roll
3. Doughnut-shaped head holder

Tips and Pearls
1. For an anterior abscess, an incision from submandibular gland to submandibular gland allows entrance into the lateral spaces and floor of mouth and creates a decompressing fasciotomy.
2. For an anterior abscess, Ludwig's angina is reflected by a brawny edema of sublingual and submental spaces, and abscess formation is late.
3. For an anterior abscess, airway control can be achieved with tracheotomy or nasotracheal intubation.
4. For a parapharyngeal space infection, palpation of the angle of the mandible may not be possible.
5. For a parotid space infection, the patient should be kept nonparalyzed, and the incisions are parallel to the facial nerve.

Pitfalls and Complications
1. Delayed diagnosis and drainage causing secondary complications
   a. Airway management
   b. Vascular rupture or pseudoaneurysm
   c. Spread to contiguous space
   d. Osteomyelitis
2. Failure to control airway in cases of Ludwig's angina
3. Failure to identify and treat an underlying cause
4. Failure to adequately drain all involved spaces

Postoperative Care Issues
1. Appropriate antibiotics
2. Patient should rapidly defervesce
3. Treatment of underlying cause, if any

References
Mosher HP. The submaxillary fossa approach to deep pus in the neck. Trans Am Acad Ophthalmol Otolaryngol 1929;34:19.

Pincus RL, Lucente FL. Cervical adenitis and deep neck infection. In: Johnson JT, ed. Antibiotic therapy in head and neck surgery. New York: Marcel Dekker, 1987:257.

Operative Procedure
Floor of Mouth Abscess

Ludwig's angina is a brawny edema involving the sublingual space and the submaxillary spaces, usually bilaterally. The patient's airway is at risk for sudden collapse. The patient's airway is first secured, often requiring an awake patient during local tracheotomy. After the airway is secured, the patient is positioned prone and in extension, and general anesthesia is induced.

An incision is made, two to three fingerbreadths below the angle of the mandible, at the level of the hyoid bone and submandibular gland (Fig. 112-1*A*). The incision is made from submandibular gland to submandibular gland, creating a wide fasciotomy. Minimal flaps are elevated. The mylohyoid muscle is split in the midline, and the incision is then brought down to the level of the inferior border of the submandibular gland. Digital dissection can then be accomplished of both submaxillary spaces and both sublingual spaces (Fig. 112-1*B*). The drainage can be extended to neighboring spaces, as indicated.

Cultures are developed to detect for aerobes, anaerobes, fungi, and mycobacteria. Abscess formation is late, and usually only a woody cellulitis is identified. Penrose drains are placed, and the wound is loosely approximated. The inciting agent, usually a mandibular molar, is extracted, if necessary.

Parapharyngeal Space Abscess

The patient is positioned prone under general anesthesia, with the neck extended and turned toward the side. The patient should not be paralyzed, if possible. An incision is outlined two fingerbreadths below the angle of the mandible and parallel to it in a natural crease (Fig. 112-2). The incision should extend at the level of the hyoid bone from approximately the anterior border of the submandibular gland to the anterior border of the sternomastoid muscle. A perpendicular limb can be made along the carotid sheath as described by Mosher for further exposure of the carotid sheath. The incision is cross-hatched to facilitate closure. The wound is then brought down in layers through the platysma, with minimal skin flap development necessary.

The space between the posterior border of the submandibular gland and the anterior border of the sternomastoid muscle is entered. The carotid sheath is identified deep to this, and vascular loops are placed around the common, external, and internal carotid arteries, if needed. Finger dissection is done within the parapharyngeal space, deep to the mandible and lateral to the superior constrictor muscle.

Appropriate cultures are taken to detect aerobes, anaerobes, fungi, and tuberculosis mycobacteria. Dissection is readily accomplished to the base of the skull and may be extended to other involved spaces if needed. The styloid is readily palpable and divides the space into the prestyloid safe compartment and the retrostyloid compartment containing the carotid sheath and cranial nerves IX, X, and XII. A large Penrose drain is placed, and the wound is closed loosely. Culture-specific antibiotic therapy is given. The retropharyngeal space may be entered and drained by retracting the carotid sheath laterally and dissecting in the space medial to the carotid artery and lateral to the trachea.

Parotid Space Abscess

The patient is positioned on the operating table in a prone position, with the next extended and turned to the side and under general endotracheal anesthesia. The patient is not paralyzed to lessen the risk of injury to the facial nerve. A temporary tarsorrhaphy is placed. An incision is outlined in a preauricular crease, as in the approach for a superficial parotidectomy (see Procedure 1) (Fig. 112-3). The skin flap is elevated in the plane superficial to the parotid fascia. Multiple linear incisions are made sharply in the fascia, parallel to the path of the facial nerve. A clamp in used to spread the fascia in the same direction (Fig. 112-3*B*). Samples are cultured to detect aerobes, anaerobes, fungi, and mycoplasma. Two large Penrose drains are placed, and the wound is closed loosely in layers. Antibiotic therapy is adjusted to the culture and sensitivity results.

ROBERT PINCUS

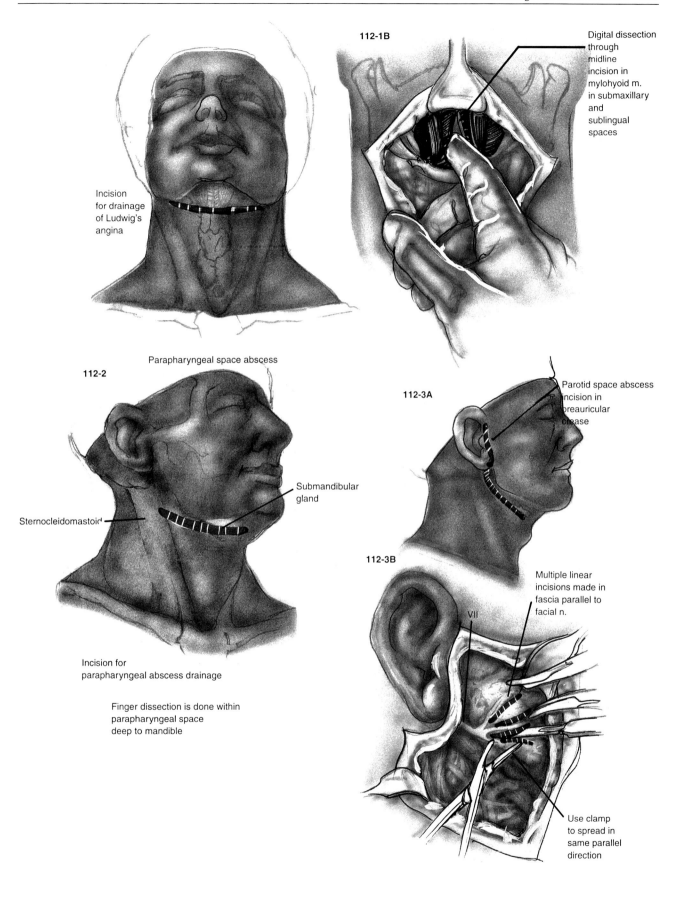

Incision for drainage of Ludwig's angina

112-1B

Digital dissection through midline incision in mylohyoid m. in submaxillary and sublingual spaces

Parapharyngeal space abscess

112-2

Submandibular gland

Sternocleidomastoid

Incision for parapharyngeal abscess drainage

Finger dissection is done within parapharyngeal space deep to mandible

112-3A

Parotid space abscess incision in preauricular crease

112-3B

VII

Multiple linear incisions made in fascia parallel to facial n.

Use clamp to spread in same parallel direction

■ 113. MAJOR VESSEL REPAIR

Repair of carotid and jugular vessels in the head and neck region

Indications

1. Blunt and penetrating trauma
2. Malignant and benign neoplasms
3. Carotid body tumors
4. Iatrogenic injury

Special Considerations

1. Prior neck irradiation
2. Coexisting oroesophageal or tracheal involvement
3. Coexisting neck infection
4. Coexisting atherosclerotic disease of the arch or carotid vessels
5. Bleeding or clotting abnormalities
6. Hemodynamic instability due to hypovolemic shock

Preoperative Preparation

1. Routine laboratory studies, including a complete blood count and coagulation tests
2. Blood typed and crossmatched
3. Aortogram and angiogram of selected vessels if the patient is hemodynamically stable
4. Perioperative antibiotics (eg, cephalosporin)

Special Instruments, Position, and Anesthesia

1. Carotid shunt (eg, Javid, Sundt, Pruitt-Inahara)
2. Cardiovascular sutures (eg, 4-0, 5-0, 6-0, monofilament polypropylene) with a tapered needle
3. Headlight
4. Loupes (optional)
5. Vascular clamps and instruments
6. General or regional (cervical block) anesthesia
7. Supine position with head extended and rotated away from side of operation

Tips and Pearls

1. Ligate and divide the common facial vein to expose the carotid bulb.
2. Dissect the lateral edge of the common and internal carotid arteries to avoid branches and nerves (eg, hypoglossal).

Pitfalls and Complications

1. Postoperative hemorrhage can be reduced by meticulous hemostasis in the operating room; drains may also help.
2. Injury to cranial nerves (eg, hypoglossal, vagus, marginal mandibular) can be avoided by staying close to the carotid artery (ie, plane of Leriche).
3. If hematoma occurs, the patient should be returned to the operating room immediately, before the trachea shifts, to avoid airway obstruction and difficult reintubation.
4. Sudden neurologic change with focal deficit indicates arterial thrombosis and requires immediate surgical reexploration.

Postoperative Care Issues

1. Neck mobility should be limited until coagulation returns to normal.
2. Intensive care monitoring for 24 hours is recommended after vascular reconstruction.
3. Postoperative pain usually is minimal.
4. Postoperative infection is rare.
5. Skin sutures can be removed in 7 to 10 days postoperatively.

References

Berguer R, Kieffer E. Special surgical problems. In: Berguer R, Kieffer E, eds. Surgery of the arteries to the head. New York: Springer-Verlag, 1992:167.

Perry MO. Injuries of the brachiocephalic vessels. In: Rutherford RB, ed. Vascular surgery, vol II. Philadelphia: WB Saunders, 1989:604.

Operative Procedure

The procedure is done under general anesthesia with orotracheal intubation, or by regional anesthesia. However, if a high carotid artery exposure is anticipated, nasotracheal intubation with or without mandibular subluxation or anterior wiring will improve visualization of the distal internal carotid artery and open angle between the mandible and the internal carotid artery. The entire neck and anterior chest should be prepped, as well as the supraclavicular region if the incisions may need to be extended. This is particularly true in trauma cases, for which proximal control may involve a neck incision and a supraclavicular or median sternotomy incision.

The neck incision is made along the anterior boarder of the sternocleidomastoid muscle if the anticipated injury or surgery involves the common carotid, internal carotid, or proximal external carotid artery (Fig. 113-1). If the patient has a deep injury to the vertebral artery or proximal subclavian artery or vein, a supraclavicular incision 1 to 2 cm above and parallel to the clavicle may provide better access. The sternocleidomastoid muscle is retracted laterally, with the remaining soft tissue retracted medially to identify the common carotid artery. If there is difficulty finding the carotid artery because of extensive hematoma, tumor, or obesity, the entire length of the internal jugular vein can be exposed and the common facial vein identified medially.

The carotid bulb is found directly below the common facial vein in most patients, and the division of this vein provides access to the carotid artery (Fig. 113-1B). The common carotid artery should be exposed first, and the internal external carotid is exposed after the common carotid artery has been mobilized. Care should be taken to dissect the artery by entering the plane directly adjacent to the artery (ie, plane of Leriche). If the surgeon stays in the plane anterior and lateral to the artery, no vessels or nerves (eg, vagus) are encountered. If the jugular vein is injured during the procedure, the vein should be compressed with a finger and clamped immediately to avoid an air embolus, particularly in the patient under regional anesthesia. The internal jugular vein, if injured, can be closed with a cardiovascular 5-0 Prolene suture.

The proximal internal carotid artery is dissected from the surrounding tissue and gradually mobilized, allowing 3 to 4 cm of the internal carotid artery to be freed. Care should be taken to avoid dissection in the crotch of the carotid artery to avoid bleeding or injury to the nerve supply to the carotid bulb.

If the carotid artery repair is required in the high internal carotid artery, the next maneuver is to fully mobilize the external carotid artery and its branches and to displace the hypoglassal nerve superiorly (Fig. 113-2). If necessary, the posterior belly of the digastric muscle may be divided. With rare exceptions, full mobilization with proximal and distal control of the arteries should be obtained before vascular repair. If distal control can not be obtained because of a tumor or bleeding, control with internal balloon occlusion (eg, Pruitt-Inahara catheter) of the distal artery may be necessary.

After the artery and vein have been fully mobilized, repair can be performed. For simple injuries to the artery or vein that have not compromised the diameter of the vessel, interrupted suture repair may be all that is necessary. For more complex lesions or repairs, it may be necessary to transect and reanastomose the vessel, perform an interposition graft with prosthetic material or saphenous vein, or transpose the external carotid artery to the internal carotid artery, maintaining arterial continuity of the internal carotid vessels (Fig. 113-3).

Cerebral monitoring or protection is necessary during carotid clamping if the artery was patent before clamping. When clamping is expected to last longer than 5 minutes, a shunt should be placed, particularly if there is contralateral carotid disease or a prior history of stroke in the ipsilateral carotid artery. Heparin (75 to 100 U/kg) is recommended before carotid clamping unless extensive trauma or bleeding is present.

PETER F. LAWRENCE
R. KIM DAVIS

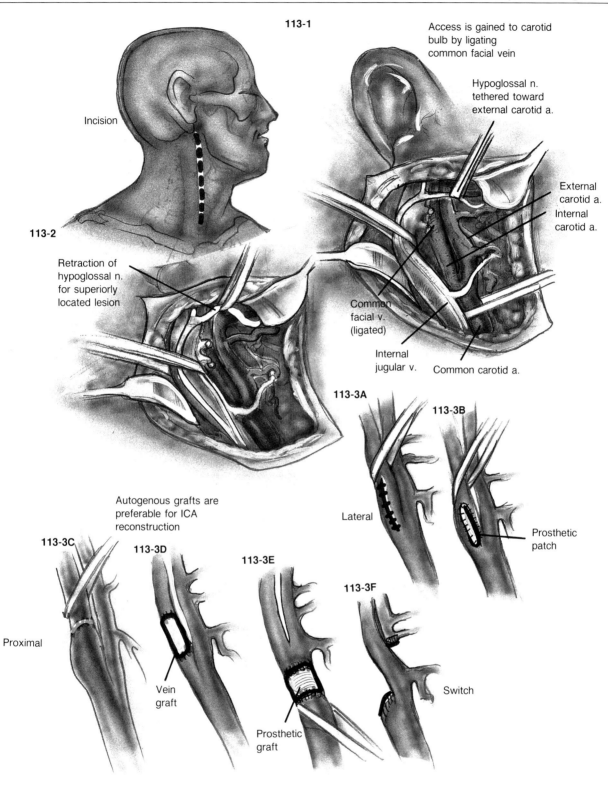

113-1

Incision

Access is gained to carotid bulb by ligating common facial vein

Hypoglossal n. tethered toward external carotid a.

External carotid a.

Internal carotid a.

113-2

Retraction of hypoglossal n. for superiorly located lesion

Common facial v. (ligated)

Internal jugular v.

Common carotid a.

113-3A

113-3B

Lateral

Prosthetic patch

Autogenous grafts are preferable for ICA reconstruction

113-3C

113-3D

113-3E

113-3F

Proximal

Vein graft

Prosthetic graft

Switch

Atlas of Head and Neck Surgery–Otolaryngology,
edited by Byron J. Bailey, J. Gail Neely, Karen H. Calhoun, and Amy R. Coffey.
Lippincott-Raven Publishers, Philadelphia © 1996.

Section Two
Otologic Procedures

Section Editor:

J. Gail Neely

External Auditory Canal and Tympanic Membrane
Middle Ear and Ossicular Chain
Mastoid
Facial Nerve
Cochlea and Labyrinth
Transtemporal Skull Base
Lateral Skull Base
Congenital Aural Atresia

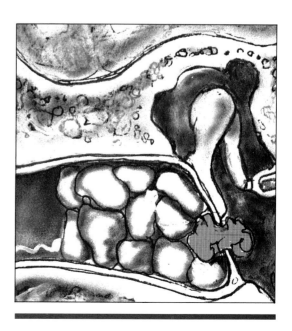

■ 114. MEATOPLASTY AND CANALOPLASTY

Canaloplasty is a procedure that removes diseased soft tissue and osseous obstructions of the external auditory canal. Meatoplasty is a procedure that widens the cartilaginous opening into the ear canal or cavity created by a canal wall down mastoidectomy.

Indications

1. Canaloplasty
   a. Stenosis of the external auditory canal
   b. Chronic otitis externa
   c. Osteoma
   d. Exostoses
2. Meatoplasty
   a. Canal wall down mastoidectomy
   b. Congenital or acquired cartilaginous stenosis or obstruction of the canal

Contraindications

1. Carcinoma medial to the osseous cartilage junction
2. Atresia of the external auditory canal

Preoperative Preparation

1. A 1.5-mm high-density bone window computed tomography scan provides visualization of the middle ear and mastoid and an assessment of the extent of external auditory canal obstruction.

Tips and Pearls

1. All drilling should be done with a diamond bur and with copious amounts of irrigation.
2. VIIth nerve monitoring should be used, especially when drilling medially and inferiorly in the external auditory canal.
3. A "postage stamp" of foil from a suture packet should be gently placed medial to the area to be drilled (lateral to the tympanic membrane) to avoid injury to canal skin flaps or the tympanic membrane.
4. The posterior canal wall can be thinned down to, but not including, the level of the mastoid air cells.
5. A skin graft taken from postauricular or anterior thigh donor sites provides excellent coverage for the new canal.

Pitfalls and Complications

1. Displaced skin grafts and hematoma can be avoided by careful packing technique.
2. Stenosis may occur because of the loss of a graft, infection, or hematoma formation.
3. Erosion of the posterior canal wall may occur from excessive thinning during the canaloplasty or mucosal invasion from the mastoid. The former may require rebuilding of the wall, and the latter can be avoided by carefully covering the mastoid cells.

Postoperative Care Issues

1. Packing is removed at 1 week.
2. Silver nitrate is applied to granulation tissue.
3. Keep the field dry.

References

Goodman WS, Middleton WC. The management of chronic external otitis. J Otolaryngol 1984;13:183.

Paparella MM, Goycoolea MV. Canaloplasty for chronic intractable external otitis and keratosis obturans. Otolaryngol Head Neck Surg 1981;89:440.

Soliman T, Fatt Hi-A, Abdel Kadir M. A simplified technique for the management of acquired stenosis of the external auditory canal. J Laryngol Otol 1980;94:549.

Operative Procedure

Canaloplasty

Canaloplasty is best performed through a postauricular approach (Fig. 114-1). To widen the bony external auditory canal medial to the cartilaginous osseous junction, the skin of the ear canal must be pedicled as a laterally based flap (Fig. 114-2). Vascular strip incisions are made lateral to the area of stenosis. The canal skin overlying the area of bony stenosis is elevated medially and laid against the tympanic membrane (Fig. 114-3). The ear drum and flap are protected by placing a small sheath of aluminum from a suture pack against the tympanic membrane.

If the bony canal requires lateral widening, a standard tympanostomy flap incision is performed. The tympanostomy flap is raised to the level of the fibrous annulus without entering the middle ear. The flap is laid against the tympanic membrane and protected with an aluminum sheath. The canal skin lateral to the tympanostomy flap is back-elevated out of the canal to expose the area of stenosis.

Under otomicroscopic visualization and with continuous suction irrigation, a diamond polishing bur is used to widen the canal (see Fig. 114-2). Posteriorly, care should be taken to avoid the mastoid air cell system, and anteriorly, the parotid bed and temporomandibular joint should remain inviolate. All bone dust is removed, and the skin flaps are returned.

If there is diseased skin or the stenosis is primarily soft tissue, this area is removed, and a split-thickness skin graft or pedicled skin flap is placed into the canal and secured with packing (Fig. 114-4). Loss of canal skin and areas of exposed bone are treated in a similar fashion.

Meatoplasty

If canal wall down surgery is planned, a Koerner's flap is performed to obtain additional skin to line the mastoid cavity. To maximize the meatal opening, conchal cartilage must be removed. The anterior and intertragic incision lines are injected with lidocaine and epinephrine. The auricle is held forward by a Weitlaner retractor, and soft tissue is removed from the posterior aspect of the conchal cartilage. Hematosis is achieved with a Bovie cautery.

An ellipse of cartilage is uncovered, with care taken not to violate the perichondrium. A crescent of cartilage is removed without injury to the skin of the concha, and hemostasis is achieved with bipolar cautery (Fig. 114-5).

Using an aural speculum, Lempert #1 and #3 incisions are cut to open the canal. Hemostasis is achieved. The #3 incision is curved into the conchal bowl and under the antihelical rim (Fig. 114-6). Avoidance of injury to the canal skin pedicled on conchal skin is imperative.

Stay sutures of 3-0 Dexon are placed from the posterior aspect of the meatal flap to the pericranium at the edge of the mastoid cavity. Three interrupted sutures are held by hemostats. The surgeon gently tightens the sutures to see the "trap door" open and assess the size of the meatus. If the auricle becomes more prominent during this maneuver, more cartilage must be removed.

At the end of the procedure, the flap is gently placed into the created opening and the sutures tied loosely. Antibiotic ointment is used to completely fill the cavity.

MYLES L. PENSAK
DANIEL J. KELLEY

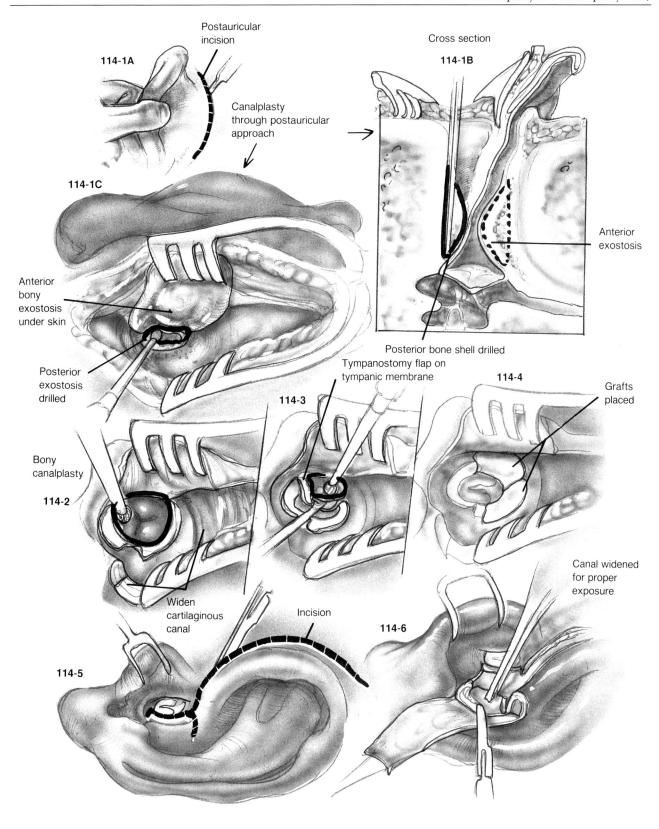

114-1A

Postauricular incision

Canalplasty through postauricular approach

Cross section

114-1B

Anterior exostosis

114-1C

Anterior bony exostosis under skin

Posterior exostosis drilled

Posterior bone shell drilled

Tympanostomy flap on tympanic membrane

Bony canalplasty

114-2

114-3

114-4

Grafts placed

Widen cartilaginous canal

Incision

Canal widened for proper exposure

114-5

114-6

■ 115. EXCISION OF EXOSTOSES OR OSTEOMA

Exostoses result from new bone growth in single or multiple areas of the osseous external auditory canal and are caused by refrigeration periostitis. Osteomas are generally unilateral, singular bone growths arising from the osseous external auditory canal. Exostoses can be differentiated histologically by the stratified lamellar growth pattern on the surface of the osseous canal, but the osteoma has no lamellar growth pattern and is attached by a small base.

Indications
1. Conductive hearing loss
2. Chronic otitis externa

Special Considerations
1. Need for skin graft
2. Packing material

Preoperative Preparation
1. Audiogram
2. Noncontrast computed tomography study of the temporal bone

Special Instruments
1. Angled otologic drill
2. Owen's gauze
3. Merocel otic sponge

Tips and Pearls
1. Careful infiltration of local anesthesia
2. Meticulous care of skin flaps
3. Remove anterior canal wall bone until annulus is visualized.

Pitfalls and Complications
1. Tympanic membrane injury
2. Ossicular chain contact with drill
3. Failure to stent the anterior sulcus
4. Scarring at skin graft site

Postoperative Care Issues
1. Compliance with water precautions
2. Use of antibiotic otic drops when packing is used
3. Timely removal of packing
4. Continuation of water precautions and of acetic acid and hydrocortisone preparations

Reference
Schuknecht HF. Pathology of the ear. 2nd ed. Philadelphia: Lea & Febiger, 1993:398.

Operative Procedure

Excision of Exostoses of the External Auditory Canal

With the patient in the supine position under general anesthesia, the head is turned to expose the involved ear. The ear is prepped and draped in the routine fashion. The ear canal is thoroughly irrigated with saline to remove any cerumen or debris. Using a 27-gauge needle, a solution of 1% lidocaine with 1:100,000 epinephrine is injected into the external auditory canal skin.

If the stenosis is severe, an incision is made from 6 to 12 o'clock, just lateral to the exostosis, using a #7200 Beaver blade. In less severe cases, the incision is carried out over the prominence of the exostosis, extending from 6 to 12 o'clock. Incisions are then made vertically, perpendicular to the initial incision, with a #6700 Beaver blade and carried to the bony external auditory meatus (Fig. 115-1). This posterior flap is elevated with a lancet knife to the limits of the incision and then folded over the meatal skin and held in place by the aural speculum. In cases of extreme exostoses, the posterior flap can be incorporated into an expanded vascular strip incision, and a postauricular incision used to allow wide exposure of the bony external canal lateral to the exostosis. The skin overlying the exostosis is then elevated toward the tympanic membrane as much as possible. Using the #7200 Beaver blade or a lancet knife (depending on the degree of stenosis), an incision is made in the anterior canal wall skin as well. The skin is elevated away from the exostosis laterally and retracted by careful reinsertion of the aural speculum. The cuff of skin medial to the exostosis is reflected toward the tympanic membrane until the fibrous annulus is reached.

An angled otologic drill with a diamond bur is used to remove the exposed exostosis. The exostosis is "cored out," leaving a thin layer of bone on the cortex to protect the canal skin (Fig. 115-2). This layer is then removed from inside out. A slightly larger bur can then be introduced to plane down the remaining exostosis posteriorly. After the bulk of the posterior exostosis has been removed, the anterior exostosis can be managed. The anterior canal wall is drilled down until the anterior fibrous annulus is identified (Fig. 115-3). During this dissection a smaller diamond bur should be used to avoid damaging the tympanic membrane or drilling on the malleus, especially the short process.

With the bony dissection complete, the remaining skin is often adequate to cover the exposed bone. A piece of Xeroform or Owen's silk impregnated with antibiotic otic drops can be placed over the skin incisions, and Merocel packing used to stent the ear canal open (Fig. 115-4). In cases of extensive exostoses, one or several small split-thickness skin grafts can be harvested from the postauricular region to cover exposed bone. If the anterior sulcus requires grafting, the medial one third of the ear canal is lined with Owen's silk, packing the canal with small cotton balls soaked in antibiotic otic drops (Fig. 115-5). The lateral two thirds of the canal can be packed similarly or stented with a Merocel wick.

Antibiotic otic drops are used for 2 to 3 weeks with packing removal in one week. Within 3 to 6 weeks, the epidermal layer of the graft often sloughs with a healthier layer remaining.

Excision of Osteoma of the External Auditory Canal

Osteomas are usually solitary and can be removed under local anesthesia. The ear canal is injected with local anesthetic circumferentially. If the osteoma is not completely filling the external auditory canal, a K-curette is applied to the osteoma in a twisting fashion. The osteoma breaks from its stalk (Fig. 115-6). The skin is elevated away from the stalk for several millimeters, and a small diamond bur is used to obliterate any remnant of the bony stalk. In cases of completely obstructive osteomas, the center of the osteoma is drilled out with a small diamond bur. The remnants of the bony capsule are then removed in a piecemeal fashion.

If extensive dissection is required, the canal can be packed with Merocel, whereas if the osteoma is localized, the ear canal may be filled with antibiotic ointment.

JOHN KVETON

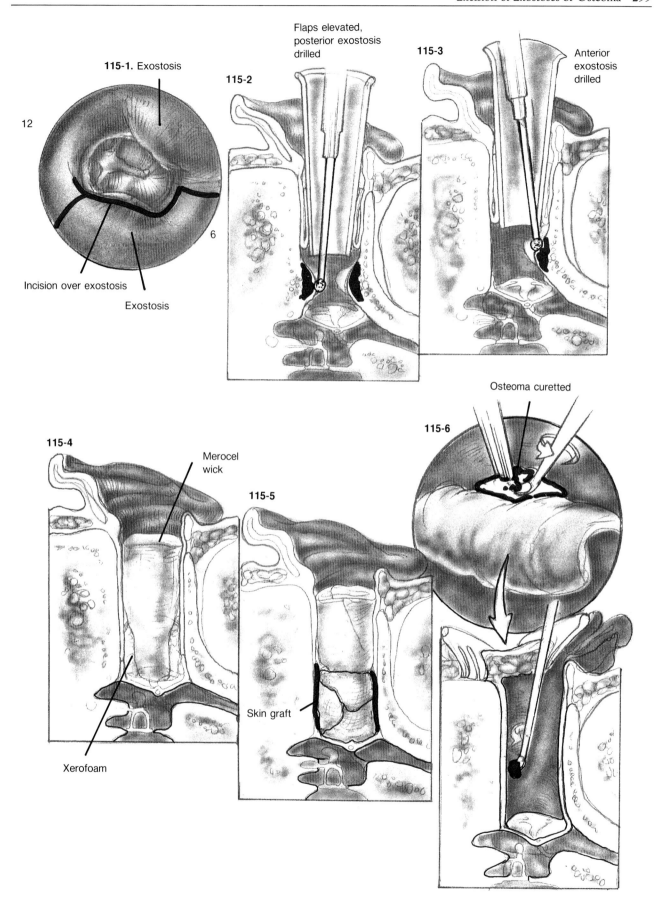

115-1. Exostosis

12

Incision over exostosis

Exostosis

6

115-2   Flaps elevated,
posterior exostosis
drilled

115-3   Anterior
exostosis
drilled

115-4

Merocel
wick

115-5

Xerofoam

Skin graft

115-6   Osteoma curetted

■ *116.* SOFT TISSUE CANAL STENOSIS

Treatment of secondary, factitious canal stenosis due to chronic external otitis or trauma to the ear canal, evidenced by a short ear canal with loss of normal landmarks and a conductive hearing loss. It can be associated with previous tympanoplasty and blunting of the anterior tympanomeatal angle.

Indications
1. Conductive hearing loss of 20 to 40 decibels (dB)
2. Aural hygiene
3. Failure to maintain adequate canal diameter

Contraindications
1. Sensorineural hearing loss of 40 dB or greater
   a. Requiring sound amplification
   b. Self-cleaning ear canal

Special Considerations
1. Audiogram, air-bone conduction, speech tests
2. Previous tympanoplasty surgery
3. Medical management
   a. Canal dilatation with expandable sponge packing for 6 to 8 weeks
   b. Steroid injection
   c. Topical steroid drops

Tips and Pearls
1. Remove all fibrous tissue.
2. Preserve the fibrous layer of the tympanic membrane and annulus.
   a. Plain of dissection the inferior annulus to the drum surface
   b. Short process of the malleus to the drum surface
3. Canaloplasty
   a. Enlarged bony ear canal
   b. Straighten anterior canal wall bulge, and enlarge the anterior tympanomeatal angle.
4. Epithelial coverage of the drum surface and ear canal with thin split-thickness skin graft
5. Prolonged postoperative packing
6. Reconstruction of the fibrous drum with medial and lateral layers of areolar fascia plus a skin graft

Pitfalls and Complications
1. Disruption of the annulus and tympanic membrane, requiring tympanoplasty
2. Failure to straighten the anterior canal wall and acute anterior tympanomeatal angle
3. Failure to cover the drum and ear canal with epithelium, leading to recurrent stenosis
4. Inadequate postoperative care and recurrent stenosis

Postoperative Care Issues
1. Packing for 6 to 8 weeks with an Owen gauze sleeve, with inner packing of ¼-in gauze saturated with antibiotic eardrops and secondary stenosis dilated with expanded sponges (eg, Pope Oto-Wick).
2. Postoperative audiogram at 2 months
3. Postoperative cleaning and maintenance with acetic acid–alcohol irrigation or 2 oz of white vinegar to 1 pint of rubbing alcohol. The area can be dried by using a hair dryer for 3 to 5 minutes.

References

Farrior JB. The anterior tympanomeatal angle in tympanoplasty: surgical techniques for the prevention of blunting. Laryngoscope 1983;93: 993.

Miglets AW, Paparella MM, Saunders WH. Surgery for infection of the ear. In: Atlas of ear surgery. St. Louis: CV Mosby, 1986:157.

Parisier SC, Weiss MH. Complications of surgery of the external auditory canal. In: Eisele DW, ed. Complications of head and neck surgery. St. Louis: Mosby, 1993:674.

Operative Procedure

Many people who develop canal stenosis secondary to chronic external otitis can be treated and maintained with office management. A narrowed ear canal can be dilated using expandable ear sponges (Pope Oto-Wicks), with repacking every 10 to 4 days for 6 to 8 weeks (Fig. 116-2). Water-soluble antibiotic eardrops are alternated with fluoridated steroid drops, such as betamethasone (Valisone), during the treatment period. In some patients, injections with Kenalog or Decadron may be a useful adjunct. After the canal is open, periodic cleaning and frequent irrigations with acetic acid–alcohol solutions help to maintain the ear. Individuals with a persistent 20-dB or greater conductive loss may wish to consider surgery.

At surgery, the patient is placed in a supine position with the head rotated away from the surgeon. The ear canal is injected with a solution of lidocaine with epinephrine.

A postauricular incision is preferred in patients with canal stenosis. The periosteum is elevated into the ear canal posteriorly. The canal skin is transected laterally to the area of fibrosis (Figs. 116-1 through 116-3).

The fibrosis is elevated circumferentially around the canal. Dissection is carried medial to the fibrous annulus. A plane of dissection over the fibrous drum can usually be established along the inferior annulus and over the short process of the malleus. Beginning a dissection posteriorly often elevates the annulus and fibrous drum, making further dissection difficult (Fig. 116-5).

A deep anterior tympanomeatal angle usually is the source of the problem. Canaloplasty with an enlargement of the ear canal, removal of the anterior canal wall bulge, and straightening of the anterior tympanomeatal angle is required (Fig. 116-4).

Thin split-thickness skin graft (0.01-in [0.2 mm] thick) is harvested from the leg or lower abdomen. The graft is 6 × 2 cm. Notches are cut on either side approximately 2 cm from one end to form the anterior tympanomeatal angle. The anterior portion of the graft may be trimmed to a width of 1.25 cm, allowing a posterior portion to fold around the ear canal (Fig. 116-6).

If the drum is perforated or the patient has had a previous tympanoplasty with graft lateralization, a sandwich graft tympanoplasty is preferred. In these cases, it often is necessary to construct a new annular shelf for fixation of the anterior drum. Thin areolar fascia is placed medial to and lateral to the annular shelf and the malleus, reconstructing the fibrous drum (see Fig. 116-5).

The skin graft is placed in the ear with the short arm over the anterior canal wall. The notched area is folded into the anterior angle; the larger area covers the drum surface and posterior canal wall. Dry roll compressed Gelfoam (1 × 5 mm) is tightly packed into the anterior angle and around the inferior annulus, holding the skin graft in position. Antibiotic-saturated Gelfoam is used over the posterior drum and to fill the ear canal. A meatal pack is formed by folding moist Merocel sponge in thirds and then rolling the piece, creating a 2 × 1.5 cm soft pack, which is covered with a nonadherent gauze. A short relaxing incision is usually made at the incisure, particularly if canaloplasty is performed.

Postoperatively, the ear canal is repacked every 2 weeks until the canal is completely healed to prevent restenosis.

JAY B. FARRIOR

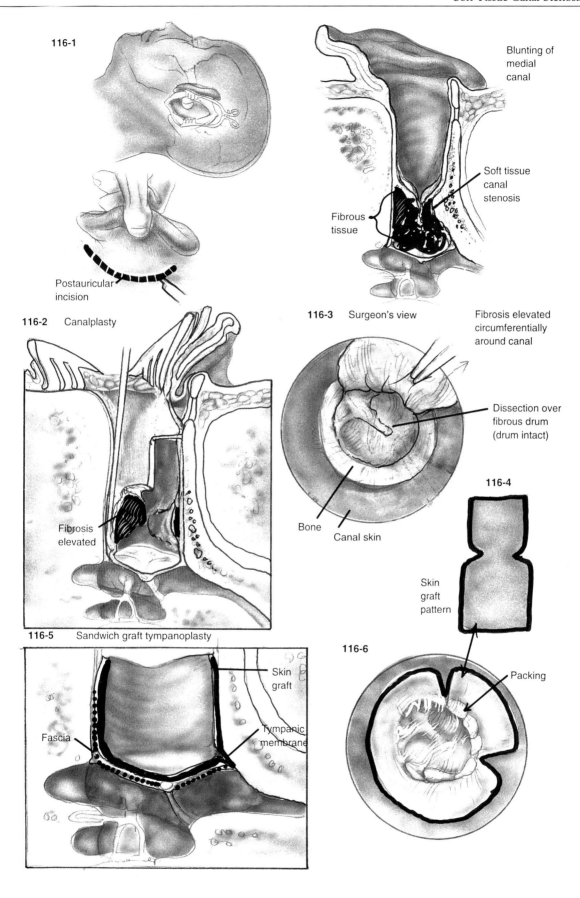

116-1

Postauricular
incision

Blunting of
medial
canal

Soft tissue
canal
stenosis

Fibrous
tissue

116-2   Canalplasty

Fibrosis
elevated

116-3   Surgeon's view

Fibrosis elevated
circumferentially
around canal

Dissection over
fibrous drum
(drum intact)

Bone

Canal skin

116-4

Skin
graft
pattern

116-5   Sandwich graft tympanoplasty

Skin
graft

Tympanic
membrane

Fascia

116-6

Packing

■ 117. MYRINGOTOMY TUBE PLACEMENT AND REMOVAL—Incision of the tympanic membrane and placement or removal of pressure-equalization tubes

Indications
1. Continuous effusion for longer than 3 months
2. Effusion persisting for more than 6 of 12 months
3. Recurrent acute otitis not responsive to antibiotic prophylaxis
4. Chronic retraction of the tympanic membrane or potential cholesteatoma pocket formation
5. Myringotomy only
   a. Relief of pain of acute otitis media or otic barotrauma
   b. Decompression or evacuation of purulent material after otic complications (eg, facial nerve paralysis with acute otitis media)

Special Considerations
1. Facial dysmorphism
2. Cleft palate
3. General medical status of the patient

Preoperative Preparation
1. Preoperative audiologic evaluation
2. Routine laboratory studies (eg, hemoglobin, hematocrit)
3. Canal preparation (eg, Betadine) has minimal effect on postoperative infection.

Special Instruments, Position, and anesthesia
1. Microscope
2. T-tubes are not the first choice of tubes because of the high rate of residual tympanic membrane perforation after extrusion and difficulty in administering otic drops if needed for postoperative otorrhea.
3. Tubes with a diameter of 1.7 mm or less may be needed for patients with very small external canals.
4. Generally, the larger the internal flange, the longer the tube is retained.
5. Supine position, with a head extension on the operating table
6. General inhalation anesthesia

Tips and Pearls
1. The myringotomy incision is placed in the anterior one half of the tympanic membrane.
2. Avoid trauma to the external canal.
3. Ensure that no blood occludes the tube.

Pitfalls and Complications
1. Atrophic tympanic membrane may dictate the location of the myringotomy (eg, very superior or anterior).
2. Mucoid effusion may plug the lumen of the pressure-equalization tube.
3. A severely inflamed tympanic membrane may hasten tube extrusion.
4. Be aware of potential middle ear vascular anomalies, such as an aberrant carotid.
5. The depth of the myringotomy incision is carefully controlled to avoid trauma to the medial wall of the middle ear cleft and potential bleeding.

Postoperative Care Issues
1. Moist, clear otorrhea is common for 24 to 48 hours.
2. Postoperative purulent otorrhea occurs in 9% of cases; the incidence not significantly changed by canal preparation or otic drops used postoperatively.
3. Postoperative otic drops may prevent the lumen from plugging in cases of mucoid effusion.
4. Postoperative audiologic evaluation at 2 weeks
5. Patients or their parents are cautioned to exclude water from the ear while pressure-equalization tubes are patent.

References
Scott BA, Strunk CL. Post-tympanostomy otorrhea: a randomized clinical trial of topical prophylaxis. Otolaryngol Head Neck Surg 1992; 106:34.

Operative Procedure
The operating microscope is examined, balanced, and appropriate tension for all movable joints is adjusted. The appropriate focal length for the distal lens is 250 mm.

The patient is placed supine on the operating table, with the head on a head extension to allow the surgeon's knees to extend below the patient comfortably. An appropriate-sized ear speculum is selected. The auricle is grasped between thumb and third finger and retracted posteriorly, and the speculum, balanced between the thumb and first finger of the same hand, is inserted into the external canal (Fig. 117-1). Operative instruments are held with the tips of the fingers and thumb to allow rotation of the instrument and to facilitate the surgeon's visualization of the operative area (Fig. 117-2). Conversely, if the operative instrument is grasped as if holding a pen, the fingers of the operating hand obscure part of the surgeon's view. The external canal is gently cleaned of cerumen. Complete and meticulous removal is suggested at this point. An added benefit is the relative lack of cerumen to obscure visualization at the first postoperative visit.

The tympanic membrane is carefully examined, and landmarks are identified. The short process and umbo of the tympanic membrane are visualized. The status of inflammation of the tympanic membrane is observed. If visualization through the tympanic membrane is possible, middle ear structures are identified and absence of vascular malformations is sought. A radial incision is made into the anterior one half of the tympanic membrane, commonly anteroinferiorly (Fig. 117-3). Occasionally, scar, atrophic portions of the tympanic membrane, or retraction pockets dictate placement. In these situations, the radial myringotomy incision is made in the high anterosuperior portion of the tympanic membrane.

After making the myringotomy incision, any middle ear effusion present is gently aspirated from the middle ear cleft. Care is taken to not suction directly on the tympanic membrane, because this may lead to bleeding. A 5-Fr suction tube is usually adequate for aspiration of the effusion, but mucoid effusion may require a 7-Fr suction tube.

The selection of pressure-equalization tubes is dictated by the patient's anatomy, expected duration of retention of the tube, and the surgeon's choice. In patients with extremely small external auditory canals, a smaller-diameter tube (≤1.7 mm) is often required. In patients in whom a longer duration of retention is desired, selection of a tube with a larger flange or a T shape may be desired. The T-tubes have a high (7%–15%) incidence of residual tympanic membrane perforation after extrusion and should be reserved for patients with recurrent otitis media despite several previous sets of pressure-equalization tubes. The tube is grasped with alligator forceps on the outer flange and inserted down the speculum (Fig. 117-4). The inner flange is placed through the myringotomy incision, and the tube is left in position (Fig. 117-5). If the angle of the canal and tympanic membrane precludes direct placement with the alligator forceps, the tube is dropped next to the tympanic membrane and manipulated into position using a straight pick.

After placement of the pressure-equalization tube, any blood that may potentially occlude the lumen of the tube is aspirated. If any blood reaccumulates, posing a potential risk for plugging the tube, otic drops are instilled to try to prevent this consequence. The routine use of otic drops is not advocated, because they have not been shown to decrease postoperative otorrhea significantly. However, the use of otic drops in the middle ear cleft in cases of mucoid effusion has been associated with increased patency rates of the tubes.

At the conclusion of the procedure, anesthesia is terminated, and the patient returned to the recovery room. Patients are discharged from the same-day surgery after they are awake and tolerating oral intake well. Patients are usually seen 1 to 2 weeks postoperatively, and the ears are examined. The postoperative audiogram is obtained at this time, and patients may be fitted with plugs to exclude water from the ears when bathing or showering.

JAY A. WERKHAVEN

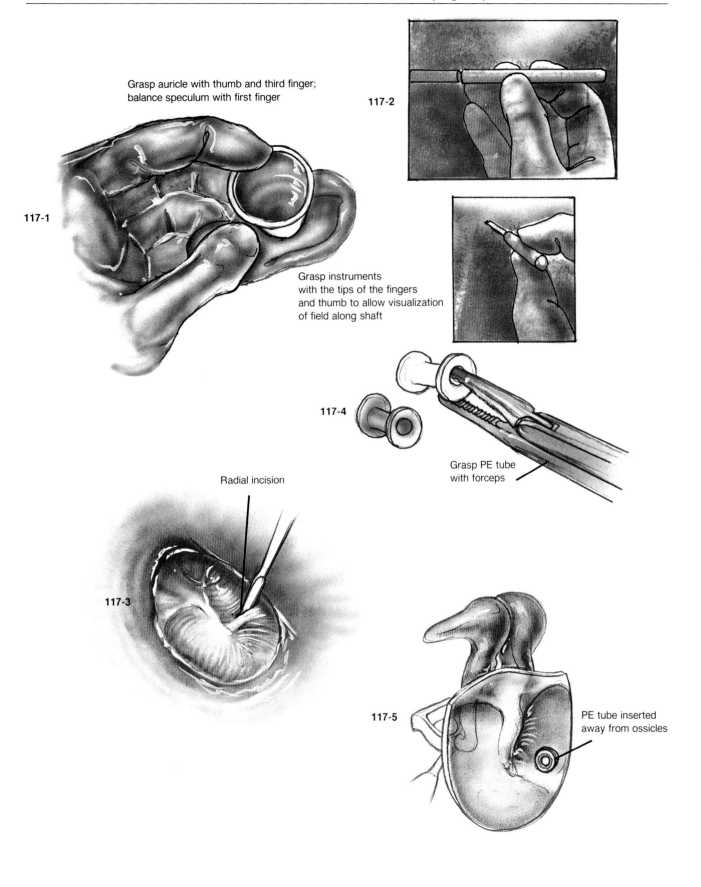

Grasp auricle with thumb and third finger; balance speculum with first finger

117-1

117-2

Grasp instruments with the tips of the fingers and thumb to allow visualization of field along shaft

117-4

Grasp PE tube with forceps

Radial incision

117-3

117-5

PE tube inserted away from ossicles

■ 118. TYMPANOMEATAL FLAP FOR EXPLORATORY TYMPANOTOMY—Direct visual inspection of the middle ear space and ossicular chain by the elevation of the canal skin flap and tympanic membrane.

Indications
1. Conductive hearing loss
   a. Otosclerosis
   b. Ossicular chain discontinuity
   c. Ossicular chain fixation, congenital or secondary to chronic otitis media
2. Perilymph fistula, oval and round window
3. Middle ear lesions with clear margins
   a. Small congenital cholesteatoma pearls
   b. Residual middle ear cholesteatoma pearls
   c. Glomus tympanic tumor, Fisch class A

Contraindications
1. Sensorineural hearing loss
2. Cerebrospinal fluid otorrhea following trauma
3. Chronic draining ear
4. Known cholesteatoma extending to the mastoid
5. Glomus tumor extending beyond tympanic annulus
6. Suspected malignancy of the ear canal or middle ear

Preoperative Preparation
1. Audiogram, air-bone conduction, and speech tests
2. Computed tomography scans of the temporal bone and middle ear to delineate ossicular abnormalities and cholesteatoma
3. Magnetic resonance imaging (MRI) scan and MRI arteriogram for suspected tumor of temporal bone

Special Instruments, Position, and Anesthesia
1. Local anesthesia with sedation
   a. General anesthesia during injection (5 minutes)
   b. Monitored sedation
2. Local anesthesia
   a. Field block for postauricular and endaural incisions, using a 2% solution of lidocaine with a 1:1000 dilution of epinephrine
   b. For the ear canal, 1 to 2 mL of 2% lidocaine 2% with 1:50,000 epinephrine
   c. For the ear canal flap, use 0.5 mL of a 2% solution of lidocaine with 1:3000 epinephrine, injected with with a tuberculin syringe

(continued)

Operative Procedure
The patient is placed in a supine position with the head rotated away from the surgeon. The hair is shaved around the ear with a margin of approximately 1 cm (0.5 in) to allow placement of an adhesive eye drape.

A small foam pillow is placed behind the patient's head to brace the surgeon's forearm. The ear is prepped and draped while the surgeon scrubs. The ear is injected with local anesthesia before the surgeon scrubs to allow adequate time for vasoconstriction. Beginning in the postauricular crease, a postauricular incision site is injected with a 2% solution of lidocaine with a 1:100,000 dilution of epinephrine. The needle is advanced forward to blanch the posterior canal skin. The needle is also advanced forward above and below the ear canal. Canal injections of 2% lidocaine with 1:50,000 epinephrine are started in the blanched portion of the canal skin, which is slowly injected with the blanching extending to the tympanic annulus. Subsequent injections are made on either side of the blanched and anesthetized area. Six to eight injections are made to fully anesthetize the ear canal without causing unnecessary discomfort to the patient.

After the ear is prepped and draped, an injection of 0.5 mL of a 1:3000 dilution of epinephrine is made in the flap area using a TB syringe. Attention is then directed behind the ear, where a 2- to 3-cm incision is made in the postauricular crease (Fig. 118-1), and areolar fascia is harvested from the postauricular muscle or mastoid cortex. After closing the incision, the fascia is pressed and dried by the scrub nurse while the surgeon gently irrigates and cleans the ear canal.

Incisions are made in the ear canal with magnifying loupes or with the operating microscope. A myringotomy or sickle knife is used for the incisions. The superior incision is made from just lateral to the short process of the malleus and directly lateral and posterior to just inside the bony cartilaginous junction. The inferior incision is made from 2 mm lateral to the inferior annulus and directed laterally and posteriorly to just inside the bony cartilaginous junction. A third incision is made connecting the superior and inferior incisions just inside the bony cartilaginous junction. The flap elevation is begun superiorly and extends inferior and medial to the annular sulcus. The annulus is elevated from the malleus inferiorly and posteriorly 180°. The flap and tympanic membrane are folded forward into the anterior tympanomeatal angle (Fig. 118-2).

It is often necessary to remove several millimeters of posterior canal wall and scutum to visualize the oval window and stapes (Figs. 118-3 and 118-4). The chorda tympani nerve is identified and elevated away from the posterior canal wall. A sharp curet is used to thin the bone lateral to the annulus (Fig. 118-3).

(continued)

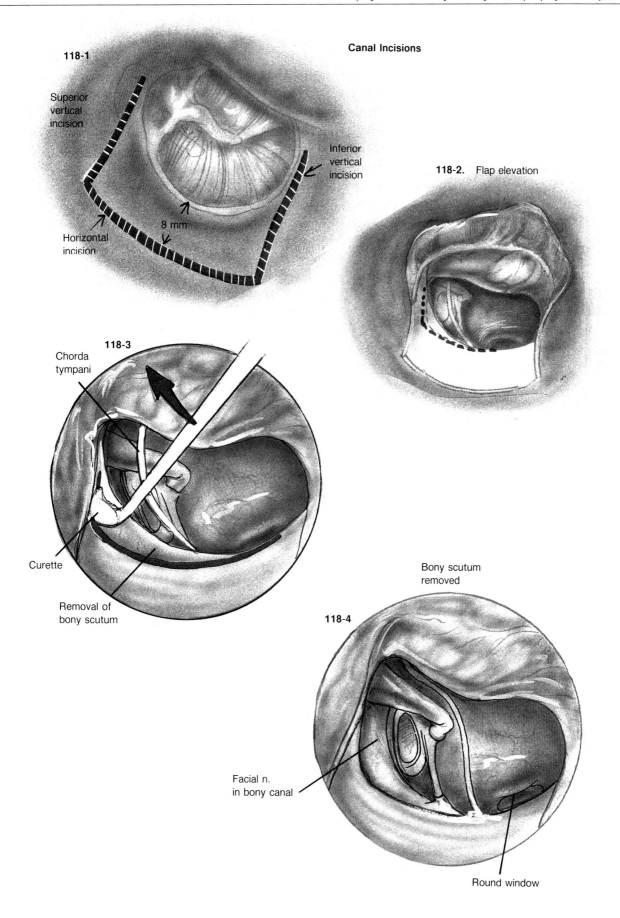

Canal Incisions

118-1

Superior
vertical
incision

Inferior
vertical
incision

Horizontal
incision

8 mm

118-2.   Flap elevation

118-3

Chorda
tympani

Curette

Removal of
bony scutum

Bony scutum
removed

118-4

Facial n.
in bony canal

Round window

■ *118.* TYMPANOMEATAL FLAP FOR EX-
PLORATORY TYMPANOTOMY *(continued)*

Tips and Pearls

1. For standard tympanomeatal flaps
   a. Sponge pillow behind the patient's head to support the surgeon's forearm
   b. Speculum holder to allow the use of both arms
   c. Postauricular fascia obtained from postauricular muscle or mastoid cortex
   d. A long tympanomeatal flap allows bone removal and perforation of the tympanic membrane
   e. The flap extends 180° from the short process of malleus to the lower tympanic annulus
2. Post-modified radical mastoidectomy incisions
   a. Posterior and superior tegmen incisions
   b. Labyrinthine incision, posterior to the facial nerve to the horizontal semicircular canal
   c. Inferior incision in the floor of the canal lateral to the facial nerve
3. Variations
   a. Superior rotation of flap pedicled at the umbo (Fig. 118-5)
   b. Inferior rotation of flap pedicled at the umbo (Fig. 118-6)

Pitfalls and Complications

1. Limited exposure
2. Bleeding
3. Facial nerve injury secondary to blind dissection
4. Sensorineural hearing loss secondary to oval window trauma
5. Taste abnormalities caused by injury to the chorda tympani nerve

Postoperative Care

1. Packing 5 for 7 days
2. Water exposure at 6 weeks
3. Postoperative audiogram at 2 months

References

Miglets AW, Paparella MM, Saunders WH. Surgery for conductive deafness. In: Atlas of ear surgery. St. Louis: CV Mosby, 1982:329.

Naumann HH. Operations for stapedial ankylosis. In: Naumann H, ed. Head and neck surgery: ear, vol 3. Philadelphia: WB Saunders, 1982: 329.

After the air cells are identified, the annulus can be safely removed to expose the posterior middle ear. After the middle ear work is completed, the eardrum and tympanomeatal flap are returned to their original positions. If a large amount of bone is removed, fascia may be needed to cover the defect. If a tear in the tympanic membrane develops, canal skin may be advanced forward for closing the defect (Fig. 118-8). The flap is packed into place with antibiotic-soaked Gelfoam. Gauze packing is used in the lateral canal.

JAY B. FARRIOR

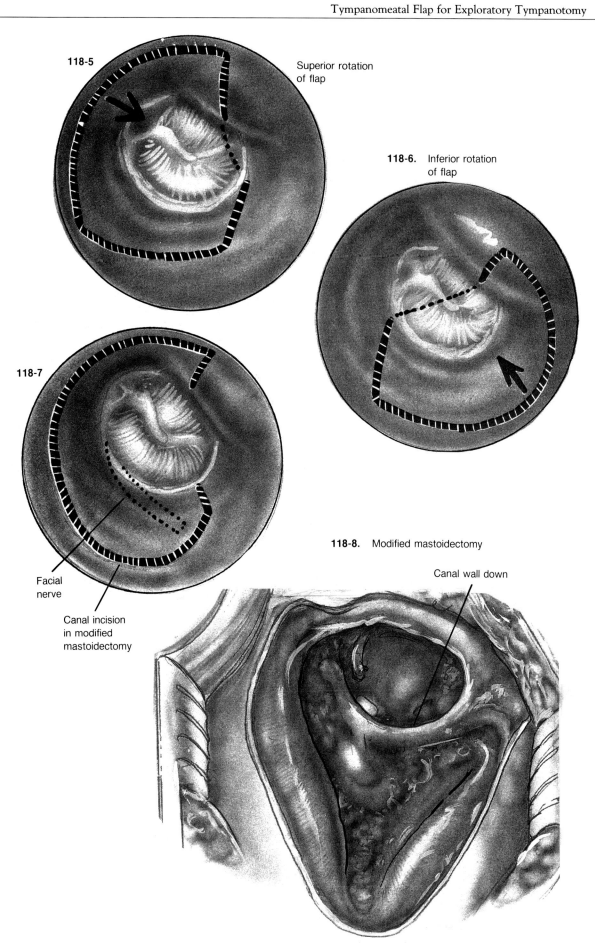

118-5

Superior rotation
of flap

118-6.   Inferior rotation
of flap

118-7

Facial
nerve

Canal incision
in modified
mastoidectomy

118-8.   Modified mastoidectomy

Canal wall down

■ 119. MYRINGOPLASTY AND TYMPANO-

PLASTY TYPE I—Myringoplasty is the surgical repair of the tympanic membrane, confined to the donor site and the drum surface. Commonly employed variations include the paper patch myringoplasty and the tissue graft myringoplasty, both of which can be performed as office procedures.

Tympanoplasty is the surgical repair of the tympanum, including the removal of diseased tissue from the mesotympanum, reconstruction of the ossicular chain, and repair of the tympanic membrane.

Indications

Myringoplasty

1. Small, dry, central perforation, usually less than 4 mm in diameter and not involving the manubrium of the malleus
2. Conductive hearing loss secondary to the loss of the round window shade effect
3. Planned removal of tympanostomy tubes
4. As a secondary procedure in conjunction with surgery on the contralateral ear
5. Residual perforation after prior tympanoplasty

Tympanoplasty

1. Conductive hearing loss due to tympanic membrane perforation
2. Conductive hearing loss due to ossicular discontinuity or necrosis
3. Conductive hearing loss due to ossicular ankylosis
4. Chronic or recurrent otitis media
5. Recurrent middle ear infections due to contamination through perforation of tympanic membrane
6. Progressive hearing loss due to chronic middle ear disease
7. Perforation or hearing loss due to trauma, infection, or prior surgery that persists for more than 3 months
8. Inability to safely bathe or participate in water activities because of perforation of the tympanic membrane, with or without hearing loss

Contraindications

Myringoplasty

1. Status of eustachian tube function in the opposite ear (ie, presence of severe adhesive otitis or effusion)
2. No hearing or extremely poor hearing in the opposite ear
3. Perforation involving the malleus or the annulus
4. Persistent otorrhea
5. Suspected cholesteatoma invading the mesotympanum
6. Clinical or radiographic evidence of pathologic conditions involving the mastoid or epitympanum

Tympanoplasty

1. Evidence of poor eustachian tube function in the opposite ear
2. No hearing or extremely poor hearing in the opposite ear
3. Unresectable cholesteatoma, including cochlear fistula, involvement of eustachian tube, or major vessels
4. Medical illness precluding surgery
5. Clinical or radiographic evidence of pathologic conditions involving the mastoid or epitympanum

Special Considerations

1. Tympanoplasty for posterior and inferior perforations can be performed through a transcanal or postauricular approach.
2. Tympanoplasty for total perforations and anterior perforations is best performed through a postauricular or endaural approach.
3. Revision tympanoplasty is best performed through a postauricular approach.
4. Commonly used graft materials include the areolar tissue overlying temporalis fascia, temporalis fascia, tragal perichondrium, fat obtained from the lobule, and homograft tissues.
5. Choice of a medial or lateral graft technique depends largely on the surgeon's training, experience, and preference, rather than any major differences in the results or outcomes. However, some surgeons use lateral graft techniques exclusively for total perforations and anterior perforations.
6. Commonly used ear canal packing includes antibiotic-soaked gelatin, antibiotic ointment, wicks, and various gauze packs.

(continued)

Operative Procedures

Myringoplasty: Tissue Graft

The lobule is injected with a solution of 1% lidocaine with a 1:100,000 dilution of epinephrine. A small fat graft is harvested through a 1- to 1.5-cm incision on the margin of the lobule.

The margins of the perforation are freshened using a small, straight micropick. The harvested fat graft is carefully inserted into the center of the perforation so that a small amount of the fatty areolar tissue extends into the middle ear and a small amount extends outside of the eardrum (Fig. 119-1). After the graft is wedged into position, it is covered with a small pledget of Gelfoam.

Tympanoplasty: Transcanal Approach

A 2- to 3-cm linear incision is made above the ear, and the incision is carried down to the temporalis fascia, and a temporalis fascia graft is harvested. The incision is closed in a subcutaneous single layer using interrupted absorbable sutures.

A speculum is then secured in place, the ear canal is suctioned, and wax and debris are removed. The margin of the perforation is carefully removed using a micropick and a cup forceps. Care is taken to remove any ingrowth of squamous epithelium (Fig. 119-2).

A tympanomeatal flap is incised 6 to 7 mm lateral to the annulus (Fig. 119-3). The tympanomeatal flap is carefully elevated, and after dissecting the fibrous annulus, the middle ear is entered. The tympanomeatal flap is elevated off of the malleus handle (Fig. 119-4). The eustachian tube and middle ear are then packed with Gelfoam sponge lightly moistened with saline.

The fascia graft is trimmed, moistened, and draped over the gelatin and onto the posterior canal wall. Using a blunt microinstrument, the fascia graft is carefully tucked under the anterior tympanic remnant (Fig. 119-5). The tympanomeatal flap is repositioned. The tympanic membrane should make good contact with the fascia graft circumferentially. The ear canal is packed with antibiotic-soaked Gelfoam or with antibiotic ointment.

Postauricular Tympanoplasty

Incisions and Grafts

The canal incisions are designed to create a laterally based canal skin flap that comprises the thicker skin of the posterosuperior canal, the so-called vascular strip (Fig. 119-6A). The horizontal incision is cut first and is begun above the short process of the malleus, some 2 to 5 mm lateral to the annulus. The horizontal incision is cut from superior to inferior, from the 12 o'clock to the 8 o'clock position (on a right ear). The vertical incisions are made next. The superior vertical limb follows the tympanosquamous suture line and the inferior vertical limb follows the tympanomastoid suture line.

The postauricular incision is made approximately 1 cm behind the postauricular crease, a location that simplifies closure (see Fig. 119-6B). A large temporalis fascia graft is harvested, cleaned of residual muscle, and placed on a ceramic block to allow drying (see Fig. 119-6C). Hemostasis is obtained on the surface of the temporalis muscle. A T-shaped incision is made in the periosteum overlying the mastoid.

The periosteum is elevated, and the periosteum overlying the mastoid is elevated anteriorly into the ear canal. The vascular strip flap is carefully elevated using a duckbill elevator. A self-retaining retractor is placed to retract the vascular strip flap and the ear forward. The blood in the canal is suctioned, and hemostasis is reestablished.

Medial or Underlay Graft Technique

A tympanomeatal flap is elevated anteriorly until the perforation is reached. The tympanomeatal flap, the fibrous annulus, and the tympanic membrane are then cut to the perforation, at approximately the 9 o'clock position. This creates two "swinging doors" or "gull wing" flaps that can be dissected and rotated anteriorly (Fig. 119-7). After rotating the flaps anteriorly, the margins of the perforation should be microdebrided to remove any squamous cellular ingrowth. Any other middle ear pathosis is usually dealt with at this point.

The eustachian tube and the middle ear are tightly packed with Gelfoam lightly moistened with saline. The packing extends up to the level of the bony annulus while leaving the malleus handle visible.

(continued)

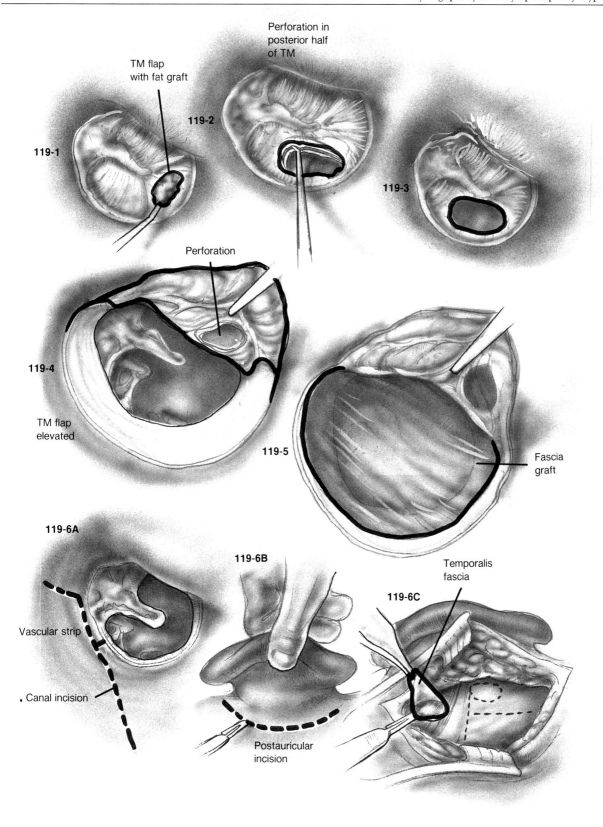

119-1

TM flap
with fat graft

119-2

Perforation in
posterior half
of TM

119-3

Perforation

119-4

TM flap
elevated

119-5

Fascia
graft

119-6A

Vascular strip

. Canal incision

119-6B

Postauricular
incision

Temporalis
fascia

119-6C

■ 119. MYRINGOPLASTY AND TYMPANO-PLASTY TYPE I (continued)

Packing is usually left in place for 2 to 4 weeks, depending on the surgeon's preference.

7. For tympanoplasty, the ear is usually dressed with sterile mastoid dressing overnight.
8. The preoperative and postoperative antibiotics used depend on the extent of drainage or inflammation.

Preoperative Preparation

1. Air- and bone-conducted audiogram with speech discrimination
2. If possible, medically control otorrhea before surgery with cleaning, acetic acid irrigations, oral and antibiotics.
3. Determine the status of eustachian tube function through a Valsalva maneuver.
4. Review benefits and risks of procedure with the patient, and obtain informed consent
5. Briefly review the postoperative care plan.

Special Instruments, Positions, and Anesthesia

1. Operating microscope with 200- or 250-mm lens
2. Patient positioned with the head turned away from the surgeon to place the head in a flat position
3. Postauricular and canal injected with a 1% solution of lidocaine with a 1:100,000 concentration of epinephrine for hemostasis
4. Facial nerve monitor not usually indicated for type I tympanoplasty or myringoplasty
5. Local or general anesthesia depends on the patient's and surgeon's preferences. Avoid nitrous oxide anesthesia, because it tends to shift the graft position. Avoid muscle relaxants.

Tips and Pearls

Tympanoplasty

1. Remove the margin of the perforation, and be certain that any squamous epithelial ingrowth is removed.
2. Carefully elevate canal skin flaps, and protect them during procedure.
3. Temporalis fascia is easier to position as a graft if it is allowed to dry and then is rehydrated.
4. The eustachian tube and middle ear should be tightly packed with moistened gelatin.
5. For medial graft technique, the undersurface of the anterior remnant should be gently abraded to promote the graft sticking to it.
6. Hemostasis using bipolar cautery, adrenaline packs, or other methods should be obtained before grafting.
7. The fascia graft should be placed to make tight contact with the anterior tympanic remnant. Multiple fascia grafts can be used.
8. For the medial graft technique, a fascia graft can be placed medial or lateral to the malleus handle. For the lateral graft technique, the fascia graft must be placed medial to the malleus handle.
9. Canal skin flaps should be replaced carefully into position before packing the ear canal.

Pitfalls and Complications

1. Postoperative graft failure can occur because the anterior mesotympanum is inadequately packed with gelatin, causing the anterior graft to fall away from the anterior drum remnant (ie, in medial graft technique).
2. Postoperative blunting of the anterior tympanic sulcus occurs because of a failure to adequately drill the anterior canal bone to open the angle of the sulcus and because of a failure to pack the canal skin tightly into the sulcus (ie, on lateral graft technique).
3. Small residual perforations can be repaired using a tissue graft or fat graft myringoplasty if performed within the first 6 weeks after surgery.

References

Kurkjian JM. Perforations of the tympanic membrane. Surgery of the ear and temporal bone. In: Nadol JB Jr, Schuknecht HF, eds. New York: Raven Press, 1993.

Schwaber MK. Postauricular undersurface tympanic membrane—some modifications of the swinging door technique. Otolaryngol Head Neck Surg 1986;95:182.

The fascia graft is shaped so that the anterior aspect can be securely placed under the anterior tympanic membrane remnant. The anterior aspect of the graft is then placed as close to the anterior tympanic membrane remnant as is possible. Using a blunt annulus dissector and small 22-gauge suction, the fascia graft is unfurled and tucked under the anterior tympanic membrane remnant (Fig. 119-8). The fascia graft is draped onto the lateral surface of the malleus and is then carefully spread out over the posterior canal wall. Specific attention is given to the spot where the fascia graft transitions from being an underlay to being an overlay. This spot is ideally covered with one of the swinging door flaps (Fig. 119-9).

It is important to inspect the swinging door flaps to ensure that they are completely unfurled and that none of the squamous lining has been inverted or rolled inward. Gelfoam is placed over the anterior tympanic membrane remnant, over the swinging door flaps, and over the fascia graft. A space is left posteriorly to allow the replacement of the vascular strip flap. The vascular strip flap is extended and is carefully placed in the ear canal. The periosteum is then reapproximated using absorbable suture. The remainder of the ear canal is then filled with antibiotic-soaked Gelfoam or with antibiotic ointment.

Lateral or Overlay Technique

A semilunar incision or circumferential incision is made at the outer third of the ear canal (Fig. 119-10). The skin of the canal is elevated lateral to medial as far as the annular ligament. Care is taken to not elevate the annulus or the middle fibrous layer of the tympanic membrane (ie, the skin of the ear canal is elevated in continuity with the squamous epithelial layer of the tympanic membrane if possible). The canal skin is kept moist in a sterile container.

The ear canal is enlarged by the removal of the anterior and inferior bony canal bulges using a drill and cutting and diamond-coated burs (Fig. 119-11). Care is taken to avoid entering the capsule of the temporomandibular joint. The anterior sulcus is completely exposed, opening the angle of the sulcus so that de-epithelialization can be completed and lessen the problem of blunting.

The margins of the perforation are carefully inspected, and any squamous ingrowth is removed. The middle ear is packed through the perforation with Gelfoam lightly moistened with saline. The fascia graft is then trimmed. The largest of the trimmed pieces of fascia is placed medial to the anterosuperior bony annulus and is extended inferiorly into the anterior mesotympanum (Fig. 119-12A).

The main portion of the fascia graft is cut to an ovoid shape that is approximately 1.5 cm larger in diameter than the size of the normal tympanic membrane. A slit is cut in the fascia graft from its edge to one third of the diameter to allow the graft to be tucked around and under the malleus handle. The graft is placed over the fibrous remnant, and using a blunt dissector and microsuction, the graft is carefully tucked under the malleus handle (see Fig. 119-12A). The fascia is then adjusted to the remnant anteriorly and inferiorly. Another small piece of trimmed fascia is placed lateral to the malleus.

The canal skin is removed from the sterile container, and frayed edges are conservatively trimmed. The skin graft is replaced to cover the anterior canal wall and the anterior sulcus and to extend for 2 to 3 mm out onto the fascia graft anteriorly (see Fig. 119-12B). The anterior sulcus is tightly packed with Gelfoam that is lightly coated with antibiotic otic suspension. The vascular strip flap is extended and is carefully placed in the ear canal. The periosteum is then reapproximated using absorbable suture. The ear canal is inspected to be certain that the vascular strip flap lies on the fascia graft posteriorly. The remainder of the ear canal is filled with antibiotic-soaked Gelfoam or with antibiotic ointment.

Closure

The postauricular incision is reapproximated using a single layer of interrupted, absorbable sutures placed in the subcutaneous tissue. A cotton ball and a mastoid ear dressing are applied to provide only light pressure and protection.

MITCHELL K. SCHWABER

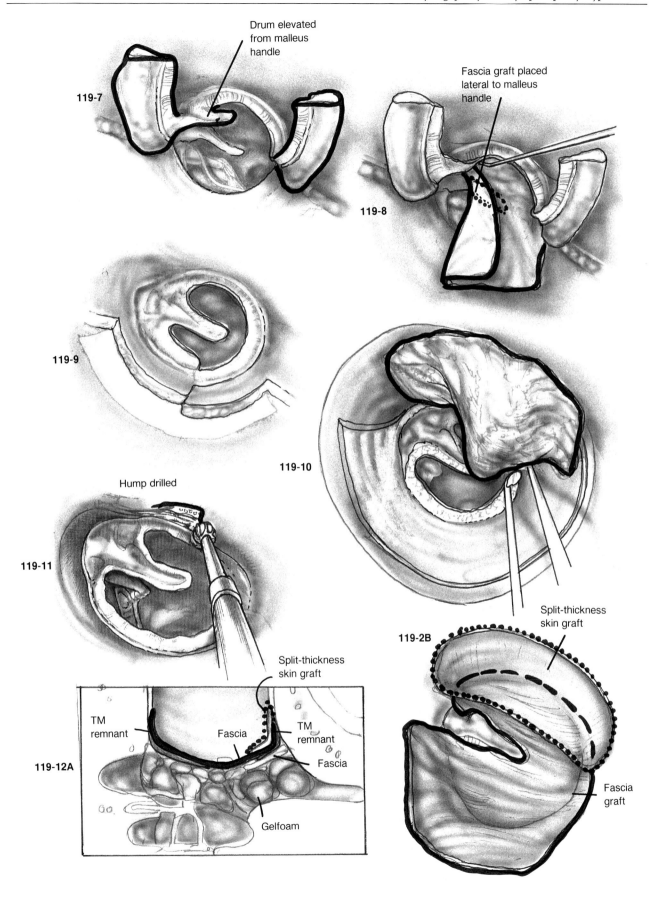

119-7 Drum elevated from malleus handle

119-8 Fascia graft placed lateral to malleus handle

119-9

119-10

119-11 Hump drilled

Split-thickness skin graft

119-12A TM remnant   Fascia   TM remnant   Fascia   Gelfoam

119-2B Split-thickness skin graft   Fascia graft

■ 120. FIRST BRANCHIAL CLEFT FISTULA

AND CYST EXCISION— Surgical removal of branchial cleft remnants from the first arch resulting from aberrant development of the external auditory canal:

Indications
1. Recurrent infections
2. Draining sinus
3. Disfiguring mass

Contraindications
1. Actively infected sinus or fistula
2. Medical contraindication to elective surgical procedure

Special Considerations
1. Management often is complicated by multiple previous excisions.
2. Successful treatment rests on safely identifying and protecting the facial nerve.
3. The surgeon must differentiate the condition from preauricular cysts and pits that originate from abnormal development and fusion of the auricular hillocks forming the external ear, which do not require extensive dissection and facial nerve exploration.
4. Often, there is an opening in the lateral external auditory canal or concha that may be overlooked.

Preoperative Preparation
1. Thoroughly treat any infections, and allow acute inflammation to resolve completely before attempting resection.
2. Document facial nerve function, especially in revision cases, and inquire about previous postoperative facial weakness.

Special Instruments, Position, and Anesthesia
1. No paralysis
2. Face exposed to visualize nerve stimulation
3. Facial nerve stimulator
4. Lacrimal probes
5. Operating microscope and ear speculum
6. Bipolar cautery

Tips and Pearls
1. Initial incisions and exposure are the same as for superficial parotidectomy.
2. In a child with a poorly developed mastoid tip, the facial nerve is more superficial. Avoid incisions below the earlobe.
3. Identification of the facial nerve using the tragal pointer as the primary landmark may result in transecting the cyst tract lying just below the external auditory canal or require dissection through extensive scar tissue. Nerve identification by approaching more inferiorly to elevate the mass off the digastric muscle, identifying the tympanomastoid suture line and styloid process, is preferable.
4. Excise the tract to the external auditory canal, and pack the canal with iodoform gauze to prevent infection or stenosis. If the excised tract is small, primary closure of the canal can be performed if the canal is not significantly narrowed by doing so.

Pitfalls and Complications
1. Incomplete excision
2. Facial nerve injury
3. Salivary fistula
4. Frey's syndrome, hematoma, flap necrosis, or great auricular nerve injury

Postoperative Care Issues
1. Drain the wound.
2. Iodoform packing is gradually removed as the wound heals. In small children, packing removal may need to be performed under general anesthesia.

References
Farrior JB, Santini H. Facial nerve identification in children. Otolaryngol Head Neck Surg 1985;93:173.
Work WP. Newer concepts of first branchial cleft defects. Laryngoscope 1972;82:1581.

Operative Procedure

The patient is placed supine, with the head away from the surgeon, and an endotracheal tube is secured in the opposite side of the mouth. Before preparing the operative site, the surgeon examines the mass and external auditory canal with the aid of the operating microscope, speculum, and probes to locate any drainage tracts into the external canal. These are often lateral, found in the floor of the canal, and a nasal speculum may ease visualization. If the tract is difficult to identify, pressing on the mass expresses the cyst's contents.

The patient is prepped and draped to allow facial movement to be observed when the nerve stimulator is used. The surgeon outlines the involved skin for excision, incorporating it as an ellipse into a standard parotidectomy incision to allow closure with a single scar (Fig. 120-1). The incision site is infiltrated with 1:100,000 epinephrine solution. Flap elevation is achieved through a subcutaneous fat plane over the parotid gland (Fig. 120-2). The surgeon identifies the great auricular nerve and preserves the anterior branches, if possible. The posterior facial vein is identified. The surgeon elevates the sterno-cleidomastoid muscle fascia, dissecting superiorly to the mastoid tip and raising the parotid and any surrounding involved tissue forward to identify the digastric muscle, taking care to avoid entering the cyst. If scar tissue involves the sternocleidomastoid fascia, dissection is achieved through the most superficial portion of the muscle to resect the scar tissue completely. Dissection is carried over the digastric muscle, and the operator elevates the fascia off the mastoid tip and the floor of the cartilaginous external auditory canal (Fig. 120-3).

If there is a tract to the external auditory canal, it is freed by dissecting to where it empties into the canal. A probe in the drainage pore aids in localizing the cyst and preventing its transection. The surgeon excises the draining tract into the external canal and retracts it inferiorly and anteriorly (Fig. 120-4). If the excised tract to the external auditory canal is small, it can be closed primarily, and a stent can be placed in the external auditory canal. If this is likely to result in stenosis, an iodoform pack can be placed in the external auditory canal at the end of the procedure and removed gradually in the postoperative period to allow secondary healing.

The styloid process and tympanomastoid suture line are palpated to delineate the position of the facial nerve. The surgeon follows the tympanomastoid suture line medially and dissects in the direction of the nerve to identify the main trunk (Fig. 120-5). Identification of the nerve from an inferior approach avoids transecting the cyst or dissecting through scar tissue to reach the nerve, as is required if the tragal pointer is used as a landmark. The facial nerve is exposed to the pes anserinus to delineate its course in relation to the cyst.

In small children, modifications of the procedure must be made to protect the facial nerve. The facial nerve in children can be located by making a more posterior and inferior incision behind the ear, over the sternocleidomastoid muscle. The sternocleidomastoid muscle is identified and freed superiorly to the mastoid tip. The digastric muscle and external auditory canal are identified, and the nerve found by blunt dissection in the triangle formed between the sternocleidomastoid muscle, the posterior belly of the digastric muscle, and the external auditory canal.

A type II cyst has no tract to the membranous external auditory canal, but there is a tract passing over or between branches of the facial nerve, paralleling the external auditory canal. The surgeon follows the mass and tracts, excising a cuff of normal parotid tissue around it, with direct visualization of the facial nerve. By working around the mass and branches of the facial nerve, the cyst is completely removed with a cuff of parotid tissue (Fig. 120-6).

After the cyst is excised, the wound is irrigated with saline, and the surgeon inspects the mass, looking for areas where the cyst may have been transected. Stimulation of the facial nerve proximal to the pes, observing for brisk motion of all areas of the face, ensures that no branches were transected or severely traumatized. A small, soft closed suction drain is placed, and the subcutaneous layer is closed in layers with 4-0 polyglycolic acid suture on a cutting needle. The skin is closed with 6-0 fast-absorbing gut or 6-0 nylon suture material. Antibiotic ointment is lightly placed on the suture line, and if a suction drain is used, no pressure dressing is necessary.

WILLIAM B. ARMSTRONG

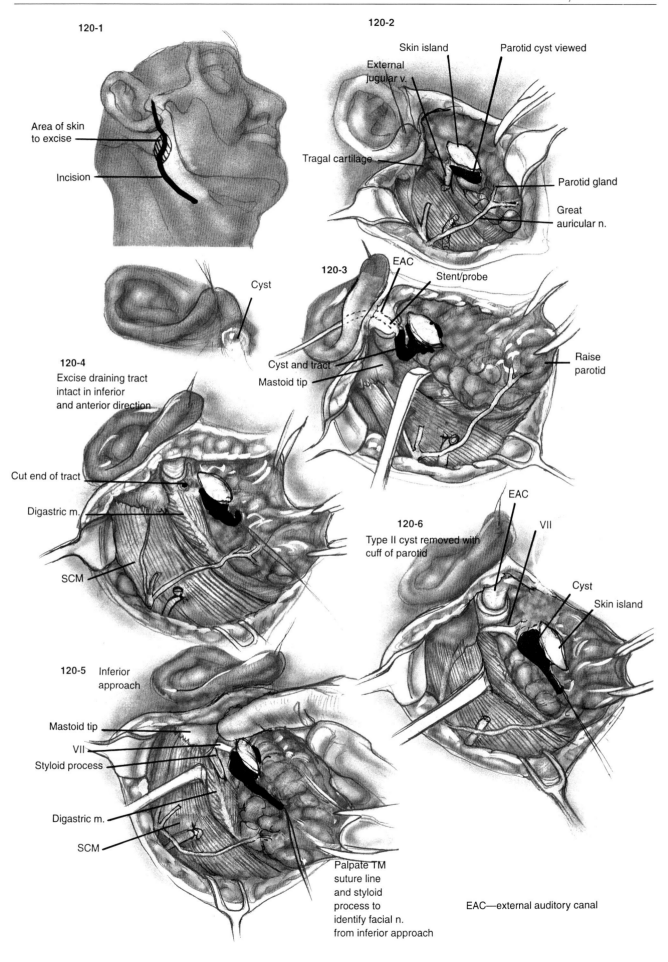

120-1

Area of skin to excise

Incision

120-2

Skin island

Parotid cyst viewed

External jugular v.

Tragal cartilage

Parotid gland

Great auricular n.

Cyst

120-3

EAC

Stent/probe

Cyst and tract

Mastoid tip

Raise parotid

120-4
Excise draining tract intact in inferior and anterior direction

Cut end of tract

Digastric m.

SCM

120-6
Type II cyst removed with cuff of parotid

EAC

VII

Cyst

Skin island

120-5 Inferior approach

Mastoid tip

VII

Styloid process

Digastric m.

SCM

Palpate TM suture line and styloid process to identify facial n. from inferior approach

EAC—external auditory canal

■ *121.* TYMPANOPLASTY TYPE II

This technique of ossicular reconstruction transmits the sound waves through prostheses of homograft ossicles or hydroxylapatite to the fluids of the inner ear by direct columellar pressure.

Indications

1. Ossicular discontinuity due to erosion or absence of the long process of the incus or the stapedial crura
2. Fixation of the malleolar head, incus, stapedial footplate, or ossicular chain (ie, all ossicles)

Contraindications

1. Infection of middle ear
2. Poor eustachian tube function
3. Extensive middle ear cholesteatoma

Special Considerations

1. Size, shape, and location of the perforation
2. Previous tympanoplasty failures
3. Type of graft material
4. Cochlear reserve
5. Tympanosclerosis

Preoperative Preparation

1. Routine laboratory studies
2. Complete audiometric studies
3. Control of infection of middle ear and mastoid
4. Control of nasal allergies

Special Instruments

1. Operating microscope
2. Complete set of delicate middle ear instruments
3. Oval ear specula in sizes 5 through 8.5 mm
4. Ear speculum holder
5. Inventory of hydroxylapatite prostheses
6. Homograft tympanic membranes with and without mallei
7. Silastic sheeting or inserts
8. General anesthesia

(continued)

Operative Procedure

Defects of the ossicular chain are repaired with homografts or the Wehrs incus or incus-stapes replacement prosthesis of hydroxylapatite. The rationale for using these prostheses is the direct columellar transmission of sound pressure to the fluids of the inner ear by the prosthesis (Fig. 121-1).[1]

I think this technique provides more efficient transmission of sound pressure than the use of a direct connection between the malleus and the stapes or stapedial footplate (Fig. 121-2). The sculptured homograft ossicular prosthesis and its commercial counterpart of hydroxylapatite are identical in size and configuration, and the following techniques apply equally to both materials.[2,3]

These operations are usually carried out with a transmeatal approach with the patient under general anesthesia. If the patient has an intact eardrum or a small posterior perforation, a tympanomeatal flap is elevated and the reconstruction carried out. For these procedures, an underlay technique is preferred. For a large perforation, the canal skin is elevated in continuity with the epithelial layer of the ear drum to be used later as a graft. Removal of the canal skin enlarges the working space in the ear canal and gives access to removal of any anterior bony overhang. The bone is removed by a diamond bur under constant irrigation.

This approach also affords good access to the posterior superior ear canal and the ossicular chain. The bony scutum is removed with a bone curette in the same manner as that used in a stapedectomy. The chorda tympani nerve is preserved if possible.

After good exposure has been obtained, the status of the ossicular chain is investigated. If there is erosion of the long process of the incus, the incudostapedial joint is separated, and the incus fragment is extracted from the ear. The malleus is palpated and should be mobile. Occasionally, the malleus head is fixed in the epitympanum and must be amputated and removed. The mucosa is stripped from the medial surface of the manubrium of the malleus to facilitate integration with the prosthesis.

Next, the stapes is evaluated. The lenticular process of the incus is often attached to the capitulum of the stapes, and it is removed if possible. If not, the hole in the prosthesis is enlarged. The stapes should be tested for mobility with a small, curved pick. After the integrity of the stapes is ensured, the location of the stapedial head in relation to the manubrium of the malleus is evaluated. If the relationship appears normal, a short or average Wehrs hydroxylapatite prosthesis with a single notch is used. If the malleus appears high and the middle ear deep, a medium prosthesis with single notch is selected. If the malleus lies far forward, the double-notched prosthesis is required. If the malleus handle is far posterior and almost directly over the stapes, the distal notch of the double-notched prosthesis is removed with a diamond bur.

The selected prosthesis is put in place on the promontory with the cup just off the head of the stapes and the notch off the tip of the patient's malleus (Fig. 121-3*A*). By means of a right-angle pick, the manubrium of the malleus is elevated, and the body of the prosthesis is engaged with a gentle curve pick and the notch slid up along the undersurface of the malleus (see Fig. 121-3*B*). The hole in the prosthesis should then engage the stapedial head (see Fig. 121-3*C*). The prosthesis is adjusted until it is vertical to the stapes and appears stable. It should be stable but loose. Gentle pressure on the body of the prosthesis should produce motion of the stapes (see Fig. 121-3*D*). Motion can be determined by observing the stapedial footplate or tendon. Occasionally, a round window reflex can be obtained.

(continued)

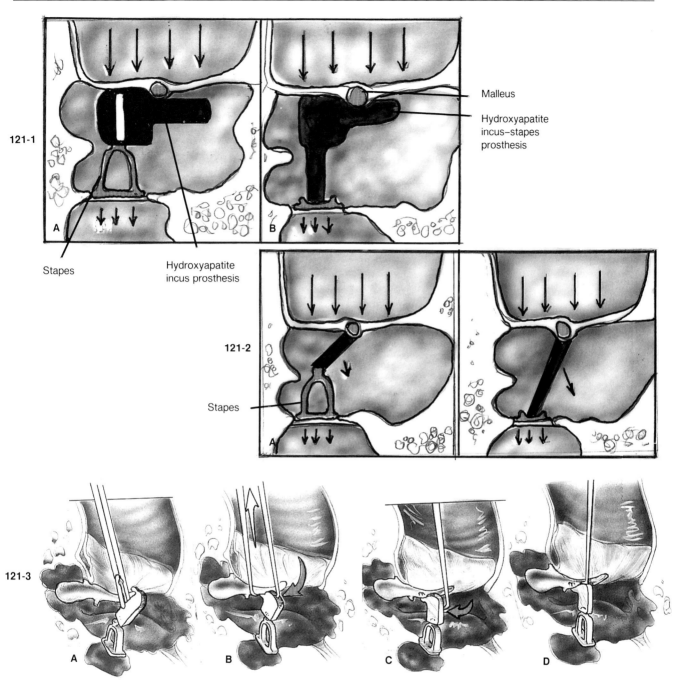

121-1

Stapes

Hydroxyapatite
incus prosthesis

Malleus

Hydroxyapatite
incus–stapes
prosthesis

121-2

Stapes

121-3

Installation of the incus replacement prosthesis of hydroxyapatite

■ *121.* TYMPANOPLASTY TYPE II *(continued)*

Tips and Pearls

1. For adequate visualization during canal skin tympanoplasty, remove the anterior bony overhang and remove the bony scutum.
2. Evaluate mucosa and remove scar tissue.
3. Silastic sheeting to prevent adhesions
4. Avoid sudden motion or rocking of the ossicular chain. If the intact ossicular chain is fixed, do not attempt to mobilize it, but remove the incus. Remove tympanosclerosis from around the ossicles before mobilizing.
5. Avoid motion or rocking of the stapes during reconstruction.
6. Avoid undue pressure by the prosthesis on the stapedial footplate during reconstruction.
7. Attempt to stabilize the prosthesis by using different sizes and locations under the malleus. Use Gelfoam packing around the prosthesis if necessary.
8. Do not remove the head of the homograft malleus in total reconstruction, because it stabilizes the manubrium and helps to hold the prosthesis in place.

Postoperative Care Issues

1. The patient must not sleep on the operated ear. He or she can wear a wire hair curler above the operated ear as a reminder.
2. The patient must not blow the nose hard, stifle a sneeze, or self-inflate.
3. Antibiotics, only if there are signs of infection
4. Remove the Gelfoam packing in 2 weeks.
5. Obtain an audiogram at 6 weeks.

References

1. Wehrs RE, White DW. Notched incus prosthesis in tympanoplasty. Op Tech Otolaryngol Head Neck Surg 1992;3:254.
2. Wehrs RE. Incus replacement prosthesis of hydroxylapatite in middle ear reconstruction. Am J Otol 1989;10:18.
3. Wehrs RE. Ossicular reconstruction in revision ear surgery. Op Tech Otolaryngol Head Neck Surg 1992;3:51.

If the superstructure of the stapes and the long process of the incus are lacking, the reconstruction is carried to the stapedial footplate. The mobility and appearance of the footplate should be evaluated. If the mucosa is thick, it should be elevated from the central footplate with a 45° pick, and a cuff of tissue should be elevated. This affords direct contact with the prosthesis for better sound transmission and helps to stabilize the prosthesis on the footplate.

If the relation of the manubrium of the malleus to the stapedial footplate is normal, a short or average prosthesis is selected. If the malleus is high or anterior, a longer or double-notched prosthesis is employed in a manner similar to that described for the incus prosthesis. The proper prosthesis is placed on the promontory with the shaft near or on the stapedial footplate (Fig. 121-4*A*).

With a right-angle pick, the manubrium of the malleus is elevated, and a gently curved pick is placed under the implant (see Fig. 121-4*B*). The notch is slid up on the malleus (see Fig. 121-4*C*). The long process should be centered on the stapedial footplate by advancing it toward the anterior crus (see Fig. 121-4*D*). This maneuver has the effect of increasing the height of the prosthesis and making a loose fit more secure. However, if the prosthesis is slightly too long, it tends to tip forward, placing the long process at the posterior part of the footplate. If this is the case, the prosthesis should be pushed back down the malleus and removed. It is replaced by a shorter prosthesis, or the shaft may be drilled down with a diamond bur. If the oval window is narrow, it may be necessary to grind down and "round" the square shaft so that it does not contact the edges of the oval window. Gelfoam may be packed around the long process and body to stabilize it in position until healing has taken place. Grafting of the perforation is carried out with a homograft tympanic membrane or dura overlaid with canal skin.

A combination defect is constituted by an intact but fixed ossicular chain. The first step in this case is separation of the incudostapedial joint. If the stapes is found to be fixed but the incus and malleus are mobile, a stapedectomy is indicated. If the tympanic membrane is intact, the procedure should be performed immediately. However, if there is a drum defect, it should be repaired first and the stapedectomy delayed for a second stage. When the stapes is mobile, the incus should be removed and the mobility of the malleus ascertained. If the malleus is mobile, reconstruction should proceed with the incus replacement prosthesis. If the malleus head is fixed, it must be amputated and removed before the reconstruction.

The ultimate combination defect consists of a loss of all ossicular tissue except the stapedial footplate. This may occur in cases with a total perforation, in extensive cholesteatoma, or if the ossicles have been removed and the drum grafted without any ossicular reconstruction. These cases are rebuilt with the homograft tympanic membrane and malleus as the main building blocks. The homograft eardrum maintains the malleus in anatomic position and reinforces the graft. If the malleus head fits well in the epitympanum and there is good middle ear mucosa, the reconstruction may be carried out in a single stage. However, if the head of the malleus must be amputated or if the mucosa is poor, the reconstruction to the footplate should be delayed for a second stage.

The dressing consists of a strip of 0.25-in (6-mm) selvage edge gauze and a cotton ball in the concha. The patients are discharged the first morning postoperatively.

The patient returns for the first postoperative visit 2 weeks after the surgery. At this time, the Gelfoam packing is removed with gentle suction. The patients then return at 2-week intervals until the ear is healed, usually 6 weeks postoperatively. At that time, an audiogram may be obtained.

ROGER E. WEHRS

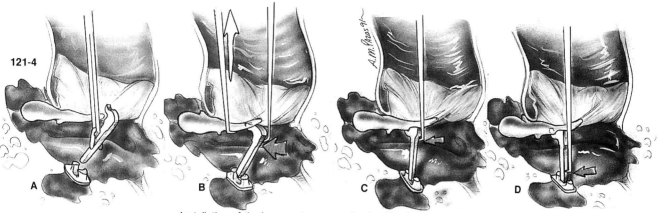

Installation of the incus—stapes prosthesis of hydroxyapatite

■ *122.* TYPE III TYMPANOPLASTY

A middle ear transformer reconstruction in which the tympanic membrane or tympanic membrane graft conducts sound directly through to the capitulum of the stapes in the fashion of a myringostapediopexy or with an interposed prosthetic device such as a partial ossicular replacement prosthesis or, if the stapes capitulum is missing, a reconstruction from the tympanic membrane graft directly to the stapes footplate using a total ossicular replacement prosthesis

Indications

1. Ossicular reconstruction because the malleus handle is absent as a result of disease or previous surgery
2. May be used in an intact canal wall tympanoplasty with mastoidectomy for the stapes footplate
3. Should be considered only in rare instances for an only hearing ear, most likely in an ear that could not otherwise be satisfactorily fitted with a hearing aid.

Contraindications

1. Not indicated for patients whose bone conduction was worse than 30 dB, because a hearing result in a serviceable range is unlikely; consideration of amplification using a hearing aid would be more appropriate.
2. Not indicated in a chronically infected ear or an ear with persistent middle ear cholesteatoma

Special Considerations

1. Has a limited effect in restoring the middle ear transformer mechanism in patients with poor eustachian tube function
2. Has limited usefulness in patients in whom air-filled middle ear cavities, providing aeration over the oval window and over the round window, cannot be obtained

(continued)

Operative Procedure

The patient is supine on the operating table, and the operated ear is prepped and draped for postauricular ear surgery. If the patient has an intact tympanic membrane or tympanic membrane graft, a transcanal posterosuperior tympanomeatal flap is created through a speculum, down to the level of the middle ear space. The tympanic membrane is rotated forward to expose the posterosuperior quadrant of the middle ear. Alternatively, a postauricular incision is made, carried down to the temporalis fascia superiorly and the mastoid cortex inferiorly. If necessary, a piece of temporalis fascia is harvested and allowed to dehydrate for later tympanic membrane grafting.

The periosteum of the mastoid is elevated forward, and the cartilaginous portion of the external canal is elevated out of the bony canal and held forward in a self-retaining retractor. If necessary, a portion of the bony canal is widened to gain access to the entire middle ear space. Care is taken not to remove excessive bony scutum, unless cartilage is to be used to obliterate this space in the reconstruction.

If the tympanic membrane is to be grafted, the edges of the perforation are stripped. Large pieces of tympanosclerosis are removed, and the result may be a near-total perforation of the tympanic membrane. Flaps are elevated posteroinferiorly to a 6 o'clock position to include the anulus, and diseased tissue is stripped from the superior aspect of the middle ear. In many cases, no malleus is present, or the malleus has been significantly foreshortened, and the remaining malleus may be removed by sectioning the tensor tympani tendon and removing the remnant of the malleus and malleus head from the epitympanum.

The area of the oval window is carefully examined. The status of the stapes is evaluated. The stapes crura are inspected, and the stapes footplate is tested for mobility. If the ear has previously been operated for cholesteatoma, meticulous examination of the middle ear, sinus tympani, epitympanic space, and mastoid is necessary to ensure there is no residual cholesteatoma.

The type of ossicular reconstruction is based on the stapes. If it is intact and freely mobile, a prosthesis sitting directly on the stapes capitulum may be selected. However, a prosthesis that extends directly to the stapes footplate may be necessary if there is some disruption of the capitulum or stapes crura.

The type of ossicular prosthesis used is the choice of the surgeon. Various synthetic materials including Plasti-Pore, Poly-Cel, bioceramics, and hydroxyapatite have been used.

For the best long-term results, two areas of the type III tympanoplasty reconstruction must be carefully performed. The first is interposition of some form of tissue barrier between the prosthetic device and the tympanic membrane or tympanic membrane graft (Fig. 122-1). The second is protection of the posterosuperior quadrant of the tympanic anulus, also known as the area of the scutum, to prevent reformation of retraction pockets and reformation of cholesteatoma disease. The most appropriate tissue for this reconstruction is the patient's own cartilage (Fig. 122-2). Cartilage can easily be accessed within the operative field by injecting local anesthesia over the tragus. An incision is made from somewhat posterior to the dome of the tragus to the perichondrium over the cartilage. A decision is made whether an isolated piece of cartilage or a piece of cartilage with the perichondrium intact is to be used for the reconstruction (Fig. 122-3). If perichondrium is also to be taken, a tunnel is created anteriorly and posteriorly to the tragal cartilage, and a portion of the cartilage is excised with sharp dissection. Hemostasis is obtained by bipolar coagulation, and the incision is closed with interrupted 5-0 subcuticular sutures.

For a large attic defect, the perichondrium is dissected free from the anterior surface of the tragal cartilage. It is dissected around the dome of the cartilage and partially dissected off the posterior surface of the cartilage to create a cartilage platform with a perichondrial attachment. The perichondrium that was on the anterior surface of the cartilage is then thinned using a sharp, curved scissors.

For maximum protection of a large attic defect, the cartilage is passed down the ear canal and extended underneath the remaining bridge in a superior direction (Fig. 122-4). It lies at almost a right

(continued)

122-1.   Myringostapediapexy

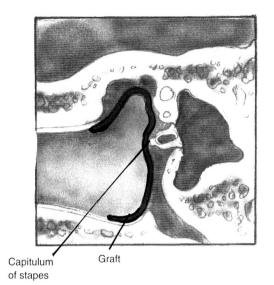

Capitulum
of stapes

Graft

Tragal incision posteriorly
on dome

122-2

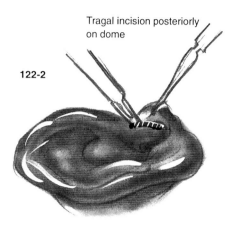

122-3A.   Dissecting anterior perichondrium

122-3B

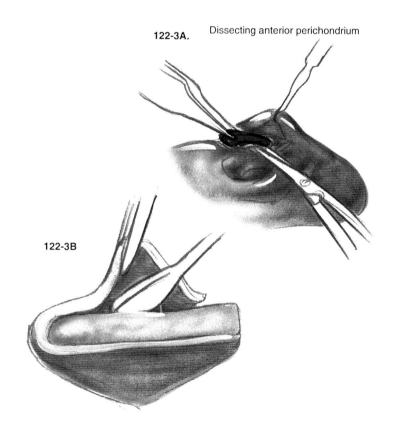

■ *122.* TYPE III TYMPANOPLASTY *(continued)*

Preoperative Preparation

1. A complete audiogram
2. Clinical assessment of eustachian tube function
3. Assessment of the presence of active inflammatory or cholesteatoma disease
4. Routine laboratory studies for local or general anesthesia

Special Instruments, Position, and Anesthesia

1. Local or general anesthesia
2. The patient is positioned supine on the operating table with the head rotated slightly to the side opposite to the ear to be operated.
3. Transcanal or postauricular incisions may be used.
   a. Transcanal surgery usually is chosen for an adult with an intact tympanic membrane or tympanic membrane graft, and transcanal surgery is performed using a standard tympanomeatal flap, as for stapes surgery.
   b. A postauricular incision is used for a patient who has had previous intact canal wall tympanoplasty with mastoidectomy and if there is a need to look for residual cholesteatoma disease in patients in whom a wider exposure of the middle ear and possibly the addition of mastoid surgery would be beneficial.

References

Kinney SE. How I do it—middle ear reconstruction using cartilage and TORP and PORP. Laryngoscope 1979;89:2004.

Wehrs RE. Aeration of the middle ear and mastoid in tympanoplasty. Laryngoscope 1981;91:1463.

angle to the bridge and may occupy the superior one third to one half of the tympanic membrane space. The perichondrium is then draped up the inside of the external auditory canal to obliterate the attic defect space (Fig. 122-5) and to support the cartilage underneath the bridge.

The appropriate prosthetic device is then chosen (Fig. 122-6). If there is an intact stapes capitulum, the cartilage is advanced forward into the middle ear. The prosthesis is then aligned directly on the capitulum, and the cartilage is rotated back posteriorly underneath the bridge, rotating the prosthesis to an upright position, with the platform of the prosthesis lying directly underneath the cartilage. This reconstruction effectively protects the top of the prosthesis from extrusion and protects the attic defect from recurrence of cholesteatoma.

After reconstruction is completed, a temporalis fascia graft can be placed underneath the drum remnant anteriorly and inferiorly and over the cartilage reconstruction and onto the posterior canal wall. The graft may be supported in the middle ear with Gelfoam impregnated with Ringer lactate solution. If there is an intact tympanic membrane or tympanic membrane graft, the tympanomeatal flap can be rotated back over the reconstruction to complete the procedure. The tympanic membrane graft or flap is then held in position using Neosporin Ointment, which is used to fill the entire bony-cartilaginous ear canal.

If the reconstruction (Fig. 122-7) is being performed in a patient with a previously completed intact canal wall tympanoplasty with mastoidectomy, the prosthetic device can more easily be placed into the middle ear underneath the cartilage using access through the facial recess. In this manner, the stapes or the stapes footplate can be more accurately seen and the prosthesis rotated out underneath the cartilage. Care should be taken to estimate the space to be occupied by the prosthesis to ensure a firm fit between the stapes, capitulum, or footplate and the cartilage. As the ear heals and the tympanic membrane or graft begins to tighten, the goal is to obtain a slight impacting of the prosthesis onto the stapes, which provides the best hearing result.

In a patient in whom an open cavity procedure has been performed, an assessment is made of the position of the stapes capitulum relative to the facial nerve. If the capitulum extends slightly lateral to the facial nerve, the tympanic membrane remnant or tympanic membrane graft can be positioned directly on top of the capitulum and then rotated out over the facial nerve, effectively creating a type III tympanoplasty. If the stapes capitulum rests medial to the lateralmost aspect of the facial nerve, the surgeon may elect to place a small piece of cartilage, obtained as previously described from the tragus, directly on top of the stapes capitulum to create a firmer attachment of the tympanic graft to the mobile stapes. In an open cavity procedure for which no stapes superstructure exists, the reconstruction becomes technically more difficult. The surgeon may chose to use a sculptured cartilage strut, which is less likely to extrude but less likely to produce accurate hearing results, or may use a prosthetic total ossicular replacement prosthesis covered by a small piece of cartilage, positioned between the top of the prosthesis to the graft or held on top of the prosthesis by a small black silk suture. The hearing results are less satisfactory for a patient with an open cavity procedure and no stapes superstructure.

On completion of the reconstruction of the type III tympanoplasty in an open cavity mastoid procedure, a tympanic remnant or tympanic membrane graft is held in place using Neosporin Ointment, which is also used to fill the remainder of the mastoid cavity. The postauricular incision is then closed with interrupted subcutaneous and subcuticular absorbable suture, with Steri-Strips placed on the skin. Remainder of the external canal in an intact canal wall procedure is filled with Neosporin Ointment. In the case of an open cavity procedure with a large meatus, a lightly packed gauze strip impregnated with Neosporin Ointment is placed within the meatus to prevent blood clot formation. This gauze strip is removed in approximately 1 week after surgery. A dressing is applied, and the patient is returned to the recovery room and may be discharged home as an outpatient or retained for 1 night in short-stay outpatient unit.

SAM E. KINNEY

122-4

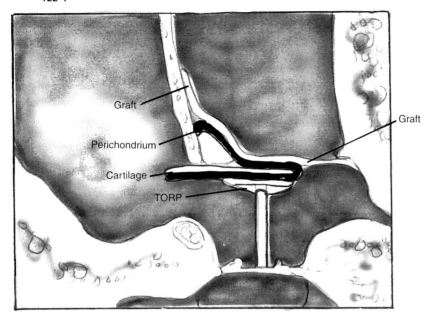

Graft

Perichondrium

Cartilage

TORP

Graft

Transcanal view showing obliteration
of large attic defect by cartilage on
top of TORP

122-5

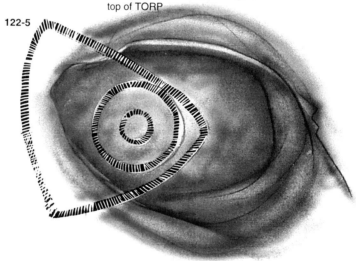

122-6

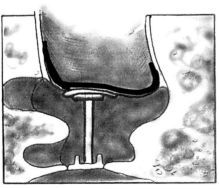

122-7 Intact canal wall
tympanoplasty with
mastoidectomy

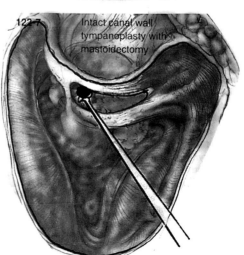

■ *123.* TYPE IV TYMPANOPLASTY

Exteriorization of the footplate with creation of cavum minor

Indications

1. Chronic tympanomastoiditis
2. Destruction of ossicles and tympanic membrane

Contraindications

1. Threatening intracranial complications
2. Recent vertigo
3. Recent sensorineural hearing loss
4. Severe loss of mucous membrane in hypotympanum
5. Blocked eustachian tube
6. Facial nerve protruding over oval window
7. High jugular bulb
8. Chronic resorptive osteitis of the bony labyrinth
9. Health problem contraindicating general anesthesia

Special Instruments, Position, and Anesthesia

1. Operation microscope
2. Full set of tympanoplasty instruments
3. Head holder
4. Sterile double-edged razor blades
5. Finely woven silk or rayon cloth
6. Teflon crescent should be available

Tips and Pearls

1. Must have a dry field to manage the placement of grafts
2. Do not compress a dehiscent nerve.
3. The skin grafts must be thin; the lettering on the razor blade should be legible through the skin as it is being shaved from the arm.
4. Leave packing 2 weeks and the cotton ball 3 or 4 weeks

References

1. Wullstein H. Theory and practice of tympanoplasty. Laryngoscope 1956;66:1076.
2. Nadol JB Jr, Schuknecht HF, eds. Surgery of the ear and temporal bone. New York: Raven Press, 1993.
3. Schuknecht HF, Chasin WD, Kurkjian JM. Stereoscopic atlas of mastoidotympanoplastic surgery. St. Louis: CV Mosby, 1966.

Operative Procedure

This operation conforms to the functional concept of the Wullstein's type IV tympanoplasty, in which the middle ear transformer mechanism (ie, tympanic membrane, malleus, incus, crura of stapes) is totally destroyed, with only an intact footplate of the stapes remaining.[1] The surgical objective is to establish a postoperative condition in which the footplate is exposed to sound energy and the round window membrane is shielded from it. The round window niche and hypotympanum (ie, cavum minor) must be pneumatized by a functional eustachian tube to secure a state of compliance of the round window membrane that allows it to perform at a physiologic level.

Application of the type IV principle is technically feasible only when a wide-field, canal wall–down approach has been accomplished, and it is prudent for the surgeon to have prepared superior and inferior pedicled muscle-fascia grafts for mastoid obliteration.

The functional success of the type IV tympanoplasty, and for other types as well, depends on the quality of the mucous membrane in the cavum minor (Fig. 123-1). Negative prognosticators are thick submucosal fibrosis, granulomatous mucosa, and areas denuded of mucosa. Another negative feature, particularly for type IV tympanoplasty, is a shallow hypotympanum; the most aggravated case is the high jugular bulb. A deep oval window niche or a facial nerve that is protruding from a dehiscence of the fallopian canal and is overlapping the footplate are negative features in the oval window area. Thickened or otherwise pathologic mucosa should be meticulously removed from the oval window niche. The epitympanum is widely exposed and denuded of mucosa and pathologic tissue in preparation for obliteration with pedicled or free grafts.

When the preparative stage of type IV tympanoplasty is completed, the reconstructive stage begins with the acquisition of autologous grafts of temporalis fascia and split-thickness skin. The skin grafts are removed from the inside of the upper arm, preferably nearer the axilla than the elbow and in a hairless area.[2] Using a very sharp double-edged razor blade that has been broken in half lengthwise and gripped at one end in a small needle holder, very thin skin is removed. The skin is mounted on silk or rayon cloth and trimmed to about 1×3 cm. Two to five such strips are usually adequate, depending on how much of the operative site needs to be surfaced. Temporalis fascia is prepared and trimmed to appropriate size to cover the mesotympanum and overlap the tympanic annulus inferiorly and anteriorly and the facial ridge posteriorly and superiorly.

A single incision is made from the center of the graft to the margin to permit exteriorization of the oval window niche through this slit. If the hypotympanum shows areas of denuded mucosa, a thin crescent of Teflon is placed in the hypotympanum, extending from the protympanum to the round window niche. The hypotympanum is filled with Gelfoam pledgets soaked in buffered saline. The temporalis graft is positioned to overlap all margins of the mesotympanum, with the slit opened sufficiently to expose the oval window niche (Fig. 123-2). One of the split-thickness skin grafts is trimmed to appropriate size to accommodate the oval window niche and to overlap the fascial graft on all sides (Fig. 123-3). The skin graft is positioned, the cloth backing is removed, and a cotton ball of appropriate size, soaked in buffered saline, is introduced into the oval window to compress the skin graft onto the footplate and walls of the oval window niche (Fig. 123-4).

The final stage consists of positioning skin grafts to cover nonepithelialized areas, positioning the pedicled grafts for obliteration of the mastoid and epitympanum, packing with rayon strips and cotton soaked in Cortisporin, suturing of the incision, and applying a head dressing. The packing is removed 2 weeks postoperatively, and the cotton ball is removed from the oval window 3 or 4 weeks postoperatively.

If the objectives of the operation—an exteriorized footplate and a shielded pneumatized cavum minor—are realized, the optimum hearing level that can be achieved is a 20-dB hearing level. In practice, about 40% of the type IV tympanoplasties achieve hearing levels of 30 dB or better.[3]

HAROLD F. SCHUKNECHT

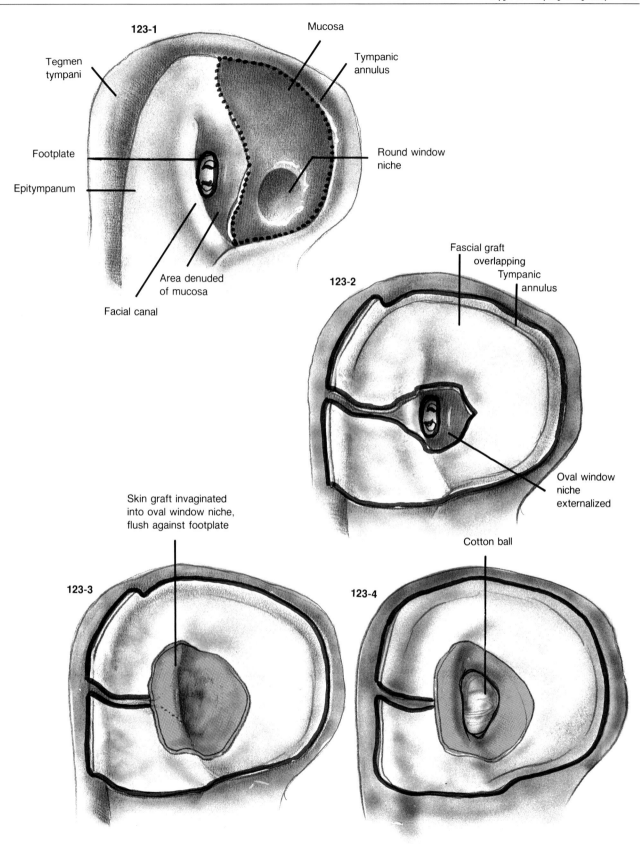

123-1

Tegmen tympani

Mucosa

Tympanic annulus

Footplate

Epitympanum

Round window niche

Area denuded of mucosa

Facial canal

123-2

Fascial graft overlapping Tympanic annulus

Oval window niche externalized

Skin graft invaginated into oval window niche, flush against footplate

Cotton ball

123-3

123-4

■ *124.* RECONSTRUCTION OF LARGE TYM-
PANIC MEMBRANE PERFORATIONS—An otologic
operative procedure for reconstruction of large tympanic membrane
perforations with a chemically modified collagen matrix of autogenous and homologous origin

Indications

1. For autogenous temporalis fascia procedure, tympanic membrane
   perforations that involve areas anterior and posterior to the intact
   manubrium of the malleus
2. For homologous tympanic membrane with malleus en bloc procedure, tympanic membrane perforations that involve anterior
   and posterior zones of the tympanic membrane and an absent
   malleus

Contraindications

1. Ears in which the scutum and posterior canal wall have been
   removed

Special Considerations

1. Ears that have had previous tympanoplasty with lateralized graft

Preoperative Preparation

1. Psychologic and chemical preparation of the patient for local
   anesthesia
2. Optimization of the external auditory canal skin and physiologic
   environment of the canal

Special Instruments, Position, Anesthesia

1. Perkins tympanoplasty elevators (90° and 120°)
2. Left and right, self-retaining Perkins tympanoplasty retractors
3. Back-action Perkins periosteal elevator
4. Double-edged sickle knife
5. Bipolar microcautery
6. For autologous temporalis fascia procedure
   a. FasciaForm kit, containing tympanic molds, solutions, and
      all graft preparation instrumentation
   b. Sharp 30° stapes pick
   c. Methylene blue dye
   d. Wooden cotton applicator
   e. #11 Bard-Parker scalpel blade
7. For homologous tympanic membrane with malleus en bloc procedure, buffered formaldehyde–processed homograft tympanic
   membrane with malleus en bloc (Earbank of Project HEAR Palo
   Alto, CA)

(continued)

Operative Procedure

With the patient in the supine position and under preoperative sedation, the postauricular and supraauricular areas are prepared. Using a 2% solution of Xylocaine with a 1:20,000 dilution of epinephrine, a classic quadratic injection is made into the external auditory
meatus. With the needle bevel parallel to the bone of the anterior
canal skin, it is inserted about 2 mm, slowly instilling the solution
to anesthetize the medial anterior wall of the canal, which is separately
innervated from the auriculotemporal branch of the fifth nerve. The
mixture of 2% Xylocaine with 1:100,000 epinephrine is injected
into the postauricular and supraauricular areas.

Transmeatally, a posterior canal skin flap is created. Incisions
are made at 6 and 11 o'clock (Fig. 124-1). The lateral extent of these
incisions are brought beyond the bony canal through the thicker
meatal tissues with a #64 Beaver blade. An incision connecting the
medial end of these is made 1 mm lateral to the annulus (see Fig.
124-1). This flap is elevated laterally 1 cm with a 120° back-angled
Perkins elevator.

A postauricular incision is made 1 cm behind the postauricular
fold. Dissection is carried between the subcuticular and periosteal
plane down to the meatus. A regular-toothed self-retaining retractor
is placed. Using a cutting monopolar electrosurgical unit, a flap of
periosteal tissue is created and elevated posteriorly with a Perkins
periosteal retractor. The posterior canal skin flap is elevated, folded
back within the lateral meatus, and retained there with a Perkins
toothed self-retaining tympanoplasty retractor.

Frequently, bone from the posterior superior meatus near the
spine of Henle is removed with a cutting bur to attain a direct view
of the anterior sulcus zone (Fig. 124-2). With a double-edged sickle
knife, an incision is made just lateral to the tympanic membrane
(Fig. 124-3). The skin is elevated laterally with a Perkins 120° back-
angled elevator to create an anterior canal skin flap (Fig. 124-4).
The flap is elevated laterally about 1 to 1.5 cm.

The posterior and inferior portions of the annulus are elevated
from the bony sulcus with a small, round knife (Fig. 124-5). An
incision is made with a sharp 45° pick in the posterior periosteum
of the manubrium Fig. 124-6). The tympanic membrane is separated
from the manubrium by dissection of the plane between the manubrial bone and the periosteum.

(continued)

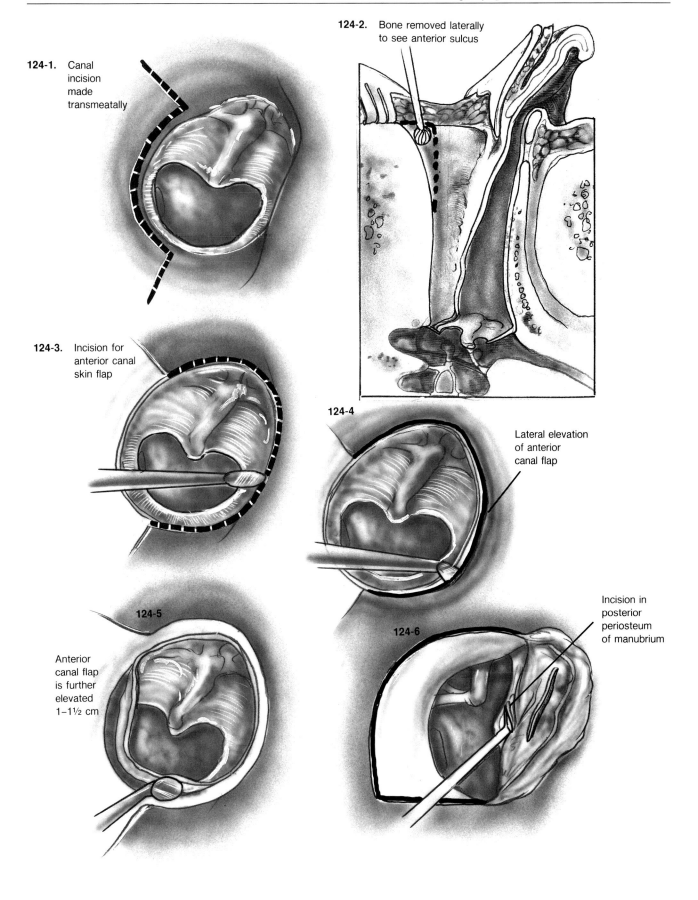

124-1. Canal incision made transmeatally

124-2. Bone removed laterally to see anterior sulcus

124-3. Incision for anterior canal skin flap

124-4

Lateral elevation of anterior canal flap

124-5

Anterior canal flap is further elevated 1–1½ cm

124-6

Incision in posterior periosteum of manubrium

■ *124.* RECONSTRUCTION OF LARGE TYMPANIC MEMBRANE PERFORATION *(continued)*

Tips and Pearls

1. For autogenous temporalis fascia procedure
   a. Harvest temporalis fascia from supratemporal area.
   b. Remove excess muscle and blood from surface of temporalis fascia.
   c. Incise umbo lateralization slit such that it does not pull the graft out of the anterior or inferior sulcus when the graft is applied to the malleus.
   d. Slit the anterior canal skin flap to prevent webbing.
2. For homologous tympanic membrane with malleus en bloc procedure
   a. Slit the anterior canal skin flap to prevent webbing.
   b. Rotate the graft 20° counterclockwise to improve the position for a second-stage ossiculoplasty.

Postoperative Care Issue

1. Remove Gelfoam with sterile instrumentation during the 1-week postoperative visit.
2. Prescribe oral antibiotics for 5 days postoperatively.
3. Prescribe antibiotic ear drops twice daily for 5 days and then every third day for 2 weeks.
4. Avoid water in the ear until the grafts are epithelialized.

References

MacDonald RR, Lusk RP, Muntz HR. Fascia form myringoplasty in children. Arch Otolaryngol Head Neck Surg 1994;120:138.
Perkins R. Formaldehyde-formed autogenous fascia graft tympanoplasty. Trans Am Acad Opthalmol Otolaryngol 1975;80:565.

The remaining tympanic annulus is elevated from its sulcus, and *the entire tympanic membrane remnant is removed* (Fig. 124-7).

If a malleus is present, a formaldehyde-formed autogenous fascia graft, prepared earlier in the procedure, is employed in the reconstructive phase of the procedure. If no malleus is present, a homograft tympanic membrane with the malleus en bloc is selected.

Preparation of the Fasciaform Graft

A 2-cm incision is made about 1 cm above the auricle using a #10 Bard-Parker blade. A 2 × 1.7 cm elliptical piece of temporalis fascia is harvested (Fig. 124-8). Blood is removed from the fascia by squeezing it in a 4 × 4 cm sponge. The fascia is placed on special molds shaped like the tympanic membrane and medial canal (Fig. 124-9). The fascia is dried with a small hair dryer by the circulating nurse. The mold and fascia are placed in a small basin containing a 4% solution of formaldehyde at pH 5.6 for approximately 12 minutes. This process causes crosslinking of the collagen and imparts a shape memory to the graft. The mold and fascia are then placed in three baths of Ringer solution for 5 minutes each to remove any nonbound formaldehyde from the tissue. The fascia is removed from the mold, and any fringed edges are trimmed. The graft has a shape that will not deform in blood or fluid.

Placement of the Formaldehyde-Formed Fascia Graft

The graft is placed into anatomic position, ensuring that the flanges of the graft are on the proximal bony wall of the ear canal while the graft contacts the malleus. Using a sharpened wooden applicator with a bent tip saturated with methylene blue dye, the position just below the midpoint of the manubrium of the malleus is marked. The graft is removed and placed on a cutting block. The point of a #11 blade is placed on the marked spot, and the graft is pulled into the blade, making a controlled slit of approximately 1 to 2 mm. The graft is placed back into position, and the lower portion of the manubrium is exteriorized through the slit (Fig. 124-10).

The anterior canal skin flap is slit to prevent webbing and placed over the anterior flange of the graft. Several pledgets of Chloromycetin-soaked Gelfoam pledgets are place over the anterior canal skin to hold it in position. No Gelfoam is placed in the middle ear. The graft maintains its position stability because of its shape memory, anchoring on the malleus and the flanges on the adjacent bony canal wall. Placement of Gelfoam in the middle ear is unnecessary and undesirable.

The postauricular incision is closed with interrupted subcuticular 4-0 Vicryl suture. Through the external meatus, the posterior canal skin flap is placed over the posterior flange of the graft, and the external canal is packed with Chloromycetin-soaked Gelfoam pledgets. A cotton ball is placed into the conchal area, Steri-Strips are placed over the postauricular incision, and a mastoid dressing is applied.

Fasciaform Graft for Revision of Lateralized Grafts

In an ear that has had lateralization of a tympanic membrane graft, the fasciaform tympanoplasty is an excellent method of revision. In these cases, an anterior canal skin flap is created from the lateralized membrane by making incisions at the inferior, posterior, and superior margins of the membrane. This anteriorly based skin flap is then placed over the anterior flange of the fasciaform graft in a manner similar to that described for the anterior canal skin flap for large, virgin perforations.

Placement of the Homograft Tympanic Membrane with Malleus En Bloc

The homograft is placed into anatomic position and rotated approximately 20° counterclockwise (Figs. 124-11 and 124-12). This maneuver optimizes the position of the manubrium lateral to the stapes for a second-stage ossiculoplasty. The remainder of the procedure is similar to that described for the fasciaform graft.

RODNEY PERKINS

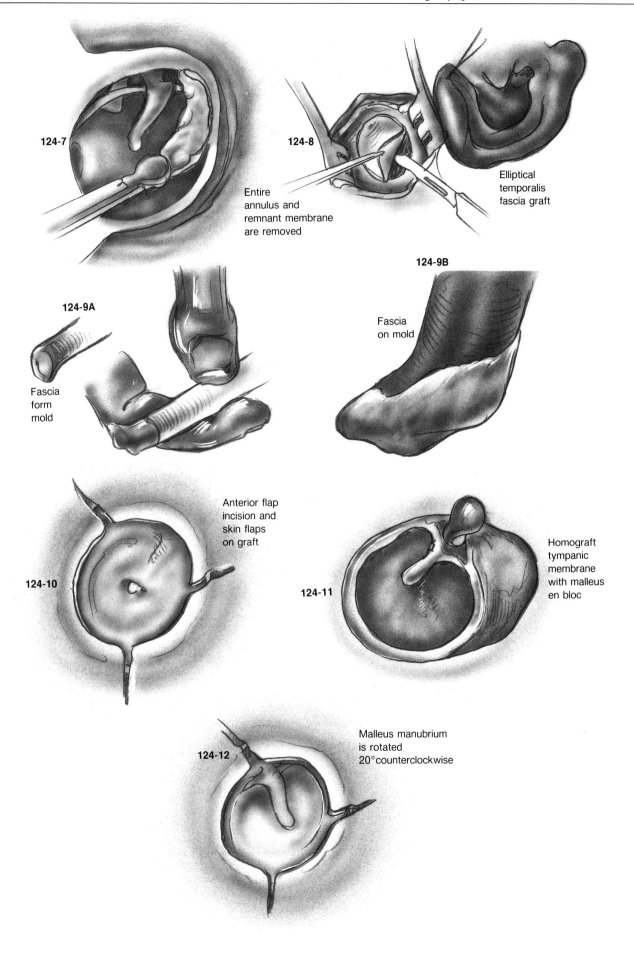

124-7

124-8

Entire
annulus and
remnant membrane
are removed

Elliptical
temporalis
fascia graft

124-9A

Fascia
form
mold

124-9B

Fascia
on mold

124-10

Anterior flap
incision and
skin flaps
on graft

124-11

Homograft
tympanic
membrane
with malleus
en bloc

124-12

Malleus manubrium
is rotated
20°counterclockwise

■ *125.* CHOLESTEATOMA REMOVAL FROM THE MIDDLE EAR

The removal of cholesteatoma from the middle ear requires a stepwise approach. Safe areas of the posterior inferior quadrant are examined first, and the dissection is carried to the more difficult areas of the posterior superior quadrant.

Indications

1. Cholesteatoma that has extended into the middle ear and cannot be managed medically under microscopic observation in the office requires surgical management unless there are medical contraindications to a patient undergoing a surgical procedure.

Contraindications

1. The patient's medical status may not allow him or her to undergo a surgical procedure.
2. Cholesteatoma may have to be removed from the middle ear in the only hearing ear, if it cannot be managed medically with a significant degree of control and safety.

Special Considerations

1. If the patient is identified as having cholesteatoma in the middle ear and is experiencing symptoms such as dizziness, significant sensorineural hearing loss, or weakness or paralysis of the facial nerve, preoperative assessment with a high-resolution computed tomography (CT) scan is advisable to counsel the patient about additional risks and potential complications that may occur with a surgical management with this type of lesion.

Preoperative Preparation

1. A complete audiogram must be performed, and a high-resolution CT scan may be performed, but it is not considered mandatory.
2. Routine temporal bone and mastoid radiographs are of limited benefit and have been replaced by high-resolution CT scans.

Special Instruments, Position, and Anesthesia

1. The patient is operated on in the supine position with the head rotated slightly away from the ear to be operated.
2. Intraoperative facial nerve monitoring may be used if there is suspected involvement of the facial nerve, but it is not relied on as the indicator for approaching the facial nerve. The facial nerve is identified anatomically.
3. The operative procedure is performed under microscopic control, using otologic middle ear instrumentation.

References

Farrior JB. Surgical approaches to cholesteatoma. [Review] Otolaryngol Clin North Am 1989;22:1015.

Marquet J. My current cholesteatoma techniques. [Review] Am J Otol 1989;10:124.

Sheehy JL. Cholesteatoma surgery: canal wall down procedures. [Review] Ann Otol Rhinol Laryngol 1988;97:30.

Operative Procedure

The initial approach is as outlined in Procedure 118 (Fig. 125-1).

In all cases of cholesteatoma in the middle ear, it is most appropriate to enter the middle ear inferiorly, away from the area of the oval window (Fig. 125-2). An immediate assessment is made of the floor of the middle ear to make sure there is no dehiscence of the jugular bulb. If the middle ear is completely filled with cholesteatoma, especially in cases of cholesteatoma intermingled with granulation tissue, resect most of the remaining tympanic membrane to gain better exposure (Figs. 125-3 and 125-4). This is performed using a small middle ear scissors in the middle ear, and the disease is gradually removed from the middle ear with cup forceps. Meticulous care is taken to remove all the disease under direct vision in the hypotympanum up to the level of the promontory, the dissection is then carried posteriorly to remove all the disease in the posterior mesotympanum, and a blunt right-angled instrument is used to gently lift the cholesteatoma from the posterior and inferior portion of the ear and rotate it over the promontory. Care is taken to maintain the integrity of the sac to ensure that all disease is being removed (Fig. 125-5).

If disease extends anteriorly up to the area of the eustachian tube, it is removed from anterior and inferior back toward the oval window. All disease is removed from the middle ear in the anterior, inferior, and posterior areas before attempting to evaluate the area of the oval window.

Once the disease is limited to the posterosuperior quadrant, an evaluation must be made to determine the status of the stapes and oval window. The surgeon gently passes a blunt, curved needle into the diseased tissue and advances it carefully from posterior to anterior, feeling with the fingertips to see if it bumps into or touches the lenticular process of the incus or the capitulum of the stapes (Fig. 125-6). This process is always performed in a posterior to anterior direction to put tension on the stapedius tendon in case the instrument does bump against an ossicular remnant. Once identified, the capitulum is uncovered. Disease is carefully stripped away from the inferior portion of the stapes until the promontory is identified. Working just superior to the stapes capitulum, the facial nerve is carefully examined. A blunt instrument is used to palpate what would be the facial nerve canal to assess if there is a bony covering. Disease can then carefully be dissected between the facial nerve and the stapes capitulum and crura. Finally, the disease can be carefully stripped off the anterior crus. In many instances, sharp dissection with a small middle ear scissors helps to remove this disease.

If the stapes capitulum or crura cannot be identified, the dissection is carried superiorly over the promontory and gently into the oval window using blunt instruments until the footplate has been identified. With care, the disease on the surface of the footplate is gently stripped away in a posterior to anterior direction, being careful to notice any remnant of the anterior crus, which can cause severe manipulation of the stapes footplate with too aggressive of dissection in this area.

The area of the sinus tympani must be carefully evaluated. The sinus tympani lies directly medial to the facial nerve and is located between the superior arch of the round window niche, known as the subiculum, and the extension from the undersurface of the pyramidal process of the stapedius tendon to the promontory, known as the ponticulus. This area cannot be examined directly with an intact canal wall or a canal wall–down procedure unless the ear is operated with an endaural incision and the auricle is pulled posteriorly, with the microscope aimed posteriorly from the patient's face.

For extensive middle ear disease, the addition of a complete mastoidectomy, with identification of the facial nerve and wide opening of the facial recess, provides supplemental access to the area of the oval window, sinus tympani, and the posterior mesotympanum (Fig. 125-7). If necessary, the facial recess opening can be extended inferiorly through the chorda tympani nerve to gain complete access to the hypotympanum.

SAM E. KINNEY

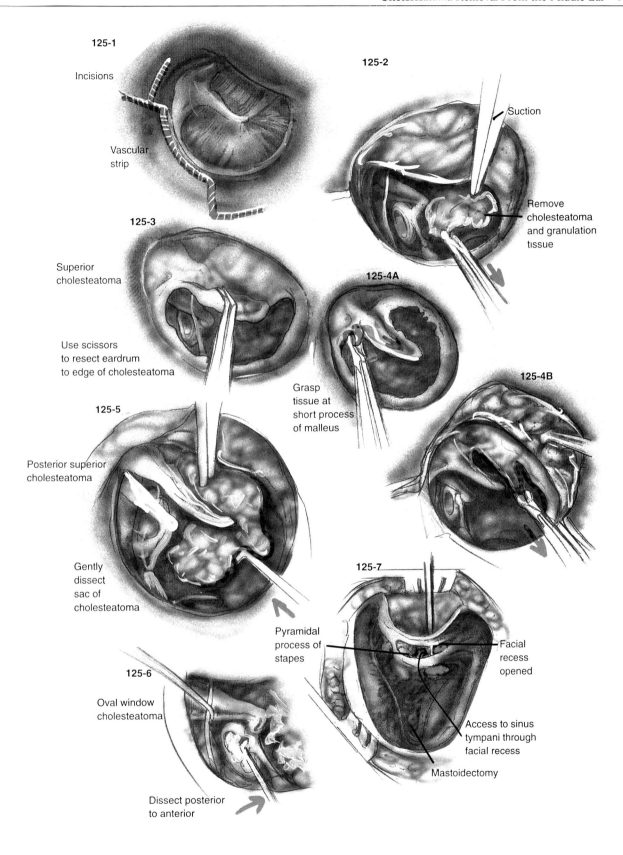

125-1

Incisions

Vascular strip

125-2

Suction

Remove cholesteatoma and granulation tissue

125-3

Superior cholesteatoma

Use scissors to resect eardrum to edge of cholesteatoma

125-4A

Grasp tissue at short process of malleus

125-4B

125-5

Posterior superior cholesteatoma

Gently dissect sac of cholesteatoma

Pyramidal process of stapes

125-7

Facial recess opened

Access to sinus tympani through facial recess

Mastoidectomy

125-6

Oval window cholesteatoma

Dissect posterior to anterior

■ *126.* STAPEDOTOMY AND STAPEDEC-

TOMY—Stapedotomy is the removal of a 0.8-mm segment of the posterior footplate to bypass otosclerotic footplate fixation and alleviate conductive hearing loss. Stapedectomy is the removal of one half or more of the footplate to position a prosthesis into the vestibule and alleviate conducting hearing loss.

Indications

1. Average patient bone conduction level of 0 to 20 dB in the speech range and air conduction of 30 to 65 dB
2. Minimum air-bone gap of 15 to 20 dB and word recognition of 60% or better
3. Unilateral or bilateral otosclerosis
4. Preferably, a negative (absent) stapes reflex
5. Criteria may be expanded for advanced otosclerosis; a patient with a bone conduction level of 45 dB or lower and an air conduction level as high as 95 to 100 dB may be a candidate.
6. Preferably, a negative Rinne on tuning forks 256 Hz and 512 Hz

Contraindications

1. Active Meniere's disease
2. Better-hearing ear or only hearing ear
3. Avoid spongiotic phase of "active" otosclerosis
4. External otitis or otitis media

Preoperative Preparation

1. Informed consent and probability of surgical success carefully explained
2. The alternative of a hearing aid is discussed.
3. Reasonable medical status for local anesthesia with sedation

Intraoperative Problems

1. Various footplate anomalies require experience in management, such as a biscuit deformity or drill out procedure for obliterative otosclerosis.
2. Surgeons performing stapes surgery should be prepared to do malleus to oval window (ie, incus bypass) techniques
3. Unexpected cerebrospinal fluid gushers may require management.
4. A floating or subluxed footplate is best left alone, with the prosthesis positioned over a mobilized footplate.

Postoperative Care Issues

1. Vertigo, which is most commonly the result of hydrops, responds to bed rest. If prolonged, consider a long prosthesis or slipped prosthesis. If delayed, evaluate the patient for a reparative granuloma or fistula.
2. Facial paralysis is unusual but can occur, usually because of an aberrant mucosa-covered nerve.
3. Cochlear hearing loss may be the result of vascular phenomena or caused by a foreign body reaction or intralabyrinthine disruption.
4. Dysgeusia secondary to chorda tympani generally is temporary and disappears in a few months.
5. Late complications may include hearing loss with incus necrosis; wire loop problems, a perilymph fistula, and others causes are rare.
6. Meningitis is rare.
7. Tympanic membrane perforation
8. Cholesteatoma may be prevented by scrupulous attention to surgical procedures.

References

Wiet RJ, Causse JB, Shambaugh GE, Causse JR. Otosclerosis (otospongiosis). Alexandria, VA: American Academy of Otolaryngology—Head and Neck Surgery, 1991.

Wiet RJ, Harvey SA, Bauer GP. Complications in stapes surgery. Otolaryngol Clin North Am 1993;26:471.

Operative Procedure

While the local anesthesia is working in the ear canal, a small amount of 1% lidocaine with 1:100,000 epinephrine is injected above the ear, and a small incision is made in the hairline and continued down to the temporalis fascia. A small amount of lidocaine is then injected underneath the fascia, and a small piece of fascia roughly the size of a pencil tip eraser is removed. This wound is closed with interrupted 3-0 Vicryl sutures in the subcutaneous tissues and a running 4-0 Vicryl subcuticular stitch. This graft is placed in a press and then dried underneath a heating lamp. This graft will be placed over the oval window before the prosthesis is put in position.

Using microscopic magnification, the ear canal incisions are made. A #64 Beaver blade is used to make a curvilinear incision, starting roughly at 6:00 o'clock, a few millimeters above the bony annulus, and reaching its apex at 3:00 o'clock, around the bony cartilaginous junction. A roller knife is used to continue the incision back down toward the bony annulus near the neck of the malleus (Fig. 126-1).

After the fibrous annulus is raised, a gimmick is used to separate any adhesions and lift the flap. If there is an overhang of the bony annulus obstructing the oval window, a "super" curette (eg, Xomed) is used to remove part of the bony annulus (Fig. 126-2). The curette is always used in the axis of the stapedial tendon to allow posterior visualization of the stapes footplate, because this is the limit of the dissection. No curetting over the incus prevents possible dislocation or subsequent depression of the tympanic membrane. A larger right-angle pick can be used to open the iter of the chorda tympani nerve to allow displacement for increased visualization. After adequate exposure is achieved, the amount of stapes fixation is assessed. This is done by palpating the underside of the malleus to ensure there is no malleolar fixation. Stapes fixation is usually made evident by a gentle rotary motion at the incudostapedial joint. This ensures that there is no malleolar fixation and that the conductive hearing loss is caused by the stapes fixation.

Using standard measuring devices, the incus to footplate distance is measured (Fig. 126-3). A controlled fenestra is opened in the oval window footplate. An argon laser set at 1.5-A intermittent pulse is used. A small rosette is made in the center portion of the oval window. A "skeeter drill" using a diamond tip is used to finish the fenestra. Care is taken to support the drill hand against the patient's head. The fenestra is enlarged using a Farrior rasp. After the controlled fenestra is achieved, the stapes superstructure is removed. Initially the incudostapedial joint is cut with a joint knife, and a laser is used to cut the stapedial tendon and to mark the anterior and posterior crura. These are then fractured, and a triangular pick and a cup forceps are used to remove the capitulum of the stapes (Figs. 126-4 and 126-5). Figure 126-4 shows that the fascia graft is then placed over the controlled fenestra. As the fascia is placed, it is initially laid in over the incus to allow it to form a cup in the oval window, allowing the prosthesis to sit nicely. A piston-type prosthesis (eg, McGee, Robinson) can be used. The usual measurement is 0.6 mm × 4.0 mm. This is placed into the oval window fenestra (Fig. 126-6). Once in place, the lenticular process is placed in the trough of the prosthesis, and the hook is pulled up over or the hook is crimped. Positioning is ensured by palpation of the prosthesis to check that it is in the oval window on fenestra. The tympanomeatal flap is then laid back down.

Because the patient is under local anesthesia, the hearing can be assessed. Usually, the hearing is tested by normal speech and a barely perceptible soft whisper.

After this is done, the ear canal is packed with strips of Owens gauze and a string of pearls, which is small cotton balls sewn onto a long silk suture. The pearls are placed in the Owens gauze, and the Owens gauze is folded over the top of these in the canal. A cotton ball then is placed in the ear. This packing is usually removed in 1 week.

RICHARD J. WIET
ALAN G. MICCO

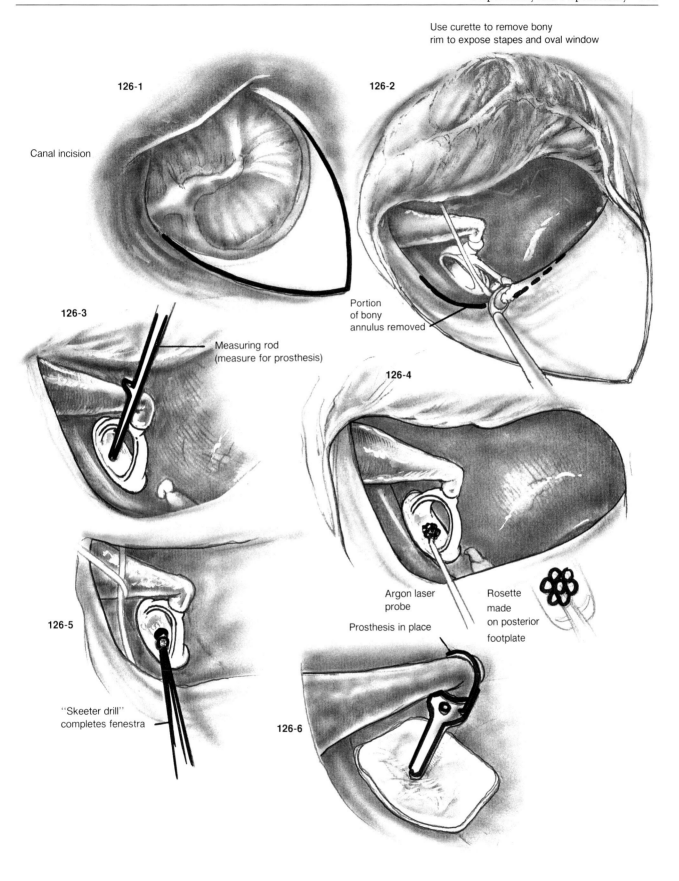

Use curette to remove bony
rim to expose stapes and oval window

126-1

Canal incision

126-2

Portion
of bony
annulus removed

126-3

Measuring rod
(measure for prosthesis)

126-4

Argon laser
probe

Rosette
made
on posterior
footplate

Prosthesis in place

126-5

"Skeeter drill"
completes fenestra

126-6

■ *127.* PERILYMPHATIC FISTULA REPAIR

Openings connecting the inner and middle ear are sealed with fine pieces of loose connective tissue. The possible sites include the fissula ante fenestram, fissure of the round window niche to the posterior canal ampulla, and stapes annulus.

Indications

1. Disorders of hearing or balance meeting the diagnostic and exclusionary criteria for perilymphatic fistulas
1. Sudden or rapidly progressive sensory hearing loss
2. Vestibular disorders with positive fistula test (Hennebert's sign or symptom), positional nystagmus or vertigo, or constant dysequilibrium (eyes closed walking)

Contraindications

1. Inflammation, neoplasia, granuloma, or anatomically related neurologic disorders with which the symptoms and signs correspond
2. The lack of a trial of conservative management

Special Considerations

1. Local anesthesia
2. Minimize blood extravasation into the middle ear.
3. Observe specific areas of anticipated fistulas.
4. Observe the source of fluid reaccumulation.

Preoperative Preparation

1. Preoperative audiograms
2. Preoperative vestibular tests
3. Recognition of allergies to local anesthesia (use injectable Benadryl)
4. No deep sedation; avoid Droperidol.

Special Instruments, Position, and Anesthesia

1. Operating microscope
2. Opposite ear down, with the face away from the surgeon, for middle ear exploration
3. Local anesthesia using a 1% solution of Xylocaine with a 1:50000 concentration of epinephrine
4. Anesthesia standby: Versed (1 mg), with or without intravenous Benadryl (10 mg), as needed, or Propofol (0.25–0.50 mg/kg loading dose; infusion of 10–30 μg/kg/min)
5. KTP 528 laser (optional)
6. Fine, angled middle ear picks
7. Use 24- and 26-gauge suction tips.

(continued)

Operative Procedure

This procedure is used for the surgical repair of so-called idiopathic perilymphatic fistulas (PLF). This type of fistula is usually the result of a developmentally formed abnormal communication between the inner and middle ear through the bony labyrinth capsule. These occur at the fissula ante fenestram or the fissure connecting the round window niche and the ampulla of the posterior semicircular canal. Infrequently, the fistula may involve the annulus of the stapes because of subluxation of this structure.

The patients cannot be considered as having an idiopathic perilymphatic fistula, even though they have the cochlear or vestibular signs and symptoms compatible with this disorder, until the presence of inflammatory, granular, neoplasia, and concomitant anatomically related neurologic defects have been excluded. After these are excluded, the presence of sudden or rapidly progressive sensory hearing loss or a vestibular disorder with the components of a positive fistula test, postural vertigo, and constant dysequilibrium constitutes the necessary criteria for this diagnosis. The physician must be careful not to be trapped by erroneously attributing to concomitant disease the symptoms and signs caused by a PLF. The mere history of trauma preceding the sensory deficit appears to be insufficient diagnostic evidence. Only when the diagnostic criteria are met should the physician consider surgery. The surgeon should initially prescribe specific nonsurgical methods of treatment. Surgery is warranted when these methods fail.

The object of the surgery is to seal the openings connecting the inner and middle ear with fine pieces of loose connective tissue and to maintain graft placement during healing. The fundamental requirements are adequate exposure, preparation of the fistula site, proper placement of the graft materials, and maintenance of the graft's position.

Local anesthesia is used, except in unusual circumstances (eg, child, overly apprehensive adult) to avoid phenomena such as coughing or straining Valsalva-like motion. If the patient is allergic to Xylocaine-like drugs, injectable Benadryl may be used. An anesthesia standby is warranted to administer short-acting sedatives when necessary (eg, 1 mg of Versed and 10 mg of Benadryl, or Propofol given intravenously). Avoid Droperidol, which frequently causes postoperative nausea and vomiting in these patients.

Before prepping and draping, the ear canal is topically anesthetized by coating with liquid benzocaine and injection of small volumes of the local anesthetic agent (Fig. 127-1).

The 1-cm postauricular incision is used for graft procurement. The loose alveolar fibrous tissue overlying the temporalis fascia is the graft material of choice. An ear canal incision parallel to the annulus (Fig. 127-2) facilitates extension for anterior middle ear exposure when necessary.

Graft material is morselized into pieces the size of the tip of a blunt middle ear pick or smaller. The material is divided into two portions, one moistened with fibrin glue component #1 and the other with component #2.

The middle ear is exposed, allowing visualization of the areas from which the fluid is expected: the annulus, the anterior edge of the stapes (ie, fissula ante fenestram area; Fig. 127-3), and the anterior

(continued)

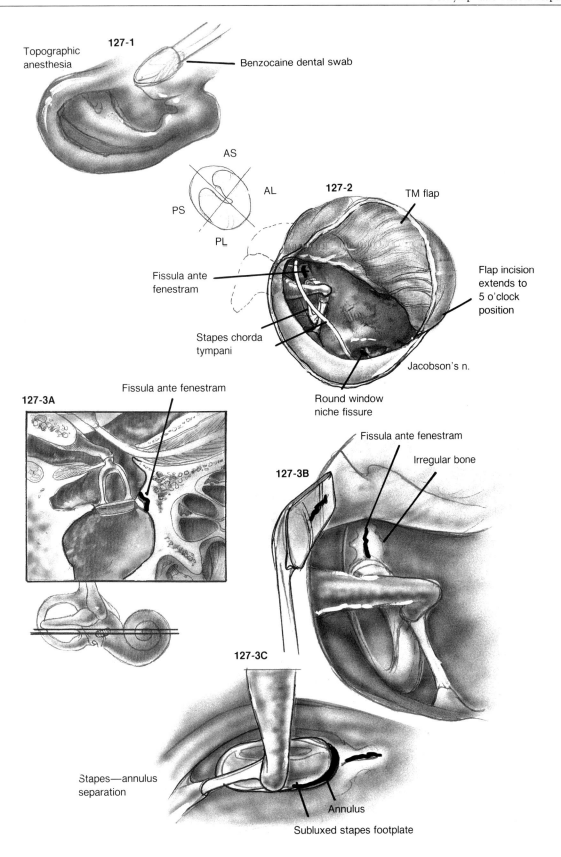

127-1

Topographic anesthesia

Benzocaine dental swab

AS

AL

PS

PL

127-2

TM flap

Fissula ante fenestram

Flap incision extends to 5 o'clock position

Stapes chorda tympani

Jacobson's n.

Round window niche fissure

Fissula ante fenestram

127-3A

Fissula ante fenestram

Irregular bone

127-3B

127-3C

Stapes—annulus separation

Annulus

Subluxed stapes footplate

127. PERILYMPHATIC FISTULA REPAIR
(continued)

Tips and Pearls
1. The overlying mucosa at the site of the leak may be opalescent and not transparent.
2. Perilymph may be contained submucosally and be ballottable.
3. The area of the fissula ante fenestram is usually at the depths of a trough, with a perimeter of irregular bone.
4. The fissure of the round window niche is located anterior superiorly within the niche.
5. The site of leakage in a subluxated stapes is defined by a widened line of demarcation of the stapes annulus.
6. Use small suction tips for the minute quantities of perilymph. Larger tips cause airflows that are desiccating. The total volume of perilymph is 73 μL.
7. The first and smallest piece of graft is critically placed, and displacement is avoided.
8. No mucosal overlay by the graft

Pitfalls and Complications
1. Mistaking extravasated local anesthesia or mucosal tissue fluid for perilymph
2. A tear of the tympanic membrane should be repaired by apposition if it is a small defect. Otherwise, graft material is inserted into the defect, followed by a partial withdrawal to evert the epithelial surface of the tympanic membrane.
3. Pain (inferior tympanic nerve) on manipulation of the mucosa anterior to the fissula ante fenestram
4. Mucosal folds of the round window niche may be mistaken for a round window membrane with a perforation.
5. Displacement of the graft by physical activities (ie, Valsalva or equivalent) is not uncommon with general anesthesia.

Postoperative Care Issues
1. Modified bed rest for 5 days
2. Bathroom with help on the first day
3. Gradual chair to ambulation activity over next 4 days
4. Five weeks of home confinement with restrictions:
   a. Head of bed elevated 10 cm (4 in)
   b. Head kept higher than the heart
   c. No lifting more than 4.5 kg (10 lb)
   d. Avoidance of activities that tighten abdominal musculature (eg, leg lifting, straining at stool); stool softeners often required
   e. Sitting or erect posture is more desirable than bed rest.
5. Patients must be warned that lowering the head to the level of the heart, straining, lifting heavy objects, and nose blowing are to be avoided.

Reference
Kohut RI. Perilymph fistulae. In: Bailey BJ, Johnson JT, Kohut RI, et al, eds. Head and neck surgery—otolaryngology. Philadelphia: JB Lippincott, 1993;1702.

superior portions of the floor of the round window niche (ie, round window niche to posterior canal ampulla fissure area; Fig. 127-4). Minimize extravasation of blood into the middle ear.

Use only small suction tips, 24 or 26 gauge. Airflow through the larger suction tips can dry the minute amounts of perilymph. The observed fluid is gently aspirated, and observation is continued for evidence of fluid reaccumulation. This process is repeated, minimizing possible false interpretations of the fluid. Misinterpretation is avoided by scrupulous observation, looking for the source of the fluid and not just the fluid accumulation. There may be minimal or no observable fluid accumulation until the area of the source (fistula site) is exposed. Occasionally, a submucosal accumulation of fluid is ballottable.

The use of a laser aids in obtaining a dry area in which the source of the crystal fluid can be identified. Without identifying this source of fluid, one can not conclude that a PLF is present.

Desiccated tissue remnants are removed from the underlying bone. Care should be taken at the round window in case of the rare occurrence of an exposed singular nerve or of damage to the membrane. If the stapes is subluxated, the surgeon observes a subtle widening of the area of the stapes annulus with a distinct contrast border (see Fig. 127-3).

The communications through the labyrinth capsule are extremely small (15 to 50 μm). It is important that the graft particles similarly be extremely small—the size of the tip of a pick. The first piece of graft is specifically placed at the identified site of the fluid source (Figs. 127-5 and 127-6). Two layers of this fine graft material composed of 6 to 12 pieces is usually adequate, taking care not to displace the original piece. Graft overlay of mucosa is avoided. If perilymph reaccumulation occurs regrafting is warranted.

The eardrum is repositioned. Canal skin junctures are adhesed using small amounts of the remaining fibrin glue components. No packing is necessary. Immediately after repair, abrupt improvement in hearing is rare, but not unusual for vestibular symptoms.

The patient is kept on modified bed rest, with head of bed elevated 30° for 5 days, gradually increasing activity to cautious ambulation. For the first 24 hours, bathroom privileges with help are permitted. Patients should be reassured that brief episodes of vestibular symptoms are not uncommon.

Daily evaluations are made for hearing (ie, tuning fork tests), nystagmus, and reports of vestibular symptoms. Ask the patient, "Are you better, worse, or the same?" After 3 days, a cautious trial of ambulation with help is initiated. The patient is discharged on the fifth day to ambulatory home confinement. Instructions are given to keep the head higher than the heart, keep the head of the bed elevated 10 cm (4 in), avoid lifting more than 4.5 kg (10 lb), and avoid straining.

At 6 weeks, the ear canal is cleared of any debris, and the patient is evaluated audiometrically and for vestibular signs (eg, nystagmus, Quix test, standing with eyes closed, gait with eyes closed). Fistula tests are not performed.

A gradual increase in activity is allowed over the next month, with the preceding restrictions on lifting liberalized to 25 pounds. The head and bed position restrictions remain.

ROBERT I. KOHUT

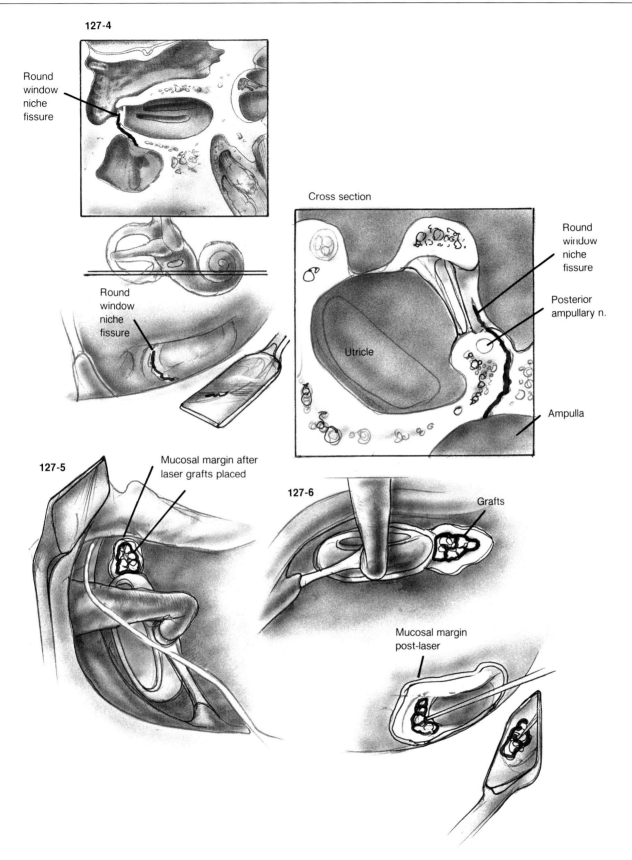

127-4

Round window niche fissure

Round window niche fissure

Cross section

Round window niche fissure

Posterior ampullary n.

Utricle

Ampulla

127-5

Mucosal margin after laser grafts placed

127-6

Grafts

Mucosal margin post-laser

■ *128.* OFFICE REPAIR OF TYMPANIC MEMBRANE PERFORATIONS—Simple outpatient methods of repairing persistent tympanic membrane perforations

Indications
1. Small (<3 mm), noninfected chronic tympanic membrane perforations
2. After removal of pressure-equalization tubes

Contraindications
1. Active ear infection
2. Squamous epithelium on the medial surface of the tympanic membrane
3. Poor eustachian tube function (relative contraindication)

Special Considerations
1. Mechanism of injury (eg, infection, explosion, head injury, barotrauma, chemical injury)
2. Location of the perforation (eg, posterosuperior quadrant, consider cholesteatoma; anterior quadrant, suspect poor eustachian tube function)
3. Degree of conductive hearing loss (>20 dB suggests possible ossicular chain disruption)

Preoperative Preparation
1. Treatment of active infection
2. Otomicroscopy
3. Audiometric evaluation
4. Cleansing of debris
5. Anesthesia with 1% lidocaine with epinephrine or iontophoresis

Special Instruments, Position, and Anesthesia
1. Rice paper or micropore strips as a scaffold membrane
2. Fine-tipped alligator forceps
3. Fine-tipped scissors
4. Myringotomy knife to rim perforation
5. Small hook (2 mm) to abrade mucosa
6. Gelfoam

Tips and Pearls
1. For paper patch, anesthesia usually is not needed.
2. Suitable only for small perforations (<25%)
3. Excise the epithelial margin.
4. Abrade medial side of tympanic membrane.
5. Fat myringoplasty requires adipose tissue four times the diameter of the defect.

Pitfalls and Complications
1. Failure of tympanic membrane closure (common with paper patch technique)
2. Premature displacement of the paper patch or fat graft caused by nose blowing
3. Postprocedure middle ear infection
4. Cholesteatoma formation (rare)
5. Thin neomembrane vulnerable to reperforation

Postoperative Care Issues
1. Maintain a dry ear.
2. Discourage nose blowing.
3. Otomicroscopic evaluation at 1 week and at 1 month
4. Audiometric evaluation at 1 month
5. Paper patch removed after 3 weeks
6. If there is no healing after 3 months, consider formal tympanoplasty.

References
Althaus SR. "Fat plug" myringoplasty: a technique for repairing small tympanic membrane perforations. Same Day Surg 1986;10:88.

Lee AJ, Jackler RK, Kato BM, Scott NM. Repair of chronic tympanic membrane perforations using epidermal growth factor: progress toward clinical application. Am J Otol 1994;156:10,18.

Saito H, Kazama Y, Yazawa Y. Simple maneuver for closing traumatic eardrum perforation by micropore strip tape patching. Am J Otol 1990;11:427.

Operative Procedure
Paper Patch

The patient may be positioned upright or reclining in the procedure room chair. The external canal and tympanic membrane surface are microscopically inspected and cleansed. The size and position of the perforation is recorded (Fig. 128-1). Removal of the epithelial margin of the perforation with a myringotomy knife or otologic needle may be performed, although this is an optional component of the procedure (Fig. 128-2). When rimming is performed, only a minimal amount of epithelium should be removed to avoid significantly enlarging the perforation. In lieu of rimming, some surgeons advocate cauterization of the perforation margin with trichloroacetic acid. We do not recommend this measure, because it tends to incite further tissue injury and may devascularize the tympanic membrane. Disruption of the mucosa on the medial aspect of the tympanic membrane is also thought to be important by some. This is accomplished with a right-angle hook that is swept circumferentially beneath the perforation margin (Fig. 128-3). Manipulation of the perforation margin typically induces a small amount of bleeding. This blood may actually provide an important stimulus for tympanic membrane healing. If on placing the paper patch the patient notices diminished hearing, an audiogram is obtained. The finding of an increased air-bone gap with the patch in place suggests an ossicular discontinuity and indicates the need for exploratory tympanotomy.

Rice paper (eg, cigarette paper from the ZigZag Corporation, Tacoma, WA) or Micropore strip tape (3M Pharmaceutical, St. Paul, MN) may be used as the patch. Using scissors, it is trimmed to a size approximately twice that of the perforation. To improve adherence to the tympanic membrane surrounding the perforation, the underside of the patch should be moistened. This may be accomplished with tap water or a topical antibiotic ointment (without steroids). The patch is placed over the perforation with fine-tipped alligator forceps (Fig. 128-4) and then smoothed against the tympanic membrane with a cerumen curette. No packing or dressing is necessary. If partial healing has occurred, the procedure may be repeated one or more times until the perforation closes or stabilizes despite continued therapy.

Fat Myringoplasty

Unlike paper patching, for which no anesthesia or iontophoresis is used, in fat myringoplasty, a 1% solution of lidocaine with a 1:100,000 dilution of epinephrine is injected into the ear canal and lobule. To harvest the fat graft, a 3- to 4-mm incision is made in the medial aspect of the earlobe (Fig. 128-5). Using fine-tipped scissors and forceps, a piece of adipose tissue approximately four times the diameter of the perforation is teased out of the earlobe. The earlobe incision is then closed with 5-0 absorbable or nylon sutures employing one or two simple, interrupted sutures.

In preparation for fat grafting, the tympanic membrane perforation is rimmed with a myringotomy knife, and the mucosa is abraded with a hook. Using fine-tipped alligator forceps, the oversized piece of fat is manipulated through the perforation. The fat should be equally distributed on each side of the perforation, in a dumbbell fashion, to maximize mechanical stability. Pledgets of antibiotic-containing Gelfoam are then laid in the medial aspect of the external canal (Fig. 128-6), and a cotton ball is placed in the meatus.

Postoperatively, the patient is advised to keep the ear dry and to avoid nose blowing. At the end of 1 week, the cotton ball and Gelfoam are removed, and the tympanic membrane is inspected. Earlobe sutures are also removed at this time. One month later, the tympanic membrane is inspected, and an audiometric evaluation is performed. For tympanic membrane perforations that are refractory to fat myringoplasty, formal tympanoplasty is recommended.

In the future, novel treatment methods, such as the application of growth factors or biomembranes conducive to epithelial growth, may be developed as office methods for inducing chronic tympanic membrane perforations to heal. Epidermal growth factor and fibroblast growth factor have demonstrated substantial efficacy in closing chronic, uninfected tympanic membrane perforations in animals models, and clinical trials are underway.

ROBERT K. JACKLER
HAYES B. GLADSTONE

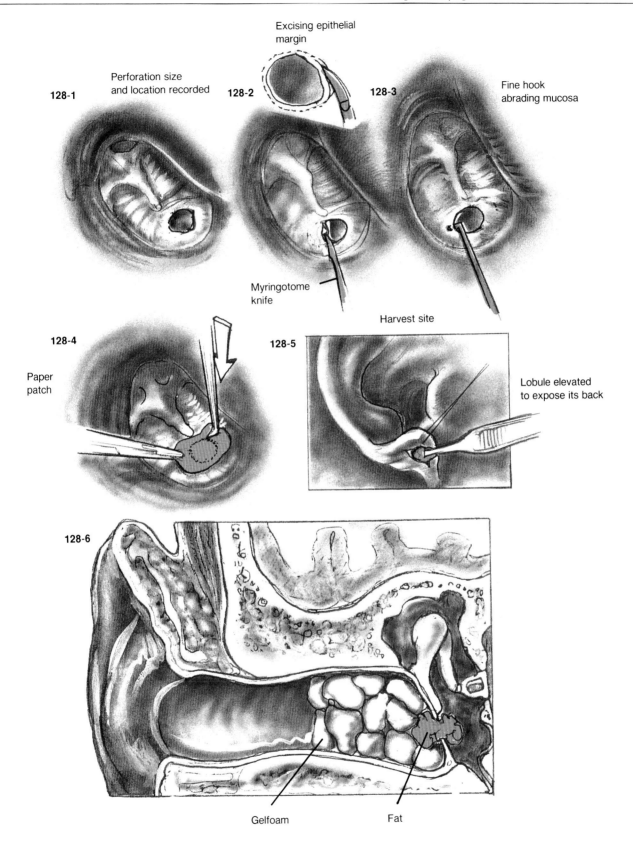

128-1 Perforation size and location recorded

128-2 Excising epithelial margin

Myringotome knife

128-3 Fine hook abrading mucosa

128-4 Paper patch

128-5 Harvest site

Lobule elevated to expose its back

128-6

Gelfoam   Fat

■ *129.* TYMPANIC NEURECTOMY

A procedure performed to decrease salivary flow by interrupting the parasympathetic fibers of Jacobson's nerve

Indications

1. Some cases of severe neurologic disorders with excessive drooling
2. Some cases of postoperative Frey's syndrome after parotid surgery

Preoperative Preparation

1. Careful discussion with the patient or the patient's family, explaining the appropriate expectations for the surgery

Special Instrumentation, Position, and Anesthesia

1. Using a transcanal tympanotomy approach, local anesthesia may be used for cooperative adult patients.
2. Using a transcanal tympanotomy approach, general anesthesia may be required for younger patients and those with severe neurologic disease.
3. The patient is in a supine position, with the head rotated slightly away from the operated ear.
4. Instrumentation is the same as transcanal stapes instruments, possibly with the addition of microbipolar coagulation and otologic laser coagulation.

References

Arnold HG, Cross CW. Transtympanic neurectomy: a solution to drooling problems. Dev Med Child Neurol 1977;19:509.

Michel RG, Johnson KA, Patterson, CN. Parasympathetic nerve section for control of sialorrhea. Arch Otolaryngol 1977;103:94.

Mullins WM, Gross CW, Moore JM. Long-term follow-up for tympanic neurectomy for sialorrhea. Laryngoscope 1979;89:1219.

Operative Procedure

With the patient supine on the operating table, the operative ear is prepped and draped in a routine fashion for transcanal surgery.

Four injections are made around the external auditory canal, with a fifth injection in the vascular strip. A posterosuperior tympanomeatal flap is created and carried down to the level of the anulus. The flap should be created so it may be extended anteriorly along the inferior canal wall to approximately the 5 o'clock position (Fig. 129-1). This extension is necessary to evaluate the inferior-most aspect of Jacobson's nerve as it enters through the floor of the hypotympanum.

The annulus is carefully dissected out of its bony annular groove and swept forward to the 5 o'clock position and superiorly to the short process of the malleus. On elevation of the tympanic membrane, the area of the middle ear is identified and the tympanic or Jacobson's nerve is identified as it crosses from inferior to superior along the promontory (Fig. 129-2). The nerve extends superiorly directly underneath the cochlear form process. Jacobson's nerve may be partially covered by bone or may have skip areas, where it is completely exposed and partially covered by bone. It is important to search the hypotympanic portion of the tympanic nerve carefully, because there may be an anteroinferior branch of the tympanic nerve; if not identified and the nerve sectioned quite inferiorly, these fibers may not be transected. After the nerves have been identified, they can be carefully dissected out of their bony groove using the small, round elevator used to separate the incudostapedial joint in a stapes operation (Fig. 129-3*A*). After the nerves have been identified, they can be carefully avulsed using the same instrument. The area of the anteroinferior branch of Jacobson's nerve should be carefully evaluated and sectioned if necessary (Fig. 129-3*B*).

If a decision has been made to include a section of the chorda tympani with the tympanic or Jacobson's nerve, this is most easily accomplished by carefully dissecting the nerve away from its position, running between the long process of the incus and malleus handle, and then gently sectioning, using middle ear scissors (Fig. 129-4). It is inadvisable to avulse the chorda tympani nerve. An avulsion technique may result in tension or traction on the facial nerve, which could result in a transient facial nerve paralysis. The tympanomeatal flap is then returned to its anatomic position on the ear canal. The flap is then held in position with a rapidly absorbable ointment preparation, a dressing is applied, and the patient is returned to the recovery room for discharge to home according to the same-day surgery protocol.

SAM E. KINNEY

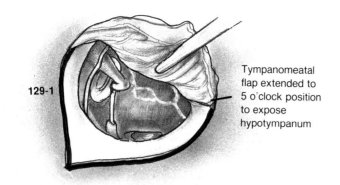

129-1

Tympanomeatal flap extended to 5 o'clock position to expose hypotympanum

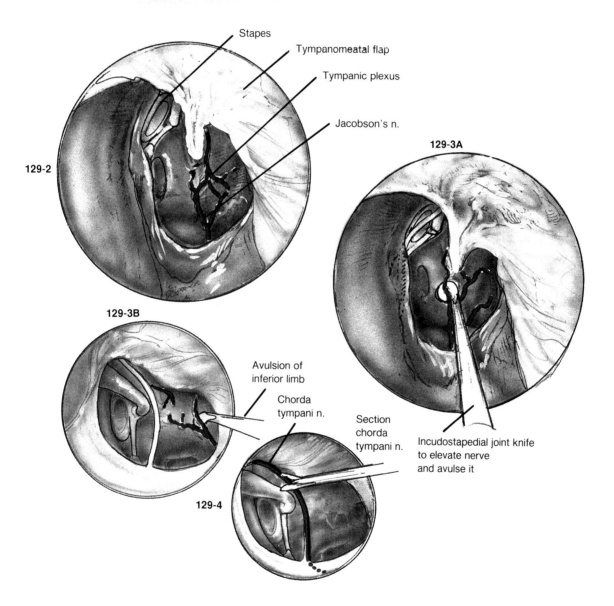

129-2

Stapes

Tympanomeatal flap

Tympanic plexus

Jacobson's n.

129-3A

129-3B

Avulsion of inferior limb

Chorda tympani n.

Section chorda tympani n.

129-4

Incudostapedial joint knife to elevate nerve and avulse it

■ *130.* SIMPLE MASTOIDECTOMY

Complete dissection of the mastoid cavity, maintaining an intact posterior canal wall. During the dissection, the tegmen mastoideum, sigmoid sinus, labyrinth, incus, and facial nerve are identified.

Indications

1. Preliminary step to otologic procedures requiring exposure of structures within and medial to the temporal bone
2. Complications of acute otitis media, including mastoiditis and subperiosteal abscess
3. Cholesteatoma
4. Chronic otitis media
5. Cerebrospinal fluid otorrhea
6. Facial nerve trauma
7. Temporal bone neoplasm

Special Considerations

1. Reconstruction of scutal defects
2. Total canal wall reconstruction
3. Mastoidectomy in children

Preoperative Preparation

1. Audiometry
2. Laboratory and radiographic studies, as indicated

Special Instrumentation, Position, and Anesthesia

1. Operating microscope
2. Otologic drill system with assorted cutting and diamond burs
3. Suction-irrigation system
4. General anesthesia

(continued)

Operative Procedures

The patient is placed in a supine position, with the operated ear facing up. Hair above and behind the ear is shaved approximately 2 cm behind the hairline for the postauricular approach; endaural incisions may also be used, but exposure is compromised. In children younger than 3 years of age, the mastoid tip may not be fully developed, and the incision must be placed more posteriorly (Fig. 130-1).

The ear is undermined at the level of the temporalis fascia, and a transverse incision is made along the inferior edge of the temporalis down to the bone (Fig. 130-2). Avoid cutting the belly of the muscle to prevent bleeding. The remaining postauricular soft tissue is divided by creating a vertical limb toward the mastoid tip. The periosteum is reflected away from underlying mastoid cortex. Weitlaner retractors are used to maintain exposure. Several bony landmarks may be identified, including the root of the zygoma and the spine of Henle. External landmarks cannot be relied on to predict the position of deeper structures. Safe mastoid surgery depends on precise identification of internal structures.

Before beginning the dissection, the surgeon should have a mental image of the completed cavity, which resembles a kidney bean (Fig. 130-3). Bone removal must proceed evenly from lateral to medial positions, across a broad plane to avoid making "potholes." Cortical bone removal requires a moderate amount of pressure to be placed on the burr. As important structures are approached, pressure on the drill is minimized to prevent injury. Dissection parallel to a given landmark facilitates its identification. The sound produced by the bur contacting bone increases in pitch as the bone is thinned, but a change in pitch cannot be recognized if the surgeon is not dissecting along a broad plane. An eggshell-thin layer of bone along the middle fossa dura, sigmoid sinus, and facial nerve should be preserved.

Begin drilling with a cutting bur that is 6.0 mm in diameter or larger and with a 12-Fr or larger suction-irrigator. Use each bur to its fullest extent before switching to a different size, and limit the number of times the bur is changed.

Landmarks within the mastoid bone should be identified in a manner that defines the borders of the cavity and allows rapid bone removal between known areas. Bone removal begins superiorly, at or above the level of the temporal line. The initial landmark is the tegmen mastoideum and the underlying dura of the middle cranial fossa. The dura is easily identified on its lateral aspect and then followed further inferiorly and medially. The dura appears white and has a lattice of small blood vessels on its surface. Continue to develop the tegmen from anterior to posterior aspects; the tegmen should form an acute angle with the sigmoid sinus at its posterior limit.

Bone removal continues inferiorly and posteriorly to identify the sigmoid sinus. The sinus sets the posterior limit of the dissection. The distance from the cortical bone to the lateral aspect of the sinus varies. The sinus appears blue and is usually readily identified. Follow the tegmen medially and posteriorly into the sinodural angle to avoid difficulty in identifying the sinus. After the sinus is found, begin to thin the bone on its lateral and anterior aspects. The sinus gently curves medially as it is followed inferiorly. The posterior semicircular canal is encountered by dissecting anterior and medial to the sinus.

The antrum is then opened (Fig. 130-4). The tegmen is followed anteriorly and medially. The air cells seem to enlarge as Korner's septum is breached and the antrum is entered. The thick, white bone of the lateral semicircular canal may be seen on the medial wall of the antrum. The incus lies more anterior. As the opening to the antrum is enlarged, the incus may be seen as a reflection in the irrigant. To fully expose the incus, open the epitympanum from lateral to medial aspects. Continue following the tegmen into the root of the zygoma while thinning the canal wall on its superior aspect. If indicated, the anterior extension may be continued to the supratubal space, anterior to the head of the malleus. If the epitympanum is approached posteriorly, damage to the incus may occur because the bur may block the path of vision.

(continued)

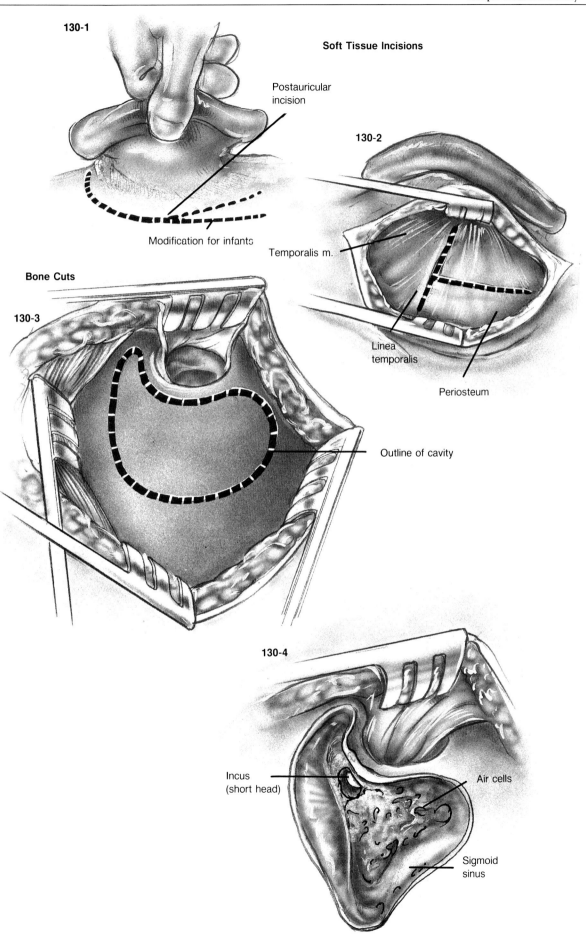

130-1

Soft Tissue Incisions

Postauricular incision

130-2

Modification for infants

Temporalis m.

Bone Cuts

130-3

Linea temporalis

Periosteum

Outline of cavity

130-4

Incus (short head)

Air cells

Sigmoid sinus

■ 130. SIMPLE MASTOIDECTOMY *(continued)*

Tips and Pearls

1. Precise identification of tegmen mastoideum, sigmoid sinus, labyrinth, ossicular chain, and facial nerve is essential.
2. Efficient dissection is facilitated by altering the pressure on the bur, not the drill speed.
3. Proper use of the suction-irrigation system allows irrigant to flow over the path of the bur, preventing bone dust from obscuring the view or collecting in the flutes of the bur.
4. Adequate epitympanic exposure

Pitfalls and Complications

1. Common areas of incomplete dissection are the sinodural angle, epitympanum, and inadequate thinning of the posterior canal wall.
2. Facial nerve injury
3. Sensorineural hearing loss or vertigo secondary to labyrinthine injury
4. Cerebrospinal fluid leak secondary to dural tear
5. Vascular injury

Postoperative Care Issues

1. Mastoid dressing overnight is advised.
2. Severe pain postoperatively is infrequent and may portend hematoma or wound infection.
3. The routine use of antibiotics is not indicated and is determined by the indication for surgery.
4. Audiometry to document outcome, usually approximately 2 months after the procedure.

References

Nadol JB Jr. Chronic otitis media. In: Nadol JB Jr, Shucknecht HF, eds. Surgery of the ear and temporal bone. New York: Raven Press, 1993.

Sheehy JL, Brackmann DE. Technique of mastoidectomy. In: English GE, ed. Otolaryngology. Philadelphia: JB Lippincott, 1993.

The inferior limit of the dissection is the digastric ridge. Follow the sigmoid sinus inferiorly on its lateral aspect to identify the digastric ridge (Fig. 130-5). The digastric ridge appears slightly lighter than the sinus and is oriented in a horizontal direction just lateral to the sinus. Mastoid tip air cells lateral to the digastric may be removed without risk to important structures. The facial nerve is found anteriorly at the level of the digastric ridge.

The canal wall may be thinned rapidly by staying lateral to the incus superiorly and the digastric ridge inferiorly. Avoid creating a defect in the canal by listening to the pitch of the burr, examining the thickness from within the canal, or placing the burr in the canal to see if its shadow is visible. A significant overhang at the lateral aspect hinders visibility during subsequent dissection.

Open the retrofacial air cell tract, dissecting anterior to the sigmoid sinus, inferior to the posterior semicircular canal, and medial to the digastric ridge. The jugular bulb soon becomes apparent.

The final objective is identification of the facial nerve (Fig. 130-6). Multiple landmarks should be available for safe and rapid identification. The tympanic segment of the nerve may be visible medial to the incus, and the second genu is just inferior to the lateral semicircular canal. The vertical segment is lateral to the retrofacial air cells and at the level of the digastric ridge. Continue thinning the posterior canal wall medially, and the nerve is encountered on its posterolateral aspect. Use a diamond bur, ample irrigation, and broad strokes parallel to the course of the nerve to ensure safety during delineation of the nerve. In patients with extensive mastoid pneumatization, it is desirable to maintain an intact canal wall.

Small defects of the canal wall or scutum may be repaired with autogenous or homograft cartilage or bone. Tragal cartilage is widely used for this purpose, because it can be harvested with ease and trimmed to fit the defect. The tragus is injected with local anesthetic. An incision is made on the medial aspect, transecting skin and cartilage. The lateral 5 mm of cartilage is preserved for better cosmesis. The skin is dissected away from the perichondrium medially and laterally, and a piece of cartilage is removed (Fig. 130-7). Minimal bleeding is encountered in most cases and controlled with bipolar cautery. The wound is irrigated and closed with interrupted, simple, 5-0 fast-absorbing plain sutures. The perichondrium is removed from one side of the cartilage. The cartilage is trimmed to fit the defect while preserving all the perichondrium on the other side. Place the cartilage into the defect with the perichondrium facing laterally, and unfurl the perichondrium onto the canal wall for support (Fig. 130-8).

Large defects are more difficult to repair. The prosthetic materials used for reconstruction are associated with the formation of granulation tissue, failure of epithelialization, and extrusion. Cartilage or bone are also suitable for this purpose but can be subject to resorption. A separate incision may be required to harvest autogenous tissue of sufficient size. In all cases, improvement of local blood supply by the concurrent use of a vascularized flap (eg, temporalis fascia flap) may improve healing.

Canal wall down surgery should be considered before performing total canal reconstruction. Review the indications as presented in subsequent chapters including techniques for cavity obliteration. A well-executed canal wall down operation frequently gives the patient a small, trouble-free cavity.

JEFFREY T. VRABEC

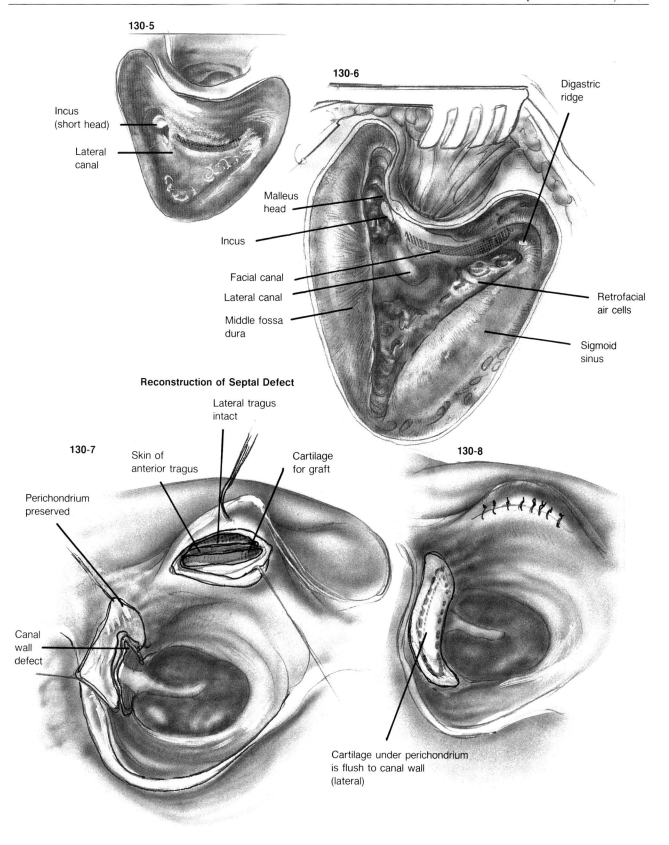

130-5

Incus
(short head)

Lateral
canal

130-6

Digastric
ridge

Malleus
head

Incus

Facial canal

Lateral canal

Middle fossa
dura

Retrofacial
air cells

Sigmoid
sinus

Reconstruction of Septal Defect

Lateral tragus
intact

130-7

Skin of
anterior tragus

Cartilage
for graft

Perichondrium
preserved

130-8

Canal
wall
defect

Cartilage under perichondrium
is flush to canal wall
(lateral)

■ 131. MODIFIED RADICAL MASTOIDEC-TOMY

—The mastoid portion of the temporal bone is exteriorized through the external auditory canal, and an attempt is made to preserve the middle ear space. Cavity obliteration and skin grafting of the mastoid bowl are rarely required.

Indications

1. Cholesteatoma with chronic or recurring otorrhea, with adequate cochlear reserve for possible future reconstruction
2. Incompletely resected or exteriorization of cholesteatoma
3. Poor compliance or follow-up
4. Unreconstructable posterior canal wall
5. Contracted mastoid (relative indication)
6. Disease in the only hearing ear or dead ear
7. Medical illness
8. Severe otologic and central nervous system complications
9. Neoplasms
10. Nonfunctioning eustachian tube
11. Neoplastic disease
12. Cavity obliteration is rarely indicated because of a high failure rate, but it is used when other forms of treatment have failed to dry mastoid bowl.
13. Skin grafting is rarely indicated. It may apply 2 to 3 weeks after a healthy granulation layer has developed.

Contraindications

1. Benign chronic mucoid, secretory, or allergic otorrhea
2. Acute otitis media with coalescent mastoiditis

Special Considerations

1. No aspirin or nonsteroidal antiinflammatory products preoperatively
2. Consider preoperative antibiotics.

Preoperative Preparation

1. Thin-cut (1.5-mm) noncontrast computed tomography scan of the temporal bone, with axial and coronal views. Check for labyrinthine fistula; position and dehiscence of the facial nerve; position, height, and erosion of tegmen and sigmoid sinus; and condition of the ossicles.

(continued)

Operative Procedure

General anesthesia is induced, and preoperative antibiotics are given, if indicated. Electrodes are applied to monitor the facial nerve. The Betadine prep includes the ear canal. Sterile drapes are applied, and the postauricular sulcus and tragus are injected with a 2% solution of Xylocaine with a 1:100,000 dilution of epinephrine. The canal is injected in a four-quadrant fashion with 2% Xylocaine and 1:50,000 epinephrine. Vascular strip incisions are made, followed by a postauricular incision 0.5 cm from the sulcus (Fig. 131-1). A large piece of preareolar fascia (or periosteum) is harvested and set aside to dry.

A T-shaped incision is made over the mastoid fascia, the tissue is elevated along with the vascular strip out of the canal and held in place with a self-retaining retractor (Fig. 131-2). If a previous mastoid defect is present, the bony rim is palpated, and the incision follows the lateral margin of the rim to avoid injury to the dura and sigmoid sinus. Canal flaps are elevated and rotated anteriorly. The middle ear is entered, and the cholesteatoma is dissected from the mesotympanum and off the ossicular chain (see Fig. 131-2). Polyps and granulation are removed, unless they are over the stapes or facial nerve. Disease in the posterosuperior quadrant of the mesotympanum is approached last. Atrophic tympanic membrane is resected.

Bone Work

A complete simple mastoidectomy is performed (Fig. 131-3). All plates are smoothed. The facial nerve is identified, leaving a thin layer of bone over it. The facial recess is opened. The cholesteatoma sac is decompressed, and dissection proceeds always from known

(continued)

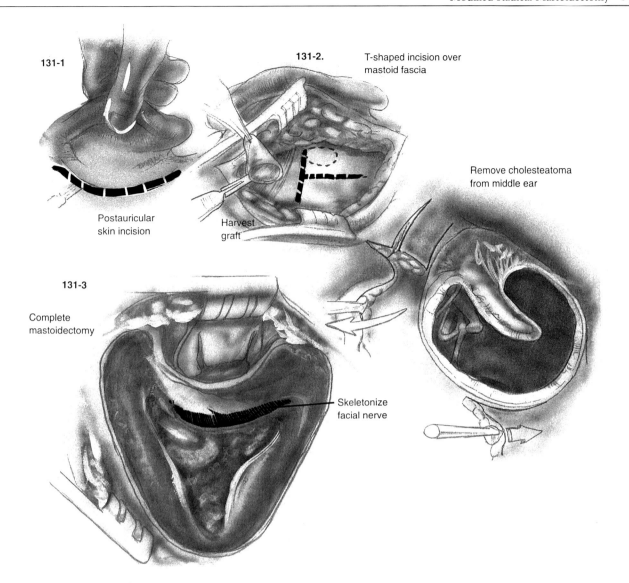

131-1

Postauricular
skin incision

131-2.   T-shaped incision over
mastoid fascia

Harvest
graft

Remove cholesteatoma
from middle ear

131-3

Complete
mastoidectomy

Skeletonize
facial nerve

131. MODIFIED RADICAL MASTOIDEC-TOMY *(continued)*

Special Instruments, Position, and Anesthesia
1. Nonparalyzed anesthesia technique
2. Xomed NIM-II facial nerve monitor

Tips and Pearls
1. Use periosteum or perichondrium (tragal or conchal) if fascia is unavailable for the graft.
2. Identify the middle fossa dura and sigmoid sinus, and enter the middle ear from the attic. Identify the facial nerve.
3. Cholesteatoma that extends onto the medial aspect of malleus head and incus requires their removal
4. Save dissection over the labyrinthine fistula or stapes for last. Dissect along the stapedial tendon from posterior to anterior.
5. Matrix firmly adherent to the dura, sigmoid sinus, or facial nerve is left exteriorized.
6. Matrix covering the footplate is left exteriorized, rather than risk opening the vestibule and causing labyrinthitis.
7. No packing is used. Fill the cavity with antibiotic ointment (eg, Polysporin).
8. Adequate meatoplasty requires a smooth, open, accessible mastoid bowl.

Pitfalls and Complications
1. Poor meatoplasty and scar bands
2. High facial ridge
3. Infection, perichondritis, and brain abscess
4. Facial nerve, dural, or sigmoid sinus injury
5. Vertigo
6. Recurrent or residual cholesteatoma
7. Mucous or chocolate cysts

Postoperative Care Issues
1. Three weeks after surgery, apply gentian violet and silver nitrate to the cavity.

Reference
Glasscock ME, Shambaugh GE Jr, Johnson GD. Surgery of the ear. 4th ed. Philadelphia: WB Saunders, 1990.

to unknown features. The malleus head is removed to expose the anterior epitympanum (Fig. 131-4A). If the incus is involved, the incudostapedial joint is separated, and the incus is removed. The lateral canal and facial nerve are palpated through the matrix to determine if a dehiscence or fistula exists. The facial ridge is lowered, and the chorda tympani is sacrificed. The inferior limit of the mastoid cavity is drilled to the level of the hypotympanum, confluent with the mastoid tip. The anterior epitympanum is drilled down to the level of the anterior external auditory canal wall (Fig. 131-4B). The tympanic membrane and malleus are removed, leaving a thin anterior rim and annulus. Cholesteatoma is dissected off the lateral semicircular canals and facial nerve last. If a fistula exists, it may be grafted quickly or left with the overlying matrix exposed into the cavity.

The final product should be a smooth-walled, rectangular cavity without ledges. The facial ridge should be low, with a smooth transition into the hypotympanum. The stapes is the only ossicular remnant, if not destroyed by disease. An anterior rim of tympanic membrane is left. Gelfoam soaked with epinephrine is placed in the middle ear and mastoid while a meatoplasty is performed.

Meatoplasty
The conchal skin is injected with a 2% solution of Xylocaine with a 1:100,000 dilution of epinephrine, and the ear is placed in retraction with dural hooks. The soft tissue medial to the conchal cartilage is removed, exposing the conchal cartilage. A 1.5- to 2-cm section of cartilage is removed, leaving the conchal skin for the Koerner flap (Fig. 131-5). The conchal skin is incised superiorly between the tragus and anterior helix and incised inferiorly. All exposed cartilage is trimmed or covered. Hemostasis of the flap is confirmed.

Grafting
Gelfilm is placed over denuded mucosal areas. Pressed Gelfoam soaked in Tis-U-Sol (Ringer lactate) is placed into the eustachian tube and middle ear. The graft is tucked firmly under the anterior annulus and draped over the stapes, facial ridge, and mastoid (Fig. 131-6). Exposed perilabyrinthine, retrofacial, zygomatic, and peritubal air cell tracts are also covered with grafts. If the stapes is lower than the facial ridge, the malleus head (autoclaved), tragal cartilage, or a partial ossicular replacement prosthesis (PORP) may be used to augment. Polysporin ointment is placed over the graft, filling the medial one half of the cavity. The Koerner flap is then tacked with a superior and inferior 3-0 Vicryl suture to maintain an adequate meatoplasty; it should not be overtightened (Fig. 131-7). The postauricular incision is closed with interrupted 3-0 Vicryl. The flap position is checked, the remainder of the cavity filled with ointment, and a Glasscock dressing is applied.

Postoperative Care
On the first postoperative day, the dressing is removed, and the cotton ball is changed. The patient is instructed to avoid nose blowing and water in the ear. Pain medication and stool softeners are dispensed. The patient returns to the office in 3 weeks and gentian violet and silver nitrate are applied during the next month, as required, on a weekly basis. The cavity is usually healed in 2 months, after which water activity is permitted.

MICHAEL E. GLASSCOCK III
DAVID G. SCHALL
JOHN D. MACIAS
MARK H. WIDICK

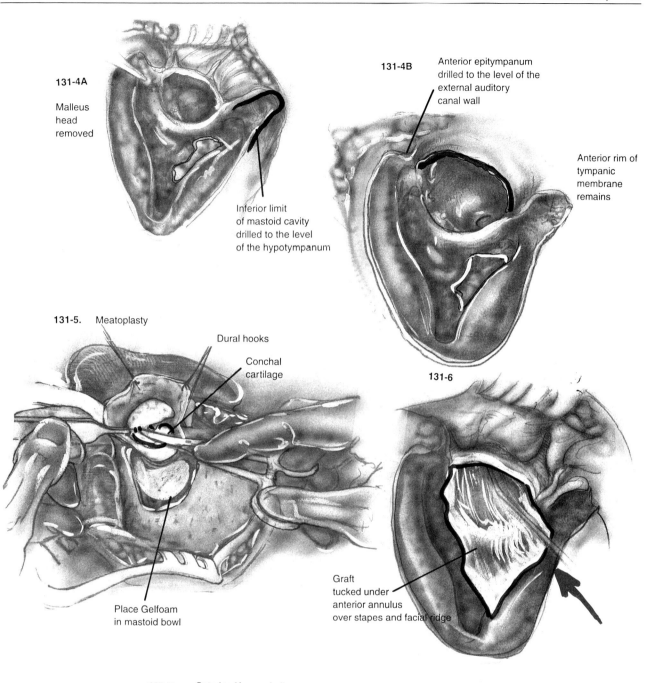

131-4A

Malleus
head
removed

Inferior limit
of mastoid cavity
drilled to the level
of the hypotympanum

131-4B Anterior epitympanum
drilled to the level of the
external auditory
canal wall

Anterior rim of
tympanic
membrane
remains

131-5. Meatoplasty

Dural hooks

Conchal
cartilage

Place Gelfoam
in mastoid bowl

131-6

Graft
tucked under
anterior annulus
over stapes and facial ridge

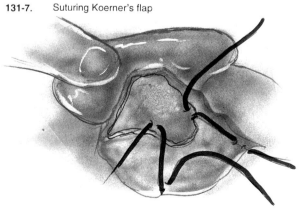

131-7. Suturing Koerner's flap

■ 132. MASTOIDECTOMY: RADICAL CAVITY AND MIDDLE EAR OBLITERATION—Radical

mastoidectomy is an operation designed to eradicate middle ear and mastoid disease by the formation of an exteriorized common cavity that includes the external auditory canal, middle ear, and mastoid cavity. This operation includes removal of the tympanic membrane and ossicles, excluding the stapes. There is no attempt to reconstruct the tympanic membrane and ossicular chain or to obliterate the mastoid cavity.

Indications

1. Radical mastoidectomy is rarely indicated except for unresectable disease.
2. Middle ear obliteration is indicated in the ear with cochlear destruction for which complete resection of disease is achieved.

Contraindications

1. Obliteration is contraindicated if there is incomplete resection of disease.

Preoperative Preparation

1. Careful patient evaluation to guide the surgical approach and patient counseling
2. High-resolution computed tomography (ie, coronal and axial views)
3. Laboratory studies, including a clotting profile if appropriate for the patient's age and history

Special Instruments, Position, and Anesthesia

1. Operating microscope
2. Otologic drill and suction irrigation system
3. Facial nerve monitor
4. Otologic instrumentation
5. Supine position secured with three safety straps and careful padding
6. Blood pressure cuff on the upper extremity opposite to the ear operated on
7. Long tubing for anesthetic delivery and intravenous fluids
8. Anesthesia is placed at the foot of the bed or in such a position as to allow placement of the microscope at the head of the bed and the scrub technician across from the surgeon at the head of the bed

(continued)

Operative Procedure

Obliteration is a controversial procedure. It is suggested as a method to reduce mastoid bowl complications after modified radical mastoidectomy, especially if there is a large cavity, by filling it with muscle, fascia, or bone pate. It is also advocated for the ear that has cochlear destruction resulting in sensorineural hearing loss and cochlear fistula. The ear is eradicated of disease, the mastoid is obliterated, and the canal is over sewn. If obliteration is deemed appropriate and is anticipated, the postauricular incision is modified to allow for a Palva flap (ie, postauricular musculoperiosteal flap). An alternative is an anteriorly based temporalis muscle pedicle or temporalis fascia flap pedicled on the superficial temporal artery. At the end of the procedure it is layered into the cavity, the canal skin is everted and oversewn in layers.

After general endotracheal anesthesia, proper positioning, and placement of the facial nerve monitor, the patient is prepared and draped sterilely, and the postauricular area and tragus is injected with a solution of 1% lidocaine and a 1:100,000 dilution of epinephrine. The ear is examined under magnification, irrigated with dilute Betadine and saline, and cleaned. If the patient has an intact posterior canal wall, the vascular strip and canal skin is injected with 1:50,000 epinephrine. Modified vascular strip incisions are made (Fig. 132-1). Attention is turned to the postauricular region, where an incision is made down to the musculofacial layer approximately 1 cm behind the postauricular crease (Fig. 132-2). The ear is reflected anteriorly.

An incision is made along the zygomaticotemporal line horizontally down to bone, with a vertical incision made at the midpoint and extending down to the mastoid tip (ie, T-shaped incision; Fig. 132-3). Hemostasis is achieved with electrocautery. Care is taken, especially in revision operations, that there is no dehiscence over the middle fossa dura or sigmoid sinus. The musculofacial tissues are reflected first posteriorly and then superiorly, with mobilization of the anterior tissue and delivery of the vascular strip. Self-retaining retractors are placed, and mastoidectomy is performed using a large cutting bur and suction irrigation in a three-dimensional anatomic fashion. The middle fossa dura and the sigmoid sinus are located, with dissection continuing medially. When diseased tissue is encountered, it is mobilized. The dissection continues, penetrating Körner's septum if it is not eroded. The mastoid tip is drilled, and the digastric ridge is identified. The digastric ridge is developed as a blunt structure, partially exposing muscle. The sinodural angle is developed. The zygomatic air cells are dissected by following the tegmen and the posterior canal wall; the incus is identified if possible. The horizontal semicircular canal is identified. Care is taken to detect fistulas.

As the bony dissection proceeds, it is important to maintain the configuration of the cholesteatoma by centrally debulking it and carefully dissecting it from the surrounding bone. This allows careful examination and detection of horizontal canal fistulas, facial nerve dehiscence, middle fossa extension, and sigmoid sinus exposure. Methodical removal in this manner maximizes the opportunity for

(continued)

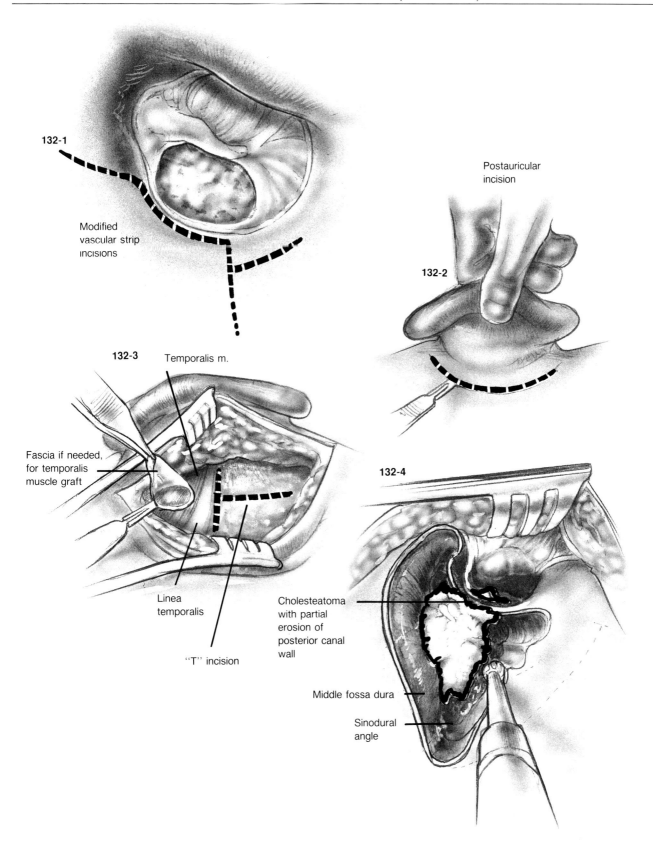

132-1

Modified
vascular strip
incisions

Postauricular
incision

132-2

132-3   Temporalis m.

Fascia if needed,
for temporalis
muscle graft

Linea
temporalis

"T" incision

132-4

Cholesteatoma
with partial
erosion of
posterior canal
wall

Middle fossa dura

Sinodural
angle

■ 132. MASTOIDECTOMY: RADICAL CAVITY AND MIDDLE EAR OBLITERATION (continued)

Tips and Pearls

1. Careful three-dimensional anatomic dissection with identification of landmarks reduces intraoperative complications.
2. Facial nerve identification is facilitated by production of an ultrathin posterior canal wall, development of the digastric ridge until it is a blunt ridge with a small amount of muscle exposed, and careful identification of the fossa incudis.
3. A large meatoplasty is maintained by preventing stenosis. This is facilitated by removal of most of the conchal cartilage instead of only a thin crescent.
4. Meticulous hemostasis and frequent irrigation of the operative field aids identification of the anatomy.
5. Bony dissection is performed with removal of as much of the mastoid air cells as reasonably possible. The limits of the cavity are dense cortical bone.

Pitfalls and Complications

1. Facial nerve injury
2. Violation of the otic capsule
3. Inadequate exteriorization and removal of disease

Postoperative Care Issues

1. Careful follow-up, with cleansing of the mastoid bowl
2. Granulation tissue is managed with silver nitrate and gentian violet
3. Vigilance for recurrent disease

References

Glasscock ME, Shambaugh GE. The open cavity mastoid operations. In: Surgery of the ear. 4th ed. Philadelphia: WB Saunders, 1990:228.

Nadol JB, Schuknecht H. Surgery of the ear and temporal bone. New York: Raven Press, 1993.

complete resection. In a poorly pneumatized temporal bone, it may be easier to identify the facial nerve in the tympanic segment after removing incus or malleus remnants and to identify the stapes superstructure, if it exits. The cochleariform process also serves as an important landmark. Facial nerve dehiscence should be kept in mind as well as the realization that this is a common area for facial nerve injury in chronic ear surgery.

In a well-pneumatized temporal bone, the fossa incudis, horizontal canal, digastric ridge, and posterior canal wall can be used as landmarks for identification of the vertical segment of the facial nerve using a #4 diamond bur. Typically, the otologist has enough information to tailor the surgical procedure, and the decision for a canal wall down procedure is made. Commonly, with this level of disease, a modified radical mastoidectomy is performed, and for the procedure to progress to a radical mastoidectomy, the disease is extensive, with destruction of middle ear landmarks and portions of the posterior canal wall (Fig. 132-4). The canal wall is taken down at this point, using a large cutting bur initially, followed by a #4 diamond bur as the fallopian canal is skeletonized (Fig. 132-5). At times, a fine rongeur speeds up the process. Large volumes of free irrigation are used throughout the procedure to maintain a clean field.

Disease is removed from the middle ear and eustachian tube as completely as possible, with care taken to maintain the integrity of the stapes superstructure, footplate, and the round window. The labyrinth and the mastoid cavity are carefully dissected with the diamond bur, removing cholesteatoma and any matrix trapped in mastoid air cells. The mucosa is stripped from the eustachian tube, with the remaining portion inverted, and the orifice is plugged with fascia or muscle (Fig. 132-6). The middle ear and mastoid are copiously irrigated with normal saline and then packed with epinephrine-soaked (1:1000) Gelfoam for hemostasis. If the middle ear is to be obliterated, the canal skin is trimmed, and mattress sutures are placed to avert the squamous epithelium sealing the ear (Fig. 132-7).

If a radical mastoidectomy is to be performed, the ear is reflected anteriorly and held in place with dural hooks. The soft tissue overlying the conchal cartilage posteriorly is dissected off with short, sharp scissors. An incision is made along the free edge of the conchal cartilage, leaving perichondrium and skin intact anteriorly, and most of the conchal cartilage is removed. An incision is made superiorly through the external auditory canal, followed by an incision inferiorly, making a large thumb-sized meatus to complete the exteriorization (Fig. 132-8). The Gelfoam is removed, and the cavity is filled with ointment. The vascular strip that was extended using the superior and inferior incisions is put into a vertical position in the mastoid cavity and held in place with three suspending 3-0 absorbable sutures. The subcutaneous tissue is then approximated using inverted 3-0 Vicryl, and the rest of the cavity is filled with antibiotic ointment. A Glasscock dressing is placed.

VINCENT N. CARRASCO

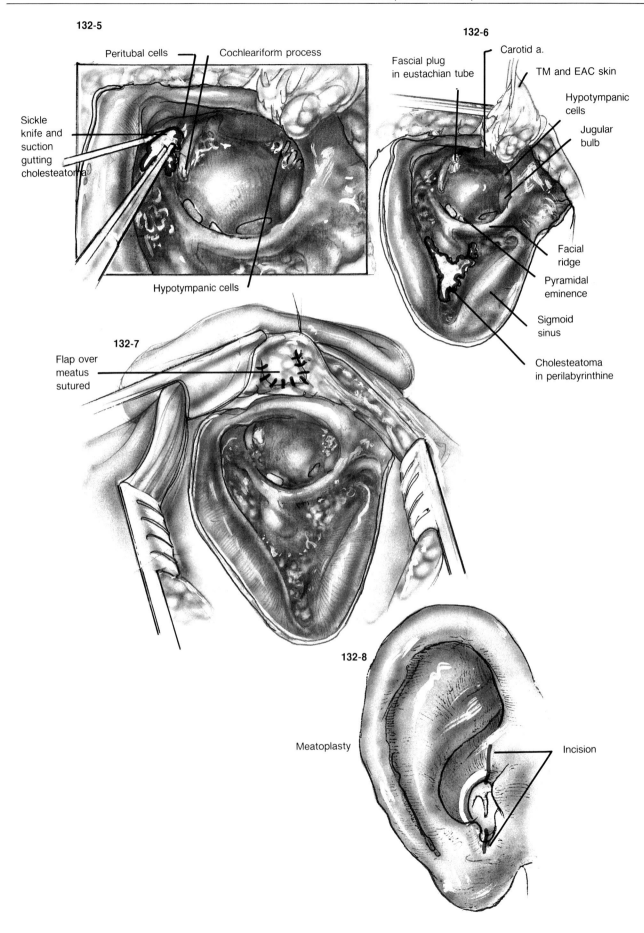

132-5

Peritubal cells   Cochleariform process

Sickle knife and suction gutting cholesteatoma

Hypotympanic cells

132-6

Fascial plug in eustachian tube

Carotid a.

TM and EAC skin

Hypotympanic cells

Jugular bulb

Facial ridge

Pyramidal eminence

Sigmoid sinus

Cholesteatoma in perilabyrinthine

132-7

Flap over meatus sutured

132-8

Meatoplasty

Incision

■ *133.* IMPLANTATION OF AN AUDIANT BONE CONDUCTOR HEARING DEVICE—Implantation into the temporal bone of the Audiant magnetic screw is accomplished by making a postauricular semilunar incision and raising the flap to expose the temporal bone. A precise double-tapping orthopedic procedure is done to create threads in the bone into which the magnet implant is firmly screwed. Careful positioning of the incision and implantation is provided by special instruments and templates.

Indications
1. Conductive hearing loss due to aural atresia (congenital or acquired); open, wet mastoid bowls; or chronic external otitis
2. Audiometric findings should include bone conduction better than 25 dB in three speech frequencies; speech reception threshold (SRT) worse than 40 dB; or discrimination better than 80%.

Preoperative Preparation
1. Physician and audiologist counseling about expectations
2. Routine laboratory studies

Special Instruments, Position, and Anesthesia
1. Local anesthesia for most adults
2. General anesthesia for children and some adults
3. Xomed Hough-Dormer set and Audiant implant kit

Tips and Pearls
1. Careful marking for implant placement
2. Watch skin thickness.
3. Do not strip bone threads.
4. Do not overtighten screw.
5. Good hemostasis

Postoperative Care Issues
1. Keep pressure dressing on the patient's head for 48 hours.
2. Do not fit the external device for 8 weeks.
3. Give careful instruction about gradually increasing the use of the device for skin tolerance.

References
Hough J, McGee M. The surgical technique for implantation of the temporal bone stimulator (Audiant ABC). Am J Otol 1986;7:315.
Hough JVD. Manual for implantation of the Xomed Audiant Bone Conductor. Jacksonville, FL: Xomed-Treece Corporation.

Operative Procedure
The Audiant, a device implanted in the postauricular area, uses the transcutaneous concept of direct bone conduction through an external electromagnetic coil and an implanted magnetic system. Implantation into the temporal bone of the Audiant magnetic screw is accomplished by making a postauricular semilunar incision and raising the flap to expose the temporal bone (Fig. 133-1). A precise double-tapping orthopedic procedure creates threads in the bone into which the magnet implant is firmly screwed (Figs. 133-2 through 133-5). Careful positioning of the incision and implantation is provided by special instruments and templates (see Figs. 133-1, 133-2, and 133-6).

The device is designed for patients with moderate to severe bilateral or unilateral conductive hearing loss with good cochlear function (better than 25dB in the three speech frequencies), who are not surgical candidates or are unable to benefit from conventional hearing aids, such as those with congenital malformations, chronic external otitis, or draining mastoid cavities.

Local anesthetic with or without general anesthetic is provided for an outpatient procedure. All special instruments are provided in the implant instrument set and disposable kit (Fig. 133-6).

The position for the incision and the location for the implant is determined by direct measurements and by using templates (see Fig. 133-1). The anteriorly based flap is elevated in the subcutaneous plane and thinned, if necessary, to approximately 5 mm. A circular area of soft tissue and periosteum slightly larger than the implant is removed, and the underlying bone smoothed with a cutting bur. With the use of the large cutting pilot collar bur (see Figs. 133-2 and 133-6), the pilot hole for the implant is precisely drilled perpendicular to the bone (see Fig. 133-2). The pilot hole is deepened with the precisely measured diamond collar bur and irrigated freely while drilling (see Fig. 133-2).

The metal guide cylinder template is used to outline the location of the three circumferential holes to be drilled in the bone for the guide cylinder pins (see Fig. 133-2). The guide cylinder pins are placed in the three guide holes, and the guide cylinder is held perpendicularly and firmly against the skull. The half-tap is screwed on the universal wrench and inserted in the guide cylinder. With firm downward pressure, the wrench is rotated clockwise, drilling the bone threads until the gap between the wrench and cylinder is closed (see Fig. 133-3). With bi-counterclockwise rotation (about 2.75 turns), the half-tap is removed from the bone, and the full-tap is placed on a universal wrench. This procedure is repeated with the full-tap to deepen the threads in the bone. Do not strip the threads. Count the turns.

The Audiant XA-II magnet implant is removed from the kit. It is fitted onto the insert tool and held by magnetic attraction. Visualize the screw tip entering the pilot hole, and with the tool held perpendicularly to the bone, the screw is rotated into the bone threads until it is fully inserted and the magnet is flush with the bone (see Fig. 133-4). Do not overtighten (see Fig. 133-5).

The wound is closed in two layers after hemostasis is achieved. A pressure dressing is applied for 1 week to prevent seroma formation. The external processor is not fitted until proper osseointegration occurs in approximately 8 to 12 weeks postoperatively.

J. V. D. HOUGH
MICHAEL MCGEE

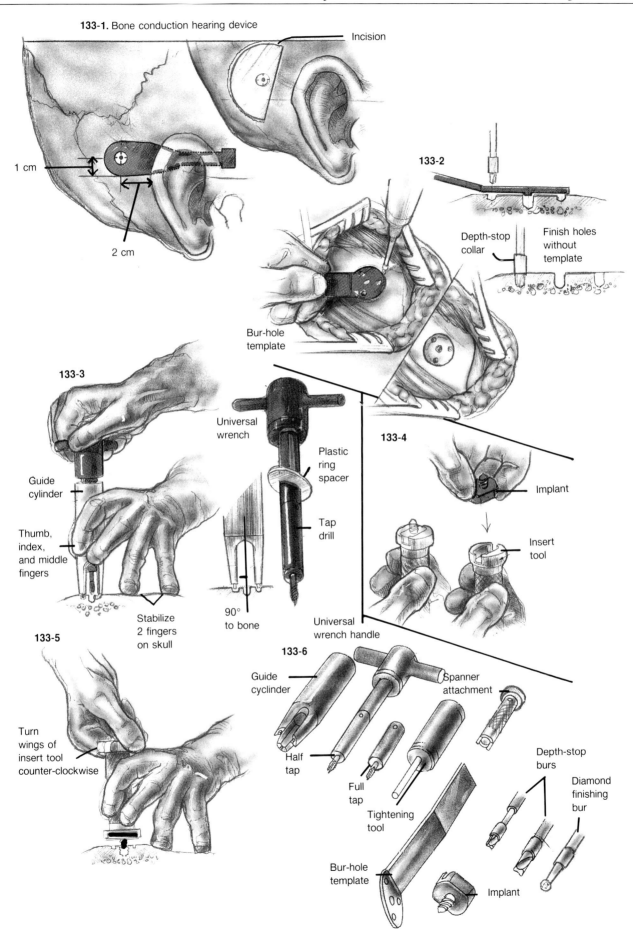

133-1. Bone conduction hearing device

Incision

1 cm

2 cm

133-2

Depth-stop collar

Finish holes without template

Bur-hole template

133-3

Universal wrench

Plastic ring spacer

Guide cylinder

Tap drill

Thumb, index, and middle fingers

Stabilize 2 fingers on skull

90° to bone

133-4

Implant

Insert tool

Universal wrench handle

133-5

Turn wings of insert tool counter-clockwise

133-6

Guide cyclinder

Spanner attachment

Half tap

Full tap

Tightening tool

Bur-hole template

Implant

Depth-stop burs

Diamond finishing bur

■ *134.* GLOMUS TYMPANICUM

Paraganglioma developing in association with Jacobsen's or Arnold's nerves, which presents as a vascular mass of the middle ear

Indications

1. Excision is advocated for symptomatic tumors that typically produce pulsatile tinnitus, hearing loss, or otalgia.
2. Small, asymptomatic lesions may be excised to prevent future disability.
3. Radiation therapy is reserved as palliative treatment for patients unwilling or unable to tolerate surgery.

Special Considerations

1. Female preponderance
2. Neuroendocrine activity is rare.
3. Rule out glomus jugulare or middle ear vascular anomaly

Preoperative Preparation

1. Coronal computed tomography (CT) to image bone overlying the jugular bulb
2. Audiometry

Special Instrumentation, Position, and Anesthesia

1. Operating microscope
2. Otologic drill system with assorted cutting and diamond burs
3. Suction-irrigation system
4. Facial nerve monitor for extended facial recess cases

Tips and Pearls

1. Complete exposure before manipulation of tumor
2. Bipolar electrocautery to control bleeding

Pitfalls and Complications

1. Excessive bleeding may obscure vision and prevent complete excision.
2. Tympanic membrane perforation
3. Tumor recurrence
4. Sensorineural hearing loss
5. Facial nerve injury
6. Cholesteatoma

Postoperative Care Issues

1. Audiometry
2. Long term follow-up

References

Jackson CG, Welling DB, Chironis P, et al. Glomus tympanicum tumors: contemporary concepts in conservation surgery. Laryngoscope 1989;99:875.

O'Leary MJ, Shelton C, Giddings NA, et al. Glomus tympanicum tumors: a clinical perspective. Laryngoscope 1991;101:1038.

Operative Procedures

Correct preoperative assessment and planning is essential in the management of vascular masses of the middle ear. Glomus tympanicum tumors must be differentiated from an anomalous artery or jugular bulb or a glomus jugulare tumor. Initial questioning should include family history and review of systems searching for neuroendocrine symptoms. The incidence of multiple tumors or catecholamine secretion is extremely rare with tympanicum tumors. Facial nerve palsy noticed during physical examination suggests significant mastoid or middle ear involvement or primary facial nerve tumor. Lower cranial nerve palsies indicate glomus jugulare tumor or other jugular foramen lesions. Audiometry most often demonstrates conductive hearing loss. A sensorineural loss may indicate otic capsule invasion.

After the lesion is suspected, imaging studies can confirm the diagnosis. CT scans in coronal and axial planes can rule out vascular anomalies and determine the integrity of the bone covering the jugular bulb. Magnetic resonance imaging is indicated if the glomus jugulare is not clearly excluded by the CT scan, for larger tympanicum tumors if inner ear or carotid invasion is suspected, or if the history and physical examination suggest multiple tumors. Open biopsy of any vascular middle ear mass should be avoided.

Local or general anesthetic may be used, although general anesthesia is preferred. Small tumors occasionally can be completely visualized after tympanotomy. Between 70% and 85% of tumors require the extended facial recess approach. The largest tumors may require radical mastoidectomy or lateral skull base dissection.

If the tumor is completely visualized preoperatively, a transcanal approach is used (Fig. 134-1). A tympanomeatal flap is elevated, carefully releasing any attachments of tumor to the tympanic membrane. The malleus may be separated from the tympanic membrane to gain additional exposure. The limits of tumor extension are then confirmed. Bipolar cautery is used to shrink the tumor and reduce vascularity (Fig. 134-2). Hypertrophied vessels supplying the tumor may be identified on the promontory, and each must be cauterized. The tumor is then separated from its medial attachment to the promontory mucosa. Nerves of the tympanic plexus are also included with the specimen. Gelfoam packing may be used to control any residual bleeding, and the tympanomeatal flap is then replaced. A small amount of Gelfoam packing is placed lateral to the flap.

If the inferior extension of the tumor is significant or unknown, the postauricular approach with standard vascular strip incisions is used. Vascular strip incisions are made first, followed by postauricular incision, undermining, and rotation of the auricle anteriorly. The tympanomeatal flap is elevated as described earlier. Tumor extension within the middle ear is determined, with attention to involvement of the ossicles, oval and round windows, protympanum, and epitympanum. If the tumor is still incompletely visualized, the extended facial recess approach is mandated (Fig. 134-3).

Simple mastoidectomy and facial recess approach are performed as described in Procedures 130 and 136. The lateral buttress of the fossa incudis must remain intact if the incus is to be preserved. The dissection proceeds with a diamond bur and continuous suction-irrigation. The chorda tympani nerve is transected, and the facial recess is enlarged. Bone is removed anterior and lateral to the vertical portion of the facial nerve. This dissection proceeds from superior to inferior aspects. The hypotympanum is widely exposed, allowing visualization of the carotid and jugular bulb. Dissection of the retrofacial air cell tract allows additional exposure of the jugular bulb. The surgeon must be cautious of the facial nerve during subsequent tumor removal.

After exposure is completed, the tumor is cauterized with the bipolar cautery and meticulously dissected from surrounding structures. Any tympanic membrane, ossicles, and middle ear mucosa that cannot be easily separated from the tumor are resected. The tumor may extend toward the petrous apex through the hypocochlear air cell tract, requiring further dissection medially after most of the tumor has been removed. Tympanoplasty and ossicular reconstruction, if necessary, are performed after tumor removal.

JEFFREY T. VRABEC

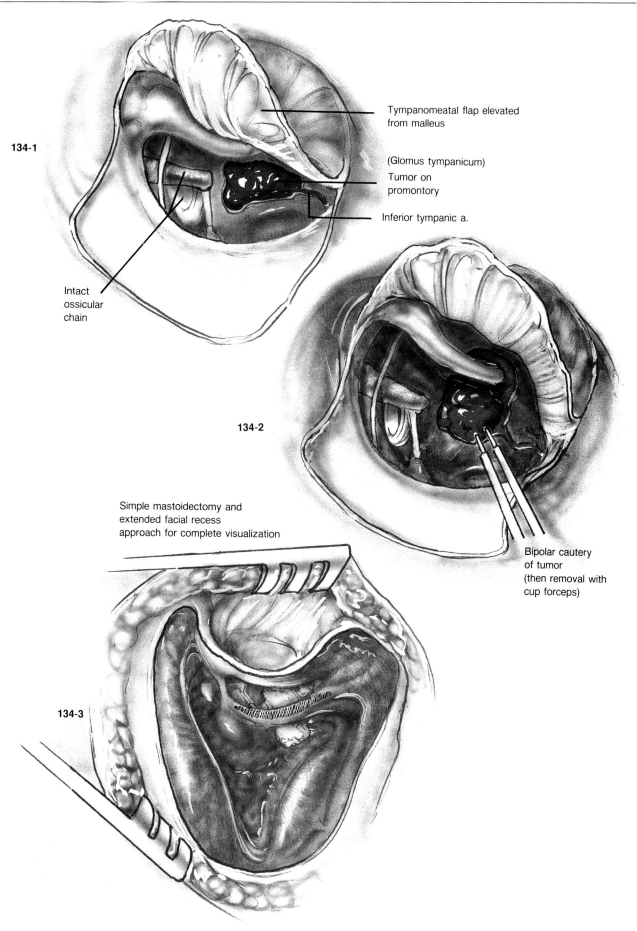

134-1

Tympanomeatal flap elevated
from malleus

(Glomus tympanicum)
Tumor on
promontory

Inferior tympanic a.

Intact
ossicular
chain

134-2

Bipolar cautery
of tumor
(then removal with
cup forceps)

Simple mastoidectomy and
extended facial recess
approach for complete visualization

134-3

■ *135.* PETROUS APICECTOMY

Surgical exenteration of perilabyrinthine and petrous apex cells through a middle fossa approach, while sparing neural, vascular, and otic capsular structures

Indications

1. Persistent or chronic infection in the petrous apex, even after a radical mastoidectomy and exenteration of cell tracts to the petrous apex. The ossicles do not necessarily have to be removed to establish the same drainage as achieved with the standard radical procedure.
2. Benign disease in the petrous apex that cannot be managed by lateral approaches, such as facial neuromas extending from the labyrinthine segment of the facial nerve.

Contraindications

1. Malignant disease
2. Failure to try lateral surgical approaches and systemic antibiotics first

Special Considerations

1. Elderly patients
2. Dominant hemisphere
3. Dehiscence of bone over the geniculate ganglion
4. Dense dural attachment to the superior petrosal nerve

Preoperative Preparation

1. Computed tomography scan of the temporal bone
2. Audiogram
3. Neurosurgical consultation and inclusion of the neurosurgeon in the surgical team

Special Instruments, Position, and Anesthesia

1. Lumbar cerebrospinal fluid (CSF) drains, if necessary
2. Anesthesia at the patient's feet (ie, head of table)

Tips and Pearls

1. Continuous drainage of spinal fluid during surgery may help reduce brain and dural risks.
2. Sharp dissection and gentle dural elevation helps to avoid facial nerve complications.
3. The surgeon should carefully read the depth within the otic capsule and avoid dissecting on the otic capsule.
4. Dissection along landmarks should extend through the middle fossa to the neck, if necessary.
5. Repair of the tegmen, if the dura has not been compromised, usually is unnecessary. If desired, conchal or tragal cartilage may be used.

Pitfalls and Complications

1. Elderly patients have thin dura that may tear and produce CSF leaks, and they may be more susceptible to temporal lobe compression.
2. The symptomatic effects of compression may be bothersome if affecting the dominant hemisphere.
3. The facial nerve may tear if the dura is tightly attached to the proximal greater superficial petrosal nerve or exposed geniculate ganglion.
4. The periotic lumen within the otic capsule may be eccentric, resulting in labyrinthine entry on the first drill pass.

Postoperative Care Issues

1. Neurologic intensive care is required for the first 24 hours.
2. Drains are not used.
3. Perioperative antibiotics are necessary.

References

Chole RA, Brodie HA. Surgery of the mastoid and petrosa. In: Bailey BJ, ed. Head and neck surgery—otolaryngology. Philadelphia: JB Lippincott, 1993:1647.

Neely JG. Intratemporal and intracranial complications of otitis media. In: Bailey BJ, ed. Head and neck surgery—otolaryngology. Philadelphia: JB Lippincott, 1993:1607.

Operative Procedure

The patient is positioned supine, with the head at the foot of the table and turned with the diseased ear up. The patient is secured to the table with tape or straps across the chest, hips, and thighs. A generous amount of temporal hair is removed, and the side of the head and ear are sterilely prepared and draped. The operation is begun with an incision reopening the radical mastoidectomy before the middle fossa is approached.

A vertical, muscle-splitting incision about 1 cm anterior to the tragus is made from the root of the zygoma superiorly to expose the squamous bone. A T-shaped muscle incision at the zygoma is usually necessary; care must be taken to incise deep to the galea extension to avoid the frontal branch of the facial nerve (Fig. 135-1).

A bone window, which is replaced later, is cut such that the complete middle fossa surface of the temporal bone may be exposed; typically, approximately two thirds of the width is anterior to the center of the external canal. The inferior cut must be flush with the floor of the middle fossa. A middle fossa retractor is placed (Fig. 135-2).

The dura is elevated medially to the petrous ridge from the foramen spinosum and middle meningeal artery to the superior petrosal sinus; extreme caution should be taken not to disrupt the petrosal sinus (Fig. 135-3).

The mastoid cavity from the previous radical procedure is opened from above, and the tegmen tympani is removed to expose the epitympanum and ossicles, if present (Fig. 135-4). The dissection is extended to skeletonize the internal carotid artery medially through thin bone, open the eustachian tube, to exenterate the petrous apex cells lying anterior to the internal auditory canal and medial to the carotid and cochlea, and to exenterate and connect the perilabyrinthine cells to the radical mastoidectomy site (Fig. 135-5). This dissection may be continued anterior and posterior to the internal auditory canal and medial to the otic capsule to connect with mastoid and hypotympanic cells (Fig. 135-6).

When all of the pneumatized spaces, diseased bone, granulation tissue, and mucosa have been removed by these combined lateral and superior approaches, a large meatoplasty is constructed, and the middle fossa and postauricular wounds are closed, leaving the cavity open.

After the infection is cleared, a tympanoplasty may be performed.

Surgical Variations

A similar combined lateral and superior approach and cavity construction may be used in one stage if a petrous apex or extradural abscess is present.

A similar combined approach with maintenance of an intact canal wall and closure at the termination of the procedure may be used for the resection of benign tumors in the apex or perilabyrinthine cells.

J. GAIL NEELY

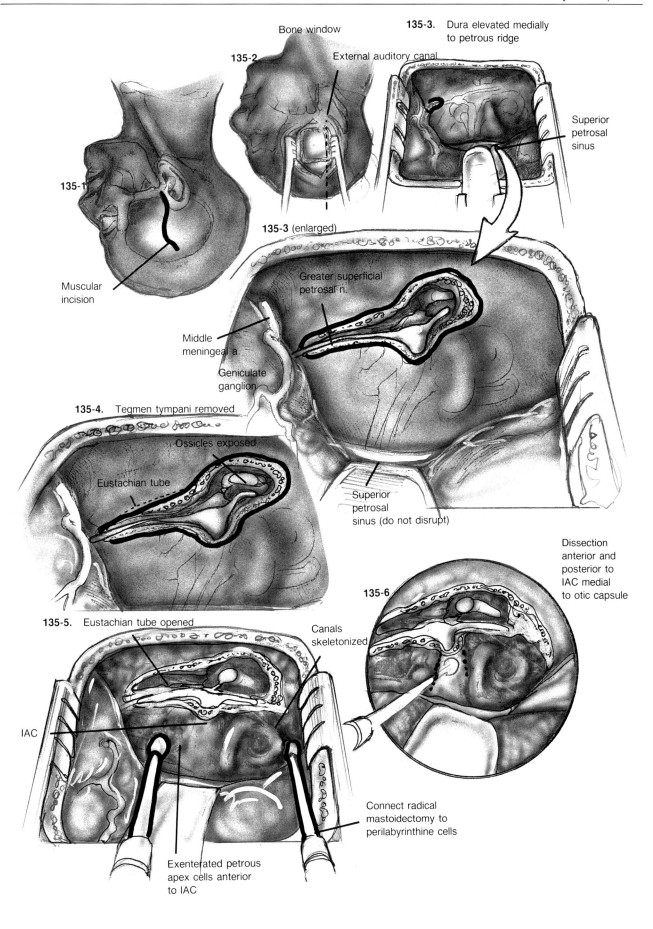

135-1.

Muscular
incision

135-2.

Bone window

External auditory canal

135-3. Dura elevated medially
to petrous ridge

Superior
petrosal
sinus

135-3 (enlarged)

Greater superficial
petrosal n.

Middle
meningeal a.

Geniculate
ganglion

Superior
petrosal
sinus (do not disrupt)

135-4. Tegmen tympani removed

Ossicles exposed

Eustachian tube

Dissection
anterior and
posterior to
IAC medial
to otic capsule

135-6.

135-5. Eustachian tube opened

Canals
skeletonized

IAC

Connect radical
mastoidectomy to
perilabyrinthine cells

Exenterated petrous
apex cells anterior
to IAC

■ *136.* FACIAL RECESS APPROACH

Access to the posterior mesotympanum by dissection of the bony triangle defined by the facial nerve posteromedially, the buttress of the fossa incudis superiorly, and the chorda tympani nerve anterolaterally

Indications

1. Visualization of posterior tympanum in intact canal wall surgery for chronic otitis media, cholesteatoma, or middle ear neoplasm
2. Exposure of the second genu for facial nerve trauma or tumor
3. Exposure of the round window niche for cochlear implantation
4. Extended facial recess approach for hypotympanic lesion and lateral temporal bone resection

Special Considerations

1. Status of incus
2. Assess the need for preservation of the chorda tympani.

Preoperative Preparation

1. Audiometry
2. Additional testing as indicated by the diagnosis

Special Instrumentation, Position, and Anesthesia

1. Operating microscope
2. Otologic drill system with assorted cutting and diamond burs
3. Suction-irrigation system
4. Facial nerve monitor (optional)

Tips and Pearls

1. Pneumatization of the facial recess varies, and accurate identification of the surrounding structures is essential.
2. Injury to the facial nerve is prevented by adequate magnification, copious irrigation to prevent thermal injury, and drilling parallel to the course of the nerve.

Pitfalls and Complications

1. Dislocation of incus
2. Facial nerve injury
3. Subluxation of stapes
4. Sensorineural hearing loss, secondary to direct labyrinthine injury, or drill contact with an intact ossicular chain
5. Tympanic membrane perforation

Postoperative Care Issues

1. Assess facial nerve function.
2. Audiometry

Reference

Sheehy JL. The facial nerve in surgery of chronic otitis media. Otolaryngol Clin North Am 1974;7:493.

Operative Procedures

A postauricular approach is required for the facial recess approach. Simple mastoidectomy is completed as described in Procedure 130. Before beginning the facial recess dissection, the incus and vertical segment of the facial recess must be fully identified. The limits of the standard facial recess dissection are the vertical segment of the facial nerve posteriorly and medially, the chorda tympani nerve anteriorly and laterally, and the buttress of the fossa incudis superiorly. The posterior wall of the fossa incudis serves as the attachment for the posterior incudal ligament. In chronic ear surgery, the status of the incudostapedial joint should also be assessed before this dissection.

The operating microscope and continuous suction-irrigation system are used. The choice of burs is left to the surgeon's discretion. Cutting burs allow faster dissection, and diamond burs provide a greater margin of safety when dissecting close to the facial nerve. The inexperienced surgeon is advised to use only diamond burs. As the degree of pneumatization is variable, 1-, 1.5-, and 2-mm sizes should be available.

Inspect the vertical segment of the facial nerve (Fig. 136-1). Usually, some air cells remain just lateral to the nerve at the superior aspect, and the inferior aspect is surrounded by dense bone. Dissection begins in this air cell tract, lateral and anterior to the facial nerve. The posterior canal wall is thinned while attempting to identify the chorda tympani. The chorda has the same light pink blush as the facial nerve. The origin of the chorda is usually from the inferior third of the mastoid segment, forming an angle with the facial of approximately 20°.

As dissection proceeds anteriorly, the tympanic cavity is entered through the facial sinus, superior to the pyramidal eminence (Fig. 136-2). Try to maintain a superior buttress 2 to 3 mm thick until the middle ear is entered. With the lenticular process of the incus in view, the buttress may be thinned, taking care not to disrupt the lateral incudal ligament. Completion of the dissection requires removal of bone to the limits of the triangle (Fig. 136-3).

Bone removal on the anterior aspect of the facial nerve is difficult but necessary to allow maximum visibility (Fig. 136-4). Maximize the lateral exposure through the recess before drilling anterior to the nerve. Rotating the patient toward the surgeon improves visibility and allows the shaft of the bur to be perpendicular to the nerve.

If the incus has been sacrificed, no attempt is made to preserve the buttress (Fig. 136-5). The fossa incudis is taken down, following the facial nerve around the second genu. Avoid drilling too far laterally during this portion of the dissection, which can produce a scutal defect.

The extended facial recess approach requires sacrificing the chorda tympani nerve and is used to improve visualization of the hypotympanum. Drill away the chorda tympani, and identify the annulus, which is slightly lateral. If a tympanomeatal flap has been elevated, identify the rim of the tympanic bone. Dissection then proceeds anterior to the facial nerve in a superior to inferior direction. The round window niche is visualized first, followed by the dome of the jugular bulb as dissection proceeds inferiorly. Continuing inferiorly to the stylomastoid foramen undermines the whole tympanic bone. To complete excision of the external canal, proceed anteriorly to define the posterolateral aspect of the carotid artery (see Procedure 55). The extent of bone removal is determined by the surgical objective.

If performing this approach in chronic ear surgery and tympanoplasty is required, be careful of retraction of the tympanic membrane graft into the facial recess. This usually can be prevented by a piece of Silastic sheeting large enough to cover the promontory and extend posterior to the facial nerve.

JEFFREY T. VRABEC

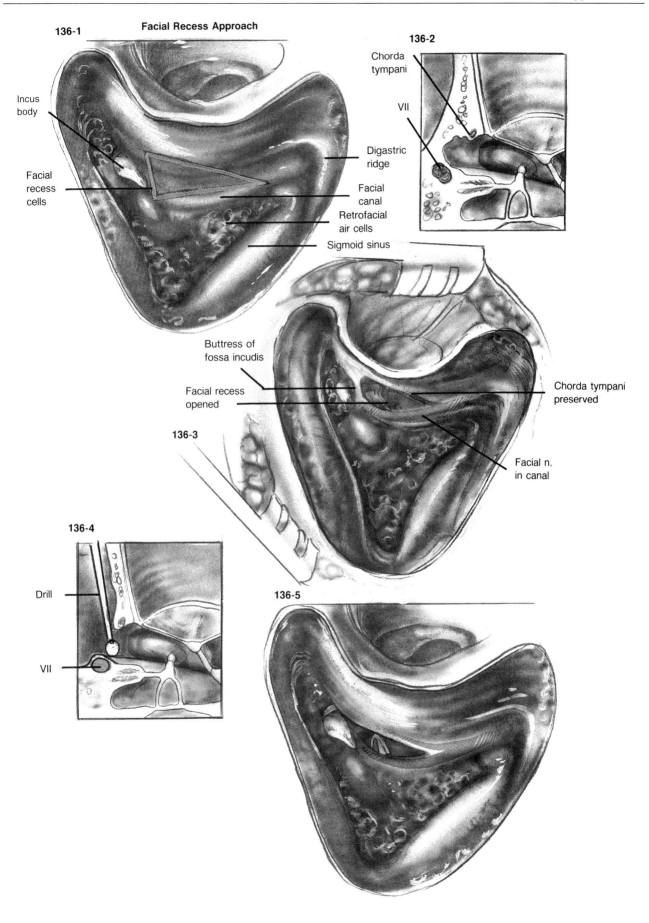

136-1   **Facial Recess Approach**

Incus
body

Facial
recess
cells

Digastric
ridge

Facial
canal

Retrofacial
air cells

Sigmoid sinus

136-2

Chorda
tympani

VII

Buttress of
fossa incudis

Facial recess
opened

Chorda tympani
preserved

Facial n.
in canal

136-3

136-4

Drill

VII

136-5

■ *137.* MANAGEMENT OF BRAIN HERNIA-TION AND CEREBROSPINAL FLUID LEAK
REPAIR—Transmastoid and middle ear repair of brain herniations and cerebrospinal fluid leaks

Indications
1. Brain herniation, meningoencephaloceles, and cerebrospinal fluid (CSF) leaks through the tegmen, roof of the eustachian tube, or posterior fossa at Trautmann's triangle
2. CSF leaks through the labyrinth into the middle ear

Special Considerations
1. Brain herniation in a cavity after a mastoidectomy
2. Meningoencephaloceles through the roof of the eustachian tube
3. CSF leaks through the labyrinth
4. CSF leaks through very small osseous holes

Preoperative Preparation
1. Computed tomography scan of the temporal bone, including coronal views
2. Audiogram
3. Neurosurgical consultation

Special Instruments, Position, and Anesthesia
1. Otologic drill, suction-irrigators, and operating microscope
2. The patient is supine, with the head at the foot of the table.
3. Sterile preparation of the lateral thigh for fascia lata donation, if necessary.

Tips and Pearls
1. Expect there to be more than one defect requiring repair.
2. CSF leaks may be associated with a Mondini deformity leak through a defect in the party wall of the lateral internal auditory canal or vestibule and subsequently through the oval window.
3. CSF leaks, meningoencephaloceles, and brain herniations through the tegmen, Trautmann's triangle, or roof of the eustachian tube occur in ears with normal hearing and conductive hearing loss.
4. Following the CSF leads to the origin of the leak.
5. Intracranial or intralabyrinthine soft and rigid tissue repairs are required to secure the closure.
6. Brain herniations in cavities after radical or modified radical procedures should be approached posterior to the cavity skin, carefully avoiding perforation of the skin into the potentially contaminated cavity.
7. Herniated brain is necrotic and nonfunctioning; it should be amputated at its dural origin.
8. Meningoencephaloceles through the roof of the eustachian tube are difficult to see.
9. A separate small opening in the squamosa to extend the middle fossa view and assist in extradural tissue placement may be useful in large or very anterior tegmen defects.
10. CSF leaks through very small osseous holes, such as Hurtle's fissure, or small perforations into a retrolabyrinthine air cell after posterior fossa acoustic tumor resection may be adequately repaired by tightly wedging a piece of fascia in a dumbbell fashion into the defect.

Pitfalls and Complications
1. Failure to establish an intracranial soft and rigid tissue repair usually leads to recurrence.
2. Failure to identify all of the lesions results in continued CSF leak.
3. Meningitis
4. Intracranial hematomas

Postoperative Care Issues
1. Elevate the head of the bed approximately 30°.
2. Short duration of perioperative antibiotics
3. Discharge from the hospital is usually possible in 48 hours.
4. The patient should avoid straining and blowing the nose for approximately 6 weeks.

References
Adkins WY, Osguthorpe JD. Mini-craniotomy for management of CSF otorrhea from tegmen defects. Laryngoscope 1983;93:1038.

Neely JG. Classification of spontaneous cerebrospinal fluid middle ear effusion: review of 49 cases. Otolaryngol Head Neck Surg 1985;93:625.

Operative Procedures
Intact Canal Wall Mastoidectomy and Repair

The patient is positioned supine, with the head at the foot of the table and turned with the diseased ear up. The patient is secured to the table with tape or straps across the chest, hips, and thighs. A generous amount of periauricular hair is removed, and the side of the head and ear are sterilely prepared and draped. The operation is begun with an incision approximately 1.5 to 2 cm posterior to the postauricular sulcus.

The mastoid periosteum is elevated to, but not beyond, the spine of Henle. No canal incisions are made. The temporalis muscle and its fascia remain intact and are elevated superiorly to expose the root of the zygoma to the plane of the anterior canal wall.

A complete transcortical mastoidectomy is performed, thinning the bone over the tegmen, sigmoid, and Trautmann's triangle. The atticotomy is extended to the anterior limit of the anterior attic compartment on a plane tangent to the anterior external auditory canal wall. The facial recess is open sufficient to view the protympanum and origin of the eustachian tube.

Meningoencephaloceles and brain herniations are identified and dissected from surrounding tissue to circumferentially expose and isolate the pedicled origin through the dural defect (Fig. 137-1). Brain herniations are evacuated and amputated at the dural plane. Meningoencephaloceles are desiccated with bipolar electrocautery; these usually are reduced sufficiently by this method to be easily elevated intracranially and do not require amputation (Fig. 137-2). The desiccated mass can assist elevation of the dura. The dura is elevated from the floor of the middle fossa circumferentially, through the osseous tegmental defect (Fig. 137-3).

Temporalis fascia and conchal cartilage with attached perichondrium, cut larger than the osseous defect, are placed through the bony defect into the prepared extradural pocket (Fig. 137-4). Additional soft tissue may be placed in the mastoid adjacent to this intracranial repair, if desired.

Surgical Variations

One surgical variation is radical or modified radical revision and repair. The postauricular incision is deepened to expose the cavity margin. The cavity skin is gently elevated, taking care not to perforate into the potentially contaminated cavity. The tegmen and Trautmann's triangle surfaces are followed to identify and isolate the pedunculed origin of the brain herniation. The "brain fungus" is evacuated using a suction-irrigator and bipolar electrocautery. The fibrous wall of the herniation may be retained on the cavity skin to assist in preserving the skin integrity. The defect is repaired as described previously.

Another variation is intralabyrinthine repair of a Mondini deformity CSF leak. Only the middle ear needs to be exposed, using a stapedectomy-type tympanomeatal flap. The thin-walled mucosal cyst originating from the oval window is opened, allowing a copious flow of CSF and exposing a footplate perforation in the deformed stapes (Fig. 137-5). After the CSF flow stops, the stapes is removed if the ear is profoundly deafened; unilateral profound sensorineural hearing loss and unilateral profound vestibular loss is the usual condition in these cases. Looking through the cavernous vestibule, a medial wall defect allows a view directly into the fundus of the internal auditory canal.

Pieces of temporalis fascia are placed in an intralabyrinthine position to occlude the flow of CSF; care must be taken not to enter the internal auditory canal and injure the facial nerve. The lateral wall of the vestibule is the fallopian canal. A piece of conchal cartilage slightly larger than the oval window is placed into the vestibule to hold the repair, as is done in repairing tegmen defects (Fig. 137-6).

Attention is directed to the round window area to ensure it is not leaking after this maneuver. More fascia may be placed in the labyrinthine area, if necessary.

J. GAIL NEELY

Figures redrawn after Neely JG, Neblett JG, Neblett CR, Rose JE. Diagnosis and treatment of spontaneous cerebrospinal fluid otorrhea. Laryngoscope 1982;92:609.

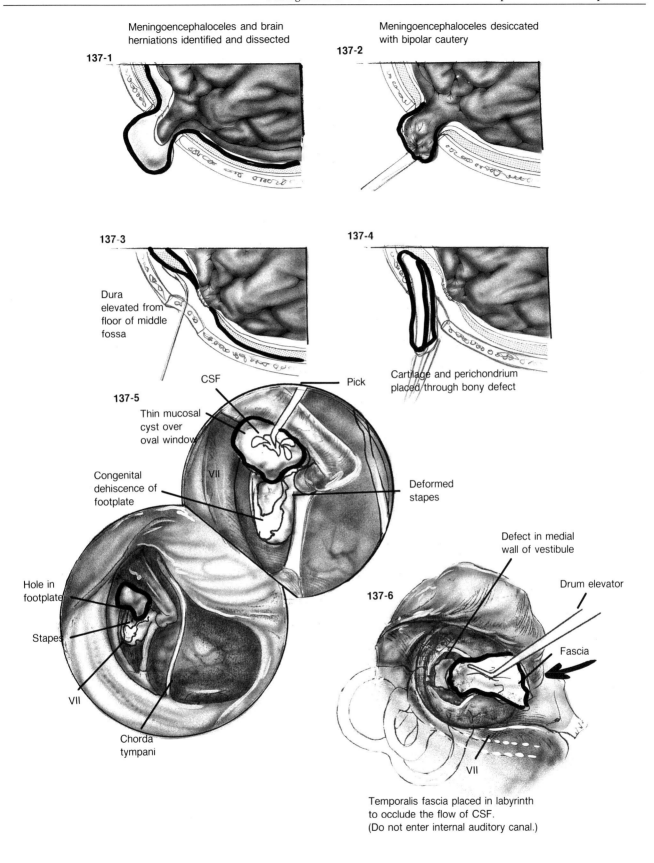

Meningoencephaloceles and brain
herniations identified and dissected

137-1

Meningoencephaloceles desiccated
with bipolar cautery

137-2

137-3

Dura
elevated from
floor of middle
fossa

137-4

Cartilage and perichondrium
placed through bony defect

CSF

Pick

137-5

Thin mucosal
cyst over
oval window

Congenital
dehiscence of
footplate

VII

Deformed
stapes

Hole in
footplate

Stapes

VII

Chorda
tympani

Defect in medial
wall of vestibule

Drum elevator

Fascia

137-6

VII

Temporalis fascia placed in labyrinth
to occlude the flow of CSF.
(Do not enter internal auditory canal.)

■ *138.* FACIAL NERVE GRAFTING

Reconstitution of a damaged segment of the facial nerve through the use of interpositional sensory nerve autografts or by rerouting and end-to-end anastomosis of the facial nerve

Indications

1. Transection of the nerve after temporal bone fractures, gunshot injuries, or iatrogenic incidents
2. Resection of the nerve for tumor extirpation
3. Severe contusion or crush injury of the nerve resulting in fibrosis and a failure of regeneration

Contraindications

1. Inaccessible proximal end of the facial nerve
2. Atrophy and fibrosis of the facial musculature from longstanding paralysis
3. Contaminated or infected wound, preventing access to the intracranial segment of the facial nerve

Special Considerations

1. When indicated, retrieve information on injured segments from preoperative imaging or operative records.
2. Knowing the status of cochlear function helps to plan surgical approaches to the intratemporal facial nerve.

Preoperative Preparation

1. Pure tone and speech audiogram
2. For traumatic injuries, high-resolution axial and coronal computed tomography (CT) scanning of the fallopian canal and neurophysiologic confirmation of complete denervation
3. For skull base tumors, CT and magnetic resonance imaging
4. Inform the patient about functional outcomes and the possible need for secondary procedures.

Special Instruments, Position, and Anesthesia

1. Otologic microscope and instrumentation
2. Neurorrhaphy instruments include neurectomy and nerve scissors, jeweler's forceps, fine-toothed forceps, and a Castroviejo needle holder.
3. Operative field preparation of donor sites in advance

(continued)

Operative Procedures

Several principles of neurorrhaphy apply to all facial nerve grafting. All neural tissue should be handled atraumatically with microinstruments designed for neural repairs. The approximation of nerve endings is performed under the illumination and magnification of the operating microscope. Exact end-to-end approximation is accomplished without tension on the anastomotic site, and an 8-0 to 10-0 monofilament suture is used for repair.

Intracranial Repair

Facial nerve injury in the posterior fossa occasionally results from tumor removal. The intracranial segment of the facial nerve is the most difficult to repair because of limited exposure, pooling cerebrospinal fluid, and brain pulsations. If avulsion or severe stretch injury occurs at the root entry zone, facial nerve grafting will not be successful. For injured intracranial, meatal, and labyrinthine segments of the facial nerve, three options exist: rerouting and end-to-end anastomosis, interpositional grafting, or rerouting and interpositional grafting.

Rerouting and End-to-End Anastomosis. Rerouting and end-to-end anastomosis is most practical for translabyrinthine or transotic approaches and requires that the dura be closed and the cavity obliterated at the conclusion of the procedure (see Procedure 151). Prerequisites to this approach include a severe sensorineural hearing loss and an injured intracranial or intratemporal section of the facial nerve.

A complete mastoidectomy is performed, exenterating all air cells in the epitympanum, zygomatic root, sinodural angle, retrosigmoid region, mastoid tip, retrofacial area, and mastoid. The posterior and superior osseous external auditory canal wall, tympanic membrane, ossicles, and air cells in the peritubal regions and hypotympanum may be removed if necessary for greater exposure (Fig. 138-1).

The facial nerve is exposed from the internal auditory canal to the stylomastoid foramen. Bone remaining over the internal auditory canal or posterior fossa dura prohibiting the identification and transposition of the intratemporal nerve should be removed. The facial nerve is skeletonized with diamond burs in the mastoid, tympanic, and labyrinthine segments of the temporal bone until one half the circumference of the nerve is uncovered. The eggshell layer of bone left on the nerve is carefully removed with a dissector to expose the nerve (see Procedure 140). The distal nerve stump is gingerly retracted and the nerve tediously dissected from the fallopian canal (Fig. 138-2). The greater superficial petrosal nerve is transected, and the fibrous attachments underlying the nerve are lysed with a sharp cutting instrument to avoid a stretch injury to the nerve. The nerve is freed to the level of the stylomastoid foramen.

The injured segment of the nerve is resected proximally and distally to viable nerve. If any doubt exists, frozen sections are obtained. The nerve ends are sharply cut at an oblique angle, and the two ends are apposed. The transposition acquires 2 to 3 cm of length to facilitate direct end-to-end anastomosis. The anastomosis requires two to three perineurial sutures of 8-0 to 10-0 monofilament, such as Ethilon (Fig. 138-3). Limitation of field exposure and pulsating CSF may hinder the ideal repair technique, in which case a single through-the-center suture must suffice.

Before repair, a new fallopian canal can be drilled between the internal auditory canal and the stylomastoid foramen in any bone remaining over the posterior fossa dura to provide additional support for the anastomosis. The intracranial segment of the facial nerve can be accessed by removing the bony plate over the posterior fossa dura and incising the dura from the porus acusticus posteriorly to the sigmoid sinus to open the cerebellopontine angle.

Rerouting and Grafting. If a long contiguous or double segment of the facial nerve is injured, rerouting and interpositional grafting may be necessary (Fig. 138-4). Grafts are used to avoid

(continued)

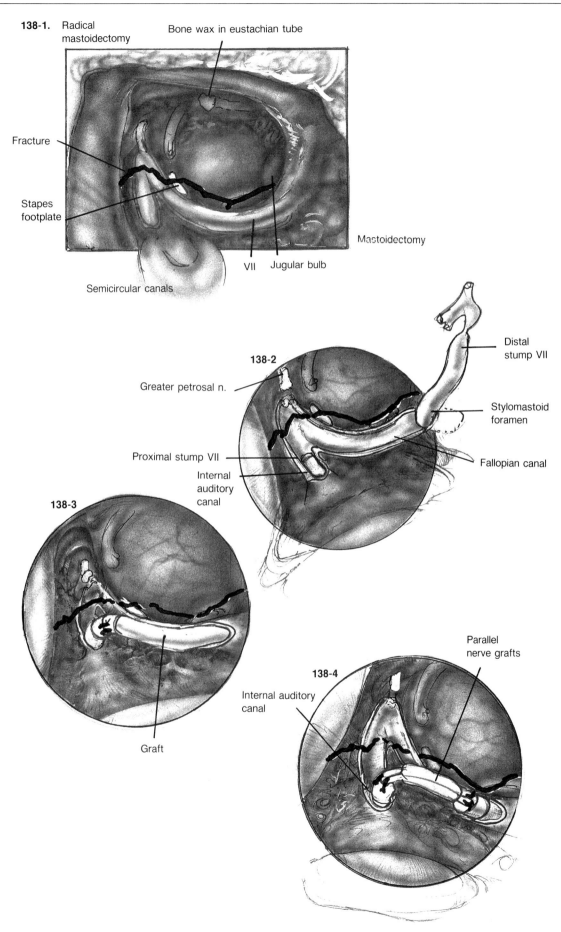

138-1. Radical mastoidectomy

Bone wax in eustachian tube

Fracture

Stapes footplate

Mastoidectomy

VII   Jugular bulb

Semicircular canals

138-2

Greater petrosal n.

Distal stump VII

Stylomastoid foramen

Proximal stump VII

Internal auditory canal

Fallopian canal

138-3

Parallel nerve grafts

138-4

Internal auditory canal

Graft

■ *138.* FACIAL NERVE GRAFTING *(continued)*

Tips and Pearls

1. Perform repairs as soon as practical.
2. The superiority of perineurial repair over epineurial repair has not been convincing; do what is practical for the situation at hand.
3. A 1-0 silk suture may be used to measure the defect in the facial nerve before harvesting and preparation of the donor graft.
4. If the caliber of the greater auricular nerve is an inadequate match for the facial nerve, harvest the sural nerve, or use the greater auricular nerve in a double-barreled grafting technique. The proximal and distal nerve stumps can be fish-mouthed to accommodate a larger sural nerve or the double-barreled graft from the greater auricular nerve.
5. One through-the-center suture may be the only end-to-end anastomosis possible in the posterior fossa or internal auditory canal.
6. Use the facial canal for stenting whenever possible; often, a new canal can be drilled to accommodate the graft.
7. The confines of surgical field may prevent the use of standard instruments. Substitute middle ear instruments; for example, use alligator forceps or jeweler's forceps to handle the needle at the graft site.
8. Never close an anastomosis under tension; use a graft.
9. Frozen sections of the injured segment may help to differentiate fibrous from viable neural tissue.
10. There is no epineurium about the intracranial, meatal, or labyrinthine segments of the facial nerve.
11. The greater auricular and sural nerves can provide as much as 7 and 30 cm of donor graft, respectively.

Pitfalls and Complications

1. The best functional outcome is grade III on the House-Brackmann scale.
2. Gunshot wounds and posterior fossa repairs have poorer prognoses.
3. Exposure keratitis
4. Sensory deficit in the distribution of the autograft

Postoperative Care Issues

1. For eye care, use ophthalmic lubricants liberally. Secondary procedures, such as tarsorrhaphy and eyelid reanimation, may provide protective and cosmetic benefits (see Procedures 141 and 142).
2. Facial message and electrical stimulation therapy are of questionable benefit for the return of facial function.
3. After an intratemporal repair, clinical evidence of the return of function may not appear for 6 to 8 months; for intracranial repairs, 12 to 18 months may be required. Judgment of the final results may require as much as 2 or 3 years after the repair.

References

Coker NJ. Management of traumatic injuries to the facial nerve. Otolaryngol Clin North Am 1991;24:215.

Fisch U, Mattox D. Microsurgery of the skull base. New York: Thieme Medical Publishers, 1988.

tension at the suture site. Rerouting is performed as previously described, and interpositional grafts are used to bridge the missing segment or gap. Grafts should be supported with newly drilled bony canals or collagen membranes (ie, lyophilized dura) when possible.

Sensory Autografts for Interpositional Repairs. The two most popular donor grafts are the greater auricular and sural nerves. Although shorter and smaller in caliber than the sural, the greater auricular nerve resides adjacent to the surgical field in most temporal bone procedures. If the caliber is inadequate, a double-barreled technique can be performed, or the sural nerve can be harvested. Figure 138-5 demonstrates the location of the greater auricular nerve coursing from Erb's point toward the external auditory canal and bisecting a line between the mastoid tip and the angle of the mandible. Approximately 5 to 7 cm of nerve can be harvested through an incision placed in the skin creases of the neck overlying the sternocleidomastoid muscle. Two stepladder incisions facilitate exposure of the proximal and distal parts of the nerve. The sural nerve courses around the fibular malleolus deep to the lesser saphenous network and is most easily identified posterior to the lateral malleolus and then traced as far proximally as needed for the appropriate length of graft (Fig. 138-6). As much as 30 cm of this nerve can be harvested for repairs. The grafts are prepared by removing excess connective tissue from the epineurial sheath and by freshening the ends with a clean cut (Fig. 138-7).

Intracranial interpositional grafting requires two anastomoses. After preparation, the graft is sewn directly to the freshened facial nerve stumps, which are void of epineurium in the posterior fossa. Three to four sutures are preferred but may not be practical, in which case a single through-the-center suture at each anastomotic site expedites the repair.

Labyrinthine Segment Repair

The labyrinthine segment repair is most applicable to injuries in the region of the geniculate ganglion, if cochlear function is intact. A middle cranial fossa approach is required to expose the meatal, labyrinthine, and proximal tympanic segments of the facial nerve. When injury occurs at the geniculate ganglion or labyrinthine segment, two options exist: interpositional grafting or rerouting of the nerve around the superior ampulla. For a very short injured segment, the nerve can be rerouted. If not affected, the geniculate ganglion is removed from the facial canal, and the greater superficial nerve is divided. Bone in the angle between the labyrinthine and tympanic segments of the nerve is then carefully removed with a diamond bur until the blue line of the superior canal and ampulla appears. A direct end-to-end anastomosis with two or three 8-0 to 10-0 monofilament sutures is performed. If tension exists, an interpositional graft is used to bridge the nerve ends. The newly created bony canal helps stent the anastomosis (Fig. 138-8).

Tympanic and Mastoid Segment Repair

Interpositional grafting is usually the most practical method of repair in the tympanic and mastoid segments. Figure 138-9 demonstrates the use of the facial canal to stent an anastomosis. One or two sutures may be added for stability.

NEWTON J. COKER

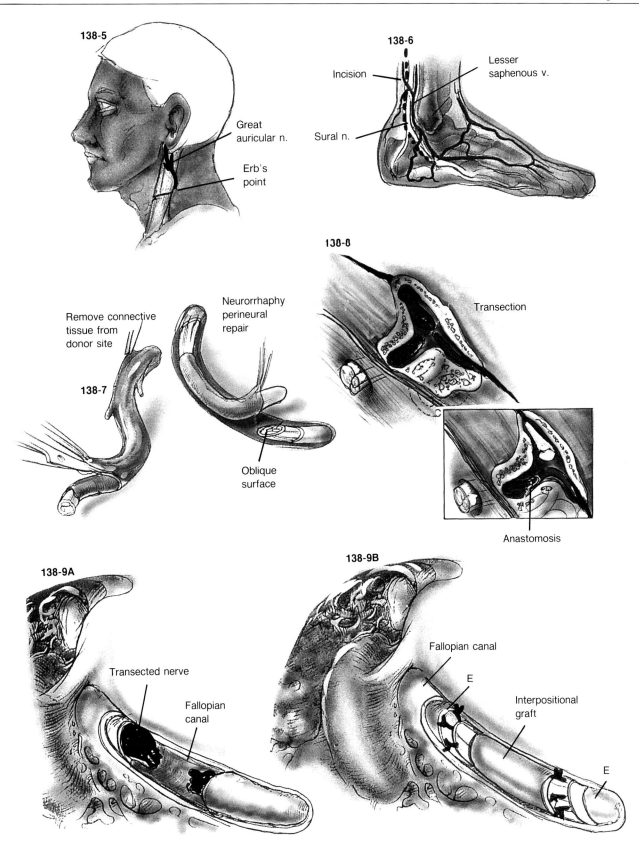

138-5

Great auricular n.

Erb's point

138-6

Incision

Lesser saphenous v.

Sural n.

138-8

Transection

Anastomosis

Remove connective tissue from donor site

Neurorrhaphy perineural repair

138-7

Oblique surface

138-9A

Transected nerve

Fallopian canal

138-9B

Fallopian canal

E

Interpositional graft

E

■ *139.* HYPOGLOSSAL-FACIAL CRANIAL NERVE CROSSOVER TECHNIQUES—Redirection of

motor axons from the hypoglossal nerve into the distal facial nerve

Indications

1. Reinnervation of the facial musculature after irreversible facial nerve injury whereby the proximal facial nerve cannot be isolated for grafting purposes

Contraindications

1. Evidence of hypoglossal denervation
2. Lower cranial nerve deficits (IX or X) on either side
3. Unavailable distal facial nerve trunk or secondary branches
4. Facial muscle atrophy and fibrosis from long-standing paralysis
5. Neurofibromatosis

Special Considerations

1. Interpositional grafts are the preferred method of reanimation when the proximal and distal stumps of the facial nerve are accessible.
2. For dynamic reanimation of paralysis of less than 2 years' duration
3. Crossover often performed in conjunction with eye rehabilitation

Preoperative Preparation

1. Cranial nerve assessment
2. Routine laboratory studies
3. Facial electromyography if the nonfunctional nerve is anatomically intact from previous surgery
4. Counsel the patient about the anticipated length of recovery and potential outcome.

Special Instruments, Position, and Anesthesia

1. Operating microscope or surgical loupes
2. Neurorrhaphy instruments: neurectomy and nerve scissors, jeweler forceps, Castroviejo needle holders
3. Supine position, with the head turned on a foam rest; shoulder roll
4. No muscle relaxants or depolarizing agents

Tips and Pearls

1. Distal dissection of the hypoglossal underneath the submandibular gland to its branching into the tongue (classic technique)
2. Dissect greater auricular nerve from Erb's point to the terminal branches before harvest (jump technique).
3. Meticulous hemostasis in parotid and neck
4. Perform anastomosis over rubber dam (Penrose)
5. Drain to upper neck
6. If there exists a mismatch in size of the nerve ends, fish-mouth the smaller end to accommodate the larger.
7. Problems with mastication and speech are less likely with the jump technique.

Pitfalls and Complications

1. Hematoma
2. Salivary fistula
3. Speech difficulties (usually temporary)
4. Mastication problems
5. Mass movement most evident in classic XII to VII technique
6. Failure of muscle reinnervation

Postoperative Care Issues

1. Drain supported with Barton's head dressing
2. Elevate head of bed 30°
3. Educate the patient in eye care

References

Conley J. Hypoglossal crossover—122 cases. Otolaryngol Head Neck Surg 1977;84:763.

May M, Sobol SM, Mester SJ. Hypoglossal-facial nerve interpositional–jump graft for facial reanimation without tongue atrophy. Otolaryngol Head Neck Surg 1991;104:818.

Montgomery WW. Facial nerve paralysis. In: . Surgery of the upper respiratory system. Philadelphia: Lea & Febiger, 1993.

Operative Procedure

Classic Technique

A Blair or modified parotid incision is made in the preauricular crease, carried under the lobule of the ear, and then extended into the neck 4 cm below the body of the mandible (Fig. 139-1). Within the subcutaneous plane beneath the level of the hair follicles, a skin flap is developed over the parotid gland. The anterior border of the sternocleidomastoid and posterior belly of the digastric muscles are identified in the neck.

The facial nerve is isolated in the triangle formed by the tragal pointer, posterior belly of the digastric muscle, and sternocleidomastoid muscle. The nerve is identified just inferior and medial to the pointer and then dissected into the parotid to the level of the temporofacial and cervicofacial bifurcation (Fig. 139-2). The nerve is dissected proximally to the stylomastoid foramen and transected.

The hypoglossal nerve is identified in the neck. The hypoglossal, vagus, and spinal accessory nerves can be located in the angle between the posterior belly of the digastric and the sternocleidomastoid muscles. The hypoglossal nerve passes lateral to the external and internal carotid arteries just superior to the carotid bulb. This nerve is followed anteriorly beneath the digastric into the submandibular triangle and transected as far distally as possible (Fig. 139-3). The descendens hypoglossi is preserved if the distal hypoglossal can be transposed without tension at the anastomotic site; otherwise, the descendens is transected, and the hypoglossal nerve is dissected free of surrounding tissues and reflected superiorly over the posterior belly of the digastric. Over a rubber dam (Penrose), an end-to-end anastomosis of the proximal hypoglossal to distal facial nerves is performed (Fig. 139-4). An epineural or perineurial repair yields satisfactory results. Excess connective tissue is removed from the nerve stumps and the ends freshened with slightly oblique cuts. The anastomosis is secured with four or five 8-0 to 10-0 monofilament sutures (Ethilon) placed in the nerve sheaths (see Fig. 139-4). The surgical field is irrigated. The anastomotic site can be protected by oversewing more superficial tissues. A Penrose drain is placed in the neck. The incision is closed with 4-0 Vicryl subcutaneous sutures and 5-0 nylon interrupted dermal sutures. A sterile pressure dressing supports the drain.

Interpositional–Jump Technique

The primary advantage of the jump graft is a satisfactory reinnervation of the facial musculature with less mass movement than is evident in the classic technique. The jump graft can be directed to the main trunk of the facial nerve or its cervicofacial division, depending on the rehabilitation plans for the eye. The jump graft preserves hypoglossal function.

The exposure is similar to the classic technique. However, the facial and hypoglossal nerves are not transected and transposed. A donor nerve graft is required (see Procedure 138). Identify the facial nerve initially to assess its size in relation to the greater auricular and hypoglossal nerves. Usually, the length and caliber of the greater auricular nerve suffices. This nerve can be found by extending the surgical exposure over the sternocleidomastoid muscle and identifying its course from Erb's point toward the auricle (see Fig. 139-2). All of the greater auricular nerve should be harvested, excluding the terminal branches in the superior aspect of the neck. The connective tissue surrounding the nerve is removed with sharp dissection and the perineurium at the ends trimmed for the side-to-end anastomosis between the hypoglossal and facial nerves.

The interpositional graft is secured to the distal facial nerve in an end-to-end manner with interrupted 8-0 to 10-0 monofilament suture (Ethilon) placed through the epineural sheaths of the two ends (see Fig. 139-4). The graft is secured to the hypoglossal distal to the descendens hypoglossi in an end-to-side fashion by partially transecting the superior one half of the nerve. Cut the epineurium first and then the nerve to prevent crushing the fibers. The end of the graft is fish-mouthed to accommodate the hypoglossal site and then secured with interrupted monofilament sutures to the epineurium. Attempts to "direct" the fibers of the hypoglossal nerve into the graft are unnecessary. Figure 139-5 demonstrates the XII to VII interpositional–jump graft technique.

NEWTON J. COKER

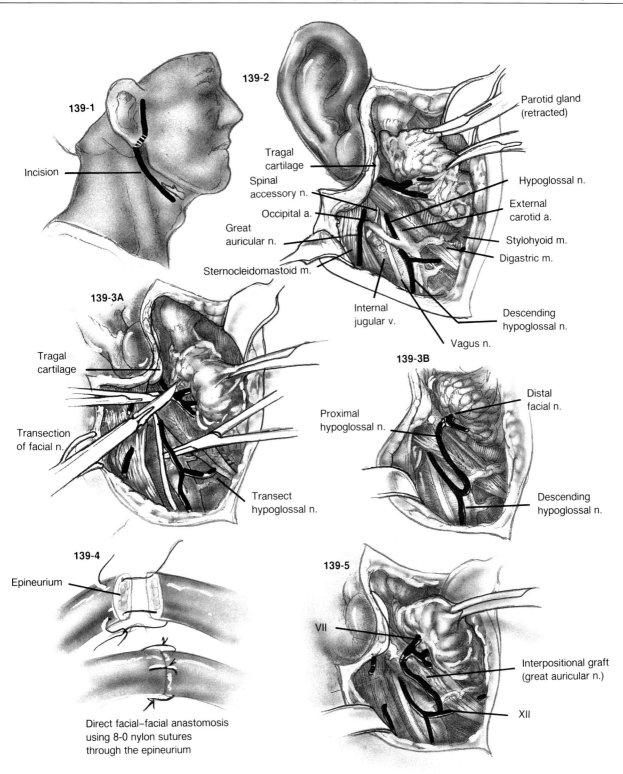

139-1

Incision

139-2

Tragal cartilage

Spinal accessory n.

Occipital a.

Great auricular n.

Sternocleidomastoid m.

Internal jugular v.

Vagus n.

Parotid gland (retracted)

Hypoglossal n.

External carotid a.

Stylohyoid m.

Digastric m.

Descending hypoglossal n.

139-3A

Tragal cartilage

Transection of facial n.

Transect hypoglossal n.

139-3B

Proximal hypoglossal n.

Distal facial n.

Descending hypoglossal n.

139-4

Epineurium

Direct facial–facial anastomosis using 8-0 nylon sutures through the epineurium

139-5

VII

Interpositional graft (great auricular n.)

XII

■ 140. FACIAL NERVE DECOMPRESSIONS

Removal of the lateral or superior 180° of the fallopian canal to expose the facial nerve sheath and the subsequent incision of the sheath through the epineurium and perineurium to expose the nerve. Facial nerve exploration without decompression may not incise the sheath.

Total facial nerve decompression is decompression from the internal auditory canal to the stylomastoid foramen.

Decompression of meatal foramen is decompression of the labyrinthine segment from the internal auditory canal to the proximal tympanic segment by middle fossa approach.

Transmastoid decompression is decompression of the tympanic and mastoid segments from the geniculate ganglion to the stylomastoid foramen by the transmastoid and facial recess approach.

Indications

1. Reduction of the transcutaneous electrically evoked compound muscle action potential, as determined by electroneuronography, or evoked electromyography, to 95% of normal or more, compared with the uninvolved side in the same patient in diseases or trauma causing acute facial paralysis
2. There is great controversy surrounding the use of this operation for several diseases. Although the reader is admonished to keep an open mind and stay informed by the emerging literature, it is not the purpose of this Procedure to review or analyze this controversy.

Contraindications

1. Young children seem to do much better than adults and may not benefit from this surgery.
2. It is proper to explore the nerve in some cases of infection-induced facial paralysis; however, it is unwise to decompress the nerve by incising the protective perineurium.
3. The middle fossa approach may not be indicated in cases of infection limited to the mastoid and requiring fallopian canal exploration.

Special Considerations

1. Removal of the incus
2. Low-lying dura
3. Chorda tympani nerve
4. Bony dehiscence proximal to the facial hiatus
5. Dural attachment to the greater superficial petrosal nerve
6. Middle meningeal artery
7. Stylomastoid foramen
8. Otic capsule
9. Order of approaches in total decompression
10. Bone removal over the facial nerve
11. Incision of the sheath, epineurium, and perineurium
12. Elderly patients
13. Dominant hemisphere

Preoperative Preparation

1. Blood studies appropriate for age, condition, and hospital standards
2. Electrocardiogram and chest radiograph
3. Magnetic resonance imaging of the eighth and seventh nerves
4. Electroneuronography
5. Audiogram
6. Neurosurgical consultation and inclusion of the neurosurgeon in the surgical team

Special Instruments, Position, and Anesthesia

1. Otologic drill, suction-irrigators, operating microscope, and craniotome
2. Lumbar cerebrospinal fluid (CSF) drain, if necessary
3. The patient is supine, with the head at the foot of the table and with the patient secured to the table with tape across the chest, hips, and thighs. No special head holders are necessary.
4. Anesthesia at the patient's feet (ie, head of the table).

(continued)

Operative Procedures

Total Facial Nerve Decompression

The patient is positioned supine, with the head at the foot of the table and turned with the diseased ear up. The patient is secured to the table with tape or straps across the chest, hips, and thighs. A generous amount of temporal hair is removed, and the side of the head and ear are sterilely prepared and draped. The operation is begun with a postauricular incision 2 cm posterior to the postauricular sulcus for mastoidectomy before the middle fossa is approached. No canal incisions are necessary.

A complete transcortical mastoidectomy is performed, extending the anterosuperior dissection transcortically to a plane tangent with the anterior wall of the external auditory canal (Fig. 140-1). Care is taken not to injure dura or enter the external auditory canal. The external posterior auditory canal wall is thinned, and the mastoid side is made parallel with the lumen (Fig. 140-2). A facial recess approach to the middle ear is performed, extending the dissection to the facial nerve, chorda, and posterior incudal ligament at the fossa incudis (Fig. 140-3).

The facial nerve is identified on a plane that bisects the horizontal semicircular canal. Dissection to the direct lateral surface of the nerve is begun approximately 4 mm inferior to the fossa incudis, and the nerve is expected to be at a depth medial to the convexity of the horizontal canal (Fig. 140-4).

Dissection along the facial nerve is extended to the stylomastoid foramen (Fig. 140-5) and through the facial recess and the epitympanum, following the lateral surface of the tympanic segment of the nerve to the geniculate ganglion approximately 2 mm anterosuperior

(continued)

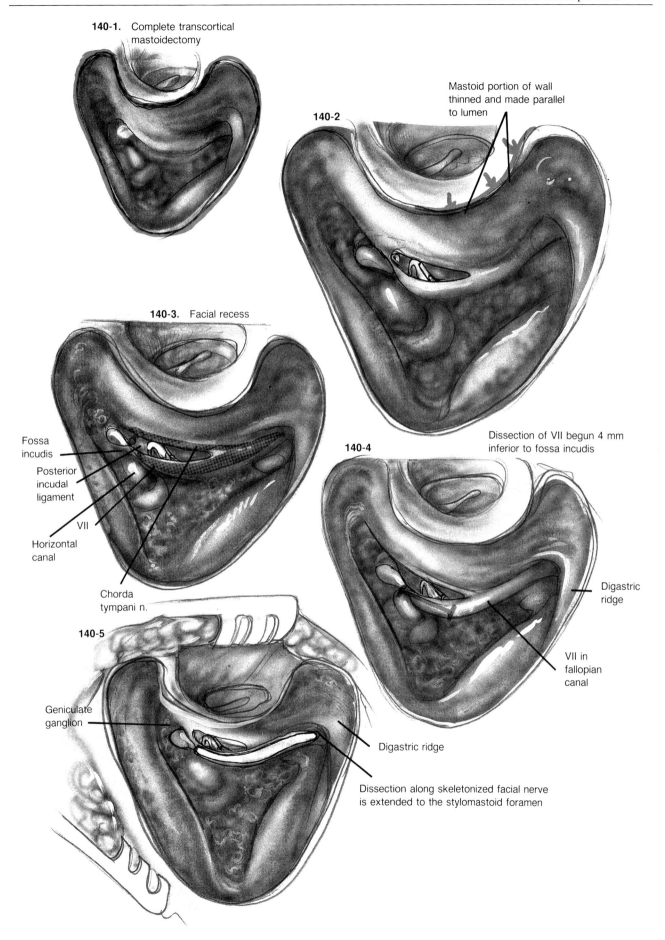

140-1. Complete transcortical mastoidectomy

140-2

Mastoid portion of wall thinned and made parallel to lumen

140-3. Facial recess

Fossa incudis

Posterior incudal ligament

VII

Horizontal canal

Chorda tympani n.

140-4

Dissection of VII begun 4 mm inferior to fossa incudis

Digastric ridge

VII in fallopian canal

140-5

Geniculate ganglion

Digastric ridge

Dissection along skeletonized facial nerve is extended to the stylomastoid foramen

■ 140. FACIAL NERVE DECOMPRESSIONS
(continued)

Tips and Pearls

1. If dissection cannot be completed without undue manipulation or drilling of the incus, the incus should be removed and replaced at the completion of the procedure.

2. Beveling the mastoid cortex to the plane of thin bone overlying the dura at the squamosa and a generous facial recess are usually sufficient to deal with low-lying dura.

3. To avoid injury to the chorda tympani, which exits the facial nerve laterally, the bony dissection may spiral along the posterior and lateral circumference of the mastoid segment.

4. Sharp dissection and gentle dural elevation helps to avoid facial nerve traction injury in cases in which a bony dehiscence proximal to the facial hiatus exposes the geniculate ganglion or in which tight dural attachment to the greater superficial petrosal nerve is appreciated.

5. If the middle meningeal artery is injured, it may be easily cauterized and the foramen spinosum packed with bone wax.

6. Decompression of the total nerve or tympanic and mastoid segments requires dissection to the stylomastoid foramen. This foramen is identified by the apparent flaring of the facial nerve sheath to become continuous with the periosteal attachment of the posterior belly of the digastric muscle.

7. Carefully read the depth within the otic capsule to avoid dissecting on the otic capsule. Remember the complex angles and depths of the fallopian canal in relation to the cochlea and superior semicircular canal in the middle fossa. Also remember that the facial nerve occupies the immediate lateral wall of the vestibule and is medial to the convex circumference of the horizontal semicircular canal in the tympanic segment.

8. When the total nerve is to be decompressed, it is helpful to complete the transmastoid approach before the middle fossa work. This avoids blood from the middle fossa interfering with the necessary clear vision of the tympanic dissection.

9. Bone over the facial nerve is thinned and microfractured (ie, "eggshelled") with a diamond bur by first thinning the bone along a line over the lateral planar surface of the nerve. With a smaller bur, a thin bone trough is created anteriorly and posteriorly, adjacent to the original plane. The last step is to connect these three planes to ensure a full 180° curvilinear exposure of the nerve sheath. With experience, the surgeon can think and dissect in a curvilinear fashion and complete all of these steps in one movement. The bone fragments are then removed with a sickle knife or angled facial nerve dissector (ie, "whirlybird").

10. Incision of the nerve sheath through the perineurium is made with sharp, pointed scalpels, the sickle knife, and very small ophthalmic knives. The sheath can be spread with the knife and a small suction tube to expose the last fine, transparent fibers and stroke through these to, but not into, the nerve fibers.

11. Continuous drainage of spinal fluid during surgery may help reduce the ill effects of brain retraction and dural tears in the elderly and minimize the effects on the dominant hemisphere.

Pitfalls and Complications

1. Sensorineural or conductive hearing loss
2. Taste paresthesia
3. Stretch injury or partial facial nerve transection
4. Vertigo
5. Cerebrospinal leak
6. Epidural hematoma
7. Speech and language disorders
8. Spinal headache

Postoperative Care

1. Neurologic intensive care is required for the first 24 hours.
2. Drains are not used.
3. Perioperative antibiotics unnecessary but occasionally used.

References

Fisch U. Surgery for Bell's palsy. Arch Otolaryngol 1981;107:1.
May M. The facial nerve. New York: Thieme, 1986.

to the cochleariform process in the anterior epitympanum. If necessary, the incus may be removed and later replaced (Fig. 140-6).

The bone is removed over the nerve, and the sheath is incised, beginning at the midtympanic segment and proceeding to the geniculate ganglion (Fig. 140-7). The dissection is continued posteroinferiorly to the stylomastoid foramen. By following this order of dissection, the arterial bleeding close to the stylomastoid foramen does not interfere with the delicate tympanic dissection.

After the transmastoid approach has been completed, the middle fossa approach for decompression of the meatal foramen is performed. A separate vertical, muscle-splitting incision about 1 cm anterior to the tragus is made from the root of the zygoma superiorly to expose the squamous bone. A craniotomy through the squamosa is performed, and the dura is elevated medially to the petrous ridge from the foramen spinosum and middle meningeal artery to the superior petrosal sinus (see Procedure 135).

The greater superficial petrosal nerve is followed to the geniculate ganglion, which is generously exposed. A limited amount of the tegmen tympani is removed to allow connection of the decompression about the ganglion with the proximal tympanic segment (Fig. 140-8).

Dissection along the labyrinthine segment of the facial nerve is carried to the first flow of CSF from the internal auditory canal (Fig. 140-9). A small piece of temporalis muscle is placed at the internal auditory canal opening to secure closure of the CSF leak, and a piece of conchal cartilage is placed over the tegmen defect of avoid CSF leaking into the middle ear and to avoid dural protrusion onto the head of the malleus and body of the incus (Fig. 140-10).

The wound is copiously irrigated with saline, hemostasis is meticulously achieved, and the wounds are closed in layers. A large mastoid dressing is applied.

J. GAIL NEELY

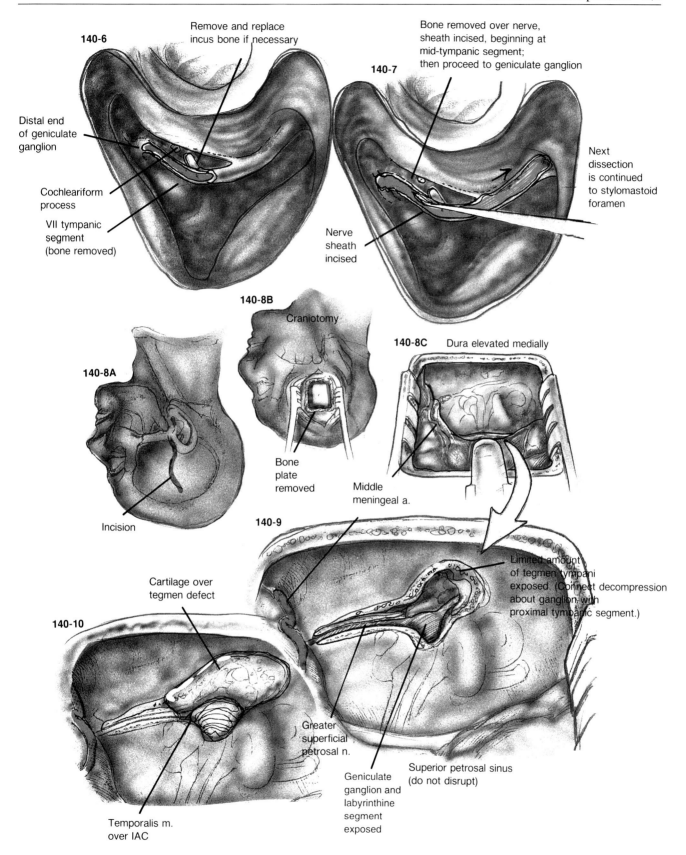

140-6

Remove and replace incus bone if necessary

Distal end of geniculate ganglion

Cochleariform process

VII tympanic segment (bone removed)

140-7

Bone removed over nerve, sheath incised, beginning at mid-tympanic segment; then proceed to geniculate ganglion

Next dissection is continued to stylomastoid foramen

Nerve sheath incised

140-8A

Incision

140-8B

Craniotomy

Bone plate removed

140-8C   Dura elevated medially

Middle meningeal a.

140-9

Limited amount of tegmen tympani exposed. (Connect decompression about ganglion with proximal tympanic segment.)

Greater superficial petrosal n.

Geniculate ganglion and labyrinthine segment exposed

Superior petrosal sinus (do not disrupt)

140-10

Cartilage over tegmen defect

Temporalis m. over IAC

■ 141. TARSORRHAPHY
Temporary or permanent joining of the upper and lower eyelids

Indications
1. Prevention of the complications of corneal exposure secondary to long- or short-term facial paralysis

Contraindications
1. Tarsorrhaphy, because of its functionally and cosmetically poor results, should be reserved for only those patients with facial paralysis who have failed more conservative management.

Special Considerations
1. Tarsorrhaphy is the gold standard for corneal protection after facial paralysis, but it should be considered only as a treatment option for patients who have failed more conservative methods of corneal protection. The procedure is strongly recommended for all patients with facial and trigeminal nerve deficits, because the loss of sensation causes the cornea to be more susceptible to keratitis and abrasions.
2. Temporary lateral tarsorrhaphy is excellent short-term treatment for patients in whom supportive eye care is difficult to accomplish.
3. Permanent tarsorrhaphy should be reserved for patients who cannot perform supportive care or do not desire to undergo procedures such as gold weight implantation, lateral canthoplasty, or palpebral spring implant.
4. For cosmetic and functional reasons, a lateral tarsorrhaphy is preferable to a medial tarsorrhaphy. For some cases, the surgeon may need to consider both forms for adequate corneal protection.

Preoperative Preparation
1. Complete ophthalmologic evaluation
2. Determination of the medial and lateral extent of the tarsorrhaphy necessary to protect the cornea with minimal visual obstruction

Special Instruments, Position, and Anesthesia
1. See the instrument list for gold weight implants (Procedure 142) for special instruments.
2. For bolster material, use a sterile cotton roll or 4-Fr soft red rubber catheter.
3. The suture for temporary tarsorrhaphy is 5-0 nylon using a tapered P-1 needle; the suture for permanent tarsorrhaphy is 6-0 nylon using a tapered P-1 needle.
4. Semi-sitting or supine position
5. Local anesthesia consists of 1% Xylocaine with 1:100,000 epinephrine, and topical anesthesia consists of a topical 4% solution of Ophthaine or 4% lidocaine.

Tips and Pearls
1. Loupe magnification is helpful but not essential.
2. Soft, 4-Fr red rubber catheters make excellent bolsters for temporary tarsorrhaphy.
3. When multiple sutures are required to achieve adequate corneal protection, it is simpler to place the tarsorrhaphy sutures if the knots are tied over the bolsters at the conclusion of the case rather than as each suture is placed.
4. Temporary tarsorrhaphy may remain in place for 4 weeks without difficulty, and in some cases, 6 weeks may pass before the temporary tarsorrhaphy is taken down or converted to a more permanent solution for eye protection.
5. Make sure no eyelashes are caught in suture or inverted into the eye.

Pitfalls and Complications
1. Infection (rare)
2. Corneal abrasion due to eyelashes

Postoperative Care
1. Topical ophthalmologic antibiotic ointment is recommended for 5 days.
2. Permanent tarsorrhaphy sutures are removed at 2 weeks.

Reference
Seiff RS, Chang J. Management of ophthalmic complications of facial nerve palsy. Otolaryngol Clin North Am 1991;24:669.

Operative Procedure
When performing a temporary lateral tarsorrhaphy, the patient is placed on the operating room table in the supine or semi-sitting position. The upper and lower eyelids are anesthetized using a 1% solution of Xylocaine with a 1:100,000 dilution of epinephrine, and the cornea is anesthetized using topical 4% ophthaine. A temporary lateral tarsorrhaphy is performed with a horizontal mattress suture of 5-0 nylon or polypropylene. Approximately 3 mm medial to the lateral canthus, the first suture is placed through a partial thickness of the upper eyelid, 6 mm from the lid margin (Fig. 141-1). The suture exits through the upper eyelid grayline. It then enters the grayline of the lower lid, passes through a partial thickness of the lower lid, and exits the skin approximately 5 mm below the lid margin. The suture is then passed through the center of a 3-mm-long, 4-Fr, soft red rubber catheter, which acts as a bolster on the lower lid (Fig. 141-2). The suture is then placed back through the lower lid skin, approximately 3 mm nasally from its previous exit point, leaving the lid at the grayline. This leaves a loop of suture with the attached bolster exposed on the lower lid. The suture then enters the upper lid grayline and exits 3 mm nasal from the original point of entry (Fig. 141-3). A 3-mm section of 4-Fr soft red rubber catheter is placed over the suture. The suture is pulled tight over the two bolsters and then tied on the upper lid (Fig. 141-4). If necessary, an additional mattress suture may be placed medially in a similar fashion.

Antibiotic eye drops are placed in the eye twice daily. The tarsorrhaphy may be left in place for as long as 4 weeks. As an alternative to a red rubber catheter bolster, a rolled piece of soft cotton or Xeroform gauze may be substituted.

A permanent tarsorrhaphy is performed by removing a 1- to 2-mm superficial layer of the upper and lower eyelid margins along the graylines from just lateral to the limbus to the lateral canthal area. A 6-0 nylon or Prolene suture is passed through the upper lid 4 to 6 mm medial to the lateral canthus, approximately 6 mm above the lid margin. The suture exits the divided grayline of the upper lid margin, and a 3-mm-deep horizontal mattress bite is taken through the tarsus at the base of the lower eyelid margin. The suture is then passed back into the base of the upper lid margin and exits the skin 3 mm nasal to the original bite. This mattress suture is then tied over a bolster as described for a temporary tarsorrhaphy. One or two additional mattress sutures may be required for adequate lateral closure of the lid. It is easier to place these sutures if the knots are all tied over the bolsters at the conclusion of the case than at the time that each individual suture is placed.

EUGENE L. ALFORD

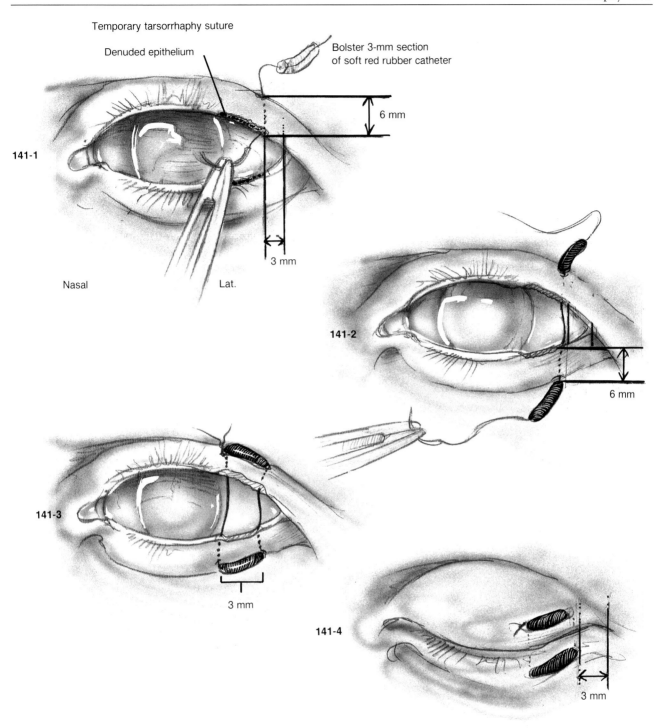

Temporary tarsorrhaphy suture

Denuded epithelium

Bolster 3-mm section
of soft red rubber catheter

6 mm

3 mm

141-1

Nasal   Lat.

141-2

6 mm

141-3

3 mm

141-4

3 mm

■ *142.* EYELID REANIMATION PROCEDURES

Operations that restore closure of the upper eyelid in cases of facial paralysis

Indications
1. Gold weight implantation
   a. Inadequate conservative measures; artificial tears, moisture chambers, and taping of the eye
   b. Chronic facial paralysis with incomplete upper eyelid closure
2. Spring Implantation
   a. Chronic facial paralysis with incomplete upper eyelid closure

Contraindications
1. Gold weight implantation
   a. Acute facial paralysis in which return of eye closure is expected
   b. Aberrant VII nerve regeneration
2. Spring implantation
   a. Previously failed spring implantation, history of upper eyelid infections, or extrusion of other upper eyelid prostheses

Special Considerations
1. Determination of corneal sensation and evaluation of Bell's phenomenon are important.
2. If lower lid ectropion or laxity is a contributing factor to corneal exposure, canthoplasty, lower tarsal wedge resection, or other lower lid procedures must be considered.
3. Gold weights rarely need to be removed after facial nerve recovery.

Preoperative Preparation
1. Gold weight implantation
   a. Determine the appropriate size and location of the gold weight necessary to achieve upper eyelid closure.

Special Instruments, Position, and Anesthesia
1. Gold weight implantation
   a. Gold weight implants are available in 0.2-ounce increments, from 0.6 to 1.8 ounces (Medev Corp.)
   b. Special instruments
      i. 2 small, smooth forceps (Bishop)
      ii. 2 small, toothed forceps (Bishop)
      iii. Castroviejo curved needle holder
      iv. Curved tenotomy scissors (5 in [12.5 cm])
      v. 6 corneal protectors
      vi. Bipolar cautery
   c. Sutures: 6-0 clear Prolene with a P-1 needle; 6-0 mild chromic with a CE-2 needle; and 6-0 fast absorbing with a PC-1 needle
   d. 2× loupes (optional)
   e. Semi-Fowler position (lounge chair or semisitting)

Tips and Pearls
1. Gold weight implantation
   a. The implant must be placed deep to the orbicularis oculi and levator muscles, inferior to the insertion of Mueller's muscle, and resting on the tarsal plate.
   b. The lower margin of the gold weight should rest 2 to 3 mm above the lash line.
   c. The midpoint of the weight should be medial to the midpoint of the upper lid.

Pitfalls and Complications
1. Gold weight implantation
   a. Care must be taken that upper lid shortening does not occur at the time of closure of the orbicularis oculi and levator muscles.

Postoperative Care Issues
1. Steri-strips (0.25 in [6 mm]) placed to make the lid slightly ptotic.
2. No antibiotics are necessary.

References

Levine R. Eyelid reanimation surgery. In: May M, ed. The facial nerve. New York: Thieme, 1986.

May M. Surgical rehabilitation of facial palsy. In: May M, ed. The facial nerve. New York: Thieme, 1986.

Operative Procedure

Placement of Upper Lid Gold Weight

Upper lid gold weight placement is performed under local anesthesia, with mild intravenous sedation. The patient is placed in the semi-Fowler position (ie, "lounge chair" position). Skin preparation using dilute Betadine solution is carried out with careful attention to avoid contact of the Betadine with the eye itself. Topical anesthesia is applied to the cornea.

The midpupillary line is marked on the upper eyelid, and the incision line is marked approximately 1 cm above the lash line and below the supratarsal fold (Fig. 142-1). Minimal amounts of local anesthesia (0.25–0.50 mL of 1% Xylocaine with a 1:100,000 dilution of epinephrine) are infiltrated just beneath the skin and subcutaneous tissue of the upper eyelid. A corneal protector is placed over the eye.

A #15 blade is used to incise the skin, and tenotomy scissors split the orbicularis oculi muscle parallel to its fibers and dissect down to the tarsal plate (Fig. 142-2). Care must be taken to not injure the levator aponeurosis or Mueller's muscle and its attachment to the tarsal plate. This tarsal plate is very thin, and great care must be taken not to penetrate or injure this structure.

The appropriate size of gold weight is placed over the eyelid to outline the exact size pocket to be created. The weight should be positioned such that approximately two thirds of the weight is medial to the midpupillary line and one third is lateral (see Fig. 142-1). The gold weight rests fully on the tarsal plate, parallel to the plane of the upper eyelid skin and globe. The inferior border of the gold weight should rest 2 to 3 mm above the upper lash line (Fig. 142-3). Often it is helpful to perform the remainder of the procedure using 2.0× loupe magnification.

The weight should be placed such that the two holes in the gold weight are inferior, with the single hole positioned superiorly. The patient is asked to open and close the eyes to demonstrate that the weight is located in the correct position to achieve eye closure. If eye closure is inadequate, the weight should be repositioned to achieve the desired result. The gold weight is fixed to the orbicularis oculi muscle and tarsal plate using 6-0 clear Prolene suture on a PS-1 needle.

Sutures should first pass through the orbicularis oculi muscle, through the tarsal plate, then beneath the gold weight, and up through the gold weight (Figs. 142-4 and 142-5). The two lower sutures should be placed first, followed by the upper suture. Ensure adequate redundancy of the orbicularis oculi muscle to cover the weight completely. The upper lid must not be shortened by excessive overlap in suturing the divided orbicularis oculi muscle. The overlying orbicularis oculi muscle is then sutured with 6-0 mild chromic suture on a CE-2 needle, and the skin is closed with 6-0 fast-absorbing gut on a PS-1 needle. Mastisol and Steri-strips should be placed so that the lid remains slightly closed and ptotic for the first 5 to 7 days.

Spring Implantation

Using 0.01-in orthodontic round wire and dental instruments, various sizes of spring implants are created preoperatively. The fulcrum loop of the palpebral spring should be approximately 5 mm in diameter and be as flat as possible. The spring is prepared and adjusted to conform to the patient's orbital rim and upper eyelid before surgery. The superior arm of the spring rests adjacent to the periosteum of the superior orbital rim, the coil is sutured to the lateral orbital rim, and the lower arm is positioned at the midportion of the upper lid. The arms of the spring should be adjusted to conform to the contour of the lid and orbital rim. The arms of the spring should be set apart 1.5 times the interpalpebral width of the normal open eye.

EUGENE L. ALFORD

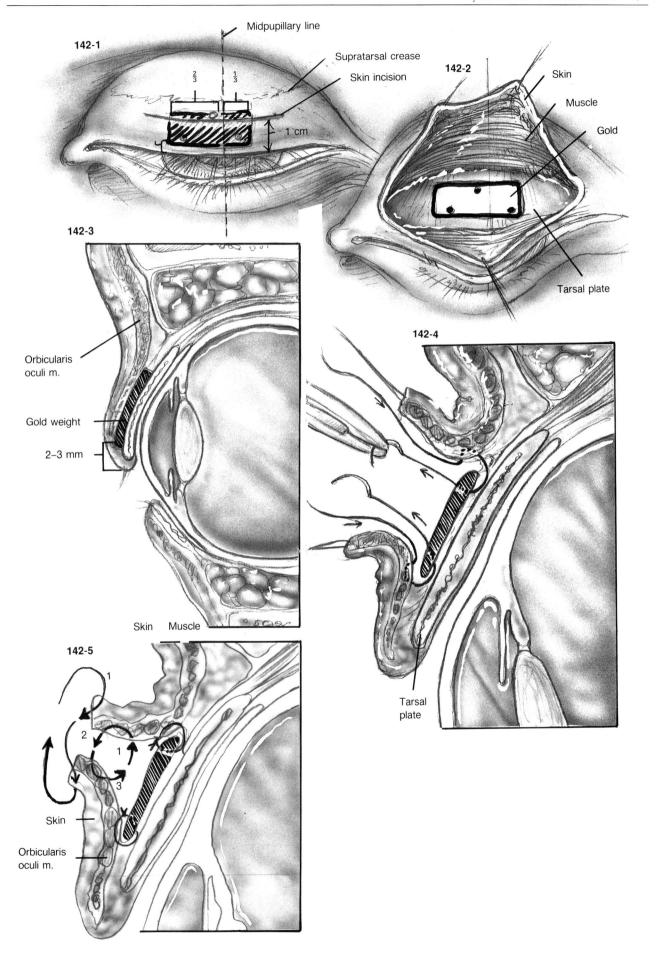

142-1

Midpupillary line

Supratarsal crease

Skin incision

$\frac{2}{3}$ $\frac{1}{3}$

1 cm

142-2

Skin

Muscle

Gold

Tarsal plate

142-3

Orbicularis
oculi m.

Gold weight

2–3 mm

142-4

Tarsal
plate

Skin   Muscle

142-5

1

2

1

3

Skin

Orbicularis
oculi m.

■ *143.* LABYRINTHECTOMY

Total destruction of the neuroepithelium of the semicircular canals, the utricle, and the saccule designed to disconnect or remove the diseased labyrinth from the remaining vestibular system, allowing the opposite side to assume full control

Indications

1. For patients with peripheral, unilateral labyrinthine involvement who remain disabled by their symptoms of vertigo despite conservative treatment. The affected ear must have severe or total loss of hearing.

Special Considerations

1. Transmastoid approach allows removal of all neuroepithelium under direct visualization.

Contraindications

1. Useful hearing (50-dB threshold or better and 50% discrimination) despite a disorder of the labyrinth
2. Only hearing ear, regardless of hearing level

Preoperative Preparation

1. Exclude nonvestibular sources of dizziness.
2. Audiogram
3. Vestibular testing: electronystagmography (eg, rotary chair, platform posturography)
4. Metabolic studies may include glucose, cholesterol, sedimentation rate, rheumatoid factor, antinuclear antibodies, thyroid function tests, and a serologic test for syphilis (FTA-ABS)
5. Magnetic resonance imaging to rule out a retrocochlear lesion

Special Instruments, Position, and Anesthesia

1. The patient is positioned supine, with the head turned away from ear to be operated.
2. Local anesthesia may be used if the preoperative vestibular function (caloric test) is profoundly depressed.
3. The procedure is usually performed under general anesthesia, because the patient may experience severe vertigo during manipulation and ablation of vestibular sense organs.

(continued)

Operative Procedure

Transcanal Labyrinthectomy

With the patient under general anesthesia, the ear is prepared and draped, and local injections of the ear canal are performed with a 1% solution of Xylocaine with a 1:100,000 concentration of epinephrine. A tympanomeatal flap is elevated and reflected anteriorly. The chorda tympani nerve is preserved. The incudostapedial joint is separated and the stapedius tendon sectioned (Fig. 143-1). The stapes is removed and the contents of the vestibule (ie, saccule and utricle) removed with a right-angle hook (Fig. 143-2). A 4- to 5-mm right-angle hook is directed superiorly and anteriorly to remove the cristae of the horizontal and superior semicircular canals (Fig. 143-3). The crista of the posterior semicircular canal is located in a separate bony recess inferior and posterior to the vestibule (Fig. 143-4). After removing all neuroepithelium, the vestibule is filled with Gelfoam impregnated with gentamycin or streptomycin (Fig. 143-5). The tympanomeatal flap is returned to its original location.

(continued)

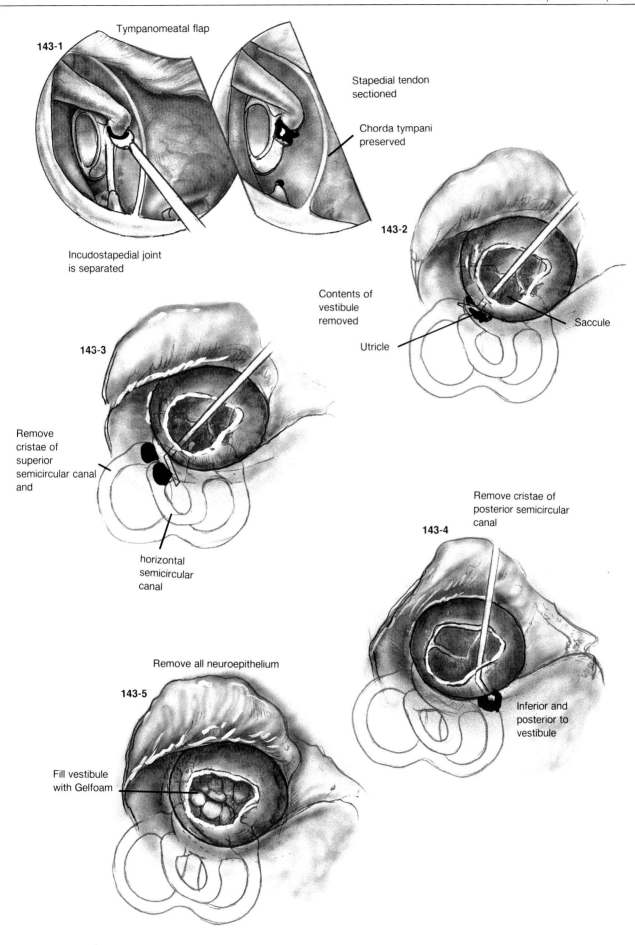

143-1

Tympanomeatal flap

Stapedial tendon sectioned

Chorda tympani preserved

Incudostapedial joint is separated

143-2

Contents of vestibule removed

Utricle

Saccule

143-3

Remove cristae of superior semicircular canal and

horizontal semicircular canal

Remove cristae of posterior semicircular canal

143-4

Inferior and posterior to vestibule

Remove all neuroepithelium

143-5

Fill vestibule with Gelfoam

■ 143. LABYRINTHECTOMY (continued)

Tips and Pearls

1. Confounding factors such as central nervous system disease or bilateral vestibular disease may compromise success.

Complications

1. The facial nerve may be dehiscent in the vicinity of the oval window niche, increasing the risk of facial nerve injury.
2. Particular care must be exercised when working in the vicinity of the cribrose areas at the fundus of the internal auditory canal to prevent a cerebrospinal leak.
3. Meningitis
4. Failure due to incomplete labyrinthectomy

Postoperative Care Issues

1. Prophylactic antibiotic therapy given for 2 days
2. Antiemetics are given as needed to control postoperative nausea and vomiting.
3. Early ambulation and exercise in bed are encouraged postoperatively to reduce risk of pulmonary embolism and to stimulate vestibular compensation.

References

Gacek RR. Surgery of the vestibular system. In: Cummings CW, ed. Otolaryngology—head and neck surgery, vol 4. St. Louis: CV Mosby, 1992.

Meiteles LZ, Telian SA. Meniere's disease: surgical therapy. In: Gates GA, ed. Current therapy in otolaryngology—head and neck surgery. 5th ed. St. Louis: Mosby-Year Book, 1994.

Vernick DM. Labyrinthectomy. In: Nadol JB, Schucknecht HF, eds. Surgery of the ear and temporal bone. New York: Raven Press, 1993.

Transmastoid Labyrinthectomy

With the patient under general anesthesia, the ear is prepared and draped, and local injections of postauricular region are performed with a 1% solution of Xylocaine with a 1:100,000 concentration of epinephrine. A postauricular incision is made, and the mastoid cortex is exposed. A complete mastoidectomy is performed, skeletonizing the middle fossa plate and the sigmoid sinus. The sinodural angle is opened to allow better exposure of the vestibule (Fig. 143-6A).

The three semicircular canals are systematically opened with a drill (Fig. 143-6B). Initially, the horizontal semicircular canal is opened, maintaining the bone inferior to its lumen to provide a bony protective barrier between the canal and the facial nerve (Fig. 143-7). The horizontal canal is followed anteriorly to its ampulla end and posteriorly toward the posterior semicircular canal. The superior semicircular canal is identified and followed from its ampulla end anteriorly to the common crus posteriorly and medially. The posterior semicircular canal is then followed from the common crus to its ampulla end (Figs. 143-8 and 143-9). Care must be exercised in exposing the ampulla end of the posterior semicircular canal, because it lies medial to the vertical segment of the facial nerve.

The neuroepithelium is completely removed from the ampulla ends of the three semicircular canals (Fig. 143-10). The vestibule is widely opened, and the utricle and saccule are removed (Fig. 143-11). Gelfoam impregnated with gentamycin is placed in the vestibule. The incision is closed in layers.

RICHARD T. MIYAMOTO
CYNTHIA L. KISH

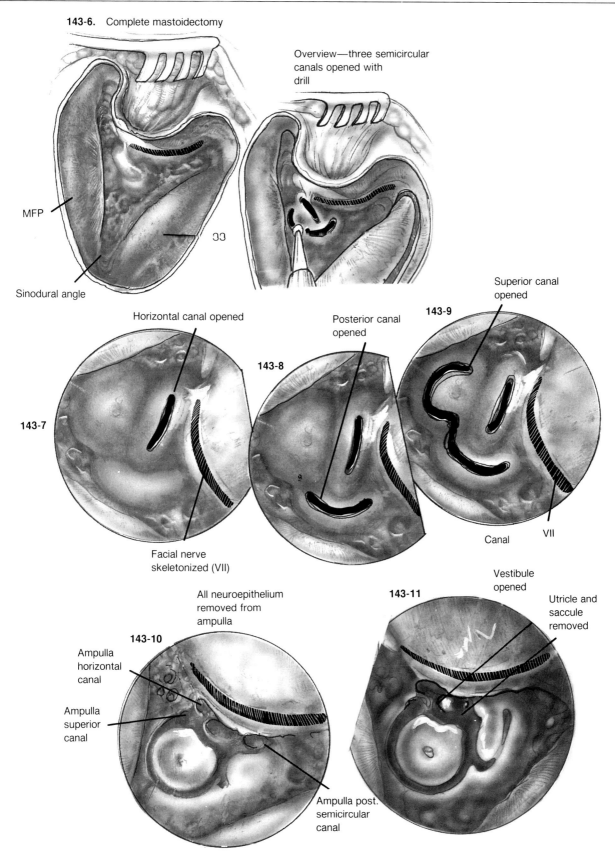

143-6. Complete mastoidectomy

Overview—three semicircular canals opened with drill

MFP

Sinodural angle

CC

143-9

Superior canal opened

Horizontal canal opened

Posterior canal opened

143-8

143-7

Facial nerve skeletonized (VII)

Canal   VII

143-10

All neuroepithelium removed from ampulla

Ampulla horizontal canal

Ampulla superior canal

Ampulla post. semicircular canal

143-11

Vestibule opened

Utricle and saccule removed

■ *144.* COCHLEAR IMPLANTS

Cochlear implants are electronic devices that convert mechanical sound energy into electric signals that can be delivered to profoundly deaf individuals. They seek to replace the nonfunctional inner ear hair cell transducer system.

Indications

1. Cochlear implants may be appropriate for children and adults with profound bilateral sensorineural hearing loss who receive no appreciable benefit from hearing aids.

Special Considerations

1. Congenitally deformed cochlea (Mondini deformity); may encounter profuse cerebrospinal fluid leak on fenestrating cochlea
2. Ossified cochlea; new bone can be drilled out and partial electrode insertion accomplished
3. Ear with previous chronic ear surgery
4. Child with frequent middle ear infections

Contraindications

1. Congenitally deaf child with deaf parents who communicate manually
2. Cochlear aplasia (Michael deformity)
3. Narrow internal auditory canal syndrome; cochlear nerve may be absent

Preoperative Preparation

1. Audiogram
2. Hearing aid trial under close observation
3. High-resolution, thin-section computed tomography scan of the temporal bone
4. Psychologic assessment

Special Instruments, Position, and Anesthesia

1. Device-specific insertion tools for introduction of the electrode into the cochlea
2. Patient in the supine position, with the head turned away from ear to be operated
3. General anesthesia

Tips and Pearls

1. Insert active electrode through the cochleostomy anterior and inferior to the round window to avoid the "hook" of the cochlea.
2. Do not seal the cochleostomy with a bone paté (may induce intracochlear bone growth).

Pitfalls and Complications

1. The skin incision must have particular attention to avoid skin breakdown over the induction coil.
2. Facial paralysis
3. Electrode extrusion

Postoperative Care Issues

1. Drain used only if needed

References

Clark G. The University of Melbourne—nucleus multi-electrode cochlear implant. Adv Otol Rhinol Laryngol 1987;38:189.

Miyamoto RT, Osberger MJ, Robbins AM, Myres WA, Kessler K, et al. Prelingually deafened children's performance with the nucleus multichannel cochlear implant. Am J Otol 1993;14:437.

Operative Procedure

Skin incisions are designed to provide access to the mastoid process and coverage of the external portion of the implant package while preserving the blood supply of the postauricular skin. The incision employed at the Indiana University Medical Center has eliminated the need to develop a large postauricular flap (Fig. 144-1). The inferior extent of the incision is made well posterior to the mastoid tip to preserve branches of the postauricular artery. From here, the incision is directed posterosuperiorly and then directed superiorly, without a superoanterior limb. In children, the incision incorporates the temporalis muscle to give added thickness. A pocket is created for positioning the implant induction coil. Well anterior to the skin incision, the periosteum is incised from superior to inferior, and a posterior periosteal flap is developed. At the completion of the procedure, the posterior periosteal flap is sutured to the skin flap, compartmentalizing the induction coil from the skin incision.

After developing the skin incision, a complete mastoidectomy is performed (Fig. 144-2). The horizontal semicircular canal is identified in the depths of the mastoid antrum, and the short process of the incus is identified in the fossa incudis. The facial recess is opened using the fossa incudis as an initial landmark. The facial recess is a triangular area bounded by the fossa incudis superiorly, the chorda tympani nerve laterally and anteriorly, and the facial nerve medially and posteriorly (Fig. 144-3). The facial nerve can usually be visualized through the bone without exposing it completely. The round window niche is visualized through the facial recess approximately 2 mm inferior to the stapes. Occasionally, the round window niche is posteriorly positioned and is not well visualized through the facial recess or is obscured by ossification. It is important not to be misdirected by hypotympanic air cells.

Entry into the scala tympani of the cochlea is best accomplished through a cochleostomy created anterior and inferior to the annulus of the round window membrane. A small fenestra slightly larger than the electrode to be implanted (usually 0.5 mm) is developed (see Fig. 144-3). A small diamond bur is used to "blue line" the endosteum of the scala tympani, and the endosteal membrane is removed with small picks. This approach bypasses the hook area of the scala tympani, allowing direct insertion of the active electrode array (Figs. 144-4 and 144-5).

After insertion of the active electrode array, the round window area is sealed with small pieces of fascia. A seat is developed in the cortical bone superior to the mastoid defect for positioning of the induction coil (see Fig. 144-2). Skin closure is performed in layers. A drain is used only if excessive drainage occurs in the incision site.

RICHARD T. MIYAMOTO

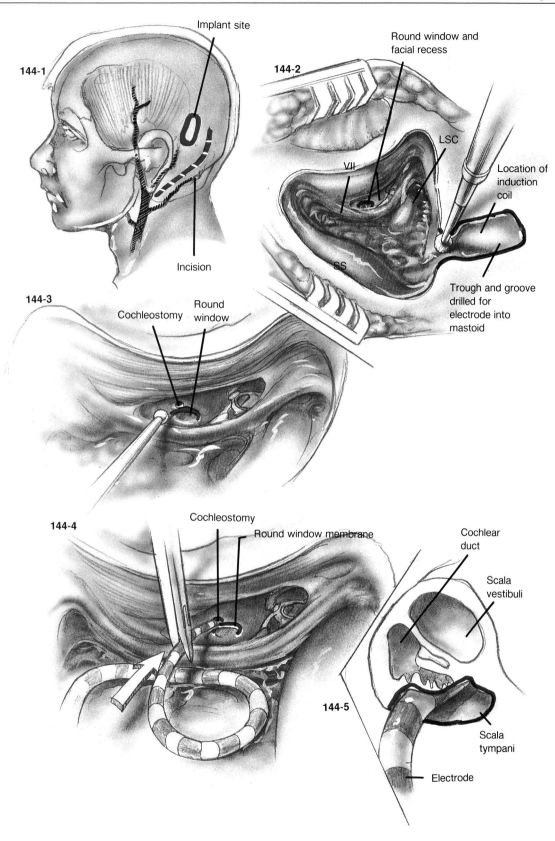

144-1
Implant site
Incision

144-2
Round window and facial recess
LSC
VII
SS
Location of induction coil
Trough and groove drilled for electrode into mastoid

144-3
Cochleostomy
Round window

144-4
Cochleostomy
Round window membrane

144-5
Cochlear duct
Scala vestibuli
Scala tympani
Electrode

■ *145.* ENDOLYMPHATIC SAC EXPOSURE, DECOMPRESSION, OR SHUNT—A nondestructive approach to the inner ear to treat endolymphatic hydrops (ELH), the underlying pathophysiologic condition of Meniere's disease. This is a transmastoid surgical identification and exposure of the endolymphatic sac (ELS) and endolymphatic duct (ELD) to facilitate long-term decompression of the hydropic labyrinth to mastoid or subarachnoid shunt of any type.

Indications
1. Episodic vertigo with symptom-free periods, fluctuating or deteriorating sensorineural hearing loss (eg, tinnitus, aural pressure; classic Meniere's disease) with persistent electrocochleography ECoG evidence of endolymphatic hydrops
2. Episodic vertigo without hearing loss: vestibular Meniere's disease, and abnormal ECoG
3. Fluctuating sensorineural hearing loss without vertigo: cochlear Meniere's disease, ELH, and abnormal ECoG

Contraindications
1. Bleeding or clotting disorders or abnormalities
2. Middle ear effusion, inflammation, or mastoiditis

Special Considerations
1. Congenital or developmental anomalies of the ELS or ELD
2. Better-hearing ear or the only hearing ear
3. Delayed endolymphatic hydrops of childhood
4. Perilymph fistula syndrome

Preoperative Preparation
1. Audiogram, ECoG, bleeding and clotting studies

Special Instruments, Position, and Anesthesia
1. Dural palpator or elevator
2. Sharp sac knife (disposable)
3. Up-angled, 30° microscissors; can also be angled to right, left, or straight

Tips and Pearls
1. Identify with certainty the real lumen of the ELS and avoid the false lumen, which is easier to get into than the real lumen.
2. If using a radiopaque capillary tipped shunt tube, the goal is to cannulate the tip into or at the external aperture of the vestibular aqueduct; check the tip position and seating with postoperative high-resolution computed tomography scan.
3. Use intraoperative ECoG to confirm that the procedure has improved the underlying hydropic condition and at what point or stage in the surgery the electrophysiologic reduction of endolymphatic hydrops occurred.

Pitfalls and Complications
1. Postoperative dizziness from opening the inner ear can be minimized by the use of intraoperative steroids (eg, 10 mg of prednisone) and postoperative use of Medrol dose pack.
2. Cerebrospinal fluid leaks

Postoperative Care Issues
1. Keep the patient's head above heart level, and counsel the patient to avoid straining, lifting, and bending.
2. Stool softener

References
Arenberg IK. Results of endolymphatic sac to mastoid shunt surgery for Meniere's disease refractory to medical therapy. Am J Otol 1987;8: 335.

Arenberg IK, Gibson WPR. Identifying the real lumen during any endolymphatic sac surgery. In: Arenberg IK, ed. Surgery of the inner ear. Amsterdam: Kugler, 1991:199.

Arenberg IK, Gibson WPR. Nondestructive surgery for vertigo. In: Pillsbury AC, Goldsmith M, eds. Operative challenges in otolaryngology—head and neck surgery. Chicago: Yearbook Publishers, 1990:93.

Arenberg IK, Rask-Andersen H, Wilbrand H, et al. The surgical anatomy of the endolymphatic sac. Arch Otolaryngol Head Neck Surg 1977;103:1.

Operative Procedure
The patient is prepped and draped to include intraoperative placement of the silver ball tip electrode in the round window niche against the round window membrane for ECoG monitoring.

A complete mastoidectomy is performed with an air drill, appropriate cutting and diamond burs, and suction irrigation while identifying the short process of the incus, the horizontal and posterior semicircular canals, tegmen, sinodural angle, descending portion of the facial nerve, and the sigmoid sinus. The dissection is carried inferiorly, and the retrofacial air cell tract is exenterated down to the jugular bulb. The posterior fossa bony plate between the posterior semicircular canals and the sigmoid sinus and from the sinodural angle down and into the retrofacial air cell tract is thinned to eggshell thickness so it can easily be removed with a dural palpator elevator.

After the ELS is uncovered from the bony eggshell of the posterior fossa bony plate, the ELS can be identified by the use of color differences, surgical anatomic findings, and the point of narrowing of the ELS into the ELD as it enters the external aperture (EA) of the vestibular aqueduct (VA).

The target of this surgery is to be able to cannulate the capillary shunt tip (radiopaque) into the VA. The postoperative position of the opaque capillary tube can readily be verified with CT. Open the ELS (Fig. 145-1) near its superior margin, which is usually the thickest area of the ELS and hence the easiest in which to find and confirm the real ELS lumen. A 120° Crabtree-type dissector can be used to palpate gently and open into the real lumen or explore for the false lumen. The false lumen is the anatomic plane between the medial wall of the ELS and the posterior fossa dura. In Meniere's disease, it is unfortunately easier to get into the false lumen than into the real lumen. After the sac is opened and the presumed real lumen identified, corroborate this by making a second incision exactly at the superior margin of the ELS at its anatomic junction with the posterior fossa dura. This allows the surgeon to follow the posterior fossa dura under the entire ELS (ie, medial and lateral ELS walls) into the false lumen. If the Crabtree-type dissector is in the false lumen, the instrument can be seen through the incision under an intact medial wall of the ELS (Fig. 145-2). The false lumen is much easier to open into and has fewer adhesions because it is only an anatomic plane.

If the first incision goes through the lateral and medial walls of the ELS, the surgeon sees the metal of the Crabtree dissector without any medial ELS wall present (Fig. 145-3). It does not help to place any type of shunt device into the false lumen. If not in the real lumen, make another incision, which is not as deep. Continue this process until it is possible to confirm surgically or anatomically the real lumen of the ELS.

After confirming the real lumen, it is helpful to rotate a lateral ELS fold inferiorly using 30° up-angled scissors (Fig. 145-4). This allows the surgeon more latitude to probe the ELS, particularly toward the ELD to find and measure the point of narrowing of the ELS into the ELD at the EA of the VA. The ELD duct probe is marked in 1-mm increments and is the same outside diameter as the capillary portion of the shunt tube. The ELD probe is passed through the ELS incision into the ELS and toward the ELD or the point of narrowing (Fig. 145-5). It is helpful to use intraoperative ECoG monitoring to enhance safety and efficacy of this inner ear decompression–type shunt surgery with confirmation of reduced endolymphatic hydrops. The best surgical or anatomic dissection may be physiologically ineffective. The capillary shunt tube, with or without a valve, can be easily inserted into the ELS or ELD along the same track produced by the same-sized ELD probe with a capillary tube introducer notched to prevent crimping (Fig. 145-6). The shunt tube should be primed with heparin. After the shunt tube is satisfactorily positioned, the inner ear opening can be sealed with autologous fibrin glue. Gelfoam soaked in dexamethasone is placed around the shunt tube. Hemostasis is confirmed and the mastoid defect is closed routinely in three layers.

I. KAUFMAN ARENBERG

145-1

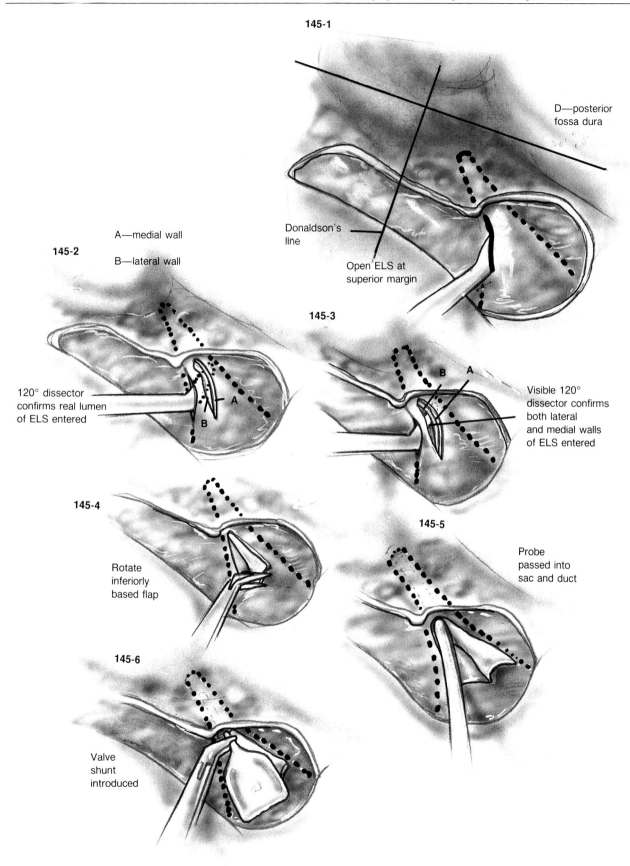

D—posterior
fossa dura

Donaldson's
line

Open ELS at
superior margin

A—medial wall

B—lateral wall

145-2

120° dissector
confirms real lumen
of ELS entered

A

B

145-3

B   A

Visible 120°
dissector confirms
both lateral
and medial walls
of ELS entered

145-4

Rotate
inferiorly
based flap

145-5

Probe
passed into
sac and duct

145-6

Valve
shunt
introduced

■ 146. POSTERIOR SEMICIRCULAR CANAL

OCCLUSION—Complete, permanent occlusion (plugging) of the bony and membranous posterior semicircular canal

Indications

1. Intractable, unilateral, benign paroxysmal positional vertigo (if bilateral, treat more troublesome side)
2. Must have all classic findings in response to Hallpike maneuver
3. Failed response to at least two particle repositioning maneuvers (alternatively, may use canalith repositioning procedure or Semont maneuver) (Fig. 146-1).

Contraindications

1. Only or significantly better-hearing ear
2. Acute or active chronic otitis media or mastoiditis

Special Considerations

1. Rule out atypical, paroxysmal, positional vertigo (eg, from central lesion).

Preoperative Preparation

1. Routine laboratory studies
2. Audiogram
3. Computed tomography scan of posterior fossa and temporal bone to rule out central lesion and check accessibility of posterior canal (magnetic resonance image fine for former but not for latter)
4. Perioperative antibiotics for history of otitis media

Special Instruments, Position, and Anesthesia

1. Standard middle ear or mastoid instruments and microdrill
2. Fibrinogen glue and bone paté "plug"

Tips and Pearls

1. Create double–blue-lined endosteal island
2. Avoid direct suction on perilymph and membranous labyrinth
3. Completely occlude lumen of bony canal
4. Ensure complete seal of fenestration site to prevent perilymph leak

Pitfalls and Complications

1. "Dead ear" may result from overzealous manipulation or suction of the membranous labyrinth or from acute postoperative infection.
2. Expect initial mixed, mild to moderate hearing loss, which should resolve within 3 to 4 weeks.
3. Expect motion sensitivity (worse in elderly) to resolve in 2 to 4 weeks.

Postoperative Care Issues

1. Early ambulation with vestibular exercises
2. Avoid excessive vestibular sedatives, which may prolong overall recovery.

References

Parnes LS. Treatment of benign paroxysmal positional vertigo. In: Myers EN, Bluestone CD, Brackman DE, Krause CJ, eds. Advances in otolaryngology-head and neck surgery, Volume 8. St. Louis: Mosby-Year Book, 1994;321.

Parnes LS, McClure JA. Posterior semicircular canal occlusion in the normal hearing ear. Otolaryngol Head Neck Surg 1991;104:52.

Parnes LS, Price-Jones RG. Particle repositioning maneuver for benign paroxysmal positional vertigo. Ann Otol Rhinol Laryngol 1993;102:325.

Operative Procedure

After induction of general anesthesia, the patient is placed in the supine position, with the head turned 45° degrees away from the operative ear. The surgical site preparation and draping are performed in a routine fashion. Intraoperative auditory and facial nerve monitoring are not routinely performed.

Through a standard postauricular incision, a limited mastoidectomy is carried out (Fig.146-2A). The antrum is opened to allow identification of the lateral semicircular canal. Thinning of the tegmen and identification of the digastric ridge are unnecessary. The sigmoid sinus is skeletonized but not bared. Bone removal proceeds anteriorly from the sinus along the cerebellar plate toward the posterior semicircular canal. The posterior canal otic capsule bone is identified, and the bone is "blue lined" with progressively smaller diamond burs and copious suction irrigation. The target zone for the occlusion is the area at or just inferior to a line extending back from the lateral posterior canal (ie, Donaldson's line). This part of the posterior semicircular canal is farthest from the ampulla and vestibule, and manipulation in this region is theoretically least likely to induce other vestibular or cochlear damage.

Using first a 1-mm and then an 0.8-mm diamond bur, a 3-mm-long segment of the canal is skeletonized 180° around the outer circumference down to endosteum, creating a 1×3 mm double–blue-lined endosteal island (see Fig. 146-2B). Bone removal should proceed evenly around the circumference of this island so that, after the endosteum is violated and perilymph is exposed, all drilling can cease. The endosteal island is removed with a fine 90° pick to expose the perilymphatic space (Fig. 146-3). Great care must be taken not to suction directly on the perilymph and especially the membranous labyrinth. The most important precaution is to not disrupt the membranous labyrinth for fear of creating a "dead ear." The membranous labyrinth is surprisingly resistant to gentle manipulation.

At this stage, the exact outline and limits of the membranous labyrinth are usually not clearly discernible. However, it was at this stage that particles were first identified within the posterior canal in several patients undergoing this procedure. Perilymph is gently wicked away with a cottonoid to expose the membranous labyrinth, at which time the membranous duct collapses. In the canals with particles, perilymph removal allows confirmation that these are indeed free-floating particles within the endolymph. Dry bone chips previously gathered from the mastoidectomy are mixed with one drop of the two-component, fast-acting human fibrinogen glue (Tisseel; Immuno, Vienna, Austria; Fig. 146-4). It sets in about 30 seconds, and it forms any easily workable, malleable plug with a firm consistency. The plug is gently but firmly inserted through the fenestra with the intention of completely filling the canal lumen and thereby compressing the membranous labyrinth closed against the opposite bony wall (Fig. 146-5). The membranous labyrinth seems to be resistant to tearing if no shearing forces are applied. The bone chips within the plug cause intracanal ossification, leading to complete and permanent occlusion of the canal.

Where commercially prepared fibrinogen glue is not available, autologous glue may be fashioned from the patient's own serum. Alternatively, some surgeons have successfully used plugs made from periosteum or fascia. I avoid using bone wax for fear of inducing an inflammatory response in the inner ear. In a variation of this technique, an argon laser applied to the blue-lined posterior canal is purported to create fibrous bands within the canal, leading to obstruction of the membranous duct and alleviation of the benign paroxysmal positional vertigo.

After completing the plug insertion, the fenestra and surrounding bone are covered with a piece of temporalis fascia, which is maintained in place by several more drops of the fibrinogen glue (Fig. 146-6). A good tissue seal is necessary to prevent a postoperative perilymph fistula. A standard closure is then carried out, followed by application of a mastoid dressing.

LORNE S. PARNES

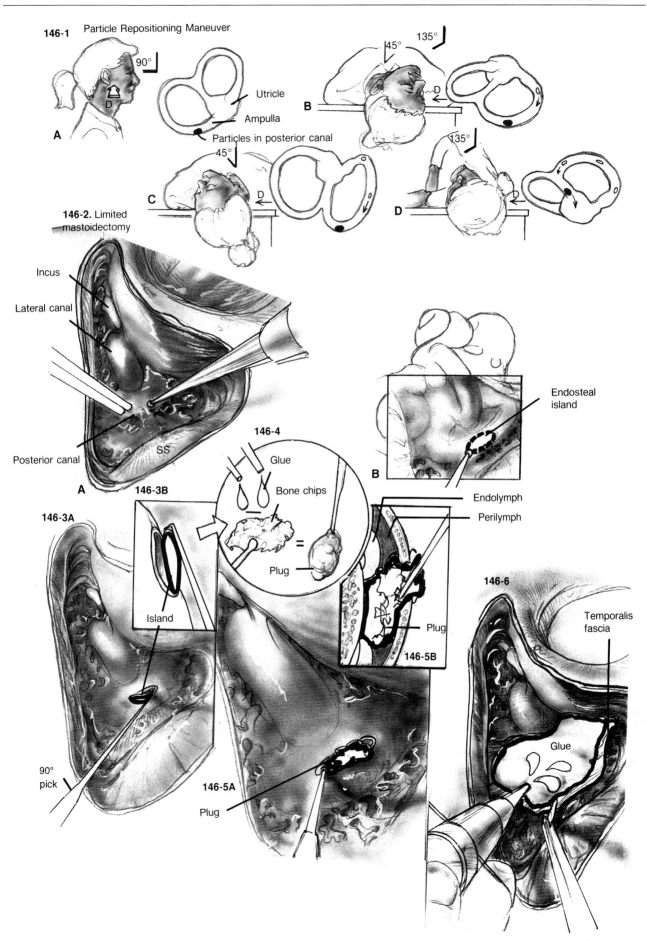

146-1 Particle Repositioning Maneuver

90°

Utricle

Ampulla

Particles in posterior canal

45°

45°

135°

135°

A

B

C

D

D

146-2. Limited mastoidectomy

Incus

Lateral canal

Posterior canal

SS

A

Endosteal island

146-4

Glue

Bone chips

Plug

=

Endolymph

Perilymph

B

146-3B

Island

146-3A

90° pick

146-5A

Plug

Plug

146-5B

146-6

Temporalis fascia

Glue

■ 147. SINGULAR NEURECTOMY

Surgical transection of the nerve to the sense organ of the posterior semicircular canal

Indications

1. Chronic benign paroxysmal positional vertigo of at least 1 year's duration that is disabling

Special Considerations

1. Fatiguing rotatory nystagmus on the Dix-Hallpike positioning maneuver
2. Negative imaging of the posterior fossa using magnetic resonance imaging (MRI) or computed tomography (CT) with contrast
3. A normal ear canal and tympanic membrane

Preoperative Preparation

1. Hearing test for speech and pure tone thresholds
2. Vestibular examination, including electronystagmography
3. Dix-Hallpike positional maneuver
4. MRI or CT scan of the posterior fossa

Special Instruments, Position, and Anesthesia

1. Supine position, with the head slightly dependent and with the operated ear upward
2. Ear speculum and instruments for transcanal ear surgery
3. Speculum holder
4. A microdrill with diamond burs of 0.5- and 1-mm diameters
5. Small 0.5-mm and 1-mm stapes hooks of up and back directions

Tips and Pearls

1. Exposure of the round window niche may require curettage of the posterior bony canal wall.
2. Exposure of the round window membrane by removal of the bony overhang of the round window niche
3. Begin the approach to the singular canal just inferior to the superior portion of the round window membrane.

Pitfalls and Complications

1. Sensorineural hearing loss from damage to the basal turn of the cochlea
2. Labyrinthitis if the ampulla of the posterior semicircular canal is entered
3. Cerebrospinal fluid leak if the singular canal is exposed proximally

Postoperative Care Issues

1. Postoperative monitoring for disequilibrium. The Dix-Hallpike maneuver is carried out on the first postoperative day and is negative for the rotatory nystagmus. However, a downbeat nystagmus is often seen, representing central compensatory mechanisms.
2. Possible infection of the middle ear is indicated by an elevation of temperature, pain in the ear, or discharge from the ear.
3. The patient is seen in 1 week postoperatively, at which time the packing is removed and hearing is tested. The next postoperative visit is usually in 4 to 6 weeks, when another hearing test is performed. Dix-Hallpike maneuvers are also performed at 1 week and at 1-month intervals.

References

Gacek RR. Transection of the posterior ampullary nerve for the relief of benign paroxysmal positional vertigo. Trans Am Otol Soc 1974;62: 73.

Gacek RR. Singular neurectomy update. Ann Otol Rhinol Laryngol 1982;91:469.

Gacek RR. Singular neurectomy, update II. Review of 102 cases. Laryngoscope 1991;101:855.

Operative Procedure

The procedure is carried out under local anesthesia with assisted sedation by the anesthesia department. The patient is placed in the supine position on an electric power operating table. The head is placed with the operated ear up toward the ceiling and in a slightly dependent position so that the ear canal lies in a vertical plane. After standard ear prepping and draping, a ear speculum is used to clean the ear canal of debris and to initiate the local anesthesia. The local anesthesia of 1% Xylocaine with a 1:100,000 dilution of epinephrine is delivered in a 5- or 10-mm syringe with a 1.5-in (3.8-cm) 27-gauge needle. The four quadrants of the external auditory meatus are injected with a local anesthetic first, and then two deep canal injections are made. To successfully complete these two deep canal injections, the needle is bent toward the beveled side of the tip so that the bevel when inserted under the skin lies against the bone of the ear canal. In this way, the local anesthetic is infused under the thin skin of the inferior and superior ear canal wall down to the tympanic annulus. The tympanomeatal flap is outlined with knives and microscissors and is elevated. The tympanic annulus is lifted out of its bony sulcus, and the drum is reflected forward.

If the round window niche is not fully visualized after tympanotomy, the posterior canal wall may require curettage to completely expose the round window niche to the subiculum (Fig. 147-1). After the round window niche has been fully exposed, a speculum holder is used to secure the speculum in position. A microdrill with a 1-mm diamond bur is used to remove the overhang of the round window niche. Usually, a mucous membrane fold covers the niche and may obscure visualization of the round window membrane. This mucous membrane fold (often with a circular defect) should be removed with hooks and picks. The overhang of the round window niche is removed in a curvilinear fashion until the entire round window membrane can be visualized clearly (Fig. 147-2). The most superior portion of the round window membrane, which parallels the long axis of the oval window, is the most difficult to visualize and may require displacement by depressing the ossicular chain. After the round window membrane has been fully exposed, a 0.5-mm diamond bur is used to begin the approach to the singular canal. This approach is initiated inferior to the attachment of the superior portion of the round window membrane, which is the portion closest to the surgeon. The drilling is carried out with intermittent irrigation to remove bone dust.

As the singular canal is approached, if the canal is in a favorable position, the white myelinated nerve bundle begins to appear as the bone over the canal is thinned (see Fig. 147-2). At this point, the patient complains of vertigo or pain. The singular canal can usually be identified at a depth of approximately 2 mm. If drilling to this depth or beyond does not expose the canal, the drilling should be directed in a superior direction, toward the round window membrane, but the drilling should be initiated at the depth of the defect, not at the level of the round window membrane attachment. The singular canal may be identified in a more superior or hidden position by the patient's response to the exposure of the canal. Periodic probing with an angled hook in this direction palpates the canal and prompts the patient's response to stimulation of the nerve.

After the nerve has been exposed, picks and small hooks are used to crush and remove nerve tissue. Only the most proximal end of the canal is probed with the hook, because the distal end of the canal may be near the ampulla. If leakage of spinal fluid occurs, Gelfoam or soft tissue (eg, earlobe fat) may be used to obliterate the defect, depending on the magnitude of the leak.

The tympanomeatal flap is replaced, and a small pack is used to hold it in its anatomic position. A small ear dressing is applied, and the patient is sent back to his or her hospital room. Prophylactic antibiotics are administered orally for 1 week.

RICHARD R. GACEK

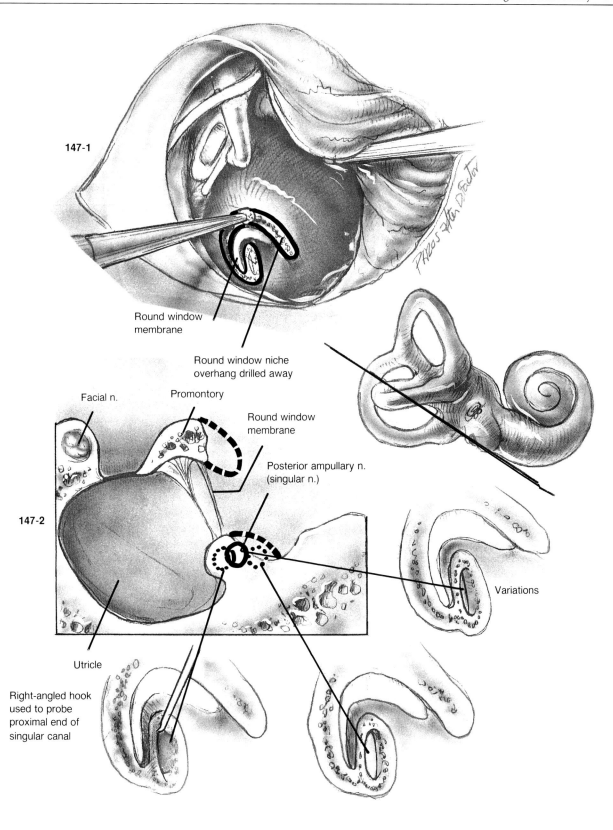

147-1

Round window
membrane

Round window niche
overhang drilled away

Facial n.

Promontory

Round window
membrane

Posterior ampullary n.
(singular n.)

147-2

Variations

Utricle

Right-angled hook
used to probe
proximal end of
singular canal

■ 148. STREPTOMYCIN PERFUSION OF THE LABYRINTH
—Perfusion of the labyrinth with streptomycin through the round window plus intravenous streptomycin to relieve the dizzy spells, fullness, and low-frequency tinnitus without making the hearing worse

Indications
1. Dizzy spells in stages II and III of Meniere's disease that are not responsive to oral dexamethasone
2. Failed endolymphatic shunt or vestibular neurectomy
3. Dizzy spells of benign paroxysmal positional vertigo not responsive to vestibular rehabilitation exercises
4. Dizzy spells of hyperlipidemia unresponsive to medical treatment

Contraindications
1. Dizzy spells from any form of labyrinthitis that prevent the streptomycin from perfusing the vestibular receptors, such as meningitis, sudden hearing loss, or head injury
2. Only hearing ear is affected.

Special Considerations
1. No allergy or hypersensitivity to streptomycin, which is rare
2. Renal failure

Preoperative Preparation
1. Complete hearing tests
2. Transtympanic electrocochleography
3. Ice water caloric electronystagmography

Special Instruments, Position, and Anesthesia
1. Operating microscope
2. Topical anesthesia for drum, such as EMLA (Astra, 50 Otis Street, Westborough, MA), which is 25% Xylocaine and 25% prilocaine in cream
3. Hyaluronate, such as VISCOAT (Viscoat, Alcon Surgical Inc., 6201 South Freeway, Fort Worth, TX), in which 120 mg of streptomycin/mL is dissolved
4. Intravenous streptomycin (1 g), administered during 4 hours

Tips and Pearls
1. Get the hyaluronate into the depths of the round window niche.

Pitfalls and Complications
1. Tearing the round window membrane loose when cleaning out adhesions and thickened membrane to allow unimpeded access to the round window membrane

Postoperative Care Issues
1. Limited activity during the 3 days of the operation

References
Norris CH, Aubert A, Shea JJ. Comparison of cochleotoxicity and vestibulotoxicity of streptomycin and gentamicin. In Filipo R, Barbara M (eds). Meniere's Disease: perspectives in the 90's. Proceedings of the Third International Symposium on Meniere's disease, Rome, Italy, October 20–23, 1993. Amsterdam/New York: Kugler Publications, 1994:485.

Shea JJ. Streptomycin perfusion of the labyrinth through the round window with intravenous streptomycin *Otolaryngol Clin North Am* 1994;27:317.

Operative Procedure
The operation begins with the installation of 1 mL of a powerful topical anesthetic, such as EMLA (25% Xylocaine and 25% prilocaine) on the posteroinferior quadrant of the drum with the patient on the operating table 20 minutes before the incision is made. An intravenous drip containing 1 g of streptomycin in 500 mL of Ringer's solution is started. After 20 minutes, the local anesthetic is wiped from the surface of the drum, and anesthesia of the drum is verified. A linear incision is made from the umbo backward, at 5 o'clock, that is long enough to expose the round window niche completely (Fig. 148-1).

The round window niche is inspected. If the round window membrane can be seen, with no adhesions or thickened membrane, nothing further is done in this area. If there are some adhesions or thickened membrane obscuring a good view of the round window membrane, a delicate 0.5-mm right-angle pick is inserted in the round window niche, and the adhesions and thickened membrane are removed. Any bleeding is controlled with Gelfoam, and blood clots are removed from the round window niche (Fig. 148-2).

Using a blunt, 1-in-long, 20-gauge needle on a tuberculin syringe, with the round window niche exposed through the incision in the drum, 0.5 mL of hyaluronate containing 120 mg of streptomycin/mL is introduced into the round window niche (Fig. 148-3).

The patient is made to lie with the operated ear up in the recovery room to keep the hyaluronate in the round window niche for 4 hours while receiving the 1 g of streptomycin intravenously.

The patient is advised that he or she may be unsteady, feeling something like seasickness, but not dizzy, and the fullness and low-frequency noise are often less pronounced. Paresthesia of the lips and face from the intravenous streptomycin are of no concern. The hearing is tested on the second and third days before the streptomycin is introduced into the round window niche to verify that the hearing is no worse.

After the third introduction of streptomycin in hyaluronate, a piece of Gelfoam is pressed onto the drum over the incision to enhance healing. The patient is allowed to resume full activity the day after the third introduction of hyaluronate with streptomycin, with no special precautions other than not to get water into the operated ear for several days. The patient is advised to begin balance rehabilitation exercises. The patient is seen 4 weeks after the operation for a hearing test and evaluation of the response. Some patients report being unsteady, with a staggering gait and loss of balance for a while, but they do not report dizzy spells. Most have less low-tone noise and fullness and some nystagmus.

In 3 months, the patients have compensated for the loss of the vestibular receptors in the operated ear. They are no longer unsteady, with no nystagmus, less fullness and low-frequency noise, no dizzy spells, no hearing loss, no caloric response to ice water, and less negative summating potential confirmed by electrocochleography.

Rarely, dizzy spells continue after streptomycin perfusion of the labyrinth through the round window, although they are less frequent and less severe than before the procedure. Most of these patients retain some caloric response to ice water and, presumably, have not had enough effect of the streptomycin on the vestibular receptors. In patients who have incomplete responses to the first streptomycin perfusion, it is possible to repeat the streptomycin perfusion for 1, 2, or 3 more days to get the desired response.

I have not done streptomycin perfusion of the labyrinth through the round window in both ears of any patient, but if I had a good response in the first ear, after a few months, I would not hesitate to apply streptomycin to the labyrinth through the round window in the other.

JOHN J. SHEA, Jr.

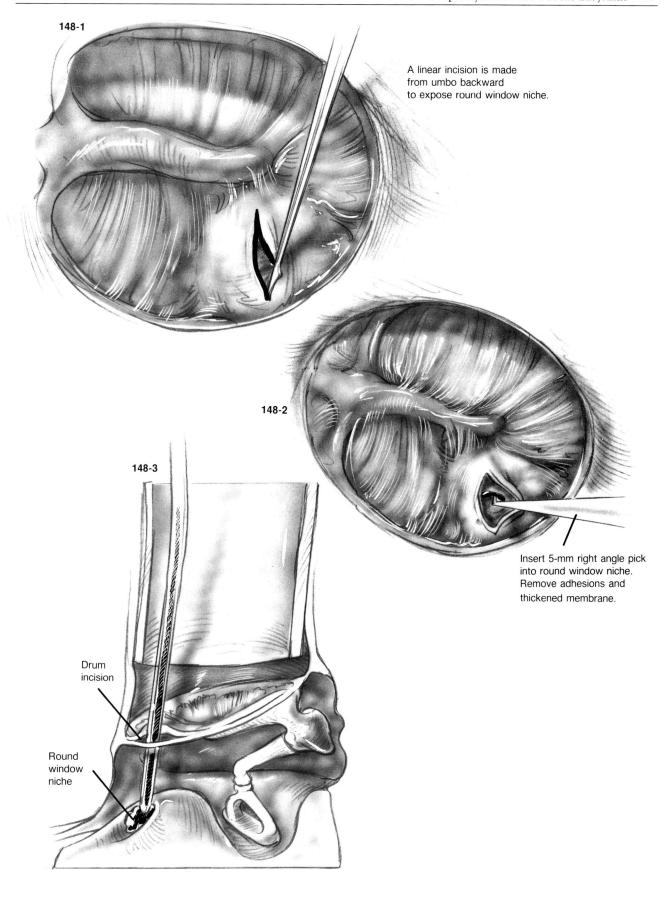

148-1

A linear incision is made
from umbo backward
to expose round window niche.

148-2

Insert 5-mm right angle pick
into round window niche.
Remove adhesions and
thickened membrane.

148-3

Drum
incision

Round
window
niche

■ 149. VESTIBULAR NEURECTOMY

Cutting the vestibular portion of the eighth cranial nerve can be performed through multiple surgical approaches:

1. In the transcochlear approach, the internal auditory canal is approached directly through the cochlea. The entire eighth nerve is severed.
2. Using the translabyrinthine method, the internal auditory canal is approached through the mastoid and labyrinth. The entire eighth nerve is cut.
3. In the middle fossa approach, the vestibular nerve is bisected in the internal auditory canal from the middle fossa. The cochlear nerve and often the saccular nerves are spared.
4. In the retrolabyrinthine approach, the posterior fossa dura is opened between the sigmoid sinus and the labyrinth. The vestibular nerve is divided in the posterior fossa.
5. In the retrosigmoid approach, the posterior fossa dura is opened posterior to the sigmoid sinus. The vestibular nerve is cut in the posterior fossa or in the internal auditory canal.
6. In the combined retrolabyrinthine-retrosigmoid approach, the posterior fossa dura is opened posterior to the sigmoid sinus. The sigmoid sinus is retracted anteriorly to give better exposure with cerebellar retraction. The vestibular nerve is cut in the posterior fossa or the internal auditory canal.

Indications

1. Objective evidence for a unilateral inner ear disorder such as classic Meniere's disease, recurrent vestibular neuronitis, traumatic labyrinthitis, or vestibular Meniere's disease
2. Attacks of vertigo severely affecting the patient's life style or attacks that occur without warning

Contraindications

1. Bilateral vestibular disease (may be relative)
2. Physiologic old age or poor medical condition
3. Vertigo from an only hearing ear
4. Ataxia, unsteadiness, or central nervous system disorder

Special Considerations

1. When hearing is better than an 80-dB speech reception threshold and 20% discrimination, a vestibular neurectomy is recommended to relieve vertigo and preserve hearing. Some patients with worse hearing may also be candidates.
2. When hearing is worse than an 80-dB speech reception threshold and 20% discrimination, an eighth nerve section or labyrinthectomy is recommended. Hearing is destroyed in this procedure.

Preoperative Preparation

1. Hearing test with an air-bone gap and discrimination score, bithermal caloric electronystagmography, electrocochleography, and brain stem auditory evoked response
2. Computed tomography scan for bony anatomy and magnetic resonance imaging with gadolinium to rule out a cerebellopontine angle mass
3. Evaluation of gait and balance function
4. Perioperative intravenous antibiotics may be given (2 g of nafcillin) in three doses of 2 g each: the first preoperatively, the second during surgery, and the third 8 hours later.
5. Intravenous mannitol (1.5 g/kg to a maximum of 100 g) is administered during posterior fossa procedures to reduce brain volume.
6. Bleeding controlled with compressed Avitene (oxidized cellulose) Gelfoam squares.

(continued)

Operative Procedures

Transcochlear Approach

A postauricular incision is made 1 cm behind the postauricular crease, and the posterior external auditory canal is incised. A large tympanomeatal flap is elevated and reflected anteriorly to expose the middle ear structures. A large bony canaloplasty is created, until the round window and horizontal and vertical portion of the facial nerve are identified.

The incus and stapes are removed. The promontory bone is removed, connecting the round and oval windows. The utricle is removed from the elliptical recess using a 3-mm right-angle pick. The posterior ampullary nerve and the singular canal (usually 4.5 mm long) are followed toward the internal auditory canal. The posteroinferior aspect of the internal auditory canal is skeletonized, and the transverse crest is removed so the superior vestibular nerve can be identified. To help the surgeon identify the cochlear nerve, the middle turn of the cochlea is opened anteriorly. When the modiolus is opened, CSF flows freely, which provides irrigation during the drilling. Bone is then removed, enabling the surgeon to see the superior vestibular nerve before it enters the internal auditory canal.

The dura is opened along the posterior aspect of the internal auditory canal over the superior vestibular nerve. The superior vestibular nerve, inferior vestibular nerve, posterior ampullary nerve, cochlear nerve, and facial nerve can be clearly seen. The cochlear nerve is transected at the modiolus. The facial nerve lies anterior, superior, and beneath the vestibular nerves, and it can be identified by electrical stimulation. A good cleavage plane is usually found between the facial and superior vestibular nerves. After the cleavage plane is clearly identified, the vestibular fibers are carefully transected, a few fibers at a time, to avoid stretching the facial nerve. A free temporalis muscle and fascia graft is obtained to obliterate the opening in the internal auditory canal. The flap is then returned to its position over the muscle and held securely in place for 2 weeks by packing the ear with round cottonoid pledgets impregnated with antibiotic ointment and polyester strips (Silverstein tympanoplasty packing, Xomed, Jacksonville, FL). A mastoid dressing is applied for 24 hours.

Translabyrinthine Approach

A postauricular incision is made 1 cm behind the postauricular crease. A complete mastoidectomy is performed with care to identify and skeletonize the sigmoid sinus. The Silverstein lateral sinus retractor is used to retract the sigmoid sinus posteriorly. The attic is opened, and the incus is extracted from the incudal fossa. The bone over the posterior fossa and endolymphatic sac is removed. The vertical portion of the facial nerve is identified in the mastoid. A bony labyrinthectomy is performed, removing the semicircular canals. The endolymphatic duct, which lies just deep to the crus commune, is followed into the vestibule of the inner ear. The internal auditory canal lies in approximately the same coronal plane as the external auditory canal. The bone is removed, skeletonizing the dura of the internal auditory canal from the vestibule to the porus acusticus. It is important to expose at least 180° of the circumference of the internal auditory canal to provide good exposure and to perform the eighth nerve section safely.

The petrosal facial nerve, superior vestibular nerve, and the vertical crest (Bill's bar) are identified at the superior aspect of the internal auditory canal, just deep to the superior and lateral semicircular canal ampulla. The superior vestibular nerve lies more superficial and distal in the bone than the facial nerve. A sharp sickle knife is used to incise the dura of the internal auditory canal, and the superior vestibular nerve is transected in its bony canal and dissected from the facial nerve. The inferior vestibular nerve and the cochlear nerve are then bisected.

Abdominal adipose tissue is harvested through a left, lower quadrant incision, and it is used to obliterate the mastoid defect. The attic and the antrum are sealed with bone wax. The wound is closed with interrupted 2-0 Dexon sutures and skin staples. No drain is placed in the wound. A mastoid dressing is applied, which is removed 2 days later.

(continued)

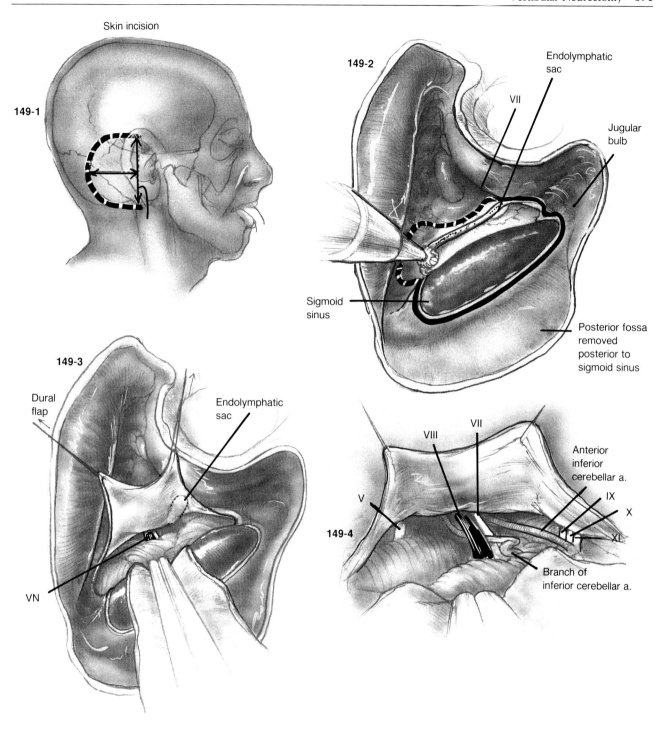

Skin incision

149-1

149-2

Endolymphatic sac

VII

Jugular bulb

Sigmoid sinus

Posterior fossa removed posterior to sigmoid sinus

149-3

Dural flap

Endolymphatic sac

VN

VIII

VII

V

149-4

Anterior inferior cerebellar a.

IX

X

XI

Branch of inferior cerebellar a.

■ *149.* VESTIBULAR NEURECTOMY *(continued)*

Special Instruments, Position, and Anesthesia

1. The facial nerve is monitored using a mechanical pressure sensor (S8 stimulator-monitor, WR Medical Electronics, Stillwater, MN) and electromyography (Brackmann monitor, WR Medical Electronics, Stillwater, MN) techniques.
2. Hearing is monitored during posterior fossa procedures using eighth nerve action potentials in combination with brain stem auditory evoked response and sometimes with electrocochleography.
3. Supine otologic position
4. Insulated neurotologic instruments (19 cm long; Storz Inc., St. Louis, MO).
5. Insulated instruments can be connected to the facial nerve stimulator.
6. Silverstein lateral venous sinus retractor (Storz, Inc.) for retrolabyrinthine and translabyrinthine approaches

Tips and Pearls

1. Practice in the temporal bone laboratory.
2. Identify the facial nerve in all cases before neurectomy.
3. Identify surrounding landmarks, the jugular dural fold (ie, in retrolabyrinthine and combined retrolabyrinthine-retrosigmoid approaches), cranial nerves IX through XI, cranial nerve V, and the tentorium cerebelli.
4. Injury to the internal auditory canal artery may result in total hearing loss. The vessel usually is located between the seventh and eighth cranial nerves.
5. Lumbar drain is the first line of treatment for a cerebrospinal fluid (CSF) leak, which is a rare complication if the middle fossa, retrosigmoid, or combined retrolabyrinthine-retrosigmoid approach is employed.
6. Use electrified instruments to stimulate the facial nerve during dissection.
7. The 90° rotation of the eighth cranial nerve, from the labyrinth to the brain stem, must be understood.

Pitfalls and Complications

1. Bleeding from a major venous sinus, usually easily controlled
2. Hearing loss is most common in middle fossa procedures.
3. CSF leaks are infrequent when dura can be closed watertight.
4. Facial paralysis is most common in middle fossa procedures.
5. Headache is most common when the internal auditory canal is drilled.
6. Meningitis is rare.

Postoperative Care Issues

1. Early ambulation and vestibular rehabilitation exercise

References

Silverstein H, Norrell H, Rosenberg SI. An evolution of approach in vestibular neurectomy. Otolaryngol Head Neck Surg 1990;102:374.
Silverstein H, Rosenberg SI. Combined retrolabyrinthine vestibular neurectomy. Operative Techniques Otolaryngol Head Neck Surg 1990;2:26.

Middle Fossa Approach

From 1963 to 1978, I used the the middle fossa approach exclusively to section the superior vestibular nerve and posterior ampullary nerve (singular nerve). Results for vertigo relief were excellent, but the procedure was formidable. Anatomic landmarks were difficult to identify, and complications, such as temporary facial nerve weakness, epidural hematoma, or deafness, occurred. This procedure is discussed and illustrated in greater detail in Chapter 152.

Retrolabyrinthine Approach

A 4 × 5 cm anteriorly based U-shaped incision is made in the postauricular skin (Fig. 149-1). The flap is elevated, keeping the skin and muscle as one layer. Sharp dissection is used to cut the muscles from the mastoid cortex. Bleeding from the mastoid emissary vein is controlled with electrocautery and bone wax. Fishhook retractors are used to hold the skin flap forward, and large Wietlaner retractors are inserted to hold the skin edges at maximal exposure.

A complete mastoidectomy is performed. The sigmoid sinus is skeletonized, and 1.5 cm of posterior fossa dura is exposed. The endolymphatic sac and posterior semicircular canal are identified. The sigmoid sinus is retracted posteriorly with a retractor (Fig. 149-2). A U-shaped dura flap is made and based anteriorly. A Penrose drain is placed over the cerebellum into the posterior fossa (Fig. 149-3). The arachnoid layer around the seventh and eighth cranial nerves is opened with a blunt instrument to allow CSF to escape from the cerebellopontine angle cistern (Fig. 149-4). The cerebellum falls away from the temporal bone allowing exposure of cranial nerves V, VII, VIII, IX, X, and XI. After the cleavage plane is visualized under high-power magnification, a longitudinal incision is made in the plane, the cochlear and vestibular fibers (superior half of eighth cranial nerve) are separated, and the vestibular nerve is transected (Fig. 149-5).

Several landmarks are helpful in finding the cleavage plane. The vestibular nerve often appears more gray, and the cochlear nerve more white than adjacent tissue. A fine blood vessel frequently courses on the surface between the cochlear and vestibular fibers. The nervus intermedius, which usually lies in the cleavage plane anteriorly, can also be seen with a mirror. The superior one half of the eighth cranial nerve is transected when a cleavage plane cannot be readily identified. Most vestibular fibers are cut and most cochlear fibers are spared using this technique. The dura is closed with three or four interrupted 4-0 silk sutures covered by temporalis fascia, and the mastoid cavity is filled with abdominal adipose tissue.

Combined Retrolabyrinthine-Retrosigmoid Approach

In the combined retrolabyrinthine-retrosigmoid approach, a limited mastoidectomy is performed to expose 3 cm of the sigmoid sinus from the transverse sinus inferiorly to the jugular bulb. The sigmoid sinus is skeletonized and the posterior fossa dura is exposed for 1.5 cm posterior to the sigmoid sinus. A 2.5-cm dural incision is made 3 mm behind and parallel to the sigmoid sinus (Fig. 149-6). The sigmoid sinus is retracted anteriorly using stay sutures placed in the dural cuff. A Penrose drain is placed against the cerebellum, and the arachnoid layer overlying the ninth cranial nerve and cerebellopontine angle cistern is opened, releasing CSF. The anterior retraction of the sigmoid sinus allows wide exposure of posterior surface of the temporal bone and posterior fossa without retraction of the cerebellum. Cranial nerves from V through XII can be seen easily. The eighth cranial nerve is examined, and a cleavage plane is identified between the cochlear and vestibular fibers. If the cochlear-vestibular cleavage plane is present, the vestibular nerve section is performed as in the retrolabyrinthine approach (Fig. 149-7). If no cleavage plane is identified, the dura is reflected off the temporal bone, the posterior internal auditory canal is opened with a diamond bur, and the superior vestibular and posterior ampullary nerves are divided. In most cases, the vestibular nerve can be successfully transected without drilling the internal auditory canal.

The dura is closed in a watertight fashion using 4-0 nylon suture. Any exposed cells are filled with bone wax, and the defect is filled with abdominal adipose tissue.

HERBERT SILVERSTEIN
SETH ROSENBERG

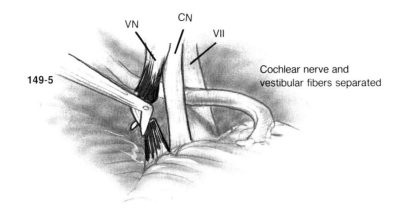

VN   CN   VII

149-5

Cochlear nerve and
vestibular fibers separated

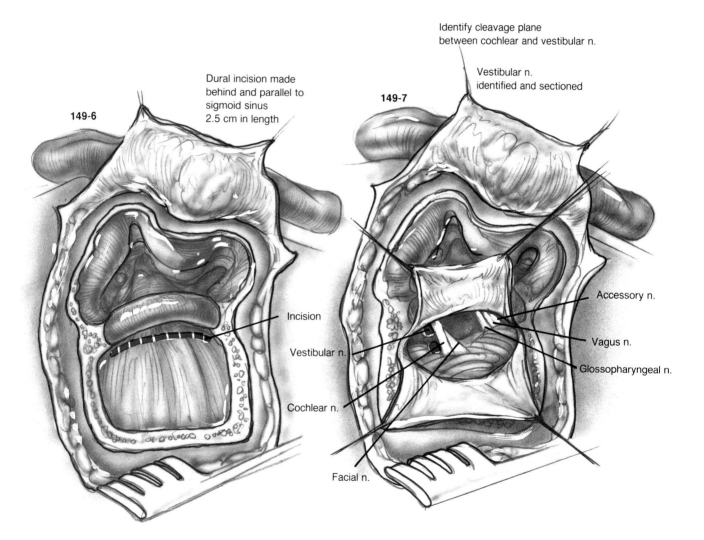

149-6

Dural incision made
behind and parallel to
sigmoid sinus
2.5 cm in length

Incision

Vestibular n.

Cochlear n.

Facial n.

Identify cleavage plane
between cochlear and vestibular n.

Vestibular n.
identified and sectioned

149-7

Accessory n.

Vagus n.

Glossopharyngeal n.

■ *150.* **TRANSLABYRINTHINE APPROACH TO ACOUSTIC NEUROMA**—Surgical removal of an acoustic neuroma by mastoidectomy, labyrinthectomy, and exposure of the internal auditory canal and posterior fossa dura

Indications

1. Intracanalicular acoustic neuroma with significant hearing loss
2. Any acoustic neuroma larger than 2.0 cm, regardless of hearing loss
3. Resection of other neoplasms involving the internal auditory canal and cerebellopontine angle (eg, meningiomas, epidermoids)
4. Complete eighth nerve section for treatment of vertigo with profound hearing loss
5. Placement of auditory brain stem implant

Special Considerations

1. Only hearing ear (may perform subtotal resection by suboccipital approach to delay deafness)
2. Concurrent chronic otitis media or tympanic membrane perforation
3. High jugular bulb

Preoperative Preparation

1. Routine laboratory studies
2. Bleeding clotting studies
3. Preoperative audiogram, magnetic resonance imaging with gadolinium, computed tomography scan to detect bone windows

Special Instruments, Position, and Anesthesia

1. Surgical microscope, with the surgeon seated
2. Otologic drill, otologic instruments, neurosurgical tumor dissection instruments, and bipolar cautery
3. Supine position, with the head turned as for mastoidectomy; shave and prep 3 in (7.5 cm) above and behind ear
4. Facial nerve monitor
5. Intravenous mannitol and furosemide administered by anesthesiologist; dexamethasone for tumors larger than 2 cm
6. No cerebellar retraction necessary

(continued)

Operative Procedure

With the patient in the supine, head-turned position on the operating table, an incision is made from 2 cm above the pinna, curving posteroinferiorly 2 cm behind the postauricular crease to the mastoid tip (Fig. 150-1). The pinna is retracted forward, and the mastoid periosteum is incised along the linea temporalis posteriorly to the sinodural angle and then inferiorly to the mastoid tip. The periosteum is elevated forward to the spine of Henle, without entering the external auditory canal, as well as posteriorly to permit drilling well behind the sigmoid sinus. Self-retaining retractors are inserted to keep the ear forward, to elevate the temporalis muscle, and to expose the mastoid tip.

An extended mastoidectomy is performed with a large cutting bur and continuous suction and irrigation (Fig. 150-2). After identification of the horizontal semicircular canal, the posterior canal wall is thinned and taken down slightly to allow better exposure of the internal auditory canal. The middle fossa dura is completely exposed, and the bone overlying the posterior fossa dura is removed to about 1 cm behind the sigmoid sinus. For large tumors, bone should be removed as far as 2 to 3 cm behind the sigmoid sinus for better tumor exposure. An island of bone is left over the dome of the sigmoid sinus to protect it from the drill. Care should be taken to avoid tearing the sigmoid sinus or emissary veins, because control of bleeding after these events is time consuming. Tears of the sigmoid sinus require packing with oxidized generated cellulose (Surgicel), and bleeding from emissary veins is controlled with bipolar cautery, Surgicel, or bone wax. Elevation and careful, complete removal of the thick bone over the superior petrosal sinus in the sinodural angle is then completed.

Labyrinthectomy is carried out by first opening the posterior semicircular canal and moving forward anteriorly to the horizontal semicircular canal, which is opened and removed. Care is taken to avoid the facial nerve, which is just lateral to the ampulla of the posterior canal and anterior to the horizontal canal (Figs. 150-3). The superior semicircular canal is opened and removed, preserving its ampulla (Fig. 150-4). All bone between the middle fossa dura and the superior canal is removed. The facial nerve is then skeletonized with the side of a diamond bur, removing bone posteriorly from the genu to the mastoid tip. This permits better visualization of the vestibule and the lateral internal auditory canal. Drilling proceeds inferiorly through the retrofacial air cells to the level of the jugular bulb, taking great care not to expose this vessel to prevent troublesome bleeding. The jugular bulb may come up into the mastoid as high as the ampulla of the posterior semicircular canal. During this part of the drilling, the vestibular aqueduct and endolymphatic duct are removed. The cochlear aqueduct is identified as the anterior limit of the dissection, protecting the ninth cranial nerve. The medial aspect of the internal auditory canal is skeletonized, with complete removal of bone between the internal auditory canal and jugular bulb, completely exposing the posterior fossa dura in this area (Fig. 150-5).

The vestibule is widely opened, and the inferior vestibular nerve is exposed inferiorly at the lateral end of the internal auditory canal. The transverse crest is identified, separating the superior and inferior vestibular nerves (Fig. 150-6). The superior vestibular nerve is identified where it joins the ampulla of the superior semicircular canal. Bone is removed superior to the internal auditory canal. The vertical crest (ie, Bill's bar) is found at the entrance of the facial nerve to the internal auditory canal, just beneath the superior vestibular nerve. The bur is rotated so that it tends to move toward the middle fossa dura and away from the facial nerve. The superior aspect of the internal auditory canal is skeletonized with great care, because the facial nerve travels superiorly in the internal auditory canal. However, it is important to completely remove the bone between the middle fossa dura and the superior aspect of the internal auditory canal to obtain adequate tumor exposure. A diamond bur is used for exposing the superior half of the internal auditory canal throughout its entire length, from the lateral end to the porus acusticus.

(continued)

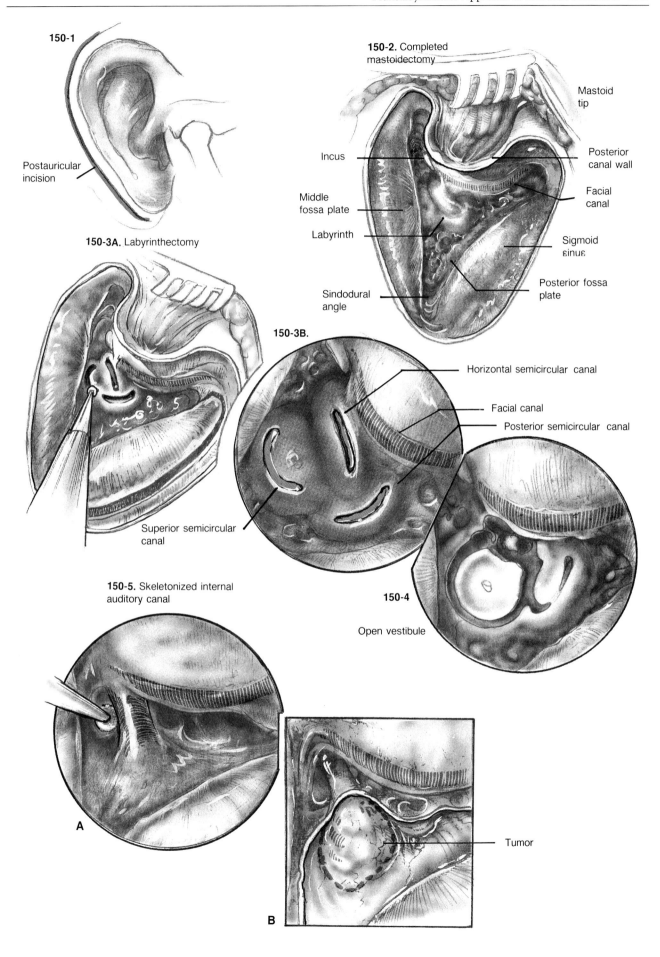

150-1

Postauricular
incision

150-2. Completed
mastoidectomy

Mastoid
tip

Incus

Posterior
canal wall

Middle
fossa plate

Facial
canal

Labyrinth

Sigmoid
sinus

Posterior fossa
plate

Sindodural
angle

150-3A. Labyrinthectomy

150-3B.

Horizontal semicircular canal

Facial canal

Posterior semicircular canal

Superior semicircular
canal

150-4

Open vestibule

150-5. Skeletonized internal
auditory canal

A

B

Tumor

■ *150.* TRANSLABYRINTHINE APPROACH TO ACOUSTIC NEUROMA *(continued)*

Tips and Pearls

1. Wide exposure of the posterior fossa dura to 1 cm behind the sigmoid sinus
2. Complete exposure of the middle fossa dura; complete removal of bone in the sinodural angle
3. Exposure of the vertical crest (ie, Bill's bar) to identify the facial nerve in the fundus of the internal auditory canal
4. Avoidance of cautery during tumor removal; peeling of vessels off the surface of tumor

Pitfalls and Complications

1. Cerebrospinal fluid (CSF) leak
2. Temporary or permanent facial paralysis
3. Meningitis

Postoperative Care Issues

1. Careful postoperative monitoring for evidence of intracranial bleeding, cerebral edema, meningitis, or CSF leak
2. Well-placed mastoid pressure dressing in place for 3 to 4 days helps prevent CSF leak
3. Ambulation with assistance within 24 to 48 hours of surgery to aid in vestibular compensation
4. Discharge 5 to 7 days postsurgically if afebrile, no CSF leak, and ambulatory

References

House WF. Evolution of transtemporal bone removal of acoustic tumors. Arch Otolaryngol 1964;80:731.

House WF, Luetje CM, eds. Acoustic tumors: management, vol II. Baltimore, MD: University Park Press, 1979.

After all bone from the middle and posterior fossa dura and the bone surrounding the internal auditory canal has been removed, an incision is made in the posterior fossa dura, anterior to the sigmoid sinus and around the porus acusticus (Fig. 150-7). The petrosal vein lies just beneath the dura superior to the internal auditory canal and should not be injured. Inferiorly, the lateral branch of the anteroinferior cerebellar artery may be pushed over the tumor and must not be cut. Microscissors are then used to cut the dura along the internal auditory canal from medial to lateral, taking care to avoid vessels.

After the dura is opened, tumor removal may begin. Small tumors may be removed by developing the superior and inferior planes of the tumor (Fig. 150-8). Medium or large tumors require intracapsular debulking with the House-Urban dissector before development of tumor planes. The posterior aspect of the tumor is inspected for nerve bundles, because the facial nerve is pushed posteriorly by tumor growth in rare cases. Then the tumor capsule is incised, and the House-Urban tumor dissector is used to debulk intracapsular tumor (see Fig. 150-8*A*). After debulking, the inferior posterior plane between the arachnoid and tumor capsule is developed with cottonoids back to the brain stem, taking care not to create traction on the facial nerve by pushing the tumor. The blood vessels surrounding the tumor may be separated from the capsule in this plane and preserved. A fenestrated suction is used to prevent damage to nerve or vessels. Inferiorly, the ninth nerve is identified and isolated from the tumor with cottonoids.

At this point, the plane between the tumor and the facial nerve is established. The superior vestibular nerve is avulsed from the lateral internal auditory canal with a hook, revealing the facial nerve anteriorly. Tumor commonly involves the lateral internal auditory canal and may be retracted posteriorly, enabling dissection with a fine hook between the tumor and the facial nerve. The inferior vestibular nerve is divided or avulsed laterally, and both vestibular nerves are removed with the tumor (Fig. 150-9). After removal of the internal auditory canal portion of the tumor with the vestibular nerves and identification of the facial nerve, superior tumor dissection may be performed by developing the plane between the tumor capsule and the arachnoid superiorly, taking care not to injure the petrosal vein. The facial nerve often becomes difficult to identify at the level of the porus acusticus because the nerve thins over the anterior tumor and because adhesions usually occur at the porus. In some cases, the facial nerve is located superiorly on the tumor. Sometimes, the facial nerve must be identified at the brain stem and followed laterally to establish a plane with the tumor at the porus acusticus. After removal of tumor from the facial nerve, any bulky fragments remaining are removed, leaving the last bit of tumor to be removed from the brain stem (Fig. 150-10).

After the tumor is removed, the wound is irrigated, and bleeding points are controlled with bipolar cautery, clips, or Avitene. Complete hemostasis is necessary and may be time consuming. The facial recess may be opened, the incus removed, and pieces of Surgicel packed into the eustachian tube and muscle in the middle ear to avoid CSF rhinorrhea. The dura may be partially sutured, and abdominal fat strips are placed between the sutures and to obliterate the mastoid cavity. The postauricular incision is closed in layers, and then subcuticular absorbable sutures and Steri-strips are placed. A mastoid pressure dressing is applied.

WILLIAM F. HOUSE
KAREN JO DOYLE

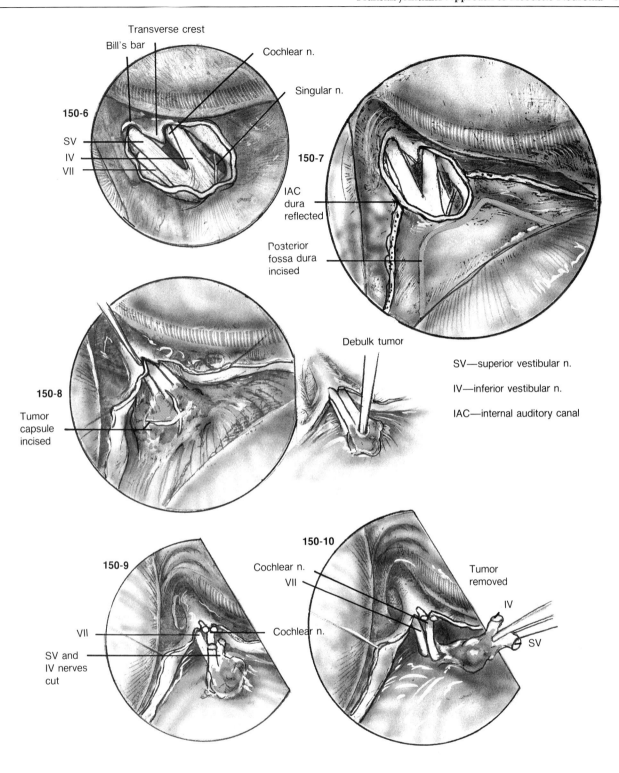

150-6

Transverse crest
Bill's bar
Cochlear n.
Singular n.
SV
IV
VII

150-7

IAC dura reflected

Posterior fossa dura incised

150-8

Tumor capsule incised

Debulk tumor

SV—superior vestibular n.

IV—inferior vestibular n.

IAC—internal auditory canal

150-9

VII
SV and IV nerves cut
Cochlear n.

150-10

Cochlear n.
VII
Cochlear n.
Tumor removed
IV
SV

■ 151. MIDDLE FOSSA RESECTION OF ACOUSTIC NEUROMA—Removal of an acoustic neuroma through a temporal craniotomy with elevation of the temporal lobe and removal of the roof of the internal auditory canal

Indications
1. Acoustic neuromas with no greater than 1.5 cm of extension into the cerebellopontine angle
2. Useful hearing in the involved ear

Contraindications
1. Total hearing loss in the involved ear
2. Tumors with greater than 1.5 cm extension into the cerebellopontine angle

Special Considerations
1. Pure tone and speech hearing level in the involved ear
2. Auditory brain stem response audiometry findings
3. Extension of tumor into the posterior fossa

Preoperative Preparation
1. Positive gadolinium-enhanced magnetic resonance image indicating an acoustic tumor
2. Routine laboratory studies, including studies of bleeding and clotting
3. Auditory brain stem response audiometry
4. Electronystagmography
5. Pure tone and speech hearing tests
6. One unit of autologous blood donation
7. Phisohex shampoo of the scalp
8. Preparation of abdomen for fat harvest
9. Insertion of Foley catheter
10. Insertion of nasogastric tube

Special Instruments, Position, and Anesthesia
1. Operating microscope
2. Intraoperative auditory evoked potential monitoring
3. Continuous intraoperative facial nerve monitoring
4. House-Urban middle fossa retractor
5. Anesthesia without muscle relaxants
6. Shaving of the hemicranium
7. Papaverine for topical application onto tumor bed

(continued)

Operative Procedure
This operation is performed under general endotracheal anesthesia using inhalation agents without muscle paralysis. Diuretics, mannitol, and hyperventilation are used to promote diuresis.

The patient is placed supine on the operating table, with the head turned so that the operated ear is facing up. The surgeon is seated at the head of the table. Hair removal and skin preparation extends almost to the top of the head and far anteriorly and posteriorly. The skin is prepared with Betadine scrub, and self-adhering plastic drapes are applied.

The middle fossa incision begins within the natural hairline, just anterior to the base of the helix, and extends superiorly approximately 10 to 12 cm, curving first posteriorly and then anteriorly (Fig. 151-1). The surgeon often encounters a branch of the superficial temporal artery, which is ligated with nonabsorbable sutures.

The initial incision extends to the level of the temporalis fascia. The temporalis muscle is incised along its insertion and freed from the temporal bone and retracted anteroinferiorly.

A 5 × 5 cm craniotomy opening is made in the squamous portion of the temporal bone two-thirds anterior and one-third posterior to the external auditory canal, near the floor of the middle fossa. A medium cutting bur and continuous suction-irrigation are used. Bone bleeders are commonly encountered and are controlled with bone wax. A joker elevator is used to separate the underlying dura, and the bone flap is removed and placed in normal saline solution during the operation for later replacement.

Dural bleeders are controlled with bipolar cautery. It is important to maintain the integrity of the dura. If a small tear is produced, it should be closed with dural silk suture. After separation of the dura from the edges of the craniotomy defect, the House-Urban retractor is locked firmly in place. The blade of the retractor is then placed, and gentle elevation of the dura from the floor of the middle cranial fossa is begun from posterior to anterior (Fig. 151-2).

The structures within the temporal bone as viewed from above are delineated in Figure 151-3. The first landmark is the middle meningeal artery at the foramen spinosum, which marks the anterior limit of the dural elevation. Venous bleeding in this area is controlled by Surgicel packing. The petrous ridge is identified posteriorly. Care is taken in this area because the petrous ridge is grooved by the superior petrosal sinus. In approximately 5% of cases, the geniculate ganglion is exposed, and care is taken not to damage it. The arcuate eminence is identified. The greater superficial petrosal nerve that passes parallel to the petrous ridge anteriorly from the geniculate ganglion is identified. At this point, the major landmarks of the middle fossa approach have been identified: the middle meningeal artery, the arcuate eminence, and the greater superficial petrosal nerve.

The area of the internal auditory canal and porus acusticus is estimated by dividing the angle formed by the greater superficial petrosal nerve and the arcuate eminence (Fig. 151-4). Bone removal

(continued)

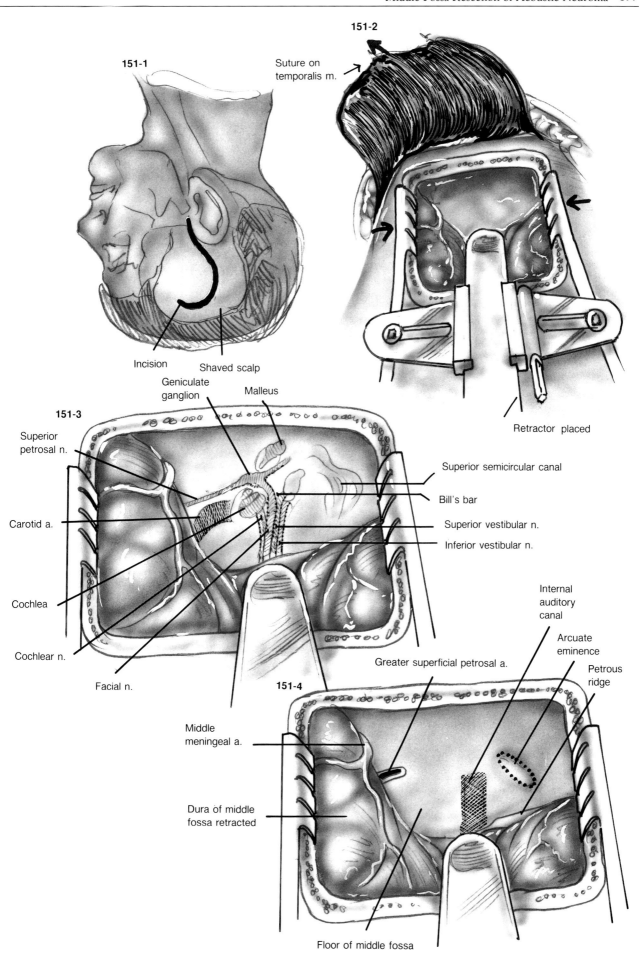

151-1

Incision

Shaved scalp

151-2

Suture on
temporalis m.

Retractor placed

151-3

Geniculate
ganglion

Malleus

Superior
petrosal n.

Superior semicircular canal

Bill's bar

Carotid a.

Superior vestibular n.

Inferior vestibular n.

Cochlea

Cochlear n.

Facial n.

Greater superficial petrosal a.

Internal
auditory
canal

Arcuate
eminence

Petrous
ridge

Middle
meningeal a.

151-4

Dura of middle
fossa retracted

Floor of middle fossa

■ 151. MIDDLE FOSSA RESECTION OF ACOUSTIC NEUROMA *(continued)*

Tips and Pearls

1. Place the craniotomy anteriorly to allow adequate exposure of the internal auditory canal.
2. Use osmotic and loop diuretics and hyperventilation to promote brain shrinkage.
3. Elevate the dura posteriorly to anteriorly to avoid injury to the geniculate ganglion.
4. Begin the dissection medially to avoid injury to the labyrinth or facial nerve.
5. Perform extensive bone removal in the area of the porus acusticus to allow adequate exposure of the cerebellopontine angle.
6. Decompress the labyrinthine segment of the facial nerve and meatal foramen.
7. Separate the tumor from the facial nerve, working in a medial to lateral direction with sharp dissection.
8. Separate the tumor from the cochlear nerve, working in a medial to lateral direction with sharp dissection.
9. Dissect within the arachnoid bed to preserve the blood supply to the cochlea.
10. Tack the dura to the lateral skull to avoid dead space and a postoperative hematoma.

Pitfalls and Complications

1. The dura may be torn while creating the craniotomy bone flap. If this occurs, it must be repaired before insertion of the retractor.
2. The geniculate ganglion may be congenitally exposed and injured during dural elevation.
3. In rare cases, the carotid artery may not be covered by bone and may be injured by rough dural elevation.
4. The labyrinth may be entered if too much bone is removed, particularly in the area of the fundus of the internal auditory canal.
5. The facial nerve may be injured with medial traction on the nerve or tumor.
6. Hearing may be lost by medial traction on the cochlear nerve or interruption of the blood supply to the cochlea.
7. Excessive fat packing may produce pressure on the facial or cochlear nerves.

Postoperative Care Issues

1. The patient is observed in the intensive care unit for 24 to 36 hours, with frequent monitoring of neurologic signs.
2. A nasogastric tube is placed for the first 24 hours.
3. A Foley catheter is placed at surgery and remains for 24 to 36 hours.
4. The head of the bed is elevated to reduce spinal fluid pressure.
5. A mastoid head dressing remains in place for 4 days.
6. Early ambulation is encouraged to promote vestibular compensation.

References

Brackmann DE, Hitselberger WE, Benecke JE, House WF. Acoustic neuromas: middle fossa and translabyrinthine removal. In: Rand RW, ed. Microneurosurgery. St. Louis: CV Mosby, 1985.

Brackmann DE, House JR, Hitselberger WE. Technical modifications to the middle fossa craniotomy approach in removal of acoustic neuromas. Am J Otol 1994;15:614.

is begun at the petrous ridge over this area until the internal auditory canal is located (Fig. 151-5). It is better to err on the side of going anteriorly and medially to locate the canal and to avoid injury to the superior semicircular canal or cochlea.

After the internal auditory canal is located, two thirds of the circumference of the porus acusticus is removed. More room is necessary posteriorly, because the tumor will be rolled out from beneath the facial nerve posteriorly. The superior semicircular canal is skeletonized. The surgeon usually is able to achieve at least 2 cm of exposure in the area of the porus acusticus.

The internal auditory canal is followed laterally. In approaching the fundus, only the superior portion of the canal can be exposed to avoid injury to the ampulated end of the superior semicircular canal and the cochlea. Follow the anterior limit of the internal auditory canal into the labyrinthine segment of the facial nerve. The labyrinthine segment of the facial nerve is then decompressed to the geniculate ganglion. Just posteriorly, the surgeon locates the vertical segment of bone (ie, Bill's bar) that separates the facial nerve from the superior vestibular nerve.

The fine eggshell layer of bone is removed, and the dura is opened along the posterior aspect of the internal auditory canal (Fig. 151-6). The dural flap is carefully elevated from the underlying tumor, and the facial nerve is identified at the lateral end of the internal auditory canal where the vertical crest of bone (ie, Bill's bar) allows positive identification.

The principle of the tumor removal is that the tumor is freed from the facial nerve and the cochlear nerve and is delivered posteriorly out from under the facial nerve. The tumor is first separated from the facial nerve by working in a medial to lateral direction. Medial to lateral dissection is necessary to avoid traction on the facial nerve where it is fixed at the labyrinthine segment (Fig. 151-7). Continuous intraoperative facial nerve monitoring greatly facilitates this dissection.

In the past, surgeons routinely avulsed the superior vestibular nerve from the fundus of the internal auditory canal. In the modern approach, surgeons leave any uninvolved nerves in place to preserve blood supply to the cochlea. The principle is to free the tumor from the arachnoid bed, always working in a medial to lateral direction to avoid tension on the cochlear nerve as it enters the cochlea. For all but the smallest tumors, a partial debulking of the tumor is performed with cup forceps. When the tumor is reduced in size, the final fragments are sharply dissected from the cochlear nerve.

After total tumor removal, the tumor bed is irrigated profusely (Fig. 151-8). Gelfoam pledgets saturated with Papaverine solution are then placed into the tumor bed to promote vasodilation.

Closure of the defect in the internal auditory canal is accomplished with a free graft of abdominal fat. The dura is tacked to the lateral skull, the temporal bone flap replaced, and the temporalis muscle resutured to its insertion. The subcutaneous tissue and skin are closed in layers over a Penrose drain, and a sterile dressing is applied.

Surgical Variations

Dr. William House originally described locating the internal auditory canal by following the greater superficial petrosal nerve to the geniculate ganglion and then the labyrinthine segment of the facial nerve into the internal auditory canal. I prefer the technique described previously.

The temporal craniotomy may be performed using a high-speed drill with a footplate attachment.

DERALD E. BRACKMANN

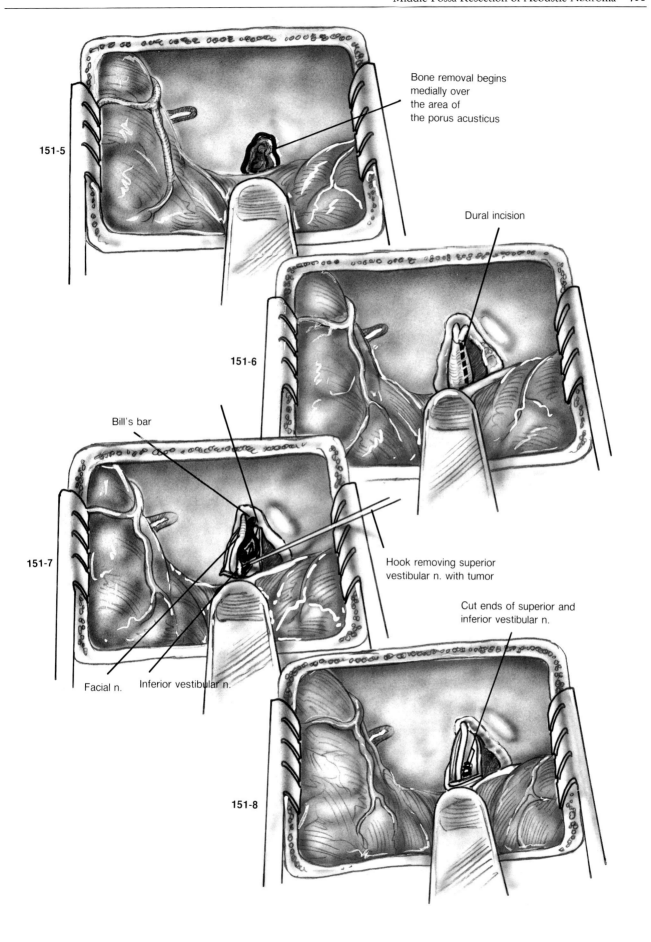

151-5

Bone removal begins
medially over
the area of
the porus acusticus

Dural incision

151-6

Bill's bar

151-7

Hook removing superior
vestibular n. with tumor

Facial n.   Inferior vestibular n.

Cut ends of superior and
inferior vestibular n.

151-8

■ *152.* ACOUSTIC NEUROMA RESECTION (RETROSIGMOID APPROACH)—This is a variant on the traditional neurosurgical suboccipital approach. The differences are

1. Conventional otologic position
2. A small inverted U retroauricular incision
3. No incision or elevation of the nuchal muscles
4. Partial mastoidectomy
5. Small (2.5-cm) bone plug craniotomy bordered anteriorly by the sigmoid sinus and superiorly by the transverse sinus
6. No cerebellar retraction
7. Drilling of posterior internal auditory canal wall to expose lateral extent of tumor
8. Preservation of cochlear nerve
9. Watertight dural closure with a temporalis fascia graft
10. Replacement of a bone plug
11. Obliteration of the mastoid cavity with abdominal fat

Indications
1. Tumor extending no farther than 15 to 20 mm from the porus acusticus
2. Serviceable hearing (ie, pure tone average of 50 dB and speech discrimination score 50% or better)
3. Reasonable anesthesia risk

Contraindications
1. Tumor larger than 2 cm in diameter
2. Nonserviceable hearing
3. Evidence of invasion of labyrinth by tumor

Special Considerations
1. Level of hearing in contralateral ear
2. Presence of tumor in contralateral ear
3. Patient's occupation (possible safety factor of binaural hearing even with poor discrimination)

Preoperative Preparation
1. Routine laboratory studies
2. Magnetic resonance imaging (MRI) with gadolinium
3. Careful recent pure tone and speech audiogram
4. High-resolution computed tomography scan of the temporal bone without contrast to visualize temporal bone anatomy (optional)

Special Instruments, Position, and Anesthesia
1. Supine otologic position with head rotated and raised
2. Facial nerve monitor
3. Ultrasonic aspirator if the tumor extends 15 mm extracanalicularly
4. Bipolar cautery forceps
5. Tympanoplasty-type dissectors, preferably with long handles

Tips and Pearls
1. Make the flap large enough so that both the craniectomy and the mastoidectomy are accessible.
2. Drill bone completely around 270° of sigmoid sinus to allow retraction.
3. Incise dura so that sigmoid sinus is compressed by dural flap.
4. Protect the cerebellum with a latex strip or Teflon drain.
5. Pack with Gelfoam above and below the tumor to prevent blood and bone dust from entering the cisterns.

(continued)

Operative Procedure

The patient is placed in the conventional otologic position, with the head rotated away from the ipsilateral ear. The table is flexed so that the head is elevated above the heart. General anesthesia is used, with paralysis avoided. A second-generation cephalosporin is used for perioperative prophylaxis. If experience shows that the surgery will take more than 4 hours, a Foley catheter is placed. Preoperatively, the patient donates 1 unit of blood to make cryoprecipitate for autologous fibrin glue production. The red cells may be used if required.

An inverted U-shaped incision is outlined and infiltrated with 1:200,000 epinephrine, followed by an incision with the cautery knife. The incision begins at the mastoid tip, extends in the postauricular crease to the upper edge of the auricle, continues 5 cm posteriorly, and finally runs inferiorly, more or less parallel to the postauricular segment (Fig. 152-1).

The incision is made in stepwise fashion, first cutting through skin into subcutaneous tissue and then extending forward approximately 1 cm to incise down to bone. This stepped incision helps to avoid a CSF leak from the wound.

The flap is then elevated off the temporalis fascia and the bone, ending at the external auditory canal. Care is taken not to incise the nuchal muscles inferiorly or the temporalis muscle superiorly.

A self-retaining retractor or barbless fishhooks are used to hold the flap inferiorly, and a large temporalis fascia graft is taken.

A partial mastoidectomy is then carried out, exposing the sigmoid sinus. The bone is drilled off the entire length of the sigmoid sinus, from anterior to posterior aspects, exposing 270°. No bony island is created. It is unnecessary to do a complete mastoidectomy. A 2.5- to 3-cm bone plug is removed after elevation of the dura using the Midas-Rex drill; the bone is preserved for replacement, and holes are drilled in the plug and the adjacent skull (Fig. 152-2).

The dura is incised, creating an anteriorly based dural flap that is sutured tightly over the sigmoid sinus, compressing it (Fig. 152-3). If there is bulging of the cerebellum, the head is elevated further. Mannitol is not used. By gently compressing the cerebellum, CSF can be released, resulting in decompression of the cerebellum. The cerebellum is then covered with a thin sheet of latex rubber (eg, split Penrose drain), and the posterior face of the petrous bone and any extracanalicular tumor are exposed (Fig. 152-4A). A cottonoid electrode is placed in contact with the undersurface, with cranial nerve VIII in the posterior fossa, to monitor the CAP. This is much more accurate than the auditory brainstem response (ABR). Gelfoam is packed above and below the tumor and VIIIth nerve, and a dural flap is then incised, based superiorly or inferiorly, exposing the posterior wall of the internal auditory canal (see Fig. 152-4B and C). The flap is based opposite the surgeon's dominant hand (ie, right-handed surgeon operating on a right ear would create a superiorly based flap). Using a cutting bur, the posterior wall is drilled approximately 7 mm, until the tumor in the internal auditory canal can be seen through the intact dura (Fig. 152-5). Smaller cutting burs and diamond burs are then used to outline at least 180° of the internal auditory canal over a length of at least 7 mm. If the tumor clearly does not extend for 7 mm, less bone is removed.

After all bone has been removed, the dura is incised, exposing the intracanalicular portion of the tumor. Dissection begins medially, attempting to establish a plane between the tumor and the cochlear division of the VIIIth nerve. The cochlear portion is inferior in the cerebellopontine angle and then rotates anteriorly within the internal

(continued)

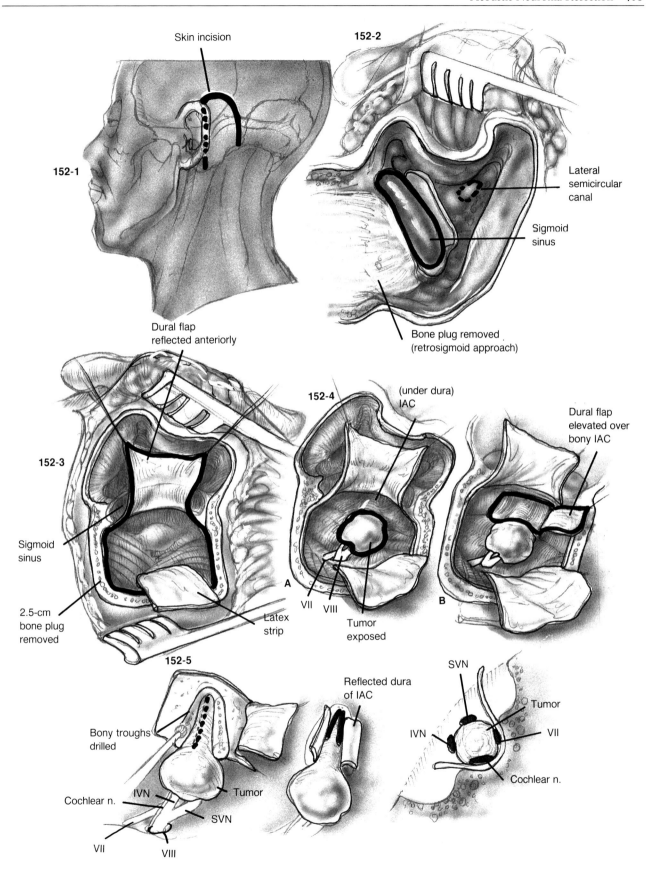

Skin incision

152-1

152-2

Lateral semicircular canal

Sigmoid sinus

Bone plug removed (retrosigmoid approach)

Dural flap reflected anteriorly

152-3

(under dura) IAC

152-4

Dural flap elevated over bony IAC

Sigmoid sinus

2.5-cm bone plug removed

Latex strip

A

VII VIII

Tumor exposed

B

152-5

SVN

Reflected dura of IAC

Tumor

Bony troughs drilled

IVN

VII

Cochlear n.

IVN

Tumor

VII

Cochlear n.

SVN

VII

VIII

■ *152.* ACOUSTIC NEUROMA RESECTION (RETROSIGMOID APPROACH) *(continued)*

6. Monitor the compound action potential (CAP) of the cochlear portion of cranial nerve VIII.
7. Drill at least 180° of internal auditory canal to the lateral end of the tumor, if not the lateral end of the canal.
8. Determine the feasibility of dissecting a plane between the tumor and the cochlear nerve medially.
9. Dissect medial to lateral and lateral to medial aspects as needed.
10. Stop dissection and add papaverine on Gelfoam if the CAP changes.
11. Avoid cautery when possible.
12. Total tumor removal is the primary goal. Hearing preservation is secondary.
13. Preserve one or both vestibular nerves if possible.
14. After tumor removal, wax petrosal air cells and fill bone defect with soft tissue.
15. Secure soft tissue with fibrin glue and a dural flap.

Pitfalls and Complications

1. Avoid injury to the sigmoid or transverse sinus. If nicked, a clip or fine suture stops the bleeding.
2. Avoid trauma to cerebellum by protecting it with rubber strip drain at all times. Retraction is not necessary.
3. Avoid trauma to the anterior and posterior inferior cerebellar arteries and to the cranial nerves.
4. Dissection of tumor on facial nerve should proceed as in other acoustic neuroma surgery.
5. Drill sufficient bone so that the lateral end of the tumor can be clearly visualized. Avoid piecemeal dissection of the tumor.
6. If the CAP is lost and dissection proceeds smoothly, continue, because hearing may still be preserved.
7. A high-riding jugular bulb may make this surgery more difficult.
8. If drilling more than 7 mm from the porus is required, watch for an opening into the labyrinth.
9. If the labyrinth is opened, do not suction, but wax immediately.
10. A cerebrospinal fluid (CSF) leak should be treated with 3 to 5 days of spinal drainage. Surgery is rarely necessary.
11. If the CSF leak persists after drainage, a craniotomy is never necessary; the leak can be stopped by reopening the mastoidectomy, drilling down to posterior fossa plate, and obliterating the defect with fascia and fat.

Postoperative Care Issues

1. Routine CSF drainage is not used postoperatively.
2. Perioperative antibiotic coverage (eg, second-generation cephalosporin) is used for 24 hours.
3. The bed remains in a 30° elevated position, and the patient has a firm mastoid dressing for 48 to 72 hours.
4. The patient should avoid bending, straining, and nose blowing.
5. Perioperative steroids are used if there has been manipulation of cerebellum or difficult dissection of cranial nerve VII.
6. Postoperative audiogram as soon as patient is able to be moved to a soundproof booth
7. Postoperative MRI in 3 months, and annually thereafter for 5 years

References

Cohen NL. Retrosigmoid approach for acoustic tumor removal. Otolaryngol Clin North Am 1992;25:295.

Jackler RK, Pitts LH. Selection of surgical approach to acoustic neuroma. Otolaryngol Clin North Am 1992;25:361.

auditory canal. Dissection then proceeds from the medial to lateral aspect, until most of the tumor has been freed. The ultrasonic aspirator is used on tumors larger than 1.5 cm in diameter (Fig. 152-6*A*).

Attention is turned to the lateral end of the tumor. If this can be visualized, the tumor is dissected off the cochlear and facial nerves under direct vision (see Fig. 152-6*B*). If the tumor extends past the area of bone removal but can be cleanly retracted into the open internal auditory canal, it is often unnecessary to remove additional bone, because the tumor arises in the medial portion of the internal auditory canal and is bound laterally only by the vestibular nerves. These are cut selectively to free the lateral end of the tumor, but they should be spared if possible.

It is usually possible to dissect the tumor cleanly off the facial and cochlear nerves and remove an intracanalicular or small extracanalicular tumor in one piece. Piecemeal dissection, especially laterally in the internal auditory canal, should be avoided. If you cannot see the clean, rounded lateral end of the tumor, remove more bone. Do not use mirrors or blind dissection.

In the case of a larger extracanalicular tumor, it may be necessary to debulk the tumor in the angle to facilitate dissection out of the internal auditory canal; we generally use the ultrasonic aspirator. Cautery should be minimized, because the most common cause of loss of hearing is probably interruption of blood supply to the cochlea or cranial nerve VIII.

If the CAP Vth wave is delayed or decreased in amplitude, stop dissection, and add Gelfoam or a cottonoid soaked in papaverine. Wait a few minutes, and then begin dissection again, preferably in another area. If the CAP does not stabilize or return after a few minutes, continue dissection.

After all tumor is removed, Gelfoam with papaverine is placed on the cochlear nerve, any visible petrosal air cells are waxed, and a free muscle graft is placed into the bony drill-out and glued in place with fibrin glue (see Fig. 152-6*C*).

The dural flap is then sutured with silk or nylon (see Fig. 152-6*D*). All blood and debris are removed from the posterior fossa, the cerebellum is checked for bleeding, and the cerebellar protection removed. A watertight dural closure is performed, using the temporalis fascia graft for reinforcement (Fig. 152-7*A*). The bone plug is replaced and sutured with heavy nylon or stainless steel. Abdominal fat is used to obliterate the mastoid cavity (see Fig. 152-7*B*).

The incision is closed in layers using Vicryl and a running nylon suture or stainless steel staples (Fig. 152-8). A mastoid dressing is placed, and the patient sent to the recovery room in the 30° head-elevated position.

Surgical Variations

If the tumor extends into the vestibule, no attempt should be made to preserve hearing; the tumor must be totally excised. Similarly, if a clean plane cannot be established between the cochlear nerve and the tumor, the cochlear nerve should be taken to achieve total tumor removal. However, if the CAP is lost, and there is a good plane of dissection, preserve the cochlear nerve, because hearing may still be preserved. If the extracanalicular portion of the tumor is 15 to 20 mm, the ultrasonic aspirator may be used to debulk that portion before removing the remainder of the tumor.

Some surgeons may prefer this approach for all tumors, regardless of size and level of hearing. I use this approach for hearing preservation and the translabyrinthine approach for all other cases.

NOEL COHEN

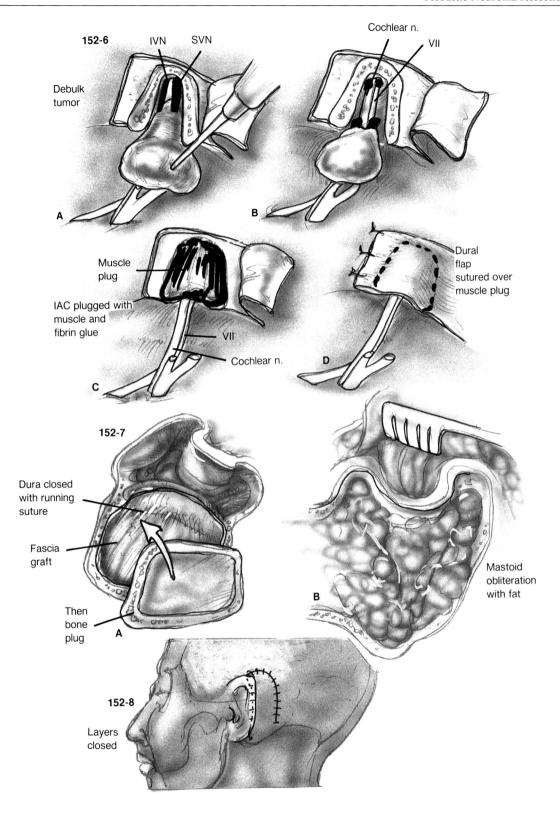

152-6   IVN   SVN   Cochlear n.   VII

Debulk
tumor

A   B

Muscle
plug

IAC plugged with
muscle and
fibrin glue

VII

Cochlear n.

C   D

Dural
flap
sutured over
muscle plug

152-7

Dura closed
with running
suture

Fascia
graft

Then
bone
plug   A

B   Mastoid
obliteration
with fat

152-8

Layers
closed

■ 153. EXTENSIVE GLOMUS TUMOR EXCISION

SION—Arising from the jugulotympanic paraganglia, glomus jugulare is predominantly a benign skull base neoplasm that derives morbidity from cranial nerve involvement and intracranial extension. Extensive resection differentiates glomus jugulare removal from the more limited excision of the glomus tympanicum lesion.

Indications

1. Imaging confirmation of a jugular foramen lesion, the growth characteristics of which have resulted or are expected to result in morbidity in the natural course of the patient's remaining years
2. Intracranial extension threatening neuraxial compression or intracranial pressure consequences
3. Progressive cranial neuropathies
4. Paraneoplastic syndromes
5. Aural bleeding
6. Progressive hearing loss or pulsatile tinnitus

Contraindications

1. If the lesion is not expected to result in morbidity during the natural course of the patient's remaining years (eg, patients older than 70 years of age)
2. Medical incapacity
3. Complicating factors associated with tumor multicentricity

Special Considerations

1. Associated lesions and paraneoplastic syndromes
2. Intracranial arterial and venous circulation
3. Intracranial extension
4. The facial nerve
5. Hemostasis
6. Conservation surgery
7. Defect reconstruction
8. Complication prophylaxis

Preoperative Preparation

1. Precise determination of the lesion type and extent
2. Identify tumor multicentricity.
3. Catecholamine secretion
4. Evaluate major vessel involvement and collateral intracranial circulation.
5. Identify the intracranial extension.
6. Comprehensive medical evaluation
7. Autologous blood donation
8. Multidisciplinary planning congress

Special Instruments, Position, and Anesthesia

1. Supine position, with the head turned and the involved side up
2. The operative site, including the hemihead, ear, and neck, is prepped, as are potential donor sites.
3. Facial nerve, electroencephalographic, cardiopulmonary (invasive) monitoring
4. Sequential compression stockings
5. Durable, powerful, reliable, rapid bone dissection drill
6. Anesthesia
   a. Maintain hemodynamic stability.
   b. Prevent intracranial pressure elevation.
   c. Maintain cerebral perfusion and oxygenation.
   d. Replace blood loss, and prevent and treat coagulopathies.

Tips and Pearls

1. Conservation surgery: increasing invasiveness as dictated by the extent of disease as the case evolves
2. Proximal and distal control of the internal carotid artery and lateral venous sinus
3. Facial nerve monitoring requires minimal manipulation and preservation of the vascular supply at the stylomastoid foramen.
4. Hemostasis by tumor isolation
5. Controlled dissection at the pars nervosa

(continued)

Operative Procedure

An approach that conserves the extended auditory canal and auditory mechanism is preferred for tumors limited to the infralabyrinthine chamber and jugular foramen, involving only the tympanic segment of internal carotid artery.

A C-shaped incision creates an anteriorly based flap (Fig. 153-1). The temporal muscle, the mastoid, and the neck anatomy are exposed. Proximal internal carotid artery and distal internal jugular vein control is established. A complete mastoidectomy, mastoid tip removal, and extended facial recess are performed (Fig. 153-2). Anterosuperior control of the tumor and distal internal carotid artery control are achieved by inferior tympanic bone removal and extended auditory canal skeletonization to expose the proximal ET (Fig. 153-3). The internal jugular vein is ligated, and the lateral venous sinus is packed intraluminally. The facial nerve is mobilized from its fallopian canal from the external genu to the face (short) to expose the jugular foramen. Skull base dissection in the infralabyrinthine chamber and posteroinferior to jugular foramen isolates the posteroinferior tumor margin. With proximal and distal internal carotid artery control, the tumor is dissected from internal carotid artery (Fig. 153-4). Once debulked and under direct vision, the tumor is resected from the jugular and hypoglossal foramina.

For larger tumors requiring distal control of the internal carotid artery in the petrous portion, the extended auditory canal and conductive hearing mechanism are sacrificed in the infratemporal fossa approach. The extended auditory canal is transected and oversewn. The bony extended auditory canal is removed with the tympanic membrane and middle ear contents lateral to the stapes. To permit anterior and inferior displacement of the mandible to access the internal carotid artery, the facial nerve is mobilized from the internal genu distally (long; Fig. 153-5). With distal control of the petrous internal carotid artery, tumor removal precedes as before (Fig. 153-6).

(continued)

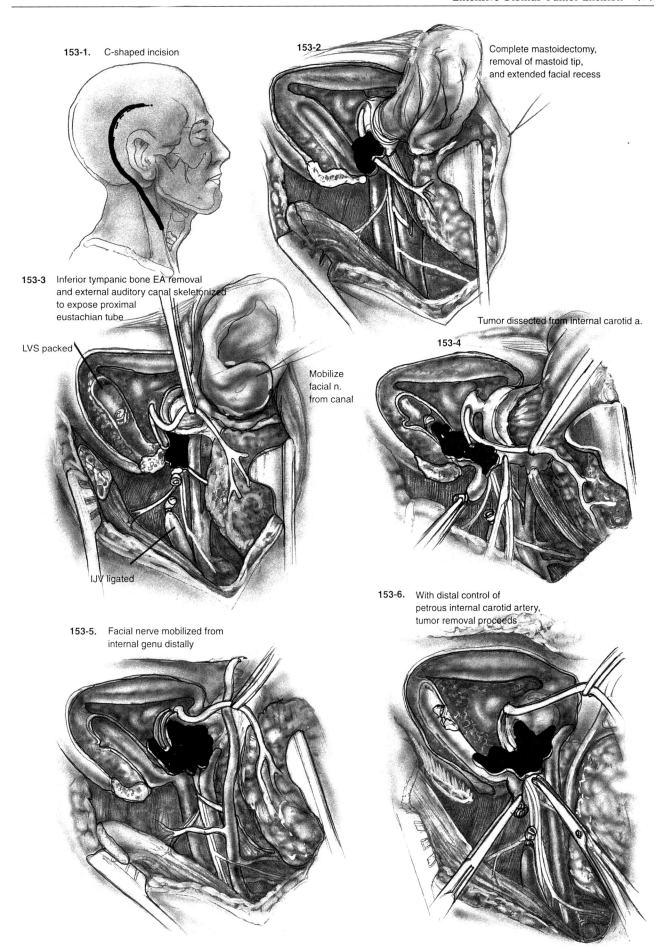

153-1.   C-shaped incision

153-2   Complete mastoidectomy, removal of mastoid tip, and extended facial recess

153-3   Inferior tympanic bone EA removal and external auditory canal skeletonized to expose proximal eustachian tube

LVS packed

Mobilize facial n. from canal

IJV ligated

Tumor dissected from internal carotid a.

153-4

153-5.   Facial nerve mobilized from internal genu distally

153-6.   With distal control of petrous internal carotid artery, tumor removal proceeds

■ *153.* EXTENSIVE GLOMUS TUMOR EXCISION *(continued)*

6. Single-stage resection of the tumor and intracranial extension
7. Vascularized defect reconstruction
8. Reconstruction that exceeds the apparent need in irradiated fields
9. Avoid tracheostomy; phonosurgery is unstaged.
10. Preoperative facial paralysis is not salvageable.
11. Revascularize sacrificed internal carotid arteries.
12. Do not sacrifice multiple cranial nerves in elderly patients.
13. Do not sacrifice both vagi.
14. Operate the life-threatening lesion first.
15. Neurotologic skull base surgery requires a multispecialty team approach.

Pitfalls and Complications

1. Unsuspected synchronous lesions foil planning.
2. Unsuspected catecholamine secretion is an anesthetic risk.
3. A grossly involved cranial nerve VII with no facial palsy is salvageable.
4. Labyrinthine invasion is not reliably detected on imaging.
5. Poor hemostasis produces complications.
6. Failure to achieve distal internal carotid artery control courts disaster.
7. Negative preoperative intraluminal test balloon occlusion does not warrant complication free internal carotid artery sacrifice.
8. Transection of the extended auditory canal transection causes stenosis.
9. Irradiation produces complications; vascularize everything.
10. Nonautologous blood may cause complications.
11. Tumor manipulation can release catecholamines and cause vital parameter instability.
12. Tumor manipulation at the pars nervosa or carotid body can cause profound bradycardia.
13. Embolization has the potential for causing complications with little benefit.
14. Tracheostomy carries the risk of complications and late glottic competency the risk of aspiration.
15. Abort the procedure if irreversible internal carotid artery spasm occurs.
16. Cover lumbar drains with prophylactic antibiotics.
17. Alpha- and beta-blockaded secretors risk deep venous thrombosis and pulmonary embolus.
18. All nerves sacrificed in elderly patients mean long-term functional dependence.
19. Ipsilateral or contralateral subclavian or internal jugular vein lines court venous disaster.

Postoperative Care Issues

1. Smooth, rapid emergence from general anesthesia to achieve neurologic baseline
2. Invasive monitoring can be performed in the neurologic intensive care unit, but postoperative lability is uncommon.
3. Slow refeeding and gastrointestinal decompression because of gastrointestinal atony.
4. Ensure early glottic competency.
5. Ensure a positive nitrogen balance.
6. Eye care
7. Delay cosmetic corrections.
8. Surveillance imaging at 1 year, 5 years, and then at 5-year intervals

References

Jackson CG, Netterville JL, Glasscock ME, et al. Defect reconstruction and cerebrospinal fluid management in neurotologic skull base tumors with intracranial extension. Laryngoscope 1992;102:1205.

Jackson CG, Poe DS, Johnson GD. Lateral transtemporal approaches to the skull base. In: Jackson CJ, ed. Surgery of skull base tumors. New York: Churchill Livingstone, 1991:141.

When extreme circumstances require distal petrous internal carotid artery or tumor margin control, the infratemporal fossa exposure can be extended. By reflecting the temporal muscle and zygoma inferiorly with extreme mandibular dislocation, the anatomy of the infratemporal fossa to the cavernous sinus can be accessed (Fig. 153-7). These exposure requirements are extreme (Fig. 153-8). The internal carotid artery can be traced to the cavernous sinus siphon. The foramen spinosum and its contents, with the eustachian tube, are sacrificed (Fig. 153-9). Cranial nerve V and the middle fossa are accessible (Fig. 153-10). The mandibular condyle and zygoma can be removed as a unit and replated to preserve joint integrity. The transcochlear approach is readily available in the event of anterior and medial tumor extension.

The management of an intracranial extension is not staged. Posterior fossa craniotomy is expedient for tumor removal (Fig. 153-11) and follows mechanics similar to those of a combined approach for acoustic neuroma removal. Wide intracranial exposures are possible (Fig. 153-12). For the unstaged removal of an intracranial extension, the surgical sequence is exposure; tumor dissection from the internal carotid artery; debulking the tumor down to dura; craniotomy and removal of the intracranial extension; and defect reconstruction.

Reconstruction of the defect depends on its size. Most glomus tumor resection defects are small or medium sized (Fig. 153-13). Basic principles include vascularized fascia reconstruction augmented by viable tissue bulk and supported by cerebrospinal fluid decompression by a lumbar drain. Vascularized free flaps are used in previously irradiated beds, even for small defects. Vascularized fascia is provided by the pericranium.

Immediate glottic competency is achieved by unstaged Silastic medialization of the vocal cord. Tracheostomy is avoided.

C. GARY JACKSON

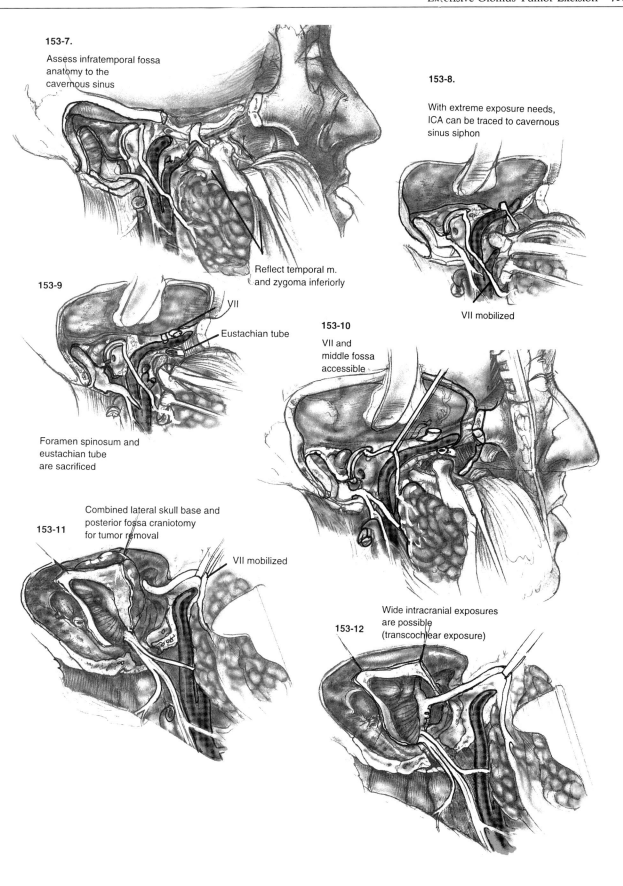

153-7.

Assess infratemporal fossa anatomy to the cavernous sinus

Reflect temporal m. and zygoma inferiorly

153-8.

With extreme exposure needs, ICA can be traced to cavernous sinus siphon

VII mobilized

153-9

VII

Eustachian tube

Foramen spinosum and eustachian tube are sacrificed

153-10

VII and middle fossa accessible

153-11

Combined lateral skull base and posterior fossa craniotomy for tumor removal

VII mobilized

153-12

Wide intracranial exposures are possible (transcochlear exposure)

■ 154. EXTREME LATERAL TRANSCONDY-LAR APPROACH—Enhanced exposure of the lower posterior cranial base to the midline through mobilization of the vertebral artery, removal of a portion of the transverse process of the first cervical vertebra, and a partial or total occipital condylectomy

Indications

1. Transcranial schwannomas of the glossopharyngeal, vagus, accessory, and hypoglossal nerves
2. Tumors of the inferior clivus and foramen magnum, such as meningiomas, neurofibromas, chordomas, chondromas, and chondrosarcomas
3. Medially based jugular foramen paragangliomas
4. Vertebral artery aneurysms

Special Considerations

1. Midline or contralateral and anterior tumor extension
2. Preexisting cranial neuropathies
3. Degree of involvement of the vertebral and basilar arteries
4. Extension of the tumor anteromedial to the carotid canal
5. Configuration and patency of the venous sinuses
6. Stability of the craniovertebral junction
7. Prior surgical or radiation therapy

Preoperative Preparation

1. Thorough history and physical examination, including a neurologic assessment of the caudal cranial nerves
2. Combined high-resolution computed tomography (CT) and magnetic resonance imaging (MRI) of the posterior cranial fossa and upper cervical spine
3. Four-vessel carotidovertebral angiography, with attention to the venous phase
4. Complete metastatic survey if the primary tumor is malignant.

Special Instruments, Position, and Anesthesia

1. Electrophysiologic monitoring of multiple modalities: somatosensory evoked responses, brain stem auditory responses, and spontaneous and evoked electromyographic activity from muscles innervated by cranial nerves VII and IX through XII
2. General anesthesia with no muscle relaxants
3. Supine position, with the head in a three-point headrest
4. Head of the operating table rotated 180° from the anesthesia station
5. Operating microscope
6. High-speed gas and electric drill systems
7. Microsurgical instruments for intracranial dissection
8. Plating instrumentation for stabilizing the craniocervical junction

(continued)

Operative Procedure

The patient is placed in the supine position, with the head fixed in a three-point headrest. The operating table is rotated 180° from the anesthesia station. The lateral aspect of the head, ear, and neck to the midline, the ipsilateral lower abdominal quadrant, and the ipsilateral iliac crest area are isolated and prepared in the standard fashion. Stimulus and response leads for electrophysiologic monitoring are placed before the final draping of the patient.

The incision is made at least 2 cm posterior to the mastoid eminence and extends inferiorly in a skin crease 3 to 4 cm below the angle of the mandible to end at the greater cornu of the hyoid bone. The cephalic portion of the incision extends at least 4 cm superior to the helical attachment. A separate curvilinear incision extending posteriorly from the nuchal line to the midportion of the postauricular part of the primary incision is outlined in the event that craniocervical fusion is subsequently required (Fig. 154-1).

To minimize bleeding and inadvertent injury to underlying neurovascular structures, the cervicofacial dissection is performed in well-defined layers. The sternocleidomastoid and splenius capitis muscles are exposed, detached from their cranial insertions, and reflected inferiorly. The jugular vein, internal carotid artery, and cranial nerves IX through XII are identified and mobilized as far cephalad as possible. The extratemporal portion of the facial nerve proximal to the pes anserinus is exposed through a parotidotomy or parotidectomy. The longissimus capitis muscle and posterior belly of the digastric muscle are detached from their insertion along the mastoid process and reflected caudally. The vertebral artery is initially identified by carefully dividing the superior capitis oblique muscle at its origin along the easily palpable transverse process of the atlas and reflecting it superiorly (Fig. 154-2). The vertebroarterial foramen is completely opened by drill curettage or with a rongeur. The vertebral artery is then mobilized to the level of its dural entry. Bleeding from the rich venous plexus that surrounds the artery is controlled with bipolar cauterization or conservative packing with Surgicel.

The amount of bone removal depends on the caudal, rostral, and anterior extent and histology of the tumor. Lesions with an epicenter at the level of the foramen magnum can be accessed through a standard retrosigmoid craniectomy bordering the sigmoid and transverse sinuses, combined with the removal of occipital bone to the foramen magnum and a part or all of the occipital condyle.

(continued)

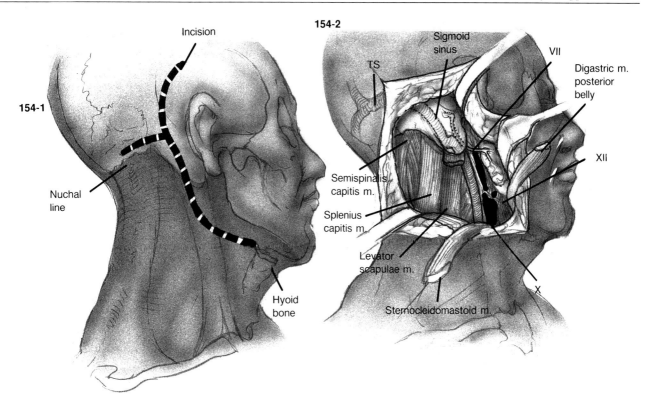

154-1

Incision

Nuchal line

Hyoid bone

154-2

Sigmoid sinus

TS

VII

Digastric m. posterior belly

XII

Semispinalis capitis m.

Splenius capitis m.

Levator scapulae m.

Sternocleidomastoid m.

X

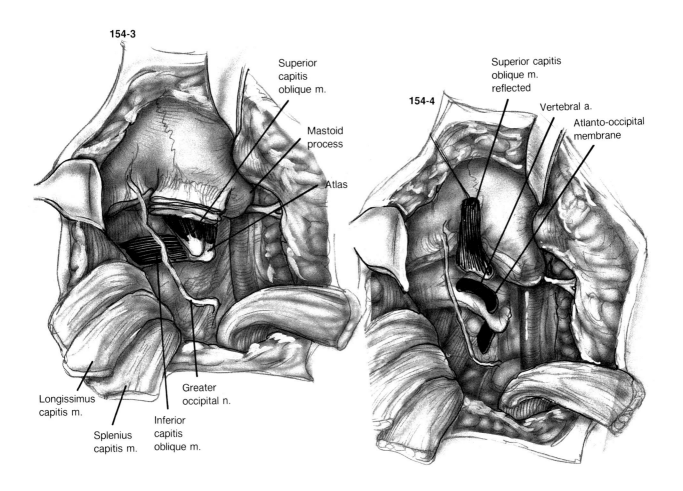

154-3

Superior capitis oblique m.

Mastoid process

Atlas

Longissimus capitis m.

Splenius capitis m.

Inferior capitis oblique m.

Greater occipital n.

154-4

Superior capitis oblique m. reflected

Vertebral a.

Atlanto-occipital membrane

■ *154.* EXTREME LATERAL TRANSCONDY-LAR APPROACH *(continued)*

Tips and Pearls

1. Tailor the degree of bone removal to the extent of disease.
2. Minimize injury to the prominent vertebral venous plexus.
3. Minimize cerebellar retraction.
4. Skeletonize the sigmoid sinus and jugular bulb to maximize exposure and prevent injury.
5. Fuse the craniocervical junction when the occipital condyle is completely removed.
6. Use a lumbar-subarachnoid drain for at least 4 days postoperatively to minimize the potential for a cerebrospinal fluid leak if dural integrity is questionable.
7. Consider a primary laryngoplasty, with or without a tracheotomy and percutaneous gastrostomy, if there is electrophysiologic evidence of irreversible injury to cranial nerves IX and X.
8. Minimize longitudinal vascular retraction, and use papaverine to minimize arterial spasm.
9. Use a team approach with overlapping responsibilities.

Pitfalls and Complications

1. New-onset cranial or spinal neuropathy
2. Craniocervical instability
3. Brain stem infarct
4. Postoperative bleeding
5. Postoperative cerebellar edema
6. Cerebrospinal fluid leak

Postoperative Care Issues

1. Intensive care monitoring of the patient until airway protection from aspiration is confirmed
2. If fusion of the craniovertebral junction is required, the patient should be immobilized in a hard collar or halo, depending on the stability rendered by the fusion.
3. Application of sequential compression stockings and early ambulation, with no chair sitting, to minimize the potential for deep venous thrombosis
4. Baseline postoperative high-resolution CT and MRI before the patient is discharged for future comparison

References

Canalis RF, Martin N, Black K, et al. Lateral approach to tumors of the craniovertebral junction. Laryngoscope 1993;103:343.

Sen CN, Sekhar LN. An extreme lateral approach to intradural lesions of the cervical spine and foramen magnum. Neurosurgery 1990;27: 197.

Optimal exposure of benign tumors that originate in the cerebellopontine angle and extend to or through the foramen magnum is achieved by combining the previously described craniectomy with an extended canal wall–up mastoidectomy, which includes identification of the vertical portion of the facial nerve canal and removal of bone over the sigmoid sinus and posterior cranial fossa dura to the posterior semicircular canal by drill curettage (Fig. 154-3). Removal of malignant lesions in this region requires additional anterolateral exposure, which can be obtained with a conventional infratemporal fossa approach.

A curvilinear durotomy extending from the junction of the transverse and sigmoid sinuses to the dural entry of the vertebral artery is performed. The dural margins are tethered to adjacent subcutaneous tissue. This allows sufficient mobilization of the vertebral artery during the remainder of the dissection. Additional anterior exposure of transcranial lesions at this level can be gained through removal of bone constituting the floor of the jugular fossa to the level of the hypoglossal canal by drill curettage. The relative positions of the glossopharyngeal, vagus, and the accessory nerves should continuously be kept in view during this portion of the dissection to avoid injuring these nerves. Further anterior exposure requires the identification and mobilization of the petrous part of the internal carotid artery, which is best performed through a different approach. After adequate exposure of the underlying tumor has been obtained, the lesion is removed by following standard microneurosurgical and oncologic principles (Figs. 154-4 and 154-5).

After tumor resection, the durotomy is closed as tightly as possible. Significant dural defects are repaired with fascial grafts. If a total occipital condylectomy has been performed, the craniovertebral junction is stabilized through the placement of a titanium plate between the occiput and decorticated laminae of C1 and C2, layered by bone from the iliac crest (Fig. 154-6). The epidural dead space and a surgically created mastoid cavity are obliterated with an abdominal fat graft. The overlying soft tissue is closed in multiple layers, and a compressive dressing is applied for 4 days. A lumbar-subarachnoid drain is inserted for 4 days if there is concern about dural integrity.

PETER G. SMITH
G. ROBERT KLETZKER
ROBERT J. BACKER

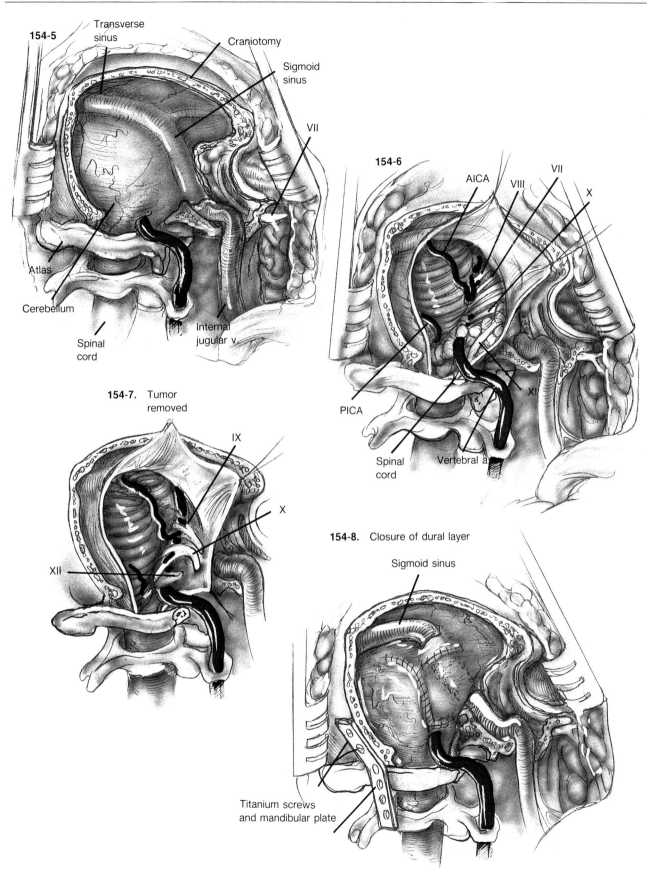

154-5

Transverse sinus

Craniotomy

Sigmoid sinus

VII

Atlas

Cerebellum

Spinal cord

Internal jugular v.

154-6

AICA

VIII

VII

X

XI

PICA

Spinal cord

Vertebral a.

154-7.   Tumor removed

IX

X

XII

154-8.   Closure of dural layer

Sigmoid sinus

Titanium screws and mandibular plate

■ 155. ACCESS TO THE NASOPHARYNX

The preauricular infratemporal middle fossa approach to the skull base for nasopharyngeal resection provides the most comprehensive anatomic exposure, preserves hearing and facial nerve function, provides low middle fossa exposure to minimize the need for brain retraction, and allows control of the carotid artery. Adequate exposure is provided for complete nasopharyngeal resection and for reconstruction with a free flap, if necessary. Extensions to the anterior or posterior cranial cavities are easily included, as are transfacial or transoral approaches.

Indications

1. Extensive benign disease and malignancy involving the nasopharynx, infratemporal fossa, or clivus
2. Malignant disease extending into the nasopharynx from the nose, paranasal sinuses, pharynx, or orbit
3. Tumors may extend bilaterally or into the nose or paranasal sinuses and may have bilateral nasopharyngeal involvement.
4. Simultaneous bilateral petrous carotid dissection and total clival exposure are possible with bilateral simultaneous infratemporal dissection.

Contraindications

1. Bilateral cavernous sinus involvement by malignant disease
2. Prepontine dural or basilar artery invasion
3. Extensive inferior cervical nodal metastasis
4. Distant metastatic disease
5. Patient physiology or psychology

Special Considerations

1. Multiple simultaneous surgical approaches to encompass disease extent
2. Carotid and cavernous sinus involvement
3. Encasement of an optic nerve or optic chiasm
4. Prepontine dural involvement
5. Need for a carotid artery graft
6. Reconstruction requiring a free flap

Preoperative Preparation

1. A complete history and physical examination, with special attention to cranial nerve testing
2. Computed tomography (CT) and magnetic resonance imaging (MRI) of the brain, skull base, paranasal sinuses, pharynx, and neck
3. CT scan of the chest and abdomen
4. Three-vessel angiography, with the carotid balloon test occlusion done with hypotension and including preocclusion and occlusion single photon emission computed tomography scan
5. Transnasal or transoral biopsy
6. Preoperative planning conference with the patient, family, and entire craniofacial team.

Special Instrumentation, Position, and Anesthesia

1. Neurosurgical, otologic, microvascular, and head and neck instrumentation
2. Operating room teams for each phase of the surgery
3. Intraoperative cranial nerve monitoring, as necessary
4. Anesthesia with balanced narcotic and inhalation technique through a tracheostomy, without muscle relaxants
5. Oximetric Swan-Ganz central venous catheter and other monitoring
6. Planned hypotension, except during carotid dissection
7. Lumbar-subarachnoid drain
8. Surgical preparation of the entire head and neck (hair shaving not necessary) and donor site areas
9. Supine position, with the head placed on sterilized Mayfield horseshoe head holder

(continued)

Operative Procedure

For the preauricular infratemporal approach to nasopharyngeal resection, the patient is positioned on the operating table in a supine position on a special alternating-pressure mattress covering a heating pad. A lumbar-subarachnoid drain is placed at the L4–L5 interspace, and Plexi-pulse venous compression boots are applied. The patient's pressure-sensitive areas are specially padded.

The incision for the craniofacial exposure is divided into three components. A bicoronal scalp incision is done through the parted hair from the vertex to the posterior aspect of the temporal line. The incision curves forward over the superior attachment of the ear and continues in a preauricular skin crease or behind the tragus and then curves around the lobule of the ear and over the mastoid to continue forward in a midcervical skin crease (Fig. 155-1). The scalp portion of the incision is made with a scalpel deep to the level of the hair follicles and then completed with cutting cautery to the depth of the periosteum and temporalis fascia. This portion of the flap is elevated from the scalp vertex to the superior orbital rim and over the temporalis muscle fascia to the zygomatic arch. The facial portion of the flap is elevated superficial to the parotid fascia, extending the dissection beyond the anterior border of the masseter muscle. The cervical skin is elevated superficial to the platysma muscle, connecting the cervical and facial portion of the flap elevation. A soft tissue envelope is created around the upper branches of the facial nerve to protect them during the subsequent soft tissue mobilization around the orbit and infratemporal fossa (Fig. 155-2).

The temporalis muscle is elevated off of the temporal squama with a cutting cautery, separating it from bone to the infratemporal fossa and along the lateral orbital wall. The periosteum is then elevated over the zygomatic arch and lateral orbital rim, and bone cuts are made with a fine-toothed oscillating saw at the frontozygomatic suture line, along the lateral orbital wall at the level of the pterion, extending the lateral orbital incision to the inferior orbital fissure. A malar exposure is obtained parallel to facial nerve branches, and a bone incision is made at the junction of the inferior and lateral orbital rim again connecting to the inferior orbital fissure. The posterior zygomatic arch is transected tangential to the glenoid fossa, and the bone complex is removed (Fig. 155-3).

To protect the facial nerve from injury due to stretching, the parotid and distal facial nerve branches are mobilized off the masseter fascia and away from the underlying structures to allow transposition of the facial skin flap and parotid below the level of the zygomatic arch. A cuff of soft tissue is maintained around the trunk of the facial nerve between the mastoid and the mandible to reduce nerve trauma (Fig. 155-4).

The infratemporal fossa dissection continues with the removal of the attachment of the pterygoid plates. An appropriate soft tissue margin is taken, the pterygoid musculature is transected with cutting cautery, the buccal fat is mobilized, and the lateral wall of the maxillary antrum is exposed. A posterior antrostomy is then created, and bone is removed from the lateral maxillary sinus with a Kerrison rongeur (see Fig. 155-4).

The cervical dissection is completed by mobilizing the sternocleidomastoid muscle and dissecting the internal jugular vein, internal carotid, and external carotid. The mandible is mobilized by dissecting the temporomandibular joint capsule out of the glenoid fossa with a periosteal elevator. By transecting the attachment at the glenoid tubercle and by dividing the sphenomandibular ligament in the infratemporal fossa and the stylomandibular ligament through a cervical approach, the mandible can be transposed anteriorly and inferiorly.

A craniotomy or infratemporal craniectomy is done for all but the most limited resections. The extent of the craniotomy is dictated by the degree of dural or petrous carotid artery involvement and varies from a 3-cm craniectomy lateral to the area of the foramen ovale to a frontotemporal craniotomy that begins at the superior orbital rim and continues posteriorly over and includes the glenoid fossa. Typically, the temporal craniotomy is accomplished between the pterion and the glenoid fossa, providing exposure of the vertical and horizontal segments of the petrous carotid artery, the tip of the

(continued)

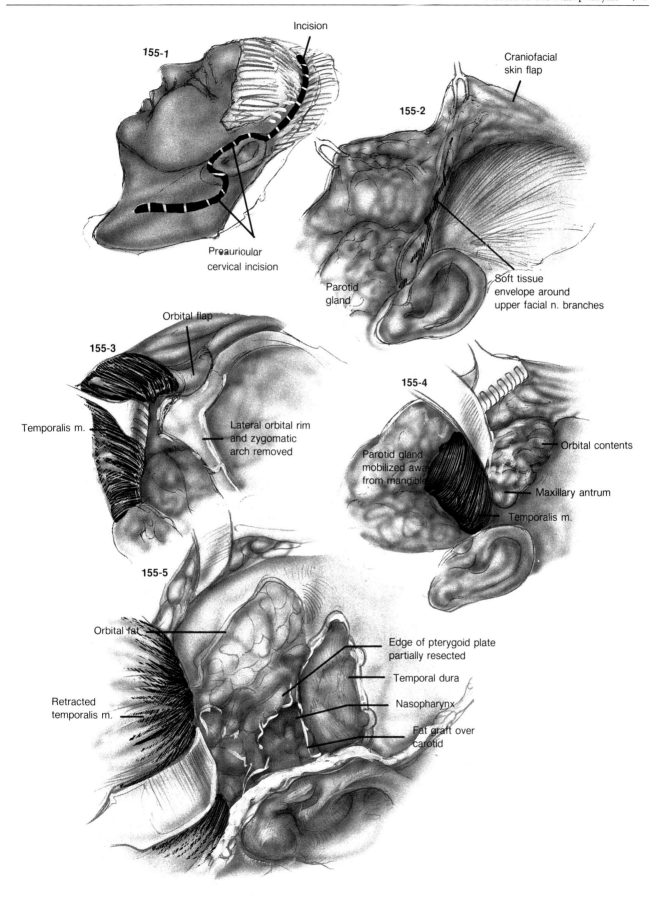

Incision

155-1

Preauricular
cervical incision

155-2

Craniofacial
skin flap

Parotid
gland

Soft tissue
envelope around
upper facial n. branches

Orbital flap

155-3

Temporalis m.

Lateral orbital rim
and zygomatic
arch removed

155-4

Parotid gland
mobilized away
from mandible

Orbital contents

Maxillary antrum

Temporalis m.

155-5

Orbital fat

Edge of pterygoid plate
partially resected

Temporal dura

Nasopharynx

Retracted
temporalis m.

Fat graft over
carotid

■ 155. ACCESS TO THE NASOPHARYNX
(continued)

Tips and Pearls

1. Plan for three-dimensional approach to difficult resection areas.
2. Lumbar-subarachnoid spinal fluid drainage is critical when craniotomy is required.
3. Do not overload the patient with fluids.
4. Do not rely on local tissue reconstruction for large defects.
5. Fine-toothed, oscillating-saw bone cuts, including the margins of the craniotomy, allow anatomically stable reconstruction.
6. Removing the lateral orbital-zygomatic bone complex and transposition of the mandible are keys to exposure.
7. Extent of the craniotomy or craniectomy depends on degree of carotid and dural involvement.
8. Mobilization of parotid and protected distal facial nerve preserves facial nerve function.
9. Take time to obtain a watertight dural closure, and consider free-flap reconstruction of all large defects and previously irradiated areas.
10. Do not try to avoid tracheostomy.

Pitfalls and Complications

1. Inadequate blood or inappropriate fluid replacement intraoperatively
2. Bleeding secondary to consumption of clotting factors or blood replacement coagulopathy.
3. Intraoperative or postoperative hypotension producing a cerebrovascular accident.
4. Cerebrospinal fluid (CSF) leak or meningitis
5. Pneumonia or hypoventilation resulting in hypoxia

Postoperative Care Issues

1. Protocols for nursing, respiratory, nutrition, and rehabilitation care
2. Ventilated respiratory support for 24 to 48 hours
3. Doppler monitoring of free-flap pulses
4. Intermittent lumbar CSF drainage if dural closure is tenuous
5. Remove the tracheostomy before starting oral feeding.
6. Hospitalization for 7 to 10 days for patients having local reconstruction and 3 to 4 weeks when free flaps are used.

References

Schramm VL. Infratemporal fossa surgery. In: Sekhar LN, Schramm VL, eds. Tumors of the cranial base, diagnosis and treatment. Mount Kisco, NY: Futura Publishing Company, 1987.

Sekhar LN, Schramm VL, Jones NF. Combined resection of large cranial base neoplasms. In: Sekhar LN, Schramm VL, eds. Tumors of the cranial base, diagnosis and treatment. Mount Kisco, NY: Futura Publishing Company, 1987.

temporal lobe, and the lateral wall of the sphenoid sinus. The anterior and posterior bone cuts are done with a fine blade and an oscillating saw, and the cuts along the infratemporal fossa are made with the drill lateral to the trigeminal nerve branches and with an osteotome across the glenoid fossa (Figs. 155-5 and 155-9A). During the elevation of the craniotomy bone flap and the subsequent intracranial dissection, dural relaxation is obtained by withdrawing spinal fluid from the lumbar subarachnoid drain.

The middle fossa dissection continues with the elevation of dura to expose the extradural portions of the second and third division of the trigeminal nerve. Bone is then removed with a rongeur to decompress both of these nerves. Sacrifice of cranial nerves V_2 or V_3 is required if the petrous carotid artery is involved or if extensive nasopharyngeal resection is to be accomplished.

The sphenoid sinus is entered at the anterior extent of the middle fossa, and the lateral wall of the sphenoid sinus is removed as the cavernous sinus and anterior temporal dura are mobilized. Ultimately, the mucosa from both sides of the sphenoid sinus is removed, and the superior nasopharyngeal margin is obtained by drilling through the floor of the sphenoid sinus.

During carotid artery resection, the patient is managed with normotensive anesthesia, and if a carotid laceration is produced or ligation is necessary, the patient is temporarily heparinized. Complete dissection of the petrous carotid artery requires sacrifice of cranial nerve V_3 and usually of V_2. Bone is removed with a rongeur across the eustachian tube and just medial to the foramen ovale. The intracranial aspect of the petrous carotid canal can be identified in the middle fossa, where a bony dehiscence usually overlies the carotid canal. The carotid artery is then mobilized within the petrous carotid canal with microsurgical instrumentation, and surrounding bone is removed with fine rongeurs. A cutting bur is used to thin bone from the carotid canal to the level of the second genu of the carotid and a lateral and inferior carotid decompression is accomplished with rongeur bone removal. The carotid artery can then be mobilized out of the petrous canal with the transection of the fibrous ring at the skull base (Fig. 155-6).

The clivus and apex of the petrous pyramid are removed with a drill as a deep margin of the nasopharyngeal resection or as part of the tumor removal if bone is directly involved. The nasopharynx can be undermined with a drill to obtain an en bloc resection. For tumors arising within the clivus, piecemeal resection has proven equally effective in curing low-grade malignancy or benign disease. Completion of the nasopharyngeal resection is accomplished by transecting the medial wall of the maxillary sinus and the posterior nasal septum and connecting this portion of the dissection with the anterior sphenoid sinus. The lateral and anterior portions of the specimen are mobilized so the nasopharynx can be visualized directly and mucosal cuts can be done with cutting cautery. Occasionally, the inferior nasopharyngeal transection is done by a transoral visualization. After the specimen has been removed, the bone margins are smoothed with a drill, and bone removal is continued to the prepontine dura, as necessary (Fig. 155-7).

Reconstruction consists of three components: dural closure, soft tissue replacement, and bone reapproximation. First, a meticulous watertight dural closure is obtained with direct dural reapproximation and with pericranial dural grafting. Soft tissue reconstruction is necessary to ensure isolation of the dura from the nasopharynx. When a small resection has been accomplished in a previously unirradiated patient, a simple closure with medialization of the temporalis muscle is sufficient. If anterior temporal dural or distal carotid exposure has been obtained, transposition of the posterior temporalis muscle may be sufficient for coverage.

For large resection defects and previously irradiated areas, a free flap is recommended. The gastric-omental free flap is the preferred technique, providing nasopharyngeal mucosal resurfacing and pliable, stable soft tissue reconstruction (Fig. 155-8). The bone flaps and zygomatic arch are anatomically repositioned and secured with titanium wire or bone plates (see Fig. 155-9). Hemovac drains are placed away from craniotomy bone cuts to prevent suction against a dural closure.

VICTOR L. SCHRAMM, JR.
ANDREW M. MARLOWE

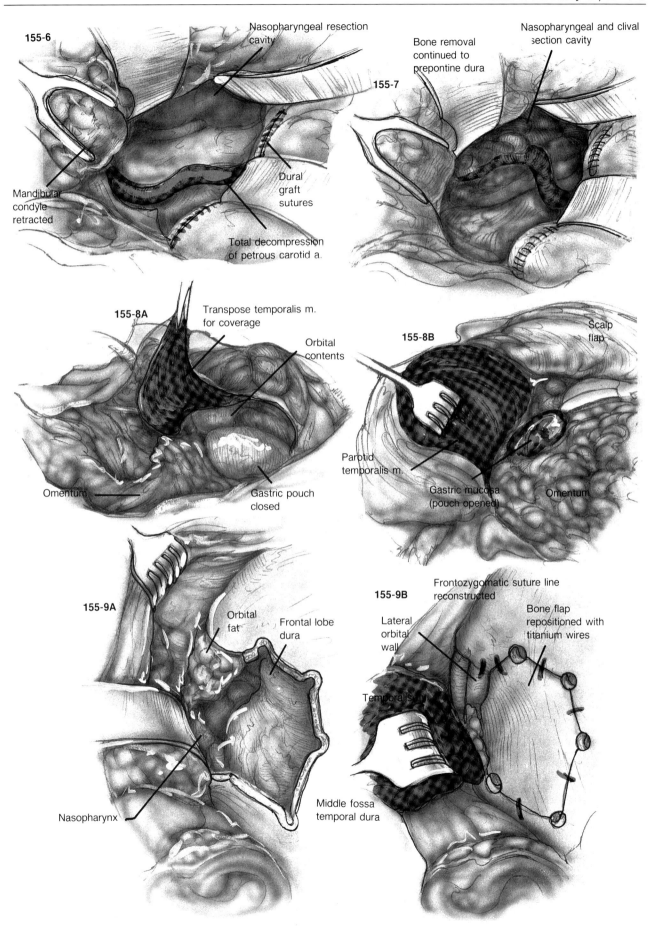

155-6

Nasopharyngeal resection cavity

Mandibular condyle retracted

Dural graft sutures

Total decompression of petrous carotid a.

155-7

Bone removal continued to prepontine dura

Nasopharyngeal and clival resection cavity

155-8A

Transpose temporalis m. for coverage

Orbital contents

Omentum

Gastric pouch closed

155-8B

Scalp flap

Parotid temporalis m.

Gastric mucosa (pouch opened)

Omentum

155-9A

Orbital fat

Frontal lobe dura

Middle fossa temporal dura

Nasopharynx

155-9B

Frontozygomatic suture line reconstructed

Lateral orbital wall

Bone flap repositioned with titanium wires

Temporalis m.

■ 156. PETROSAL APPROACH

A lateral approach to the posterior cranial fossa that is centered on the petrous portion of the temporal bone. Presigmoid intradural exposure is obtained after a standard complete mastoidectomy combined with a temporal and a retrosigmoid single-flap craniotomy. Because the otic capsule is preserved, the petrosal approach is most useful for patients with preoperatively intact and serviceable hearing.

Indications

1. Benign clival tumors, such as meningiomas, chordomas, epidermoids, and neuromas
2. Benign tumors of the petrous ridge
3. Medially based cerebellopontine angle tumors
4. Medially based jugular foramen tumors

Contraindications

1. Malignant tumors of the clivus or temporal bone
2. Nonconfluent venous sinus system

Special Considerations

1. Extensive supratentorial tumor extension
2. Midline prepontine and contralateral tumor extension
3. Vertebrobasilar arterial anatomy
4. Venous sinus anatomy
5. Mastoid and petrous bone anatomy
6. Preoperative hearing
7. Status of the lower cranial nerves

Preoperative Preparation

1. Complete history and physical examination
2. Special attention to cranial nerve testing
3. Full audiologic assessment
4. Computed tomography (CT) scans and magnetic resonance imaging of the temporal bones and posterior fossa, respectively
5. Four-vessel angiography, with special attention to the vertebrobasilar system and the venous system

Special Instruments, Position, and Anesthesia

1. Intraoperative monitoring of cranial nerves V, VII, VIII, X, and XI, as well as cranial nerves III and VI if the tumor involves the cavernous sinus
2. General anesthesia without muscle relaxants
3. Supine positioning, shoulder roll, three-point Mayfield headrest fixation
4. Cerebellar and temporal lobe retractors
5. High-speed air drill or electric drill
6. Craniotome
7. Operating microscope

(continued)

Operative Procedure

The patient is placed in the supine position, with the head turned away and fixed in a three-point Mayfield headrest. The head and ipsilateral shoulder are slightly elevated, and operative exposure is altered as needed by side-to-side table rotation (Fig. 156-1).

A preauricular incision is carried posterosuperior to the auricle in a reverse question mark fashion, and it is extended into the postauricular scalp behind the mastoid process. The temporalis muscle is elevated superiorly while the musculoperiosteal tissue over the mastoid process and occipital bone is elevated posteroinferiorly. These flaps must be preserved to ensure a layered closure.

A temporal-occipital bone flap is removed; it straddles the transverse sinus after the connection of bur holes positioned above and below the transverse sinus (Fig. 156-2). Extreme caution must be exercised in elevating this bone flap away from the delicate dura at the junction of the transverse and sigmoid sinuses.

After exposure of the transverse and sigmoid sinuses, a complete canal wall–up mastoidectomy is performed. The semicircular canals are isolated, the facial nerve is skeletonized in the vertical segment, and the sigmoid sinus is completely decompressed (ie, bone removed) from the sinodural angle above to the jugular bulb below (Fig. 156-3). All of the bone anterior to the sigmoid sinus is removed from the sinodural angle to the jugular bulb, taking care not to fenestrate the posterior semicircular canal.

Intradural exposure is accomplished by opening the presigmoid posterior fossa dura above the jugular bulb and extending the vertical durotomy to the superior petrosal sinus (Fig. 156-4). The superior

(continued)

156-1. Patient in 3-point Mayfield headrest

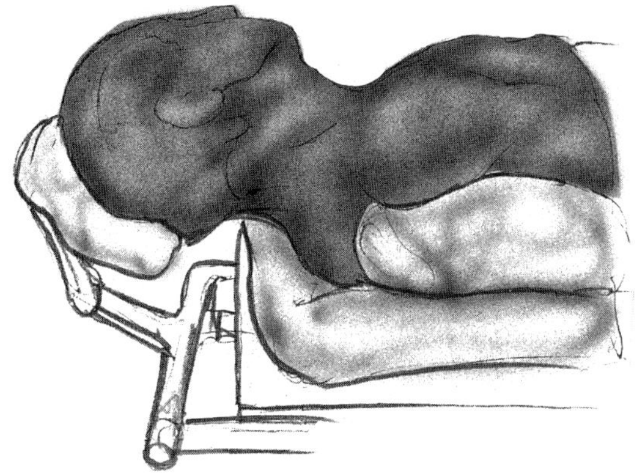

156-2. Skin incision

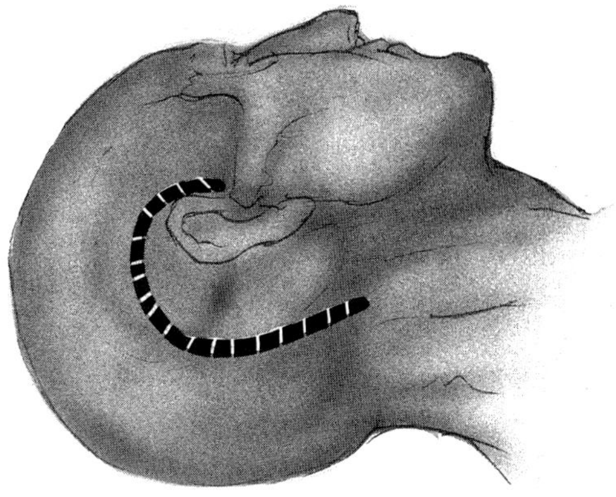

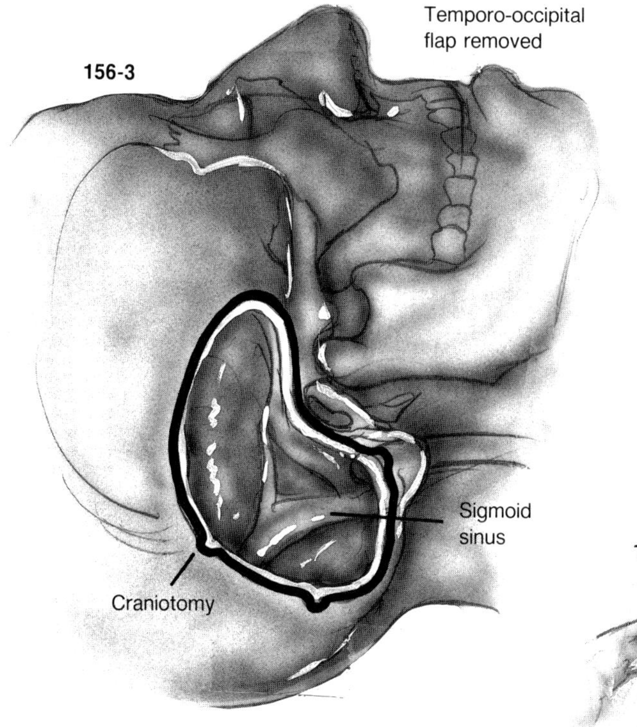

Temporo-occipital
flap removed

156-3

Sigmoid
sinus

Craniotomy

156-4

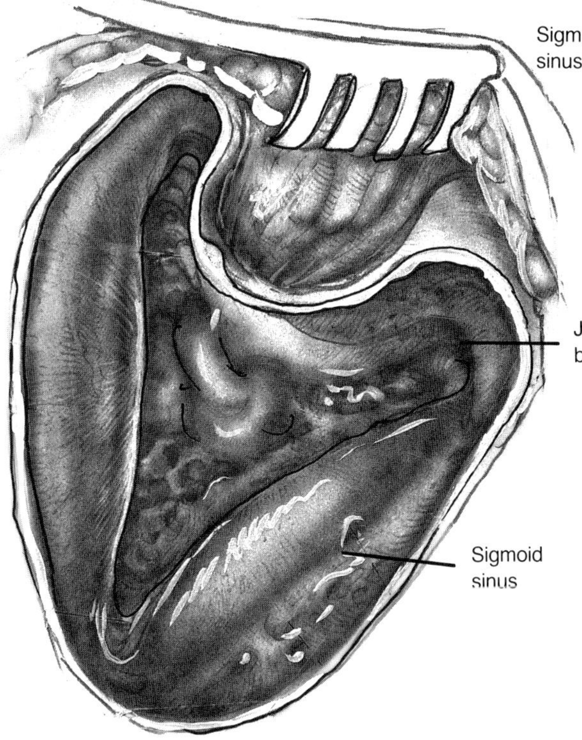

Mastoidectomy
(canal wall up)

Sigmoid
sinus

Jugular
bulb

Sigmoid
sinus

■ 156. PETROSAL APPROACH *(continued)*

Tips and Pearls

1. Inspect the degree of pneumatization of the temporal bone on the CT scan.
2. Identify the position of the sigmoid sinus preoperatively.
3. Perform the mastoidectomy with sigmoid sinus decompression first if the temporal-occipital flap is adherent to the underlying dura.
4. Preserve the presigmoid dura during the mastoidectomy to ensure a watertight dural closure.
5. Minimize brain retraction by maximizing bone removal.

Pitfalls and Complications

1. Facial paralysis due to stretch injury during tumor dissection
2. Sensorineural hearing loss
3. Aspiration and voice change may result after lower cranial nerve dissection.
4. CSF fistula, with or without meningitis
5. Occipital headache, neck stiffness, and facial pain may occur.

Postoperative Care Issues

1. Neurosurgical intensive care monitoring for 24 to 28 hours
2. Mastoid compressive dressing for 4 to 5 days
3. Use a lumbar-subarachnoid drain with bed rest if a CSF leak occurs. Surgical wound repair is indicated if these conservative measures fail to seal the CSF leak.
4. Liquid diet on the third postoperative day and advance as tolerated
5. Ambulation on fourth postoperative day
6. Uncomplicated discharge from the hospital in 7 to 10 days
7. Lower cranial nerve palsies may require voice and swallow therapy.

References

Al-Mefty O, Fox JL, Smith RR. Petrosal approach for petroclival meningiomas. Neurosurgery 1988;22:510.

Rosomoff HL. The subtemporal transtentorial approach to the cerebellopontine angle. Laryngoscope 1971;81:1448.

petrosal sinus is clipped and transected, and the presigmoid dural opening is joined with a supratentorial dural incision. The anterior incision of the tentorium, parallel to the petrous pyramid, is extended through the incisura. A retractor is placed in such a way as to medially and posteriorly displace the sigmoid sinus, cerebellum, and the cut edge of the tentorium (Fig. 156-5).

Enhanced tumor visualization is achieved after penetration of the cerebellomedullary cistern and cerebrospinal fluid drainage. Significant supratentorial tumor extension may necessitate posterior temporal lobe elevation after the identification and protection of the vein of Labbé (see Fig. 156-5).

Devascularization of the tumor can be accomplished by the bipolar coagulation of meningeal feeding vessels and the tumor insertion on the petroclival ridge. Tumor debulking is achieved with extreme caution between cranial nerves V, VII, and VII above and cranial nerves IX through XII below. Medial tumor removal often requires brain stem dissection with preservation of the posterior inferior cerebellar artery (PICA), the anterior inferior cerebellar artery, and cranial nerves IV and VI.

After tumor removal, the presigmoid durotomy is closed primarily or with the use of a pericranial patch. The temporalis muscle is turned into the mastoid defect and the musculoperiosteal flaps are reapproximated. The soft tissues are closed in multiple layers, and a compressive mastoid dressing is applied for 4 to 5 days.

JOHN P. LEONETTI
OSSAMA AL-MEFTY

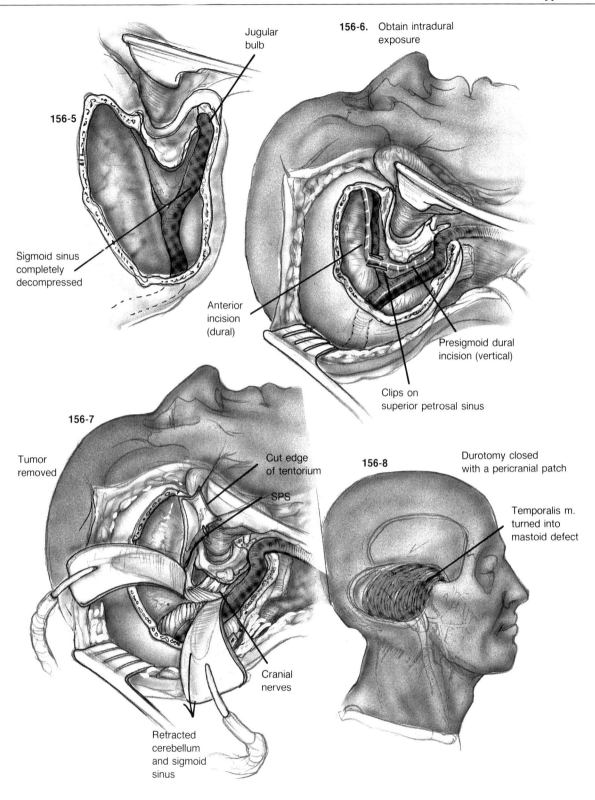

Jugular bulb

156-6. Obtain intradural exposure

156-5

Sigmoid sinus completely decompressed

Anterior incision (dural)

Presigmoid dural incision (vertical)

Clips on superior petrosal sinus

156-7

Tumor removed

Cut edge of tentorium

SPS

156-8

Durotomy closed with a pericranial patch

Temporalis m. turned into mastoid defect

Cranial nerves

Retracted cerebellum and sigmoid sinus

■ 157. REPAIR OF CONGENITAL AURAL ATRESIA—Removal of atretic bone to create an external ear canal with tympanoplasty, meatoplasty, and possible ossicular reconstruction, employing an anterior surgical approach

Indications
1. Unilateral or bilateral atresia in patients older than 4 years of age
2. Normal or near-normal sensorineural function bilaterally
3. Adequate middle ear development, as assessed by computed tomography (CT) scan
   a. Middle ear space of at least one half to two thirds of the normal size
   b. Good definition of the deformed ossicular chain
4. Cholesteatoma delineated by CT or clinical examination is an absolute indication for surgery.
5. Only approximately 60% of patients with aural atresia meet these criteria for surgical intervention.

Contraindications
1. Unilateral or bilateral moderate or more severe sensorineural hearing loss
2. Poorly developed middle ear space, as delineated by CT
3. Absence of ossicular mass, as delineated by CT
4. Parental decision to allow the child with unilateral atresia to reach young adulthood for his or her input regarding surgery

Special Considerations
1. Selection of patients with unilateral or bilateral aural atresia
2. Assessment of cochlear reserve in bilateral atresia cases
3. Risk of cholesteatoma in cases of severe canal stenosis or canal atresia
4. Timing of otologic surgery with regard to auricular reconstruction
5. Other craniofacial anomalies
6. Developmental status of the inner ear

Preoperative Preparation
1. Physical examination, with attention to the development of first and second branchial arch structures
2. Audiometric evaluation, including bone conduction auditory brain stem response testing in bilateral atresia cases
3. Temporal bone CT scans in axial and coronal planes

Special Instruments, Position, and Anesthesia
1. Monitor the facial nerve, including use of a stimulation probe.
2. No neuromuscular blockade after induction of anesthesia

(continued)

Operative Procedure
The operative ear is exposed by positioning the patient supine, with the head rotated approximately 45° toward the contralateral side. Electromyographic electrode needles are placed in the orbicularis oculi and orbicularis oris muscles for continuous facial nerve monitoring.

A postauricular incision is made approximately 1 cm behind the reconstructed auricle. Superiorly, the temporalis fascia is exposed, and inferiorly, the incision is carried down to the mastoid bone. A piece of temporalis fascia is harvested and set aside to dehydrate. A periosteal incision is extended posteriorly from the zygomatic root along the temporal line. A second periosteal incision perpendicular to the first is made over the mastoid bone. Periosteum and the overlying soft tissues are elevated anteriorly until a depression in the bone is encountered; these tissues and the auricle are held forward with a self-retaining retractor. In most major malformations, this depression is the glenoid fossa, although a stenotic bony canal may be encountered.

A tympanic bone remnant may be identified posterior to the glenoid fossa in atretic ears (Figs. 157-1 and 157-2). With a cutting bur, drilling is begun at this tympanic bone remnant or just posterosuperior to the bony depression. The middle cranial fossa dura is identified and used as a superior landmark. The posterior wall of the glenoid fossa is thinned and serves as an anterior landmark. Care is taken to limit opening into the mastoid ear cells posteriorly (Figs. 157-3 and 157-4). Drilling is confined to the area just lateral to the middle ear space. Bone is removed medially along the middle cranial fossa dura until the epitympanum is entered.

The fused heads of the malleus and incus are the first middle ear structures identified (Fig. 157-5). The external canal is enlarged inferiorly, taking care to avoid injury to the facial nerve, which is vulnerable in the posteroinferior portion of the new bony canal. In this area, the nerve may lie lateral to the middle ear space and be anteriorly displaced. A diamond bur is used to thin the bone over the ossicular mass.

After a thin shell of bone has been created, the ossicular chain is exposed using a small hook or incudostapedial joint knife (Fig. 157-5). Fusion of the ossicular chain typically occurs at the neck of the malleus. The periosteum in this area should be sharply excised with a microknife or microscissors. Exposure around the ossicular chain is obtained using smaller burs so that the ossicular mass is centered in the new bony canal (Figs. 157-6 through 157-8).

The status of the ossicular chain is assessed. The stapes may be partially obscured because of the contracted middle ear cavity, the malformed lateral ossicular mass, or an overlying facial nerve. Usually, enough of the suprastructure can be seen to assess its continuity with the incus and its mobility. The superstructure of the stapes is usually small, with delicate, misshapen crura. Despite these deformities and the fused malleus and incus, the ossicular chain, if mobile, is left intact.

The dehydrated fascia graft is cut to the appropriate size and placed over the mobilized ossicular chain; no attempt is made to anchor the graft to the malleus-incus complex. To prevent lateralization, the graft is tucked beneath the anterior and superior bony ledges of the canal wall. Posteriorly, the graft extends for several millimeters up the canal wall. Occasionally, no canal ledge exists anteriorly, and a sulcus several millimeters deep is drilled into the anterior canal wall medial to the level of the ossicles. The edge of

(continued)

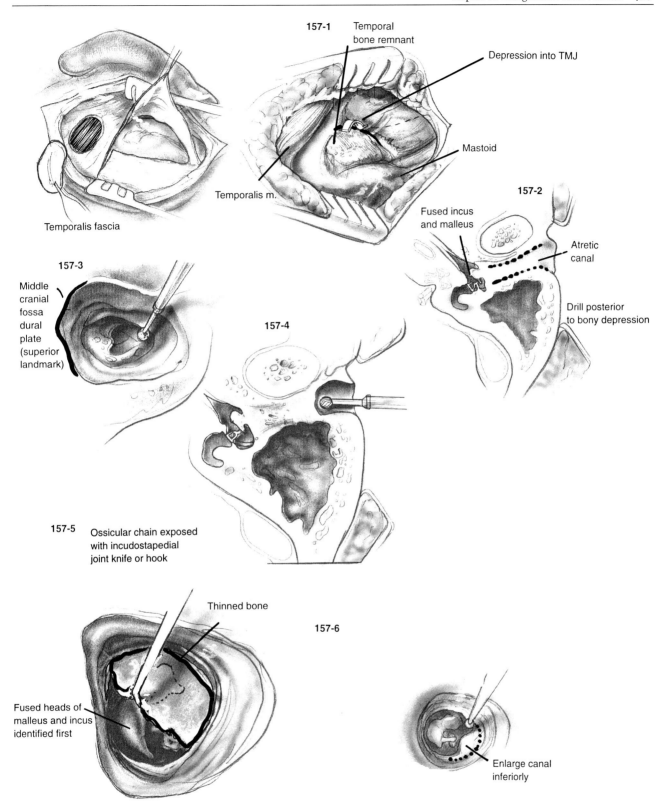

157-1   Temporal bone remnant
Depression into TMJ
Mastoid
Temporalis m.
Temporalis fascia

157-2   Fused incus and malleus
Atretic canal
Drill posterior to bony depression

157-3   Middle cranial fossa dural plate (superior landmark)

157-4

157-5   Ossicular chain exposed with incudostapedial joint knife or hook

Thinned bone   **157-6**
Fused heads of malleus and incus identified first
Enlarge canal inferiorly

157. REPAIR OF CONGENITAL AURAL ATRESIA (continued)

Tips and Pearls

1. Identify and use the glenoid fossa as an anterior landmark for the external canal.
2. Identify and use the middle cranial fossa dura as a superior landmark for the external canal.
3. Limit the exposure of mastoid air cells.
4. Enter middle ear space in epitympanum, identifying the fused heads of malleus and incus.
5. Ossicular fixation most commonly occurs at the malleus neck.
6. Although the stapes superstructure is frequently deformed, anticipate a mobile footplate.
7. If intact and mobile, the ossicular chain should be maintained, despite deformity.
8. Anticipate an abnormal facial nerve: dehiscence of the tympanic segment and/or anterior and lateral displacement of mastoid segment.

Pitfalls and Complications

1. Sensorineural hearing loss from ossicular chain trauma can be minimized by careful bone removal around ossicular chain.
2. The facial nerve is particularly vulnerable when drilling in the posterior and inferior portion of the new external canal.
3. Postoperative granulation tissue in the ear canal can be avoided by meticulously lining the bony canal with the split-thickness skin graft and carefully approximating the skin graft to the meatal skin.
4. Stenosis of the lateral canal can be limited by creating a large meatus and properly aligning the membranous and bony external canals.
5. Regular follow-up examinations may be necessary to remove desquamated epithelium within the external canal.

Postoperative Care Issues

1. Perioperative antibiotics are not used.
2. The Nu-Gauze packing in the external canal is removed at 10 to 14 days, and the canal is repacked with Cortisporin-soaked Gelfoam.
3. Healing of the ear canal and tympanic membrane is anticipated by 2 months, at which time the first audiogram is obtained.

References

Jahrsdoerfer RA. Congenital atresia of the ear. Laryngoscope 1978;88(Suppl 13):1.
Lambert PR. Congenital aural atresia. In: Bailey BJ, Johnson JT, Kohut RI, Pillsbury HC III, Tardy ME Jr, eds. Head and neck surgery—otolaryngology. Philadelphia: JB Lippincott, 1993:1579.

the fascia graft is then packed into this sulcus and stabilized with Cortisporin-soaked Gelfoam (Fig. 157-9).

The reconstructed auricle is undermined as an initial step for the meatoplasty. The deep soft tissues are debulked from the area of the meatus, and a through-and-through circular meatal opening about twice the normal size is made. Limiting the thickness of subcutaneous tissue around the meatus shortens the membranous canal and helps prevent postoperative stenosis. The auricle is then returned to its normal anatomic position to check for alignment of the meatus and the bony canal. Frequently, the meatus appears to be offset anteriorly or inferiorly. In such cases, further undermining of the auricle is necessary so it can be positioned more posteriorly and superiorly without tension. To accomplish this alignment, a strip of skin can be excised from the postauricular incision. Alternatively, permanent sutures between the mastoid periosteum (or through a suture tunnel drilled in the mastoid bone) and the cartilage framework of the auricle may be necessary to maintain proper position of the external ear. The facial nerve is vulnerable to injury if extensive undermining of the auricle is necessary, because prior auricular reconstruction may have caused scarring and tethering of the extratemporal facial nerve in a more superficial position.

A split-thickness skin graft (0.012 in [0.3 mm]) is taken from the upper thigh and used to line the external ear canal. To determine the proper configuration of the skin graft, a 2-0 silk suture is used to measure various dimensions of the canal. Circumferential measurements are made at the external meatus, at the lateral opening of the bony canal, and at the level of the tympanic membrane. Two longitudinal measurements are taken, one of the length of the bony canal and another of the length of the membranous canal (Fig. 157-10). The split-thickness skin graft is configured to these measurements. Typically, the graft is shaped like a hexagon and is approximately 4×6 cm. To facilitate graft placement at the level of the tympanic membrane and to ensure eversion of the skin edges, multiple small wedges are excised from that portion of the graft; the graft is also fashioned in a pie-crust pattern (Fig. 157-11).

With the ear retracted forward, the split-thickness skin graft is positioned in the bony canal so it overlaps the fascia graft by 2 to 3 mm. A layer of Cortisporin-soaked Gelfoam is placed over the fascia graft and adjacent split-thickness skin graft. The skin graft is stabilized within the ear canal by a 6-mm (0.25-in) layer of Nu-Gauze impregnated with an antibiotic ointment placed into the canal (Fig. 157-12).

After the bony canal has been fully packed, the ear is returned to its normal anatomic position, and the postauricular incision is closed with subcuticular sutures. Working through the meatus, the lateral end of the split-thickness skin graft is grasped and pulled through the meatal opening. It is trimmed as necessary and carefully sutured to the meatal skin. A second piece of Nu-Gauze packing is layered in to fill the lateral, soft tissue portion of the canal (Fig. 157-13). Packing of the split-thickness skin graft in the bony canal prevents it from being dislodged during the final step of suturing it to the meatus. The initial placement of the split-thickness skin graft in the bony canal with the ear reflected forward provides maximum exposure, ensuring that all the canal is covered and that the graft has been positioned accurately relative to the fascia graft. A mastoid dressing is applied.

PAUL R. LAMBERT

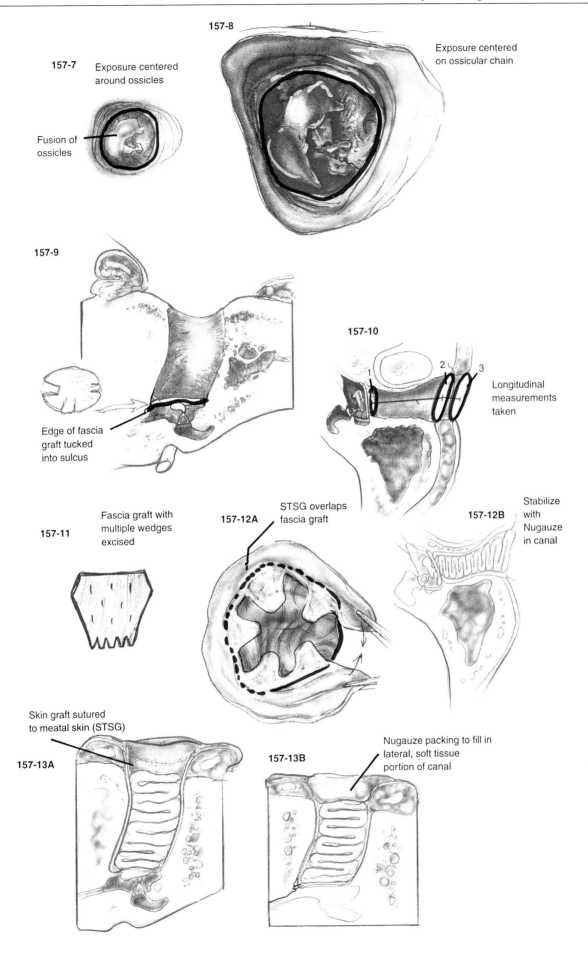

157-7   Exposure centered around ossicles

Fusion of ossicles

157-8

Exposure centered on ossicular chain

157-9

Edge of fascia graft tucked into sulcus

157-10

Longitudinal measurements taken

Fascia graft with multiple wedges excised

157-11

157-12A   STSG overlaps fascia graft

157-12B   Stabilize with Nugauze in canal

Skin graft sutured to meatal skin (STSG)

157-13A

157-13B   Nugauze packing to fill in lateral, soft tissue portion of canal

Atlas of Head and Neck Surgery–Otolaryngology,
edited by Byron J. Bailey, J. Gail Neely, Karen H. Calhoun, and Amy R. Coffey.
Lippincott-Raven Publishers, Philadelphia © 1996.

Section Three
Plastic and Reconstructive Surgery

Section Editor:
Karen H. Calhoun

Otoplasty and External Ear
Rhinoplasty
Mentoplasty and Malarplasty
Rhytidectomy and Related Procedures
Blepharoplasty
Facial Trauma
Laryngoplasty and Tracheoplasty

Local and Regional Flaps
Grafts and Free Flaps
Facial Reanimation and Fascial Sling
Mandibular Surgery, Cleft Lip
   and Palate, TMJ Surgery
Excision of Skin Lesions
   and Scar Revision
Aesthetic Reconstruction

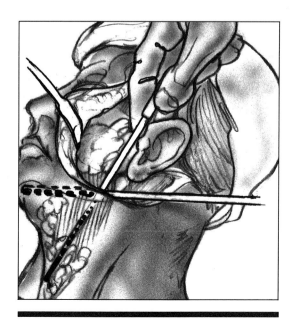

■ 158. OTOPLASTY FOR THE DEEP CONCHAL BOWL—Repair of prominauris or congenitally prominent ears, also called protruding ears, bat ears, elephant ears, Dumbo ears, or jug ears

Indications
1. Greater than a 20-mm maximal lateral projection of the helical rim from the mastoid skin or scalp due to a deep conchal bowl
2. Asymmetrically projecting ears
3. Associated psychologic distress

Contraindications
1. Children younger than 5 years of age
2. Radical or modified radical mastoidectomy bowls

Special Considerations
1. Consider if the antihelical fold also needs correction and perform simultaneously (see Chap. 159)
2. Observe ear asymmetries
3. Seek perfection; accept improvement.

Preoperative Preparation
1. Photography: frontal, full right, left lateral, and close-up right and left lateral views
2. Measurements of the lateral helical projection, degrees of conchal depth and of antihelical unfurling, areas of cosmetic concern of the helical rim, and lobe or scapha abnormalities

Special Instruments, Position, and Anesthesia
1. Headlight, cat's paw retractors, 4-0 Mersilene suture, bipolar cautery
2. Local infiltration with 1:1 mixture of 1% lidocaine hydrochloride (Xylocaine) with 1:100,000 epinephrine and of 0.5% bupivacaine hydrochloride (Marcaine) with 1:200,000 epinephrine
3. General anesthesia for children; local anesthesia with intravenous sedation for adults

Tips and Pearls
1. Soft tissue removal, not cartilage cutting, provides the ideal setback of the prominent conchal bowl.
2. The horizontal mattress sutures must secure the anterior conchal perichondrium and mastoid periosteum to prevent pull-through.
3. Avoid over correction of the middle third.

Pitfalls and Complications
1. A hematoma should be drained immediately to prevent subsequent deformity.
2. Pain is unusual. Beware of hematoma or infection.
3. Hypertrophic scar or keloid formation may occur with overly aggressive skin excision. Steroid tape (Cordran), 20 mg/mL of triamcinolone (Kenalog) injected intradermally, or both may control scarring.

Postoperative Care Issues
1. Remove dressing and inspect the wound on the first postoperative day. For adults, the dressing may be left off. For children, replace the dressing for 3 to 4 more days.
2. A head band is worn continuously for 2 weeks and at night only for an additional 4 to 6 weeks.
3. Measure the ears at the end of the procedure and postoperatively. Expect some loss of correction. A difference between the two ears of less than 3 mm is usually insignificant.

References
Adamson PA, McGraw BL, Tropper GJ. Otoplasty: critical review of clinical results. Laryngoscope 1991;101:883.

Adamson PA, McShane DP, Feldman RI. Otoplasty: an update. J Otolaryngol 1987;16:258.

Operative Procedure
A dose of broad-spectrum antibiotic and steroid is administered before skin incision. Our choice for adults is 300 mg of clindamycin hydrochloride (Cleocin, Dalacin C) and 125 mg of methylprednisolone (Solu-Medrol). For children, a proportionately smaller dose is used. If the ears are asymmetric, the more deformed ear is approached first.

An eccentric fusiform incision is planned around the postauricular sulcus, with more skin removed from the posterior surface of the auricle than the mastoid. The inferior aspect of the incision is carried onto the postauricular surface. As the ear is set closer to the head, the eccentric excision allows the final scar to lie in the postauricular sulcus (Fig. 158-1). Exposure of the posterior conchal and helical surfaces is also improved. At least 1 cm of the superior and inferior sulcus is left undisturbed so no scar is visible when the ear is viewed laterally.

To determine the width of the excised fusiform, the concha is set back manually when planning the skin excision, and the amount of redundant skin after conchal setback is estimated. Usually, the fusiform area is about 10 to 12 mm at its widest point. Excess skin excision increases the risk of hypertrophic scarring.

The skin fusiform is incised, and the skin and soft tissue deep to the conchal bowl are excised, leaving the perichondrium intact. The soft tissues of the postauricular sulcus (ie, fat and postauricular muscle) are elevated with the overlying skin (Fig. 158-2). The depth of the soft tissue excision varies with the prominence of the conchae cymba and cavum. Little to no soft tissue excision is needed inferior to the level of the antitragus. Care is taken to remain 1 cm posterior to the external auditory canal, avoiding canal injury.

The remaining skin and soft tissue of the posterior aspect of the helix, antihelix, and conchae is undermined with scissors.

White 4-0 Mersilene suture is used for conchal setback. The conchomastoid horizontal mattress sutures are placed at the lateral third of the concha cavum and concha cymba in an arc paralleling the normal curve of the cartilage (Fig. 158-3A). The sutures are placed at the projected position of the junction of the horizontal floor and vertical wall of the conchae. The precise location for the suture in the cartilage is determined by palpating the anterior aspect of the cartilage with the index finger (Fig. 158-3B), locating the optimal position for conchal setback, and then everting the ear with the thumb, keeping the index finger in place. A full-thickness bite of cartilage and lateral perichondrium, but not lateral skin, is taken. The lie of the suture should parallel the outer conchal rim.

The ear is then set back the desired amount, the location for the bite on the mastoid surface is determined, and the horizontal mattress throw is completed. Anchoring of the suture to the mastoid periosteum is essential for long-term correction. At least three such sutures are required for adequate setback. Sutures are tied after they have all been placed, with the middle suture tied last to reduce the chance of overcorrection of the middle third of the ear with a subsequent "telephone ear" deformity (Fig. 158-3C).

With overly thick cartilage or excessively high conchal walls, the cartilage may be weakened with vertical shaves. Adult cartilage in particular tends to be stronger and more brittle. A cartilage island is shaved at the point where the floor of the concha will meet the new lateral sweep of the wall (Fig. 158-4). Conchomastoid sutures are tied after shaving.

With properly placed conchomastoid sutures, the overly prominent conchal wall is reduced by extending the relative length of the floor. The conchal cartilage must be set back, not just set in, to prevent buckling of the posterior aspect of the external auditory canal.

Hemostasis is obtained with bipolar cautery to minimize injury to the medial perichondrium. The wound is irrigated with clindamycin hydrochloride solution and closed with interrupted, inverted 4-0 chromic catgut sutures (Fig. 158-5). Antibiotic ointment is applied to the closed wound, and cotton saturated with mineral oil and peroxide is molded to the lateral surface of the ear and into the postauricular sulcus. A mastoid pressure dressing is applied. No drain is used.

PETER A. ADAMSON
MINAS S. CONSTANTINIDES

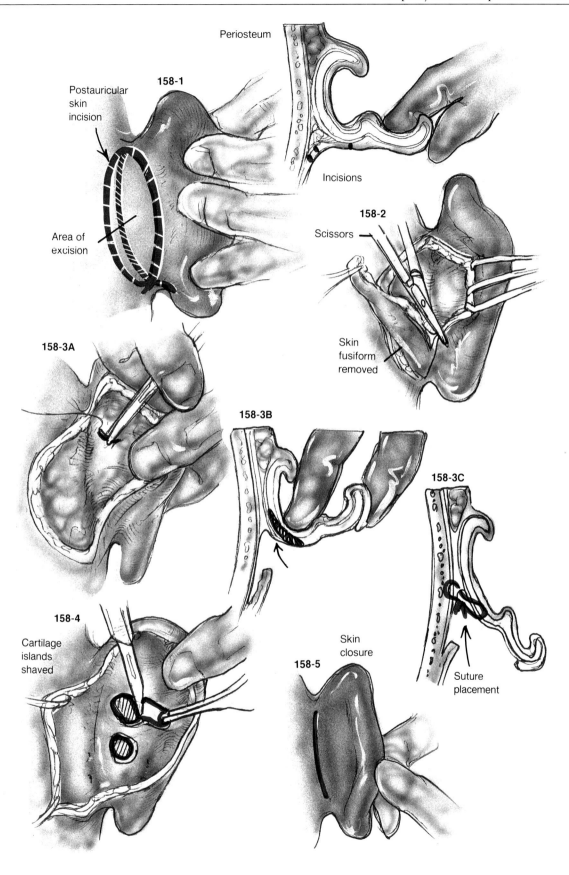

Periosteum

158-1

Postauricular
skin
incision

Area of
excision

Incisions

158-2

Scissors

Skin
fusiform
removed

158-3A

158-3B

158-3C

Suture
placement

158-4

Cartilage
islands
shaved

Skin
closure

158-5

■ *159.* OTOPLASTY FOR THE ANTIHELICAL

FOLD—Technique for correcting prominauris, also called protruding ears, bat ears, elephant ears, Dumbo ears, or jug ears

Indications
1. Abnormal unfurling of the antihelical fold
2. Asymmetrically projecting ears
3. Associated psychologic distress

Contraindications
1. Children younger than 5 years of age
2. Bleeding dyscrasias
3. Previous chondritis
4. Brittle insulin-dependent diabetes
5. Unrealistic expectations

Special Considerations
1. Protruding ears with abnormal unfurling of the antihelical fold is an autosomal dominant trait with variable penetrance.
2. Often bilateral, protruding ears are caused by an overly deep conchal bowl, unfurled antihelical fold, or both.
3. Normal parameters include an average lateral projection of the helical rim from mastoid skin of 15 to 20 mm. It is considered less than ideal if the projection is greater than 22 mm.
4. The average prominent ear projects 26 mm at the point of maximal projection. Surgery can reduce the lateral projection by about 10 mm immediately and by 6 mm at 1 year after surgery.
5. Conchal setback should be completed before the creation of an antihelical fold.
6. A white, permanent suture should be used. Our choice is 4-0 Mersilene.
7. Asymmetries in ear sizes are usual and should be pointed out preoperatively.
8. As in any cosmetic procedure, the goal is improvement, not perfection.

Preoperative Preparation
1. Photography: frontal, full right, left lateral, and close-up right and left lateral views, with a headband holding the hair back
2. Measurements of the lateral helical projection, degrees of conchal depth and of antihelical unfurling, areas of cosmetic concern of the helical rim, and lobe or scapha abnormalities

(continued)

Operative Procedure

In most otoplasties, conchal setback is desirable. This is performed, if required, before creating the antihelical fold. The conchal bowl setback alone draws in the superior helical pole, lessening the degree of furling required to correct a prominent antihelical fold (see Procedure 158).

The patient is placed supine, and the face and both ears are prepped and draped into the sterile field so the head can be turned easily and both ears observed simultaneously. Local anesthetic solution is injected into the posterior auricular surface. A dose of broad-spectrum antibiotic and steroid is administered before skin incision. Our choice for adults is 1 g of cefazolin (Ancef) and 125 mg of methylprednisolone (Solu-Medrol). For children, a proportionately smaller dose is used. If the ears are asymmetric, the more deformed ear is approached first.

An eccentric fusiform incision is planned around the postauricular sulcus. More skin is removed from the posterior auricle than from the mastoid. The inferior aspect of the incision is carried onto the postauricular surface. As the ear is set closer to the head, the eccentric excision guarantees a final scar in the postauricular sulcus and improves exposure of the posterior conchal and helical surfaces (Fig. 159-1). At least 1 cm of the superior and inferior sulcus is left undisturbed so no scar is visible when the ear is viewed laterally.

To determine the width of the excised fusiform, the helix (and concha, if it is being set back as well) is set back manually when planning the skin excision, and the amount of redundant skin after setback is determined. Usually, the fusiform area is about 10 to 12 mm at its widest point. Excess skin excision increases the risk of hypertrophic scarring due to wound tension.

The skin fusiform is incised. Using scissors, the skin to be excised is undermined, leaving perichondrium intact. The remaining skin of the posterior aspect of the helix, antihelix, and conchae is undermined with scissors (Fig. 159-2). The helix is completely mobilized by cutting the anterior helical ligament at the anterior root of the helix. Soft tissues overlying the temporalis fascia and the posterior root of the zygoma are debulked to allow adequate medialization and set back of the fossa triangularis. Care is taken to remain directly on the perichondrium at the root of the helix to avoid injury to branches of the superficial temporal artery and vein. Such wide undermining ensures adequate intraoperative exposure and good redraping of the skin over the posterior auricle at closure.

After the concha is set back, attention is turned to the antihelix. First, the amount of folding necessary is determined by placing an index finger on the anterior surface of the auricle and furling the antihelix to determine the optimal position for the helical fold (Fig. 159-3). The ear is then everted without moving the index finger, and a 4-0 Mersilene horizontal mattress suture is placed in the helical cartilage, parallel to the helical rim at the lateral extent of the desired antihelical fold. The index finger on the lateral surface serves as a guide. Care is taken to include the full thickness of helical cartilage and lateral perichondrium, but not the lateral skin. Skin retraction with cat's paw retractors aids in suture placement (Fig. 159-4). A releasing incision may be necessary for exposure of the upper helix. This incision can be placed at right angles to the initial elliptical skin excision, at the junction of the upper and middle thirds of the incision.

(continued)

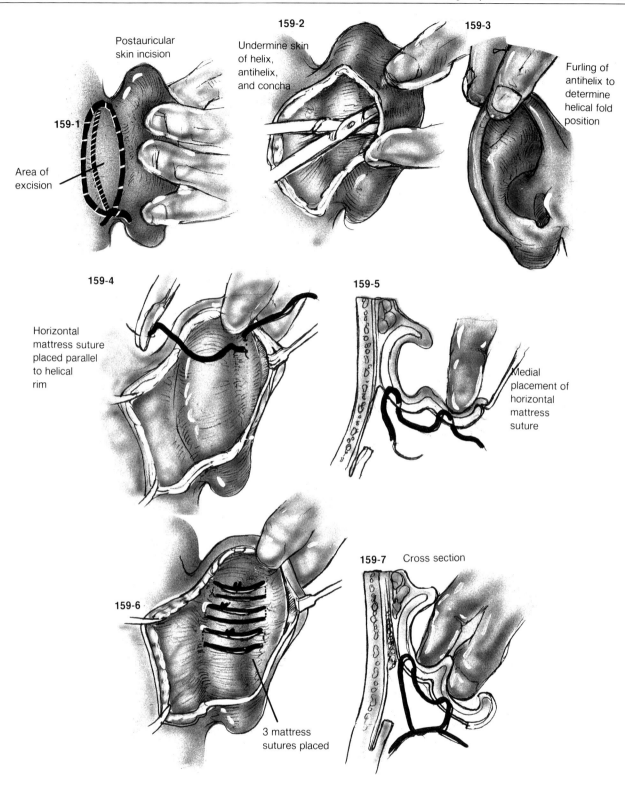

159-1

Postauricular skin incision

Area of excision

159-2

Undermine skin of helix, antihelix, and concha

159-3

Furling of antihelix to determine helical fold position

159-4

Horizontal mattress suture placed parallel to helical rim

159-5

Medial placement of horizontal mattress suture

159-6

3 mattress sutures placed

159-7 Cross section

■ **159.** OTOPLASTY FOR THE ANTIHELICAL FOLD *(continued)*

Special Instruments, Position, and Anesthesia

1. Headlight, cat's paw retractors, 4-0 Mersilene suture, bipolar cautery
2. Local infiltration with 1:1 mixture of 1% lidocaine hydrochloride (Xylocaine) with 1:100,000 epinephrine and of 0.5% bupivacaine hydrochloride (Marcaine) with 1:200,000 epinephrine
3. General anesthesia for children; local anesthesia with intravenous sedation is possible for adults

Tips and Pearls

1. A graduated approach is mandatory, with correction a continuum between conchal setback, antihelical fold creation, and refinement techniques.
2. The ideal aesthetic position of the antihelical fold is medial to the helical rim on anterior view.
3. Avoid cartilage cutting and scoring techniques to maintain smooth contours. Cartilage bends away from the side on which it is scored.
4. The horizontal mattress (Mustardé) stitch must secure the anterior perichondrium to prevent later pull-through and loss of correction.
5. Middle-third antihelical sutures are tied last to prevent overcorrection and a "telephone ear" deformity.

Pitfalls and Complications

1. Hematoma, often heralded by unusual pain, should be drained immediately. Otherwise, subsequent fibrosis may produce deformity, infection, chondritis, or cartilage necrosis.
2. Pain is unusual. Beware of hematoma or infection.
3. Mersilene suture extrusion, usually antihelical, is reported in as many as 8% of cases. Careful technique and antibiotic wound irrigation can reduce the incidence.
4. Hypertrophic scar or keloid formation can occur with overly aggressive skin excision in predisposed patients. Triamcinolone acetonide, (Kenalog; 20 mg/mL) injected intradermally may control the amount of collagen deposited.
5. Antihelical ridging may follow posterior cartilage scoring or misplacement of an antihelical suture.

Postoperative Care Issues

1. Remove dressing and inspect wound on the first postoperative day. Any small hematoma may be expressed by releasing a skin suture. The dressing may be left off in adults but should be replaced for 3 to 4 more days in children.
2. After the dressing is removed, a head band is worn continuously for 2 weeks and at night only for an additional 4 to 6 weeks.
3. Measure the ears with the patient on the table at the end of the procedure and postoperatively. Expect an average loss of correction of 4 to 5 mm at the upper pole. A difference between the two ears of less than 3 mm is usually not perceived as an asymmetry.

References

Adamson PA, McGraw BL, Tropper GJ. Otoplasty: critical review of clinical results. Laryngoscope 1991;101:883.

Adamson PA, McShane DP, Feldman RI. Otoplasty: an update. J Otolaryngol 1987;16:258.

Adamson PA, Tropper GJ, McGraw BL. Otoplasty. In: Krause CJ, ed. Aesthetic facial surgery. Philadelphia: JB Lippincott, 1991.

After the helical portion of the horizontal mattress has been placed, the pull of the suture is varied from superior to inferior to determine the best line of tension for creation of the antihelical fold. Any tendency toward ridging of the helical cartilage is determined, and that line of pull is avoided. The location for optimal helical furling is marked by the index finger, and the ear is everted. The medial placement of the horizontal mattress is near the junction of the conchal wall and conchal floor, creating the antihelical fold (Fig. 159-5). A full-thickness bite of cartilage and lateral perichondrium is taken.

The first antihelical suture is usually placed at the level of the helical root to create the superior crus of the antihelical fold. The second suture, if needed, is placed just inferior to the junction of the superior and inferior crura of the antihelix. Third and fourth sutures can be placed as needed (Fig. 159-6).

Sutures are cinched and tied after they are all in place. The most superior suture is secured first, the more inferior sutures last. The degree of correction is maintained during suture tying by an assistant, who pinches the antihelical fold while the suture is being secured (Fig. 159-7). Care is taken not to overcorrect the antihelix, because this may give an unnatural appearance, with the antihelix lateral to the helical rim. Overtightening of the middle-third antihelical suture can produce a "telephone ear" deformity.

Some overcorrection is necessary at the upper pole, because a loss of as much as 40% of the initial correction may occur during the first postoperative year. Inherent tensile forces within the conchal wall and antihelical fold cause the loss. There is less loss of correction at the middle and lower thirds. To help maintain the correction, a suture placed between the fossa triangularis and the deep temporalis fascia or temporal periosteum is helpful. This suture is placed after all other sutures have been tied. The surgeon's index finger marks the optimal spot for suture placement in the fossa triangularis, and a 4-0 Mersilene suture is driven through the cartilage and lateral perichondrium. The horizontal mattress is then completed by driving a deep bite through the temporalis muscle into the deep temporal periosteum, and the suture is tied.

A special problem occurs with overly projected ear lobes. The ear lobe position may improve somewhat with conchal setback, but it can be worsened by overcorrection of the middle third of the ear. Occasionally, further medialization is desirable. In this case, the cauda helix can be incised sharply (Fig. 159-8), and a 4-0 Mersilene horizontal mattress suture placed between the cauda helix and the inferior concha cavum (Fig. 159-9). For a technique to reduce the size of the lobe, see Procedure 160.

After correction of prominent ears, the anterior portion of the postauricular skin excision may need tailoring to minimize standing tissue cones (ie, dog-ear defects). Burow's triangle excisions effectively trim the redundant skin (Fig. 159-10).

Hemostasis is obtained with bipolar cautery to minimize injury to the perichondrium. The wound is irrigated with a gentamycin solution and closed with interrupted, intradermal 4-0 chromic catgut sutures. Antibiotic ointment is applied to the closed wound, and cotton saturated with mineral oil and peroxide is molded to the lateral surface of the ear and into the postauricular sulcus (Fig. 159-11). A mastoid pressure dressing is applied. No drain is used.

PETER A. ADAMSON
MINAS S. CONSTANTINIDES

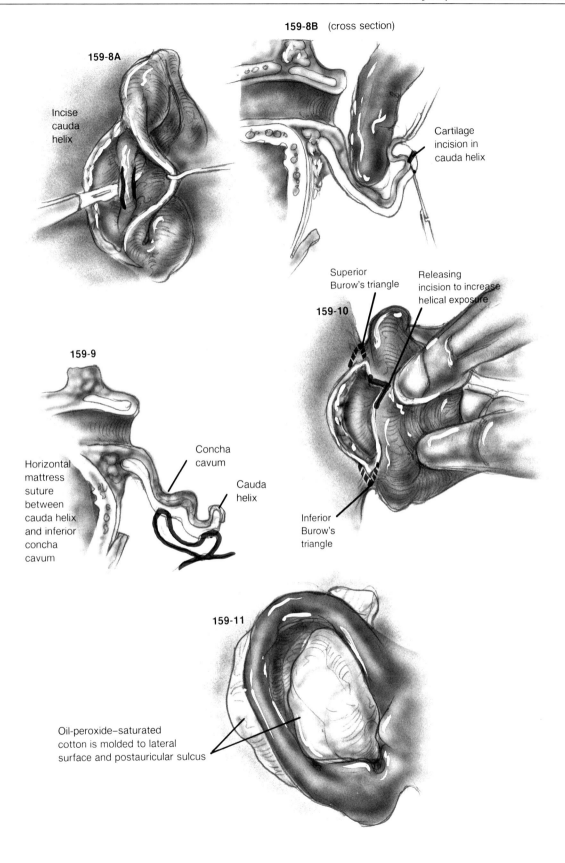

159-8B (cross section)

159-8A

Incise
cauda
helix

Cartilage
incision in
cauda helix

Superior
Burow's triangle

Releasing
incision to increase
helical exposure

159-10

159-9

Horizontal
mattress
suture
between
cauda helix
and inferior
concha
cavum

Concha
cavum

Cauda
helix

Inferior
Burow's
triangle

159-11

Oil-peroxide–saturated
cotton is molded to lateral
surface and postauricular sulcus

■ *160.* OTOPLASTY REFINEMENT TECH-
NIQUES—Surgical remodeling of gross asymmetry or bilateral, unappealing excesses of the helix, auricle, or lobe

Indications
1. Helical prominences
   a. Superior outer helical rim cartilage excess (ie, elf ears, Spock ears)
   b. Superior helical fold cartilage excess (ie, lop ear)
2. Deficient helical fold
   a. Cartilage present but not furled, so no groove exists between the helical fold and the scapha
   b. No helical fold due to cartilage deficiency
3. Large ear lobe; fibrofatty laxity causes increased lobe ptosis with aging
4. Large auricle

Contraindications
1. Minor asymmetries are common and aesthetically acceptable.
2. Antihelical sutures may prevent scaphal reductions.
3. History of keloids
4. Unrealistic expectations

Special Considerations
1. Cartilage cutting techniques and cartilage scoring may lead to visible irregularities.

Preoperative Preparation
1. Careful measurements of auricular size and deformities
2. Photography: full frontal, full right, left lateral, and close-up right and left lateral views
3. Construction of a model of the "normal" ear with exposed x-ray film for easy intraoperative comparison and accurate determination of the amount of reduction desired

Special Instruments, Position, and Anesthesia
1. Face and both ears are draped into the sterile field.
2. General anesthesia for children, and local anesthesia with intravenous sedation for adults
3. Local infiltration anesthesia with epinephrine

Tips and Pearls
1. Mark twice; cut once.
2. Suture meticulously.
3. Seek perfection; accept improvement.

Pitfalls and Complications
1. Follow the wound closely for hematoma, infection, or chondritis. Treat problems aggressively with drainage and antibiotics.
2. Treat hypertrophic or keloid scars with topical steroid tape (Cordran) or intradermal triamcinolone acetonide (Kenalog; 20 mg/mL).
3. Meticulous surgery avoids irregularities and asymmetries.

Postoperative Care Issues
1. Antibiotic ointment improves epithelial migration.
2. Inspect the wound on the first postoperative day. For children, the dressing is replaced for 3 more days.

References
Adamson PA, Tropper GJ, McGraw BL. Otoplasty. In: Krause CJ, ed. Aesthetic facial surgery. Philadelphia: JB Lippincott, 1991;707.
Tanzer RC. Deformities of the auricle: congenital deformities. In: Converse JM, ed. Reconstructive plastic surgery. Philadelphia: WB Saunders, 1977;1703.

Operative Procedure
Reduction of Helical Prominences
The helical rim may contain excess cartilage that alters the smooth rim contour and distorts the symmetry achieved by setback otoplasty (see Procedures 158 and 159). Most refinements are performed as the final step in otoplasty, or they can be performed independently. The patient is placed supine, and the face and both ears are prepped and draped into the sterile field. The helix is injected with local anesthetic containing epinephrine.

A helical prominence on the outer helical rim causes the rim to be angulated (ie, Spock ears). A fusiform incision is made on the outer helical rim directly over the prominence. The skin is undermined over the prominence, the excess cartilage shaved (Fig. 160-1), and excess skin trimmed.

Excess helical cartilage may distort the helical fold on the lateral aspect of the helix (ie, Darwin's tubercle). An incision is made under the fold to allow dissection up over the helical rim. The skin is elevated and excess cartilage trimmed (see Fig. 160-1). Skin is trimmed from the upper flap to allow adequate draping over the helical rim. The incision is closed with interrupted 6-0 nylon. No pressure dressing is required.

Improvement of a Deficient Helical Fold
An effaced helical rim can be rolled to provide better definition. If there is adequate cartilage length, an incision is made on the medial surface of the auricle, the medial skin is undermined, and the medial cartilage is scored to bend it into the desired shape. The skin is closed with 5-0 fast-absorbing catgut. A dental roll is placed into the new groove on the lateral surface and tied with a 2-0 nylon to another roll placed opposite it on the medial surface with a through-and-through horizontal mattress suture. The rolls are removed in 7 days.

If there is a helical cartilage deficiency, simply scoring the medial cartilage may not provide sufficient improvement. An incision is made on the medial surface of the scapha parallel to the helical rim. The skin is undermined to the rim and just onto the lateral surface of the cartilage. This skin flap is then advanced and doubled onto itself, reforming the helical rim (Fig. 160-2). A buried 4-0 polyglycolic acid suture (Dexon, Vicryl) apposes both dermal surfaces. For more severe deficiencies, a cartilage graft may provide stability to the new helical rim. The donor area of the medial scapha is left to heal secondarily if small, or it is covered with a full-thickness skin graft from a postauricular donor site. Apposing dental rolls maintain the correction for 7 days.

Reduction of the Large Ear Lobe
The large ear lobe is refined best with a simple fusiform wedge excision and closure (Fig. 160-3). The new lobe size is marked on the ear lobe anteriorly and posteriorly in a curvilinear fusiform fashion. The lobe is injected with local anesthetic. The skin and soft tissue excision is executed in a V-shaped wedge. Simple 6-0 Nylon sutures are used for closure and removed in 6 days.

Reduction of a Large Scapha
Careful preoperative measurements, augmented by construction of a model of the smaller ear with exposed x-ray film for easy intraoperative comparison, allows accurate determination of the amount of scaphal reduction desired. An offset pentagonal wedge excision is marked near the junction of the upper third and middle third of the helical rim (Fig. 160-4). A through-and-through excision is made, removing lateral skin, full-thickness cartilage, and medial skin. The cartilage is cut back slightly more than the skin to allow a tension-free closure. The step at the junction of the helical rim and scapha breaks up the incision, which is important for scar camouflage and prevention of scar contracture across the helical rim. The wound is closed with one or two polyglycolic acid (Dexon, Vicryl) cartilage sutures to decrease wound tension. Interrupted 6-0 nylon sutures are used laterally and interrupted 5-0 fast-absorbing catgut sutures medially. A light pressure dressing is placed.

Other techniques for reducing the size of a large scapha include excisions of various portions of the helical rim coupled with crescent-shaped excisions of the scapha (see Fig. 160-4*B*).

PETER A. ADAMSON
MINAS S. CONSTANTINIDES

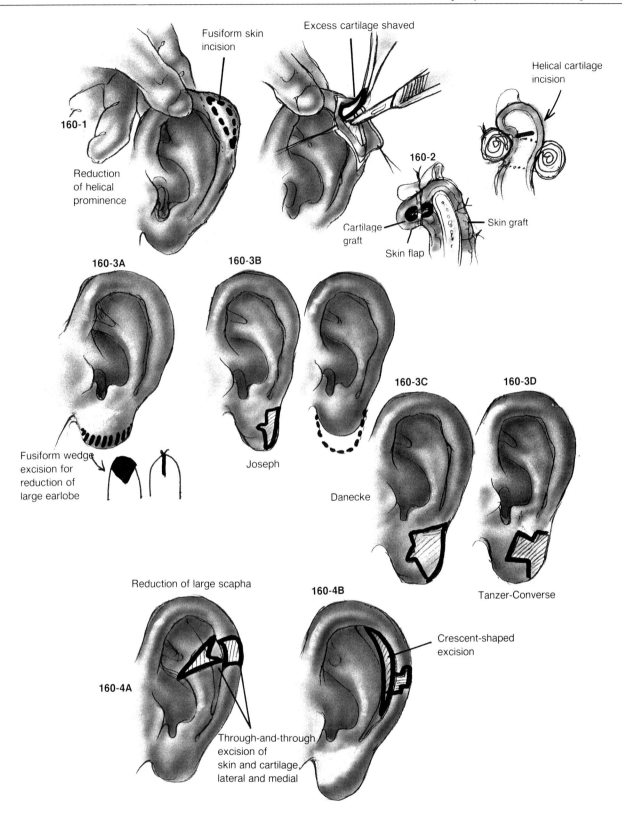

160-1 Reduction of helical prominence

Fusiform skin incision

Excess cartilage shaved

160-2

Helical cartilage incision

Cartilage graft

Skin flap

Skin graft

160-3A

Fusiform wedge excision for reduction of large earlobe

160-3B

Joseph

160-3C

Danecke

160-3D

Tanzer-Converse

Reduction of large scapha

160-4A

160-4B

Crescent-shaped excision

Through-and-through excision of skin and cartilage, lateral and medial

■ 161. PARTIAL AND TOTAL AVULSIONS OF THE AURICLE—

For preserving tissue and reconstituting the ear after a partial avulsion, tunnel, pocket, and fenestration approaches are used. Total avulsion of the auricle can be approached by suturing of the auricle back into position, a pocket technique, microvascular replantation, and the use of a turnover flap from the temporoparietal area.

Indications
1. Abnormal placement, proportion, and contour of the ear
2. Primary repair of the traumatized ear

Contraindications
1. None, although the same technique may not work for all patients.

Special Considerations
1. Tissue preservation is paramount.
2. Auricular segments should be kept in clean saline for later use in surgery.
3. Preoperative and posttreatment photographs should be obtained.

Preoperative Preparation
1. Meticulous cleaning and removal of dirt and foreign materials to prevent infection or tattooing
2. Antibiotic and tetanus prophylaxis

Special Instruments, Position, and Anesthesia
1. Anesthesia varies, with some patients requiring general anesthesia and others managed with a field block around the ear.

(continued)

Operative Procedure

The patient is brought to the operating room, and general or sedation anesthesia is obtained. Field blocks around the ear with a 1% solution of lidocaine, with or without a 1:100,000 dilution of epinephrine, are also placed. The operative site is meticulously cleaned with antibiotic soap and painted with Betadine or benzalkonium chloride solution. The field is then draped sterilely, including enough surrounding area for any flap or grafts that may be needed.

Partial Avulsions

Partial avulsions of the ear typically involve a loss of part of the helix and surrounding tissue. Techniques for preserving this tissue and reconstituting the ear are the tunnel, pocket, and fenestration approaches. All of these aim to support the avulsed segment by placing it in contact with subcutaneous tissue of the mastoid and temporal area while new vascular channels develop at the reattached margins.

For the tunnel procedure, all epithelium of the avulsed segment is removed down to the perichondrium by dissection or with a dermabrasion unit. A postauricular incision is made and the tissues undermined, creating a pocket (Fig. 161-1A). The anterior edge of the incision is sutured to the posterior aspect of the auricular wound, creating a tunnel, and the denuded segment then sutured to the auricular stump (Fig. 161-1B). The posterior edge of the incision is then sutured to the anterior margin of the wound to cover the replanted segment (Fig. 161-1C). In 3 to 6 weeks, the posterior aspect of the new lateral skin can be released and a skin graft applied to the back of the ear and the mastoid-temporal area.

When the pocket procedure is used, the epithelium is not completely removed, as in the tunnel procedure, and the mastoid skin is not transferred onto the anterior ear surface. In this approach, the epidermis alone is removed from the amputated segment by dermabrasion. The avulsed segment is reattached to the auricular stump with 5-0 clear Prolene through the cartilage and 6-0 Prolene or 5-0 Vicryl in the skin (Fig. 161-2A). A postauricular subcutaneous pocket is created as in the tunnel procedure (Fig. 161-2B). The postauricular skin is then advanced over the denuded segment and sutured to the anterior wound margin, burying the segment in the pocket (Fig. 161-2C).

The ear remains in the pocket for 10 days to 4 weeks. The lateral or anterior surface of the ear is then exposed by pushing back the covering skin. The auricular surface is kept coated with antibiotic ointment as it epithelializes from the dermis that remains. The posterior or medial attachment of the ear is not disturbed during this procedure; it is allowed to remain in place for another week and then it is released by blunt dissection. The postauricular skin flap can then be replaced into its anatomic position. The advantages of this approach are that the skin-cartilage relation is not disturbed and the delicate contour of the ear is well preserved.

Another approach to partial avulsion is to remove the skin from the posterior surface of the avulsed auricle and create several 1-cm fenestrations in the cartilage, as described by Baudet. The segment is sutured back into position on the auricle. A flap of retroauricular skin is raised, and the denuded posterior surface of the auricle is secured to the periosteal and subcutaneous recipient bed. This area supplies nourishment to the segment while revascularization occurs along the suture line. The auricle can be released after about 3 to 4 weeks, taking the postauricular flap with it to supply coverage to the posterior surface of the helix. A skin graft is then applied to the donor area.

Total Avulsion

Total avulsion of the auricle presents a much more difficult problem and can be approached in four ways. Simple suturing of the auricle back into position is successful only in rare cases and cannot be recommended as a useful technique. The previously described pocket technique can salvage the ear when microvascular replantation is not available or impossible, but it is not as reliable for the entire

(continued)

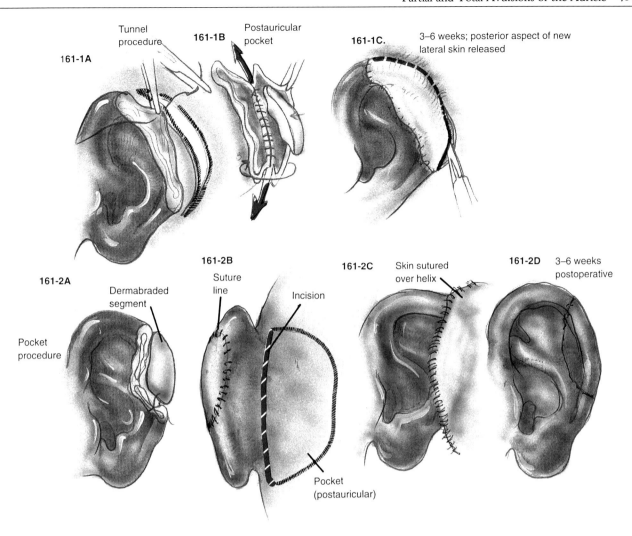

Tunnel
procedure

161-1A

161-1B   Postauricular
pocket

161-1C.   3–6 weeks; posterior aspect of new
lateral skin released

161-2A

Pocket
procedure

Dermabraded
segment

161-2B

Suture
line

Incision

Pocket
(postauricular)

161-2C   Skin sutured
over helix

161-2D   3–6 weeks
postoperative

■ 161. PARTIAL AND TOTAL AVULSIONS OF THE AURICLE *(continued)*

Tips and Pearls

1. Avoid overly compressive dressings that may cause ischemia.

Pitfalls and Complications

1. Necrosis of the reattached tissue
2. Infection
3. Secondary cosmetic deformity caused by thickening and other changes in the ear after reconstruction

Postoperative Care

1. Basic postoperative care includes routine wound care with prophylactic antibiotics, as indicated, and with close observation of the reattached segment for viability.

References

Baudet J. Successful replantation of a large severed ear fragment. Plast Reconstr Surg 1973;51:82.

Jenkins AM, Finucan T. Primary nonmicrosurgical reconstruction following ear avulsion using the temporoparietal fascial island flap. Plast Reconstr Surg 1989;87:148.

Mladick RA, Carraway JH. Ear reattachment by the modified pocket principle. Plast Reconstr Surg 1973;51:584.

Turpin IM. Microsurgical replantation of the external ear. Clin Plast Surg 1990;17:397.

auricle as it is for smaller segments. Microvascular repair of the ear and use of a turnover flap from the temporoparietal area are other alternatives.

Successful microvascular reanastomosis provides the best long-term results. It recreates a normal-appearing ear, avoiding the contractures and distortions sometimes caused by other techniques. Unfortunately, failure of a microvascular replantation usually results in total loss of the autogenous cartilage and creates a significant secondary reconstruction burden. The major limiting factors preventing more successful microvascular repairs have been technical difficulties, the small size of the auricular vessels, and the overall condition of the avulsed segment, with skin and subcutaneous tissue loss or damaged vessels precluding microvascular repair.

The amputated auricle must be kept clean in cold saline while a search for suitable vessels on the ear and in the donor area is undertaken. The vascular supply to the auricle derives from the superficial temporal artery through one or two anterior auricular arteries into the ascending helix and posterior auricular arteries that course around the inferior part of the concha. These vessels follow the nerves to the ear, which are often easier to find. Frequently, only arteries can be identified during the initial search, and veins become apparent after arterial inflow is reestablished.

Using the microvascular technique, as described in Procedure 262, vessels are repaired using 11-0 nylon sutures under the microscope with a 150-mm lens. Size discrepancy is common and can be overcome by using the "fish-mouth" or "spatula" techniques. Interposition vein grafts are sometimes needed and can be obtained from other sites. Postoperative monitoring includes frequent visual inspection with the use of flow indicators such as thermocouple probes or laser Doppler flow measurements.

The major cause of graft failure remains venous congestion and thrombosis. A loading dose of 5000 units of heparin is followed by 1000 units/hour to keep the partial thromboplastin time between 1.5 to 2 times the control. Treatment with heparin, aspirin, dextrans, and dipyridamole continues for 4 to 10 days to minimize the chance of graft failure. Medicinal leeches or relaxing incisions may sometimes be needed. Reexploration is usually not effective and can lead to further vascular damage. Prophylactic antibiotics, such as a first-generation cephalosporin, are strongly recommended, or if leeches are required, ciprofloxacin or Septra to prevent *Aeromonas* infection.

The temporoparietal fascia flap is an axial flap based on the superficial temporal artery. It is frequently used to cover rib cartilage grafts and to supply vascular support to skin grafts in congenital auricular atresia cases. After the patient is prepared, the direction of the superficial temporal artery is traced with the Doppler probe. The flap is marked out with wide margins to ensure coverage of the medial and lateral surfaces of the cartilage (Fig. 161-3*A*). The cranial margin must be high enough to allow the flap to be turned without kinking the vascular pedicle and to avoid blunting the superior auricular sulcus as much as possible. An incision is made up into the the temporal area, and the skin and subcutaneous tissue are elevated, exposing the temporoparietal fascia. The fascia is elevated off the muscle preserving the veins that lie on the outer surface and is then ready to be turned over (Fig. 161-3*B*).

The skin of the amputated ear may be dissected free and saved if it is in good condition to cover the cartilage and flap. Otherwise, a postauricular graft from the opposite side or a split-thickness graft from another site can be used, using fine Vicryl or Prolene sutures. The fascial flap is draped over the replanted cartilage and sutured into position. The skin that was saved is then sutured into position as a free graft and secured with bolsters or a foam stent (Fig. 161-3*C*). Long-term results of this approach are fairly good, and the risk of failure is low. Aggressive splinting ensures good contour with less bulkiness and distortion.

BRIAN F. GIBSON

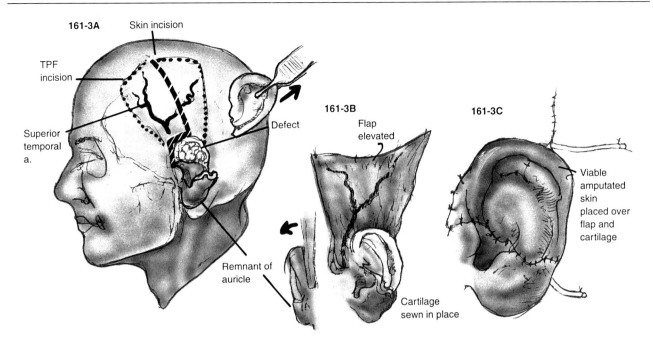

161-3A

TPF incision

Skin incision

Superior temporal a.

Defect

Remnant of auricle

161-3B

Flap elevated

Cartilage sewn in place

161-3C

Viable amputated skin placed over flap and cartilage

■ 162. AURICULAR HEMATOMA

Collection of fluid between the auricular perichondrium and cartilage, most commonly seen in competitive wrestlers, boxers, and victims of falls, motor vehicle accidents, or assaults

Indications

1. Drainage of the hematoma is necessary to prevent compromised blood flow to cartilage, inflammation, and eventual neocartilage formation (ie, cauliflower ear).

Contraindications

1. Untreated bleeding disorders may be the only contraindication to open drainage of an auricular hematoma. In these cases, aspiration and placement of a pressure dressing could be substituted.

Special Instruments, Position, and Anesthesia

1. Fine forceps including Adson, Griffiths-Brown, Bishop-Harman, and Castroviejo; #15 scalpel; small curved hemostats; and a needle holder such as a Halsey or Webster type.
2. Local anesthesia with 1% lidocaine and 1:100,000 epinephrine; some surgeons prefer not to use epinephrine on the auricle because of possible ischemia.
3. Common sutures include 3-0 silk and 3-0 or 4-0 Prolene.

Tips and Pearls

1. Complete evacuation of the hematoma is essential to avoid inflammation and infection.

Pitfalls and Complications

1. Incomplete drainage
2. Reaccumulation of fluid
3. Infection

Postoperative Care

1. Local wound care with the application of antibiotic ointment several times a day
2. Systemic antibiotics, such as cephalexin, for 7 days
3. Removal of the bolster dressing in 10 days to 2 weeks

References

Giffin CS. Wrestler's ear: pathophysiology and treatment. Ann Plast Surg 1992;28:131–139.

Schuller DE, Dankle SD, Strauss RH. A technique to treat wrestlers' auricular hematoma without interrupting training or competition. Arch Otolaryngol Head Neck Surg 1989;115:202–206.

Starck WJ, Kaltman SI. Current concepts in the surgical management of traumatic auricular hematoma. J Oral Maxillofac Surg 1992;50: 800–802.

Operative Procedure

Drainage of auricular hematomas can be easily performed in the office setting. The patient is brought to the procedure room and placed in supine position on the operating chair. A plastic fenestrated ear drape or towels are used to keep hair out of the field, and skin preparation is performed with Betadine or other antibacterial solution. Local anesthesia is obtained by infiltrating the skin of the lateral and medial sides of the pinna with a 1% solution of lidocaine with or without a 1:100,000 dilution of epinephrine.

Some physicians advocate needle aspiration of the fluid under aseptic conditions followed by application of a compressive dressing. This approach is complicated by reaccumulation of fluid in many cases. Definitive care for these injuries is best accomplished by incision and drainage. The hematoma is most often drained through a 0.5- to 1-cm incision in the conchal skin curved to parallel the antihelical fold. Depending on where the hematoma is found (Fig. 162-1), the incision for drainage can be camouflaged by placing it anterior to the helical rim, within the cymba concha, or on the posterior surface (Fig. 162-2).

The hematoma can be expressed through the incision, and a hemostat is used to ensure that any loculated areas are broken down (Fig. 162-3). If the perichondrium overlying the hematoma is thickened and inflamed, it should be debrided before closure to prevent later deformity of the ear. Neocartilage formation may begin about 7 to 10 days after injury. When draining hematomas that have been present for some time, it may also be necessary to curet or dermabrade the underlying cartilage to sculpt a more normal-appearing ear. After the hematoma is drained, the cavity is irrigated with saline solution and the skin replaced into position.

Dental rolls are placed as a compressive dressing (Fig. 162-4). The first roll is cut to overlie the area of skin in the concha undermined by the hematoma. A smaller piece is used on the medial surface of the auricle. A 3-0 or 4-0 Prolene suture is passed through the lateral dental roll and then through the auricular skin, near the superior edge of the hematoma cavity. It is brought through the cartilage and medial skin and then through the medial roll. The suture is passed back through the medial roll, auricle, and lateral roll, creating a mattress suture (Fig. 162-5). A similar suture is placed inferiorly. If the area is too large for a single pair of rolls to cover, a second pair can be placed in a similar fashion.

The wound and ear are dressed with antibiotic ointment and a mastoid-type dressing that is left in place overnight and then removed. Patients can resume exercise on the same day that the hematoma is drained. A systemic antistaphylococcal antibiotic is taken for 7 days. Local wound care with reapplication of the ointment several times a day is done at home. The patient returns to have the dressing removed in 10 days to 2 weeks.

F. BRIAN GIBSON

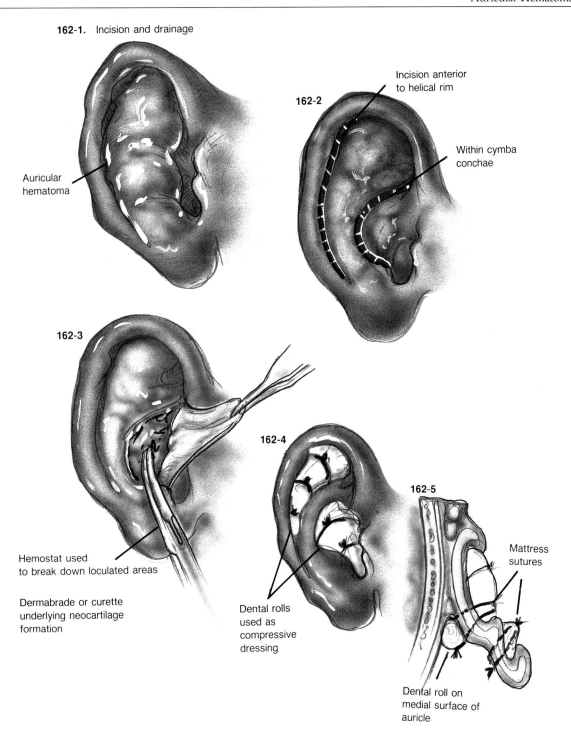

162-1. Incision and drainage

Auricular hematoma

162-2

Incision anterior to helical rim

Within cymba conchae

162-3

Hemostat used to break down loculated areas

Dermabrade or curette underlying neocartilage formation

162-4

Dental rolls used as compressive dressing

162-5

Mattress sutures

Dental roll on medial surface of auricle

■ 163. NASAL–FACIAL ANALYSIS

Evaluation of the aesthetic parameters of the nose and their proportions in relation to the remainder of the face. A method of objective measurements rather than subjective assessment is important for surgical planning and for postoperative evaluation of results.

Indications

1. Preoperative assessment for rhinoplasty or nasal reconstruction
2. Preoperative planning for orthognathic surgery
3. Preoperative planning for genioplasty or chin augmentation

Special Considerations

1. Cleft lip rhinoplasty
2. Occlusal or bite abnormalities
3. Facial malformations or significant asymmetries

Preoperative Preparation

1. Clinical examination of overall facial symmetry and proportion
2. Assessment of modifiers of aesthetic parameters, such as age, sex, race, and body habitus
3. Photographic documentation for soft tissue analysis, including full face frontal, laterals, obliques, and base views of the nose
4. Cephalometric analysis for orthognathic or occlusal abnormalities
5. Video-computer analysis useful for assessment and visualization of potential effects of proposed changes in parameters

Tips and Pearls

1. Special parameters
   a. Facial thirds for vertical facial symmetry
   b. Facial width to length ratio
   c. Facial angles: nasofrontal, nasofacial, nasolabial, mentocervical
   d. Nasal tip projection, rotation, nasal length, nasal length to width ratio
   e. Alar base width, lobule to columellar ratio, alar to lobule ratio, alar–columellar relationship
2. Mark anatomic reference points on the anterior and lateral facial views before assessment.
3. On the frontal view, consider facial symmetry, facial shape, and facial third proportions, and notice nasal deviations. Measure the basal width of the nasal bones and nasal base, and the width to length ratio of the nose.
4. On the profile view, evaluate the overall facial contour and occlusal relations. Assess the nasion position, the nasofrontal angle, and the dorsal nasal profile. Measure the nasal tip rotation, projection and nasal length, and the nasofacial and nasolabial angles. Look at the alar to lobule ratio of the nasal base and the degree of columellar show.
5. On the basilar view of the nose, look at the shape of the nose and the nostrils. Measure the columellar to lobule ratio and the lobule width to alar width ratio.

References

McGraw-Wall BL. Facial analysis. In: Bailey BJ, ed. Head and neck surgery—otolaryngology. Philadelphia: JB Lippincott, 1993:2070.

Powell N, Humphries B. Proportions of the aesthetic face. New York: Thieme-Stratton, 1984.

Operative Procedure

Thorough nasal–facial analysis allows the surgeon to identify and define specific facial disproportions and to establish surgical goals for their correction. Nasal–facial analysis for rhinoplasty requires assessment of soft tissue proportions and the relation of the major facial aesthetic masses to the nose. Computer imaging also allows the surgeon to estimate the effects of surgical changes without the tedious tracing and outlining required when using patient photographs or cephalograms. Reference points should be identified and marked on anterior and lateral views of the face for the analysis (Fig. 163-1).

Overall facial balance is first assessed on the frontal view of the face by evaluating for asymmetries between the two sides. Assess the length and proportion of the face by dividing it into thirds from the trichion to the glabella (G), the glabella to the subnasale (Sn), and the subnasale to the menton (M). Each third should be approximately equal (Fig. 163-2). The width of the face may be divided into fifths, and each one fifth should equal one interpalpebral distance. The facial profile is measured relative to the Frankfurt horizontal, which passes through the nasion (N). The subnasale and pogonion (Pg) of the chin should rest on or slightly posterior to a perpendicular line (ie, 0° meridian line) dropped from this horizontal (see Fig. 163-1). A general evaluation of the occlusion using Angle's classification is done at this time.

Specific assessment of the nose begins by considering the frontal view. The overall facial shape, gender, race, and body habitus affect the ideal proportions of the nose. Asymmetries and any dorsal nasal curvatures or deviations are noted. The widths of the nasal bones and the nasal base are assessed. The base of the nose between alar grooves should approximate the interpalpebral distance. Wider alar widths are acceptable in Asian and black populations. The bony base width should be about 2 mm less than the interalar. The ratio of nasal base width to length (from nasion to tip defining point [Tp]) on frontal view ideally equals 70% (Fig. 163-3).

On the nasal profile, the nasion should be located at the upper eyelid lash line, and it should lie 4 to 6 mm posterior to the glabella. The nasofrontal angle (NFA) should be measured at the nasion (N); optimally, the NFA should be 115° to 130° (see Fig. 163-4). Any dorsal hump deformities or deficiencies should be identified. The height of the nasal dorsum should ideally lie 1 to 2 mm below a line drawn from N to Tp.

Nasal tip rotation is the degree of inclination of the columella from the upper lip. It is measured as the nasolabial angle (NLA), which has the subnasale as its vertex (Fig. 163-4). The NLA has one arm through the superior vermilion border (Sn-Vs) and the other arm through the columellar point (Sn-Cm), which is the anteriormost projecting point of the columella. Ideally, the NLA measures 90° to 105° in men and 100° to 120° in women.

Projection is the extent of anterior protrusion of the nasal tip from the anterior facial plane. This can be indirectly measured using the nasofacial angle (NFcA). The NFcA is measured by intersecting a line drawn from the glabella to pogonion with a line tangent to the nasal dorsum (see Fig. 163-4). A value of 36° is considered optimal. A quick way to estimate the ideal nasal tip projection is to compare it with the length of the upper lip. Nasal length is defined as the distance along the nasal dorsum to the Tp. Tip projection, rotation, and nasal length interact such that increasing rotation effectively increases projection but decreases nasal length.

On the lateral view of the alar base, the alar to lobule proportion should be evaluated; a 1:1 ratio is most desirable (Fig. 163-5). The degree of columellar show should be approximately 2 to 4 mm. The cause of excess or deficiencies of columellar show should be evaluated. On the basilar view, the nasal base should resemble an equilateral triangle, with the columella dividing it into two right triangles (see Fig. 163-5). Vertically, the columella to lobule ratio should be 2:1. The width of the lobule should measure about 75% of the width of the entire nasal base.

BECKY L. MCGRAW-WALL

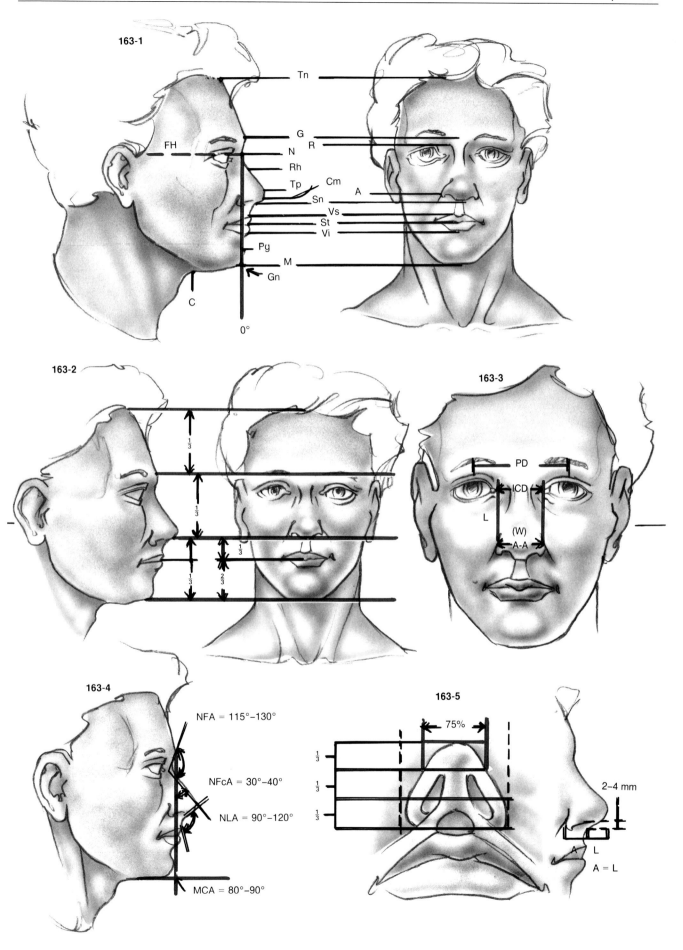

163-1

Tn
G
R
FH — N
Rh
Tp   Cm
Sn
A
Vs
St
Vi
Pg
M
Gn
C
0°

163-2

$\frac{1}{3}$
$\frac{1}{3}$
$\frac{1}{3}$
$\frac{1}{3}$
$\frac{2}{3}$

163-3

PD
ICD
L
(W)
A-A

163-4

NFA = 115°–130°

NFcA = 30°–40°

NLA = 90°–120°

MCA = 80°–90°

163-5

75%

$\frac{1}{3}$
$\frac{1}{3}$
$\frac{1}{3}$

2–4 mm

A
L
A = L

■ 164. LOCAL ANESTHESIA FOR NASAL SURGERY

—Technique of obtaining transient control of sensation to a defined portion of the nose

Indications

1. Rhinoplasty and nasal reconstruction
2. Septoplasty, with submucous resection
3. Transnasal surgical approaches

Contraindications

1. History of adverse reaction to local or topical anesthetic agents
2. Poorly cooperative patients or patients with panic disorders or claustrophobia

Special Considerations

1. May be used as sole anesthesia, with intravenous sedation, or as an adjunct to general anesthesia
2. Caution in patients with hypertension, cardiac abnormalities, hyperthyroidism (ie, hypersensitive to epinephrine), or liver disease (ie, slowed metabolism of agents)
3. Local anesthetic with epinephrine may produce severe, prolonged hypertension in patients on monoamine oxidase inhibitors (eg, Parnate), tricyclic antidepressants (eg, Elavil), carbamazepine (eg, Tegretol) or cyclobenzaprine (eg, Flexeril).

Preoperative Preparation

1. Lessen patient anxiety by explaining all details of local anesthesia and the planned procedure in advance.
2. Premedication with analgesic and antianxiety agents
3. Establish intravenous line for emergency access and medication delivery.

Special Instruments

1. Flat cotton pledgets or thin strip (0.5-in [1-cm]) gauze
2. Use of 27-gauge, 1.5-in (3.8-cm) needles and 5- or 10-mL syringe.
3. Continuous monitoring of cardiac rhythm, oxygen saturation, respiratory rate, and blood pressure

Tips and Pearls

1. Use the lowest concentration and volume that provides satisfactory anesthesia.
2. Ensure correct place of injection to minimize volume and prevent distortion of anatomy.
3. Plan incisions, and mark important anatomic details before injection.
4. Allow adequate time, at least 5 to 10 minutes, for the anesthetic and vasoconstrictive effect.
5. Careful monitoring of the level of sedation and pain control, with additional medication as necessary

Pitfalls and Complications

1. Overdose may occur from excessive dosing, rapid infusion, or inadvertent intravascular injection. Symptoms of lidocaine overdose include confusion, excitability, apprehension, tremor, convulsion, and respiratory disturbances. Symptoms of epinephrine toxicity include anxiety, restlessness, throbbing headache, pallor, and palpitations.
2. Inadequate injection or poor pain control
3. Allergic or idiopathic reaction (rare)
4. Prolonged procedure, with loss of effectiveness

Postoperative Care Issues

1. Continued monitoring until the patient is fully awake
2. Continued postoperative pain control with oral or parenteral medication as the local anesthetic effect declines

References

Calhoun KH. Introduction to rhinoplasty. In: Bailey J, ed. Head and neck surgery—otolaryngology. Philadelphia: JB Lippincott, 1993: 2113.

Hodges JM, Tierney MB. Local anesthesia guidelines for ambulatory surgery, vol 5. In: Johnson JT, Derkay CS, Mandell-Brown MK, Newman RK, eds. Current concepts in otolaryngology. St. Louis: Mosby-Year Book, 1992:25.

Operative Procedure

The surgeon must be familiar with the pharmacologic properties of any agent used for local anesthesia, including the maximum safe volume for any patient. Lidocaine, the most commonly used injectable local anesthetic, is effective in even low concentrations (0.5–1.0%). The addition of epinephrine results in decreased blood flow to the affected area, producing desired vasoconstriction and prolonging the anesthetic's effect. Because absorption is slowed, the addition of epinephrine increases the maximum safe dosage. Topical cocaine provides vasoconstriction and an anesthetic effect. Used in low concentrations (4%) and controlled volumes (≤4 mL), it is a safe topical anesthetic. Some surgeons prefer to use combinations of agents to obtain this same effect. The surgeon should personally check the contents and concentration of all agents used.

Sensory innervation to the nasal dorsum and tip is provided by the fifth cranial nerve through the external ramus of the ophthalmic nerve. The nerve passes deep to the nasal bones and then becomes superficial between the nasal bones and upper lateral cartilages (Fig. 164-1). The infraorbital nerve, a branch of the maxillary division of cranial nerve V, innervates the alae and lateral wall. The external nose is best anesthetized by a field block at the base of the nostrils and dorsum, along with infiltration of the area of the infraorbital foramen. Sensation to the superior lateral intranasal mucosa is supplied by the anterior ethmoidal nerve. The sphenopalatine ganglion, lying just behind and above the posterior end of the middle turbinate, sends sensory fibers from the maxillary division of the fifth cranial nerve to the inferior aspect of the lateral intranasal mucosa. The inferior septal mucosa is innervated by the medial branch of the nasopalatine nerve. Control of pain in these areas depends on careful placement of topical anesthetic agents.

With the patient in a supine position, with the head positioned on a foam doughnut and the neck gently flexed, visualization is obtained with a nasal speculum and focused beam headlight. Four to six flattened cotton pledgets are moistened with a 4% cocaine solution (4 mL total) and then gently slid into the nose with Bayonet forceps (Fig. 164-2). The superior pledget should be placed high in the apex of the triangle formed by the septum and the lateral walls of the nose. Other packs should be placed to maximize contact with the posterior aspect of the middle turbinate and the floor of the nose beneath the inferior turbinate. Time is allowed for the anesthetic effect, while other preparations, including trimming of vibrissae and anatomic marking, are carried out.

Infiltrative anesthesia is begun (Fig. 164-3), placing approximately 1 mL of the lidocaine and epinephrine solution as a field block just lateral to the piriform aperture on each side. The 1.5-in (3.8-cm), 27-gauge needle is advanced up toward the infraorbital foramen, and approximately 1 mL is delivered into this area. It is not necessary to inject directly into the infraorbital canal, because infiltration of the general area is sufficient. The base of the nose near the nasal spine is then injected with less than 1 mL. The dorsum of the nose is anesthetized by advancing the needle from the intercartilaginous area on each side of the nose to the region of the glabella. A small volume (0.5 mL) is injected as the needle is withdrawn. A similar technique is used to inject the lateral osteotomy sites through the piriform aperture area. Injections are performed in the immediate area of the planned incisions. With careful needle placement and controlled volume (<10 mL total), there should be minimal distortion of the nose. Tissue distortion may be further minimized by gentle massage of the soft tissues.

The septal mucosa is anesthetized by a series of submucoperichondrial injections. With correct applications of topical agents and adequate elapsed time, these injections should be relatively well tolerated. The surgeon should see a vascular blanching as the mucosa is infiltrated. It is necessary to infiltrate both sides of the septum and along the floor of the nose.

The cotton pledgets moistened with cocaine are then gently returned to their positions within the nose, and time is allowed to elapse for the anesthetic and vasoconstrictive effect. The diligent surgeon is rewarded with a comfortable patient and an almost bloodless field.

BRUCE A. SCOTT

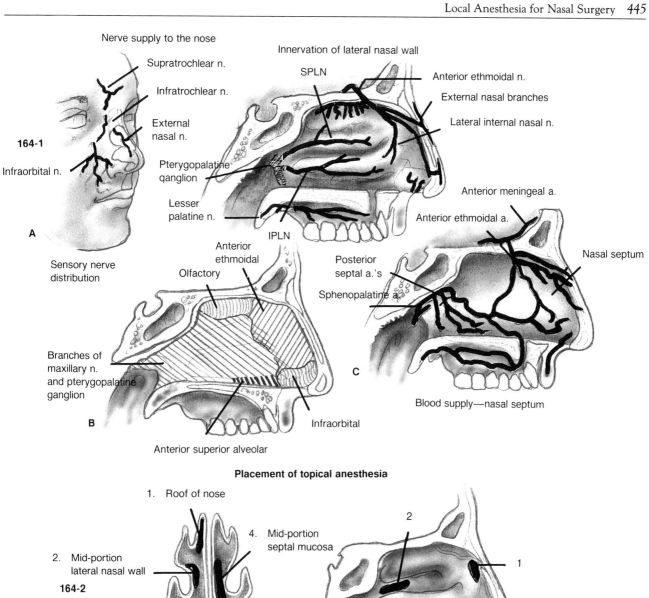

164-1

Nerve supply to the nose

Supratrochlear n.

Infratrochlear n.

External nasal n.

Infraorbital n.

Pterygopalatine ganglion

Lesser palatine n.

IPLN

A

Sensory nerve distribution

Innervation of lateral nasal wall

SPLN

Anterior ethmoidal n.

External nasal branches

Lateral internal nasal n.

Anterior meningeal a.

Anterior ethmoidal a.

Nasal septum

Posterior septal a.'s

Sphenopalatine a.

C

Blood supply—nasal septum

Anterior ethmoidal

Olfactory

Branches of maxillary n. and pterygopalatine ganglion

B

Anterior superior alveolar

Infraorbital

Placement of topical anesthesia

1. Roof of nose

2. Mid-portion lateral nasal wall

164-2

4. Mid-portion septal mucosa

A

3. Floor of nose

2

1

B

3

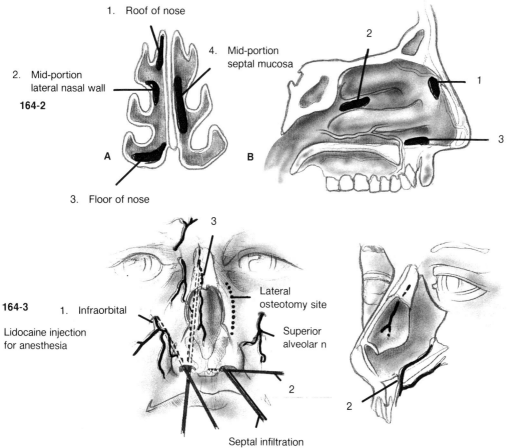

164-3

Lidocaine injection for anesthesia

1. Infraorbital

3

Lateral osteotomy site

Superior alveolar n

2

2

Septal infiltration

■ 165. NASAL SEPTOPLASTY AND SUBMUCOUS RESECTION—Surgical alteration, selective removal, and repositioning of nasal septal cartilage. Submucous resection is a form of septoplasty in which a large amount of obstructing septal cartilage and bony perpendicular plate is removed rather than repositioned.

Indications
1. Nasal obstruction secondary to deviated or obstructing nasal septal cartilage or bone
2. Sleep apnea with contributing nasal obstruction
3. Relief of recurrent septal epistaxis
4. Cosmetic correction of the deviated or twisted nose in conjunction with rhinoplasty.
5. Chronic sinusitis in cases of septal deviation
6. Septal neoplasms (rare)

Special Considerations
1. Patients with rhinitis medicamentosa (must first be treated medically)
2. Patients who abuse cocaine (should not be operated on)
3. Previous septal or nasal surgery
4. Specific sites of deviation: quadrilateral cartilage, vomer, perpendicular plate of ethmoid, anterior nasal spine, and various combinations
5. Whether one or both sides are obstructed
6. Posterior deflection, anterior deflection, or both
7. Concomitant nasal disease (eg, sinusitis)
8. Bleeding or clotting abnormalities
9. Other causes or contributing factors to nasal obstruction, such as nasal valve collapse or enlarged turbinates
10. Prior septal perforations or trauma

Preoperative Preparation
1. Routine laboratory studies
2. Consider allergy studies if allergic disease exists.
3. Consider sleep study if the history suggests sleep apnea.
4. Consider computed tomography scan if sinus disease exists.

(continued)

Operative Procedure
We prefer the technique of septoplasty whenever possible rather than a submucous resection (SMR) for several reasons. Septoplasty better preserves the septal support system and makes the nose more resilient to trauma. The septoplasty technique minimizes the complication of postoperative septal perforation. After SMR, the lack of cartilage support may allow the septal mucosa to move during inspiration toward the side with the highest flow (ie, Bernoulli effect) and may produce obstruction.

This does not mean that all septal cartilage, no matter how deviated, should be straightened and not removed. In many cases, an SMR is much faster and easier than septoplasty and may be the preferred procedure. We routinely remove portions of the quadrilateral cartilage adjacent to the vomer and ethmoid plate and cartilage that cannot be easily straightened or shaved. In this narrative, we use the terminology shown in Figure 165-1.

Most of our septal surgery is performed on an outpatient basis, using local anesthesia and intravenous sedation. The nose is first sprayed with a combination of 2% lidocaine and 1:100,000 epinephrine. After waiting several minutes, two 1 × 3 in (2.5 × 7.5 cm) neurosurgical pledgets soaked in the same anesthetic solution are inserted on each side to provide topical anesthesia and shrink the turbinates. Occasionally, three pledgets are necessary, and some surgeons prefer to use a 4% cocaine solution on the pledgets for topical anesthesia. These are left in place for 5 minutes, and then the septum is infiltrated with a 1% lidocaine and 1:100,000 epinephrine anesthetic solution using a ring syringe with a 2-in (5-cm) 25- or 27-gauge needle. Because the nerve supply to the septum comes equally from both sides, both sides must be injected; 10 mL is usually adequate. The injection should be under the mucoperichondrium so that the mucosa is elevated (ie, hydrodissection) from the bone and cartilage. This approach makes the dissection much easier.

Septal deflections can be classified as anterior to the nasal valve, posterior to the valve, or mixed. To adequately expose and mobilize a deviated anterior nasal septum, the incision must be placed ahead of the obstruction. In this case, a transfixion incision is used (Fig. 165-2). The incision can be made through the mucosa on both sides, or it may be made only on one side and is called a hemitransfixion incision. The incision is made with a #15 blade scalpel in the membranous septum. It should expose the caudal septum from the superior septum down to the nasal spine inferiorly. Using a small Stevens scissors, gentle dissection is performed to locate the cartilaginous end of the septum. A Cottle or Freer elevator is used in a sweeping upward and downward motion to gently elevate the mucoperichondrium of the septum (Fig. 165-3). The proper plane for elevation of the flap is directly on the quadrilateral cartilage, under the perichondrium. The proper layer over the bony septum is under the periosteum, directly on bone. The mucoperiosteal layer is not contiguous with the mucoperichondrium, and raising the septal flap in this junctional area is difficult, and perforations are common.

One technique to avoid this problem is to raise the vomer mucoperiosteal flap as a separate procedure after the quadrilateral cartilage mucoperichondrium has been elevated. After the two flaps have been elevated, the compartments are joined using a #15 blade or the Freer elevator (Figs. 165-4 and 165-5). The remainder of the operation is performed working under this mucoperichondrial-mucoperiosteal flap, which can be raised on one or both sides of the septum.

In anterior deflections, the septum commonly lies on one side of the midline, producing obstruction. Working underneath the mucoperichondrial flaps, we attempt to shave the deviated portion of the septum. Sometimes, it is also necessary to detach the inferior portion of the septal cartilage, weaken or resect a small wedge of cartilage approximately 1 to 1.5 cm posterior to the anterior edge of the cartilage, and swing the cartilage into the midline. The cartilage must be sutured in the midline to the periosteum and soft tissue of the nasal spine with a slowly absorbable stitch, usually 3-0 Vicryl (Fig. 165-6). It may be necessary to drill a small hole in the bony

(continued)

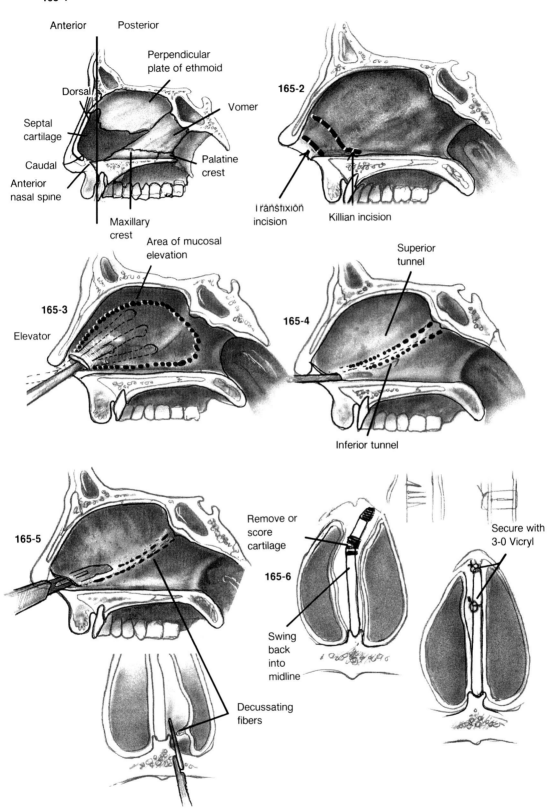

165-1

Anterior   Posterior

Perpendicular
plate of ethmoid

Dorsal

Vomer

Septal
cartilage

Caudal

Palatine
crest

Anterior
nasal spine

Maxillary
crest

165-2

Transfixion
incision

Killian incision

Area of mucosal
elevation

165-3

Elevator

165-4

Superior
tunnel

Inferior tunnel

165-5

Remove or
score
cartilage

165-6

Swing
back
into
midline

Decussating
fibers

Secure with
3-0 Vicryl

■ **165.** NASAL SEPTOPLASTY AND SUBMUCOUS RESECTION *(continued)*

Special Instruments, Position, and Anesthesia

1. Headlight
2. Septorhinoplasty tray should include Freer elevator, Cottle elevator, swivel knife, small 6- to 10-mm Frazier suction tips, 4-mm straight osteotome, Takahashi biting forceps, scalpel, double-action biting Jansen-Middleton forceps, bayonet forceps
3. Slight reverse Trendelenburg position
4. Preoperative vasoconstriction: cocaine, oxymetazoline, or another decongestive agent 10 minutes before beginning the operation

Tips and Pearls

1. Take the time to get in the correct surgical plane, which is bloodless, white, and has a slightly gritty feel. In the correct plane, the operation can be performed extremely rapidly and without mucosal tears.
2. If the mucoperichondrial flap does not elevate easily, the surgeon is in the wrong plane.
3. Small unilateral tears in the mucoperichondrial flap usually heal without sequelae and need not be repaired

Pitfalls and Complications

1. Through-and-through mucosal tears must be avoided and should be repaired when they occur.
2. Septal perforation
3. Loss of septal support and saddle nose deformity
4. Postoperative bleeding may occasionally require packing
5. Cerebrospinal fluid (CSF) rhinorrhea can occur from damage to the cribriform plate during resection of the bony septum.
6. Recurrent or persistent nasal obstruction
7. Septal hematomas should be drained and the nose packed.

Postoperative Care Issues

1. Persistent clear rhinorrhea suggests a CSF leak.
2. Persistent obstruction may be caused by enlarged turbinates.
3. Nasal packing may be required for 24 hours.
4. Splints, when used, are usually removed 5 to 7 days postoperatively.
5. Antistaphylococcal antibiotics should be prescribed if packing or splints are used.

References

Goode RL. Nasal septal surgery. In: Krause CJ, Mangat DS, Pastorek N, eds. Aesthetic facial surgery. Philadelphia: JB Lippincott, 1991.

Price JC. Septoplasty. In: Johns ME, Mattox DE, Miller MM, eds. Atlas of head and neck surgery. Philadelphia: BC Decker, 1990.

anterior nasal spine using a 1-mm microdrill. The suture can then be passed through this hole and the cartilage secured.

If it is difficult to bring the cartilage into the midline, the cartilage can be further weakened by scoring the cartilage on the concave side (Fig. 165-7). This is done by using a cartilage knife or #15 blade to incise the cartilage under the mucoperichondrial flap almost through the cartilage, taking care to leave a small amount of cartilage on the convex side intact. When this is performed, the cartilage straightens, as shown in Figure 165-7. In general, this maneuver of scoring the septal cartilage on the concave side can be used to assist in straightening the cartilage anywhere in the deviated septum. The scoring occasionally must be performed in both horizontal and vertical directions to straighten a septal cartilage that is deviated in more than one plane. This is called crosshatching (Fig. 165-8).

In a patient with an isolated posterior deflection, a Killian incision is made 1 to 1.5 cm behind the end of the caudal septum on the concave side. The mucoperichondrial flap is elevated, and a septoplasty is performed using the techniques of shaving, scoring, and crosshatching described previously. The swinging door technique involves excising any overriding cartilage along the nasal spine and bony perpendicular plate and then swinging the septum into the midline, where it is sutured in place (Fig. 165-9). This is often used in combination with scoring or crosshatching. Any severely deviated cartilage that resists repositioning can be resected safely as long as at least 1 cm of cartilage remains dorsal and anterior (Fig. 165-10).

It is often easier to perform these maneuvers if a mucoperichondrial flap has been elevated on both sides of the septal cartilage. If a transfixion incision is made, the surgery is easily performed by elevating on both sides, as previously described. If a Killian incision has been used, the opposite side is reached by incising the cartilage at an angle and then elevating on the opposite side with the Freer elevator (Fig. 165-11).

Nasal spine deviations are treated by removal of the deviated bone with a 4-mm straight osteotome. The deviated portion of the spine is shaved using the osteotome in a fashion similar to that for fine deviations of the caudal septum. Rarely, when the spine is extremely deviated, it is best to use the chisel to fracture the base of the spine off the premaxilla and move it back into the midline. When this is done, it must be held in position with permanent sutures.

Deviations of the bony perpendicular plate of the septum (ie, vomer and ethmoid) can usually be handled by removing the deviation using Takahashi or biting forceps after elevating bilateral mucoperiosteal flaps (Fig. 165-12). Excessive twisting during this maneuver can fracture the cribriform plate and cause a CSF leak.

The SMR is performed in a manner similar to that described for the septoplasty. Bilateral mucoperichondrial-mucoperiosteal flaps are elevated as described using a transfixion incision or a Killian incision. The deviated portions of the cartilaginous septum and bony septum are removed using a swivel knife, Takahashi forceps, or biting forceps. Most of the cartilaginous septum can be removed if the surgeon is careful to leave at least 1 cm of cartilage dorsal and anterior for support (see Fig. 165-11). Although the nose does not collapse when this is done, the nasal support is weakened, and the risk of septal perforation is increased. However, when properly performed, a SMR is sometimes the best operation for extremely deviated septums, which would be difficult to correct with the standard septoplasty techniques.

At the end of the procedure, the incisions are closed with 4-0 chromic sutures. Magnet-containing silicone rubber splints (Magnesplints) are placed on each side. The magnets in the splints attract each other and hold the septal flaps together without the need for packing. The splints are held in the proper position with a 4-0 silk suture. The splints are removed in 5 to 7 days. The flaps may also be sutured together with a running mattress stitch. Occasionally, the nose may require light packing postoperatively. These packs can usually be safely removed after 24 hours.

RICHARD L. GOODE
LANE F. SMITH

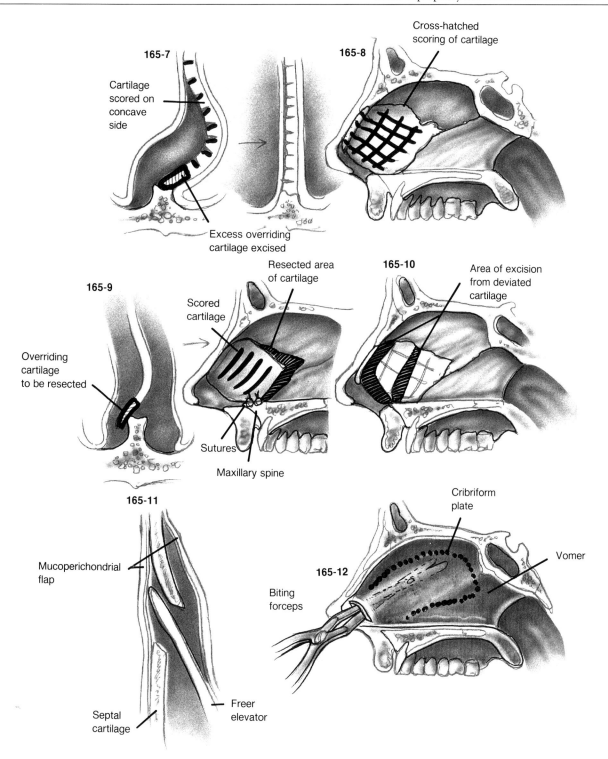

165-7
Cartilage scored on concave side
Excess overriding cartilage excised

165-8
Cross-hatched scoring of cartilage

165-9
Overriding cartilage to be resected
Scored cartilage
Resected area of cartilage
Sutures
Maxillary spine

165-10
Area of excision from deviated cartilage

165-11
Mucoperichondrial flap
Septal cartilage
Freer elevator

165-12
Cribriform plate
Vomer
Biting forceps

■ 166. RHINOPLASTY

The surgical rearrangement of the soft tissue, cartilage, and bone of the nose to provide a better nasal airway, a more pleasing appearance, or both. Various skin and mucosal incisions can be used to access the deeper tissues of the nose. The four main variations are the intercartilaginous, intracartilaginous, bipedicle delivery, and open approaches.

Indications

1. Need for access to the cartilage or bone of the nose for rhinoplasty
2. Occasionally useful as part of larger approach for tumor removal

Contraindications

1. Use skin incisions with caution in keloid-forming patients.

Special Considerations

1. Discontinue all aspirin and nonsteroidal antiinflammatory agents at least 2 weeks before surgery.

Preoperative Preparation

1. Routine laboratory studies
2. High-quality photographs

Special Instruments, Position, and Anesthesia

1. Nasal instrument tray
2. Use local anesthesia with epinephrine injections, even if the patient is under general anesthesia, to decrease blood loss.

Tips and Pearls

1. Be sure the patient understands and accepts the columellar incision of the external approach.
2. Careful suturing of nasal incisions promotes rapid healing.
3. External approach gives best visualization for posttraumatic or otherwise complicated nasal anatomy.

Pitfalls and Complications

1. Making the intercartilaginous incision so that less than 7 or 8 mm of the lower lateral cartilage remains permits later buckling and scarring.
2. If rhinoplasty incision is joined to a transfixion or hemitransfixion incision for septoplasty, webbing can occur in the nasal valve area. Gentle tissue handling and careful suturing minimize this problem.

Postoperative Care Issues

1. Use packing only if needed.
2. Local wound care to discourage crust formation at the suture lines

References

Anderson JR, Ries R. Rhinoplasty, emphasizing the external approach. American Academy of Facial Plastic and Reconstructive Surgery monograph. New York: Thieme, 1986.
Sheen J. Aesthetic rhinoplasty, 2nd ed. St Louis: CV Mosby. 1987.

Operative Procedure

The mucosa of the nose is anesthetized and vasoconstricted with topical cocaine, and the soft tissues of the nose then are infiltrated with lidocaine (usually 1% with 1:100,000 epinephrine).

Intercartilaginous Approach

The intercartilaginous approach (Fig. 166-1) is most useful for access to the nasal dorsum when little tip alteration is needed. A short nasal speculum exposes a bulging ridge where the lower lateral cartilages (LLC) and the upper lateral cartilages (ULC) abut. This ridge is accentuated by finger pressure on the outside of the nose. The intercartilaginous incision is made here, between the LLC and ULC. It can be carried just onto the septum medially or can be joined with a hemitransfixion approach if greater cartilage exposure is desired. Blunt-pointed or Foman scissors undermine the plane between the ULC and the skin, hugging the cartilage. A Joseph elevator undermines between the nasal bones and the periosteum. Further visualization for resection of the cephalic LLC can be obtained by undermining between the LLC and the skin. The upper edge of the LLC can be pulled down, everting it into the nostril. This retrograde delivery puts the LLC inside out and upside down from its normal anatomic position, making the effect of cartilage changes difficult to predict accurately.

Intracartilaginous Approach

The intracartilaginous approach (Fig. 166-2) resembles the intercartilaginous, but is made nearer the nostril, splitting the LLC. It is placed so the remaining caudal LLC is at least 7 to 8 mm high, preventing later buckling. The divided upper segment of the LLC is freed from soft tissue and removed. Thus a cephalic trim of the LLCs and access the nasal dorsum are performed through the same incision. Exposure for further tip refinement is not optimal.

Bipedicle delivery begins with an intercartilaginous incision (Fig. 166-3). A second incision hugs the caudal border of the lower lateral cartilage, extending from the medial crus, around the dome, to about three-quarters of the way out the lateral crus. The LLC is freed from external nasal skin. Freed in its central portion but remaining attached on either side, the LLC is delivered as a bipedicled flap through the nares, like pulling down a bucket handle. When delivered, a skin hook or Freer elevator is slipped under the "bucket handle," providing good visualization and allowing comparison for symmetry between the two sides. This approach requires an additional incision, but provides better exposure of the LLC in a more nearly normal anatomic relationship.

The open approach affords the best exposure of the lower lateral cartilages in their normal anatomic positions (Fig. 166-4). The incision can be performed medial-to-lateral OR lateral-to-medial. If begun medially, a #64 Beaver blade is used to incise a "V" over the columella. The incision is made over the medial crura, rather than beyond the feet of the crura, so that the crura provide a firm platform against which the columella scar contracture can take place without notching. Great care is taken to avoid cutting into the medial crura, because the skin is very thin here. Columellar skin is elevated, and the domes of the LLCs identified. The incision and undermining are carried laterally, just inside the rim of the nose, following the inferior border of the LLC like the inferior incision for a bipedicled flap. If begun laterally, the inferior border of the LLC is identified at the lateral-most extent of the proposed incision. Undermining is carried out from here medially between the LLC and the nasal skin. The incision is gradually lengthened medially to "catch up" with the undermining, which is carried over the domes and down the columella. A closed scissors or other instrument is passed between the undermined columellar skin and the medial crura, and the columellar incision is made onto the instrument, eliminating the possibility of accidentally cutting into the crura.

KAREN H. CALHOUN

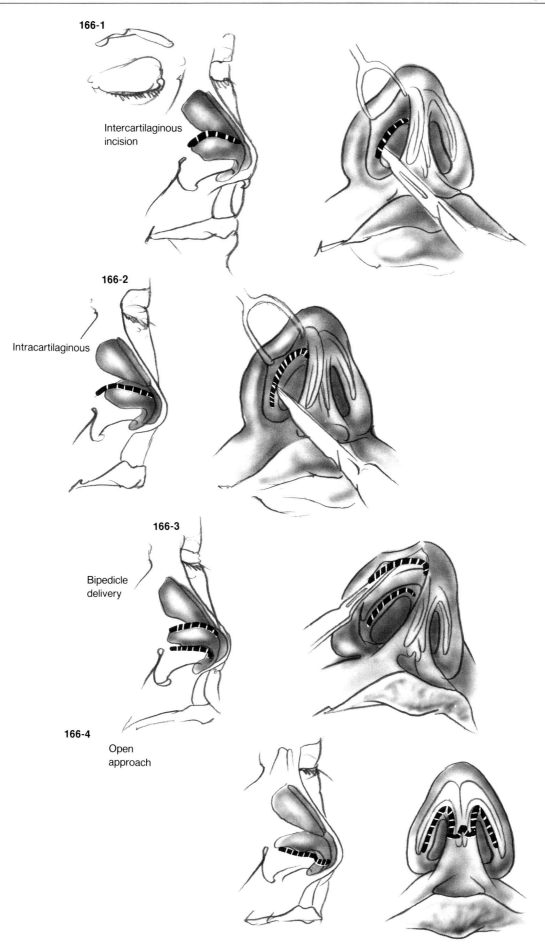

166-1

Intercartilaginous
incision

166-2

Intracartilaginous

166-3

Bipedicle
delivery

166-4

Open
approach

■ 167. OSTEOTOMIES

Surgical cutting of the nasal bones. A high osteotomy is closer to the dorsum, and a low osteotomy is farther away.

Indications

1. Closing an open roof deformity after removal of nasal hump (Fig. 167-1)
2. Straightening an asymmetric nasal pyramid, usually after trauma

Contraindications

1. Possibly contraindicated after a comminuted nasal-frontal-ethmoid fracture
2. Contraindicated in cases of bleeding disorders or systemic anticoagulation
3. Generally contraindicated in patient whose cardiac or other pathology precludes the use of epinephrine in the local anesthetic

Special Considerations

1. Usually results in periorbital ecchymosis and swelling

Preoperative Preparation

1. No aspirin, nonsteroidal antiinflammatory drugs, or medications containing these drugs for 2 weeks before surgery
2. Good-quality photographs

Special Instruments, Position, and Anesthesia

1. Use the smallest osteotome that can fracture the bones. This minimizes soft tissue trauma. For a thin-skinned, 16-year-old girl, this may be a 2- or 3-mm osteotome; for an older man with thick skin and a multiply traumatized nose, a 7- or 8-mm osteotome may be required.

Tips and Pearls

1. Reinject the stab incision site anterior to the inferior turbinate and the course of the lateral osteotomy 5 to 10 minutes before performing the osteotomy.
2. Draw the proposed course of the osteotomy on the skin with a surgical marking pen to provide a clear visual reference.
3. If an osteotomy results in an incomplete fracture or a small triangular spicule of bone remains immobile at the superior end of the osteotomy, a 2-mm osteotome can be passed directly through the overlying skin and used to complete the fracture.
4. Apply iced saline-soaked gauze pads to the periorbital regions before the osteotomies. This reduces ecchymosis and swelling.
5. Ecchymosis and swelling are minimized by periorbital iced saline-soaked pads in the recovery room and during the first night and by elevation of the head of bed to about 30°.

Pitfalls and Complications

1. Asymmetry is decreased by careful planning of the osteotomy lines, especially on the already traumatized, asymmetric nose.
2. Keep the osteotome perpendicular to the midsagittal plane of the head (Figs. 167-2 and 167-3).
3. Reduce the chance of bleeding from the angular artery by pretunneling along the osteotomy course, using a small instrument that does not disrupt the overlying soft tissue, or use a guarded osteotome with the guard turned out to protect the overlying soft tissue.
4. Start the lateral osteotomies at the attachment of the inferior turbinate, not lower in the nose. This prevents narrowing of the inferior-most part of the piriform aperture and consequent narrowing of the airway (Figs. 167-4 and 167-5).

Postoperative Care Issues

1. Surgical adhesive and tape applied to the nose at the end of surgery and a plaster cast or other splint applied to hold the repositioned nasal bones in their optimal position during early healing
2. If plaster cast is used, make a template for cast sizing and shape from paper, allowing the plaster to be cut and wetted before applying it to the nose. This avoids getting plaster dust in the eyes.

Operative Procedure

The nasal dorsum is undermined, with the periosteum elevated over the nasal bones. Medial osteotomies are usually performed first. If a large hump has been removed, medial osteotomies are unnecessary. The osteotome is placed through the nasal incisions and positioned perpendicular to the bone at the caudal end of the nasal bone, just lateral to the septum. Gentle hammer taps are used to advance the osteotome in a cephalic direction, tapering outward. Intermediate osteotomies, if required, are performed next. For the lateral osteotomies, a stab incision is made in the soft tissue just anterior to the anterior end of the inferior turbinate. This is carried down to the bone of the pyriform aperture. If desired, a Joseph elevator can be used to elevate periosteum from the bone along the proposed course of the osteotomy. The osteotome is engaged in the bone with an initial horizontal course, which then turns upward, progressing anteromedially to the lacrimal fossa. As the top end of the osteotomy is approached, the osteotome is twisted inward to complete the osteotomy.

Alternatively, a 2- or 3-mm osteotome can be pushed directly through the skin and used to make postage-stamp osteotomies (ie, each skin incision is used to make three or four bone perforations). The osteotomy is completed by firm inward pressure with the fingers.

KAREN H. CALHOUN

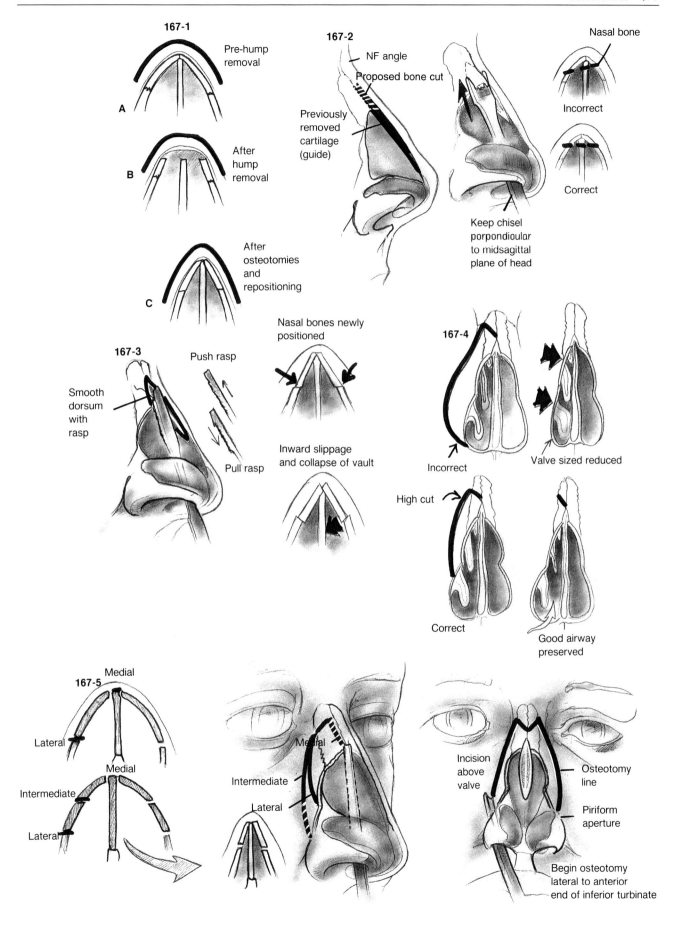

167-1

A — Pre-hump removal

B — After hump removal

C — After osteotomies and repositioning

167-2

NF angle

Proposed bone cut

Previously removed cartilage (guide)

Keep chisel porpondioular to midsagittal plane of head

Nasal bone

Incorrect

Correct

Nasal bones newly positioned

Inward slippage and collapse of vault

167-3

Smooth dorsum with rasp

Push rasp

Pull rasp

167-4

Incorrect

High cut

Correct

Valve sized reduced

Good airway preserved

167-5

Medial

Lateral

Medial

Intermediate

Lateral

Medial

Intermediate

Lateral

Incision above valve

Osteotomy line

Piriform aperture

Begin osteotomy lateral to anterior end of inferior turbinate

■ 168. NASAL TIP PROCEDURES

The functional and aesthetic repair, reorientation, reconstitution, and refinement of the nasal tip during rhinoplasty

Indications

1. Functional and aesthetic anatomic abnormalities of the nasal tip structures, including hypertrophy, asymmetry, overprojection, underprojection, dependency, incomplete development, and deviation.

Contraindications

1. Because surgery of the nasal tip is acknowledged to be the most difficult aspect of rhinoplasty, inexperience with the procedure constitutes a relative contraindication.

Special Considerations

1. The surgeon must thoroughly appreciate tip anatomy, tip support mechanisms, and the long-term dynamics of healing on the ultimate tip appearance.
2. Refined skills of analysis and the ability to visualize an ideal intended result are required for accurate judgment. Artistic skills are necessary to sculpture an ideal normal appearance.
3. No single technique suffices to correct the myriad anatomic variants encountered, requiring knowledge and mastery of a wide range of reconstructive maneuvers.

Preoperative Preparation

1. Careful analysis of the patient's general and detailed facial features, with evaluation of standardized photographs, is required.
2. A review of the patient's wishes and expectations is mandatory.
3. Detailed informed consent, with a mutual understanding of the goals and limitations of tip surgery, must precede correction.

(continued)

Operative Procedure

Nasal tip anatomy can vary profoundly among patients, and no single surgical technique may be employed routinely in successful nasal tip refinement. The objective in tip surgery is to construct a defined, stable, symmetric, and properly projecting nasal tip, which is roughly triangular on the base view and blends harmoniously with the remainder of the nasal anatomy (Fig. 168-1). Commonly, cephalic rotation of the tip is desirable, but it must be avoided when not indicated. The emphasis once placed on tissue excision, with more radical division of the tip cartilages and supporting structures, has gradually been replaced by more conservative reconstructive techniques of tip sculpture. The long-term results are improved when the supporting structures of the tip are preserved or strengthened. An exacting presurgical plan must be devised, based on skin thickness, strength and shape of the alar cartilages, tip-lip angulation, requirements for tip projection and rotation, and patient requests.

Every rhinoplasty procedure inevitably results in preservation of the existing tip projection, reduction of projection, or if indicated, enhancement of tip projection. Preservation of the existing projection is the desired surgical goal, if the preoperative tip projection is satisfactory, as is true in most Caucasian patients. Certain patients require an increase in the projection of the tip relative to the intended new profile line. A predictable variety of reliable operative methods exists for creating or augmenting tip projection. In a limited, clearly definable group of patients with overprojecting tips, a calculated intentional reduction of excessive tip projection is desirable.

In assessing the need for tip remodeling, the surgeon must determine whether the tip requires a reduction in the volume of the alar cartilages, a change in the attitude and orientation of the alar cartilage, a change in the projection of the tip, and a cephalic rotation with a consequent increase in the columellar inclination (ie, nasolabial angle). Once these factors are accurately assessed, the most favorable incisions, the approach and the tip sculpture technique may be chosen (see Fig. 168-1).

An unusual tip deformity may require an entirely new or unusual series of individual surgical steps, based on a sound knowledge of sound rhinoplasty principles, to achieve a satisfactory outcome. The surgeon must become thoroughly familiar with the broad scope of traditional techniques and be prepared to improvise with sound technical innovation when required by variant anatomy. Suturing techniques, cartilage grafting techniques, and methods of reliable rotation must be mastered.

Nondelivery Approaches

When the anatomic situation encountered (ie, minimal bulbosity, symmetry, no bifidity) requires only conservative or minimal tip refinement and rotation, a nondelivery approach, such as cartilage splitting or retrograde eversion, is preferred. Most of the lateral crus is left intact as a complete strip, resecting only a few millimeters of the medial-cephalic portion of the lateral crus to effect refinement. This operation is useful in many patients, because it tends to mimic nature, disturbs very little of the normal anatomy of the tip, and consistently heals with symmetry and minimal scarring (Figs. 168-2 and 168-3).

The transcartilaginous approach is the preferred nondelivery approach because of its simplicity; similar tip modifications can be accomplished through the retrograde approach. These approaches are most effective in patients demonstrating minimal nasal tip bulbosity that would only require modest volume reduction of the cephalic margin of the alar cartilages.

(continued)

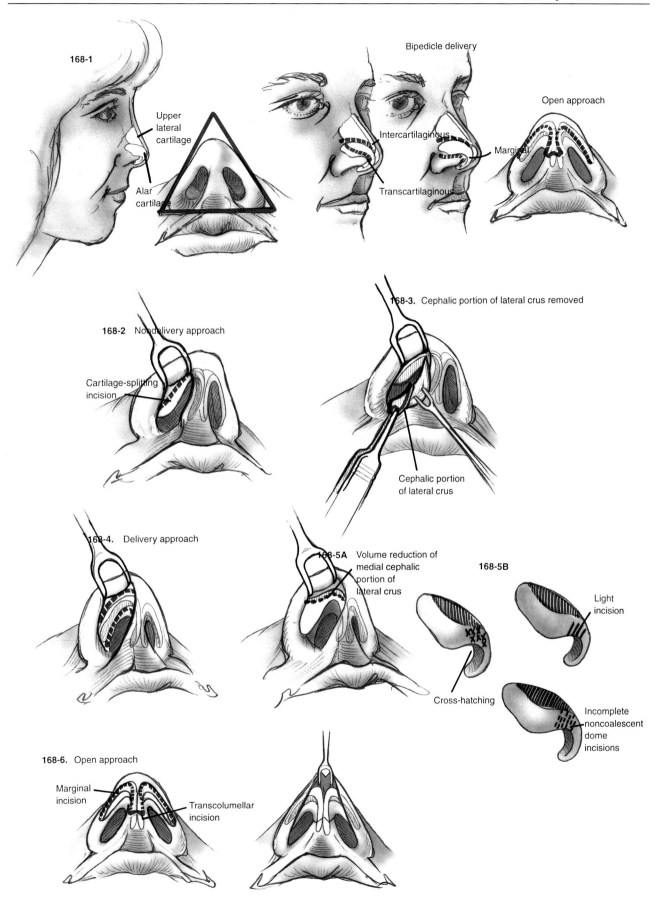

168-1

Upper lateral cartilage

Alar cartilage

Bipedicle delivery

Intercartilaginous

Transcartilaginous

Marginal

Open approach

168-2   Nondelivery approach

Cartilage-splitting incision

168-3. Cephalic portion of lateral crus removed

Cephalic portion of lateral crus

168-4.   Delivery approach

168-5A Volume reduction of medial cephalic portion of lateral crus

168-5B

Light incision

Cross-hatching

Incomplete noncoalescent dome incisions

168-6. Open approach

Marginal incision

Transcolumellar incision

■ *168.* NASAL TIP PROCEDURES (continued)

Special Instruments, Position, and Anesthesia

1. The usual standard instruments for rhinoplasty, with small dissecting scissors, fine hooks, and delicate #15c Bard-Parker knife blades, are required.
2. Local anesthesia with a 1% solution of Xylocaine with a 1:50,000 dilution of epinephrine, complemented by monitored intravenous analgesia or general anesthesia, provides freedom from pain and the intense vasoconstriction needed for absolute hemostasis. After infiltration, 12 to 15 minutes should pass before initiating surgery.

Tips and Pearls

1. A graduated anatomic approach is ideal, selecting minimally invasive surgery if the existing tip anatomy requires only modest change, and gradually selecting more involved (and more risky) procedures if the tip anatomy is more abnormal or asymmetric.

Pitfalls and Complications

1. Because tip surgery is a bilateral operation on a midline organ feature, ultimate asymmetry represents a common complication.
2. The loss of tip support, ultimately causing tip ptosis, can result when tip support mechanisms are violated and not reconstituted.
3. The combination of thin skin and strong alar cartilages may set the stage for visible irregularities years after surgery.
4. Overreduction or vertical interruption of the residual complete strip may lead to inspiratory alar collapse if sufficient alar sidewall support is lost.

Postoperative Care Issues

1. Compression taping of the entire tip aids in early edema reduction.

References

Tardy ME. Aesthetic rhinoplasty. In: Bailey BJ, Johnson JT, Kohut RI, Pillsbury HC III, Tardy ME Jr, eds. Head and neck surgery—otolaryngology. Philadelphia: JB Lippincott, 1993.
Tardy ME, Patt BS, Walter MA. Transdomal suture refinement of the nasal tip: long-term outcomes. Facial Plast Surg Monogr 1993;9:275.

Delivery Approaches

As the tip anatomy becomes more abnormal or asymmetric, more complex surgical techniques are gradually employed. In these patients, a delivery approach is required, allowing visual presentation of the alar cartilages as bipedicled chondrocutaneous flaps for further modifications of various designs to be executed symmetrically (Fig. 168-4). Greater volume reduction of the medial-cephalic portion of the lateral crus is usually necessary, while maintaining a complete strip with a width of at least 7 to 8 mm. If judged necessary, further tip refinement may be achieved by weakening the complete strip convexity with conservative cross-hatching, using gentle morselization, or with incomplete noncoalescent dome incisions.

Delivery approaches are indicated almost exclusively if significant defatting or scar resection is required, if the alar cartilages are asymmetric, and if an abnormal bifidity of the tip exists.

Open or External Approaches

For correcting cleft lip and nose deformities, severely asymmetric tips, and some markedly overprojecting or underprojecting tips with eccentric anatomy, an open or external approach to the tip through a transcolumellar incision may be helpful, particularly if the variant anatomy is not clear preoperatively. Although more operative edema and scarring results from this approach, the advantages of a precise direct-vision diagnosis, bimanual surgery, and extraordinary exposure render this approach useful in selected cases (Fig. 168-6). No major tip supports are routinely divided during the open approach. Significant restructuring of the nasal tip contours with sutured-in-place tip grafts and columellar struts are facilitated through the open approach.

Tip-Refinement Techniques

Because of the variations in tip anatomy encountered, numerous techniques must be mastered to achieve predictable refinement. If the tip anatomy is almost normal, only a moderate reduction in the bulk of the supratip lateral crura suffices, and a volume reduction with a residual complete strip is ideal (Fig. 168-7).

In patients presenting with a wide, trapezoid, boxy tip configuration, volume reduction accompanied by transdomal suture narrowing of the residual complete strip (Fig. 168-8) produces a natural-looking refinement, with narrowing of the boxy configuration and preservation of existent tip projection.

Overprojection of the nasal tip due to hypertrophy of the alar cartilages may be normalized by amputation or cartilage excision of domal regions with fine suture repair (Fig. 168-9). Transdermal or interdomal suture narrowing is often combined with this technique.

Significant and calibrated rotation of the tip is achieved in certain patients with highly dependent tips by triangular excision of the lateral portion of the lateral crura and reconstituting the cut edges with 6-0 nylon suture to effect predictable cephalic rotation by reorienting the alar axis of the cartilages (Fig. 168-10). When less profound rotation is required, various adjunctive techniques are employed (Fig. 168-11).

If substantial tip projection is necessary, tip asymmetries require camouflage, or contouring of the infratip lobule is planned, cartilage tip grafting becomes necessary (Fig. 168-12). Tip grafts may be placed in precisely dissected pockets or sutured in place for complete stabilization. Multiple grafts are commonly employed for tip recontouring.

M. EUGENE TARDY, JR.
ERIC O. LINDBECK
JAMES A. HEINRICH

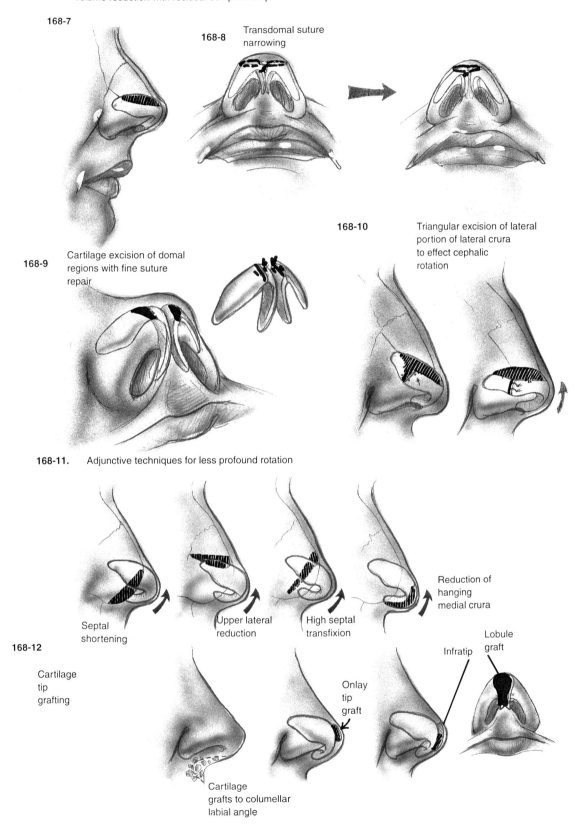

Volume reduction with residual complete strip

168-7

168-8 Transdomal suture narrowing

168-9 Cartilage excision of domal regions with fine suture repair

168-10 Triangular excision of lateral portion of lateral crura to effect cephalic rotation

168-11. Adjunctive techniques for less profound rotation

Septal shortening

Upper lateral reduction

High septal transfixion

Reduction of hanging medial crura

168-12

Cartilage tip grafting

Cartilage grafts to columellar labial angle

Onlay tip graft

Infratip

Lobule graft

■ 169. NASAL BASE PROCEDURES

Narrowing of the alar base and lateral alar sidewalls is a refinement step in rhinoplasty designed to bring the alar base into proportion with the newly designed nose.

Indications

1. Flaring alar sidewalls that fall outside a perpendicular line dropped from the inner canthi
2. Excessively horizontally oriented nostrils
3. An excessively wide nostril sill and floor
4. Unsightly eversion of the nostrils and flaring nostrils after retroprojection of the significantly overprojected tip

Contraindications

1. Unwillingness of the patient to accept a potentially visible scar near the alar-facial junctions. Informed consent is essential.

Special Considerations

1. Alar base reduction is best performed as the final or near-final step in the rhinoplasty sequence.

Preoperative Preparation

1. Exacting analysis of the nasal aesthetic and photographic proportions, with elaboration of an operative plan to symmetrically reduce or reorient the nostril anatomy.

Special Instruments, Position, and Anesthesia

1. The delicate soft tissue hooks, scissors, and #15c knife blade found in the typical rhinoplasty set suffice for alar base surgery.
2. Suture placement is aided by the use of magnification and the small Castroviejo needle holder.

(continued)

Operative Procedure

During the course of many rhinoplasties, modification of the alar anatomy may become necessary by some form of reduction, repositioning, reorientation, or sculpturing. Aesthetic narrowing of the nasal skeleton and tip should be balanced by concomitant reduction and refinement of the alar base, or the nose appears "bottom heavy." In general, a vertical line dropped from each inner canthus alongside the nose should define the lateral limits of the alae for an ideal appearance (Figs. 169-1 and 169-2). Wider or more flaring alae merit consideration for alar reduction techniques, which are best executed in a graduated fashion, based entirely on the anatomy encountered and the aesthetic appearance desired. Retropositioning tip techniques employed to correct overprojecting noses inevitably result in alar sidewall flaring, inviting alar reduction of the width and overall alar sidewall length.

The exact technique to be employed depends on the anatomy encountered, the aesthetic outcome desired, and the need to camouflage resultant epithelial scars. Alar modifications are consistently required to balance the nasal anatomy in certain ethnic anatomic types, such as Negroid, Asian, and Mestizo noses, but the need to perform alar reduction in the more typical Caucasian nose is less common. Nonetheless, alar modifications are indicated when alar flaring, bulbosity, or excessive width of the nasal base is present, or when retropositioning of excessive tip projection results in a displeasing postoperative alar flare. Excessively wide nostril floor dimensions may also dictate the need for alar sill or nostril floor modifications.

Alar modifications are usually most accurately performed as one of the final steps in aesthetic rhinoplasty, after all major and adjunctive procedures have been completed. The general appearance of the modified tip may be assessed, and the indicated method of alar sculpturing may be selected and carried out. If doubt exists about nasal proportions, it is best to defer alar reduction until the nasal tip is healed and more accurate evaluation of the modified surgical anatomy is possible. Alar reduction of any type must be carried out in a conservative and symmetric manner to prevent one deformity being substituted for another.

Although the surgeon's aesthetic judgment ultimately determines the site and degree of resection, a more precise surgical approach may be determined if several anatomic guidelines are assessed and integrated. Conservatism is mandatory to avoid overreduction and asymmetry, conditions almost impossible to correct satisfactorily. To determine the planned approach and site of incisions, several anatomic factors are evaluated:

The internal (medial) length, shape, thickness, and flare of the alar margin

The external (lateral) length, shape, thickness, and flare of the alar margin

The width and shape of the nostril floor and sill

The shape of the nostril aperture

The shape of the columella and related medial crural footplates, including the length of the medial crura and lateral flare of the medial crural footplates

The length of the lateral sidewalls of the nose, determined by the site of insertion of the alae into the face

After determining which factors need modification, a graduated surgical scheme is employed to achieve the desired aesthetic result.

(continued)

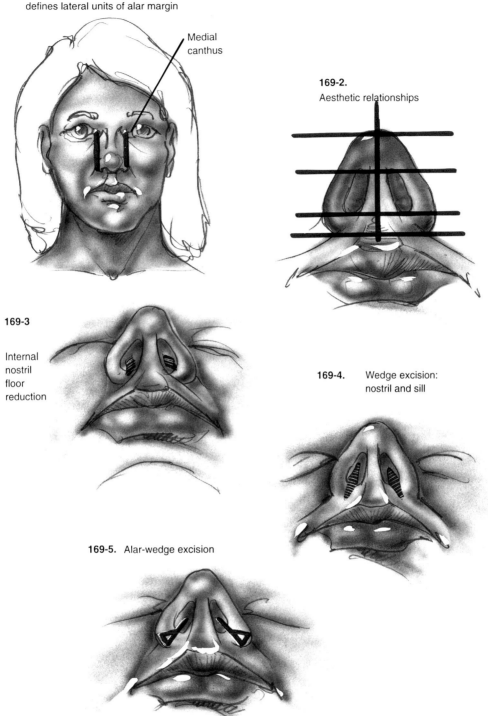

169-1. Vertical line from inner medial canthus
defines lateral units of alar margin

Medial
canthus

169-2.
Aesthetic relationships

169-3

Internal
nostril
floor
reduction

169-4. Wedge excision:
nostril and sill

169-5. Alar-wedge excision

■ 169. NASAL BASE PROCEDURES (continued)

Tips and Pearls

1. Placement of the visible external alar base incision 1.5 to 2 mm above the alar-facial crease (not within the crease itself) facilitates accurate suture placement and improved scar camouflage.
2. Sealing the wound edges with Histoacryl tissue glue provides immediate hemostasis and prevents annoying postoperative seepage from the highly vascular alae.
3. Scar camouflage is facilitated by closing the internal wound with 5-0 chromic catgut and the visible external wound with 5-0 or 6-0 fast-absorbing catgut suture.

Pitfalls and Complications

1. Asymmetrical reduction
2. Overreduction or underreduction
3. Unnatural vertical notching of the nostril sill
4. Unsightly suture marks

Postoperative Care Issues

1. Neo-Decadron ophthalmic ointment is applied to the alar base incision twice daily for 5 to 7 days, after which the sutures and dried glue fall away spontaneously.

Reference

Tardy ME, Walter MA, Patt BS. Alar reduction and sculpture: anatomic concepts. Facial Plast Surg Monogr 1993;9:295.

Internal Nostril Floor Reduction

In patients requiring minimal alar reduction, excision of a wedge of epithelium and soft tissue from the nostril floor only (Fig. 169-3). reduces the slight alar flare by reducing the dimension of the internal (medial) border. Although the outward curve of the ala is altered, no medial repositioning of the alar-facial junction is effected. The scar is effectively hidden within the nostril floor if the nostril sill is not violated. The shape of the nostril sill sometimes determines whether this approach is appropriate. Subtle, conservative but effective improvements are possible with this approach. The dimension of the lateral alar border remains unchanged.

Wedge Excision Nostril Floor and Sill

Further reduction of alar flare is accomplished by carrying the incision across the sill into the alar-facial junction. Reduction of flare and a slight reduction of the alar bulk is effected (Fig. 169-4).

Alar Wedge Excision

If the alar development is excessive and bulbous, excision of a wedge of ala at the alar-facial junction reduces the overall bulkiness of the alar anatomy (Figs. 169-5 and 169-6). Some medial repositioning of the alae may be effected with this maneuver. Reduction of the overall length of the alar sidewalls occurs when generous wedges are excised, which is ideal in the overall reduction of the over-projecting tip.

Sheen Alar Flap

Minimal alar reduction and slight medial repositioning of the alar-facial junction with excellent scar camouflage is accomplished with the approach advocated by Sheen (Fig. 169-7). In this approach the incision does not traverse the nostril sill, avoiding a "notched" appearance. Only modest changes are possible with this technique.

Sliding Alar Flap

Maximal alar reduction with medial repositioning is effected with a generous incision near the alar-facial junction and various degrees of alar excision (Fig. 169-8). Reduction of the volume, curve, and flare of the internal and external alar margins results from this procedure; the extent of each depends on the angulation of the alar incision. A back cut placed 2 mm above the alar-facial junction allows the alar flap to slide medially, narrowing the alar base significantly.

The key to avoiding a visible nostril sill scar lies in exacting approximation of the cut edges with fast-absorbing 5-0 catgut sutures, supplemented by Histoacryl tissue adhesive (Fig. 169-9). If the excised tissue gap is large, buried interrupted sutures of 5-0 polydioxanone are initially placed subcutaneously to appose the wound edges and relieve tension on the delicate catgut sutures. External suture marks may be largely eliminated with this closure sequence. Nonabsorbable sutures should be avoided, because suture marks almost inevitably result.

Effective camouflage of the scar just above the alar-facial junction may be facilitated by positioning incisions 1 to 2 mm above the alar-facial crease, avoiding the thick sebaceous glands located in this junction (Fig. 169-10). The 1- to 2-mm cuff of skin remaining facilitates exact edge-to-edge closure, which may be facilitated by magnification. This simple but critical approach to incision sitting almost completely eliminates visible scars, suture marks, and widened, visible sebaceous gland openings.

M. EUGENE TARDY, JR.
ERIC O. LINDBECK
JAMES A. HEINRICH

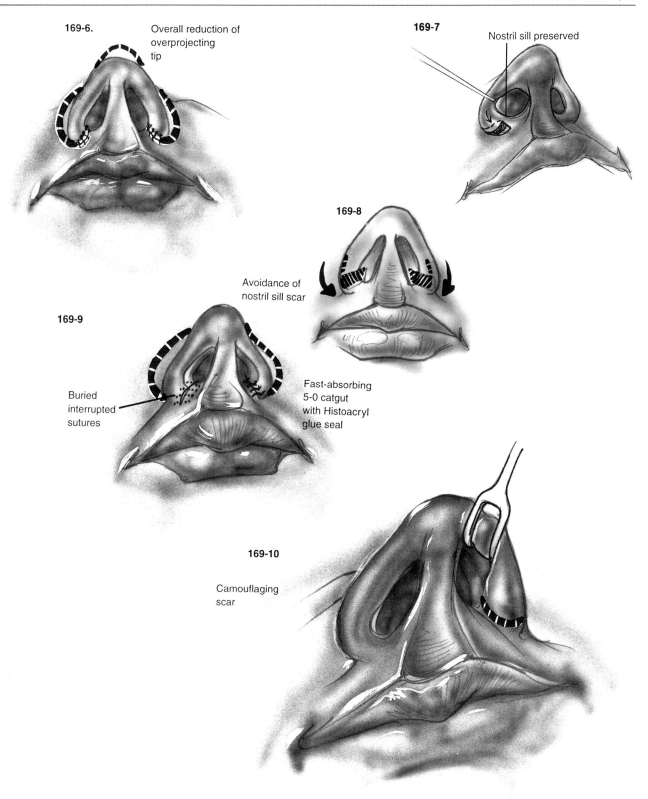

169-6. Overall reduction of overprojecting tip

169-7 Nostril sill preserved

169-8 Avoidance of nostril sill scar

169-9 Buried interrupted sutures

Fast-absorbing 5-0 catgut with Histoacryl glue seal

169-10 Camouflaging scar

■ 170. NASAL DORSAL CHANGES

Alteration of the bony and cartilaginous contour and height of the nasal dorsum

Indications

1. Reduction of prominent bony or cartilaginous profile
2. Augmentation of a low radix and saddle type deformities

Special Considerations

1. Inadequate septal and nasal bone support
2. Obtuse nasofrontal angle
3. Low radix
4. Inadequate tip projection

Preoperative Preparation

1. Routine laboratory studies
2. Bleeding and clotting studies, if th history is questionable
3. Complete preoperative photographic analysis

Special Instruments, Position, and Anesthesia

1. Headlight
2. Nasal speculum, dorsal nasal retractor, and bayonet forceps
3. Right-angle scissors, 13-mm-plane osteotome, and rasps
4. Supine position, with the neck slightly extended
5. Deep intravenous sedation, titrated and monitored by the anesthesiologist
6. Local anesthesia consisting of a 1% solution of lidocaine with a 1:100,000 dilution of epinephrine

Tips and Pearls

1. Larger dissection is required for reduction.
2. Soft tissue completely separated from cartilaginous framework
3. Subperiosteal plane over nasal bones raised with elevator
4. Use a conservative approach.
5. For augmentation, a precise pocket and more limited dissection are desirable.
6. Contour implants smoothly to avoid irregularities.
7. Soak the implant in antibiotic solution before implantation.

Pitfalls and Complications

1. Inadequate exposure due to bleeding or poor illumination
2. Overzealous reduction of bone or cartilage
3. Failure to close an open roof
4. Improper placement of the graft, causing asymmetries and irregularities
5. Inflammation, infection, or graft rejection

Postoperative Care Issues

1. Intraoperative and postoperative antibiotics with implants
2. Adequate external taping and splinting for 5 to 6 days.
3. Internal Telfa dressing for 24 hours
4. Clean the internal nares daily with hydrogen peroxide, and lubricate with Vaseline.
5. Remove tapes carefully to avoid lifting skin off the nasal dorsum.
6. The patient should avoid nose blowing for 10 days and avoid vigorous exercise for 3 weeks.

References

Meyer R. Secondary and functional rhinoplasty. In: The difficult nose. San Diego: Grune & Stratton, 1990.

Rees T. Aesthetic plastic surgery, vol I. Philadelphia: WB Saunders, 1980.

Operative Procedure

Access is gained through an apical incision outlined at the junction of the upper lateral cartilages and the septum. A nasal speculum is used to retract the lobular cartilages to allow identification of the apex. Careful scalpel dissection enlarges the apical incision as needed, extending inferiorly along the caudal edge of the septum and laterally at the inferior border of the upper lateral cartilages (Fig. 170-1). To gain better mobility and exposure of the nasal dorsum, a similar incision is outlined on the contralateral side. A Fomon scissors incises the remaining attachments of the septocolumella membrane and soft tissues overlying the dorsal cartilaginous framework.

The dissection proceeds superiorly to the rhinion. A Joseph periosteal elevator is insinuated beneath the periosteum of the nasal bones and carefully raised toward the radix, lateral enough to be able to insinuate an osteotome without traumatizing the skin or injuring the periosteum. Junction tunnels are made to separate the upper lateral cartilages from the septum. A Cottle septal elevator is used to create a subperichondrial pocket at the apex, which is raised to the rhinion by sweeping the mucosa off the dorsal septum. A scalpel can often facilitate the beginning attempts to find the proper subperichondrial plane of dissection. A similar maneuver is performed on the opposite side, effectively denuding and exposing the nasal septal and bony framework.

Dorsal Reduction

The cartilaginous dorsal septum is reduced under direct vision. An Aufricht dorsal nasal retractor is placed, and with adequate illumination, a Joseph right-angle scissors is used to lower this structure. The approach to the rhinion should be conservative. The anterior borders of the upper lateral cartilages are lowered to the level of the septum by judicious trimming before proceeding with the bone work (Fig. 170-2). Small bony nasal humps can be rasped, but more prominent ones require osteotomies. A 13-mm-plane nasal osteotome is usually wide enough to remove most humps. The chisel is engaged at the rhinion, lying flush and along the cartilaginous dorsal septum. An assistant taps the osteotome with a mallet. The angle is determined and controlled by the surgeon (Fig. 170-3). The angle of the chisel must be carefully controlled to prevent too much bone from being inadvertently removed. Any soft tissue attachments are separated and the freed bony hump removed with a clamp. The new bony profile is smoothed with appropriate rasps. If the nasofrontal angle is somewhat obtuse, it can be deepened by lowering the nasal process of the frontal bone with a Parkes gouge (Fig. 170-4).

The open nasal roof is closed by individualized lateral osteotomies made along the nasomaxillary groove. The nasal bones are infractured to close the open roof and to reapproximate the nasal bones into their normal, but lowered anatomic position (Fig. 170-5). Fine adjustments in the dorsal profile line are made by judicious rasping of bone and cartilaginous trimming under direct vision.

Dorsal Augmentation

The patient is given intravenous antibiotics. Dorsal augmentation is facilitated by placement of autologous or alloplastic implants in precise pockets overlying a deficient nasal framework. A unilateral limited apical septal incision is outlined. Scissors dissection is kept to a minimum, and an attempt is made to raise the periosteum with a Joseph elevator. The midline pocket is made just large enough to admit the graft like a hand in a glove (Fig. 170-6). Careful contouring of the graft minimizes postoperative irregularities and asymmetries. The grafts are soaked in an antibiotic solution, and with a smooth bayonet forceps, they are carefully implanted into the pocket. External manipulation and judicious dissection ensures proper placement.

The apical incision is closed with a 4-0 chromic catgut. A 5 × 7.5 cm (2 × 3 in) ophthalmic Telfa pad is folded and cut in half, and each of the pieces is folded and inserted into a nostril to act as an internal dressing for the first postoperative day. An external tape dressing and splint are applied to promote stability during the first postoperative week.

FRANK M. KAMER

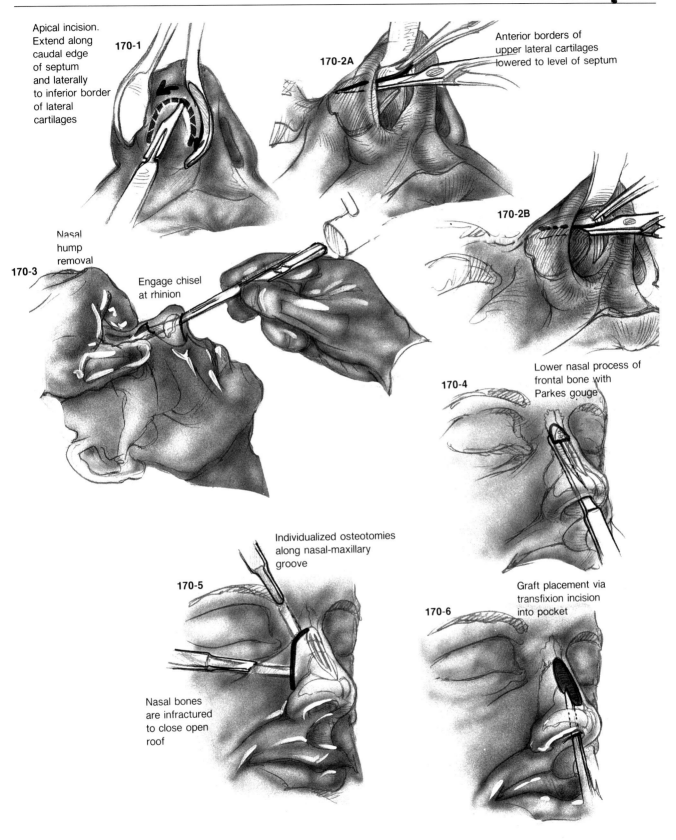

Apical incision. Extend along caudal edge of septum and laterally to inferior border of lateral cartilages

170-1

170-2A

Anterior borders of upper lateral cartilages lowered to level of septum

170-2B

Nasal hump removal

170-3

Engage chisel at rhinion

170-4

Lower nasal process of frontal bone with Parkes gouge

Individualized osteotomies along nasal-maxillary groove

170-5

Nasal bones are infractured to close open roof

Graft placement via transfixion incision into pocket

170-6

171. MAJOR NASAL RECONSTRUCTION

Any nasal defect that involves more than one subunit of the nose or requires a regional flap.

Indications

1. Subtotal loss of the nose secondary to trauma, resection for cancer, or infection.

Contraindications

1. Persistent or recurrent cancer
2. Persistent infection or autoimmune process
3. Unavailable forehead flap or cartilage grafts

Special Considerations

1. Smoking tobacco causes a significantly greater risk for flap loss.
2. Patients with previous surgery in the orbit and glabellar regions may have compromised local vasculature.
3. Significant resections of the nasal septum or mucosa may require modified techniques.
4. Patients with squamous cell carcinoma primaries should be evaluated for possible nodal metastases.

Preoperative Preparation

1. Anticoagulants or aspirin must be discontinued preoperatively.
2. For smokers, a 10- to 14-day delay of the forehead flap

Special Instruments, Position, and Anesthesia

1. Headlight
2. Fine plastic surgical instruments
3. Nasal instruments
4. A Mayfield head holder or other narrowed headrest
5. General anesthesia is usually preferred.

Tips and Pearls

1. Approach each nasal defect with the goal of restoring each component (eg, lining, skeleton, external coverage) as completely and accurately as possible.
2. If local septal cartilage is not available, the next best alternative is conchal cartilage.
3. Attach the cartilaginous skeletal components to the mucosal lining with plain gut mattress sutures.
4. The correct outline of the forehead flap is critical. A foil template is fashioned by placing it over the defect. If the defect is heminasal, the remaining opposite side of the nose is used as a model.
5. The paramedian forehead flap is clearly superior to the classic median forehead flap and allows the design of a narrow pedicle with sufficient arc of rotation to reach anywhere on the nose without having to angle it obliquely across the forehead.

Pitfalls and Complications

1. Failure to provide adequate inner lining for nasal reconstructions
2. The forehead flap is designed with the exact amount of tissue required to replace the defect. Extra tissue causes an amorphous, poorly defined nose.
3. The forehead flap is thinned of all frontalis muscle and as much subcutaneous tissue as possible.

Postoperative Care Issues

1. Any nasal packing is removed on postoperative day 1 or 2.
2. The forehead defect is kept moist with occlusive dressings.
3. The forehead flap pedicle is kept moist by wrapping with Vaseline gauze or a thin split-thickness skin graft over the raw surface of the pedicle.
4. Careful suctioning of the nose is performed as necessary.
5. Peroxide and Polysporin ointment are used on the suture lines to keep crusting at a minimum.
6. The pedicle of the forehead flap is divided at 2 to 3 weeks postoperatively.
7. Minor revisions of the reconstruction as necessary, particularly thinning and insetting of the superior portion of the flap.

References

1. Burget GC, Menick FJ. Nasal support and lining: the marriage of beauty and blood supply. Plast Reconstr Surg 1989;84:189.
2. Burget GC, Menick FJ. Nasal reconstruction: seeking a fourth dimension. Plast Reconstr Surg 1986;78:145.
3. Shumrick KA, Smith TL. The anatomic basis for the design of forehead flaps in nasal reconstruction. Arch Otolaryngol Head Neck Surg 1992;118:373.

Operative Procedures

Before major nasal reconstruction, the nose is decongested with Neo-Synephrine, and local anesthesia consisting of Xylocaine and epinephrine is injected.

The inner lining of the nose is reconstituted. Adequate lining can usually be obtained from the mucosa of the nose, mainly from the septum and upper vault. Mucosa can be removed from these areas without serious consequence because the rigid underlying skeletal structure resists scar contraction as remucosalization takes place. A nasal septal mucosal flap is developed, with superior and inferior incisions extending posteriorly into the nose.[1] A vertical cut is make posteriorly, and the mucosal flaps are elevated anteriorly in a supraperichondrial plane. The mucosal flap is based anteroinferiorly on a pedicle at the inferior part of the nasal vestibule (Fig. 171-1). This mucosal flap is folded into the defect to form the new lining of the nose and sutured to any remaining soft tissue at the margins of the defect.

Cartilage is obtained for reconstitution of the nasal skeleton. Septal cartilage is easily obtainable, provides good support, conforms to the desired shape, and is minimally resorbed.[2] The cartilage graft is secured to the remaining cartilage with clear nylon. The cartilage grafts are attached to the mucosal lining with through-and-through mattress sutures of 6-0 plain gut (Figs. 171-2). If septal cartilage is not available, auricular conchal cartilage is used.

The final part of reconstruction is recreation of external skin coverage with sufficient tissue that is a reasonable match for nasal skin. The forehead is the first choice as a donor site for skin defects greater than 1.5 to 2.0 cm in diameter.[3] A paramedian forehead flap is more versatile than the classic midline forehead flap. The paramedian flap is centered over the supratrochlear artery, which exits the orbit in the superomedial quadrant, passes over the corrugator muscle, passes under the orbicularis muscles, pierces the frontalis muscle at the level of the medial eyebrow, and ascends the rest of the forehead in the subcutaneous tissues external to the frontalis muscle.

The forehead flap is designed by using an exact template of the defect that is fashioned from a foil suture pocket in an anatomically accurate, three-dimensional form. The supratrochlear artery on the side to be used is identified with a Doppler monitor; for predominantly unilateral defects, the ipsilateral artery is employed, and for midline or large defects, the choice of which side to use is less critical. The artery consistently ascends the forehead in a paramedian position corresponding to the medial part of the eyebrow. The foil template is smoothed out and centered over the course of the artery, and the pattern for the flap traced around it. The flap is designed with a narrow pedicle (ie, 0.5 cm on either side of the artery) and is most pleasing if not extended into the hairline (Fig. 171-3A). Instead of extending into the hairline or obliquely across the forehead to gain length, it is better to continue the inferior incisions below the eyebrow and even past the orbital rims. By extending the incisions inferiorly and keeping the pedicle narrow, a flap of sufficient length to reach almost anywhere on the nose can be developed. The outline of the flap is then incised and raised in a plane just deep to the frontalis, leaving periosteum and overlying loose areolar tissue; it is important to leave vascularized tissue to support the growth of granulation tissue.

After elevating the flap, the underlying frontalis muscle and as much as possible of the subcutaneous tissue is removed (Fig. 171-3B). If the flap has been extended into the hairline, individual hair follicles on the undersurface of the flap are clipped with a scissors. The forehead flap is then rotated into position and sutured to skin at the margins of the defect and the margins of the mucosal flap (Fig. 171-4). The forehead flap may be coapted to the underlying soft tissue by quilting sutures or close suction. The forehead defect is closed primarily if possible. Any area that cannot be closed is allowed to granulate and heal secondarily, usually yielding amazingly good results. The forehead flap is divided and inset at 3 weeks. The unused portion of the flap pedicle is trimmed to allow primary closure in the eyebrow area.

KEVIN A. SHUMRICK

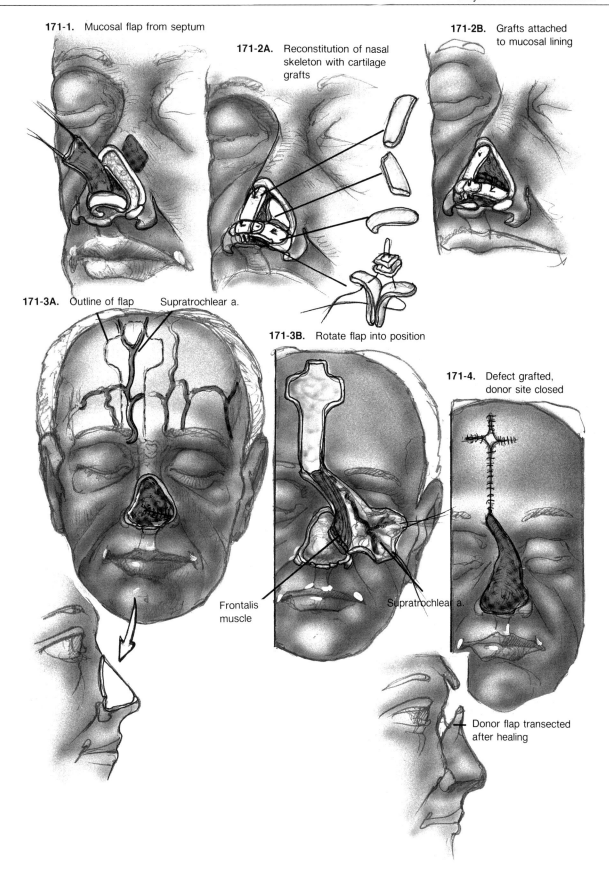

171-1. Mucosal flap from septum

171-2A. Reconstitution of nasal skeleton with cartilage grafts

171-2B. Grafts attached to mucosal lining

171-3A. Outline of flap   Supratrochlear a.

171-3B. Rotate flap into position

171-4. Defect grafted, donor site closed

Frontalis muscle

Supratrochlear a.

Donor flap transected after healing

■ 172. OUTLINE REVISION RHINOPLASTY

Reconstruction and repair of an aesthetic or functional nasal deformity. The tailored surgical responses include reduction, which is the judicious excision of offending excesses of bone, cartilage, septum, or skin, and augmentation, which is the addition of tissue to the septum, bony pyramid, midcartilaginous area, or tip.

Indications

1. Inadequate or inappropriate resection of bone or cartilage
2. Nasal tip bossa or asymmetries
3. Pinching of the lateral alar wall, with or without airway compromise
4. Alar retraction, with or without external valvular dysfunction
5. Columella retraction
6. Supratip fullness (ie, polly-beak deformity)
7. Midnasal deformities and asymmetries

Contraindications

1. Significant local or systemic infections or inflammatory disorders
2. Significant emotional, behavioral, or psychologic disorders
3. Insufficient healing time since the previous procedure
4. Insufficient or inadequate donor tissue available
5. Surgeon's limitations or inexperience

Special Considerations

1. Redundant skin requiring an external dorsal skin excision
2. Scarified or insufficient skin blanket requiring skin grafting
3. Prior harvesting of grafts compromising available donor sites
4. Strength, shape, and consistency of the grafts
5. Alloplastic implants for dorsal augmentation
6. A litigious patient with a severe deformity

Preoperative Preparation

1. Complete history and perusal of prior surgical records
2. Routine laboratory studies
3. Bleeding and clotting studies, if the history is questionable
4. Careful preoperative functional and aesthetic analysis
5. Preoperative photographic documentation
6. Thorough patient education for proper informed consent

(continued)

Operative Procedures

Excessive Reduction

Errors of inadequate resection are corrected by the judicious excision of the excesses of bone, cartilage, or skin. Overresection produces deformities that require grafting to fill, contour, or elevate the defects. Revision rhinoplasty requires tailored surgical responses for each offending problem. The most frequent ones include knuckling (ie, bossa), pinching, alar retraction, columellar retraction, supratip fullness (ie, polly-beak), and midnasal asymmetries. It is best to wait 1 year after the primary rhinoplasty.

Bossa

For bilateral, asymmetric bossa, the surgeon must decide whether to lower the high side, raise the lower side with a graft, or perform a combination. A small slot incision is made, allowing the area to be visualized (Fig. 172-1). If a unilateral prominence provides the more pleasing profile line, a small alar graft of septal cartilage can be layered over the opposite dome to provide symmetry. Conversely, the unnatural knob can be removed by simple shave excision.

One or two 4-0 catgut sutures close the wound. Antibiotic ointment–impregnated cottonoid wadding is placed in the nostril, and no external dressing is necessary.

Pinching

Treatment for pinching is replacement with cartilage carved to a proper shape, thickness, and dimension. Septal cartilage is easily molded into the desired shape, and possesses a consistency and elasticity that compares well with the normal lateral crural elements. An incision is outlined 2 to 3 mm superior to the nostril rim (Fig. 172-2). Thick scar tissue between vestibular and external skin is often encountered. Dissection is facilitated by hydrodissection with a local anesthetic. A precise pocket is created just large enough to admit the graft, which should fit like a hand in a glove. The graft and pocket should be long enough to extend inferiorly toward the sesamoids and wide enough to simulate the normal lateral crural shape as it approaches the dome area (Fig. 172-3). Gentle morselization or crushing can slightly soften the graft, but enough stiffness must be maintained to allow the graft to act like a collar stay and restore the integrity of the external nasal valve.

Two or three 4-0 catgut sutures are used to close the incision, and a light internal packing and external dressing are applied.

Alar Retraction

Alar retraction with a normal nasolabial relation requires lengthening, using a septal cartilage or an auricular cartilage minicomposite graft. Minimal retraction of 1 to 2 mm can be improved with autogenous septal cartilage. A composite is used if the cartilage and vestibular skin have been sacrificed. The cymba concha best simulates the shape, curve, and consistency of the normal lateral crus. Ideally, the left alar should be replaced with the contralateral right cymba concha and vice versa (Fig. 172-4). The graft should be wide enough to lengthen the ala appropriately, allowing 10% to 15% for shrinkage, (Fig. 172-5).

An incision is outlined 2 to 3 mm from the nostril rim. Freeing adhesions allows the retracted alar to be inferiorly displaced, creating a defect that can be filled with contralateral composite auricular graft.

Careful approximation of the skin with fine catgut sutures anchors the graft in place (Fig. 172-6).

Columella Retraction

If lengthening of the columella is needed, inferior traction on the columella with the thumb and index finger tests its mobility. If relatively stiff, a composite graft is required. If the membranous lining is not deficient, cartilage replacement alone can suffice.

A pocket is created through an incision at the caudal septum. A retrograde pocket is dissected between the septocolumellar membranes to mobilize the septocolumellar complex and scar tissue. The

(continued)

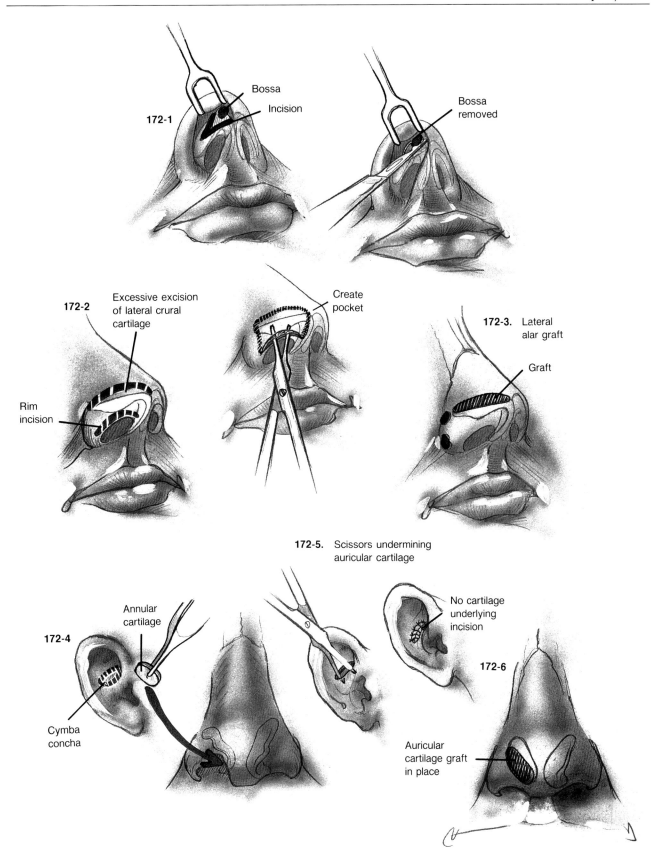

172-1   Bossa   Incision   Bossa removed

172-2   Excessive excision of lateral crural cartilage   Create pocket   172-3.   Lateral alar graft   Graft   Rim incision

172-5.   Scissors undermining auricular cartilage

172-4   Annular cartilage   No cartilage underlying incision   172-6   Cymba concha   Auricular cartilage graft in place

172. OUTLINE REVISION RHINOPLASTY
(continued)

Special Instruments, Position, and Anesthesia
1. Headlight
2. Nasal speculum
3. Septal and periosteal elevators, nasal osteotomes, and rasps
4. Fine, delicate plastic surgery instruments
5. Supine position, with the head slightly extended
6. Monitored intravenous sedation or general anesthesia
7. Local infiltration of a 1% solution of lidocaine with 1:100,000 epinephrine

Tips and Pearls
1. Hydrodissect the tissue planes with local infiltration.
2. Avoid "buttonholing" the skin.
3. Dissect precise pockets for graft placement to fit like a glove.
4. Use autologous cartilage grafts to fill, elevate, or contour defects.
5. Soften, morselize, and bevel the graft edges.
6. Carefully suture and close all incisions with fine catgut.

Pitfalls and Complications
1. Skin necrosis
2. Inflammation, infection, or shrinkage of the grafts
3. Prominent palpable or visible graft edges
4. Persistent asymmetries, irregularities, and deviations
5. Septal flaccidity or perforation

Postoperative Care
1. Light Telfa pack for 24 hours and daily lubrication for 7 to 10 days
2. External bandage and splint removed in 5 to 7 days
3. Follow-up assessments at 6, 12 and 24 months
4. Minor revisions possible after 1 year

References
Kamer FM, McQuown SA. Revision rhinoplasty, analysis and treatment. Arch Otolaryngol Head Neck Surg 1988;114:257.

Meyer R. Secondary and functional rhinoplasty. The difficult nose. San Diego: Grune & Stratton, 1990.

graft is shaped and placed into the pocket (Fig. 172-7). Slight overcorrection allows for shrinkage. This technique is helpful in the correction of a defect due to lack of adequate caudal septal cartilage, causing a retracted columella, a condition that often affects the non-Caucasian nose.

If the membrane and cartilage are deficient, a composite graft can lengthen the retracted columella. Posterior conchal skin is less adherent to the cartilage, easier to manipulate and leaves a minimal scar. A staggered technique with retrograde dissection of the septocolumella is accomplished by a hemitransfixion incision a few millimeters superior to the old, retracted scar. The scar is freed from its attachments to the nasal spine and caudal septal remnants by sharp scissors dissection. A parallel septal hemitransfixion incision is made on the contralateral side 1 to 1.5 cm superior to the first incision. Wide subperichondral dissection allows the inferior septocolumellar complex to be mobilized. The distance separating the two contralateral incisions and the degree of submucosal dissection needed are determined by the width of the graft required to augment the retracted septocolumellar complex (Fig. 172-8).

The composite is placed into the defect. A few sutures of 4-0 catgut help stabilize the graft and anchor the postauricular skin to the septal mucosa. A light internal nasal packing is applied overnight.

Supratip Fullness
Treatment for supratip fullness is tailored to the specific problem. A high cartilaginous septum or exuberant scar tissue in the supratip area can be corrected by trimming excessive tissue through a unilateral intercartilaginous and complete septocolumellar incision. Scissors dissection separates the dermal elements from the underlying scar. If the tip is adequately supported and projection is adequate, this approach suffices to improve the problem.

If tissue must be replaced, cartilage grafts harvested from the septum or concha are fashioned to augment the deficient pyramid or tip. Auricular composite grafts can be used if the mucosal lining and cartilage require replacement. Septal cartilage can be carved and shaped into an appropriate shield graft to gain added projection while maintaining dorsal height. The graft is placed through a small slot incision into a pocket just large enough for the graft (Fig. 172-9). Lateral alar grafts add stability to deficient nostril walls and improve support and projection. They are shaped and placed in a pocket, as described for treatment of the pinched tip. Dorsal cartilaginous grafts increase the cantilever effect of the pyramid on the tip and improve the aesthetic result by raising the dorsal profile. Dissection is facilitated by a small apical septal incision to allow submucoperichondrial elevation and proper pocket formation in this area (Fig. 172-10).

Some cases require combined dorsal pyramid replacement, lateral alar grafting, and tip shield grafting in addition to supratip scar tissue excision to treat a polly-beak deformity because of deficient tissue after a poorly performed primary rhinoplasty. Open rhinoplasty is an appropriate alternate approach if direct visual correction of these asymmetries seems necessary.

Midnasal Deformities
Bony disparities contributing to midnasal asymmetry are corrected by appropriate nasal bone restructuring and refracturing to restore the nasal pyramid. Septal deformities in the middle portion of the nose are straightened. If an upper lateral cartilage is subluxed, onlay grafts can camouflage the deformity (Fig. 172-11).

Placement is facilitated by a precise pocket dissection through a unilateral intercartilaginous incision. Spreader grafts can improve the function of the internal valve and the appearance of the collapsed or overresected midnasal area. Cartilage strips from the septum are trimmed and placed in a precise pocket at the junction of the septum and collapsed or overexcised upper lateral cartilage. Dissection is facilitated by a small apical septal incision to allow submucoperichondrial elevation with a Cottle elevator. It is best to leave an adequate bridge of mucoperichondrium between this pocket and the donor septal area to ensure proper placement and fixation of the spreader graft in its pocket (Fig. 172-12).

FRANK M. KAMER

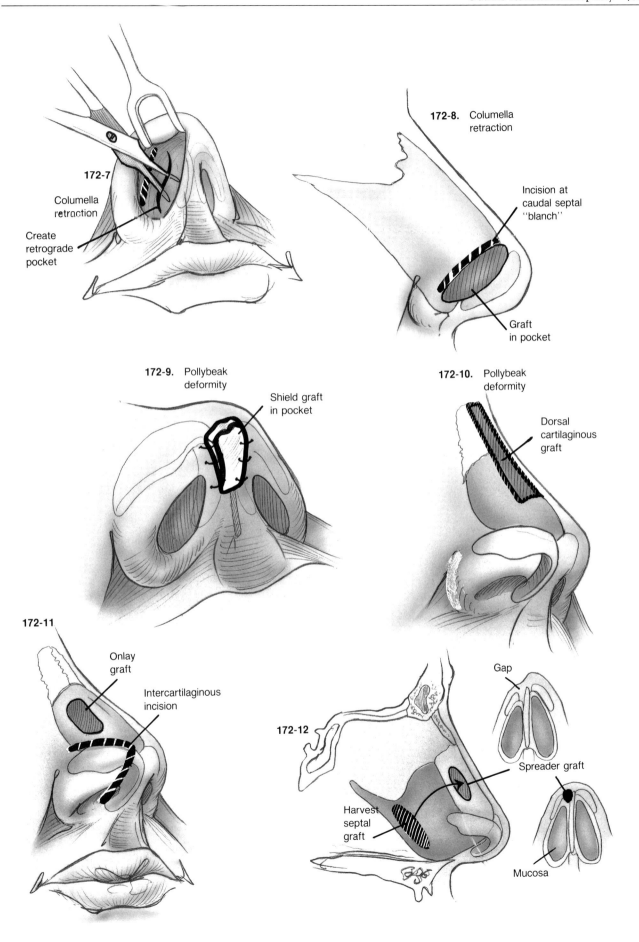

172-7

Columella retraction

Create retrograde pocket

172-8.   Columella retraction

Incision at caudal septal "blanch"

Graft in pocket

172-9.   Pollybeak deformity

Shield graft in pocket

172-10.   Pollybeak deformity

Dorsal cartilaginous graft

172-11

Onlay graft

Intercartilaginous incision

172-12

Harvest septal graft

Gap

Spreader graft

Mucosa

■ 173. NASAL VALVE SURGERY

Surgery to repair nasal obstruction due to collapse or incompetence of the nasal valve.

Indications

1. Nasal obstruction due to collapse in the nasal valve area
2. Nasal obstruction due to cicatricial scarring or synechiae in the nasal valve area
3. Facial paralysis leading to loss of function of the nasal dilator muscles and subsequent nasal valve collapse

Contraindications

1. Physiologic nasal valve collapse; some collapse of the nasal valve due to heavy breathing or exercise is normal, and these patients should not be operated on.
2. The "chronic sniffer" is a form of nasal neurosis.
3. Patients who abuse cocaine should not be operated on.

Special Considerations

1. Nasal obstruction due to other causes such as high septal deviation, thick septums, ptotic nasal tips, and enlarged turbinates should be corrected before valve surgery.
2. True nasal valve collapse is rare in patients who are not elderly or have not had previous nasal trauma or nasal surgery (eg, rhinoplasty).
3. If the patient does not give a history of nasal surgery or trauma, the diagnosis of nasal valve incompetence should be made with caution.
4. Patients with rhinitis medicamentosa should be treated medically before to surgery.
5. Geriatric patients may develop nasal valve collapse.

Preoperative Preparation

1. Routine laboratory studies
2. Operative reports of any previous nasal surgeries should be reviewed before valve surgery.

Special Instruments, Position, and Anesthesia

1. Headlight
2. Septorhinoplasty tray should include Freer elevator, Cottle elevator, cartilage knife, small 6- to 10-mm Frazier suction tips, 4-mm straight osteotome, Takahashi biting forceps, double-action biting Jansen-Middleton forceps, bayonet forceps
3. Slight reverse Trendelenburg position
4. Preoperative vasoconstriction: cocaine, oxymetazoline, or another decongestive agent 10 minutes before beginning the operation

Tips and Pearls

1. Replace what is missing with like material.
2. When correcting the valve collapse with a strut, it is important that the strut extends all the way from the septum medially down to the nasofacial groove laterally.
3. Every effort must be made to decrease the nasal resistance elsewhere in the nose so that the negative pressure required to provide adequate inspiratory airflow through the nose is as low as possible. This helps prevent collapse of the valve.

Pitfalls and Complications

1. Persistent nasal valve stenosis
2. Persistent nasal valve collapse
3. Cicatricial scarring or synechiae in the nasal valve area
4. Polybeak deformity
5. Enlargement of the tip area of the alae

Postoperative Care Issues

1. Packing is used for 1 to 2 weeks postoperatively.
2. Antistaphylococcal antibiotics should be used until the splints are removed.
3. Careful cleaning of nasal valve area helps prevent stenosis.

References

Goode RL. Surgery of the incompetent nasal valve. Laryngoscope 1985;546.
Kern EB. Nasal valve surgery. In: Krause CJ, Mangat DS, Pastorek N, eds. Aesthetic facial surgery. Philadelphia: JB Lippincott, 1991.

Operative Procedure

The nasal valve is the area of nose formed by the distal inferior border of the upper lateral cartilage laterally, nasal septum medially and upper border of the anterior inferior turbinate inferiorly.

Inadequate Vestibular Skin

The scar tissue producing the contracture is completely excised, and the size and shape of the defect are measured. The skin graft should be about 20% larger than the defect to allow for shrinkage. This can usually be done endonasally without an external incision, but occasionally, placement of the graft can be facilitated by performing an alotomy incision (Fig. 173-1). Three or four absorbable 4-0 chromic sutures are first placed through the medial and lateral borders of the defect and then sewn into the medial and lateral borders of the edge of the graft before it is inserted into the defect. The graft is then inserted and the sutures tied. A piece of Xeroform is placed over the graft, and the vestibule is generously packed with 1-cm Vaseline or Adaptic gauze impregnated with tetracycline ointment.

Inadequate Cartilage

The cartilage graft may be taken from the quadrilateral cartilage of the septum or the ear concha laterally. If the graft is too short (a common error), nasal valve collapse will occur (Fig. 173-2). We try to obtain a 3-cm-long graft, which can be shortened as needed. The cartilage should be thin, strong, slightly convex, and about 4 to 7 mm in diameter. A marginal incision, just inside the alar rim, is favored for placement of the cartilage graft (Fig. 173-3). The graft is inserted into a pocket made just under the vestibular skin at the site of collapse (ie, the nasal valve). It is held in place by passing the absorbable sutures used to close the incision through the caudal edge of the graft. The graft must extend from the superior nasal septum medially down to the floor of the nose and to the nasofacial groove laterally (see Fig. 173-3B).

Occasionally, the patient may also have alar floor narrowing or stenosis that require correction. We prefer to excise a crescent-shaped wedge of skin just lateral to the alae and place this as a skin graft just medial to the alae, widening the nasal alae as needed (Fig. 173-4).

Inadequate Vestibular Skin and Cartilage

Inadequate vestibular skin and cartilage is the most common defect and requires treatment with a composite graft of cartilage and skin from the ear or a two-stage repair consisting of vestibular skin grafting and insertion of a cartilage batten 2 months later. The best donor site is the upper concha just below the inferior crus.

The scarred area in the valve area is excised. The composite donor graft is trimmed to fit the defect, allowing for some contraction. The composite graft can be placed endonasally without external incisions or with the help of an alotomy incision as described for the skin grafts (see Fig. 173-1). The graft is stabilized with a 5-0 chromic mattress suture passing through the graft and external skin and tied over a bolster. This is left in place for 1 week and then removed (Fig. 173-5).

When bilateral valvular insufficiency exists, another solution is to take one large composite graft, trim it to an oval shape, and remove a 3-mm-wide strip of skin and cartilage from the center so that only the perichondrium holds the two pieces together (Fig. 173-6). This type of graft is more stable than two separate grafts. It acts to open the roof of the valve, pushing the upper lateral cartilages laterally (Fig. 173-7).

The skin over the nasal dorsum is elevated by connecting the marginal incision of each nostril with a transcolumellar incision (ie, standard external rhinoplasty approach). The skin is elevated over the recipient sites using small plastic or Stevens scissors so that a pocket is formed over the septum and between the upper lateral cartilages and skin. The graft is positioned over the septum and nasal cartilage, extending from the upper lateral cartilages down to the lower lateral cartilages (see Fig. 173-7). The upper lateral cartilages are cut from the septum on each side and sewn to the lateral aspect of the composite graft on each side, opening the roof of the valve.

RICHARD L. GOODE
LANE F. SMITH

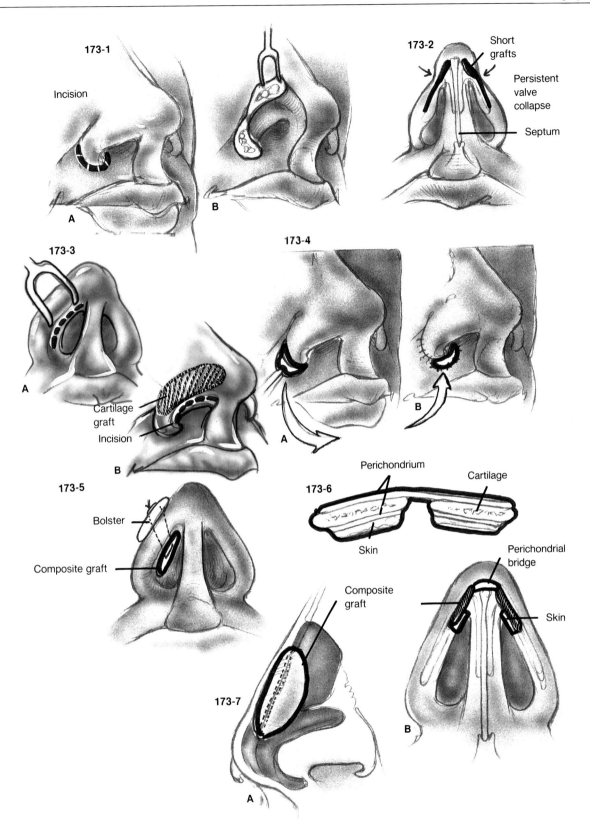

173-1

Incision

A

B

173-2

Short grafts

Persistent valve collapse

Septum

173-3

A

B

Cartilage graft

Incision

173-4

A

B

173-5

Bolster

Composite graft

173-6

Perichondrium

Cartilage

Skin

Composite graft

173-7

A

Perichondrial bridge

Skin

B

■ *174.* CLEFT-LIP NASAL REPAIR

Repair of the congenital abnormalities associated with unilateral or bilateral cleft lip.

Indications (Fig. 174-1)

1. Unilateral deformity
2. Bilateral deformity
3. Nasal alar collapse
4. Septal deviation
5. Oronasal fistula
6. Nasal obstruction
7. Cosmetic deformity

Special Considerations

1. Completion of major revisions of the cleft lip deformity
2. Age of patient for nasal surgery related to functional airway needs and psychologic benefits
3. Absence of nasal or sinus infection
4. Patient's desire to have surgery to improve function and appearance

Preoperative Preparation

1. Review of preoperative photographs with the patient and family to discuss pathology, goals, and risks
2. Fiberoptic nasal endoscopy to identify coexisting intranasal or sinus disease

Special Instruments, Position, and Anesthesia

1. Secure an oral endotracheal tube in a midline position to prevent distortion of the lips.
2. Fiberoptic headlight
3. Low-power loupes
4. Fine ophthalmic forceps and small, double skin hooks

(continued)

Operative Procedure

The repair of the cleft-lip nasal deformity is usually one of multistaged procedures, with their timing appropriate to the child's age and functional problems. One of the first procedures to consider is septal surgery for deviation and obstruction that produces mouth breathing and complicates dental arch growth and development. Septoplasty can be performed on a child as young as 8 years of age if there are good clinical indications. This procedure should be performed under general anesthesia and with the addition of calculated, safe dosages of associated topical and locally injected anesthetic agents.

Only one mucoperichondrial flap need be elevated enough to visualize the septal abnormalities. If a palatal cleft is still present or if closure has been accomplished only recently, the maxillary crest should be left alone. Where the septum is deviated or dislocated, a small strip can be excised; just enough is removed to accomplish the task. In a few cases, the cartilaginous septum requires mobilization from its attachment to the vomer bone and ethmoid plate to center it within the nasal cavity. It is wise to stay low on the septum if possible and not violate the superior position where it contacts the upper lateral cartilages. This type of minor and conservative septal reconstruction usually suffices to reestablish a better nasal air flow.

When necessary, a deflection of the vomer bone and perpendicular plate of the ethmoid can be refractured into a straighter position, taking care not to injure the region of the ethmoid perpendicular plate. Conservative resection of major bony deflections can also be carried out but should be minimized to avoid injuring the abnormal hard palate.

Columellar abnormalities often coexist with septal abnormalities and may restrict the degree of improvement desired with septoplasty. Because the columella is uniformly shortened in this deformity, it must be lengthened in some fashion.

The V-Y advancement flap is a simple, effective means of achieving increased vertical height to the columella (Fig. 174-2). Several conditions direct the use of this flap, including adequate width of the existing columella and sufficient upper lip tissue from which to "borrow" new columellar soft tissues. The apex of the V-shaped incision should be placed at the region of greatest tissue width to minimize visible narrowing when primary closure occurs. The increased height of the columella may not support the nasal tip well without insertion of a narrow, strong piece of cartilage to serve as a columellar strut. This cartilage could be donated from the septum if a strip resection septoplasty was carried out.

Another method of lengthening the columella is to outline a rectangular flap based superiorly on the dome region of the lower lateral cartilages and to advance this flap upward (Fig. 174-3). The lateral segments of the columella are sutured together in the region where the rectangular flap used to be, and the columella is lengthened. In this case, an elevation and projection of the entire tip of the nose is achieved through the concomitant advancement of the domes of the lower lateral cartilages. This technique is a more generous variation of the V-Y advancement flap previously described.

The Brauer-Foerster technique of columellar lengthening involves the development of two sickle-shaped flaps along the medial and superior alar rims and based inferiorly on the columella (Fig. 174-4). Essentially, they become a bilateral pedicle flap. Part of the inferior margin of the lower lateral cartilage can be included in the flap to give more support to the structure. This is not a full-thickness alar rim excision, because the vestibular skin is left intact to become the new alar rim. These flaps are then rotated medially and sutured together, resulting in increased columellar height. Gentle handling of these small flaps is important, because any tip necrosis will compromise the ultimate result.

Because a deformity of the columella often occurs in conjunction with an abnormality of the rest of the nostril, many techniques have been developed to repair both deformities concomitantly. One of the most common is the Ivy modification of the Blair procedure (Fig. 174-5). The constricted nostril is incorporated into a flap based on the lateral ala and advanced medially and superiorly. The apex

(continued)

174-1

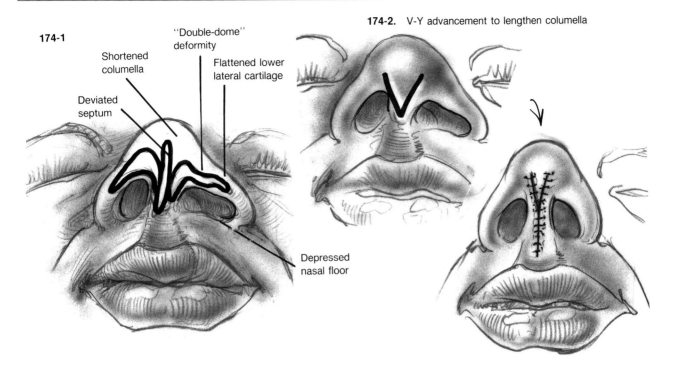

Shortened columella

Deviated septum

"Double-dome" deformity

Flattened lower lateral cartilage

Depressed nasal floor

174-2. V-Y advancement to lengthen columella

174-3. Columellar flap to lengthen columella

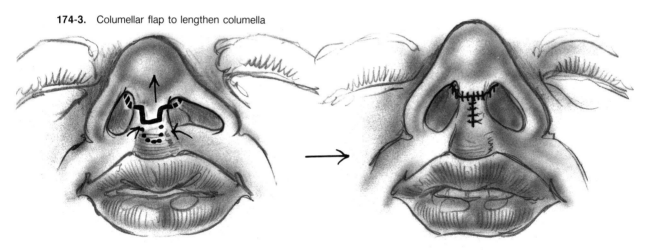

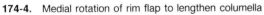

174-4. Medial rotation of rim flap to lengthen columella

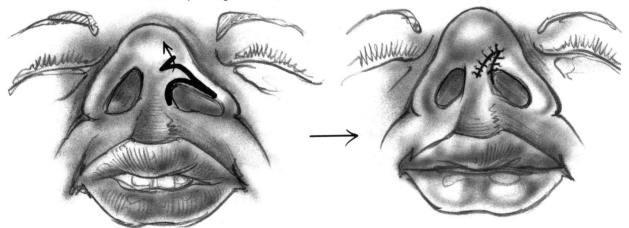

■ *174.* CLEFT-LIP NASAL REPAIR *(continued)*

Tips and Pearls

1. Caution in elevating scarred or abnormal skin at the columella and floor of the nostril
2. Possible anatomic abnormalities of the cleft lip nose (Fig. 174-1)
   a. Nostril floor depressed on the affected side
   b. Ala more inferior and posterior on the affected side
   c. Shorter columella on the affected side
   d. Narrow and collapsed anterior nares on the affected side
   e. Double dome of lower lateral cartilage's lateral crus on the affected side
   f. Deviated septum
   g. Possibility of small oronasal fistula of the floor of the nose on the affected side
3. Have a good surgical plan based on knowledge of the pathophysiology.
4. Have the photographs and surgical plan posted in operating room near the surgeon.

Pitfalls and Complications

1. Loss of skin on ala or columella
2. Reopening previously closed oronasal fistula with too-vigorous septoplasty
3. Infection and bleeding
4. Undercorrection of deformities

Postoperative Care Issues

1. Soft intranasal packing to support incisions, compress vessels, and reduce edema
2. If an external approach is used, avoid taping the columella to reduce the risk of tissue loss.
3. Use oral broad-spectrum antibiotics with good antistaphylococcic coverage, saline nasal spray, gentle peroxide cleaning of incisions, and topical Bactroban ointment.
4. Hematoma of septum, ala, or columella

References

Brattstrom V, McWilliam J, Larson O, et al. Craniofacial development in children with unilateral clefts of the lip, alveolus and palate treated according to three different regimes: assessment of nasolabial appearance. Scand J Plast Reconstr Hand Surg 1992;26:313.

Holt GR. Management of cleft lip nasal deformity. Facial Plast Surg 1986;3:161.

Koltai PJ, Hoehn J, Bailey CM. The external rhinoplasty approach for rhinologic surgery in children. Arch Otolaryngol Head Neck Surg 1992;118:401.

of the nostril is advanced into a defect created by the excision of a full-thickness wedge of tissue just below the soft tissue facet. Small soft tissue Burow triangles can be removed at the inferior alar base to reduce the length disparity of the two sides of the alar base. This technique also repositions an alar that is located too far laterally on the maxilla.

The Dingman technique is another excellent method of reorienting the nostril and lengthening the ipsilaterally shortened columella (Fig. 174-6). Two flaps are formed in the nostril, one based superiorly on the medial crus and the second based laterally on the alar base. The medial flap is rotated first in a superior direction. Then the lateral-inferior flap is rotated medially to close the nostril defect. This technique reorients the nostril but may also narrow the nostril base. The anatomic deformity determines if this is a favorable goal. The skin defect is closed with 6-0 chromic catgut sutures in younger children and 6-0 Prolene in older children.

If the nostril is short but has a normal width to its alar base, the easiest technique to effect the simple elevation of the apex of the nostril entails excising a full-thickness wedge of tissue at the apex. A thin rim of skin is left intact at the top of the apex of the nostril to prevent webbing. The apex is advanced superiorly and sutured into its new position. If the nostril is severely constricted, a full-thickness skin or composite graft can be inserted where the wedge has been removed to broaden the width of the apex.

One of the major deformities found in the cleft-lip nasal deformity is the atrophic lower lateral cartilage, which is flattened and positioned lower in the nostril (or nasal tip) than the opposite side. Several procedures can be used to correct or improve this deformity. In the Thomas Rees technique, the lower lateral cartilages are delivered through intercartilaginous and marginal incisions, and the abnormal lateral crus is severed from its lateral attachment (Fig. 174-7). The lateral crus and its attached skin are advanced medially and superiorly into a more favorable position. The abnormal dome is then sutured to the normal dome to ensure their symmetric position postoperatively. Clear polypropylene suture can be used to suture the domes to create a longer-lasting connection. The lateral nostril defect is closed primarily using chromic catgut sutures. This technique can correct mild to moderate deformities of the flattened ala.

When the flattening of the nasal apex and ala is caused by the dorsal displacement of the dome of the involved lower lateral cartilage, the Farrior repair is useful (Fig. 174-8). The lateral alar sulcus is incised, creating a near-triangular flap that can be advanced laterally. This technique is a variation of the V-Y advancement, using the lateral alar base as the advancing segment. The defect in the upper lip is closed primarily using 4-0 chromic catgut suture and 6-0 Prolene for the skin. A variation on this technique involves the development of an upper lip flap horizontal to the alar base that is advanced into the floor of the nose, transposing tissue from the upper lip into the nasal floor. This allows the lateral alar base to be moved laterally to a more favorable and symmetric position.

Onlay cartilage grafts, obtained preferably from the auricular concha or from the nasal septum, may be used to augment insufficient areas of soft tissue or cartilage in the deformity. If the grafts are placed along the depressed lateral crus of the lower lateral cartilage, an external rhinoplasty approach may be used for exact placement, or a marginal rim incision of the ala can provide an entrance for an onlay cartilage graft. The former approach is commonly used in conjunction with a columellar lengthening procedure. Whatever the technique, the graft can be laid on the insufficient area, used to bolster tip projection, or used as a columellar strut. A cartilage graft can also be placed through a small sublabial or lateral alar incision to elevate the floor of the affected nostril and depressed lateral alar base. Additional anterior maxilla augmentation can be accomplished by inserting a "mustache" cartilage graft through a sublabial incision, fixing the graft directly to the periosteum and septolabial muscle with 4-0 Vicryl sutures. The mucosal incision may be closed with 4-0 chromic catgut sutures.

G. RICHARD HOLT

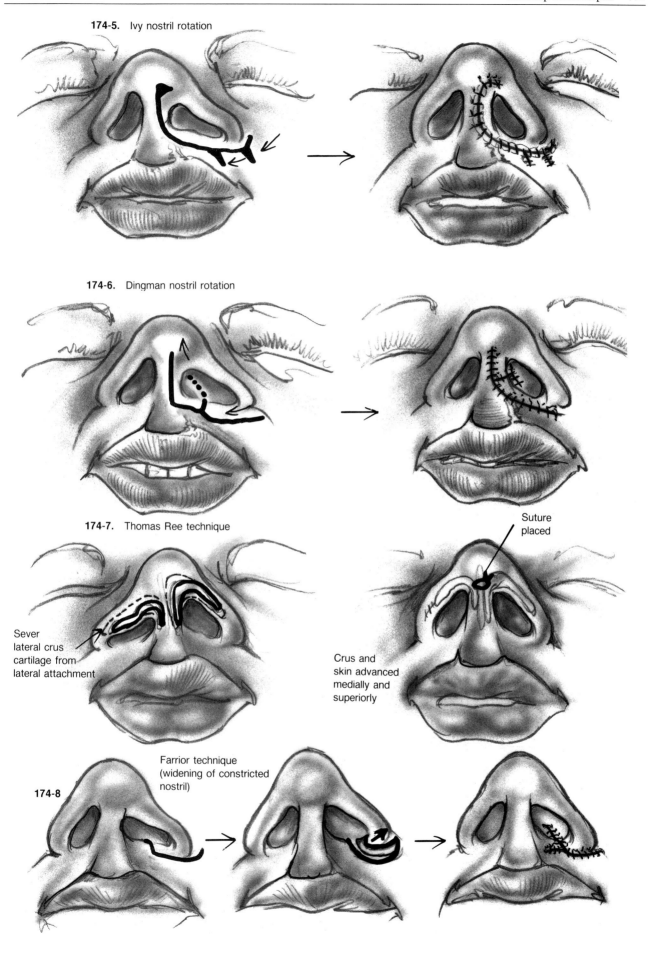

174-5. Ivy nostril rotation

174-6. Dingman nostril rotation

174-7. Thomas Ree technique

Suture placed

Sever lateral crus cartilage from lateral attachment

Crus and skin advanced medially and superiorly

Farrior technique (widening of constricted nostril)

174-8

■ *175.* RHINOPHYMA SURGICAL TECH NIQUES— Rhinophyma is a sebaceous overgrowth of nasal skin with redness and nodular swelling, resulting in marked deformity

Indications

1. Rosacea of nasal skin
2. Functional and aesthetic impairment
3. Not related to alcohol consumption
4. Male predominance
5. Primarily affects lower portion of the nose
6. Vascular dilatation and nonspecific dermal lymphatic infiltrates; foci of epithelioid and giant cells
7. Incidence of basal cell carcinoma of nose not increased in rhinophyma

Special Instruments, Position, and Anesthesia

1. Lounge chair position
2. Headlight (optional)
3. Weck-blade knife and argon beam coagulator
4. Intravenous sedation; local anesthesia with 0.5% Xylocaine and 1:200,000 epinephrine
5. Copious amounts of vitamin A and D ointment for raw nasal surface after the procedure

Preoperative Preparation

1. Routine laboratory studies
2. Bleeding and clotting studies, if the history suggests problems

Tips and Pearls

1. Careful dissection with preservation of basal appendages
2. Particular attention to alar rim dissection
3. Copious amount of local anesthetic agents (10 to 15 mL) for hemostasis achieved by the epinephrine effect and tamponading of tissue by local anesthetic and for hydrodissection of tissue to separate the rhinophyma from the basal layer
4. Dissection of rhinophyma from superior to inferior direction
5. Argon beam coagulator set at 60 watts, with exposure to tissue of less than 3 seconds

Pitfalls and Complications

1. Careful analysis of the depth of rhinophyma, especially a large, amorphous tumor; err on the side of more superficial dissection.
2. Too-deep dissection leads to scar contracture, especially in the alar region.
3. Hypertrophic scar on the nasal dorsum is a rare but possible sequela of the healing process. If scarring occurs, inject on a weekly basis with Kenalog 10 until the scar softens.
4. Antibiotic ointments can induce an atopic reaction. Nonantibiotic ointment is just as effective for epithelization.
5. If scar contracture occurs, composite graft reconstruction is necessary as soon as the problem is identified.

Postoperative Care Issues

1. Postresection, the nose appears charred; this is not an abnormality.
2. No dressing is used postoperatively; apply copious amounts of vitamin A and D ointment.
3. If stable, the patient can be discharged to his or her home the same day as surgery.
4. Instruct the patient to clean wound every 4 to 6 hours with hydrogen peroxide and reapply vitamin A and D ointment for the next few weeks. Epithelialization is complete in about 3 weeks.
5. Avoid sun exposure until re-epithelialization has completed. Protect the nose with a hat and sun block for the next 6 months.

References

Freeman BS. Reconstructive rhinoplasty for rhinophyma. Plast Reconstr Surg 1970;46:265.

Stucker FJ, Hoasjoe DK. Rhinophyma: a new approach for hemostasis. Ann Otol Rhinol Laryngol 1993;102:925.

Operative Procedure

The patient is taken to the operating room and put in the lounge chair position (Fig. 175-1*A*). Intravenous sedation is initiated. One cotton pledget soaked in 4% cocaine is inserted in the superior buccogingival sulcus, and two cotton pledgets are inserted into each nostril. A nerve block is initiated using 0.5% Xylocaine with 1:200,000 epinephrine (Fig. 175-1*B*). The infraorbital nerve on either side is anesthetized, along with the nasociliary. Under pressure, another 10 to 15 mL of local anesthetic agent is injected into the rhinophyma. This helps with hydrodissection of the tumor and tamponading of the vessels within it.

After the patient has been prepped and draped in the sterile fashion, and 10 minutes have elapsed after the local anesthetic injection, the rhinophyma is removed. This is done from a superior to inferior direction (Fig. 175-2). Care is taken, especially around both alar rims, to prevent the level of the dissection from being too deep. The alar resection is performed after the bulk of the rhinophyma has been resected. The basal appendages are observed during the shaving of the rhinophyma to make sure that re-epithelialization can be achieved without any difficulties (Fig. 175-3*A*). A wet sponge is put on the nose for temporary hemostasis.

Final hemostasis is achieved. Using the argon beam coagulator set at 60 watts, the hemostasis is achieved by passing the coagulator over the excised portion of the rhinophyma (Fig. 175-3*B*). With proper manipulation, the total passage time of the coagulator on the excision bed is less than 3 seconds. One or two passes of the coagulator are adequate for achieving proper hemostasis (Fig. 175-4*A*). Care is taken around the rim of the alar on either side to prevent deep tissue damage. After final hemostasis has been achieved, copious amounts of vitamin A and D ointment are applied to the nose (Fig. 175-4*B*). No additional dressing is required. The usual estimated blood loss for this procedure is in the range of 5 to 15 mL.

FRED J. STUCKER
DENIS K. HOASJOE

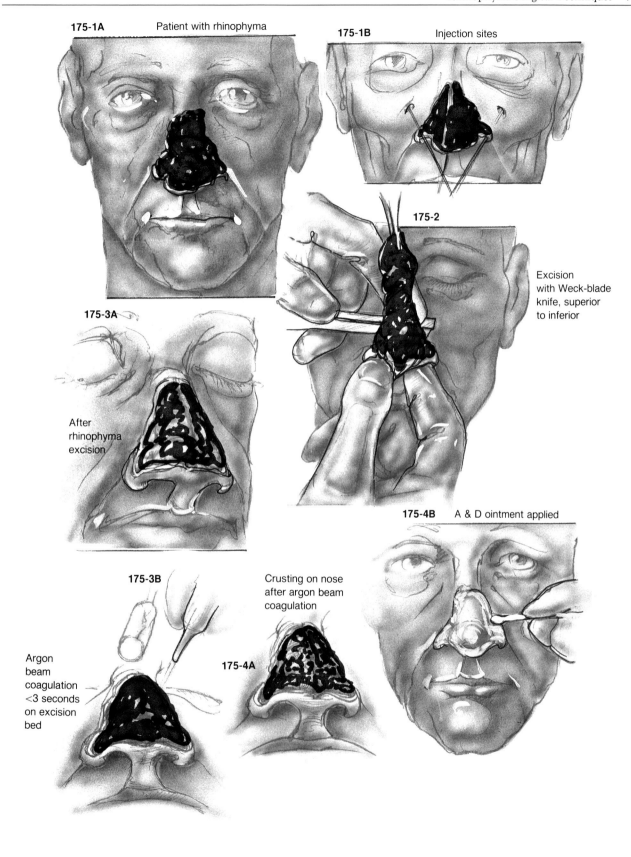

175-1A   Patient with rhinophyma

175-1B   Injection sites

175-2

Excision
with Weck-blade
knife, superior
to inferior

175-3A

After
rhinophyma
excision

175-4B   A & D ointment applied

175-3B

Argon
beam
coagulation
<3 seconds
on excision
bed

Crusting on nose
after argon beam
coagulation

175-4A

■ *176.* NON-CAUCASIAN RHINOPLASTY

Correcting the broad, flat nasal appearance characteristic of certain black and Asian populations

Indications

1. Broad, flat bridge with shortened nasal bones at an increased obtuse angle to each other
2. Broad base with a flattened alar and marked alar groove
3. Amorphous, rounded, flat tip, lacking projection
4. Deepened and inferiorly placed nasofrontal area having an increased obtuse angle
5. Acute nasolabial angle
6. Saddle deformity
7. Enlarged piriform orifice, with flared alae and large horizontally aligned nostrils
8. Large alae extending beyond the alar attachment to the cheek and covering the columella in profile
9. Shortened columella
10. Increased (open) angle between the medial and lateral crura of the alar cartilages
11. Upper lateral cartilages are small and triangular.
12. Anterosuperior border of the septal cartilage is recessed, with an anterior septal angle more obtuse and cephalically placed.
13. Anteroinferior border of the septal cartilage is recessed.
14. Quadrilateral septal cartilage is relatively smaller and considerably thinner than in Caucasians.
15. Underdeveloped anterior nasal spine

Tips and Pearls

1. The septum is rarely deviated.
2. All cartilages are soft, lacking firmness.
3. Augmentation of profile
   a. Medial and lateral osteotomies
   b. Dorsal grafts
4. Tip narrowing refinement and projection
   a. Debride fibrofatty tissue
   b. Vertical alar division lateral to the dome
   c. Medial crura apposition
   d. Columellar strut
   e. Layered shield graft
5. Additional refinements
   a. Weir resection to moderate the alar flare, nostril size, and alignment
   b. Plumping graft to improve the nasolabial angle and maxillary projection
   c. Alar base may be narrowed with a bunching suture.

References

Rees TD. Nasal plastic surgery in the Negro. Plast Reconstr Surg 1969;43: 13.

Stucker FJ, Bryarly RC, Shockley WW. Plastic and reconstructive surgery of the head and neck. In: Ward PH, Berman WR, eds. Proceedings of the 4th International Symposium. St. Louis: CV Mosby, 1984.

Stucker FJ. Non-Caucasian rhinoplasty and adjunctive reduction cheiloplasty. Otolaryngol Clinic North Am 1987;20:877.

Operative Procedure

The preferred open rhinoplasty approach uses an inverted V-shaped incision in the columella just above the feet of the medial crura, or a V-type incision can be used at the base of the columella, permitting a V-Y closure for lengthening the columella. Incisions are then made bilaterally along the caudal margin of the lower lateral cartilages, connected to the columella incision, and extended slightly beyond so an exact closure can be made (Fig. 176-1).

A sharp iris scissors is used to begin the dissection over the dorsum of the lower lateral cartilages, and a blunted, flat-tipped scissors is used to elevate the soft tissues off the dorsum of the nose, up to the glabella and laterally as needed for skin draping. The dissection is carried out across the tip of the nose to the other side and then brought over the tip, down along the columella, such that the entire nasal dorsum is elevated with minimal dissection when the columella is released. The fibrofatty tissue overlying the nasal cartilages is dissected off in one piece and set aside for later use as filler and to soften any dorsal implants that are made (Fig. 176-2).

The lower lateral cartilages are separated in the midline until the nasal septum is encountered, and any fibrofatty tissue is dissected away. The mucoperichondrium is elevated off the nasal septum, and this separation may be extended back over the mucoperiosteum of the bony septum and down over the maxillary crest to the floor of the nose. Any septal deformities can be corrected at this point.

A submucous resection of the cartilaginous septum leaves dorsal and caudal struts and obtains tissue for later grafting. With the tip cartilages well-exposed, a minimal cephalic strip of lower lateral cartilage may be removed and any excess scrolling of the upper lateral cartilages may also be excised. After making submucoperichondrial tunnels, the upper lateral cartilages are separated from the nasal septum (Fig. 176-3). The lower lateral cartilages are vertically divided at a level lateral to the domes that can accomplish the gain in projection hoped for. The lateral portion of the lower lateral cartilages are then dissected from the underlying vestibular skin such that they may be projected superiorly, forming a more acute angle at the new area of the dome (Fig. 176-4). A strut of cartilage taken from the nasal septum along the maxillary crest where it is thickest is fashioned and placed between the medial crura of the lower lateral cartilages for a caudal columella strut.

The medial crura and columella struts are sutured together with 4-0 Prolene, starting from the bottom to the top and taking care to bury the knots. Shield grafts are formed from the remaining harvested cartilaginous septum or auricular cartilage. Two or more grafts usually are necessary to obtain the projection and refinement needed (Fig. 176-5). These are sutured into place anterior to the columella strut and apposed medial crura.

Osteotomies usually are needed to narrow the nose and to add some dorsal projection. Vertical medial osteotomies are performed with very low lateral osteotomies, and the nasal bone is reduced. A horizontal medial osteotomy is used to lower a dorsal hump, and the reduced hump may be remodeled to fill in the dorsum (Fig. 176-6). Most patients have deficits in the dorsum, and various graft materials can be used to correct the saddle nose deformity. Any remaining septal cartilage, tip cartilage, or auricular cartilage may be used, or if necessary, irradiated cartilage or an alloplastic implant with Gore-Tex, Mersilene mesh, or other material may be used.

A premaxillary pocket is undermined, and a plumping graft is placed to soften the nasolabial angle and fill out the deficient maxilla. The dorsal skin flap is then rotated back into position, and the undersurface of the skin flap may also be cross-hatched to enable better draping. The columella is closed with interrupted 6-0 nylon suture, and the margin incisions are closed with interrupted 5-0 Vicryl suture. The mucoperichondrial flaps overlying the septum can then be reapproximated using a 5-0 chromic basting stitch.

Weir resections are made to decrease the alar flare and nostril size, reorienting the axis of the nostrils in a more vertical direction. Benzoin is then applied to the nose and 1-cm paper tape is placed, followed by a plaster of Paris cast.

FRED J. STUCKER
ROBERT F. AARSTAD

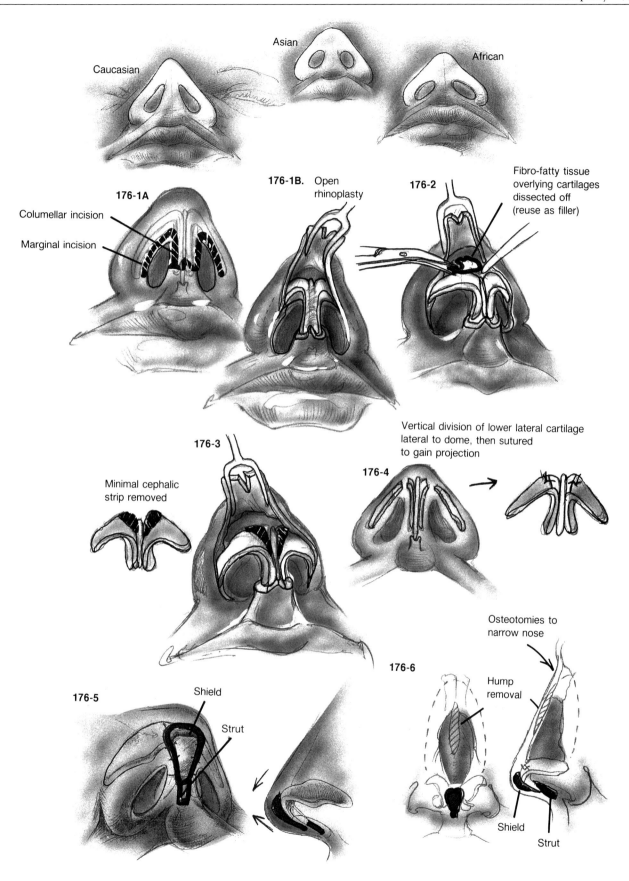

Caucasian

Asian

African

176-1A

Columellar incision

Marginal incision

176-1B. Open rhinoplasty

176-2

Fibro-fatty tissue overlying cartilages dissected off (reuse as filler)

176-3

Minimal cephalic strip removed

Vertical division of lower lateral cartilage lateral to dome, then sutured to gain projection

176-4

176-5

Shield

Strut

176-6

Osteotomies to narrow nose

Hump removal

Shield

Strut

■ *177.* MENTOPLASTY OUTLINE

Analysis of the lower third of the face, especially the chin relative to the rest of the facial profile, and operative planning

Indications
1. Large nose with apparent small chin
2. Lower face disproportion

Special Considerations
1. Occlusal relationship, class II
2. Planned orthognathic surgery
3. Moderate to severe retrognathia
4. Micrognathia
5. Severe microgenia

Preoperative Preparation
1. Patient made aware of chin deficiency
2. Adjunctive procedure to rhinoplasty
3. Intraoral or extraoral approach to augmentation

Special Instruments, Position, and Anesthesia
1. A computer imaging system is useful.
2. Photographs for discussion
3. Local or general anesthesia

Tips and Pearls
1. Augmentation excellent for most patients
2. Complex technique requires photographs and radiographs

Pitfalls and Complications
1. Severe retrusion or protrusion of subnasale affects perception of the chin projection.
2. Class II occlusion may make augmentation difficult.

References

Gibson FB, Calhoun KH. Chin position in profile analysis: comparison of techniques and introduction of the lower facial triangle. Arch Otolaryngol Head Neck Surg 1992;118:273.

Gonzalez-Ulloa M, Stevens E. The role of chin correction in profileplasty. Plastic Reconstr Surg 1968;41:477.

Maas CS, Merwin GE, Wilson J, Frey MD, Maves MD. Comparison of biomaterials for facial bone augmentation. Arch Otolaryngol Head Neck Surg 1990;116:551.

TABLE 177-1. Properties of Alloplastic Chin Implants

Property	Silicone Gel Bag With Dacron Backing	Supramid	Proplast	Porous Polyethylene	Acrylics
Firmness	Soft	Soft	Firm	Firm	Hard
Shapability	Fixed	Good	Fair	Good	Fair
Tissue reaction	Minimal	Slightly more than minimal	Moderate	Minimal	Minimal
Fixation	Good	Excellent	Excellent	Excellent	Poor
Trauma	Good	Good	Fair	Good	Poor
Removal	Easy	Difficult	Difficult	Fair	Easy

Mentoplasty Profile Analysis and Operative Planning

The facial plastic surgeon can glance at a facial profile and determine whether there is a deficiency of the chin. The assessment of the facial profile requires consideration of the overall size, shape, and mass of the entire face, especially the nose. Most often, the patient with a large nose seeks correction for this problem without considering the remaining facial structures that influence the perception of the nose, and it is the facial plastic surgeon who includes the chin in the overall plan for profile correction.

The deficiency in the chin can take several forms. If the chin is underdeveloped but the mandible is otherwise normal, the condition is called microgenia. In retrognathia, the deficient chin is caused by the class II occlusal abnormality with a normal mandible that is retrusive. Micrognathia is the most severe abnormality in this category because of the hypoplastic mandible, which is retruded, and because the teeth are in class II occlusion. By definition, less deficient chins are microgenic, and these can be corrected using simpler methods; the more severe forms of deficiency may require more sophisticated and involved procedures to correct the chin and possibly correct the mandible. Evaluation of the chin is primarily performed in the profile, but many patients need evaluation and correction in the frontal plane as well.

Several techniques are available. The Frankfurt horizontal line is used in the zero meridian of Gonzalez-Ulloa and in the alar crease method of Goode. The Gonzalez-Ulloa approach drops a line from the nasion perpendicular to the Frankfurt horizontal line (Fig. 177-1). The ideal position of the chin for males and females is at or just behind this perpendicular. Goode uses a perpendicular from the Frankfurt plane that is tangential to the alar crease (Fig. 177-2). The ideal position of the chin would be at or just behind this line. Others use angles to define the optimal position of the chin. Legan's angle is formed by lines from the glabella and the pogonion to the subnasale (Fig. 177-3). The ideal angle is said to be 12°. Another technique employing angles is the lower facial triangle formed by the tragion, subnasale, and the pogonion (Fig. 177-4). The ratio of the sides of the triangle and the angle formed at the chin is used to determine the ideal positions of the chin and the subnasale.

All of these techniques require a photograph and identification of certain anatomic landmarks. Establishing the Frankfurt horizontal line can be difficult if the photograph taken does not lend itself to this analysis. Cephalometric analysis can be done to determine the correct Frankfurt horizontal line and, from this analysis, determine the amount of deficiency present (Fig. 177-5). This is somewhat cumbersome and requires a radiograph.

A simpler technique for establishing the deficiency in the chin is to use the lips as reference points. This technique should be used in patients whose occlusion and mandibular development are reasonable (ie, mild to moderate cases of deficiencies). A line drawn vertically from the lower lip or a line drawn tangential to the upper and lower lips, as with a small straight edge ruler held against the lips, can rapidly determine a deficiency (Fig. 177-6). The degree of correction (ie, augmentation needed to correct the deficiency) can be established during the first examination of the patient, facilitating the overall approach to the correction of the facial profile.

There is little operative planning required in addition to the profile analysis except for choosing the appropriate alloplastic material for the chin augmentation. The selection of material is a matter of the surgeon's preference. As is demonstrated in Table 177-1, there are favorable and unfavorable properties of each implant. The surgeon must decide which of the characteristics is more significant and which is not. All of the listed materials are in use today. The preformed shapes and sizes of the Silastic implants are probably the most widely used. Silicone gel implants, which were once used extensively, have been taken off the market because of the concerns raised about extrusion of the silicone gel and its effects on the body.

KWEON I. STAMBAUGH

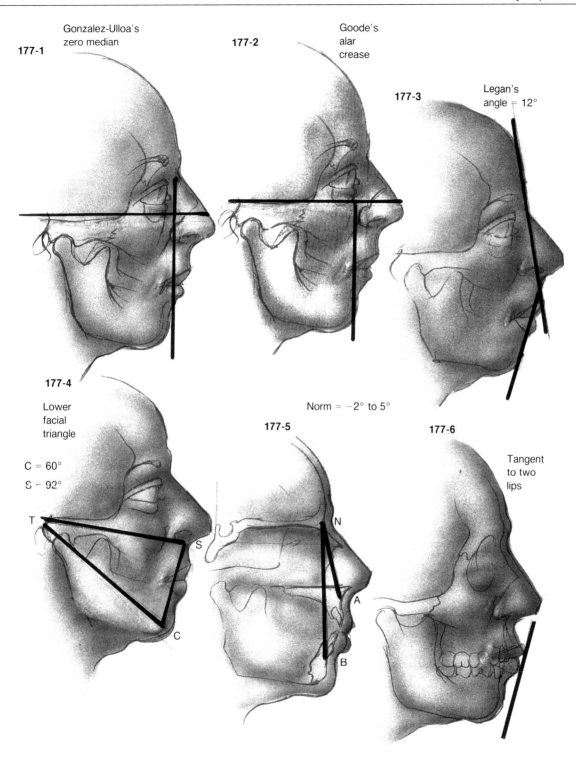

177-1 Gonzalez-Ulloa's zero median

177-2 Goode's alar crease

177-3 Legan's angle = 12°

177-4 Lower facial triangle

C = 60°

S = 92°

Norm = −2° to 5°

177-5

177-6 Tangent to two lips

■ *178.* CHIN IMPLANT
Surgical augmentation of the anterior portion of the chin

Indications
1. Microgenia
2. Retrognathia (mild to moderate)
3. Micrognathia (mild)

Special Considerations
1. Retrognathia (moderate to severe) requiring orthognathic correction
2. Micrognathia (moderate to severe) requiring orthognathic correction
3. Dental occlusion problems and anticipated corrective surgery
4. Limited correction with augmentation (<10 mm)

Preoperative Preparation
1. Routine and medically indicated laboratory tests

Special Instruments, Position, and Anesthesia
1. Headlight
2. Aufricht retractor and Lempert periosteal elevator
3. Implant soaked in antibiotic solution
4. 1-cm (0.5-in) Steri-Strips and 5-cm (2-in) foam tape

Tips and Pearls
1. Extend the periosteal pocket beyond the inferior border of the mandible.
2. The pocket size is a little larger than the implant.
3. Place implant as low along the mandible as possible.
4. Relaxing incisions in periosteum

Pitfalls and Complications
1. Implant displacement due to pocket size
2. Implant asymmetry
3. Implant riding high on the chin
4. Hematoma
5. Infection
6. Inadequate correction of the deficiency

Postoperative Care Issues
1. Keep the original tape and dressing on for 1 to 3 days.
2. Remove fluffy dressing on day 1 to 3, and remove tape on day 7.
3. Keep the patient on antibiotics for 7 to 10 days.

References
Flowers RS. Alloplastic augmentation of the anterior mandible. Clin Plast Surg 1991;18:107.

McCarthy JG, Ruff GL, Zide BM. A surgical system for the correction of bony chin deformity. Clin Plast Surg 1991;18:139.

Stambaugh KI. Chin augmentation: an important adjunctive procedure to rhinoplasty. Arch Otolaryngol Head Neck Surg 1992;118:682.

Operative Procedure
This operation, alone or in conjunction with a rhinoplasty, can be performed with the patient under local or general anesthesia. A 1% solution of Xylocaine with a 1:100,000 concentration of epinephrine solution is infiltrated about the premarked 2- to 2.5-cm incision line.

The external incision (2 to 2.5 cm long) is made in the first submental crease area down into the subcutaneous fat plane (Fig. 178-1). Two wide double hooks are applied for exposure. Sharp dissection through this fatty layer is carried down to the periosteum overlying the inferior border of the mandible. Further exposure of the anterior inferior border is obtained by sharp dissection laterally. Retraction at the corner with a Senn retractor facilitates dissection.

The periosteal incision, which extends 2 to 3 cm from the midline, is placed precisely at the inferior border of the mandible (Fig. 178-2). The tendency is for this incision to be placed superiorly as it is carried laterally toward the mental foramen. The #15 knife blade should be stroked firmly through the periosteum and into the bone to cut the periosteum.

Elevation of the periosteum anteriorly is difficult because of the extensive muscular attachments, and the use of a Lempert periosteal elevator is helpful. The remainder of the periosteal elevation is easy, and a Freer elevator is sufficient (Fig. 178-3).

The subperiosteal pocket formation should be precise and is facilitated by the use of the Aufricht retractor along with the headlight. The lateral pocket should extend slightly below the level of the inferior margin of the mandible and should extend superiorly enough to admit the implant. The size of the pocket overall should be sufficient to place the implant properly, but the pocket should not have enough excess space for the implant to shift easily with only slight manipulation. Depending on the size and shape of the implant, the mental foramen and and its neurovascular bundle may have to be carefully exposed during the pocket formation (Fig. 178-4). Most of the implants with lateral extensions are designed to fit inferior to the bundle, and the dissection of the pocket is less risky if the dissection proceeds along the inferior border of the mandible. If necessary, direct visualization of the bundle can be done to prevent injury to it. Along the midportion of the periosteal pocket, two parallel relaxing incisions are placed to allow the periosteum to be closed over the implant at the conclusion of the procedure.

The implant is soaked in antibiotic solution before implantation. It is oriented and its midline identified to align it correctly after insertion into the pocket. The Aufricht retractor is used to retract one side of the pocket, and the implant is grasped longitudinally along the corresponding half and carefully inserted into the pocket as far as it will go. The Aufricht is rotated to the opposite side, and the implant is grasped and the end of it inserted into the pocket. A Freer elevator is used to manipulate below the implant to ensure that it is placed flat against the bone and aligned properly. Recheck the midline alignment and overall balance of the chin by looking at the external appearance and making the final corrections before closure (Fig. 178-5). Some implants have a location where a tacking stitch can be placed to stabilize the implant to the periosteum.

Closure of the wound is begun by tacking the periosteal edges together using 4-0 Vicryl. Two or three interrupted sutures are sufficient. The skin is closed in a layered plastic manner by placing modified Halsted sutures in the subcuticular layer with 4-0 Vicryl. The final skin closure is accomplished by placing locked, running 6-0 fast-absorbing gut.

A small amount of bacitracin ointment is placed on the incision line. A small Telfa strip is placed on top of this. Benzoin ointment is applied to the entire chin area, and 1-cm (0.5-in) Steri-Strips are placed around the point of the chin (like a doughnut) to keep the implant in a stented position. A small, fluffy dressing is applied and taped with foam tape.

Figure 178-6 depicts the intraoral approach to the placement of a chin implant. The incision is placed further inferior to the sulcus to ensure adequate mucosa for closure. The remainder of the procedure is essentially the same as the external approach.

KWEON I. STAMBAUGH

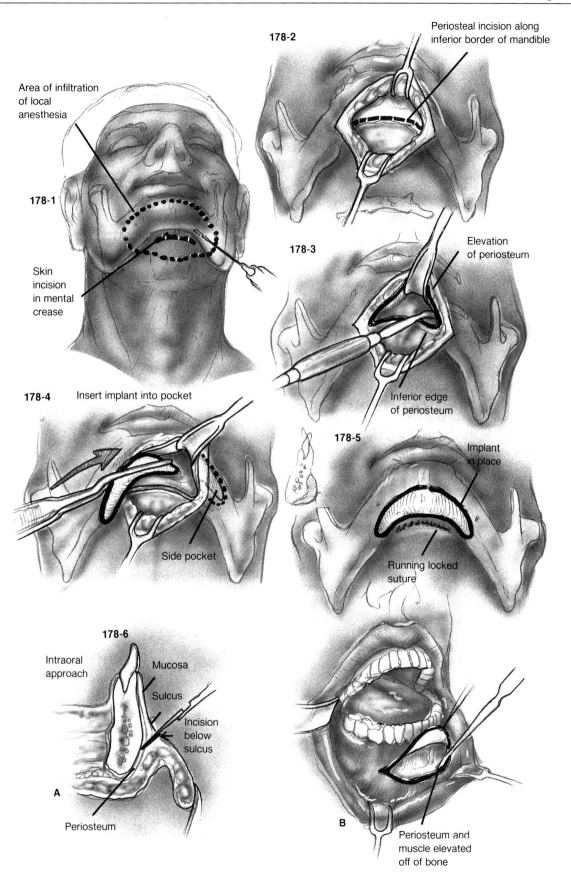

178-1

Area of infiltration of local anesthesia

Skin incision in mental crease

178-2

Periosteal incision along inferior border of mandible

178-3

Elevation of periosteum

Inferior edge of periosteum

178-4 Insert implant into pocket

Side pocket

178-5

Implant in place

Running locked suture

178-6

Intraoral approach

Mucosa

Sulcus

Incision below sulcus

A

Periosteum

B

Periosteum and muscle elevated off of bone

■ 179. GENIOPLASTY: HORIZONTAL POSITION CHANGES—A horizontal osteotomy of the mandibular symphysis and parasymphyseal areas that allows movement of the chin relative to the mandibular body to correct a variety of deformities of the chin area

Indications

1. As an isolated procedure for the correction of microgenia or macrogenia
2. For a class I occlusion if the deformity lies solely within the chin area
3. Genioplasty may accompany orthognathic operations for combined deformities.

Contraindications

1. Genioplasty is contraindicated when the chin area is normal and the actual deformity lies in the relationship of the mandible to the maxilla, as in retrognathia or prognathism. Such problems are best treated by orthognathic surgery.

Special Considerations

1. Evaluation of the patient's motivation and emotional stability is beneficial for the patient and physician, as for any cosmetic operation.

Preoperative Preparation

1. Treatment planning consists of clinical and cephalometric evaluation. Prediction cephalometric tracings allow precise preoperative planning of the amount of movement required to correct the deformity.

Special Instruments, Position, and Anesthesia

1. Reciprocating saw
2. Rotary bur
3. Rigid plating equipment
4. Patient in the supine position, with the head elevated
5. General nasal endotracheal anesthesia and deep intravenous sedation are anesthetic options.

Tips and Pearls

1. The osteotomy must pass at least 5 mm beneath the mental foramina to avoid injury to the mental nerves.
2. Expect several months of numbness in the mental nerve distribution, and prepare the patient for this preoperatively.
3. A degree of indentation is unavoidable at the osteotomy site along the inferior border of the mandibular body.

Pitfalls and Complications

1. Be aware of the patient who habitually and subconsciously postures the retrognathic mandible forward, improving the deficient mandibular profile and simulating a normal occlusion. Such patients appear to require only genioplasty, but they actually require mandibular advancement.

Postoperative Care Issues

1. A supportive tape or facial sling dressing improves comfort and minimizes hematoma formation.

References

Park HS, Ellis E, Fonseca RJ, Reynolds ST, Mayo KH. A retrospective study of advancement genioplasty. Oral Surg Oral Med Oral Pathol 1989;67:481.

Putman JM, Donovan MG. Modified reduction genioplasty. J Oral Maxillofac Surg 1989;47:203.

Spear SL, Kassan M. Genioplasty. Clin Plast Surg 1989;16:695.

Operative Procedure

Osseous genioplasty is performed by means of a horizontal osteotomy of the mandibular symphysis area, extending posteriorly to the mid-mandibular body. The amount and direction of movement is determined by preoperative clinical and cephalometric assessment. Osseous genioplasty is often performed in conjunction with other orthognathic procedures, as dictated by the preoperative surgical plan.

The osteotomy is performed through an intraoral incision placed on the labial aspect of the lower mucobuccal fold, extending from first premolar to first premolar. The incision passes obliquely through the mentalis muscle and through the underlying periosteum. The periosteum is then reflected inferiorly to the inferior border of the mandible, and the mental foramina are identified (Fig. 179-1).

A vertical midline reference mark long enough to cross the osteotomy site is scribed with a rotary bur on the anterior mandibular cortex. A reciprocating saw is used to make the osteotomy, beginning at the inferior mandibular border about 2 cm posterior to the mental foramen. The osteotomy extends anteriorly in an oblique fashion, tapering superiorly to pass no closer than 5 mm beneath the mental foramen (Fig. 179-2). The opposite osteotomy is then performed, and the two are joined in the midline. Care is taken to avoid excessively stretching the mental nerves. The lingual muscle attachments on the posterior aspect of the mobilized segment are preserved.

After completion of the osteotomy, the mobilized segment is repositioned appropriately to correct the anteroposterior or lateral deformity, in accordance with the preoperative plan (Fig. 179-3). The mobilized segment can be split, shifted laterally (Fig. 179-4), or designed asymmetrically to correct any type of three-dimensional deformity. After the final position is established, it may be necessary to remove minor irregularities from the osteotomy site to ensure adequate approximation of the cut surfaces. One or more titanium miniplates are contoured and applied to fix the segment rigidly in its new position (Fig. 179-5). A final check of the contour of the inferior mandibular border may reveal excessive notching at the osteotomy site, although some depression at the osteotomy site is expected. A power reciprocating rasp or rotary bur can be used to improve this contour.

Wound closure is performed in two layers to ensure adequate reapproximation of the chin soft tissues to the underlying bone. The mentalis muscle is reapproximated with interrupted 3-0 chromic gut and mucosal closure is performed with running, locking 3-0 chromic gut suture. Placement of an external pressure dressing is helpful for the first 24 to 48 hours.

ERIC J. DIERKS

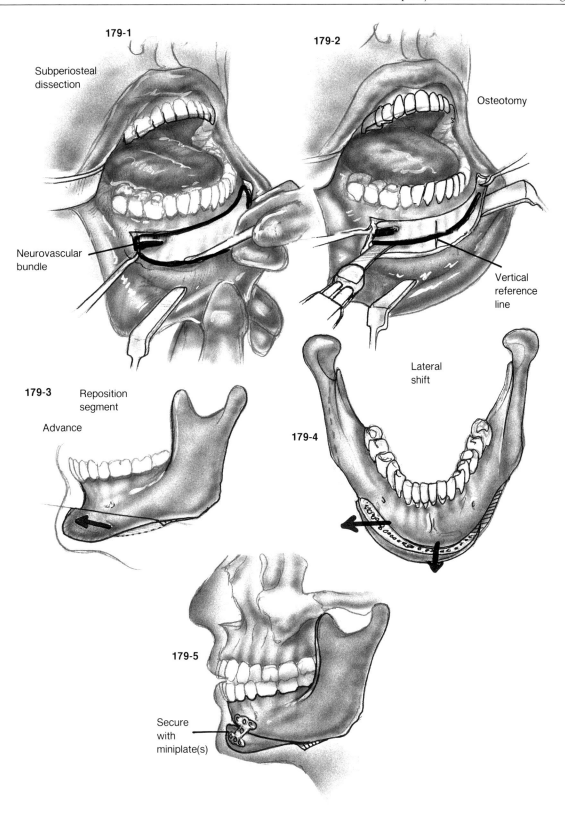

179-1

Subperiosteal
dissection

Neurovascular
bundle

179-2

Osteotomy

Vertical
reference
line

179-3   Reposition
            segment

Advance

Lateral
shift

179-4

179-5

Secure
with
miniplate(s)

■ 180. GENIOPLASTY: VERTICAL POSITION
CHANGES— A horizontal osteotomy of the mandibular symphysis and parasymphyseal areas that allows removal of bone or addition of grafted bone to produce movement of the chin relative to the mandibular body to correct a variety of deformities of the chin area

Indications
1. As an isolated procedure for the correction of microgenia or macrogenia
2. For a class I occlusion if the deformity lies solely in the chin area
3. May accompany orthognathic operations for combined deformities

Contraindications
1. Genioplasty is contraindicated if the chin area is normal and the deformity instead lies in the relation of the mandible to the maxilla (eg, retrognathia, prognathism).

Special Considerations
1. Evaluation of the patient's motivation and emotional stability is beneficial for the patient and physician, as for any cosmetic operation.

Preoperative Preparation
1. Treatment planning consists of clinical and cephalometric evaluation.
2. Prediction cephalometric tracings allow precise preoperative planning of the amount of chin movement and the amount of bone removal or graft addition required to correct the deformity.

Special Instruments, Position, and Anesthesia
1. Reciprocating saw
2. Rotary bur
3. Rigid plating equipment
4. Patient in the supine position, with the head elevated
5. If bone grafting is required, the iliac crest is prepared.
6. General nasal endotracheal anesthesia is preferred.

Tips and Pearls
1. The osteotomy must pass at least 5 mm beneath the mental foramina to avoid injury to the mental nerves.
2. Expect several months of numbness in the mental nerve distribution, and prepare the patient for this preoperatively.
3. An irregular contour is unavoidable at the osteotomy site along the inferior border of the mandibular body, particularly if a bone graft has been placed.

Pitfalls and Complications
1. Be aware of the patient who habitually and subconsciously postures the retrognathic mandible forward, improving the deficient mandibular profile and simulating a normal occlusion. Such patients appear to require genioplasty only, but they actually require mandibular advancement.

Postoperative Care Issues
1. A supportive tape or facial sling dressing improves comfort and minimizes hematoma formation.

References
Bell WH, Gallagher DM. The versatility of genioplasty using a broad pedicle. J Oral Maxillofac Surg 1983;41:763.

Wessberg GA, Wolford LM, Epker BN. Interpositional genioplasty for the short face syndrome. J Oral Surg 1980;38:584.

Operative Procedure
The osteotomy design for the reduction of a vertically excessive chin is similar to that described in Procedure 179 (Fig. 180-1), but a second parallel osteotomy must be placed beneath the first (Fig. 180-2) to allow removal of bone. In most instances, the lines of osteotomy tend to converge posteriorly, describing a wedge-shaped crescent of bone to be removed (Fig. 180-3). The anterior height and orientation of this bone excision is determined by preoperative clinical and cephalometric analysis. The overly large chin is usually excessive in the vertical and horizontal planes, and adaptation of the shape and orientation of the bone wedge allows accurate correction of the deformity. Combined vertical and horizontal reduction of the chin may accentuate submental fullness. Concomitant liposuction of the submental fat can be performed directly through the osteotomy site, before fixation of the chin fragment.

The dissection and exposure of the chin is performed as described in Procedure 179. Care is taken to keep the superior osteotomy at least 5 mm beneath the mental foramen, because the mental nerve descends several millimeters beneath the mental foramen as it courses into the mandibular canal. Both osteotomies are outlined and are nearly completed before mobilization of the chin element. The repositioned chin is rigidly fixated with one or two miniplates, as needed to achieve stability. Wound closure is performed as described in Procedure 179. As with other chin surgery, a pressure dressing helps in controlling postoperative edema.

The infrequently encountered problem of a vertically deficient chin requires the interposition of an iliac crest wedge graft of appropriate height (Fig. 180-4). Two to three miniplates are needed to provide adequate rigid fixation for the mobilized chin segment and the bone graft. Such vertical deficiency is usually associated with concomitant horizontal deficiency, and the native chin element may be horizontally advanced beneath the bone graft, according to the surgical plan. Combined vertical and horizontal chin repositioning may require carefully contoured miniplate fixation to achieve absolutely rigid fixation. Careful, watertight mucosal closure minimizes the risk of postoperative infection.

ERIC J. DIERKS

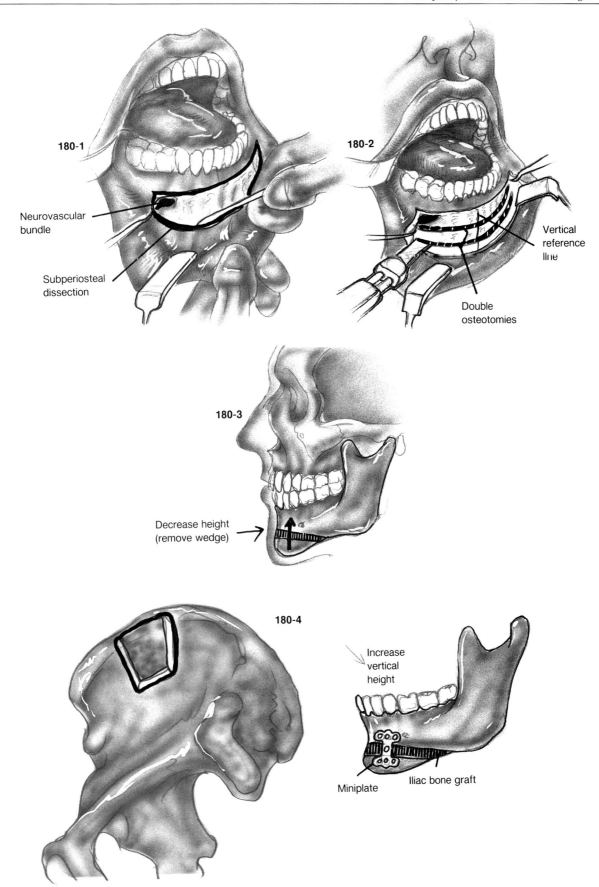

180-1

Neurovascular bundle

Subperiosteal dissection

180-2

Vertical reference line

Double osteotomies

180-3

Decrease height (remove wedge)

180-4

Increase vertical height

Miniplate

Iliac bone graft

■ 181. MALAR IMPLANTS

Insertion of an alloplastic prosthesis over the cheek bone to add prominence to the malar bone

Indications

1. Aesthetic considerations
2. A malar prominence that is more than 5 mm posterior to the nasolabial groove on a true lateral projection

Special Considerations

1. Define the area to be augmented, usually the malar prominence triangle.
2. Selection of material, such as Proplast, Gore-Tex, or Silastic
3. Special handling of material, such as antibiotic pressure loading for Proplast or Gore-Tex

Preoperative Preparation

1. Photographic analysis
2. Malar prominence triangle
3. Size of implant
4. Intravenous administration of antibiotics 30 minutes before surgery

Tips and Pearls

1. Incision placed 2 cm above the papillae of the upper teeth
2. Subperiosteal dissection for a large pocket if using Proplast and a smaller pocket if using Silastic
3. A Silastic implant must be stabilized for 24 to 48 hours with a guide suture.
4. Use two-layer closure.

Pitfalls and Complications

1. A hematoma, which is an early complication, should be drained.
2. Infection requires implant removal.
3. Tissue reactions may occur some time after the procedure.

Postoperative Care Issues

1. Ice packs postoperatively
2. Antibiotics for 4 days

References

Binder W. Submalar augmentation: a procedure to enhance rhytidectomy. Ann Plast Surg 1991;24:200.

Kent J. Chin and zygomaticomaxillary augmentation with Proplast. J Oral Surg 1981;39:912.

Operative Procedure

One gram of Cefalosporin is given 30 minutes before the procedure to avoid any bacterial infection. The patient is placed in the supine position, and initially, the infraorbital nerve is blocked on both sides with 2% solution of Xylocaine with epinephrine. If using general anesthesia, a 1% solution of Xylocaine with epinephrine is used. The gingival buccal sulcus just lateral to the canine fossa is then injected with the Xylocaine, and the malar area is carefully infiltrated up to the lateral orbital rim. This is completed on both sides. Fifteen minutes is allowed for vasoconstriction.

Using a #15 blade, the mucosa is carefully cut 2 cm above the dental papillae. The muscle layer is cut, and the wound is retracted superiorly with an Army-Navy retractor. The #15 blade is used to cut the periosteum, after which a Joseph elevator is used to elevate the periosteum carefully over the anterior lateral portion of the maxillary sinus wall (Fig. 181-1). The dissection is carried posteriorly as the maxillary sinus begins to turn posteriorly. The surgeon carries the dissection superiorly to the orbital rim, keeping in mind the location of the infraorbital nerve. A finger compresses the infraorbital rim to avoid periosteal elevator slippage and injury to the eye. The infraorbital nerve is carefully identified, and care is taken to avoid stretching this area to prevent postoperative paresthesia. The periosteum is elevated over the lateral portion of the orbital rim toward the zygomatic arch. Hemostasis is maintained with bipolar cautery. Using the periosteal elevator, the inferior part of the initial incision is carefully elevated inferiorly. The same procedure is repeated on the opposite side.

After complete hemostasis is achieved, the preformed, presized malar implant is carefully inserted into the pocket, as the surgeon keeps in view the most prominent portion of the implant so it will coincide with the most central portion of the malar prominence triangle (Figs. 181-2 and 181-3). If a Silastic implant is used, a stay suture of 2-0 silk is passed using a Stamey needle passer, going through the posterior lateral portion of the pocket into the deep tissues and out into the hairline. The implant is gently pulled and pushed into place. After it is in the appropriate position, as determined by visual evaluation, the silk tie is tied over a small cotton bolster (Fig. 181-4). The muscle layer is closed with 3-0 chromic interrupted sutures, and the mucosal layer is closed with interrupted 2-0 sutures.

Using the preformed Proplast or Gore-Tex implant avoids the problem of fixation in the tissues, because it does not slide around. However, the pocket must be made larger for the Proplast implant than for the Silastic implant to avoid compression of the pores of the Proplast. Before inserting the Proplast, it has been pressured loaded with Cleocin.

Before closing the second incision, care is taken to ensure that both implants are placed in symmetric positions. The second wound then is closed in two layers. Ice pads are applied to both cheek areas, with only a minimal wrap of Kling to hold the ice pads in place.

WILLIAM SILVER

181-1. Subperiosteal elevation

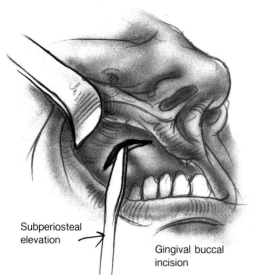

Subperiosteal
elevation

Gingival buccal
incision

181-2. Malar prominent triangle

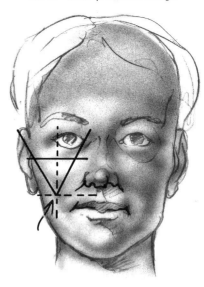

Cotton bolster

2-0 silk suture

Silastic
implant

181-4

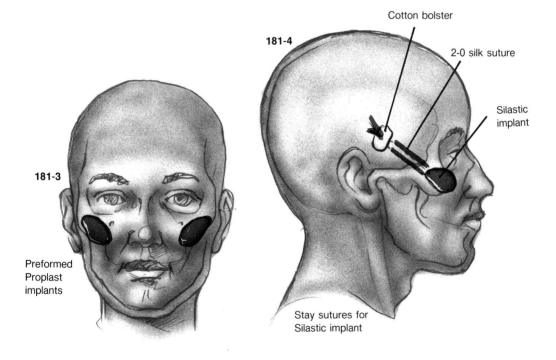

181-3

Preformed
Proplast
implants

Stay sutures for
Silastic implant

■ *182.* RHYTIDECTOMY INCISIONS
The incisions needed to perform a rhytidectomy

Indications
1. Access for forehead, brow, cheek–jowl, and cervical lifting
2. Access to subgaleal, subplatysmal, and superficial musculoaponeurotic system planes of dissection

Special Considerations
1. Intratrichial incision used to best camouflage the scar
2. Subtrichial incision used to avoid raising the hairline
3. Pretragal incision in males and in females with a tragal prominence
4. Posttragal incision used to better camouflage the scar

Preoperative Preparation
1. Routine preoperative studies
2. Bleeding and clotting studies
3. Complete preoperative photographic analysis
4. Discontinue cigarette smoking and aspirin 2 weeks before surgery
5. Betadine preparation to hair, face, and neck
6. Intended incisions outlined with surgical markers
7. Hair arranged and parted with water-soluble surgical gel
8. Towel drapes sutured to scalp

Special Instruments, Position, and Anesthesia
1. Adequate overhead or headlight illumination
2. #15 scalpel blade; fine plastic surgery instruments
3. Supine position, with the neck slightly extended and turned to one side
4. Solution of 0.75% lidocaine with a 1:150,000 concentration of epinephrine

Tips and Pearls
1. Bevel the incision parallel to the hair shafts
2. Superficial incision around the ear to avoid injuring the perichondrium
3. Do not cauterize skin bleeders.
4. Outline and mark incisions with the patient sitting upright.

Pitfalls and Complications
1. Postoperative wound separation
2. Postoperative scarring (hypertrophic or keloid)
3. Pigmented scarring

Postoperative Care Issues
1. Bacitracin ointment applied to incisions
2. Drain usually removed in 24 hours
3. Moderately bulky protective dressing for 3 days
4. Staples and all sutures removed in 8 days

References
Pitanguy I. Aesthetic plastic surgery of head and body. New York: Springer-Verlag, 1981:174.
Rees T. Aesthetic plastic surgery, vol 2. Philadelphia: WB Saunders, 1980.

Operative Procedures
The patient's face, neck, and hair are prepared with Betadine solution. The location of the incisions can be best determined and outlined with the patient sitting upright. The intended face, neck, and hair incision sites are marked with a surgical marker. The patient then reclines and is appropriately sedated and monitored by the anesthesiologist. After the patient is adequately sedated, the hair is parted along the intended incision lines, matted with water-soluble surgical jelly, and arranged with rubber bands. The intended surgical field is adequately anesthetized by subcutaneous injection of a local anesthesia. Deep nerve blocks can be considered if deeper levels of dissection are required. Towel drapes are secured to the scalp with surgical clips or sutures, and the remaining loose hairs are smoothed with surgical jelly. No hair is shaved or clipped.

For optimal camouflage, the location of the incisions vary according to the patient's anatomic characteristics, gender, and aesthetic goals. In the upper face, an infratrichial incision is used (Fig. 182-1) if the patient has a relatively high temporal or frontal hairline; otherwise, the intratrichial incision is the preferred method to lift the forehead and brows (Fig. 182-2). The incision is outlined 4 to 5 cm from the hairline and deepened to the subgaleal level, beveling the scalpel and avoiding cautery in the subcutaneous plane to minimize injury to the hair follicles. The superficial temporal artery and vein commonly are transected and must be ligated or adequately cauterized. The inferior incision becomes more superficial in the subcutaneous plane, avoiding injury to the temporal branch of the facial nerve, which lies deeper and runs from the tragus to the lateral brow. The incision emerges from the hair and hugs the superoanterior helical fold in a natural crease posterior to the sideburn.

If a posttragal incision (Fig. 182-3) is used, it is outlined at an angle determined by the individual characteristics of the tragus. The incision continues into the tragal groove and then descends just posterior to the tragal prominence to blend into the cheek-lobular crease. Care must be taken not to disturb the tragal perichondrium while incising this thin-skinned area. If a pretragal incision is indicated, it follows the intratragal groove a few millimeters anterior to the tragus in the malar-tragal junction, merging with the cheek-lobular crease inferiorly toward the earlobe (Fig. 182-4). The incision continues superiorly onto the posterior concha, close to the earlobe and a few millimeters anterior to the postauricular sulcus, taking care not to injure the posterior conchal perichondrium. The incision extends superiorly over the mastoid bone then arches posteriorly. The angle of the incision depends on whether an infratrichial or intratrichial incision is indicated. The subtrichial incision (Fig. 182-5) is used if raising or rotating the posterior scalp is not indicated. The incision is best placed at or just within the hairline, taking care that a not too acute angle is not created at the apex of the flap.

In most cases, the better hidden intratrichial incision is used (Fig. 182-6). The incision should be beveled and not cauterized to prevent injury to the hair follicles. The subcutaneous scalp incision is outlined at a higher level, creating a more obtuse angle at the apex of the flap. After the flaps have been adequately mobilized and advanced, the incisions are closed with interrupted and continuous 5-0 and 6-0 nylon sutures. Subcutaneous sutures are placed in all areas of possible tension. Stainless steel staples are used to close the hair-bearing incisions. Drains should be considered if there is a question of persistent or probable postoperative bleeding. To avoid disturbing the incision, the drains are best brought out by a separate postoccipital stab incision and should be connected to the negative-pressure reservoir before removing the drapes and manipulating the dressings.

After the drapes are removed, all the hair, face, and neck incisions are washed with hydrogen peroxide to remove surgical debris and blood. The area is dried gently, and Bacitracin ointment is applied to the incisions. A moderately bulky protective dressing is lightly compressed by an elasticized bandage and secured with tape. The drain reservoir is attached to the dressing by a safety pin. The dressings are removed the day after surgery, and the incisions are examined. The drains are also removed if the drainage is not excessive; otherwise, they remain another day.

FRANK M. KAMER

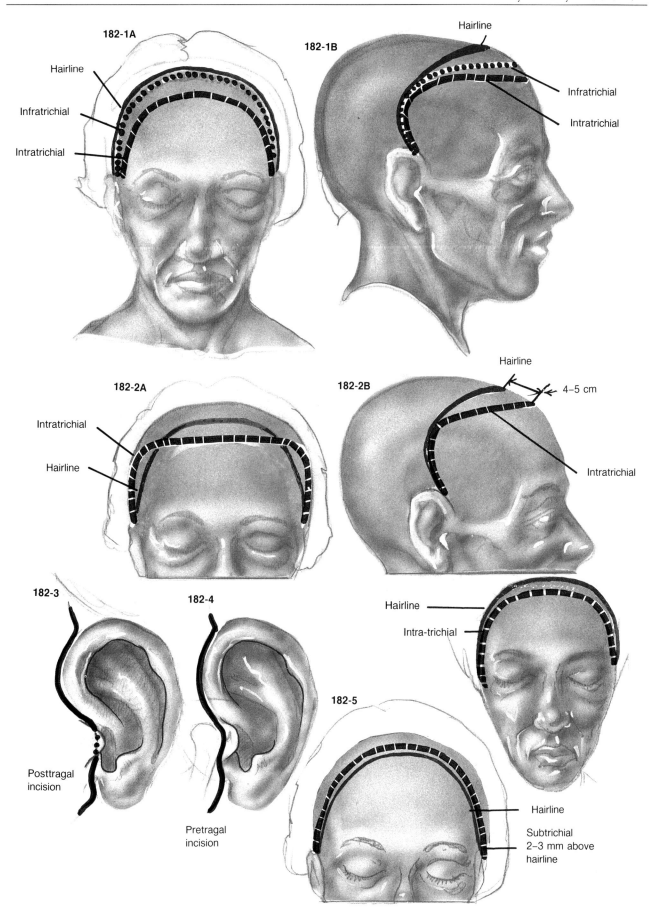

182-1A

Hairline

Infratrichial

Intratrichial

182-1B

Hairline

Infratrichial

Intratrichial

182-2A

Intratrichial

Hairline

182-2B

Hairline

4–5 cm

Intratrichial

182-3

Posttragal
incision

182-4

Pretragal
incision

Hairline

Intra-trichial

182-5

Hairline

Subtrichial
2–3 mm above
hairline

■ *183.* RHYTIDECTOMY USING SUPERFICIAL MUSCULOAPONEUROTIC SYSTEM PLICATION AND A SHORT FLAP OR LONG FLAP—

A surgical procedure to diminish the effects of aging caused by senile skin laxity and gravitational pull

Indications

1. Facial aging
2. Facial nerve rehabilitation

Special Considerations

1. Smoking, with its increased complications
2. General medical condition, with attention to disorders such as diabetes, bleeding disorders, and hypertension
3. Recent aspirin or nonsteroidal antiinflammatory drug use
4. Patients with unrealistic expectations

Preoperative Preparation

1. General medical review
2. Aesthetic evaluation should assess the degree of laxity and specific areas of concern, with attention to the position of the hairline in planning incisions and the quality of the skin. The stage of facial aging determines the need for a short or long flap rhytidectomy procedure. Superficial musculoaponeurotic system (SMAS) plication and platysma modification have become a standard fixture in rhytidectomy, increasing the longevity of the surgical result (Fig. 183-1 and Table 183-1).
3. A psychologic evaluation may be necessary if the patient's expectations do not seem realistic.
4. Evaluate preexisting facial and body scars to observe the potential for hypertrophic scars and keloid formation.

(continued)

Operative Procedure

The patient is placed in a supine position, with the head in a holder that provides access to the posterior cervical area bilaterally. The intravenous anesthesia is initiated, and the first hemifacial area is infiltrated with local anesthetic. The field is extended past the midline to facilitate treatment of the anterior neck and submental areas early in the procedure. After the local anesthetic is infiltrated, the entire head and neck area is prepped with an antiseptic soap, and the drapes are applied.

The incisions are made on one side, and the skin flap is carefully elevated, preserving a thin layer of fat on the underside of the flap. The choice of incisions dictates whether the temporal area is elevated in a subcutaneous or subgaleal plane. The skin flap is thinnest over the sternocleidomastoid muscle, with the greater auricular nerve just under the muscle fascia. The submental incision is made in a natural crease, and the skin is elevated for a short distance.

A 3- or 4-mm facial round liposuction cannula is used to tunnel from the facial and submental incisions. Fat is removed from the cervical, submental, and jowl areas, as necessary for contouring. The flat spatula-type cannula can be used to clean fat off of the platysma muscle at the anterior and posterior borders. If a long-flap rhytidectomy is planned, the tunnels can be connected with scissors dissection to complete the elevation (Figs. 183-2 and 183-2).

(continued)

183-1

I

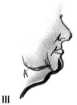

II

III

TABLE 183-1.   Classification of Cervical Abnormalities

Class I

Minimal deformity. Well-defined cervical mental angle, good platysma tone, no accumulation of fat (younger patient).

Class II

Laxity of the cervical skin. Begins to hang like a curtain. No fat accumulation, no platysma weakness.

Class III

Fat accumulation.

Class IV

Muscle accentuation (banding present in repose or on contraction).

Class V

Congenital or acquired retrognathia.

Class VI

Low hyoid.

From Dedo DD: A preoperative classification of the neck for cervicofacial rhytidectomy, *Laryngoscope* XC(11):1895, 1980.

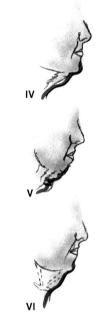

IV

V

VI

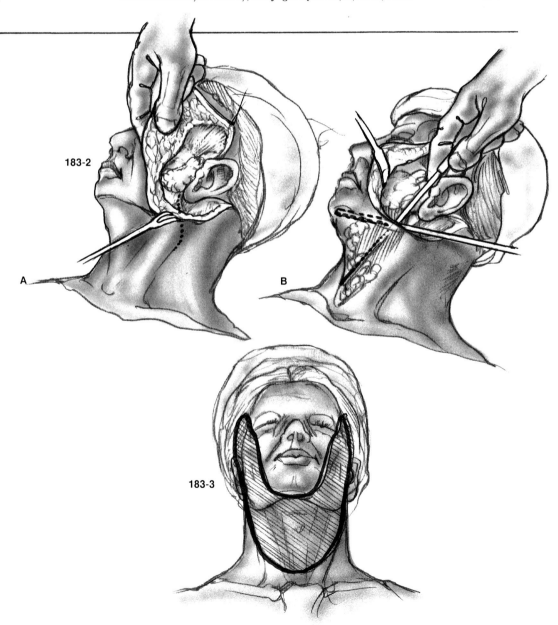

183-2

A

B

183-3

■ *183.* RHYTIDECTOMY USING SUPERFICIAL MUSCULOAPONEUROTIC SYSTEM PLICATION AND A SHORT FLAP OR LONG FLAP

(continued)

Special Instruments, Position, and Anesthesia

1. Most rhytidectomy procedures are performed with intravenous sedation and local anesthesia. The incision areas and face are widely infiltrated with 1% lidocaine with 1:100,000 epinephrine. Sedation with Diprovan, Versed, and Fentanyl usually ensures that the patient has little memory of the procedure.
2. The patient is placed in the supine position, with a head-holding attachment on the operating room table to allow access to the posterior cervical dissection area bilaterally.
3. Special instruments include appropriate rhytidectomy scissors for easy dissection of the facial flap. These scissors have semisharp outer edges. Liposuction equipment is also helpful in defatting the appropriate submental and masseteric jowl areas. Nontraumatizing retractors and adequate lighting are essential. Bipolar cautery helps to limit thermal damage and decrease edema.

Tips and Pearls

1. A careful preoperative evaluation should include cautioning the patient against unrealistic results. Meet with patient just before surgery to discuss goals and incisions.
2. Attention to planes of dissection avoids necrosis of the skin flaps and preserves the greater auricular nerve.
3. Meticulous hemostasis prevents hematoma and subsequent infection or skin necrosis. Men seem to have a more prominent subdermal plexus, with a higher incidence of bleeding.
4. Avoid dull instruments to decrease tissue trauma.
5. Assess the heat from the operating room lights, because the resulting thermal injury has caused flap necrosis in extended operations.
6. Postoperative dressings should be firm but not constricting enough to compromise flap circulation.

References

Hilger J. Rhytidectomy. In: Papel ID, Nachlas NE, eds. Facial plastic and reconstructive surgery, St. Louis: Mosby-Year Book, 1992.

Mitz V, Peyronie M. The superficial musculoaponeurotic system (SMAS) in the parotid and cheek area. Plast Reconstr Surg 1976;58:80.

The anterior platysmal bands are isolated and resected sharply. Hemostasis is performed with bipolar cautery, as indicated. The platysma muscles are then plicated with interrupted 4-0 polydioxanone sutures (PDS) from the mandible to the level of the thyroid cartilage. Care must be taken not to "bunch" the muscle and create uneven contours (Fig. 183-4).

The SMAS layer is located in the preauricular area, and a strip is removed by scissors from the zygomatic arch to the level of the inferior earlobe. The SMAS flap is then elevated bluntly along this incision for a distance of 5 to 6 cm. The substance of the parotid gland is plainly visible beneath the flap, and the branches of the facial nerve are exposed if the flap is dissected past the anterior border of the parotid gland. As the dissection moves inferiorly, the posterior border of the platysma muscle is elevated in conjunction with the SMAS flap, and the dissection continues deep to the cervical platysma muscle. The facial nerve must be avoided over the midportion of the zygomatic arch and at the facial notch of the mandible. The elevated flap is advanced in a posterosuperior direction, and the excess fascia is excised in the preauricular region. The flap is sutured under tension to the preauricular SMAS posterior to the dissection, with a Burow's triangle excised just below the zygomatic arch. The platysma muscle is plicated to the fascia over the posterior sternocleidomastoid muscle and mastoid area with interrupted inverted 4-0 PDS sutures (Fig. 183-5).

Hemostasis is again confirmed, and any fat depositions are contoured before closure. The skin flaps are draped in a posterosuperior direction, and tension sutures are placed just above the ear and at the height of the postauricular incision. The cervical skin is positioned to maintain a normal hairline, and the excess skin is excised. A similar technique is used to align the temporal hair and remove the excess skin. The earlobe is then exposed by incising parallel to the helix of the ear, and the preauricular skin is trimmed to allow a tension-free closure. If a retrotragal incision has been used, the skin draping over the tragus must be thinned. The hair-bearing areas can be closed with staples, and the preauricular area is closed with running 6-0 nylon or Prolene. The postauricular sulcus is closed with 4-0 nylon running suture. The earlobe is carefully positioned and closed with 6-0 mattress sutures to ensure eversion of the skin edges (Fig. 183-6). Drains are optional and usually placed in the posterior incision within the hairline. The local anesthetic for the second hemifacial unit is infiltrated just before closure of the initial dissection.

After all incisions have been closed, bacitracin is applied, and fluffy gauze is placed around the ears and along the facial and cervical dissection areas. A firm but forgiving elastic dressing is placed to provide gentle pressure to the neck and face. The patient is then transferred to the recovery area in a semisitting position.

IRA D. PAPEL

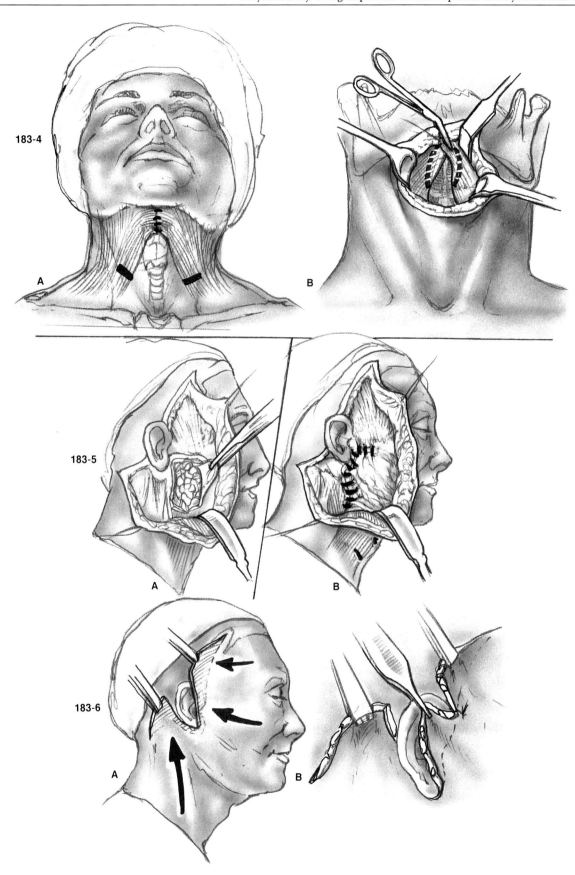

183-4

A

B

183-5

A

B

183-6

A

B

■ *184.* LIPOSUCTION OF THE NECK WITH FACELIFT PRETUNNELING— Removal of cervical subcutaneous fat and preliminary undermining of the face

Indications
1. Class III neck
2. A pathologic collection of subcutaneous fat causing poor definition of the normal youthful topographic landmarks of the neck (eg, mandible border, thyroid cartilage, obtuse cervicomental angle)

Special Considerations
1. Ptotic submandibular glands
2. Previous facelift
3. Presence of a deep submental fat pad

Preoperative Preparation
1. Bleeding and clotting studies

Special Instruments, Position, and Anesthesia
1. Liposuction cannula (4 to 6 mm)
2. Vacuum pump that can deliver as close to one atmosphere of pressure as possible with a high flow rate
3. Supine position, with hyperextension of the neck
4. Local anesthesia is preferred for closed liposuction of the neck; when combined with a facelift, general anesthesia is used with local infiltration of the neck for hemostasis

Tips and Pearls
1. Dissection in proper plane
2. Insert the cannula with the vacuum off.
3. Begin deep, and work subcutaneously.

Pitfalls and Complications
1. Uneven contouring and scarring results if the opening of the cannula is turned so the dermis is puckered into the opening.
2. Secondary and revision facelifts must be undermined carefully, because the skin is densely adherent to the sternocleidomastoid muscle, and the cannula can easily slip under the greater auricular nerve with subsequent injury as the tunnels are connected.

Postoperative Care Issues
1. Closed vacuum drains are placed if the cervical skin has been completely undermined from angle to angle of the mandible during the facelift. No drains are used for closed liposuction.
2. A bulky Barton head dressing is placed to reduce edema and keep pressure on the undermined area. This is changed daily for a facelift until the drain is removed (usually on the third postoperative day). The dressing for closed liposuction of the neck, after it is changed on the first postoperative day, is removed on the fourth day.

References
Dedo DD. Liposuction. In: Lee KJ, ed. Atlas of aesthetic facial surgery, vol III. New York: Grune & Stratton, 1983.

Dedo DD. Liposuction and the platysma muscle. Arch Otol 1986;112: 306.

Operative Procedure
The area of undermining and incisions are marked on the face and neck with the patient in the sitting position. Key landmarks for cervical liposuction are the mandible border superiorly, the anterior edge of the sternocleidomastoid muscle laterally, and the inferiormost horizontal crease to be corrected in the neck inferiorly (usually just inferior to the cricoid cartilage). Symmetric tunnels originating at the submental incision are outlined on the neck. If the jowl fat is prominent and ptotic, it too is outlined (Fig. 184-1).

The face and neck are infiltrated with a dilute solution of 100 mL of 0.25% Marcaine with 1:200,000 epinephrine in 200 mL of normal saline. For closed liposuction of the neck, incisions are made beneath each ear lobule and in the first submental crease. A short pair of scissors is placed in each incision and spread to the correct plane and level. The skin below each ear is particularly adherent to the fascia, and by spreading the scissors tips about 0.5 cm (1 in) inferiorly, the liposuction cannula insertion is greatly facilitated (Fig. 184-2).

With the vacuum off, the palpating hand of the surgeon lifts the cervical skin up while the cannula is pushed to the end of the tunnel (Fig. 184-3). Care is taken to stay as deep as possible in the tunnel. After the vacuum is turned on, the liposuction cannula is pushed back and forth in short strokes in the tunnel, using the cannula as a battering ram to remove the subcutaneous fat held between the thumb and fingers of the opposite hand. Rotating of the cannula within the tunnel ensures adequate fat removal. After the fat has been removed from this short section of the tunnel, the palpating hand moves up the tunnel toward the incision to repeat the maneuver until the tunnel has been completely treated. With the vacuum off, the first lateral tunnel is suctioned. By gently threading and feeling for the anterior border of the platysma muscle with the tip of the cannula, the surgeon tries to position the cannula on the floor of the tunnel on top of the platysma muscle (Fig. 184-4). The distal end of the tunnel is treated as before, working gradually back to the incision. Care is taken to treat symmetric areas on the neck. No attempt is made to connect the tunnels with a sweeping motion. This interrupts the vascular supply to the skin and causes bleeding.

After the fat has been removed from the submental incision, a second set of tunnels that run diagonally across the neck from each lobule is created (Fig. 184-5). If there are prominent ptotic jowls, the cannula is threaded into each from the submental incision. By grasping the jowl fat and pulling it laterally, the cannula tip is threaded into the middle of it. The vacuum is turned on, and several short strokes are made within the fat to try and reduce the bulk of it. When the surgeon attempts to suction the jowl fat by going between the skin and fat, irregular contouring may result.

After the cervical area has been treated, the incisions are closed with a subcutaneous absorbable suture. A bulky Barton dressing is applied.

The liposuction cannula can be used to pretunnel and facilitate the flap undermining in a facelift. After the neck has been treated, the incisions are made as outlined. In the temple, the cannula is inserted at the root of the auricle, and multiple tunnels are created in a fan-like manner over the preauricular area (Fig. 184-6). Similarly, from the infralobular area the cannula is directed superiorly over the preauricular area to create a cross-hatching effect (Fig. 184-7). As the cannula sweeps over the mandible, fanning out from the ear, it connects with the previous tunneling of the neck liposuction. Care is taken to be on top of the superficial musculoaponeurotic system in the face. The pretunneling is continued over the posterior cervical areas and into the occiput from the infraauricular incision. The last pretunneling is done from the posterior cervical incision anteriorly into the neck. The facial, cervical, and occipital flaps are then elevated by cutting the septa between these tunnels with a knife or scissors.

After the flaps are elevated, open liposuction is done in the face and neck areas by rubbing the opening of the cannula on the fat with the vacuum turned on. This maneuver beautifully skeletonizes the superficial musculoaponeurotic system, posterior border of the platysma, and sternocleidomastoid fascia.

DOUGLAS D. DEDO

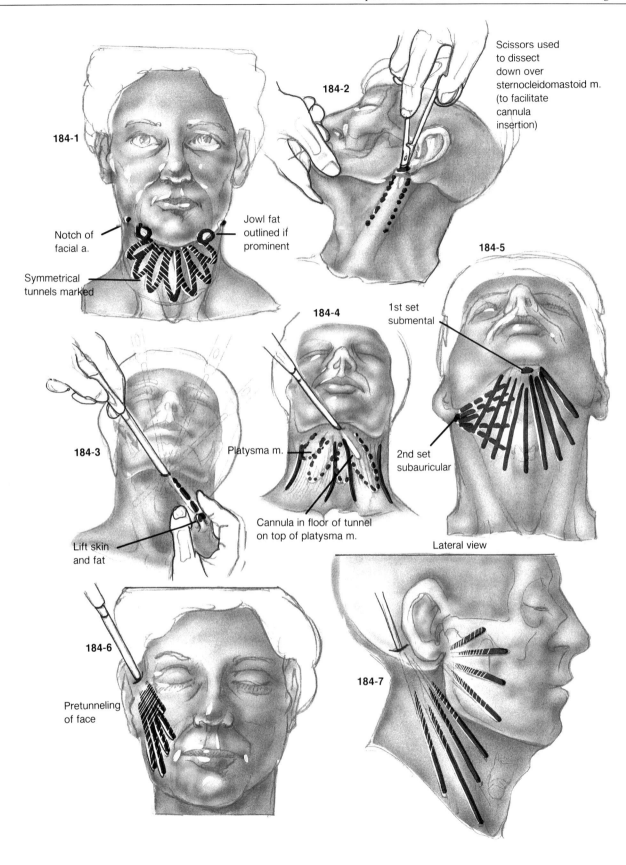

184-1

Notch of facial a.

Symmetrical tunnels marked

Jowl fat outlined if prominent

184-2   Scissors used to dissect down over sternocleidomastoid m. (to facilitate cannula insertion)

184-5

184-4

1st set submental

2nd set subauricular

184-3   Platysma m.

Lift skin and fat

Cannula in floor of tunnel on top of platysma m.

Lateral view

184-6   Pretunneling of face

184-7

■ 185. SUBMENTAL TUCK FOR THE AGING

NECK—The aging neck and the "turkey wattle" deformity can be surgically corrected using either a midline excision of skin, affording also a direct approach to the midline neck structures, or a submental incision to approach the midline neck structures with a concomitant facelift.

Indications

1. An obtuse cervicomental angle
2. Vertical banding of the platysma muscle
3. Lax platysma accentuated by voluntary contraction of the muscle
4. A "full"-appearing neck not corrected with liposuction

Special Considerations

1. The patient must accept a midline zigzag vertical scar for direct skin excision with platysma tuck.
2. Ptotic submandibular glands are not helped.
3. Smokers are at risk for skin necrosis, so if extensive undermining is planned they should not smoke for 2 weeks before and after surgery.

Special Instruments, Position, and Anesthesia

1. General anesthesia local infiltration for hemostasis is best for a full facelift; local alone is adequate for a direct midline approach.
2. Headlight, Aufricht-style retractor.
3. Patient supine; surgeon at patient's head.

Tips and Pearls

1. First identify the platysma fibers as they decussate in the midline near the pogonion to be at the correct level. Keep the platysma visible beneath the scissors to avoid undermining laterally. Leave fat attached to the skin. Avoid cutting the muscle: this reduces bleeding, increases support of the resuspended muscle, and reduces the chance of facial nerve injury.
2. Because the cervical dissection is tedious and time-consuming, perform this before undermining the facial flaps.
3. Using braided, double-looped suture reapproximates the cut edge of the platysma and distributes tension over a larger area.

Pitfalls and Complications

1. Uneven contouring with lumpiness
2. Overexcision, Z-plasty, horizontal sectioning, or improper redirection of the platysma muscle results in masculinization of the neck by accentuating the thyroid cartilage or produces unnatural folds.
3. The platysma may adhere to the skin, causing abnormal folds on swallowing. This occurs because the normal fat layer is removed.
4. Simply suturing platysma muscle edges without excising a midline strip of muscle and fascia produces a midline ridge that blunts the acute cervicomental angle.

Postoperative Care Issues

1. Dressings changed daily while checking for seromas and hematomas. Drain removed on third postoperative day.
2. If a small seroma or hematoma develops postauricularly, remove a suture and express the fluid.
3. A major hematoma causes unilateral pain unrelieved by analgesics. Such patients are returned to the operating room and the wound explored; usually a discrete bleeding point is not found.
4. Dusky skin with compromised circulation may not be seen until postoperative day 5 or 6. Needling the flap to reduce venous congestion and application of nitroglycerin paste can sometimes save a flap. If necrosis occurs, see the patient daily, assuring him or her that sequential scar excision or tissue expansion can be done in a year to reduce scarring.

Operative Procedure

Hair is placed in rubber bands, with trimming confined to the area of anticipated scalp excision. With the patient sitting, landmarks are outlined: incisions, platysma edge, mandible border, facial artery notch, and undermining extent. After general anesthesia is induced, the face and neck are infiltrated with 300 mL of 0.08% Marcaine with 1:500,000 epinephrine (100mL of 0.25% Marcaine with 1: 200,000 epinephrine in 200 mL of saline) using tumescent technique. A curved 2-cm (0.75 in) submental incision is made, apex in the first submental crease and laterally paralleling the mandible (Fig. 185-1). Submental muscle is identified by blunt dissection and followed inferiorly to find the decussating platysma fibers and fascia (Fig. 185-2).

Platysma edges are followed inferiorly as outlined on the skin. The flap is tented by the retractor, and Metzenbaum or Rees facelift scissors peel muscle fibers from the fat layer. With skin countertraction, dissection continues laterally to the sternocleidomastoid muscle. Inferiorly, undermining is carried at least to the cricoid cartilage (sometimes to within 1 cm of the clavicle), and superiorly, to the mandible. Superior skin is undermined to the pogonion, and a chin implant placed if necessary. The mentalis muscle is incised, and platysma muscle and midline fascia are excised to the thyroid notch. Mandibular periosteum is preserved, and initial excision of muscle should not exceed 1 cm. Muscle bleeding is controlled with electrocautery. The deep submental fat pad is not reduced unless it causes a bulge when the facial flaps are pulled superiorly. This occurs primarily in obese patients, and is corrected with gentle open liposuction. Preserving a fat layer between the platysma and mylohyoid prevents a concavity.

A 4-0 braided permanent suture is placed through the lateral cut edge of platysma just below the mandible to mandibular periosteum superiorly, reconstructing the submental triangle (Fig. 185-3). The submental tuck continues with reapproximation of midline to the thyroid notch (Fig. 185-4). Excess muscle is excised before suturing. This area is packed with moist sponges while the facelift is completed.

To complete the reconstruction of the cervical sling and allow redraping of the cervical skin, the facial and occipital flaps are elevated and connected with the midline cervical undermining. Open liposuction over the sternocleidomastoid muscle and superficial musculoaponeurotic system identifies the posterior border of the platysma. This is plicated with double looped 3-0 PDS suture to the fascia of the sternocleidomastoid muscle (see Fig. 185-4). Because the platysma is continuous with the superficial musculoaponeurotic system of the face, this plication continues superiorly to the pretragal area.

The direct midline excision of skin and muscle begins with preoperative marking of the seated patient: the first submental crease, platysma muscle anterior borders, suprasternal notch, and estimated width of skin excision (pinch the redundant skin into a midline fold). After infiltration of local anesthetic, a midline incision is made from the first submental crease to the suprasternal notch. The skin flaps are elevated from the platysma, just beyond the markings of anticipated skin excision. Open liposuction is used in the midline to delineate the fascia and platysma. Do not overexcise fat and create a trough. Feather laterally over the platysma with the liposuction cannula to contour the neck. The superior skin is undermined from the submental crease to the mandible. The mentalis muscle is incised to mandibular periosteum. Midline muscle and fascia are excised to the thyroid cartilage notch. Redundant fat deep to platysma is gently suctioned. Muscle tuck is completed as described previously (Fig. 185-5).

After reconstitution of the muscle in the midline to the mandible, a horizontal incision is made in the submental crease along one edge of the flap. Skin is sutured with 5-0 polyglycolic acid suture subcutaneously to the opposite corner of the submental crease. The remaining incision is closed by excising the redundant skin as large Z-plasty flaps are created from each flap. Progressively smaller flaps are used as the inferior end of the incision is approached.

DOUGLAS D. DEDO

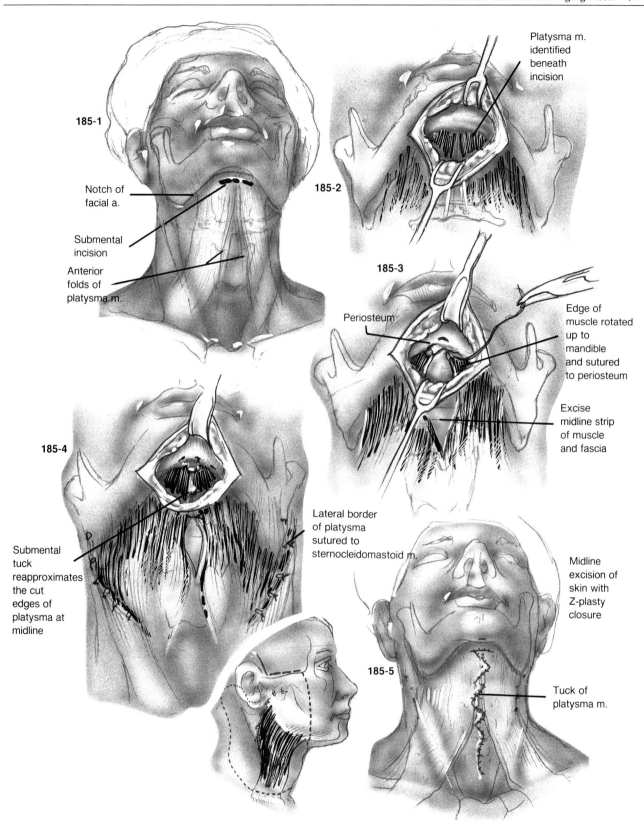

185-1

Notch of
facial a.

Submental
incision

Anterior
folds of
platysma m.

185-2

Platysma m.
identified
beneath
incision

185-3

Periosteum

Edge of
muscle rotated
up to
mandible
and sutured
to periosteum

Excise
midline strip
of muscle
and fascia

185-4

Submental
tuck
reapproximates
the cut
edges of
platysma at
midline

Lateral border
of platysma
sutured to
sternocleidomastoid m.

185-5

Midline
excision of
skin with
Z-plasty
closure

Tuck of
platysma m.

■ 186. ANALYSIS OF THE UPPER ONE THIRD OF THE FACE AND NECK

Neck Analysis—Critical evaluation of fat distribution; position of the anterior mandible, submandibular glands, hyoid and larynx; and laxity and contour of the platysma and excess skin.

Indications
1. Evaluation before liposuction, rhytidectomy, mentoplasty

Tips and Pearls
1. Palpate position of hyoid
2. Note position of anterior platysma bands
3. Evaluate occlusion and mandible (with cephalometrics as needed)

Pitfalls and Complications
1. Failure to recognize anteriorly placed hyoid
2. Failure to recognize ptotic submandibular glands
3. Failure to recognize underlying orthognathic problems

Analysis of the Neck
The youthful neck has a well-defined cervicomental angle, a sharp mandibular line, a well-supported chin, and no visible platysma banding. With age, the chin descends in much the same manner as the nasal tip and the brows. The well-defined angle between the submandibular line and the neck is lost with age. The hyoid bone and the larynx gradually descend, making the larynx look more prominent. The cervical appearance with aging is a combination of changes in the skin, fat distribution, in platysma muscle, and the underlying bony skeleton.

Analysis of the Upper One Third of the Face—Critical evaluation of the upper vertical one third of the face, including hairline location, presence of rhytids, and brow position

Indications
1. Evaluation before blepharoplasty or rhytidectomy
2. Brow ptosis or forehead rhytids

Special Considerations
1. Relations among lower, middle, and upper vertical facial thirds
2. Temporal facial nerve paralysis
3. Location of eyebrow in relation to superior orbital rim
4. Location of highest point of eyebrow
5. Location of the hairline and evidence of hair thinning or balding

Tips and Pearls
1. Female brows should be located on the supraorbital rim medially and arch above the rim laterally.
2. The location of highest point of the female eyebrow varies, ranging between vertical lines drawn tangent to lateral limbus and lateral canthus. The most aesthetic position is thought to be closer to the lateral canthus than the lateral limbus of the iris.
3. Male brows should be located on the supraorbital rim in most cases.

Pitfalls and Complications
1. Failure to appreciate the contribution of ptotic brows to excessive upper eyelid skin and subsequent overresection of upper eyelid skin during blepharoplasty, drawing the brows down further
2. Browplasty resulting in arching of male eyebrows, with subsequent feminizing effect
3. Bony prominence of the supraorbital rim can masquerade as lid fullness.
4. A low or poorly defined lid fold can give the appearance of excess skin on the upper lid.

References
Johnson CM, Toriumi DM. Forehead deformities. In: Krause CJ, Mangat DS, Pastorek N, eds. Aesthetic facial surgery. Philadelphia: JB Lippincott, 1991:545.
Larrabee WF Jr, Makielski KH. Forehead and brow. In: Surgical anatomy of the face. New York: Raven Press, 1993:123.

Upper One-Third Facial Analysis
The vertical facial thirds of Leonardo Da Vinci are useful for determining facial proportions. The upper third comprises the forehead, temple, eyebrow, and glabella. The middle third is occupied by the eyes and nose. With aging, the effect of gravity causes lengthening or laxity of the forehead, temple, and glabella, with ptosis of the eyebrow. The ptotic eyebrows change the proportions of the vertical thirds by reducing the length of the middle third and increasing that of the upper third.

Ideally, the female eyebrow is positioned on or above the supraorbital rim or glabella medially and arches above the supraorbital rim laterally (Fig. 186-2). The highest point of the arch should be between vertical lines through the lateral limbus and lateral canthus. The arch usually occurs one third to one half of the distance from the lateral limbus to the lateral canthus but may occur anywhere between these two lines (Fig. 186-3). Laterally, the brow arches downward and ends just lateral to a line drawn from the alae to the lateral canthus. At its lateral termination, the eyebrow should lie at or above a horizontal line drawn through the medial termination of the eyebrow.

Male eyebrows are ideally positioned on the supraorbital rim and are usually more prominent in their lateral third than female brows (see Fig. 186-2). Minimal arching is typical, giving the brow, orbital rim, and nasal bones a T-shaped configuration.

Evaluation of the brow is important for accurate analysis of the upper and middle vertical facial thirds. Sagging of the lateral portion of the forehead and temple often leads to the lateral hooding seen as the initial sign of aging. If a blepharoplasty alone is performed to correct this problem because of the mistaken belief that it involves only redundant upper lid skin, the brow may be incarcerated in an unnatural inferior position and the hooding left uncorrected. A brow lift should precede the blepharoplasty in this situation. An appearance of lateral hooding and fullness may be exacerbated by the eyebrow fat pad, which contributes to eyebrow mobility and is found deep to the muscle layer. Occasionally, this fat pad extends inferiorly between the orbicularis oculi muscle and the orbital septum to form the lateral "preseptal fat" seen in blepharoplasty.

Many patients unconsciously adapt to ptotic brows by tonic contraction of the frontalis muscle, which interdigitates with the orbicularis oculi muscle and the skin of the eyebrows. Having the patient close his or her eyes and gently open them after gentle downward massage of the forehead relaxes the brows to their resting state.

Rhytids of the upper one third of the face are the result of aging and action of three sets of muscles, resulting in three patterns of rhytids. Recurrent action of the paired frontalis muscle results in horizontal rhytids across the forehead. Vertical rhytids may form in the glabella region as a result of the activity of the corrugator supercilii muscle, and the procerus activity results in horizontal glabellar rhytids. Knowledge of the muscles responsible for a particular group of rhytids is required for accurate surgical treatment of the aging forehead.

WAYNE F. LARRABEE, JR.

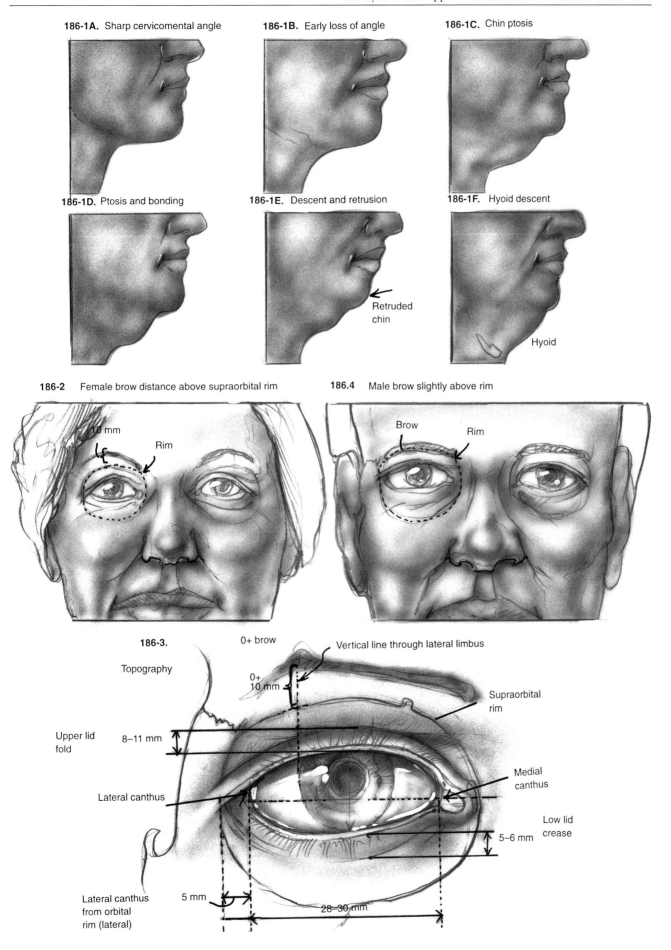

186-1A. Sharp cervicomental angle

186-1B. Early loss of angle

186-1C. Chin ptosis

186-1D. Ptosis and bonding

186-1E. Descent and retrusion

Retruded chin

186-1F. Hyoid descent

Hyoid

186-2   Female brow distance above supraorbital rim

10 mm

Rim

186.4   Male brow slightly above rim

Brow   Rim

186-3.

Topography

0+ brow

Vertical line through lateral limbus

0+
10 mm

Supraorbital
rim

Upper lid
fold

8–11 mm

Lateral canthus

Medial
canthus

Low lid
crease

5–6 mm

Lateral canthus
from orbital
rim (lateral)

5 mm

28–30 mm

■ 187. BROWLIFTS

Coronal, trichophytic, pretrichial, and endoscopic forehead lift and surgical elevation of eyebrows with or without treatment of forehead ptosis or rhytids through an incision located at or behind the hairline

Indications

1. Brow ptosis
2. Lateral eyelid hooding due to brow ptosis
3. Forehead and glabellar rhytids

Special Considerations

1. Coronal lifts are best for women with medium or low forehead hairlines.
2. Trichophytic or pretrichial lift is indicated for women with higher hairlines or males with higher hairlines to avoid lengthening of the forehead.
3. Endoscopic forehead procedures are excellent for treating rhytids and can also be used to elevate brows with minimal incisions.

Preoperative Preparation

1. Routine laboratory studies
2. Preoperative assessment of facial nerve function

Special Instruments, Position, and Anesthesia

1. Headlight
2. Bipolar cautery
3. Infiltrate with a solution of 1% lidocaine with 1:100,000 epinephrine along the superior orbital margin, including the supraorbital and supratrochlear nerves, laterally paralleling the zygomatic arches and along proposed incision lines.
4. Local with intravenous sedation or general anesthesia acceptable
5. Endoscopic equipment as indicated

Tips and Pearls

1. Allow time for vasoconstriction.
2. Bevel incisions parallel to the hair follicles for coronal incisions.
3. Avoid electrocautery as much as possible in subcutaneous plane to avoid damage to the hair follicles.
4. Laterally, avoid injuring the temporal branch of the facial nerve by elevating the flap with gentle blunt dissection just above the superficial layer of the deep temporalis fascia.
5. Endoscopic procedure ideal for treatment of corrugations

Pitfalls and Complications

1. Postoperative bleeding
2. Injury to temporal branch of facial nerve
3. Alopecia
4. Excessive elevation or asymmetries of eyebrows
5. Hyperesthesia or paraesthesia of the forehead

Postoperative Care Issues

1. Wound dressing for 24 hours
2. The patient may gently wash hair 24 hours after surgery.
3. Hypesthesia or paresthesia posterior to the incision line improves somewhat over time.

References

Adamson PA, Cormier R, McGraw BM. The coronal forehead lift: modifications and results. J Otolaryngol 1992;21:1.
Brennan HG. The frontal lift. Arch Otolaryngol Head Neck Surg 1978;104:26.
Kerth JD, Toriumi DM. Management of the aging forehead. Arch Otolaryngol Head Neck Surg 1990;116:1137.

Operative Procedures

Confirm the degree of brow ptosis and the location of forehead or glabellar rhytids with the patient sitting upright. The patient is then placed supine, and a curvilinear incision is marked 6 cm behind the hairline for a coronal lift and 2 to 3 mm behind the hairline for the trichophytic modification of the pretrichial lift (Figs. 187-1 and 187-2). Local infiltration with a solution of 1% lidocaine with 1:100,000 epinephrine begins with the supraorbital and supratrochlear nerve notches or foramen and is then extended along the supraorbital rim and laterally, paralleling the zygomatic arch. The proposed incision line is injected with a local anesthetic with the addition of some infiltration into the subgaleal plane. Allow 5 to 10 minutes for vasoconstriction.

The coronal incision is beveled parallel to the hair follicles, observing the change in direction of the follicles from the frontal to temporal region. Trichophytic incisions are beveled in an open Z-configuration to allow the de-epithelialized portion of the posterior flap to regrow hair through the scar (Fig. 187-3). This results in a superior camouflage of the scar compared with the pretrichial incision. Incise an 8- to 10-cm section, and then obtain hemostasis with bipolar cautery before going on the next section. The galea can be freely cauterized, but cautery in the subcutaneous plane should be minimized to avoid damage to the hair follicles.

After the incision is completed, the flap is elevated anteriorly in the subgaleal plane by using a scalpel or scissors while keeping the pericranium intact. Elevation of the flap laterally is accomplished in the plane just above the superficial layer of the deep temporalis fascia, superior to the region of the zygomatic arch. Elevation in this region is best done with gentle blunt dissection to avoid injury to the branches of the facial nerve. After exiting the parotid, branches of the facial nerve run subcutaneously with the superficial musculoaponeurotic system between the brow and the temporal hairline. The nerves then enter the frontalis muscle on its deep aspect about 1 cm above the supraorbital rim.

Approximately 2 cm above the supraorbital rim, blunt scissors dissection of the corrugator supercilii muscles is performed. The supraorbital and supratrochlear nerves and vessels are identified and preserved. To free the brow for elevation, the flap is dissected over the orbital rim ending before exposing orbital fat. Bleeding is controlled with bipolar cautery. Sections of the corrugator and procerus muscles are incised, or small strips are removed with unipolar electrocautery to reduce the activity of these muscles. The frontalis muscle is incised in regions of prominent forehead rhytids in the central portion of the forehead only. Hemostasis is obtained, with particular attention paid to the superficial temporal vessels.

The flap is then advanced posteriorly, and an appropriate amount is excised to place brows in the desired position. The excess can be excised posterior to the incision, which places the closure farther from the hairline and makes the flap easier to elevate. More skin can be excised from the central or temporal regions, depending on the needs of the patient.

The techniques of endoscopic forehead lifting are still evolving. Most surgeons use 3–5 small hairline incisions and prefer a subperiosteal dissection. Specialized instruments and/or lasers are used to section corrugators and procerus muscles. Dissection is performed posteriorly to vertex and the repositioned forehead temporarily stabilized with titanium screws. Wound closure is accomplished with deep 2-0 absorbable suture for the galea, followed by staples for the coronal flaps. Trichophytic incisions are accurately closed with 4-0 absorbable subcutaneous sutures and interrupted nylon skin closure. Antibiotic ointment and a light dressing are applied. The dressing is removed on the first postoperative day, and sutures or staples are removed at days 7 and 9.

WAYNE F. LARRABEE, JR.

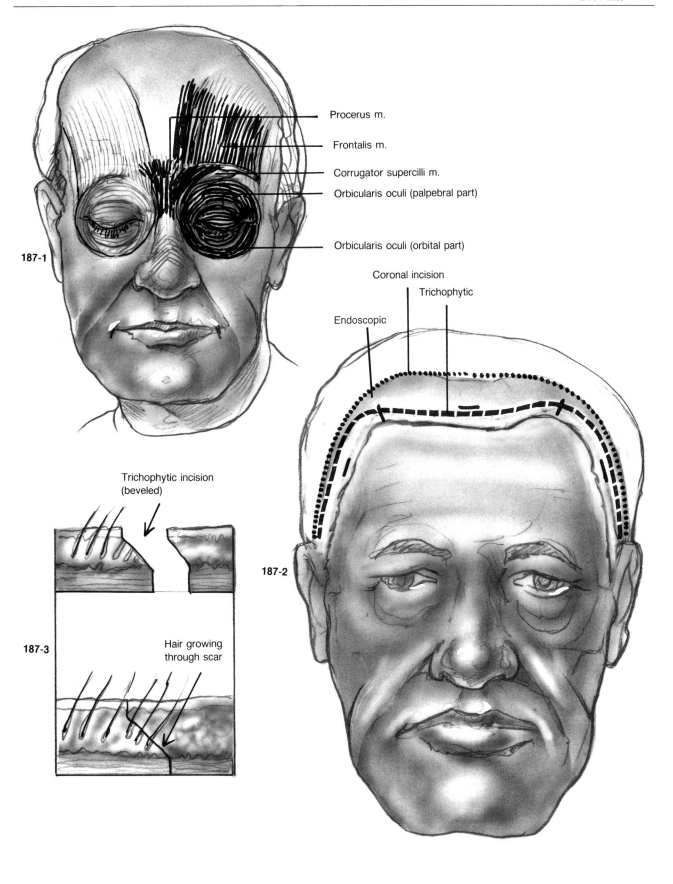

Procerus m.

Frontalis m.

Corrugator supercilli m.

Orbicularis oculi (palpebral part)

Orbicularis oculi (orbital part)

187-1

Coronal incision

Trichophytic

Endoscopic

Trichophytic incision
(beveled)

187-3

Hair growing
through scar

187-2

■ 188. BROWLIFTS

Direct, indirect, midforehead, and temporal browlifts are achieved by surgical elevation of the eyebrow with an incision placed just above the eyebrow or in a selected forehead rhytid. In many cases similar results can be obtained with an endoscopic forehead lifts.

Indications

1. Lateral brow ptosis (direct and temporal endoscopic lifts)
2. Generalized brow ptosis (indirect and midforehead endoscopic lifts)
3. Glabellar ptosis and rhytids (midforehead endoscopic lift).
4. Facial paralysis (direct lift)

Special Considerations

1. A direct browlift works best in male patients with bushy eyebrows, and can be used in cases of unilateral brow ptosis, such as from facial paralysis.
2. Direct browlift can be used for selected female patients in whom a coronal or trychophytic is contraindicated and avoidance of a midforehead incision is desired.
3. An indirect browlift is excellent for male patients with asymmetric or marked brow ptosis, forehead furrows, or in patients in whom a coronal browlift is contraindicated, such as those with baldness.
4. A midforehead lift is good for men with brow ptosis, glabellar ptosis, high or sparse hairlines, and marked preexisting furrows in which to place incisions.
5. A temporal browlift is useful in women with only lateral brow ptosis.
6. An endoscopic browlift involves the least morbidity.

Preoperative Preparations

1. Preoperative photographs
2. Careful discussion with the patient about scar visibility
3. Preoperative assessment of facial nerve function

Special Instruments, Position, and Anesthesia

1. Inject supraorbital and supratrochlear nerves first.
2. Bipolar cautery
3. Local anesthesia with sedation unless other ancillary procedures are planned
4. Endoscopic browlift requires specialized instruments and endoscopes.

Pitfalls and Complications

1. Noticeable scar in midforehead lifts
2. Unnatural sharp superior border of brows in males (direct browlift)
3. Injury to sensory nerves

References

Adamson PA, Johnson CM, Anderson JR, Dupin CL. The forehead lift. Arch Otolaryngol Head Neck Surg 1985;111:325.

Cook TA, Brownrigg PJ, Wang TD, Quatela VC. The versatile midforehead browlift. Arch Otolaryngol Head Neck Surg 1989;115:163.

Rafaty FM, Brennan HG. Current concepts of browpexy. Arch Otolyngol Head Neck Surg 1983;109:152.

Operative Procedure

Confirm the degree of brow ptosis and glabellar rhytids or ptosis with the patient sitting upright. To mark incisions in the sitting position, first mark the inferior incision with the patient relaxed, and then manually elevate the brow to the desired position, hold the marking pen at the new brow height, release the brow, and mark the vertical height to be excised. In direct browlifts, the incision is placed primarily over the lateral three quarters of the brow, and it should result in an appropriately designed brow arch in female patients.

For direct browlifts, an ellipse of skin corresponding to the degree of desired brow elevation is marked just above the eyebrows (Fig. 188-1). The supraorbital and supratrochlear nerves are then injected with a 1% concentration of lidocaine with a 1:100,000 dilution of epinephrine, followed by infiltration of the proposed excision site. After waiting for vasoconstriction to occur, the ellipse is excised, sparing the underlying frontalis muscle. The inferior incision is beveled to spare eyebrow hair follicles. The eyebrow is then suspended using a 4-0 permanent suture from the orbicularis muscle to the periosteum of the frontal bone at the superior edge of the incision to fix the brow in its new position (Fig. 188-2). The incision is then closed with a 5-0 absorbable subcutaneous suture, and the skin is closed with 6-0 nylon.

For indirect browlifts, the proposed fusiform excisions are placed in the forehead rhytids instead of in the immediate suprabrow region (see Fig. 188-1). This allows greater resection of skin medially for medial brow ptosis if desired. Fusiform excisions are planned so that the resulting scar is aligned with the original rhytid. This usually involves placing about two thirds of the excision above and one third of the excision below the level of the rhytid. Excisions can be drawn at slightly different levels on each side to assist in camouflage. Anesthesia and hemostasis are obtained using a 1% solution of lidocaine with a 1:100,000 dilution of epinephrine. After removal of the skin ellipse, moderate undermining of the inferior skin flap in the plane above the frontalis muscle is required. As in the direct browlift, permanent horizontal mattress suspension sutures are placed through the orbicularis oculi muscle immediately underlying the brows. The brows are then suspended to the periosteum at the level of the incision using a 4-0 nonabsorbable suture. The wound is then carefully closed with 5-0 absorbable subcutaneous suture and a 5-0 subcuticular suture.

The midforehead browlift involves one incision based in a centrally located horizontal rhytid (see Fig. 188-1). After the amount of brow and glabellar ptosis or rhytid is evaluated with the patient sitting, the proposed incision is marked. A single incision is marked in a prominent forehead rhytid, with a staggered line at the midportion to provide added camouflage (see Fig. 188-1). After infiltration with a solution of 1% lidocaine with 1:100,000 epinephrine, the incision is made and an inferior flap is developed above the plane of the frontalis muscle. If desired, glabellar and forehead rhytids can be treated by division or excision of a portion of the corrugator supercilia, procerus, and lower central frontalis muscles. The eyebrows are then suspended in a manner similar to the direct and indirect forehead lifts. The inferior flap is then draped superiorly, and the excess is trimmed. Closure is achieved with 5-0 absorbable and 5-0 subcuticular suture. Sutures are removed at 5 days.

The temporal lift involves fusiform skin excision and plication of fascia without significant undermining of the flaps. Closure is done with 4-0 permanent sutures in the fascia, 5-0 absorbable in the subcutaneous tissues, and 5-0 nylon in the skin.

Endoscopic browlift is usually performed through 3 to 5 incisions at the hairline or just posterior to it. Dissection is either subgaleal or subperiosteal. Special endoscopic instruments are used to free the soft tissue from the orbital rim and to treat the muscles. Various fixation techniques are used to fix the galea to outer cortex and thus maintain brow elevation after wide undermining of the scalp.

WAYNE F. LARRABEE, JR.

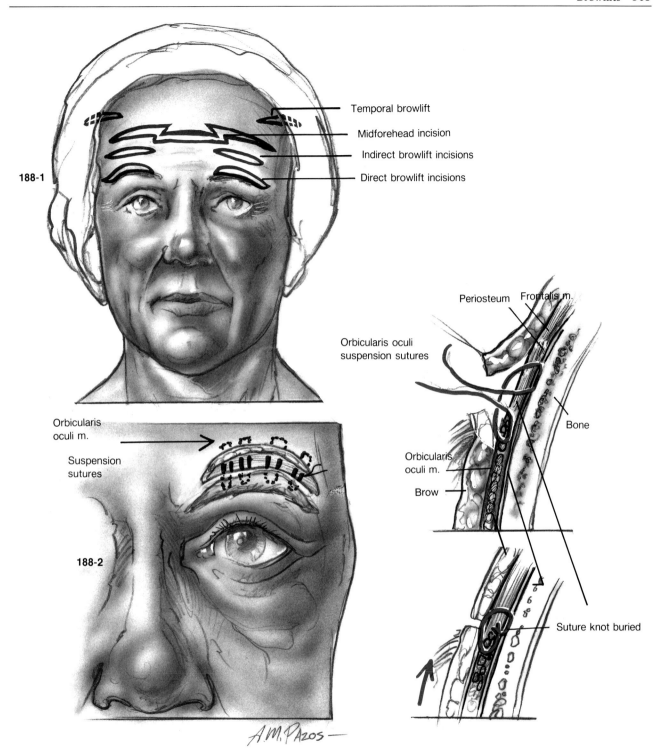

Temporal browlift

Midforehead incision

Indirect browlift incisions

Direct browlift incisions

188-1

Orbicularis
oculi m.

Suspension
sutures

188-2

Periosteum   Frontalis m.

Orbicularis oculi
suspension sutures

Bone

Orbicularis
oculi m.

Brow

Suture knot buried

A.M. PAZOS —

■ 189. INJECTIONS OF COLLAGEN OR FAT

Injections of autografts, xenografts, and placement of synthetic material subcutaneously to correct depressions, scarring, and wrinkles

Indications

1. Subcutaneous deficiencies that produce an overlying depression in the skin (eg, acne scars, lacerations)
2. Lines of aging as the skin loses its elasticity and the tension lines from contraction of the facial muscles create the predictable relaxed skin tension lines.
3. Folds and large atrophic areas amenable to subcutaneous augmentation

Contraindications

1. Allergic reaction to the collagen skin test or subsequent development of an allergic reaction may occur after treatment is begun. A relative contraindication is a history of an autoimmune disease.
2. Patient unwilling to accept the temporary nature of the soft tissue augmentation that lasts 3 months to 1 year
3. Patient unwilling to accept the possibility that the Gore-Tex graft may be palpable under the skin

Special Considerations

1. Autograft fat, collagen, and xenograft collagen are temporary.
2. Skin tests are required, with a 4- to 8-week hiatus if one or two tests are administered before beginning treatment with xenograft collagen.
3. A maximum of 2 cc of xenograft collagen are injected at one sitting.
4. Lines from active animation (eg, lips, corner of the mouth, cheek lip folds) absorb the injectable graft quicker than those areas of less movement (eg, forehead, cheeks).
5. Gore-Tex (polytetrafluoroethylene) graft material is treated with an antibiotic solution by displacement in a syringe.

Preoperative Preparation

1. No laboratory studies are necessary if the patient is healthy and taking no special medications.

Special Instruments, Position, and Anesthesia

1. Xenograft collagen comes in prefilled syringes with supplied 30-gauge needles. Zyplast collagen is the most concentrated and lasts the longest. Zyderm collagen is more dilute, and as the solution is absorbed, less of a correction is achieved.
2. Autograft fat injection is harvested with a 10-cc syringe and 14-gauge needle, and it is injected with an 18-gauge needle.
3. Garamycin, lincomycin, or bacitracin antimicrobials are suspended in normal saline in a 20-cc syringe to displace the Gore-Tex graft material before implantation.

References

Elson ML. Update on soft tissue augmentation. Am J Cosmet Surg 1992;9:267.
Mole B. The use of Gore-Tex implants in aesthetic surgery of the face. Plast Reconstr Surg 1992;90:200.

Operative Procedure

Collagen Injection

The facial rhytids to be treated are identified by the patient, and the site of injection is prepped with alcohol. If the patient has a particularly low pain threshold, covering the areas to be treated with Emla cream 1 hour before treatment greatly reduces the pain of injection. The 30-gauge needle is placed in the dermis (Fig. 189-1) with the bevel up at the end of the wrinkle (Fig. 189-2). After a wheal is created and the depression corrected, the needle is withdrawn, and coalescent wheals of collagen are injected as the operator "walks up" the wrinkle (Fig. 189-3). Injection too deeply into the subcutaneous fat reduces the length of time the correction lasts and can be avoided by holding the syringe at a 30° to the skin. The collagen squirts out of prominent adjacent pores, and in these patients, insertion of the needle with the bevel down reduces this problem. The physician can usually treat the glabellar, procerus, cheek lip fold, and circumoral rhytids with 2 cc of material. By having the patient hold a mirror during treatment, there is no question about not treating the correct area. No makeup is applied for 4 hours after the treatment.

Acne scars are particularly difficult to treat, because the thin, atrophic, depressed skin usually splits open during the injection process. Similarly, depressed facial scars from trauma do not tolerate ballooning of the dermis with the collagen, and the material usually extrudes into the adjacent tissue.

Autograft Fat and Collagen Injection

The fat is harvested from the abdomen (Fig. 189-4), which is anesthetized with a local solution. The 14-gauge needle is attached to the 10-cc syringe, and once inserted into the subcutaneous layer, the plunger is withdrawn to create a vacuum. The opposite hand holding the skin squeezes it (Fig. 189-5) while the syringe is moved back and forth between the fingers. Multiple strokes are required as the syringe fans out from the corner of the donor area. After 8 cc of material are withdrawn, the syringe is placed with the needle end down to allow the supernatant to settle and the fat to collect on top. The number of syringes to be filled depends on the areas to be treated. An 18-gauge needle is placed on the syringe and the supernatant discarded. The fat graft is then placed in the subcutaneous layer (Fig. 189-6) beneath the rhytids to be corrected. Facial nerve blocks may increase patient comfort, but these injections are painful. Overcorrection by 20% is recommended, and any lumpiness is reduced by squeezing and manipulating the treated skin.

Autograft collagen processed from the patient's skin removed at the time of surgery is expensive and does not last any longer than xenograft collagen or autograft fat. It requires a 27-gauge needle for injection and can be infiltrated into the dermis similar to Zyplast.

Gore-Tex Graft Augmentation

A more permanent subcutaneous augmentation material is Gore-Tex. Lip, cheek lip folds, chin, and malar and nasal dorsum have been treated with this material. It comes in 1- and 2-mm thicknesses of various sizes. The area to be treated is marked and anesthetized. The lips are augmented by cutting the graft into 1-mm strips and displacing the pores with an antibiotic solution in a syringe (see Fig. 189-1). A tunnel is created beneath the orbicularis muscle with a hemostat (see Fig. 189-2). The graft is sutured with a 2-0 silk on a Keith needle. It is passed in the tunnel from one side of the lip to the other (see Fig. 189-3). The end of the graft is cut to release the suture and allow it to lie beneath the muscle. The opposite end is cut so it too falls beneath the muscle. The opening is closed with a 4-0 chromic suture. The lower lip can similarly be threaded with Gore-Tex.

The cheek lip folds are undermined with a scissors from the alar crease. A triangular piece of antibiotic-treated Gore-Tex is sutured to a Keith needle and passed into the pocket by bringing the needle out the bottom of the fold (see Fig. 189-4). The alar incision is closed with a Prolene suture. Layered grafts of Gore-Tex have been placed in the cheeks and along the nasal dorsum. Care must be taken to make sure the edges are flat and not rolled up.

DOUGLAS D. DEDO

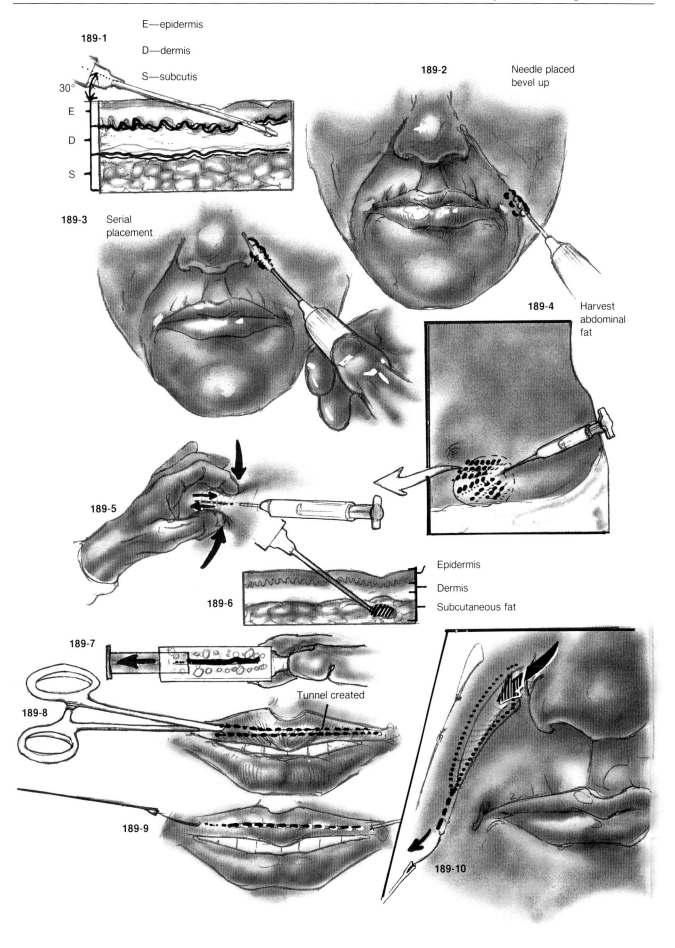

189-1

E—epidermis

D—dermis

S—subcutis

30°

E

D

S

189-2   Needle placed bevel up

189-3   Serial placement

189-4   Harvest abdominal fat

189-5

189-6   Epidermis

Dermis

Subcutaneous fat

189-7

189-8   Tunnel created

189-9

189-10

■ 190. DERMABRASION

Removal of epidermis and upper level of dermis by means of manual or power-driven abrasion, usually to reduce surface irregularities

Indications

1. Postacne scarring
2. Elevated or depressed scars
3. Fine facial rhytids
4. Surgical scars at least 4 to 6 weeks old

Special Considerations

1. History of herpes simplex infection
2. Previous use of isotretinoin (Accutane)
3. Infection with human immunodeficiency virus (HIV), hepatitis, or syphilis
4. Discoid lupus erythematosus, scleroderma, chronic radiodermatitis
5. Hypertrophic scarring with active acne

Preoperative Preparation

1. Complete blood count, hepatitis screen, and tests for venereal disease and HIV as indicated
2. Preoperative photographs
3. For a previous history of herpes simplex (ie, "fever blisters"), administer acyclovir (three 800-mg tablets t.i.d.) for 2 days before surgery and 14 days postoperatively.

Special Instruments, Position, and Anesthesia

1. Bell hand engine or other high-speed dermabrader
2. Diamond fraises, standard and coarse grits, or wire brushes
3. A liquid refrigerant containing Freon
4. Local anesthesia for abrasion of limited areas; general anesthesia or heavy sedation for full-face dermabrasion
5. Protective masks and eyeware for operating room personnel

Tips and Pearls

1. Angle dermabrader so that it tracks away from the eyes.
2. Pear-shaped fraise allows easier feathering around the nose and pretragal and periorbital regions.
3. Wide scars are better treated by surgical scar excision, with revision followed by dermabrasion at 6 weeks.
4. Localized acne scarring in the aging patient can be treated with dermabrasion of the involved areas plus a chemical peel (35% trichloroacetic acid) of the remainder of the face.

Pitfalls and Complications

1. Diamond fraises remove tissue at a slower rate than brushes and are best for novice use.
2. Excessive dermabrasion results in scarring where abrasion is too deep. Use care in the danger areas: mandibular ramus, zygomatic arch, malar eminence, bossing of chin, and bossing of forehead.
3. Herpes simplex activation treated with oral and topical acyclovir
4. Persistent, localized postoperative erythema may be an early scar. Treat with topical 2.5% hydrocortisone cream applied three times daily.

Postoperative Care Issues

1. Small regions of dermabrasion are maintained moist with antibacterial ointment; larger regions benefit from Adaptic or Vigilon dressings initially.
2. Gentle washing without scrubbing is important to avoid scarring.
3. Early sun exposure may result in hyperpigmentation.
4. Pruritus can be treated with topical 2.5% hydrocortisone applied three time daily.
5. Healing usually requires 7 to 10 days.

References

Alt TH. Dermabrasion facial plastic surgery. Facial Plastic Surgery Clinics of North America 1994;2:43.

Alt TH. Dermabrasion. In: Krause CJ, ed. Aesthetic facial surgery. Philadelphia: JB Lippincott, 1991.

Farrior RT. Dermabrasion in facial surgery. Laryngoscope 1985;95:534.

Fulton JE. The prevention and management of postdermabrasion complications. J Dermatol Surg Oncol 1991;17:421.

Operative Procedure

Dermabrasion is a mechanical removal of the epidermis and various layers of the dermis. Limited areas of dermabrasion can be performed using local anesthesia, supplemented with intravenous sedation as required. General anesthesia is recommended for full-face dermabrasion. Local anesthesia is obtained using a 1% solution of lidocaine with a 1:100,00 dilution of epinephrine for regional nerve blocks, avoiding "ballooning" of regions to be dermabraded.

The limits of regions to be dermabraded are marked. Depressions are marked with the marking pen, and raised scars are highlighted with the pen. Deep-pitted acne scars may benefit from removal by punch biopsy and replacement with a postauricular plug that is 0.5 mm larger 4 weeks before dermabrasion. Skin pretreatment with 0.05% tretinoin (Retin-A) or 10% glycolic acid twice daily for 4 to 6 weeks before dermabrasion may increase the healing rate and decrease the incidence of postoperative milia.

Dermabrasion for localized scars is performed by manually fixing the surrounding tissue lightly and dermabrading at a 45° angle to the scar. Excessive traction on the skin overly flattens the scar and leads to uneven dermabrasion. After the initial abrasion is performed, a second abrasion is performed at right angles to the initial abrasion, with the result of a "micro Z-plasty" effect on the scar in addition to the dermabrasion. The dermabrader is moved at a right angle to the direction of the spinning fraise or wheel (Figs. 190-1 and 190-2), with the abrader spinning in a direction that takes it away from the eyes, in case it catches.

Attention is kept constantly on the level of abrasion to avoid excessive depth, with texture and appearance used as guides. The change from the upper dermis to deeper dermis is delineated by increasing coarseness of the fibrous collagen. The epidermis reepithelializes from the skin appendages, which must not be damaged (Fig. 190-3). Bleeding is controlled by pressure with a sponge soaked with a solution of 1% lidocaine with 1:100,000 epinephrine.

For larger dermabrasions, as is often the case in acne scarring, abrasions should be extended to include the entire aesthetic unit of the region. Freezing with an agent containing Freon is recommended for best results, particularly for acne scarring and pock marks. This agent may be applied approximately 6 in (15 cm) from the skin acne and in an area about 2 cm in diameter. Several blasts of spray lasting 3 to 4 seconds are usually required to obtain a solid surface.

Full-face dermabrasions begin with the forehead, followed by cheeks and the perioral, nose, and chin regions. Care is taken to protect hair, eyes, and mouth from injury by using surgical towels and the hand. Minimal feathering (1–2 mm) onto the lip vermilion, over the jaw line, and into the hairline prevents sharp demarcation of dermabrasion regions.

Postoperative dressing with Vigilon, Adaptic, or bacitracin ointment with Telfa is changed at 24 hours and removed at 48 hours. After 48 hours, the patient is directed to shower twice daily with water gently running over the face. After gentle drying, bacitracin or polymyxin ointment is applied to nonhealed areas.

WAYNE F. LARRABEE, JR.

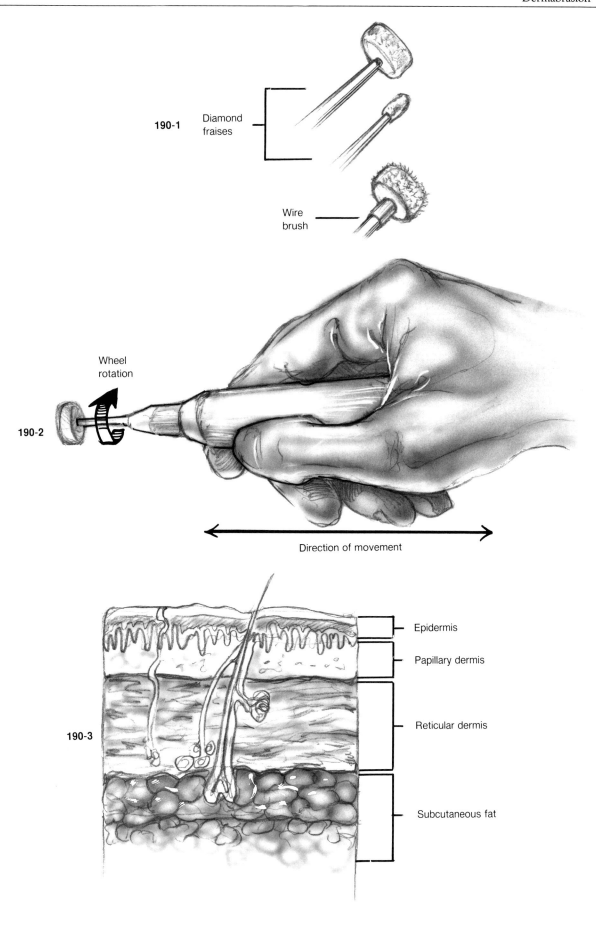

190-1 Diamond fraises

Wire brush

190-2 Wheel rotation

Direction of movement

190-3

Epidermis

Papillary dermis

Reticular dermis

Subcutaneous fat

■ 191. CHEMICAL PEELS

Application of a desquamating agent that improves the skin's character and appearance. Light peels refresh the skin at the epidermal level, medium-depth peels penetrate to the upper dermis, and deep peels penetrate to the midreticular dermis.

Indications
1. Photoaging, rhytids, and poor skin texture
2. Active acne (superficial peels only)
3. Melasma, postinflammatory pigmentation, and lentigines
4. Actinic changes and keratoses

Contraindications
1. Phenol peels should not be used for active herpetic lesions; in cases of renal, hepatic, or cardiac disease; and with estrogen-containing medications.
2. No absolute contraindications for light and medium peels

Preoperative Considerations
1. Assessment of skin quality by Fitzpatrick's scale of sun reactivity and Glogau's classification of photoaging
2. Education of the patient about the possibilities of different peels
3. Careful evaluation of the patient's health, lifestyle, and work.

Preoperative Preparation
1. Pretreatment with Retin-A or α-hydroxy acid creams before light and medium-depth peels improves the penetration and the rate of healing.
2. Laboratory studies needed before phenol peels include an electrocardiogram, sequential multiple analyzer-18 profile test, and urinalysis to evaluate liver and kidney functions.

Special Instruments, Position, and Anesthesia
1. No anesthesia needed for superficial peels
2. Medium peels may require oral sedation or nerve blocks with local anesthetic
3. Intravenous sedation and local nerve blocks with anesthetist monitoring for phenol peels
4. Premedication with 1 g of aspirin and 10 mg Decadron to reduce the inflammatory response

Tips and Pearls
1. Adequate skin preparation is essential for an even peel. The agent must be applied carefully to avoid leaving untreated areas.

Pitfalls and Complications
1. Hypopigmentation or hyperpigmentation
2. Milia
3. Persistent erythema for more than 3 months
4. Sun sensitivity (most common with deep peels)
5. Phenol toxicity (eg, ventricular arrhythmias, hypotension, headache, central nervous system depression, nausea, liver or renal failure)
6. Hypertrophic scarring, often around the mouth, chin, or neck
7. Herpetic outbreak or infection

Postoperative Care
1. Beginning on the first day, the patient washes his or her face 3 to 6 times each day using a cotton ball or fingertips to help remove any coagulum (ie, phenol peels) and speed desquamation. A moisturizer such as Eucerin or Aquaphor creams is applied.
2. Water-based cosmetics can be used about 5 days after a light peel, 10 days after a medium peel, and 14 days after a phenol peel.
3. Exposure to sunlight should be minimized, and non–para-amino benzoic acid (PABA) sunscreens should be used whenever the patient is outdoors.

References
Baker TJ, Gordon HL. Surgical rejuvenation of the face. 1986.
Brody HJ. Chemical peeling. St. Louis: CV Mosby, 1992.
Monheit GD. The Jessner's + TCA peel: a medium-depth chemical peel. J Dermatol Surg Oncol 1989;15:945.
Van Scott EJ, Yu RJ. Alpha hydroxy acids: procedures for use in clinical practice. Cutis 1989;43:222.

Operative Procedures

Oils, dirt, and other debris on the skin surface must be removed to avoid an uneven peel. Patients first wash thoroughly with a low-residue soap, such as Septisol. The limits of the peel are marked out with the patient in a sitting position. The skin is then cleaned with acetone on a 2 × 2 sponge (Fig. 191-1).

Light Peels

The patient is positioned on the operating chair or table, with the heads elevated about 30°. The peeling solution is applied with cotton-tipped applicators to each aesthetic unit (Fig. 191-2), carefully working the solution into deeper rhytids and folds. The cotton is moistened just enough to wet the skin without any excess runoff. Limited peels can be done for specific aesthetic units, usually the upper lip or lower eyelids.

The trichloroacetic acid (TCA) is neutralized by serum in the dermal vessels and causes no systemic toxicity. A 15% to 35% solution is used, with the depth of peeling controlled by the amount and concentration of solution applied and by the preoperative skin preparation. When peeling, an even redness or slight whitish frosting is sought. Light exfoliation similar to a mild sunburn begins on day 2 and continues for 3 to 6 days.

α-Hydroxy acid treatment consists of weekly to monthly application of 30% to 70% glycolic acid or glycocitrate solutions. The solution is left in place for 1 to 3 minutes and then washed off carefully. Erythema develops and fades within 8 to 24 hours, possibly followed by mild epidermal flaking and peeling.

Supplemented Medium Peels

Preparations are performed as for light peels. One to two coats of Jessner's solution are applied to the entire face. A mild erythema appears, followed by a faint frosting. The thicker frosting seen with TCA acid does not appear. After about 1 minute, a 35% solution of TCA is applied in the same fashion as for other TCA peels. The frosting gradually fades to a deeper erythema, and the skin becomes dry, with minimal or no swelling. Desquamation begins on day 2 or 3, and healing normally occurs over the next 7 to 10 days. Postoperative erythema fades during the next month.

Phenol Peels

Intravenous lines are started before the peel, and the Ringer's lactate solution is infused at about 500 mL/hour to a total of at least 1500 mL, which promotes excretion of the phenol. Cardiac, blood pressure, and pulse oximetry monitors are used. Supplemental oxygen maintains oxygen saturation above 90%. A "crash cart" with emergency medications and equipment is kept available.

A fresh batch of peel solution is prepared for each patient according to the Baker and Gordon formula of 3 mL of 88% USP liquid phenol, 2 ml of water, 8 drops of liquid soap (eg, Septisol), and 3 drops of croton oil. After the skin is prepared and the solution is applied, the skin frosts to a gray-white patina, and the patient experiences a burning sensation that subsides in a few minutes. Major aesthetic units are treated in turn, allowing about 15 minutes to elapse between each unit to prevent phenol toxicity.

The solution must be applied so that it overlaps the zone of erythema, which extends outward about 5 to 8 mm beyond previously treated areas. Feathering of the solution into the hairline and just below the jaw line prevents unsightly demarcation (Fig. 191-3). Applicators should be changed frequently to ensure that no surface oils become mixed with the solution.

The lower lids are treated to within 2 mm of the lid margin with almost dry applicators (Fig. 191-4). Assistants should stand by with dry applicators to catch any tears that may leak out. This prevents dilution of the solution and overpenetration. If any peel solution gets into the eyes, they should be copiously irrigated with saline. Around the mouth, care is taken to carry the solution 2 to 3 mm onto the vermilion to reduce the radiating perioral rhytids and avoid a line of demarcation (Fig. 191-5).

Patients are observed in the recovery area for 1 to 2 hours. Beginning about 20 to 30 minutes after application of the peel, the patient again experiences a burning sensation, which may be quite intense, but it can be relieved with analgesics.

BRIAN F. GIBSON

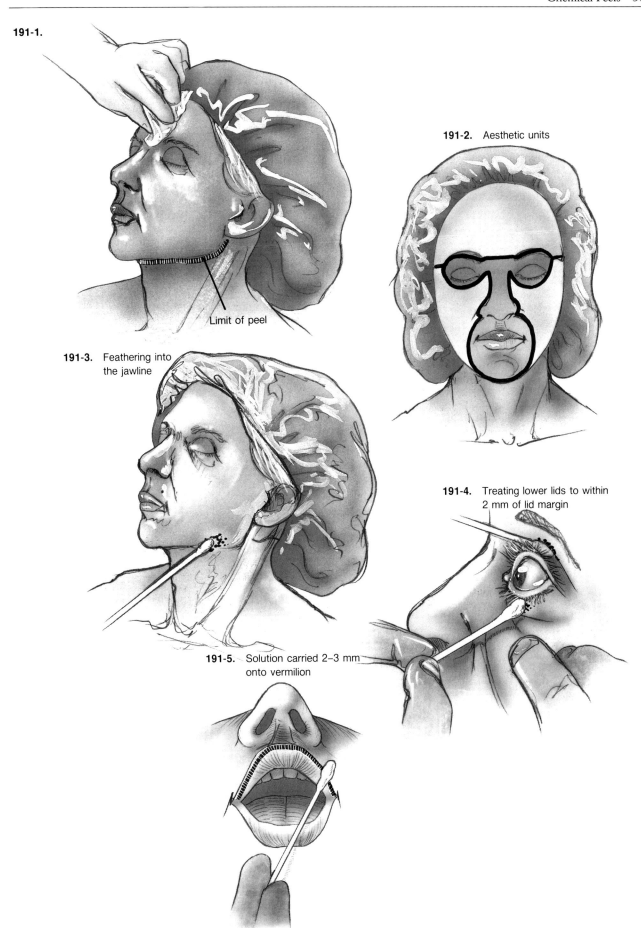

191-1.

Limit of peel

191-2.   Aesthetic units

191-3.   Feathering into the jawline

191-4.   Treating lower lids to within 2 mm of lid margin

191-5.   Solution carried 2–3 mm onto vermilion

■ 192. UPPER EYELID BLEPHAROPLASTY

Surgical excision of redundant eyelid skin and underlying orbicularis oculi muscle with or without excision or cautery of herniated orbital fat

Indications

1. Dermatochalasia, in which excessive eyelid skin is the result of laxity, aging, and sun exposure
2. Blepharochalasia, a rare inherited eyelid disorder causing swelling and laxity
3. Correction of ptosis through elevation of the eyelid usually requires excision of redundant skin.
4. Donor site for skin graft to replace lost eyelid skin
5. Visual field loss due to redundant skin

Special Considerations

1. History of aspirin, nonsteroidal antiinflammatory drugs, or other anticoagulant agents
2. Myocardial infarction within the last 6 months
3. Sensitivity to sympathomimetics
4. Smoking history

Preoperative Preparation

1. Photographs
2. Complete ophthalmologic examination, including Schirmer's test
3. Visual field examination

Special Instruments, Position, and Anesthesia

1. Fine ophthalmic plastic surgery instruments
2. Head of operating room table elevated slightly
3. Anesthetic mixture of 5 mL of 0.25% Marcaine, 5 mL of 2% lidocaine, 0.1 mL of 1:1000 dilution of epinephrine, and one ampule of hyaluronidase
4. Monopolar and bipolar cautery

Tips and Pearls

1. Do not let the excised eyelid skin leave the sterile operating field until you are certain you will not need to replace some due to excessive removal.
2. The upper eyelid should be elevated enough to display about 3 mm of pupil after suturing the wound with the patient in the supine position.
3. Skin and muscle should be excised.

Pitfalls and Complications

1. It is relatively easy to cauterize the upper eyelid fat tissue in lieu of excision; however, do not use oxygen near the face during cautery.
2. Remember that the lacrimal gland, not fat, occupies the lateral third of the upper eyelid; do not remove, or a dry eye condition will ensue.
3. Meticulous hemostasis must be performed on any fat excision to prevent a retroorbital hematoma.

Postoperative Care Issues

1. Careful postoperative monitoring of vital signs in older patients in recovery area
2. Cool compresses to eyelids for as long as 48 hours
3. Use of eye lubricants and artificial tears until eyelids fully close again, usually 1 to 2 days
4. Watch for red eyelids as a sign of topical antibiotic allergic reaction; switch to entirely different chemical group if occurs.
5. For retroorbital hematoma, open the wound, and evacuate clots. If necessary, perform lateral canthotomy, and always call an ophthalmology consultant.

References

Beeson WH, McCollough EG. Blepharoplasty. In: Aesthetic surgery of the aging face. St. Louis: CV Mosby, 1986:37.

Holt JE, Holt GR. Blepharoplasty—medications and preoperative assessment. Arch Otolaryngol 1985;111:394.

Kohn R. Blepharoplasty. In: Textbook of ophthalmic plastic and reconstructive surgery. Philadelphia: Lea & Febiger, 988:178.

Operative Procedure

In most cases, upper lid blepharoplasty is performed under local anesthesia, usually with intravenous sedation and close monitoring, particularly of the oxygen saturation. A local anesthetic combination that has proven effective includes equal parts by volume of 0.25% marcaine, 2% lidocaine, one ampule of hyaluronidase, and sufficient 1:1000 epinephrine to obtain a final concentration of 1:100,000 in the injection. It is wise to inject the upper eyelids before prepping the patient so that the epinephrine is effective at the start of the procedure (Fig. 192-1).

With the patient's head elevated approximately 20° with respect to the floor, the upper eyelid crease is identified and marked with a fine, sterile marking pen (Fig. 192-2). If the incision is to be made medial to the punctum of the upper lid, an M-plasty should be incorporated to prevent scar web formation (Fig. 192-3). The lateral portion of the incision is marked beyond the lateral canthus, curving the incision to fall within a lateral wrinkle line.

Several methods are available for excising the redundant skin. One way is to use the Van Graefe fixation forceps and pinch up the excessive tissue, based on the lid crease incision (Fig. 192-4). As the tissue is pinched, it quickly becomes obvious how much extra skin can be removed without exposing the entire cornea; the superior base of that pinch becomes the superior incision. The surgeon can use curved tenotomy scissors and excise the extra skin while it is still bunched up or one can stretch the eyelid again and use the skin dimpling to mark the superior incision.

A second way to determine the extent of the skin excision is to incise the skin and orbicularis muscle at the skin crease incision, followed by undermining elevation of a skin-muscle flap. As the flap is redraped over the margin of the eyelid, extra tissue can be excised with the tissue scissors (Fig. 192-5). This technique is particularly helpful for patients with thickened skin (ie, smokers) or for low-set eyebrows.

I excise muscle with the skin; if the muscle is left behind, the new eyelid crease often appears blunted and not as well defined (Fig. 192-6). Hemostasis of the skin margins and base is achieved with a pencil-type monopolar electrocautery or bipolar electrocautery with fine ophthalmic forceps.

If orbital fat is protruding into the wound, it can safely be reduced through the use of low-current monopolar cautery; the fat is essentially dissipated and "shriveled" until it is reduced in size. The cautery tip is not introduced directly into the periorbital fat; the orbital septum and surface of the fat are instead "painted" until dissipation has occurred. If too much fat is present for electrocautery dissipation, the fat can be exposed by bluntly opening the orbital septum and "teasing" the fat into view. Each 1 to 2 cm section of fat can be clamped with a straight hemostat and cut sharply at its base with scissors. Some additional intravenous analgesia may be required. The fat stump, still held in the hemostat, is cauterized, taking care not to allow the hemostat to touch any skin. Slowly opening the hemostat, the fat stump is visualized to make sure there is no further bleeding; if so, the bipolar cautery forceps can be used to grasp the bleeder and cauterize it.

After the major steps in blepharoplasty have been accomplished, including skin and muscle excision, hemostasis, and fat removal or dissipation, the wound is ready to be closed. In most upper eyelid blepharoplasties, the wound may be closed in a single layer with 6-0 Prolene or mild chronic catgut interrupted or running suture (Fig. 192-7). I prefer interrupted Prolene to chromic catgut because of the lower local tissue reaction observed in patients. When an M-plasty is used medially, it should be sutured well by slightly advancing the center "V" of the design and placing a stitch to keep it from retracting medially.

After completion of the closure, the eyelid should be slightly open, with perhaps 2 to 3 mm of pupil visible in the recumbent position. Too much pupillary show could lead to inability to close the eye, and it is wise not to remove the resected eyelid skin from the surgical field until it is clearly shown whether an excessive amount has been excised and some needs to be replaced.

G. RICHARD HOLT

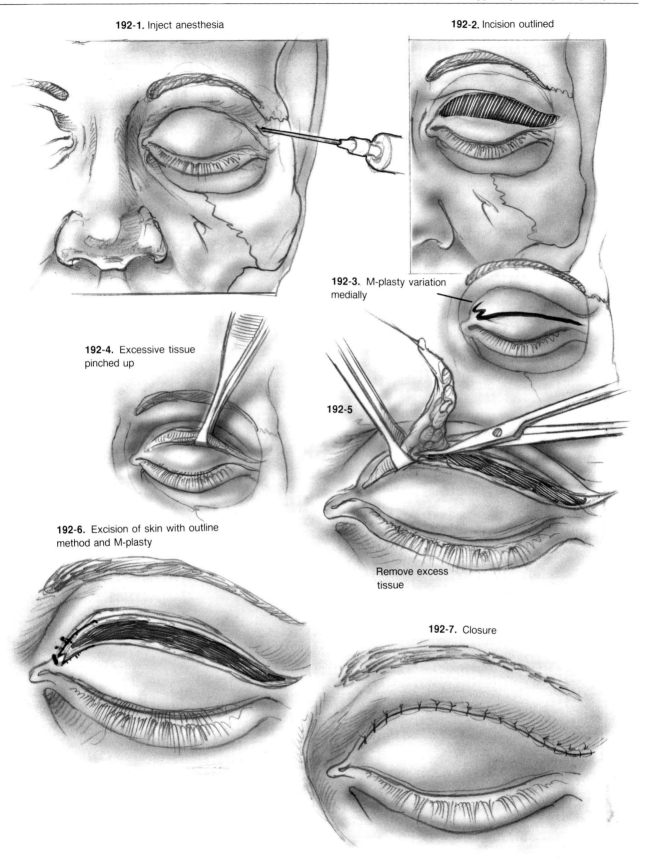

192-1. Inject anesthesia

192-2. Incision outlined

192-3. M-plasty variation medially

192-4. Excessive tissue pinched up

192-5

Remove excess tissue

192-6. Excision of skin with outline method and M-plasty

192-7. Closure

■ 193. LOWER LID BLEPHAROPLASTY

Surgical rejuvenation of the lower eyelid, involving excision of appropriate amounts of skin, orbicularis muscle, and periorbital fat

Indications

1. Dermachalasis or elastosis of the lower lid skin
2. Protrusion of periorbital fat
3. Hypertrophy of orbicularis oculi muscle

Special Considerations

1. Accurate preoperative assessment of the relative contribution of the skin, orbicularis, and periorbital fat to the lower lid deformity
2. Assessment of the lower lid tone and relative prominence of the globe
3. Tear function is assessed by the patient's history and a physical examination. Routine use of Schirmer's test is controversial; the history and periorbital morphology examination may be more accurate predictors of dry eye syndrome.
4. Hyperostosis of the medial aspect of the infraorbital rim may produce fullness medially and is often confused with protrusion of the medial fat pad. Fat resection in such cases exacerbates this bony prominence.

Preoperative Preparation

1. Visual acuity assessment
2. Visual field assessment if preoperative evaluation suggests temporal encroachment
3. Lower lid distraction and displacement tests to assess lid tone
4. Ophthalmologic consultation if abnormalities are noted or for a high-risk patient

Special Instruments, Position, and Anesthesia

1. Kaye scissors
2. Castroviejo forceps
3. Fine hemostats
4. Fine skin hooks
5. Webster needle holder
6. Hyfrecation or bipolar cautery
7. Supine position
8. Local anesthesia is preferred to minimize intraoperative bleeding.
9. Freshly prepared anesthetic-epinephrine solution provides better hemostasis than commercially prepared solution; 2 mL of 1:1000 epinephrine in 10 mL of local anesthetic equals a 1:50,000 concentration.

(continued)

Operative Procedures

Skin and Muscle Flap Blepharoplasty

A transverse incision is made through skin and orbicularis muscle in a periorbital line beginning 2 mm lateral to the external canthus, extending laterally (Fig. 193-1). This incision is made horizontally, avoiding extension in an infralateral direction, which would predispose to postoperative lateral canthal rounding. Using Kaye scissors, the entire skin–muscle flap is dissected through the lateral incision. The pretarsal skin is undermined 3 to 4 mm inferiorly, beginning 2 mm below the ciliary margin (Fig. 193-2). Pretarsal skin is incised from the lateral canthus to 1 mm lateral to the punctum. The orbicularis muscle separating the skin–muscle flap and abbreviated skin flap is incised, beveling the scissors at a 45° angle, which ensures that 3 to 4 mm of orbicularis muscle remains attached to the tarsal plate (Fig. 193-3). Final dissection of the skin–muscle flap is completed.

The thin, filmy orbital septum is incised, allowing access to the periorbital fat. By applying gentle digital pressure on the globe through the upper lid, periorbital fat in the medial and middle compartments is displaced into the wound, and an appropriate volume, estimated by removal of all fat protruding anterior to the infraorbital rim when digital pressure is applied, is excised (Fig. 193-4). Before excision, the pedicle of fat to be removed is gently clamped with a fine hemostat, and the pedicle is severed anterior to the hemostat with scissors or cutting current. The fat pedicle is cauterized before its release into the periorbital space. Although classic anatomy teaches that a distinct lateral fat pad is not present in the lower eyelid, lateral extension of the medial fat pad often produces sufficient fullness to warrant removal. Each lower lid should be examined for such extensions before completion of lipectomy.

The entire periorbital space is inspected to assess hemostasis, with particular attention directed to the medial fat pad, through which traverse substantial branches of the ethmoidal vessels. The orbital septal defect is not repaired. Pretarsal orbicularis may be thinned by judicious excision of the anterior surface.

With the patient gazing superiorly and the mouth opened approximately 75% of its maximal excursion, the skin–muscle flap is draped superiorly and medially, and sufficient tissue is excised to allow approximation of flap and ciliary margin without tension (Fig. 193-5). A small triangle of the skin–muscle flap is excised to facilitate proper insetting (Fig. 193-6). The orbicularis oculi at the superior aspect of the trimmed flap is grasped with a fine-toothed forceps, and approximately 2 mm is removed along the entire infraciliary extent of the flap, equalizing the tissue thickness at the suture line.

Orbicularis oculi suspension is accomplished by placing a 5-0 nylon suture through periosteum 2 mm lateral to the external canthus at the level of the canthus (Fig. 193-7). This suture is directed medially to laterally, with the periosteum engaged through a tacked orbicularis (ie, an orbicularis tunnel is not fashioned). The suspension suture is directed laterally to medially through the orbicularis muscle, just inferior to the superior margin of the flap, with care taken to avoid engaging the undersurface of the dermis. The skin–muscle flap must be engaged at a point more lateral than initial inspection would suggest; as the lateral aspect of the flap is drawn slightly medially, the lateral extent of the incision is closed without a dog-ear formation.

The skin edges are approximated with a continuous suture of 6-0 plain gut. Steri-Strips are used such that lower lid traction is applied in a superolateral direction. No dressings are used. The patient is transported to the recovery area and positioned with the head elevated 45° above the plane of the bed, and ice compresses are placed on the orbit.

Transconjunctival Blepharoplasty

The major indication for this surgical variation is protruding periorbital fat without substantial skin excess or orbicularis hypertrophy. Patients undergoing secondary blepharoplasty, who exhibit residual or recurrent periorbital fat protrusion without substantial skin excess,

(continued)

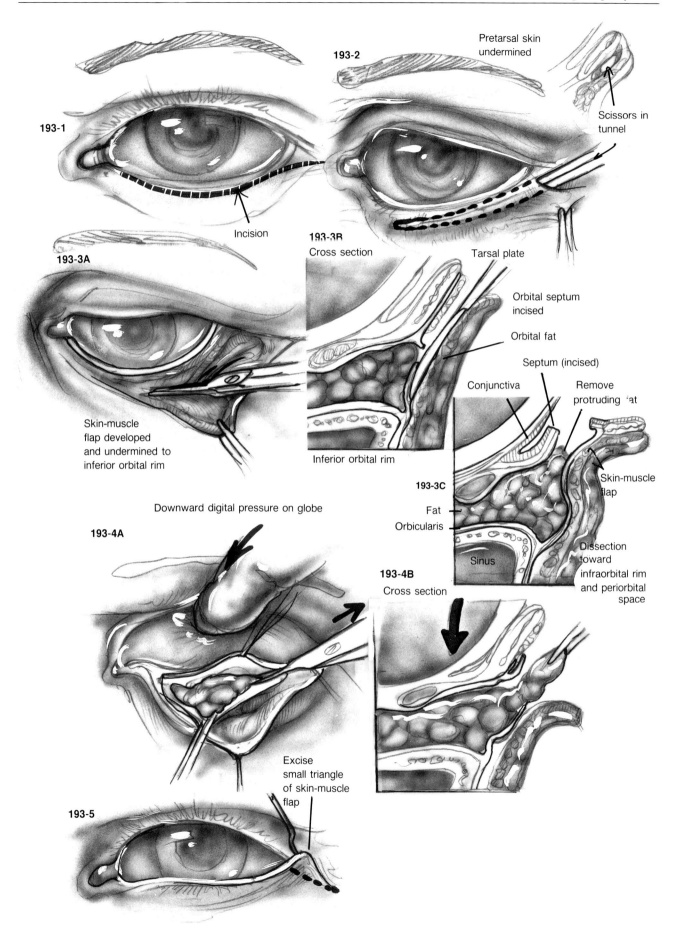

193-1

Incision

193-2

Pretarsal skin
undermined

Scissors in
tunnel

193-3A

Skin-muscle
flap developed
and undermined to
inferior orbital rim

193-3B
Cross section

Tarsal plate

Inferior orbital rim

Orbital septum
incised

Orbital fat

Septum (incised)

Conjunctiva

Remove
protruding fat

193-3C

Fat

Orbicularis

Sinus

Skin-muscle
flap

Dissection
toward
infraorbital rim
and periorbital
space

Downward digital pressure on globe

193-4A

193-4B

Cross section

Excise
small triangle
of skin-muscle
flap

193-5

■ *193.* LOWER LID BLEPHAROPLASTY

(continued)

Tips and Pearls

1. Preserve anatomic lower lid support.
   a. Place the lateral aspect of the incision as horizontal as possible.
   b. Preserve a 3- to 4-mm strip of the pretarsal orbicularis oculi on the tarsus.
   c. Rotate and advance the skin–muscle or skin flap superiorly and medially.
   d. Orbicularis oculi suspension suture
2. Meticulous hemostasis is mandatory. The medial fat pad is considerably more vascular than the middle fat pad.
3. Injection of 10 mg of triamcinolone per 1 mL of solution (0.2 mL) in the plane of the middle lamella to reduce cicatricial activity predisposing to postoperative lower lid retraction
4. Postoperative tape support of the lower lids
5. Absorbable suture (6-0 plain gut) in the infraciliary wound obviates the need for uncomfortable postoperative suture removal.

Pitfalls and Complications

1. Postoperative hemorrhage predisposes to increased intraocular pressure and possible visual impairment.
2. Retraction secondary to cicatricial activity in the plane of the middle lamella (eg, orbital septum, lower lid retractors, capsulopalpebral fascia) is a more common cause of lower lid malposition than ectropion (ie, anterior lamellar shortening) secondary to excessive skin muscle excision.
3. Excessive lipectomy may produce "hollowness," and overzealous resection of the medial fat pad may accentuate the "tear trough" deformity.

Postoperative Care Issues

1. No occlusive dressings
2. Swelling accompanied by pain suggests hematoma and requires immediate evaluation regarding increased intraocular pressure.
3. Institute lower lid massage after suture removal.
4. Triamcinolone (10 mg/mL) injections into the middle lamellar plane at the first sign of induration or impending fixation of the lower lid postoperatively

Pitfalls and Complications

1. Intraoperative bleeding may obscure the anatomy, impairing surgical manipulation and predisposing to postoperative lower lid malposition.
2. Hematoma
3. Visual impairment
4. Lower lid malposition
5. Lid "hollowness" secondary to excessive periorbital lipectomy
6. Dry eye syndrome
7. Suture granuloma (eg, orbicularis suspension suture)
8. Scarring in the lateral canthal region is minimized by placing the incision as far horizontally as possible.

References

Furnas DW. The orbicularis oculi muscle. Clin Plast Surg 1981;8:687.
Rees T, Tabbal N. Lower blepharoplasty. Plast Surg Clin North Am 1981;8:643.

or those with lower lid laxity are candidates for this procedure, often in conjunction with lateral canthopexy. An increasing number of surgeons recommend fat removal through the transconjunctival approach in conjunction with a simultaneous trichloroacetic acid or phenol peel as treatment for skin rhytidosis. Transconjunctival fat removal may also be combined with skin flap blepharoplasty, avoiding the middle lamella (ie, orbital septum, lower lid retractors, capsulopalpebral fascia), reducing the incidence of postoperative lower lid malposition.

The lower lid margin is retracted anteriorly with two fine skin hooks, and a conjunctival incision is made using a cutting current 4 to 5 mm inferior to the ciliary margin extending from the punctum to the lateral canthus (Fig. 193-8). The incision is carried through the lower lid retractors and capsulopalpebral fascia, and a 5-0 nylon suture is placed through the midpoint of the inferior conjunctival edge, weighted with a hemostat, and draped over the forehead such that the inferiorly based conjunctival flap is retracted over the cornea, protecting this structure (Fig. 193-9).

Dissection is directed toward the infraorbital rim, and the periorbital space is entered, avoiding the more anterior orbital septum (Fig. 193-10). Periorbital fat is gently released from the medial and middle fat pads, and the appropriate amount is resected, using the anterior margin of the orbital rim as a guide. The medial fat pad is more granular and aponeurotic when encountered from the transconjunctival approach. Attention should be directed toward removing the lateral extension of the middle fat pad. Such extensions are more difficult to identify from the transconjunctival approach.

After completing the lipectomy, the periorbital space is inspected and adequate hemostasis ensured. The conjunctival incision is then approximated with a single suture of 6-0 plain gut placed at the middle part of the wound. General superiorly directed traction is applied to the ciliary margin to discourage incipient adhesions that could cause postoperative lower lid malposition.

Skin Flap Blepharoplasty

Although most surgeons use the skin–muscle flap for transcutaneous blepharoplasty, patients with excess skin without periorbital fat protrusion may benefit from skin flap blepharoplasty. The fat is accessible through the skin flap approach. Total elimination of lower lid rhytids cannot be effected by skin resection. Overzealous excision of skin, muscle, and fat must be avoided to minimize the possibility of postoperative lower lid malposition. Skin flap blepharoplasty is sometimes advocated in conjunction with fat resection through the transconjunctival approach or as a secondary procedure after transconjunctival blepharoplasty in patients who subsequently request skin excision.

The incision for skin flap blepharoplasty is identical to that described for the skin–muscle flap operation, although only skin is incised, and the lower lid skin is separated from underlying orbicularis oculi by scissors dissection. This dissection is more tedious than the skin–muscle flap dissection but is facilitated by directing the scissors in a lateral to medial direction paralleling the fibers of the orbicularis muscle. Skin flap elevation is continued to the level of the infraorbital rim. If periorbital lipectomy is indicated, the orbicularis muscle and underlying orbital septum are buttonholed at two to three points along the muscle, allowing the fat to be displaced into the wound by gentle pressure on the globe through the upper lid. The amount of necessary fat excision is estimated as previously described. The buttonhole orbicularis defects are not repaired.

The skin flap is draped in a superior and medial direction, and the skin is excised. An orbicularis oculi suspension suture is not used. Before skin closure, trimming of the anterior surface of the pretarsal orbicularis oculi may be performed if indicated for treatment of orbicularis hypertrophy (Fig. 193-11). The wound is closed with 6-0 nylon laterally and 6-0 plain gut in the infraciliary region.

JOHN A. MCCURDY, JR.

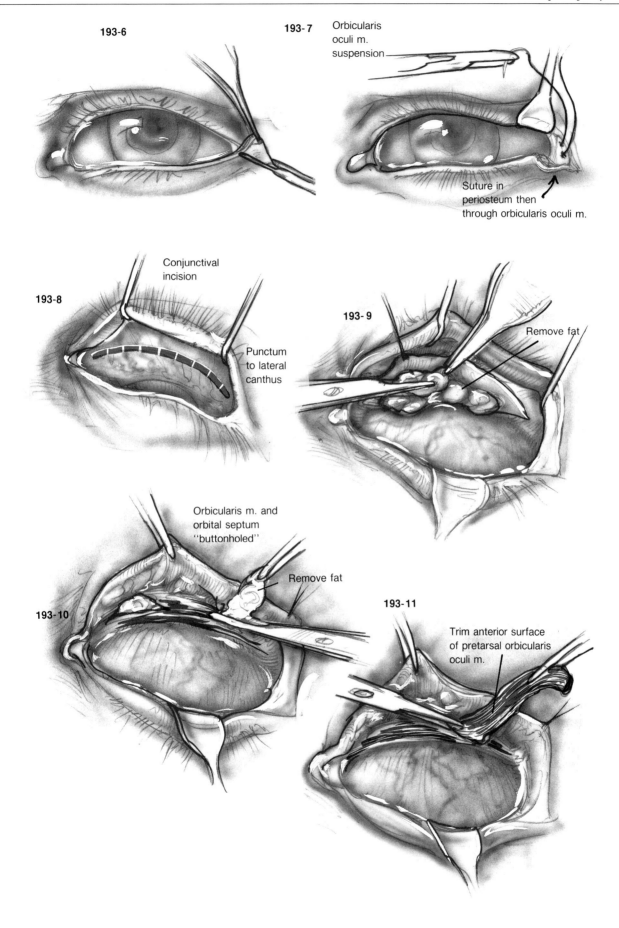

193-6

193-7 Orbicularis oculi m. suspension

Suture in periosteum then through orbicularis oculi m.

193-8 Conjunctival incision

Punctum to lateral canthus

193-9 Remove fat

193-10 Orbicularis m. and orbital septum "buttonholed"

Remove fat

193-11 Trim anterior surface of pretarsal orbicularis oculi m.

■ *194.* UPPER LID BLEPHAROPLASTY FOR THE ASIAN EYE

A variation of upper lid blepharoplasty in which the major goal is creation of a well-defined superior palpebral fold.

Indications

1. Absence of a superior palpebral fold
2. Accentuation of a poorly defined superior palpebral fold
3. Alteration of the height of an existing superior palpebral fold
4. Effacement of an epicanthal fold

Special Considerations

1. Careful preoperative evaluation stressing the type of eyelid transformation (eg, the size and shape of fold, disposition of epicanthus) desired by each patient.
2. Photographically document preexisting asymmetries of the brows and lids. Ensure that patient is aware of the preexisting asymmetry.

Preoperative Preparation

1. Visual acuity
2. Tear function is assessed by history and physical examination.
3. Ophthalmologic consultation if indicated

Special Instruments, Position, and Anesthesia

1. Kaye scissors, Castroviejo forceps, fine hemostats, fine skin hooks, Webster needle holder, hyfrecation or bipolar cautery
2. Local anesthesia is preferred to minimize intraoperative bleeding.

Tips and Pearls

1. Proper symmetric preoperative marking of the planned skin excision is essential to achieving the desired result.
2. Enter the periorbital space near the upper skin edge to avoid injury to the levator aponeurosis.
3. The orbital septum is more substantial in the Asian eyelid and may be confused with the levator aponeurosis. A prominent layer of suborbicularis fat may be misidentified as periorbital fat. Accurate identification of the levator aponeurosis is essential to proper placement of fixation sutures.
4. The extent of periorbital lipectomy depends on the type of eyelid transformation desired by each patient. The levator aponeurosis must be completely defined and particular attention directed toward clearing fat and overlying tissue from the lateral aspect of the aponeurosis.
5. Injection of triamcinolone (10 mg/mL) in the epicanthal region reduces postoperative induration and hypertrophic scarring.
6. Symmetry is best achieved by placing the lateral fixation suture first in the right lid, and then the corresponding fixation suture (lateral) in the left lid. This process is repeated for the middle and medial fixation sutures.
7. Use of external fixation sutures (rather than buried internal fixation sutures) allows more accurate intraoperative determination of lid symmetry.

Pitfalls and Complications

1. Excessive edema or hematoma may result in failure of the fixation sutures.
2. Hypertrophic scar in the epicanthal region
3. Excessive hollowness of the upper lid from overzealous lipectomy
4. Patients may be dissatisfied by creation of a "too large" upper lid. When in doubt, create a smaller, more conservative lid.
5. Temporary ptosis secondary to supratarsal fixation is more common after creation of a large eyelid.

Postoperative Care Issues

1. No occlusive dressing
2. Pretarsal lid edema renders the eyelid somewhat larger than the anticipated final result. Frequently, edema is asymmetric (usually greater on the side on which the patient sleeps). The surgeon must resist requests by patients for surgical revision until the edema has resolved.
3. Use of cosmetics 7 days postoperatively.

References

Flowers RS. The art of eyelid and orbital esthetics: multiracial considerations. Clin Plast Surg 1987;14:703.

Hin LC. Unfavorable results in oriental blepharoplasty. Ann Plast Surg 1985;14:523.

Operative Procedure

Proper preoperative markings are essential in Asian blepharoplasty. The most important factor in determining the level of the superior palpebral fold is the distance from the ciliary margin, at which the inferior lid incision is drawn, ranging from 6 to 10 mm (Fig. 194-1). For creation of a small "double eyelid," the incision is placed 6 to 7 mm above the ciliary margin; for a medium-sized lid, 8 mm; and for a large eyelid, 9 to 10 mm. An initial mark is placed at the desired height at the level of the lateral limbus, after which the entire inferior incision is drawn.

To create an eyelid with an oval shape, the incision is approximately 2 mm more inferior at the medial canthus, remaining at the same level at the lateral canthus. The incision extends superiorly and laterally to fall in a periorbital line. If a round eyelid shape is desired, the lateral aspect is 1 to 2 mm more inferior at the lateral canthus than at the lateral limbus. Individual desires regarding the epicanthal region determine the location of the lid incision. If an "inside" fold (ie, no epicanthal modification) is requested, the incision is lateral to the existing epicanthus. If an "outside" fold (ie, epicanthal effacement) is desired, the incision terminates medial to the epicanthal web.

The level of the superior incision is determined by pinching the skin with forceps and asking the patient to open and close the eyes. The amount of skin excised is 3 to 10 mm. The amount of skin removed is important in determining the amount of pretarsal "show." For a small double eyelid, only 2 to 3 mm of skin are excised; for a medium-sized lid, half of the maximal amount of skin that can be removed is removed; and for a large, Westernized lid 2 mm less than the maximum amount of skin that could be removed is excised. The superior incision is marked so it courses parallel to the previously marked inferior incision, joining it at the medial and lateral canthal areas (see Fig. 194-1).

Skin and subcutaneous tissues are excised, exposing the orbicularis muscle. A 3- to 5-mm strip of orbicularis is excised above the tarsal plate. The orbital septum is incised, exposing periorbital fat (Fig. 194-2). If a deep palpebral sulcus is desired, removal of all visible fat in the central and lateral compartments is performed to completely clear the levator expansion. Removal of medial fat is more conservative, because creation of a deep hollow in the medial aspect of the lid does not produce an aesthetically desirable effect. Excessive fat removal medially also predisposes to hypertrophic scarring because more tension is placed on the skin closure. Little or no fat is excised if a small double lid is desired; the fat is carefully separated so the levator expansion can be identified (Fig. 194-3).

Before placement of fixation sutures, a 2- to 3-mm strip of muscle is removed from beneath the skin near the inferior skin incision. This maneuver provides a wider base of adhesion for formation of the palpebral fold (Fig. 194-4).

Three fixation sutures of 5-0 nylon are placed, incorporating the skin edge of the inferior incision, the levator aponeurosis, and the superior skin incision (Fig. 194-5). Buried "internal" fixation sutures of permanent or absorbable suture, incorporating only the inferior skin edge and levator, may be substituted for the "external" fixation suture, but including the upper skin edge in the fixation enhances intraoperative determination of symmetry. Three fixation sutures are used: laterally (one half of the distance between the lateral canthus and lateral limbus), centrally (midpupillary level), and medially (medial limbus) (Fig. 194-6). The lateral fixation suture is placed, followed by the middle and medial sutures. Assessment of symmetry is enhanced if the sutures are placed sequentially in the right and left eyelids; the lateral fixation suture is placed in the right eyelid, after which the lateral fixation suture is placed in the left lid. With the eyes open, symmetry is assessed by inspection and direct measurement, after which the middle fixation sutures are placed. One or two additional medial fixation sutures are often placed in the medial aspect of the lid to efface the epicanthal fold, if desired.

Occasionally, more advanced techniques of epicanthoplasty are necessary. The entire incision is then approximated with a running suture of 6-0 plain gut.

JOHN A. MCCURDY, JR.

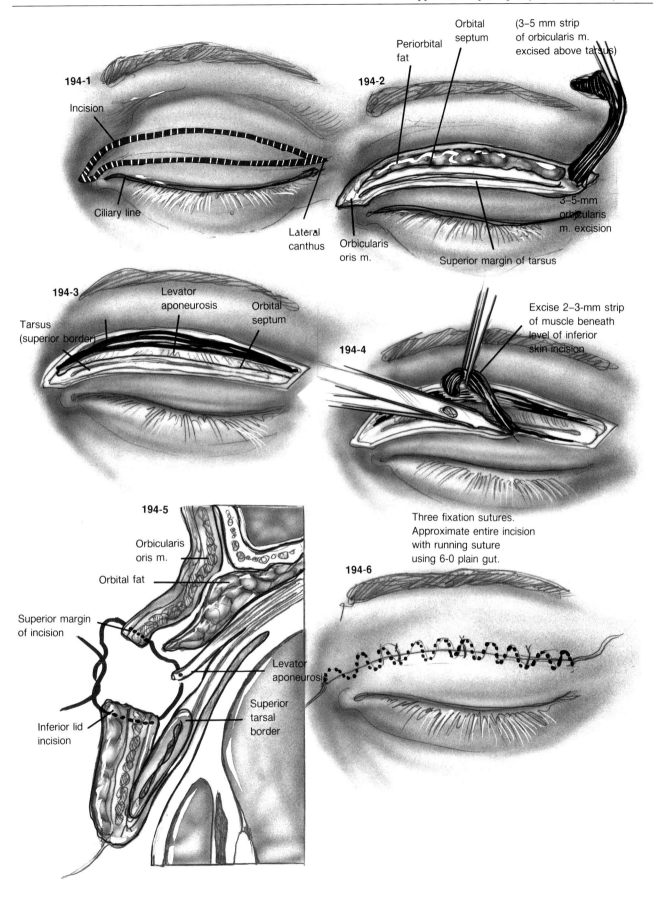

194-1

Incision

Ciliary line

Lateral canthus

194-2

Periorbital fat

Orbital septum

(3–5 mm strip of orbicularis m. excised above tarsus)

3–5-mm orbicularis m. excision

Orbicularis oris m.

Superior margin of tarsus

194-3

Tarsus (superior border)

Levator aponeurosis

Orbital septum

194-4

Excise 2–3-mm strip of muscle beneath level of inferior skin incision

194-5

Orbicularis oris m.

Orbital fat

Superior margin of incision

Levator aponeurosis

Superior tarsal border

Inferior lid incision

Three fixation sutures. Approximate entire incision with running suture using 6-0 plain gut.

194-6

■ 195. EYELID LACERATION REPAIR—Repair may

involve all layers of the eyelids, the medial canthus, the lacrimal drainage system, and the orbital contents

Indications

1. Exploration required for full evaluation of depth of penetration
2. Vertical lacerations
3. Horizontal lacerations
4. Eyelid avulsions

Special Considerations

1. Ophthalmologic examination if risk of penetration, globe injury, and decreased vision exist
2. Visual acuity
3. Range of motion of globe
4. Integrity of levator muscle
5. Pupillary response
6. Direct ophthalmoscopy

Preoperative Preparation

1. Routine laboratory studies appropriate for age and if general anesthesia will be required
2. Ophthalmologic tests
3. Betadine solution to prep eyelids
4. Tetanus prophylaxis

Special Instruments, Position, and Anesthesia

1. Most simple eyelid lacerations can be repaired under local anesthesia
2. Children may require general anesthesia
3. Although many lacerations can be repaired in the emergency room, some may require the formal surgical suite.
4. Loupe magnifying glasses
5. Fine ophthalmic plastic surgery instruments
6. Topical anesthetic for cornea and conjunctiva

Tips and Pearls

1. Check for levator function before the patient is anesthetized.
2. If the levator appears to be transected, perform surgery under local anesthesia, if possible, to enlist the patient's active assistance in finding the proximal stump of the muscle.
3. Ask an ophthalmologist to help if there is any doubt about the extent of injury.
4. A thorough knowledge of eyelid and orbital anatomy is mandatory.

Pitfalls and Complications

1. Missed injury to globe, levator, or lacrimal system
2. Missed foreign body in the orbit
3. Retroorbital hematoma
4. Preexisting ocular disorder not diagnosed preoperatively

Postoperative Care Issues

1. Ophthalmic topical antibiotic and ocular lubricant
2. Cool compresses to eyes for 48 hours
3. Perioperative intravenous and oral antibiotics
4. Follow-up ophthalmology examination
5. Visual checks for acuity and motion

References

Holt GR. Concepts of soft tissue trauma repair. Otolaryngol Clin North Am 1990;23:1019.

Holt JE, Holt GR. Ocular and orbital trauma. Washington, DC: American Academy of Otolaryngology—Head and Neck Surgery, 1983:30.

Kohn R. Basic principles. In: Textbook of ophthalmic plastic and reconstructive surgery. Philadelphia: Lea & Febiger, 1988:28.

Operative Procedure

Eyelid lacerations need not undergo extensive debridement, even with an avulsive injury, because of the excellent blood supply. However, the wound should be copiously irrigated and inspected for retained foreign bodies. If orbital fat is found in the wound, the orbital septum has been penetrated, and the risk is increased for orbital or globe involvement.

Horizontal eyelid lacerations, if not deeper than skin and muscle, usually can be repaired by a single-layer closure, using 6-0 Prolene or 6-0 mild chromic catgut suture, as in a blepharoplasty closure. If orbital fat has herniated into the wound and no other complicating injury is present, then the orbital septum may be gently reapproximated with 5-0 or 6-0 chromic catgut interrupted sutures to keep the fat in its proper location.

If the levator muscle has been cut from its attachment to the superior tarsus and skin anterior to the tarsus, it must be located and reattached (Fig. 195-1). With the patient awake and the wound open, the surgeon can ask the patient to "look up." This maneuver causes the cut end of the levator muscle to retract upward. This movement enables identification of the stump of the muscle; it can be grasped with fine ophthalmic forceps and brought down to its natural location. The aponeurosis is then reattached to the anterior tarsus and dermis using 4-0 Vicryl sutures along its entire length (Fig. 195-2). The horizontal laceration is then closed in one layer with 6-0 Prolene (Fig. 195-3).

A vertical laceration of the eyelid margin is repaired after trimming the wound edges (Fig. 195-4). The eyelid margin is brought into initial apposition with a 6-0 silk suture placed through a meibomian gland orifice about 1 mm from one wound edge and passed through a similar orifice on the opposite margin (Fig. 195-5). If the margin does not align well, the suture should be replaced. A posterior marginal suture of 6-0 silk is placed at the junction of the skin and conjunctiva (Fig. 195-6). Care should be taken not to place the suture too far posteriorly, causing the knot to abrade the cornea. These two sutures are left long and tied beneath the knot of the third anterior marginal suture. Before tightening these marginal sutures, one or more 5-0 Vicryl sutures are used to close the tarsal layer from the anterior side, not penetrating the conjunctiva. The remainder of the skin incision is closed with 6-0 interrupted Prolene sutures sufficiently deep to reapproximate the orbicularis muscle. Antibiotic ointment is usually applied, and the skin sutures are removed in 3 to 5 days; the marginal sutures should remain in place for 10 to 14 days. The detailed and correct realignment of a lacerated eyelid margin is necessary to prevent lid notching, which can cause misdirected eyelashes and poor tear film movement with blinking.

If there has been loss of tissue but the defect is less than one half of the eyelid, primary closure usually may be performed. A lateral canthotomy allows the lateral portion of the remaining eyelid to advance into the defect if excessive tension develops. Extensive avulsion of one or both eyelids requires the composite replacement of all the lamellae of the eyelid: mucous membrane, skeletal support (ie, tarsus or its replacement), skin, and muscle. The use of a full-thickness transposition flap from the other eyelid is one method for accomplishing this. However, the upper eyelid should not be sacrificed to repair the lower eyelid; surgical compromise of the upper eyelid function may result, which can be disastrous.

Other methods of repair of tissue loss of the eyelids can be found in Procedures 196, 197, and 210.

Close follow-up by an ophthalmologist for visual symptoms or after a globe injury is mandatory.

JEAN EDWARDS HOLT

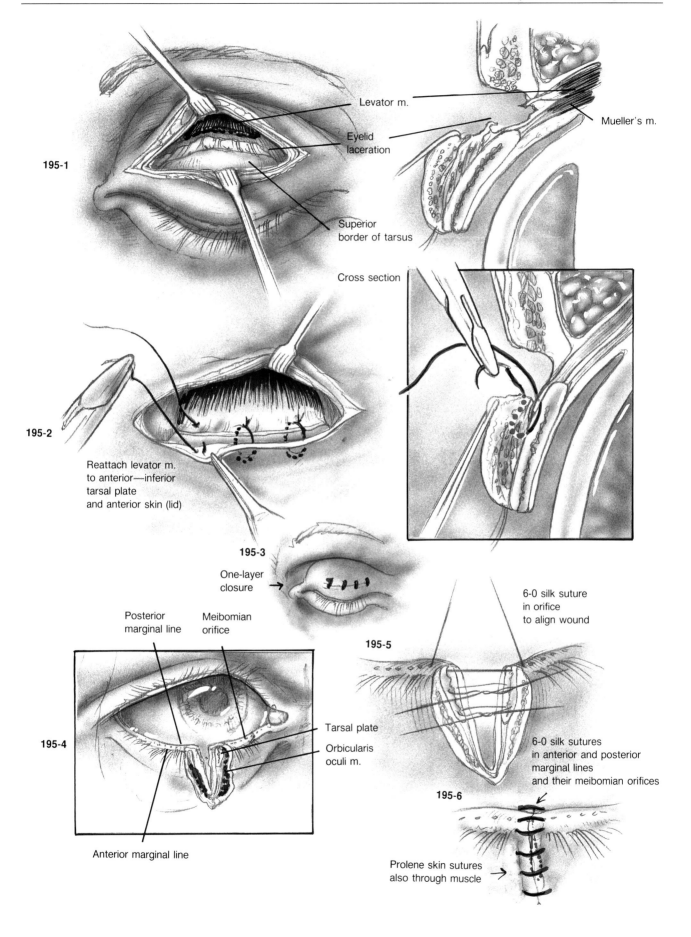

195-1

Levator m.

Eyelid laceration

Superior border of tarsus

Mueller's m.

Cross section

195-2

Reattach levator m. to anterior—inferior tarsal plate and anterior skin (lid)

195-3

One-layer closure

Posterior marginal line

Meibomian orifice

Tarsal plate

Orbicularis oculi m.

195-4

Anterior marginal line

195-5

6-0 silk suture in orifice to align wound

6-0 silk sutures in anterior and posterior marginal lines and their meibomian orifices

195-6

Prolene skin sutures also through muscle

■ 196. UPPER EYELID DEFECT REPAIR

Reconstruction and repair of the functional integrity of the upper eyelid after trauma or surgery

Indications

1. Traumatic injury
2. After neoplasm extirpation

Special Considerations

1. Repair depends on the depth of the defect and the eyelid structures missing:
   a. Outer lamella
      i. Skin
      ii. Orbicularis oculi muscle
   b. Inner lamella
      i. Tarsus
      ii. Levator muscle
      iii. Conjunctiva
2. Visual acuity
3. Extraocular muscle activity
4. Status of adjacent forehead, nasal, and cheek skin
5. Skill of surgeon

Preoperative Preparation

1. Complete ophthalmologic examination
2. Schirmer's tear test
3. Head and neck examination with close inspection of facial skin
4. Routine laboratory studies
5. Preoperative photographs (close-up)

Special Instruments, Position, and Anesthesia

1. Loupe magnifying glasses
2. Camera for intraoperative photographs
3. Preparation for skin graft from neck or postauricular region
4. Exposure of both eyes for comparison

(continued)

Operative Procedure

Most upper eyelid defect repairs can be performed under local anesthesia with intravenous sedation. For extensive facial flap repairs and for children younger than 16 years of age, general anesthesia is preferable. If local anesthesia is used, it is helpful to inject the eyelid before the face is prepped and draped; this is particularly helpful when a traumatic defect requires cleaning. The use of epinephrine in the local injection solution helps maintain hemostasis during the excision or repair. If the procedure on the primary defect will require a long time, as in waiting for frozen-section analysis, injection of the donor sites for flaps or grafts with local anesthesia can be delayed until that procedure is needed.

If a neoplasm is to be resected, the planned excision should be outlined with a sterile marker. It may not be necessary to obtain full 1-cm margins around squamous carcinomas initially because of the relative small size of the eyelids. Additional tissue can be resected as required. As with traumatic defects, all devitalized tissue should be debrided. The surgeon should search for foreign bodies or deeper penetrating injuries to the globe. Foreign bodies should be removed, if possible, and the wound should be irrigated with saline to complete the cleaning. The repair of global injuries has precedence over the eyelids.

For a simple defect involving nonmarginal eyelid skin or eyelid skin and underlying muscle, repair by flap or graft is recommended (Fig. 196-1). The best tissue for outer lamellar replacement is contralateral upper eyelid skin, harvested under local anesthesia through a blepharoplasty-type skin excision (Fig. 196-2). Muscle need not be removed, although it facilitates closure of the donor site and equalization of the thickness of the upper eyelids after repair.

The donor site can be closed with 6-0 Prolene or 6-0 mild chromic catgut interrupted sutures. The graft can be sutured in place with the same suture material. The graft undersurface can be secured to the recipient site by the placement of chromic catgut sutures or by the application of a stent to the graft. The stent is constructed by placing interrupted 5-0 or 6-0 silk sutures along the graft–recipient site margin and leaving one end about 4 to 6 in (10 to 15 cm) long (Fig. 196-3). An equal number should be placed along both margins, because these are tied together over a bolster in pairs. The bolster can be made up of Adaptic gauze wrapped around a cotton ball; the entire ball is covered with ophthalmic antibiotic ointment and placed over the graft. The long silk suture ends are tied over the bolster, effectively compressing the graft against its recipient bed. The bolster is kept moisturized with ointment and can be removed as long as 7 days after placement.

Other donor sites for grafts include postauricular skin, non–hair-bearing skin of the neck, and thin skin of the inner upper arm. Because of the fibrous tissue that forms beneath the graft dermis, a connection forms that reestablishes the continuity of the orbicularis muscle.

Another method of repair of an outer lamellar defect is to use a thin, skin-only pedicle or transposition flap from the upper nose, glabella, forehead, or lateral cheek (Fig. 196-4). The pedicle flap may be based medially or laterally, and the blood supply is usually random, occasionally axial. The flap should be outlined after the defect size is finalized (ie, after all margins are confirmed to be tumor free by frozen-section analysis) and elevated in the subdermal plane, taking care to leave adequate soft tissue beneath the dermis to protect the vascular arcade in this area. If possible, a flap length-to-width ratio of 2:1 should be maintained, although an axial flap and one based in the well-vascularized periorbital tissues can probably support a 4:1 ratio. As the flap is elevated toward the vase, its thickness should increase, providing added safety to the blood supply entering

(continued)

196-1

Defect of muscle
and skin
of upper eyelid

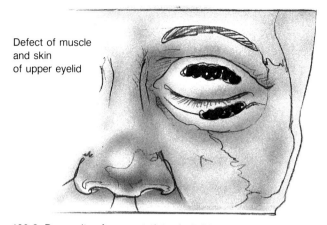

196-2. Donor sites from contralateral eyelids

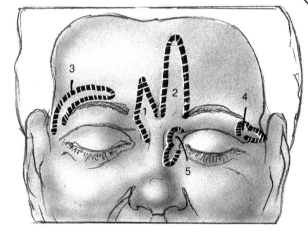

6-0 silk suture
tied over stent
to compress graft

196-3

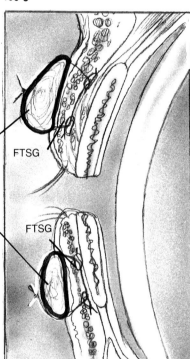

FTSG

FTSG

FTSG—full-thickness skin graft

Possible sites
of donor grafts

196-4

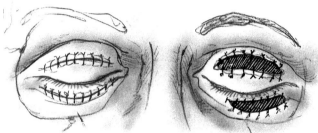

■ 196. UPPER EYELID DEFECT REPAIR

(continued)

Tips and Pearls

1. A thorough knowledge of eyelid anatomy is mandatory.
2. Excessive skin from the opposite upper eyelid may be used as a graft for the involved eyelid if the defect is on the outer lamella.
3. The levator muscle can be reattached but not replaced with another muscle.
4. Reconstituting the circumferential orbicularis oculi muscle is important.
5. A temporary tarsorrhaphy may be necessary for a bilamellar defect.
6. Have multiple options available for reconstructing the defect.

Pitfalls and Complications

1. Corneal abrasion due to exposure of cornea or injury during surgery
2. Suture irritation due to malpositioned sutures close to the cornea or conjunctiva
3. Hematoma beneath the flap or graft
4. Loss of the flap or graft
5. Ptosis due to failure to resuspend tarsus

Postoperative Care Issues

1. Copious eyeball and eyelid lubrication and moisturizing through the use of eye ointments and artificial tears
2. Do not remove eyelid margin sutures before 2 weeks.
3. Frequent evaluation of visual acuity and corneal integrity is mandatory.
4. Consider perioperative antibiotics with the use of flaps and grafts.
5. Watch for hematoma development beneath the flap or graft; expose and drain if one develops.

References

Shumrick KA, Smith TL. The anatomic basis for the design of forehead flaps in nasal reconstruction. Arch Otolaryngol Head Neck Surg 1992;118:373.

Spinelli HM, Jelks GW. Periocular reconstruction: a systematic approach. Plast Reconstr Surg 1993;91:1017.

the base. The flap may be sutured into the defect with dermal sutures of 5-0 chromic catgut and the skin closed with 6-0 Prolene (Figs. 196-5 and 196-6).

For a pedicle flap, the base cannot be sutured to the defect and it requires separation and fitting into place approximately 3 weeks after surgery. A transposition flap can be sutured completely into place, because there are no overlapping margins. Skin sutures may be removed in 5 to 7 days.

For defects also involving the inner lamella (ie, tarsus, conjunctiva), a flap reconstruction with a cartilaginous-perichondrial graft is recommended (Fig. 196-7). The graft can be obtained from the auricular concha, keeping the perichondrium on the concave surface of the cartilage. The graft's natural curvature closely follows that of the eyelid, and the perichondrium becomes rapidly mucosalized as it lies in contact with the conjunctiva at its margins. The perichondrial-conjunctival interface need not be sutured. The first sutures to be placed are those joining the cartilage graft with the tarsal plate, usually employing 6-0 Vicryl with the knot superficial to the conjunctiva. After the graft is secured in place, it is covered by a full-thickness pedicle or transposition flap. It is not wise to apply a harvested skin graft over the cartilage graft, because each requires a vascular nourishment and cannot give nourishment to the other. The flap is secured as described previously.

If the defect is in the central eyelid and requires a cartilage graft to replace the lost tarsus, the levator muscle must be reattached to the flap under the surface anterior to the graft, similar to its attachment to a normal eyelid. Proper placement of 5-0 Vicryl sutures from the end of the levator muscle to the skin reestablishes the proper muscle insertion and recreates a new eyelid skin crease (Fig. 196-8).

JEAN EDWARDS HOLT

196-5. Glabellar and forehead flaps in place

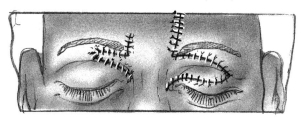

196-6. Lateral and medial flaps in place

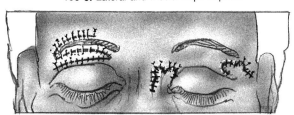

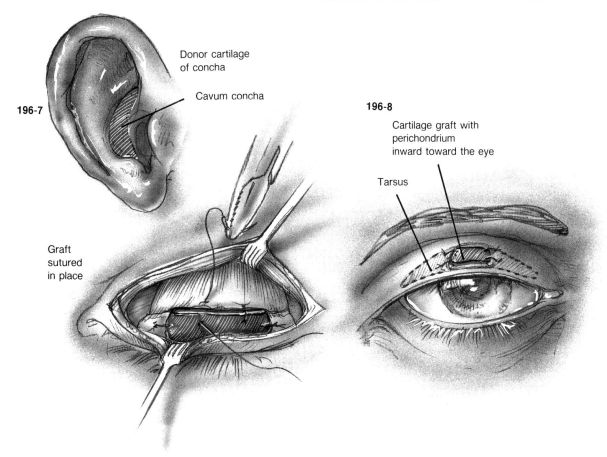

196-7

Donor cartilage
of concha

Cavum concha

Graft
sutured
in place

196-8

Cartilage graft with
perichondrium
inward toward the eye

Tarsus

■ 197. LOWER EYELID DEFECT REPAIR

Reconstruction and repair of the functional integrity of the lower eyelids after trauma or surgery

Indications

1. Traumatic injury
2. After neoplasm extirpation

Special Considerations

1. Repair depends on the depth of the defect and the eyelid structures missing:
   a. Outer lamella
      i. Skin
      ii. Orbicularis oculi muscle
   b. Inner lamella
      i. Tarsus
      ii. Levator muscle
      iii. Conjunctiva
2. Visual acuity
3. Extraocular muscle activity
4. Status of adjacent forehead, nasal, and cheek skin
5. Skill of surgeon

Preoperative Preparation

1. Complete ophthalmologic examination
2. Schirmer's tear test
3. Head and neck examination, with close inspection of facial skin
4. Routine laboratory studies
5. Preoperative photographs (close-up)

Special Instruments, Position, and Anesthesia

1. Loupe magnifying glasses
2. Camera for intraoperative photographs
3. Preparation for skin graft from neck or postauricular region
4. Exposure of both eyes for comparison

Tips and Pearls

1. A thorough knowledge of eyelid anatomy is mandatory.
2. Excessive skin from opposite lower eyelid may be used as a graft for the involved eyelid if the defect is in the outer lamella.
3. The eyelid retractor muscles are not of great physiologic importance and their continuity is unnecessary.
4. Reconstituting the circumferential orbicularis oculi muscle is important.
5. A temporary tarsorrhaphy may be necessary for a bilamellar defect
6. Have multiple options for reconstructing the defect

Pitfalls and Complications

1. Corneal abrasion due to exposure of cornea or injury during surgery
2. Suture irritation due to malpositioned sutures close to cornea or conjunctiva
3. Hematoma beneath the flap or graft
4. Loss of the flap or graft
5. Ectropion with exposure keratitis and conjunctivitis due to scar contraction or inadequate lower eyelid suspension

Postoperative Care Issues

1. Copious eyeball and eyelid lubrication and moisturizing through the eye of ointments and artificial tears
2. Do not remove eyelid margin sutures before 2 weeks.
3. Frequent evaluation of visual acuity and corneal integrity is mandatory.
4. Consider perioperative antibiotics with the use of flaps and grafts.
5. Watch for a hematoma beneath the flap or graft; expose and drain if one develops.

References

Becker FE. Eyelid reconstruction. In: Facial reconstruction with local and regional flaps. New York: Thieme-Stratton, 1985:79.

Ellis DS, Toth BA, Stewart WB. Temporoparietal fascial flap for orbital and eyelid reconstruction. Plast Reconstr Surg 1992;89:606.

Holt JE, Van Kirk M, Holt GR. Use of temporalis fascia in eyelid reconstruction. Ophthalmology 1984;91:89.

Operative Procedure

For a simple defect involving nonmarginal eyelid skin or eyelid skin and underlying muscle, repair by flap or graft is recommended (Fig. 197-1). The best tissue for outer lamellar replacement is contralateral upper eyelid skin, harvested under local anesthesia through a blepharoplasty-type skin excision (Fig. 197-2). Muscle need not be removed, although it facilitates closure of the donor site and equalization of the thickness of the upper eyelids after repair.

The donor site can be closed with 6-0 Prolene or 6-0 mild chromic catgut interrupted sutures. The graft can be sutured in place with the same suture material. The graft undersurface can be secured to the recipient site by the placement of chromic catgut sutures or by the application of a stent to the graft. The stent is constructed by placing interrupted 5-0 or 6-0 silk sutures along the graft–recipient site margin and leaving one end about 4 to 6 in (10 to 15 cm) long (Fig. 197-3). An equal number should be placed along both margins, because these are tied together over a bolster in pairs. The bolster can be made up of Adaptic gauze wrapped around a cotton ball; the entire ball is covered with ophthalmic antibiotic ointment and placed over the graft. The long silk suture ends are tied over the bolster, effectively compressing the graft against its recipient bed. The bolster is kept moisturized with ointment and can be removed as long as 7 days after placement.

Another method of repair of an outer lamellar defect is to use a thin, skin-only pedicle or transposition flap from the upper nose, glabella, forehead, lateral cheek, or nasolabial flap (Fig. 197-4). The pedicle flap may be based medially or laterally, and the blood supply is usually random, occasionally axial. The flap should be outlined after the defect size is finalized (ie, after all margins are confirmed to be tumor free by frozen-section analysis) and elevated in the subdermal plane, taking care to leave adequate soft tissue beneath the dermis to protect the vascular arcade in this area. If possible, a flap length to width ratio of 2:1 should be maintained, although an axial flap and one based in the well-vascularized periorbital tissues can probably support a 4:1 ratio. As the flap is elevated toward the base, its thickness should increase, providing added safety to the blood supply entering the base. The flap may be sutured into the defect with dermal sutures of 5-0 chromic catgut and the skin closed with 6-0 Prolene.

For a pedicle flap, the base cannot be sutured to the defect, and it requires separation and fitting into place approximately 3 weeks after surgery. A transposition flap can be sutured completely into place, because there are no overlapping margins. Skin sutures may be removed in 5 to 7 days.

For defects also involving the inner lamella (ie, tarsus, conjunctiva), a flap reconstruction with a cartilaginous-perichondral graft is recommended. The graft can be obtained from the auricular concha, keeping the perichondrium on the concave surface of the cartilage. The graft's natural curvature closely follows that of the eyelid, and the perichondrium becomes rapidly mucosalized as it lies in contact with the conjunctiva at its margins. The perichondrial-conjunctival interface need not be sutured. The first sutures to be placed are those joining the cartilage graft with the tarsal plate, usually employing 6-0 Vicryl with the knot superficial to the conjunctiva. After the graft is secured in place, it is covered by a full-thickness pedicle or transposition flap. It is not wise to apply a harvested skin graft over the cartilage graft, because each requires a vascular nourishment and cannot give nourishment to the other. The flap is secured as described previously.

Perhaps the best transposition flap for 50% to 100% defects is the Mustarde cheek flap, using lateral orbital and zygomatic skin to provide some muscularized and some skin-only tissue to fill in a defect (Fig. 197-5). Care must be taken to keep the skin flap dissection superficial to the zygomatic branch of the facial nerve at the region of the zygoma. A key to preventing ectropion is to suture the flap securely to the lateral orbital periosteum with 4-0 Vicryl suture. The skin-conjunctiva margin or skin-perichondrium margin (if a graft is first inserted) can be closed with 6-0 silk sutures brought out long over the new lower eyelid and taped or sutured to the skin (Figs. 197-6 and 197-7).

JEAN EDWARDS HOLT

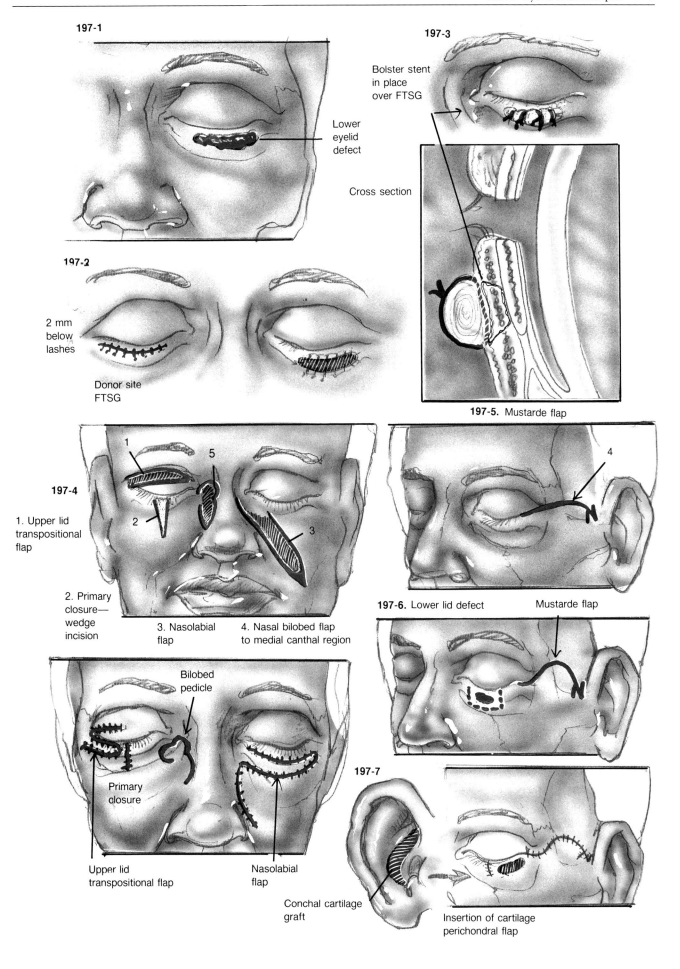

197-1

Lower eyelid defect

197-2

2 mm below lashes

Donor site FTSG

197-3

Bolster stent in place over FTSG

Cross section

197-5. Mustarde flap

197-4

1. Upper lid transpositional flap

2. Primary closure—wedge incision

3. Nasolabial flap

4. Nasal bilobed flap to medial canthal region

5

197-6. Lower lid defect   Mustarde flap

Bilobed pedicle

Primary closure

Upper lid transpositional flap

Nasolabial flap

197-7

Conchal cartilage graft

Insertion of cartilage perichondral flap

■ 198. SURGICAL TREATMENT OF LOWER LID MALPOSITION AFTER BLEPHARO-PLASTY

—The cause and extent of lower lid malposition dictate which surgical procedure is indicated for correction:

Lateral canthopexy is used if middle lamellar adhesions are responsible for retraction. This procedure reduces horizontal laxity and elevates the lower lid.

Lid shortening by means of pentagonal or wedge resection is the classic method to tighten without elevating the lid margin.

Full-thickness skin grafting is used for treatment of ectropion or coexisting retraction and ectropion.

Indications

1. Postblepharoplasty lid malposition
2. Lateral canthopexy is indicated in conjunction with lower lid blepharoplasty in patients with poor lower lid tone or other anatomic factors predisposing to lower lid malposition.

Special Considerations

1. Precise determination of the cause of the lid malposition is necessary before successful surgery can be planned.

Preoperative Preparation

1. Accurate preoperative photographs
2. Ophthalmologic consultation for tear function, visual acuity, intraocular pressure, and associated postblepharoplasty upper lid abnormalities

Special Instruments, Position, and Anesthesia

1. Kaye scissors
2. Castroviejo forceps
3. Fine hemostats
4. Fine skin hooks
5. Webster needle holder
6. Hyfrecation or bipolar cautery
7. Supine position
8. Local anesthesia is preferred to minimize intraoperative bleeding.

Tips and Pearls

1. Most cases of mild lower lid malposition respond to nonsurgical management, such as lid massage, tape support, and intralesional triamcinolone, and operative intervention usually is deferred for at least 3 to 6 months.
2. Complete release of middle lamellar adhesions allows full release and mobilization of the lower lid.
3. Middle lamellar "spacer grafts" are used for treatment of severe retraction or recurrence of lid malposition after attempted lateral canthopexy.
4. Shortening of the tarsal strip is not indicated except for extreme lower lid laxity, because extra length is generally required for suspension to the periosteum. Tarsal strip shortening may predispose to tethering of the lower lid beneath the curvature of the globe.
5. Tarsal strip fixation must be posterior to the lateral orbital rim in the region of Whitnall's ligament. Creation of a small, anteriorly based periosteal flap facilitates accurate and secure suspension.

Pitfalls and Complications

1. Recurrent lower lid malposition
2. Conjunctival cyst
3. Suture granuloma
4. Hematoma
5. Visual impairment
6. Dry eye syndrome

Postoperative Care Issues

1. Inferior traction on the suspended lower lid, as could be inadvertently performed in conjunction with wiping of tears, must be avoided for at least 6 weeks postoperatively.

References

Lisman RD, et al. Experience with tarsal suspension as a factor in lower lid blepharoplasty. Plast Reconstr Surg 1987;79:897.

Neuhaus RW, Baylis HI. Complications of lower eyelid blepharoplasty. In Putterman A (ed). Cosmetic oculoplastic surgery. New York: Grune and Stratton, 1982.

Operative Procedures

A lateral canthotomy is performed with Kaye scissors, dividing the lateral canthus into superior and inferior segments (Fig. 198-1). The Kaye scissors are placed between the conjunctiva and skin, and the inferior segment of the lateral canthal tendon is completely released (Fig. 198-2). Usually, this maneuver does not completely mobilize the middle lamellar scar tissue producing lid fixation. This scar tissue is released by undermining the lower lid skin through the canthotomy incision. The middle lamellar scar tissue layer is palpated with the scissors and lysed at about the level of the infraorbital rim (Fig. 198-3). This lysis is continued medially until the lower eyelid is freely mobile.

The lateral tarsal strip is fashioned by dividing the lateral 3 to 4 mm of the eyelid into anterior (ie, skin and muscle) and posterior (ie, tarsus and conjunctiva) lamellae, after which the conjunctiva is scraped from the tarsus using a #15 blade. The lid margin overlying the tarsal strip is excised, and skin and orbicularis muscle immediately anterior to the strip are removed, leaving a completely denuded strip of tarsus (Fig. 198-4).

The site of periosteal fixation is determined by rotating the tarsal strip superiorly such that the lid margin lies 2 to 3 mm above the inferior limbus. This overcorrection is necessary to compensate for a slight loosening of the fixation that occurs during healing. At the determined level, a stab wound is made on the lateral surface of the orbital periosteum about 2 mm posterior to the orbital rim. Using a 5-0 braided suture, the lateral orbital periosteum is engaged through the stab wound, and the security of the suture is checked by gentle traction on the stitch before engaging the tarsal strip (Fig. 198-5). The suture is slowly tightened, being careful not to strangulate the periosteum or tarsal strip, which would cause suture failure. If lateral canthopexy is performed bilaterally, care must be taken to ensure symmetry before final closure. The orbicularis muscle is then closed over the tarsal periosteal suture, and the skin is closed with 6-0 silk.

If this procedure is performed in conjunction with lower lid blepharoplasty, the steps described are undertaken after dissection of the skin or skin-muscle flap and appropriate lipectomy. The fixation is accomplished before determining the amount of skin or skin and muscle to be excised.

Lateral Canthopexy in Conjunction With Levator Recession

In cases of severe retraction or recurrence of lower lid malposition after lateral canthopexy, additional lower support may be achieved with a graft (cartilage, sclera, or hard palate mucoperiosteum). The lower lid is mobilized and a tarsal strip fashioned as described previously. The conjunctiva is incised at the lower border of the tarsus, and the lower eyelid retractors are separated from the inferior tarsal margin. A recipient bed is created on the posterior surface of the orbicularis muscle, and a graft of appropriate size is sutured into place (Fig. 198-6). The conjunctiva is loosely approximated, and fixation of the tarsal strip is accomplished as described earlier.

Correction of Ectropion by Full-Thickness Skin Grafting

An infraciliary incision is made along the entire length of the lower lid, and a skin flap is created, releasing the lid margin in a superior and posterior direction. When the lid margin has returned to its normal position, the defect is measured, and a full-thickness skin graft is harvested and sutured into place. Meticulous hemostasis is obtained to minimize the chance of hematoma formation.

JOHN A. MCCURDY

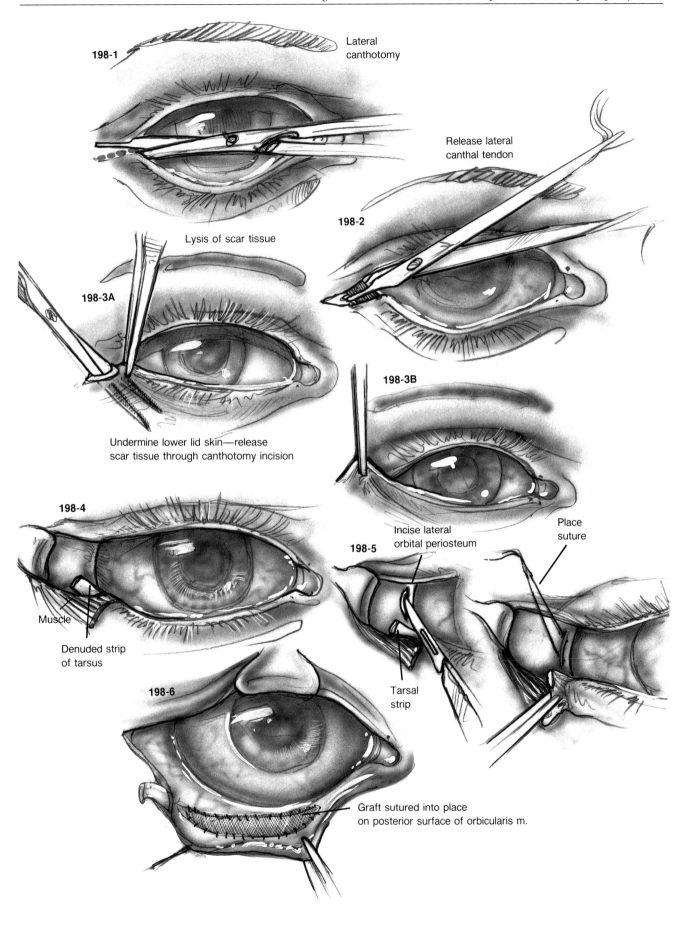

198-1 Lateral canthotomy

Release lateral canthal tendon

198-2

Lysis of scar tissue

198-3A

Undermine lower lid skin—release scar tissue through canthotomy incision

198-3B

198-4

Muscle

Denuded strip of tarsus

Incise lateral orbital periosteum

198-5

Tarsal strip

Place suture

198-6

Graft sutured into place on posterior surface of orbicularis m.

■ 199. CLOSED REDUCTION OF NASAL FRACTURES—Reduction of nasal fractures using digital pressure combined with instruments inserted gently into the nose to push fragments into proper position

Indications
1. Displaced nasal fracture

Special Considerations
1. Associated nasal lacerations
2. Crepitus of the nasal bones[1]
3. Other facial fractures
4. Systemic injuries
5. Type of anesthetic
6. Age of patient (eg, child or adult)
7. Radiographs if other fractures are suspected

Preoperative Preparation
1. None for adults undergoing topical and local anesthesia
2. Routine laboratory studies for a patient needing general anesthesia

Special Instruments, Position, and Anesthesia
1. Sitting, semireclining, or supine position
2. Topical and local anesthesia in cooperative patients without other serious injuries
3. Headlight
4. Freer or Ballenger elevator and Asch fracture forceps
5. External nasal splint
6. Internal nasal packing occasionally needed

Tips and Pearls
1. Examine a preinjury photograph to help determine the premorbid appearance.
2. If swelling is excessive, wait a few days for the swelling to subside.

Pitfalls and Complications
1. If the septum appears swollen, consider the possibility of a septal hematoma.
2. Question the patient to make certain that the deviated nose was not the result of an old injury.

Postoperative Care Issues
1. Taping and splinting the external nose decreases edema and helps protect the nose.
2. After 10 days, the bony skeleton has healed sufficiently to preclude further manipulation.

References
1. Goode RL, Spooner TR. Management of nasal fractures in children: a review of current practices. Clin Pediatr 1972;11:526.
2. Murray JAM, Maran AGD, Mackenzie IJ. Open v closed reduction of the fractured nose. Arch Otolaryngol 1984;110:797.
3. Stucker FJ, Bryarly RC, Shockley WW. Management of nasal trauma in children. Arch Otolaryngol 1984;110:190.

Operative Procedure
The patient is placed in a sitting or semireclining position when performing the procedure in the clinic or in the minor surgical suite. The internal nose is sprayed with a topical decongestant and an anesthetic solution. In addition, cotton or cottonoids impregnated with the decongestant-anesthetic solution are placed into the nose if intranasal manipulation is anticipated. A 1% solution of lidocaine with a 1:100,000 concentration of epinephrine is injected intranasally between the upper and lower lateral cartilages and advanced subcutaneously along the bony dorsum bilaterally using a 25- or 27-gauge 1.25- or 1.5-in (3- or 3.75-cm) needle. The surgeon should wait at least 5 minutes for the anesthetic agent to take affect before manipulating the nose.

If a general anesthetic is needed, the patient is placed in a supine position. A topical decongestant solution is applied intranasally to decrease bleeding, and a throat pack is inserted to prevent blood from entering the larynx.

The fracture commonly can be reduced using pressure from the surgeon's thumb (Fig. 199-1). If the nasal bones are comminuted and displaced medially toward the nasal cavity, an instrument such as a Freer or Ballenger elevator is inserted gently into the nose to push the fragments into proper position while the surgeon's finger rests on the fracture site to determine whether the fracture is adequately reduced. If, after reduction, the comminuted fragments tend to displace toward the nasal cavity, an intranasal pack consisting of 0.5- or 0.25 in (1.3- or 0.6-cm) gauze impregnated with antibiotic ointment is inserted high in the nose in the region of the nasal bones to help hold the fractured bones in place. The packing is maintained for 5 days.

Occasionally, an Asch forceps is needed to disimpact or realign the fractured segments. The forceps is gently inserted into the nose, and steady force is applied to bring the fractured nasal bone fragments into proper alignment (Fig. 199-2).

Usually, bleeding is minimal, and no packing is used. If bleeding is a problem, intranasal packing may be needed for 24 to 48 hours. Telfa pads, covered with an antibiotic ointment and folded into three or four thicknesses, or 0.5-in (1.3-cm) gauze impregnated with antibiotic ointment is inserted into each nostril.

The external nose is taped, and a thermoplastic splint is applied. The patient is instructed to keep the head of his or her bed elevated for several days and to use cold compresses around the eyes if edema exists or is anticipated. One week later, the tape and splint are removed. At this time, the surgeon can correct minor asymmetries by applying digital pressure. Occasionally, the patient is instructed to apply gentle pressure to a localized area of the bony nasal skeleton several times each day for 1 week to mold the nose into a better shape.

Open reduction may be necessary for patients with severe deformities. Murray and colleagues reported a 30% failure rate in achieving optimal cosmetic and functional results in patients undergoing closed nasal reduction.[2] Their cadaver studies showed that a concomitant C-shaped septal fracture dislocation occurred at the junction of the septal cartilage and bone if the nasal bones were deviated more than one-half of the bridge width of the nose (Fig. 199-3). By performing a limited septoplasty in patients with severe external nasal deformities, they were able to obtain a better cosmetic result than with closed reduction.

Treatment of nasal fractures in children usually requires a general anesthetic. Open reduction is usually unnecessary. If, however, a satisfactory appearance cannot be achieved by closed reduction, a 2-mm osteotome can be used to perform a conservative osteotomy of the nasal bones to allow proper alignment of the nose (Fig. 199-4).[3]

STEPHEN J. WETMORE

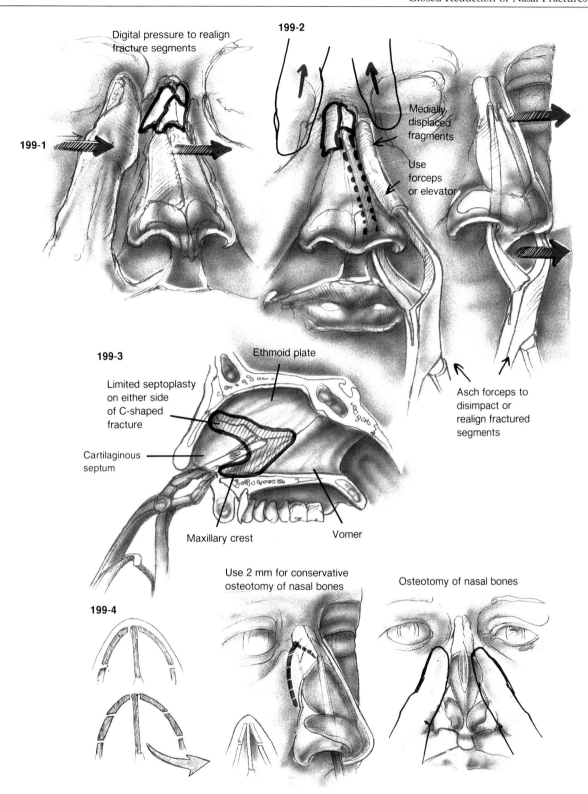

199-1

Digital pressure to realign fracture segments

199-2

Medially displaced fragments

Use forceps or elevator

Asch forceps to disimpact or realign fractured segments

199-3

Ethmoid plate

Limited septoplasty on either side of C-shaped fracture

Cartilaginous septum

Maxillary crest

Vomer

199-4

Use 2 mm for conservative osteotomy of nasal bones

Osteotomy of nasal bones

■ 200. NASAL SEPTAL FRACTURE-

DISLOCATION—Septal fracture-dislocations are treated either with closed reduction or open reduction, depending on the severity of the injury, the extent of associated injuries, and the philosophy of the surgeon.

Indications

1. Displaced septal fracture

Special Considerations

1. Associated external nasal fracture
2. Intranasal lacerations
3. Other facial fractures
4. Systemic injuries
5. Type of anesthetic
6. Age (eg, child or adult)
7. Radiographs if other fractures are suspected

Preoperative Preparation

1. None for an adult or child undergoing topical and local anesthesia
2. Routine laboratory studies for a patient needing general anesthesia

Special Instruments, Position, Anesthesia

1. Sitting, semireclining, or supine position
2. Topical and local anesthesia in cooperative patients without other serious injuries
3. Headlight
4. Freer or Ballenger elevator and Asch fracture forceps
5. Internal nasal splint
6. Internal nasal packing is usually needed.

Tips and Pearls

1. Examine a preinjury photograph to help determine the premorbid appearance.
2. If swelling is excessive, wait a few days for the swelling to subside.
3. Use an otoscope to examine the neonatal nose to visualize a subluxated septum.[1]

Pitfalls and Complications

1. If the septum appears swollen, consider the possibility of a septal hematoma.
2. Question the patient to make certain that the deviated nose was not the result of an old injury.

Postoperative Care Issues

1. Intranasal packing for 24 to 48 hours
2. Intranasal splinting for 1 week

References

1. Jazbi B. Subluxation of the nasal septum in the newborn: etiology, diagnosis, and treatment. Otolaryngol Clin North Am 1977;10:125.
2. Holt GH. Nasal septal fractures. In: Otolaryngology, vol 4. English GM, ed. Philadelphia: JB Lippincott, 1992:1.
3. Murray JAM, Maran AGD, Mackenzie IJ. Open v closed reduction of the fractured nose. Arch Otolaryngol 1984;110:797.

Operative Procedure

Nasal septal fracture-dislocations present with swelling and deviation of the septum. Septal hematomas may accompany or mimic fracture-dislocations. Hematomas should be incised and drained and the nose packed. Septal fracture-dislocations are treated with closed reduction or open reduction, depending on the severity of the injury, the extent of associated injuries, and the philosophy of the surgeon. Most septal fractures are accompanied by fractures of the external nasal skeleton. Generally, the severity of the internal nasal injury mirrors the extent of the external nasal injury.

Minimal septal injuries in cooperative patients can be treated using topical and local anesthesia. An Asch forceps is gently inserted with one prong in each nostril, and force is applied perpendicular to the face (Fig. 200-1). The nose is packed with folded Tefla pads or 0.5-in (1.3-cm) gauze. Antibiotic ointment is applied liberally to either type of pack before intranasal insertion.

Septoplasty should be considered in the treatment of moderate and severe nasal septal fracture-dislocations (Fig. 200-2). Studies have demonstrated that open treatment leads to better functional and cosmetic results for this group of injuries.[2,3] Septoplasty is performed using an incision on the caudal edge of the septal cartilage on the side of the nose with the greatest convex deflection. Muco-perichondrial flaps are elevated, and the fracture sites are exposed. Murray and colleagues described a C-shaped fracture that is frequently seen in patients with severe nasal septal injuries (Fig. 200-3).[3] This type of fracture occurs at the junction of the septal cartilage with the vomer and the perpendicular plate of the ethmoid bone and is treated by excising a strip of cartilage at the fracture site and along the maxillary crest. This is essentially the swinging door technique that is commonly used when performing a septoplasty. Intranasal splints and packing are used.

Some fracture dislocations of the septum are associated with intranasal lacerations. If accessible, a few absorbable stitches can be placed; if inaccessible, the mucosal edges are reapproximated, and septal splints and packing are inserted intranasally.

Septal dislocation in the newborn due to birth trauma is uncommon. This injury can be treated in the nursery without anesthesia. A deviation of the nasal tip to the left side means that the septum is dislocated along the right floor of the nose. A small, blunt instrument is placed along the floor of the nose, and the septum is elevated back into its groove while the surgeon applies traction with her or his other hand to lift the nose away from the face.[1] The tip of the nose and the columella often remain somewhat deviated immediately after closed reduction, but this deformity usually corrects itself in 1 to 2 weeks (Fig. 200-4).[1]

STEPHEN J. WETMORE

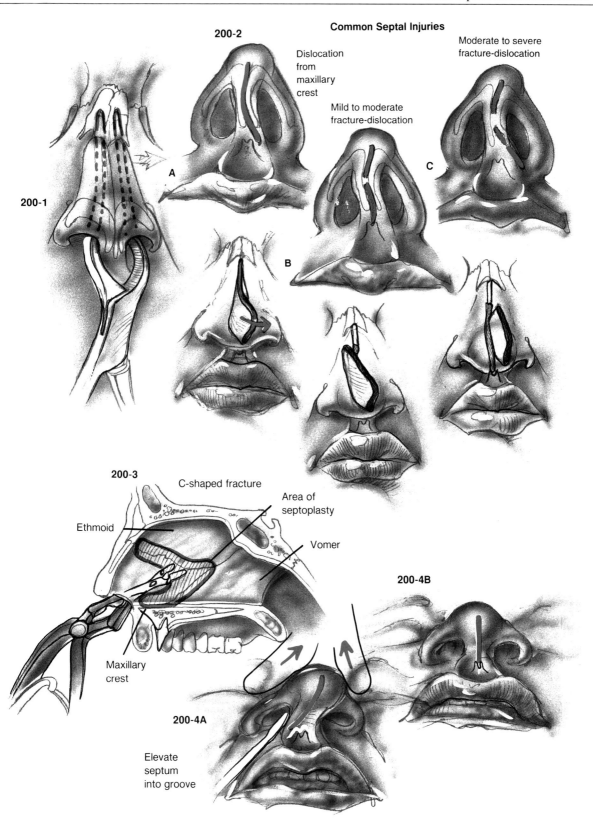

Common Septal Injuries

200-2

Dislocation from maxillary crest

Mild to moderate fracture-dislocation

Moderate to severe fracture-dislocation

A

B

C

200-1

200-3

C-shaped fracture

Ethmoid

Area of septoplasty

Vomer

Maxillary crest

200-4B

200-4A

Elevate septum into groove

■ *201.* ZYGOMATIC ARCH REDUCTION

Elevation of a displaced fracture of the arch of the zygoma

Indications

1. Cosmetic deformity of the arch
2. Depressed fracture causing interference with the function of the temporalis muscle at the coronoid process insertion

Special Considerations

1. Look for a coronoid process fracture of the mandible.
2. Examine the frontal branch of the facial nerve.

Preoperative Preparation

1. Preoperative plain radiographs or computed tomography scan
2. Shaving the scalp is unnecessary.
3. Unless using the oral approach, perioperative antibiotics are unnecessary.

Special Instruments, Positions, and Anesthesia

1. General or local anesthesia
2. Gilles elevator
3. Packing with gauze or placing a Penrose drain is occasionally helpful.

Tips and Pearls

1. Ensure the elevation is performed deep to the temporalis fascia.
2. Measure the distance from the incision to the arch, and mark the distance on the elevator to ensure that the instrument is under the arch.
3. Lift the arch; do not pry it against the skull.

Pitfalls and Complications

1. After the arch "pops up," do not continue to move it around. This action mobilizes the arch, creating a floppy segment that will not stay up.
2. Elevation superficial to the temporalis fascia can result in injury to the frontal branch of the facial nerve.
3. Persistent postoperative trismus despite a good reduction may indicate an undiscovered coronoid process fracture.

Postoperative Care Issues

1. Use of a protective device made from a bent aluminum finger splint can help avoid postoperative trauma and subsequent depression of the arch.
2. Postoperative radiographs should be obtained to document the reduction.

References

Dingman RO, Natvig P. Surgery of facial fractures. Philadelphia: WB Saunders, 1964.
Ellis III E. Fractures of the zygomatic complex and arch. In: Fonseca RJ, Walker RV, eds. Oral and maxillofacial trauma. Philadelphia: WB Saunders, 1991.
Rowe NL, Killey HC. Fractures of the facial skeleton, 2nd ed. Edinburgh: E & S Livingston, 1970.

Operative Procedure

The patient is placed in the supine position, with the head rotated away from the involved side, exposing the depressed arch in the operative field. The entire side of the face and head are prepped and draped to allow an appropriate incision for reduction and allow palpation of the arch during the surgical procedure.

After injection with a solution of 1% lidocaine with a 1:100,000 concentration of epinephrine, an incision is made in the temporal region, approximately 2 to 3 cm behind the hairline. This incision is approximately 1.5 to 2.0 cm long and is extended deeply to the level of the superficial fascia of the temporalis muscle. The muscle is carefully incised, avoiding injury to the superficial temporal artery (Fig. 201-1). A Freer elevator is used to elevate the tissue plane deep to the fascia while staying superficial to the temporalis muscle.

The distance from the incision to the depressed segment of zygoma is measured and marked on the Gilles elevator. The elevator is introduced into the fascial incision and directed toward the depressed arch segment (Fig. 201-2). For a severely depressed arch, it is occasionally difficult to insinuate the elevator under the depressed fragment, but with care and attention to placement, this can usually be successfully accomplished. After the elevator is properly positioned, the depressed arch segment is firmly lifted into its normal anatomic position. This movement is usually accompanied by a distinct popping sensation. The skull should not be used as a fulcrum to lever the fragment.

When the reduction seems to have been achieved, the appearance of the arch should be carefully scrutinized. The temptation to continually move the segment up and down to ensure that it has moved should be avoided, because this action invariably results in a free-floating arch fragment, ultimately requiring packing or an open approach for rigid plate fixation.

Postoperative protection of the fracture site can be provided by shaping a malleable aluminum finger splint to form a protective bridge over the zygomatic arch and taping this in place. Although not actually splinting the fracture, it acts as a reminder for the patient to avoid accidentally compressing and subsequently depressing the arch (Fig. 201-3).

An alternate approach through the buccogingival sulcus can be used for access and elevation of the depressed arch fragment (Fig. 201-4).

THOMAS A. TAMI

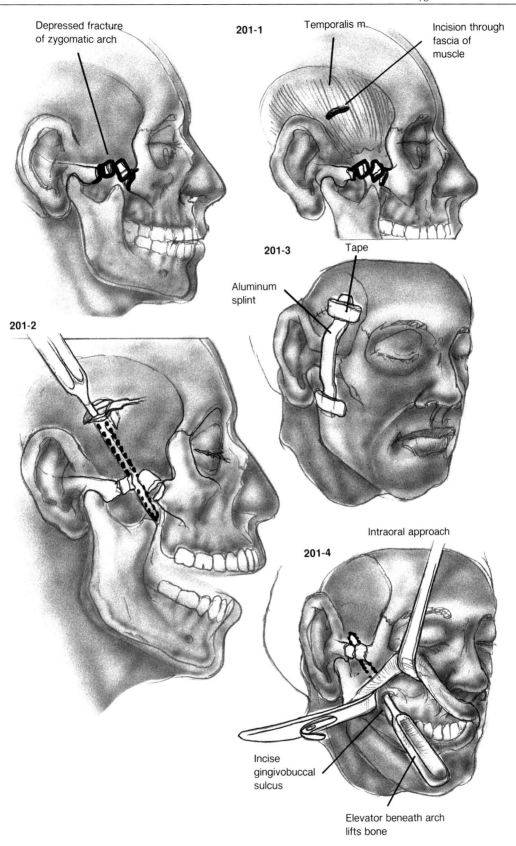

Depressed fracture of zygomatic arch

201-1

Temporalis m.

Incision through fascia of muscle

201-2

201-3

Tape

Aluminum splint

201-4

Intraoral approach

Incise gingivobuccal sulcus

Elevator beneath arch lifts bone

■ *202.* ZYGOMATIC-TRIMALAR REDUCTION AND FIXATION—Elevation and fixation of a displaced fracture of the zygomatic complex (ie, trimalar fracture)

Indications
1. Cosmetic deformity of the malar eminence
2. Depressed fracture causing interference with function of the temporalis muscle

Special Considerations
1. Always consider a possible orbital floor fracture.
2. Is the globe intact and vision normal?

Preoperative Preparation
1. Preoperative computed tomography is vital to evaluate the zygoma and the orbit.
2. A formal ophthalmology consultation can help ensure that a subtle orbital, retinal, or other eye injury has not been overlooked.
3. Shaving the scalp is unnecessary.
4. Perioperative antibiotics should be considered.
5. The entire face is included in the surgical field so that postreduction facial symmetry can be assessed.

Special Instruments, Positions, and Anesthesia
1. General anesthesia
2. Gilles or other appropriate elevator
3. Midfacial plating system.

Tips and Pearls
1. Exposure of the maxillary buttress through a sublabial incision clearly shows the degree of fracture reduction.
2. If exploration of the orbital floor is unnecessary, single plate fixation through the sublabial approach usually is adequate.
3. Reduction of the trimalar segment can often be accomplished through a 1- to 2-cm Gilles incision placed behind the hairline. Reduction can be achieved and maintained through this approach while a plate is placed on the buttress through the sublabial exposure.
4. In severely displaced and comminuted fractures, a hemicoronal incision provides excellent exposure.
5. The use of perioperative corticosteroids (ie, 8–10 mg of intravenous dexamethasone) reduces postoperative edema to allow visual assessment of alignment and reduction.

Pitfalls and Complications
1. Poor reduction produces an asymmetric postoperative result.
2. Overzealous elevation and stripping of the subcutaneous tissue and skin from the underlying facial bones causes poor draping and a poor postoperative appearance.
3. Injury to the infra orbital nerve can occur from elevation and retraction during the sublabial exposure.

Postoperative Care Issues
1. A protective device fashioned from a bent aluminum finger splint can help avoid postoperative trauma and subsequent depression of the arch.
2. Postoperative radiographs should be obtained to document the reduction.

References
Dingman RO, Natvig P. Surgery of facial fractures. Philadelphia: WB Saunders, 1964.
Ellis E III. Fractures of the zygomatic complex and arch. In: Fonseca RJ, Walker RV, eds. Oral and maxillofacial trauma. Philadelphia: WB Saunders, 1991.
Rowe NL, Killey HC. Fractures of the facial skeleton. 2nd ed. Baltimore: Williams & Wilkins, 1968.

Operative Procedure

The patient is placed in the supine position, with the head positioned in the midline. The entire face is exposed to provide visual comparison with the uninvolved side.

After injection of a solution of 1% lidocaine with 1:100,000 epinephrine, an incision is made in the sublabial region, as for a Caldwell-Luc operation. The mucosa and periosteum is elevated from the face of the maxilla, revealing the fracture through the maxillary buttress. This elevation is continued to allow visualization of the orbital rim and piriform aperture. Careful protection of the infraorbital nerve must be provided throughout (Fig. 202-1).

Fracture reduction can be attained through this incision by passing an elevator superior and posterior to the zygoma; however, reduction is often difficult and awkward to maintain.

After injection with a solution of 1% lidocaine with 1:100,000 epinephrine, a Gilles incision is made in the temporal region, as described for reduction of the zygomatic arch. By introducing an elevator into this fascial incision and directing it toward the depressed and rotated trimalar complex, reduction can be easily achieved and maintained, while fixation of the buttress is performed through the sublabial incision (Fig. 202-2). Manual palpation of the frontozygomatic suture and the infraorbital rim further ensure that the reduction is adequate.

With severely depressed fractures, it is occasionally difficult to establish the appropriate relation at the frontozygomatic suture line with confidence. In those instances, a lateral brow incision to expose and plate this suture line is indicated. This incision is placed lateral and inferior to the brow, directly overlying the fracture line.

After reduction is achieved, the cosmetic appearance and symmetry should be carefully scrutinized. By aligning the fractures by means of the sublabial view, while palpating the infraorbital rim and frontozygomatic suture line, precise anatomic reduction can be attained.

If a single maxillary buttress plate is used for stabilization of the fracture, it should be anchored in regions of thick bone. The areas best suited are near the margin of the piriform aperture medially and in the substance of the zygoma laterally. Although bone grafting can bridge areas of bony loss, metal plates alone often offer an acceptable alternative (Fig. 202-3).

Adequate reduction is assessed intraoperatively by comparing the operated to the nonoperated malar eminence. Palpation of the infraorbital rims and frontozygomatic suture lines further ensures that proper anatomic alignment has been achieved.

For severely comminuted and displaced fractures, an alternate approach through a frontal hemicoronal incision can be helpful for access and visualization of the arch, frontozygomatic suture, zygoma, and the lateral aspect of the infraorbital rim. This approach is rarely indicated for otherwise uncomplicated trimalar injuries.

THOMAS A. TAMI

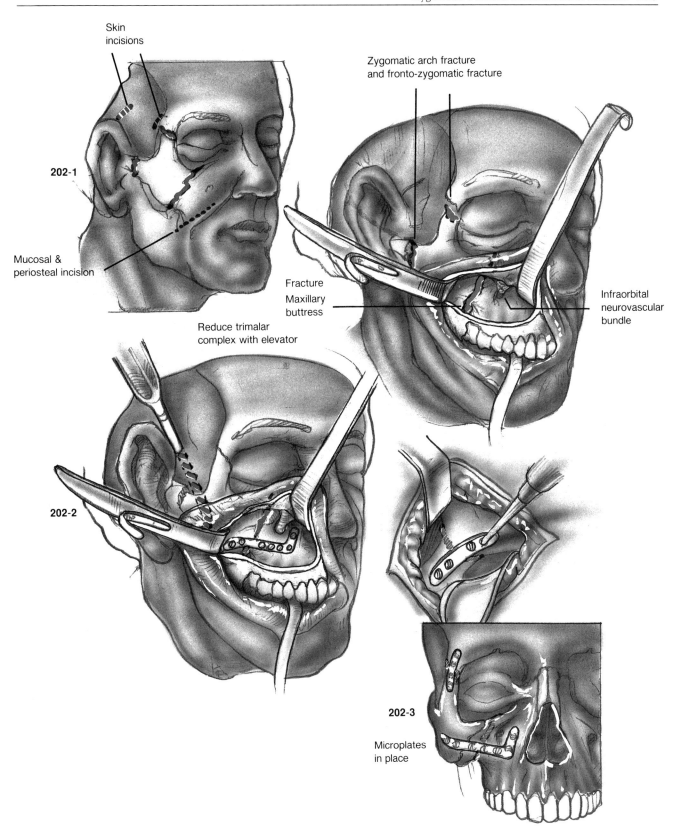

Skin incisions

202-1

Mucosal & periosteal incision

Zygomatic arch fracture and fronto-zygomatic fracture

Fracture
Maxillary buttress

Infraorbital neurovascular bundle

Reduce trimalar complex with elevator

202-2

202-3

Microplates in place

■ *203.* WIRING AND PLATING OF A PALATAL FRACTURE—

The fracture of the palate, usually midline, extends into the nasal floor and commonly is associated with a LeFort I fracture

Indications
1. Repair of fracture
2. Stabilization of the occlusal relation

Contraindications
1. Medically unstable trauma patient
2. Bleeding dyscrasia

Special Considerations
1. Stabilization of associated fractures
2. Attention to the patient's dentition and occlusal relation
3. Status of palatal and nasal mucosal
4. Status of nasal septum

Preoperative Considerations
1. Adequate dentition
2. Preparation of existing dentures or manufacture of splints when necessary

Special Instruments, Position, and Anesthesia
1. Arch bars
2. Cheek and lip retractors
3. Miniplates and microplates
4. Anesthesia is delivered by a nasal tube when possible, so it does not interfere with intermaxillary fixation (IMF).

Tips and Pearls
1. Anterior maxilla may be a guide to proper positioning.
2. When the palate is lacerated, use the laceration for the incision.
3. When the palate is not lacerated, a U-shaped palatal flap decreases the likelihood of later fistulization.

Pitfalls and Complications
1. Avoid injury to the nerves and vessels of the greater palatine foramen.
2. Because the arch bars are buccally positioned, the IMF tends to divert dentition lingually.
3. A symphyseal mandibular fracture makes proper occlusal positioning difficult.

Postoperative Care Issues
1. Keep the oral mucosa clean.
2. Airway concerns if IMF is needed

Reference
Kellman RM, Marentette LJ. Atlas of cranio-maxillofacial fixation. New York: Raven Press, 1995.

Operative Procedure
With the patient in the supine position on the operating table, the maxillary and mandibular arch bars are applied to the teeth (Fig. 203-1*A*). If a mandibular fracture exists, it is repaired first. In some severe, complex fracture cases, bone fragments may need to be tentatively repositioned and readjusted as each succeeding area is realigned and stabilized. In this situation, fragments are wired together loosely, readjusted throughout the procedure, and ultimately rigidly fixed with plates when the ideal positions have been obtained. IMF is then established with wires. Because the palate is fractured, great care must be taken to avoid lingual version of the teeth. Tension on the arch bars tends to cause rotation inward of the fractured fragments.

When a maxillary denture or splint is available, it helps position the alveoli, decreasing the likelihood of rotation around the palatal fracture (Fig. 203-1*B*). The splint, however, is not wired to the zygomatic arches or frontal bones at this time.

Sublabial and palatal exposure may be needed. The sublabial incision extends from above the maxillary molars on one side, across the midline, and to the molars on the opposite side, usually 5 to 10 mm above the gingival margin (Fig. 203-2*B*). Using a small periosteal elevator, such as a Freer elevator, the maxillary bone is exposed bilaterally, taking care not to elevate bone fragments with the flap (Fig. 203-1*A*). Associated LeFort fractures are addressed. Palatal fractures typically occur in the midline, although through-and-through fractures of the maxillary alveolus traverse the palate laterally. The maxillary component is exposed through the sublabial elevation. If there is significant distraction and the exact position is uncertain, interosseous wiring is used to bring the fragments together. A hole is drilled on either side with a 1.5-mm drill bit, and a 24- or 26-gauge wire is looped through the fragments and tightened by twisting clockwise.

Palatal exposure is typically accomplished through an existing laceration by elevating the mucoperiosteum on either side of the fracture. The laceration usually corresponds to the fracture. If no laceration is present, a U-shaped palatal flap can be elevated, taking care to avoid the neurovascular bundle on either side.

With the fracture reduced, the teeth are held in IMF while a miniplate is applied across the maxillary portion of the fracture (Fig. 203-3). When a denture is used, it provides the spacing between the alveoli. Otherwise, extreme care must be used to maintain their proper position. If the fracture is unstable, a second plate may be placed across the palate. A microplate or a geometric (ie, three-dimensional) microplate suffices for the second plate. If the palatal plate is the only means of fixation, a miniplate is advised (Fig. 203-4). Care should be taken to minimize penetration of screw tips into the nose. All screws should be tight. Mucosal incisions and lacerations are carefully reapproximated using permanent or absorbable sutures, depending on the surgeon's preference.

If adequate plate fixation has been applied, the IMF can be released. If the fracture has been repaired with interosseous wires only or the rigidity of plate fixation is in doubt, the IMF is left in place postoperatively for stabilization, usually for 3 to 6 weeks. If dentures or splints were used and IMF is required, they are wired to the zygoma and frontal bone, as needed.

ROBERT M. KELLMAN

203-1A. Arch bars applied

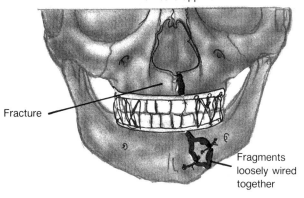

Fracture

Fragments
loosely wired
together

203-1B. Maxillary denture or splint to position alveoli
to decrease rotation around palatal fracture

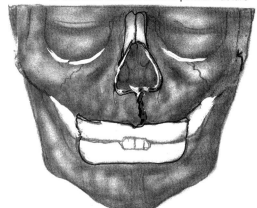

203-2A. Elevate mucoperiosteum;
expose maxillary bone bilaterally;
address fractures

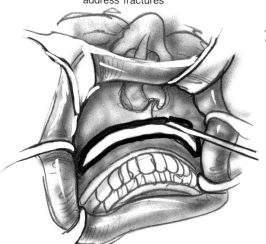

203-2B. Sublabial incision to
expose maxillary fractures

Interosseous wiring
to approximate
fragments

203-3. Fracture reduced; IMF in place;
miniplate applied

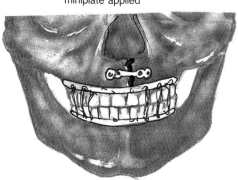

203-4A

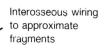

If palatal plate is
only means of fixation,
a miniplate is advised.

203-4B

Alternate plate for
additional stabilization

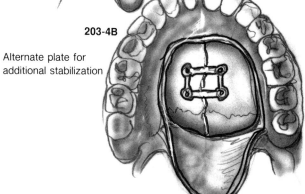

■ 204. LEFORT I FRACTURE REPAIR (GUERIN'S FRACTURE REPAIR)—Intermaxillary fixation to repair a midfacial fracture involving the piriform aperture, lateral wall of the maxillary sinus below the zygomatic arch, pterygoid plates, and septum

Indications

1. Any fracture of the facial skeleton involving the piriform aperture, lateral wall of the maxillary sinus below the zygomatic arch, pterygoid plates, and septum that gives mobility to the midface and that, if not stabilized, would result in future functional impairment and cosmetic deformity (Fig. 204-1).
2. Repair should occur within the first 10 to 14 days, after the facial swelling has decreased and before the beginning of a fibrous or osseous union of the fracture fragments.

Special Considerations

1. Associated injuries:
   a. For laryngotracheal injuries, assess the need for tracheotomy.
   b. Cervical spinal injuries are associated with 1% to 4% of all facial fractures.
   c. Dental injuries, including fractured or missing teeth; rule out aspiration
   d. Head injury
   e. Ocular injury
   f. Facial soft tissue lacerations or avulsion
   g. Infraorbital nerve praxia or disruption
2. Preinjury occlusion
3. Timing of intervention during first 10 to 14 days
4. Possible sagittal palate fracture
5. Edentulous patient

Preoperative Preparation

1. Routine laboratory studies
2. Ophthalmology consultation if ocular injury suspected
3. Assess need for tracheotomy
4. Facial computed tomography scan
5. Evaluate for open bite deformity from posterior impaction
6. Physical examination to identify "floating" maxilla

Special Instruments, Position, and Anesthesia

1. Nasotracheal or orotracheal intubation or tracheotomy
2. Titanium plating system
3. Cervical spine immobilization, if indicated

Tips and Pearls

1. Adequate disimpaction and reduction
2. Fixation to stable component
3. Reestablish occlusion
4. Avoid injury to infraorbital nerve

Pitfalls and Complications

1. Malocclusion
2. Malunion or nonunion
3. Postoperative sinusitis
4. Cosmetic deformities

Postoperative Care Issues

1. Adequate immobilization with intermaxillary fixation for 4 to 6 weeks
2. Elevate the head of the bed, and use ice to decrease swelling.
3. "Wired jaw diet," and oral care
4. Antibiotic coverage

References

Fonseca RJ, Walker RV. Oral and maxillofacial trauma. Philadelphia: WB Saunders, 1991.

Mayer MH, Manson PN. Plate and screw fixation in craniomaxillofacial skeletal fractures. In: Serafin D, Manson PN, eds. Problems in plastic and reconstructive surgery: craniomaxillofacial trauma. Philadelphia: JB Lippincott, 1991.

Operative Procedures

The patient is placed on the operating table in a supine position, with cervical spine immobilization as necessary. LeFort I fractures do not have a cranial base component that precludes nasotracheal intubation. This method is preferred because it facilitates placement of the intermaxillary fixation and plating. If nasotracheal intubation cannot safely be accomplished, orotracheal intubation or awake tracheotomy under local anesthesia may be used to secure the airway.

After airway management has been safely accomplished, the face is prepped with Phisohex or Betadine, avoiding any exposure of the eyes to the solution. Arch bars are then placed, extending from tooth #2 to #15 and from #18 to #31. Twenty-four–gauge wire is used on the molars and premolars, and 26-gauge wire is used for wiring the canines (Fig. 204-2). The incisors need not be wired to the arch bar unless the teeth are injured and stabilization is required or unless it is necessary to further stabilize the arch bar because of missing or injured molars or premolars.

Accurate occlusion is obtained by careful inspection of the wear facets. The occlusion is maintained by the assistant while the surgeon places a minimum of two 24-gauge wire loops on the both the right and left sides to achieve intermaxillary fixation. If adequate occlusion cannot be obtained as the result of an impacted fracture or a fibrous union, reduction should be accomplished using the Rowe disimpaction forceps. One flange is placed in the nares, and the other placed in the mouth; a gentle rocking motion is used in conjunction with a distracting force to move the palate forward and downward (Fig. 204-3). After adequate reduction of the fragment and occlusion have been established, the fracture is stabilized with rigid plating or interosseous wiring (Fig. 204-4).

A sublabial incision is made in the superior gingivobuccal sulcus with a #15 knife. The Bovie cautery is then used to carry this incision deeply to the face of the maxilla (Fig. 204-5). Care must be taken to place the incision superiorly so that there is an inferior 3- to 4-mm rim of mucosa to allow adequate closure. A Freer elevator is used to elevate the periosteum off the face of the maxilla superiorly. Carefully identify and preserve the infraorbital nerve. The fracture lines are delineated, and the soft tissue is removed to facilitate reduction. The procedure is repeated on the contralateral side (Fig. 204-6).

After the fractures are delineated and the medial and lateral buttresses are exposed, a 1.5- to 2.0-mm titanium plate is made to span the fracture. It enables the placement of two screws on either side of the fracture. These plates should be placed on the medial and on the lateral buttresses (Fig. 204-7).

If plating cannot be accomplished or is unavailable, interosseous wiring may be used. A hole is drilled superior to the fracture line, and a 24-gauge wire is passed to stabilize the fracture. Two such wires are placed on each buttress. In either technique, four-point fixation of the palate is accomplished (ie, medial and lateral buttress on each side), which is mandatory for adequate immobilization (Fig. 204-8).

The operative site is irrigated. Closure is achieved by using 3-0 chromic suture in a running horizontal mattress fashion. The intermaxillary fixation is maintained for 4 to 6 weeks.

WM. RUSSELL RIES
MARK A. CLYMER

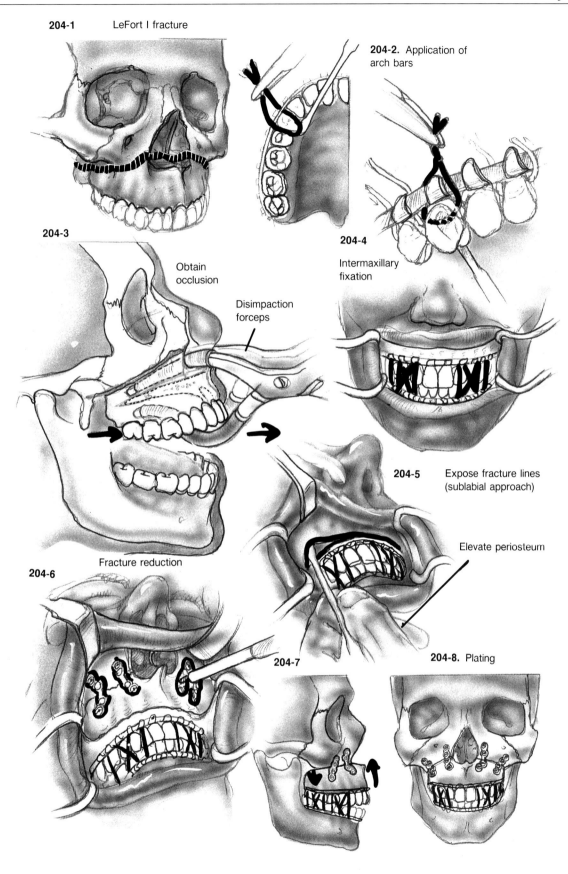

204-1   LeFort I fracture

204-2. Application of arch bars

204-3

Obtain occlusion

Disimpaction forceps

204-4

Intermaxillary fixation

204-5   Expose fracture lines (sublabial approach)

Elevate periosteum

Fracture reduction

204-6

204-7

204-8. Plating

■ *205.* LEFORT II REPAIR OF PYRAMIDAL

FRACTURE—Midfacial fracture involving the nasal bones (ie, apex of the fracture), maxillary antrum, and the inferior orbital rims, usually at the infraorbital foramen, orbital floor, or pterygoid plates

Indications

1. Any fracture of the facial skeleton involving the previously described suture lines that gives mobility to the midface and that, if not stabilized, would result in future functional impairment and cosmetic deformity (Fig. 205-1)

Special Considerations

1. These fractures should be repaired within the first 10 to 14 days, when the facial swelling has decreased and before the beginning of a fibrous or osseous union of the fracture fragments.
2. Associated injuries
   a. Laryngotracheal (assess need for tracheotomy)
   b. Cervical spine injuries are associated with 1% to 4% of all facial fractures.
   c. Fractured or missing teeth; rule out aspiration
   d. Head Injury
   e. Ocular injury, including lens subluxation or retinal detachment
   f. Epiphora and disruption of the canalicular apparatus
   g. Diplopia; entrapment or edema of the extraocular muscles, orbital fat, and periorbita
   h. Infraorbital nerve praxis and disruption are common with LeFort II fractures.
3. Avoid confusion with preexisting class III occlusion and open bite deformity from posterior impaction.
4. The incidence of cerebrospinal fluid (CSF) leak is as high as 25% in cases of severe facial fractures.

Preoperative Preparation

1. Routine laboratory studies
2. Ophthalmology consultation if ocular injury is suspected
3. Axial facial computed tomography scan and coronal images.
4. Evaluate the status of the infraorbital nerve.
5. Evaluate for an open bite deformity.

Special Instruments, Position, and Anesthesia

1. Nasotracheal, orotracheal intubation, tracheotomy
2. Titanium plating system
3. Corneal protection with lubrication, corneal shield, or tarsorrhaphy suture
4. Cervical spine immobilization, if indicated
5. Rowe disimpaction forceps

Tips and Pearls

1. Adequate reduction and fixation
2. Reestablish occlusion
3. Avoid injury to infraorbital nerve
4. Adequate closure of periosteum over plates
5. Avoid injury to lacrimal duct; if lacerated, marsupialize to avoid postoperative epiphora.
6. Carefully inspect the medial canthal ligament; if injured, suture it to the periosteum.

Pitfalls and Complications

1. Malocclusion, malunion, nonunion
2. Cosmetic deformities, blindness, epiphora
3. CSF leak, dacryocystitis, hypertelorism

Postoperative Care Issues

1. Immobilization for 4 to 6 weeks with intermaxillary fixation
2. Elevate the head of the bed, apply ice to decrease swelling, and follow visual acuity closely.

References

Fonseca RJ, Walker RV. Oral and maxillofacial trauma. Philadelphia: WB Saunders, 1991:515.
Mayer MH, Manson PN. Plate and screw fixation in craniomaxillofacial skeletal fractures. In: Serafin D, Manson PN, eds. Problems in plastic and reconstructive surgery: craniomaxillofacial trauma. Philadelphia: JB Lippincott, 1991:290.

Operative Procedure

The patient is placed on the operating table in the supine position, using cervical spine immobilization as indicated. Corneal protection is achieved by using an ophthalmic ointment such as Lacri-Lube, followed by placement of tarsorrhaphy sutures or corneal shields.

Arch bars are applied as described for LeFort I fractures. Careful inspection of the dental ware facets is mandatory to reestablish adequate occlusion. Care must be taken to avoid mistaking a preexisting class III occlusion for a posteriorly displaced fracture. However, if an impacted fracture is encountered, as is often the case, reduction may be achieved by digital distraction or by the use of Rowe disimpaction forceps. When using the Rowe disimpaction forceps, one blade is placed in the nares, and one is placed in the mouth to grasp the hard palate. A gentle rocking motion is performed with a downward and forward distraction force to reduce the fracture (Fig. 205-2). Care must be taken to avoid injury to the optic nerve and intraorbital contents, remembering that the LeFort II fracture involves the orbital floor.

After adequate reduction of the fracture is accomplished and normal occlusion is restored, attention is then turned to exposure of fracture lines and plating. The components of the LeFort II fracture that require fixation are the lateral buttress and the infraorbital rim. The lateral buttress is approached through an intraoral incision in the gingivobuccal sulcus. A solution of Xylocaine with epinephrine (1:100,000) is injected, and a sublabial incision is made with a #15 scalpel, extending from the region of the central incisor posteriorly approximately 3 cm, avoiding inadvertent entry into the piriform aperture or the buccal fat pad. The incision is carried deeply to the face of the maxilla using Bovie electrocautery. The periosteum is then elevated using a Freer elevator, while carefully preserving the infraorbital nerve. The fracture line is identified, and any residual soft tissue is delivered (Fig. 205-3).

Attention is directed to exposure of the infraorbital rim. The subciliary incision is first marked in a preexisting skin crease 2 mm below the palpebral margin and carried laterally in a natural crease (ie, crow's foot line). The lateral orbital rim is palpated, and the incision is then carried deeply through the subcutaneous tissues to the level of the orbicularis oculi. The subciliary incision is then made using a #11 scalpel held with the cutting edge directed upward. With the tip in the subcutaneous tissue, the blade is advanced along the previously marked line. An iris scissors is used to spread the fibers perpendicular to the orientation of the muscle fibers (which at that point are oriented in a superoinferior direction) to the level of the lateral orbital rim. It is important to palpate the lateral orbital rim at all times when spreading these fibers to avoid injury to the periorbita and entry into the orbit. A curved iris scissors or curved Metzenbaum scissors is used, with the tips directed downward along the infraorbital rim, to dissect bluntly in a plane just superficial to the periosteum. A skin-muscle flap is then created by placing one blade of the scissors in the newly created tunnel and placing one blade externally along the previously made skin incision to divide the orbicularis oculi. It is imperative to bevel the scissors as shown in Figure 205-4. This helps avoid postoperative ectropion.

The periosteum is then incised along the infraorbital rim. This incision is placed approximately 1.5 to 2 mm inferior to the superior edge of the rim, which facilitates closure of the periosteum. The periosteum is elevated using the Freer elevator in the usual fashion. As the periosteum is elevated, the orbital contents are gently delivered from the maxillary sinus (Fig. 205-5).

The medial orbital wall and nasal bones are inspected closely. If a large fragment is attached to the medial canthal tendon, the fragment should be plated to the larger infraorbital rim. The infraorbital rim is plated using a 1.0- to 1.5-mm plate that is placed along the inferior aspect of the rim. When drilling holes in the infraorbital rim, a Teflon-coated malleable retractor is used to protect the orbital contents. Plating of the lateral buttress is accomplished in the same manner as LeFort II fractures, using a 1.5- to 2.0-mm plate (Fig. 205-6).

WM. RUSSELL RIES
MARK A. CLYMER

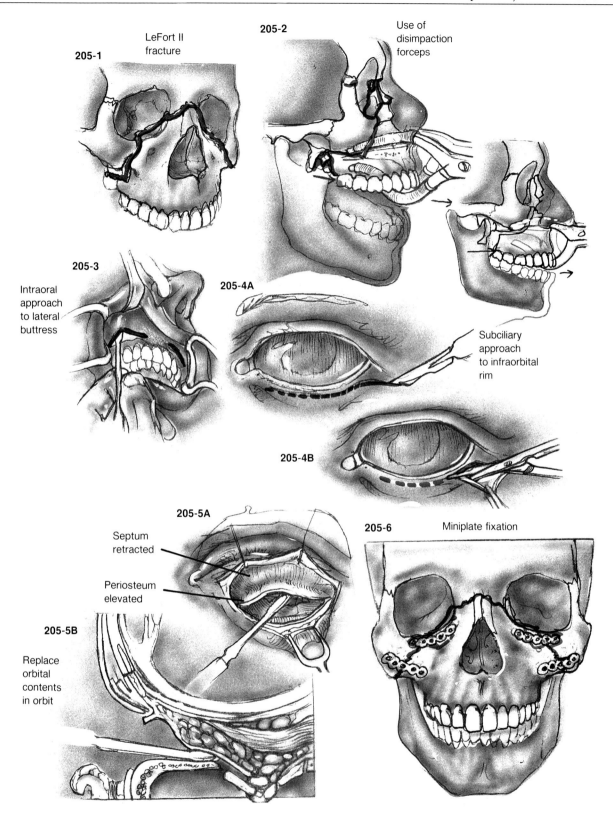

205-1 LeFort II fracture

205-2 Use of disimpaction forceps

205-3 Intraoral approach to lateral buttress

205-4A

205-4B Subciliary approach to infraorbital rim

205-5A Septum retracted / Periosteum elevated

205-5B Replace orbital contents in orbit

205-6 Miniplate fixation

■ 206. LEFORT III FRACTURE REPAIR (CRANIOFACIAL DISJUNCTION)

—The most complex of the maxillary fractures results from a force directed at the orbital level. The fracture lines extend from the zygomaticofrontal and zygomaticotemporal suture lines through the lateral orbital wall and inferior orbital fissure and across the midline at the nasofrontal suture. Posteriorly, the fracture extends through the pterygoid plates and ends in the pterygomaxillary fissure.

Indications

1. Any fracture of the facial skeleton involving the previously described suture lines that gives mobility to the midface and that, if not stabilized, would result in future functional impairment and cosmetic deformity (Fig. 206-1).
2. Repair should occur within the first 10 to 14 days, after the facial swelling has decreased and before the beginning of a fibrous or osseous union of the fracture fragments.

Special Considerations

1. Associated Injuries
   a. For laryngotracheal injuries, assess the need for tracheotomy, especially if there is a concomitant mandible fracture.
   b. Cervical spinal injuries are associated with 1% to 4% of all facial fractures.
   c. Dental injury, such as fractured or missing teeth; rule out aspiration
   d. Head injury
   e. Ocular injury caused by lens subluxation or retinal detachment
   f. Epiphora due to disruption of the canalicular apparatus
   g. Diplopia caused by entrapment and edema of the extraocular muscles, orbital fat, and periorbita
2. Preinjury occlusion, such as an open bite deformity from posterior impaction, which should not be confused with preexisting class III occlusion
3. Intervention should occur during the first 10 to 14 days.
4. Cerebrospinal fluid leak caused by an injury to the cribriform plate, which occurs in 25% of patients with severe facial fractures

Preoperative Preparation

1. Routine laboratory studies
2. Ophthalmology consultation if ocular injury is suspected
3. Axial facial computed tomography scan and additional coronal images if obtainable
4. Evaluate the status of the infraorbital nerve.
5. Evaluate for an open bite deformity.

(continued)

Operative Procedures

The patient is placed on the operating table in the supine position with appropriate cervical spine immobilization. If the patient is not yet intubated, securing the airway with orotracheal or nasotracheal intubation may be attempted. However, LeFort III fractures involve the nasofrontal suture. With an injury as extensive as this, injury to the cribriform plate must be suspected, and nasotracheal intubation should be avoided if possible. Options for obtaining the airway are awake tracheotomy or orotracheal intubation followed by tracheotomy. Although not all patients with LeFort III fractures require tracheotomy, this is often the safest way to manage the airway, because the patients have marked facial edema postoperatively. An alternative is to leave the patient intubated postoperatively until the facial edema resolves and extubation may be accomplished safely.

As with LeFort II fracture repair, corneal protection is provided by ophthalmic ointment and corneal shields or tarsorrhaphy sutures. The face is then prepped and draped.

Occlusion is established as described for LeFort I and II fractures. If a concomitant mandible fracture exists, it is reduced, and rigid fixation is applied. After the midface component is placed in normal configuration with the mandible by establishing preinjury occlusion and intermaxillary fixation, attention is directed toward establishing the correct anteroposterior and lateral relation of the midface component to the cranium. It may be necessary to disimpact the midface, as described for LeFort II fractures (see Procedure 205) to establish adequate occlusion and restore the anteroposterior relation of the midface to the cranium (Fig. 206-2). In the classic LeFort III fracture, the areas that must be addressed are the zygomaticofrontal suture, the infraorbital rim, the nasofrontal suture, and the orbital floor. When there is a force severe enough to result in craniofacial disjunction, an associated maxillary fracture usually occurs, and the medial or lateral buttress need to be approached. This is done through the standard intraoral incision described for LeFort II (see Procedure 205).

The classic LeFort III fracture lines may be approached through a bicoronal flap or a combination of subciliary, lateral brow, and nasofrontal (ie, external ethmoid) incisions. A subciliary incision or a transconjunctival approach is used in conjunction with a bicoronal approach to expose the infraorbital rim and allow exploration of the orbital floor (Fig. 206-3).

(continued)

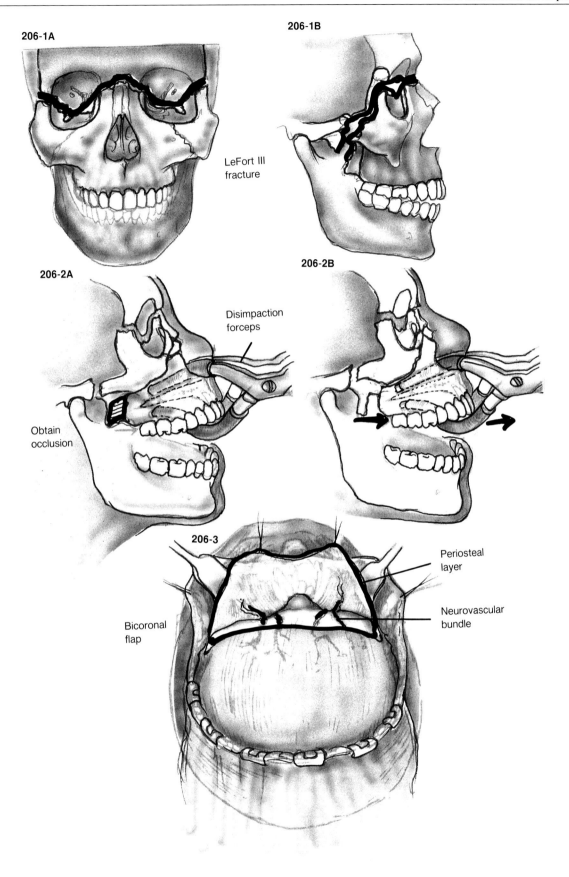

206-1A

206-1B

LeFort III
fracture

206-2A

206-2B

Disimpaction
forceps

Obtain
occlusion

206-3

Periosteal
layer

Neurovascular
bundle

Bicoronal
flap

■ 206. LEFORT III FRACTURE REPAIR (CRANIOFACIAL DISJUNCTION) *(continued)*

Special Instruments, Position, and Anesthesia

1. Nasotracheal tube, orotracheal tube, or tracheotomy tube
2. Titanium plating system
3. Corneal protection with lubrication, corneal shield, or tarsorrhaphy suture
4. Cervical spine immobilization, if indicated
5. Rowe disimpaction forceps

Tips and Pearls

1. Adequate disimpaction and reduction
2. Fixation to stable component, the cranium
3. Reestablish occlusion
4. Adequate closure of the periosteum over plates
5. Avoid injury to the lacrimal duct; if the duct is lacerated, marsupialize to avoid postoperative epiphora.
6. Carefully inspect the medial canthal ligament; if it is injured, suture to the periosteum.
7. Bicoronal or lateral brow approach, combined with subciliary and sublabial incisions
8. Allow resolution of the edema before definitive fracture repair
9. Establish stable outer framework and proceed medially, working from the superior, most-stable component

Pitfalls and Complications

1. Malocclusion
2. Malunion or nonunion
3. Postoperative sinusitis
4. Cosmetic deformities
5. Blindness
6. Epiphora
7. Cerebrospinal fluid leak
8. Dacryocystitis
9. Hypertelorism

Postoperative Care Issues

1. Adequate immobilization through intermaxillary fixation for 4 to 6 weeks
2. Elevate the head of the bed, use ice to decrease swelling, and follow visual acuity status closely.

References

Fonseca RJ, Walker RV. Oral and maxillofacial trauma. Philadelphia: WB Saunders, 1991:535.

Putterman AM, Smith BC, Lisman RD. Blowout fractures. In: Smith B, Della Rocca RC, Nesi FA, Lisman RD (eds). Ophthalmic plastic and reconstructive surgery. St. Louis: CV Mosby, 1987:477.

Schultz RC. Facial injuries. 3rd ed. Chicago: Year Book Medical Publishers, 1988:264.

The bicoronal incision extends from the preauricular crease on either side of the face, extending over the cranium approximately 4 to 5 cm behind the hairline. A "widow's peak" or point should be made in the midline to assist in relocation at the time of closure. The flap is extended anteriorly in a subgaleal plane and laterally approximately 1 cm above the temporal line. The plane is developed just superficial to the deep layer of the deep temporal fascia to avoid injury to the frontal branch of the facial nerve. Approximately 2 cm above the supraorbital rims, the periosteum is incised, and it is elevated with the flap. This allows exposure to the supraorbital nerves and their foramina (Fig. 206-3). The surgeon can then gently chisel the bone of the inferior aspect of the supraorbital foramen to release the nerve, allowing greater reflection of the flap and better exposure of the nasofrontal and lateral orbital rim regions.

After adequate exposure of the fracture lines is obtained, gentle manipulation of the fracture fragments to attain reduction is performed. If a comminuted nasal fracture is present, careful inspection of the medial canthal ligament is warranted. If this is avulsed from its insertion, it should be reattached using a 5-0 Prolene suture.

Plating is then performed as described for LeFort II fractures, using 1.5- to 2-mm plates for the lateral orbital rim (ie, zygomaticofrontal suture) and inferior orbital rim and 1- to 1.5-mm plates for the nasofrontal suture fracture. If a comminuted nasoethmoid fracture exists, a 0.6- to 1-mm plating system may be used to stabilize the small fragments of the root of the nose (Fig. 206-4).

If a plating system is not available, interosseous wiring may be used for rigid fixation. Regardless of the system used for fixation, bilateral two-point fixation is mandatory to avoid the late complication of medial and inferior migration of fracture fragments.

A second but seldom used technique is that of external fixation. It has been used in delayed treatment of retrodisplaced fractures that have undergone fibrous malunion. Combined bilateral mandibular condyle fractures have been treated in the past with external fixation to prevent posterior drift secondary to lateral pterygoid activity. With the availability of modern plating techniques, these methods are primarily of historical interest.

WM. RUSSELL RIES
MARK A. CLYMER

206-3 (continued)

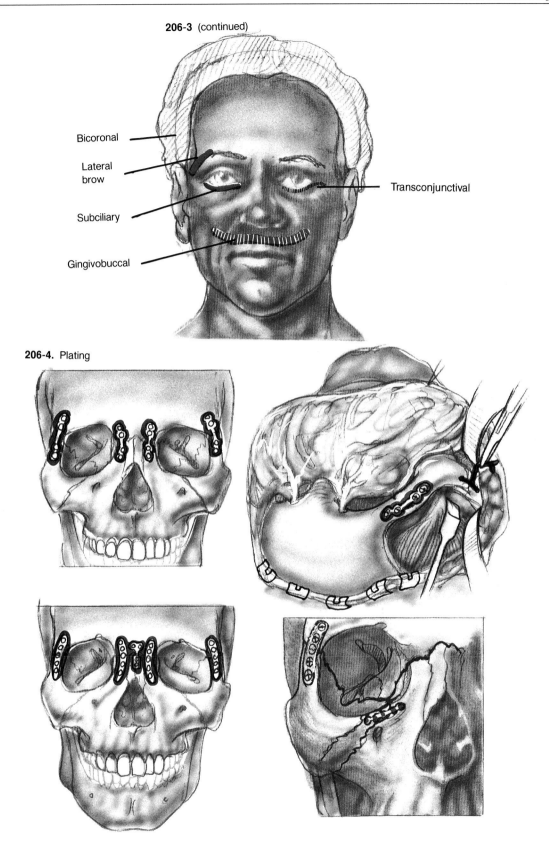

Bicoronal

Lateral brow

Subciliary

Gingivobuccal

Transconjunctival

206-4. Plating

■ 207. ORBITAL BLOWOUT FRACTURE

The classic orbital blowout fracture involves the thin bone of the orbital floor, without a concomitant infraorbital rim fracture.

Indications

1. All orbital blowout fractures that have clinical or radiographic evidence of diplopia, restricted extraocular motion, enophthalmos, hypophthalmos, or a large orbital floor defect.
2. Some surgeons allow 10 to 14 days for resolution of intraorbital edema and subsequent resolution of diplopia.

Special Considerations

1. Timing of intervention
   a. Allow swelling to resolve, and repair within the first 10 days.
   b. Repair 1 to 2 weeks after injury if diplopia or enophthalmos is persistent.
   c. Monitor diplopia and enophthalmos, and repair when measurements stabilize.
2. Forced duction testing to assess entrapment acutely
3. Associated injuries to the globe
   a. Corneal abrasion or laceration
   b. Subconjunctival hemorrhage
   c. Hyphema
   d. Retinal detachment
   e. Lens subluxation and dislocation
   f. Vitreous hemorrhage
   g. Scleral rupture
   h. Optic nerve injury and blindness
   i. Infraorbital nerve contusion and transection
   j. Retrobulbar hemorrhage
   k. Posttraumatic ptosis and disinsertion of levator aponeurosis
4. Ophthalmic examination
   a. Visual acuity testing, with correction if possible
   b. Visual field testing
   c. Pupillary reactivity
   d. Extraocular movements
   e. Cornea, conjunctiva, anterior chamber, retina, iris, and lens
   f. Intraocular pressure assessed with Schiotz tonometry

Preoperative Preparation

1. During the complete head and neck examination, notice associated soft tissue injuries and concomitant midfacial or mandibular fractures.
2. For edema resolution, use ice packs and elevate the head of the bed.
3. Prophylactic antibiotics until time of definitive repair
4. Axial and coronal computed tomography scans

Special Instruments, Position, and Anesthesia

1. Corneal shield or tarsorrhaphy; Lacri-Lube (Fig. 207-1)
2. Malleable retractor
3. Gelfilm, titanium mesh, hydroxyapatite, Silastic, and bone grafting for reconstruction
4. Caldwell-Luc approach for visualization of the orbital floor, if needed
5. Headlight
6. Suction elevator

Tips and Pearls

1. Subciliary or transconjunctival approach
2. Gentle retraction of the globe
3. If an implant is used, placement of anterior edge should be posterior to the infraorbital rim to decrease the likelihood of extrusion.

Postoperative Care

1. Visual acuity checks
2. Ice packs and elevation of the head of the bed
3. Erythromycin ophthalmic ointment to subciliary incision

References

Holt GR, Holt JE. Management of orbital trauma and foreign bodies. Otolaryngol Clin North Am 1988;21:35.
Nesi FA, Spoor TC. Orbital fractures. In: Smith BC et al (eds). Ophthalmic plastic and reconstructive surgery. St. Louis: CV Mosby, 1987:473.

Operative Procedure

Our preferred approach is a subciliary incision (Fig. 207-2*A*). The incision is marked in a preexisting skin crease 2 to 3 mm below the palpebral margin and carried laterally in a natural crease or "crow's foot." This area is injected with a 1% solution of Xylocaine with a 1:100,000 concentration of epinephrine. The lateral orbital rim is palpated, and the incision is then carried deeply through the subcutaneous tissues to the level of the orbicularis oculi. Iris scissors are used to spread fibers perpendicular to the orientation of the orbicularis oculi muscle fibers (ie, superoinferior direction) to the level of the lateral orbital rim. It is important to palpate the lateral orbital rim at all times when spreading these fibers to avoid injury to the periorbita and entry into the orbit. The subciliary incision is made using a #11 scalpel, held with the cutting edge directed upward. With the tip in the subcutaneous tissue, the blade is advanced along the previously marked line (Fig. 207-2*B*). Curved iris scissors or cured Metzenbaum scissors are then used, with the tips directed downward along the infraorbital rim, to dissect bluntly in a plane just superficial to the periosteum (Fig. 207-2*C*). A skin–muscle flap is created by placing one blade of the scissors in the newly created tunnel and one blade externally along the previously made skin incision; the orbicularis oculi is divided. It is imperative to bevel the scissors (Figs. 207-2*D* and -2*E*) to avoid postoperative ectropion.

A nylon traction suture is placed through the orbicularis fibers on the lower lid to retract the lid superiorly. The periosteum is then incised along the inferior aspect of the infraorbital rim (Fig. 207-3*A*). The incision should not be made at the junction between the infraorbital rim and the orbital floor, because this would preclude adequate closure of the periosteum at the completion of the procedure.

A Freer elevator or suction elevator is used to elevate the periosteum from the infraorbital rim. Care should be taken to follow the rim closely, because it dives inferiorly to meet the orbital floor. Delicate elevation of the periosteum allows identification of the fracture lines. The globe is gently retracted with a malleable retractor (Fig. 207-3*B*).

The herniated periorbital fat, periosteum, and possibly the inferior rectus and inferior oblique are delivered from the maxillary sinus using the Freer elevator (Fig. 207-4). If necessary, a Caldwell-Luc approach may be used to obtain a transmaxillary view of the orbital floor. Complete fracture reduction through this approach without simultaneous exposure of the orbital floor superiorly should be avoided, because manipulation of bone fragments may result in optic nerve impingement or injury, laceration or entrapment of inferior rectus or inferior oblique, or injury to the globe. Some surgeons have used this approach and employed gauze packing or a Foley catheter balloon to support the orbital floor. With the available alloplastic materials and the concomitant risks associated with packing or Foley use, these technique are seldom necessary.

After all soft tissue has been delivered from the maxillary sinus, the globe should move without restriction. An implant is then selected to support the globe and orbital contents (Fig. 207-5). Minimally comminuted fractures with negligible bone loss may be treated by placement of a sheet of Gelfilm. Some surgeons use Silastic or Teflon. If a severely comminuted fracture exists with extensive bone loss, titanium mesh or orbital floor reconstruction plates are available for reconstruction of the orbital floor defect. Another alternative is bone grafting with iliac crest, split calvarium, or rib grafts.

The implant chosen should span the fracture lines and be placed 2 to 3 mm posterior to the anterosuperior edge of the infraorbital rim. The implant placement and closure of the periosteum reduce the likelihood of graft extrusion. The graft should be fashioned to conform with the natural curvature of the orbital floor, because any dead space between graft and remaining orbital floor fragments serves as a potential site for hematoma accumulation and infection.

Closure is obtained by using 4-0 Vicryl to close the periosteum and interrupted 6-0 fast-absorbing plain gut is to close the skin. No muscle layer or subcutaneous closure is performed, because this may lead to postoperative ectropion.

WM. RUSSELL RIES
MARK A. CLYMER

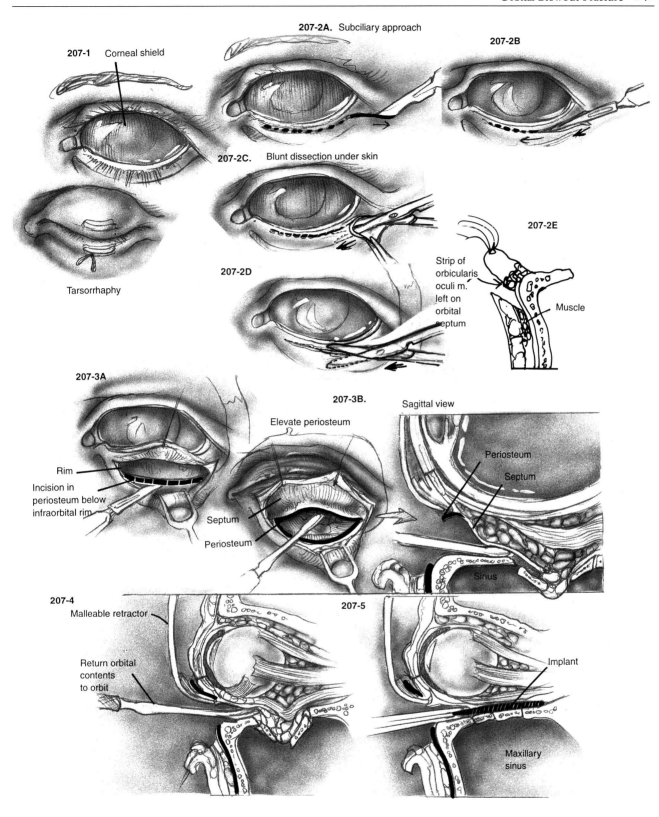

207-1 Corneal shield

Tarsorrhaphy

207-2A. Subciliary approach

207-2B

207-2C. Blunt dissection under skin

207-2D

207-2E

Strip of orbicularis oculi m. left on orbital septum

Muscle

207-3A

Rim

Incision in periosteum below infraorbital rim

207-3B.

Elevate periosteum

Septum

Periosteum

Sagittal view

Periosteum

Septum

Sinus

207-4

Malleable retractor

Return orbital contents to orbit

207-5

Implant

Maxillary sinus

■ 208. NASOETHMOID FRACTURE

Repair of a fracture involving the components of the nose and medial orbits: the bony and cartilaginous framework of the nose, frontal process of the maxilla, lamina papyracea, lacrimal bones, medial orbital wall and floor, medial canthal tendons, and lacrimal draining system

Indications

1. Unilateral injury to the nasal pyramid in combination with medial orbital wall fracture and canthal displacement
2. Bilateral injury to the nasal pyramid in combination with medial orbital wall fracture and canthal displacement

Contraindications

1. Globe injury (eg, salvageable rupture, hyphema)
2. Optic nerve injury

Preoperative Preparation

1. Coronal and axial computed tomography scans of maxillofacial skeleton
2. Ophthalmologic evaluation and clearance for surgery
3. Diagnosis of associated craniomaxillofacial fractures
4. Preoperative counseling of patient regarding incisions, scars, visual disturbance (eg, diplopia, visual acuity impairment), and postoperative asymmetries

Special Instruments, Position, and Anesthesia

1. Headlight
2. Orbital instrumentation (eg, flap retractors, Wright or wire passing needle)
3. Microplating set
4. A 26- or 28-gauge wire or large (2-0) permanent sutures
5. Drills, osteotomes, saws for calvarial bone grafting
6. Delicate bipolar cautery

Tips and Pearls

1. Oral intubation, if possible
2. Palpation of nasal framework
3. Bimanual palpation of canthal tendons with intranasal instrumentation
4. Transcoronal incision preferred
5. Careful medial dissection of the orbital region; do not dissect tendon from medial orbital bone.
6. Precise repositioning of bony fragments
7. Ethmoidectomy, as required
8. Calvarial bone graft to the nasal dorsum, if indicated

Pitfalls and Complications

1. Unacceptable scars caused by external nasal incisions
2. Inadequate medialization of nasal and medial orbital fragments
3. Inadequate attention to the proper orientation of the medial orbital rim fragment
4. Improper plate positioning
5. Lack of recognition of nasal comminution (ie, bone and cartilaginous structure)
6. Improper recognition of a canthal attachment to the central bony fragment (see Chap. 209)
7. Improper repositioning of medial canthus (see Chap. 209)

Postoperative Care Issues

1. External nasal splint
2. Frequent visual acuity examinations during the first 24 hours
3. Care to observe for cerebral spinal fluid leaks

References

Markowitz BL, Manson PN, Sargent L, et al. Management of the medial canthal tendon and nasoethmoid orbital fractures: the importance of the central fragment in classification and treatment. Plast Reconstr Surg 1991;87:813.

Mathog RH. Nasal ethmoid fractures. In: Mathog RH, ed. Atlas of craniofacial trauma. Philadelphia: WB Saunders, 1992:317.

Operative Procedure

After intubation, the incisions are performed. I prefer a transcoronal approach to the medial orbital region (Fig. 208-1). Extension of existing lacerations may, in some cases, provide adequate exposure.

Using the transcoronal approach to the medial orbital region, careful release of the supraorbital neurovascular bundle from their respective medial supraorbital notches or foramina is required to enable adequate medial dissection.

Limiting this discussion to the nasoethmoid component, attention is first focused on the limits of dissection in the medial orbital region. Deep medial orbital dissection is usually required, and this may involve isolation and ligation of the ethmoidal vessels. During the anterior aspect of the medial orbital dissection, it is essential to determine whether the medial canthal tendon is attached to a bony fragment. This is most commonly the case, and the surgeon must carefully limit the dissection of this region to refrain from elevation of the properly anatomically positioned medial canthal tendon, particularly the superior limb of this tendon. This so-called central fragment, when properly isolated with its attached tendon, may be reapproximated using microplate fixation, producing a normal-appearing medial canthus postoperatively (Fig. 208-2). Additional dissection includes dissection anteriorly over the nasal dorsal framework, including exposure of the cephalic aspect of the upper lateral cartilages. For bilateral involvement, similar dissection of the medial orbit is carried out on the contralateral side.

The repair begins by careful reduction of all bony fragments and microplating them into position (Figs. 208-2 through 208-4). The central fragment must be properly oriented with respect to canthal positioning (see Procedure 209) and medial inferior orbital rim positioning. The latter is important, because the inferior aspect of the bony fragment usually encompasses the lacrimal fossa and the most medial aspect of the inferior orbital rim. Proper positioning is critical for the medial inferior eyelid position and because the remainder of the orbital rim fragments must be secured in the proper upward slant in the medial aspect of the infraorbital rim. A common mistake in such repairs is inferior displacement of the infraorbital rim, leading to poor rim position and globe malposition. Microplating of the various bony fragments with care limits the total number of plates and screws, which should be placed with care so they are minimally palpable through the skin.

After reconstruction of the nasal framework with microplates, attention is turned to the repair of the medial canthal apparatus. This is described in Procedure 209.

After fixation of the bony fragments, structural nasal integrity is reassessed by external dorsal palpation. If there is a residual lack of stability in the dorsal bony support or cartilaginous support of the nose, particularly when there is significant comminution and bone loss in the bony dorsum, further support should be added with a cantilevered bone graft (Figs. 208-5 and 208-6). This bone graft is usually calvarial in origin, although rib has been used by many surgeons, and it is sarcophagus-shaped, which is the normal shape of the nasal dorsum, with the widest point at the rhinion. Keys to graft positioning include careful cantilevering of the graft and care to position the distal portion of the graft deep to the lower lateral cartilages. The graft is secured with lag screw fixation when a stable bony segment exists at the nasion and there is a deep nasofrontal angle. More practical is the use of a small miniplate anchored approximately into a groove drilled into the glabella, with distal placement of the plate on the undersurface of the bone graft.

After the reconstruction of the nasal dorsal framework and medial canthal tendon repair, the wounds are closed in a standard fashion. External nasal splinting can assist the medialization of comminuted nasal bones. Occasionally, transnasal splints can be applied to assist in this narrowing. If the latter is performed, care must be taken not to overtighten these splints, because excessive edema is common in such cases, and it may lead to excessive pressure and subsequent necrosis of the underlying skin.

JOHN L. FRODEL

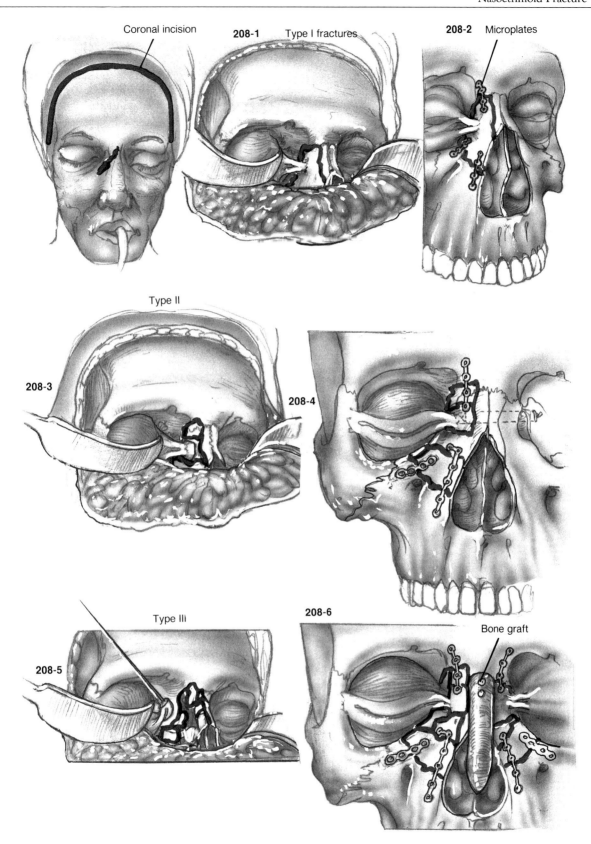

Coronal incision

208-1 Type I fractures

208-2 Microplates

Type II

208-3

208-4

Type III

208-5

208-6

Bone graft

■ 209. MEDIAL CANTHAL TENDON REPAIR

The repair of unilateral or bilateral medial canthal tendons when malpositioned as part of a nasoethmoidal complex fracture:

Type I injury: unilateral or bilateral fracture with a large, central medial orbital segment with an intact medial canthal tendon

Type II injury: increased comminution of the medial orbit with complete attachment of the medial canthal tendon to a central fragment

Type III injury: fractures extending into the osseous region of the tendon attachment or avulsion of the medial canthal tendon from the underlying bone

Indications

1. Unilateral or bilateral acute traumatic telecanthus associated with a nasoethmoid fracture

Contraindications

1. Globe injury
2. Optic nerve injury

Preoperative Preparation

1. Preoperative intercanthal and interpupillary distance measurements
2. Computed tomography (CT) evaluation
3. Ophthalmologic evaluation and clearance

Special Instruments, Position, and Anesthesia

1. Headlight
2. Orbital retractors
3. Wright or wire-passing needle
4. Stainless steel wire, 26- to 28-gauge
5. Permanent 2-0 suture

Tips and Pearls

1. Preoperative bimanual palpation with an intranasal hemostat
2. Recognition of canthal attachment to a central bony fragment
3. Adequate exposure (coronal approach recommended)
4. Upward, posterior, or medial overcorrection of the medial canthal tendon position
5. Repair bilateral injuries independently.

Pitfalls and Complications

1. Dissection of the medial canthal tendon from the central fragment during exposure
2. Poor bony reconstruction before canthal tendon repair
3. Inferior and anterior positioning of the tendon
4. Inadequate fixation of the tendon
5. Postoperative traumatic telecanthus

Postoperative Care

1. Frequent examinations of visual acuity during the first 24 hours

References

Mathog RH. Nasoethmoid fractures. In: Mathog RH, ed. Atlas of craniofacial trauma. Philadelphia: WB Saunders, 1992;317.

Markowitz BL, Manson PN, Sargent L, et al. Management of the medial canthal tendon and nasoethmoidal orbital fractures: the importance of the central fragment in classification and treatment. Plast Reconstr Surg 1991;87:813.

Operative Procedure

The early evaluation of the medial canthal region in a patient with a central facial injury is critical. Initial measurements of intercanthal and interpupillary distances should be performed. In the adult, the intercanthal distance is approximately 35 mm. The diagnosis of fragmentation of the medial canthal region also is important. Axial and coronal CT scans are useful. With the patient under anesthesia, assess the fragmentation by placing a large hemostat intranasally and placing a finger over the medial canthal region, allowing bimanual palpation. This maneuver usually allows the surgeon to diagnose whether there is fragmentation in this region and whether the tendon is attached to a bony fragment.

Canthal repair follows repair of the bony-cartilaginous framework. Recognition of the canthal attachment to a central medial orbital fragment is critical. Most patients have type I or type II injuries, in which the tendon remains attached. Repositioning and plating of these fragments generally leads to the most anatomic-appearing result in the medial canthal region. The most common error is inadequate medialization of the posterior or intraorbital portion of this large fragment. It is occasionally useful to apply transnasal wiring to the posterior portion of the central fragment in addition to the microplating that has been used to position this fragment. The transnasal wiring becomes particularly important when progression into type II (ie, more comminuted) fractures occurs.

The most difficult scenario is that of the type III fractures, in which the canthal tendon attachment is torn or the bony attachment is disrupted. Typically, it is not possible to delineate the exact location of the normal anatomic landmarks for canthal positioning (ie, anterior and posterior lacrimal crests). Accordingly, the tendons need to be located and positioned as posteriorly, superiorly, and medially as possible. The choice of fixation materials varies, but 26- to 28-gauge stainless steel wire; a large, nonabsorbable suture (2-0 or greater); or a combination of the two are commonly used.

One technique is to locate the medial canthal tendon and place a figure-of-eight suture through the canthal tendon. A knot is then tied, securing the tendon. If uncertain about the location of the tendon, another method is to create an approximately 2-mm, vertical skin incision over the region of the medial canthus. A double-needled suture is placed with each end of suture positioned at the respective superior and inferior aspects of the vertically oriented incision. This enables "capture" of the medial canthal tendon by looping the subcutaneous tissue and underlying canthal apparatus with the transcutaneous suture. This suture is then grasped internally and secured.

Next, the tendon must be pulled into position superiorly, posteriorly, and medially. A transnasal hole is created using a Wright fascial needle or a long wire-passing needle. This needle is directed toward the opposite medial orbit such that it perforates the perpendicular plate of the ethmoid and the involved opposite medial orbital region. Ideally, this creates a hole such that the contralateral pull is posterior, medial, and superior. The suture or wire attached to the medial canthal tendon is placed through the hole in the transcanthal needle, which is then withdrawn to the contralateral side. A small microscrew is placed along the superior medial aspect of the orbit to secure the suture or wire.

If there is inadequate support in the ipsilateral or contralateral medial orbit or in the perpendicular plate of the ethmoid to allow for proper posterior and superior positioning of the medial canthus, a bone graft may be necessary within the medial orbit to allow a proper pulley effect in that region. This calvarial graft should be thin, inset medially to the lamina papyreacea, and have holes drilled posteriorly and superiorly for wire placement. Alternatively, a plate can be cantilevered posteriorly for the same purpose.

For bilateral nasal canthal injuries, the contralateral tendon is repaired in a fashion identical to that of the opposite side, but independently. Transcanthal fixation is suboptimal. In the bilateral situation, the external appearance of the canthi should be observed repeatedly, and the distance from the presumed midline should be measured. It is not uncommon that one or both repairs must be released and performed again to ensure adequate symmetry postoperatively.

JOHN L. FRODEL

209-1.   Tendon prepared

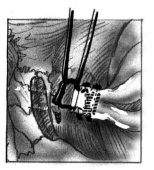

209-2.   Needle passed with wire posterior to lacrimal crest

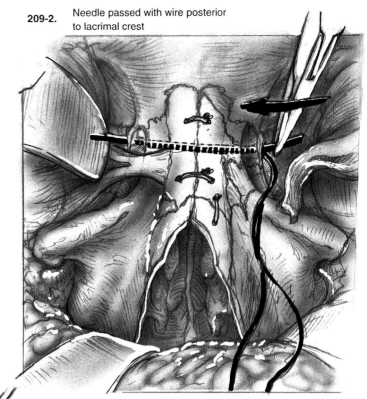

209-3.   Wire pulled through

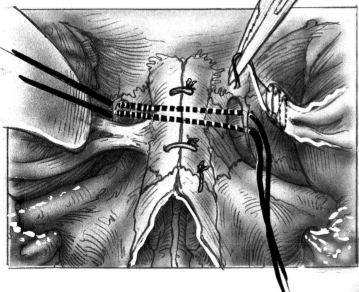

209-4.   Wires twisted

Screw

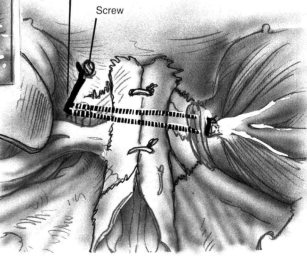

■ *210.* NASOLACRIMAL SYSTEM EVALUATION AND REPAIR—Nasolacrimal system abnormalities that have congenital, traumatic, cancer ablation, or inflammatory origins

Indications

1. Epiphora of obstructive origin
2. Laceration or traumatic discontinuity of lacrimal drainage system
3. After cancer ablation in the region of the medial canthus or medial eyelids, usually in conjunction with eyelid and medial canthal reconstruction
4. Congenital blockage or stenosis
5. After partial maxillectomy
6. After inflammatory stenosis
7. Secondary to sinus and nasal allergic or polypoid disease

Special Considerations

1. Most infants and young children clear the blockage after probing and irrigation of the lacrimal drainage system.
2. Many older patients do not require reconstruction after resection of the lacrimal drainage system because of poor tear production (ie, dry eye) and subsequent failure of epiphora to occur.

Preoperative Preparation

1. Complete ophthalmologic examination
2. Schirmer's testing
3. Slitlamp examination of lacrimal puncta
4. Eyelid snap-back test
5. Flexible or rigid nasal endoscopy
6. Irrigation of lacrimal drainage system

Special Instruments, Position, and Anesthesia

1. Magnifying loupe glasses
2. Fiberoptic headlight for intranasal visualization
3. Lacrimal probes
4. Lacrimal irrigation syringe and special needle
5. Lacrimal intubation catheters
6. Local anesthetic composed of equal parts of 2% Xylocaine and 0.50% Marcaine plus enough 1:1000 epinephrine to make a final concentration of 1:100,000.
7. Children and patients with more significant injuries are likely to require general anesthesia.
8. Topical ophthalmic anesthetic drops
9. Topical anesthetic and decongestant for the nose
10. Nasal packing if dacryocystorhinostomy is performed

(continued)

Operative Procedure

The lacrimal system has distinct secretory and excretory components. The secretory portion is responsible for formation of the film, composed of a mucous layer supplied by the conjunctival goblet cells, a watery layer supplied by the lacrimal and accessory lacrimal glands, and an oily layer supplied by the tarsal glands. Abnormalities in tear production, whether excessive, reflex, or inadequate, may be tested with the Schirmer and basic secretion tests.

The Schirmer I test is performed with filter paper strips (5 × 35 mm) folded at the notched indentation, draping the short end over the lower eyelid margin (Fig. 210-1). The degree of wetness of the strip is usually measured at 5-minute intervals; however, a 1-minute measurement multiplied by three is approximately equivalent. This test measures basic and reflex tear production. The basic secretion test is performed in a similar way after the conjunctiva and cul-de-sac have been anesthetized with topical anesthetic.

Performance of the Jones dye tests is the next step in the patient's evaluation. The primary Jones dye test consists of instilling 2% fluorescein dye into the conjunctival cul-de-sac and, after 5 minutes, attempting to retrieve the dye within the nose on a previously placed cotton pledget (Fig. 210-2). The retrieval of dye is probably the most difficult problem in this test and can be the cause of a false-negative result. The opening of the nasolacrimal duct, the lacrimal fold, lies anteriorly beneath the inferior turbinate. Under direct visualization, a cotton-tipped applicator soaked in 5% cocaine or 1% Neo-Synephrine and 4% Xylocaine is placed under the inferior turbinate to shrink the nasal mucosa and to obtain anesthesia. A positive Jones I dye test, which is a yellow-tinged cotton pledget from the fluorescein, proves there is no anatomic or physiologic blockage and points to hypersecretion as the cause of the epiphora. This is rare, unless related to allergy, irritants, or other types of ocular diseases.

If the Jones I dye test result is negative, some form of lacrimal drainage obstruction is suggested. The eyelid position should be examined for ectropion or telecanthus, which can cause an abnormal punctal position, not allowing the tears to be properly collected. A complete nasal examination should be performed.

Functional or anatomic obstruction and an estimation of the level of the blockage may be diagnosed using the Jones II dye test (Fig. 210-3). This is accurate in more than 80% of the cases; approximately 20% of normal persons exhibit a negative Jones I test result and a subsequent positive Jones II test result without evidence of a pathologic condition. The remaining dye in the cul-de-sac from the Jones I test is irrigated from the eye. The punctum is anesthetized with a cotton-tipped applicator soaked in tetracaine and then dilated with a punctal dilator. An irrigation cannula, attached to a 3-mL syringe filled with normal saline, is inserted through the inferior punctum and canaliculus, and the patient is instructed to tilt his or her head forward so that fluid irrigated through the system can be retrieved from the nose.

There are four possible findings from this test. A positive Jones II test result (ie, colored fluid from the nose after irrigation) indicates a false-negative Jones I test result (ie, normal) or partial stenosis of the lower drainage system (ie, nasolacrimal sac or duct); a normal punctal and canalicular pumping mechanism (ie, upper system) gathered the fluorescein from the instillation, but complete excretion was prohibited. The appropriate therapy is dacryocystorhinostomy. A negative Jones II test result (ie, clear fluid retrieved from the nose) indicates a physiologic obstruction of the upper collecting system; the pumping mechanism is nonfunctional, but passive irrigation is possible. These patients require a complete canalicular intubation or a Jones tube conjunctivodacryocystorhinostomy. If no fluid can be irrigated through, complete anatomic obstruction is the diagnosis. Backflow through each canaliculus during irrigation indicates complete upper system blockage, requiring a Jones tube for bypass of the system. Reflux through the one canaliculus when the other is irrigated indicates a blockage distal to the common canaliculus and may be treated with a dacryocystorhinostomy.

Repair of lacerations through one or both puncta or canaliculi is no different from repairing an eyelid laceration under other cir-

(continued)

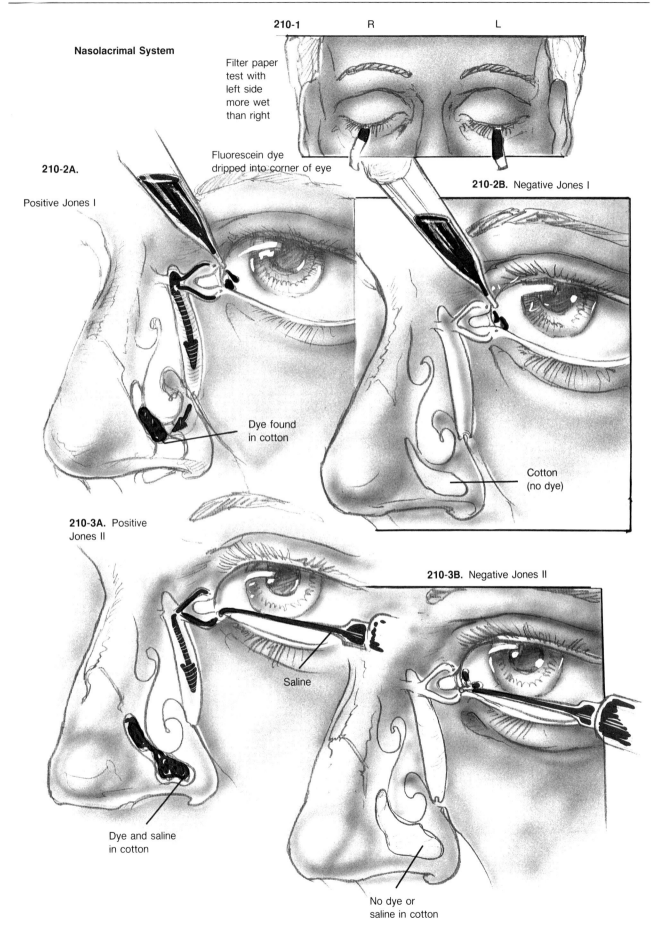

210-1   R   L

Nasolacrimal System

Filter paper test with left side more wet than right

Fluorescein dye dripped into corner of eye

210-2A.

Positive Jones I

210-2B. Negative Jones I

Dye found in cotton

Cotton (no dye)

210-3A. Positive Jones II

210-3B. Negative Jones II

Saline

Dye and saline in cotton

No dye or saline in cotton

■ 210. NASOLACRIMAL SYSTEM EVALUATION AND REPAIR (*continued*)

Tips and Pearls

1. Be careful not to injure an uninvolved punctum and canaliculus by overaggressive or repeated attempts to pass a probe or catheter.
2. Protection of the cornea is essential.
3. Decongest the nasal mucosa in sufficient time before attempting to pass and retrieve catheters to decrease bleeding.
4. Be prepared to perform a dacryocystorhinostomy if standard cannulation cannot be performed.

Pitfalls and Complications

1. Excessive bleeding in patients who are taking aspirin, nonsteroidal antiinflammatory drugs, or other anticoagulant medications
2. Do not to create a false passage when probing or cannulating the lacrimal drainage system (unless performing dacryocystorhinostomy).
3. Retrieve the metal pullout wires for the lacrimal stents in the nose as atraumatically as possible.

Postoperative Care Issues

1. Saline nasal spray to decrease crusting around catheter ends intranasally; use as long as tubes are in place.
2. Ophthalmic antibiotic ointment to eyelid laceration repair or drops if only tubes are in place
3. Perioperative intravenous or oral antibiotics may be used, especially in the face of a traumatic wound or dacryocystitis.
4. Canalicular tubes may be left in place indefinitely, but 6 months is a good minimal requirement.
5. If the canalicular tube loop in the corner of the eye accidentally extrudes with sneezing or rubbing, the patient or surgeon can replace it easily. It occasionally requires pulling the loop inward from the nose.
6. When it is time to remove the tubes, visualize the tied ends in the nose. Grasp the end with a small nasal forceps (usually using an endoscope), cut the inner eyelid loop, and remove it through the nose.

References

Holt JE, Holt GR. Nasolacrimal evaluation and surgery. Otolaryngol Clin North Am 1988;21:119.

Holt JE, Holt GR. Reconstruction of the lacrimal drainage system. Arch Otolaryngol 1984;110:211.

Kohn R. Lacrimal system. In: Textbook of ophthalmic plastic and reconstructive surgery. Philadelphia: Lea & Febiger, 1988:251.

cumstances (see Procedure 195), except that the punctum and canaliculus must be stented (Fig. 210-4). The most commonly used method is to insert a silicone canalicular tube in each canaliculus, find the sac and nasolacrimal duct, and bring both ends out into the nose through the inferior meatus (Fig. 210-5). These maneuvers are facilitated by the incorporation of metal guidewires into the ends of the silicone catheters. The metal ends are removed after both are brought out the nose and the free ends of the catheters are tied, secured with a 6-0 Prolene suture tied around the knot and replaced in the nose. The loose catheter end inside the nose should be neither too loose (easy for eye loop to occur) nor too tight (difficult to find at retrieval time). The eyelid laceration is then repaired as previously described.

In cases of blunt trauma to the nasoethmoid complex, the lacrimal system may be injured by avulsion of the common canaliculus from the sac or by fracture or separation of the sac from the duct. For the former, the medial canal tendon should be explored for avulsion, and if found, it may be resutured to its proper position using 4-0 Vicryl suture. The lacrimal drainage system then can be cannulated in the usual manner.

In the case of a severe nasoethmoid complex fracture, I prefer to first perform an open reduction of the fractures, using transcanthal wiring to narrow and reposition the splayed bones, including the lacrimal fossa. Because of the almost uniform separation of the sac from the lacrimal duct (in the maxilla) due to the fractures, it is necessary to cannulate the sac, followed by placement of the catheters into the nose in a new location, usually by maneuvering the guidewires through fracture planes into an area just beneath the middle turbinate. The end result is a new lacrimal sac or rhinostomy opening several millimeters in diameter, sufficient to carry tears if the medial canthal tendon and eyelid integrity have been properly reestablished.

In many adults, because of senile cicatricial or postinflammatory changes, the sac may become fibrotic and blocked. After ensuring that any acute infection has been treated, the patient's site of obstruction is identified as previously described. For sac blockage, dacryocystorhinostomy is required. In this procedure, a small, curvilinear incision is made in the medial canthal region, similar to that of an external ethmoidectomy (Fig. 210-6). The medial canthal tendon is deflected laterally by incising and elevating the nasal periosteum. Care must be taken to avoid the angular vein of the nose. The anterior lacrimal crest is encountered, and the sac is elevated out of the fossa (Fig. 210-7). The fossa is then entered with a Freer elevator and a 5- to 8-mm opening made into the nose. The sac is opened using a laterally based flap, and the contents are evacuated and cultured (Fig. 210-8). The canalicular tubes are placed through the puncta into the sac and then into the neorhinostomy opening, tying them in the nose as previously described (Fig. 210-9). The lateral sac flap is then sutured to the periosteum, and the medial canthal tendon is replaced with 4-0 chromic catgut sutures (Fig. 210-10). The skin is closed with 6-0 Prolene (Fig. 210-11).

Cool compresses are used on the eyelids for 48 hours postoperatively to reduce swelling and bruising. Intranasal packs may be necessary for overnight tamponade of the neorhinostomy area. The tubes can be left in place for at least 6 months to establish a mature lacrimal opening or indefinitely if the patient has no trouble.

In rare cases in which the canaliculi are stenotic or nonpatent, it is necessary to place a glass Jones tube in the corner of the eye. After anesthetizing the medial palpebral area and nasal interior with topical and local anesthesia, a small incision is made in the region of the caruncle of the eye. A large-bore, hollow needle (approximately 14 gauge) is then inserted into the medial palpebral fissure through the lacrimal sac and fossa and into the nasal cavity. Some force may be required to do this. The needle hub is then cut off, and a glass Jones tube is threaded onto the needle and slid down into place (as a sheath) into the nose. The needle is then withdrawn, and the glass tube maintains the position in the new conjunctivodacryocystorhinostomy. After maturation of the tract, the tube may be changed periodically. Abundant care is required of the patient to keep the tube clean and patent.

JEAN EDWARDS HOLT

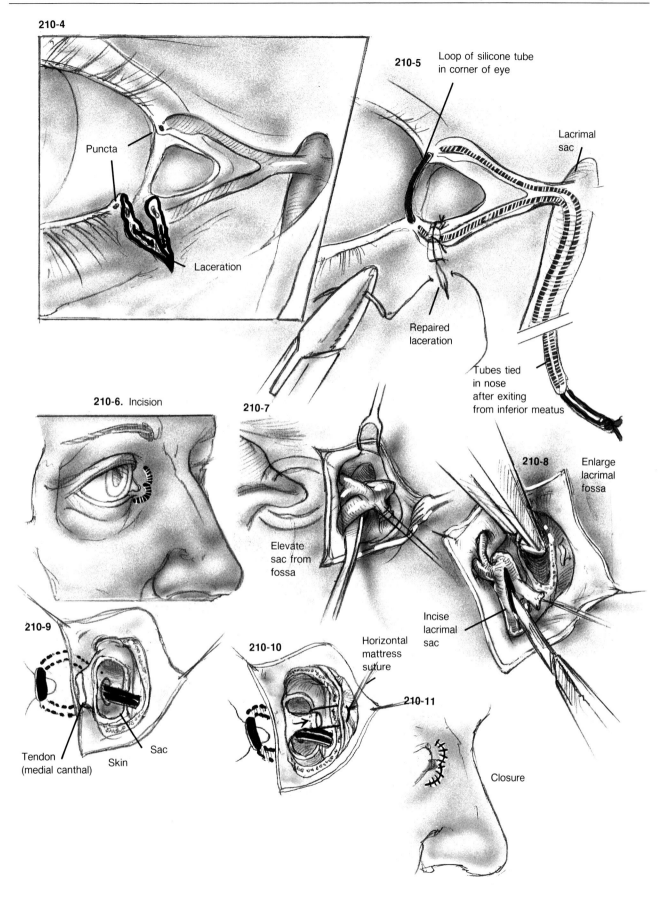

210-4

Puncta

Laceration

210-5

Loop of silicone tube
in corner of eye

Lacrimal
sac

Repaired
laceration

Tubes tied
in nose
after exiting
from inferior meatus

210-6. Incision

210-7

Elevate
sac from
fossa

210-8

Enlarge
lacrimal
fossa

Incise
lacrimal
sac

210-9

Tendon
(medial canthal)   Skin

Sac

210-10

Horizontal
mattress
suture

210-11

Closure

■ *211.* ANTERIOR WALL FRONTAL SINUS
FRACTURE—A disruption of the bony integrity of the frontal sinus limited to the anterior wall

Indications
1. Blunt or penetrating trauma that results in a displaced fracture of the anterior table of the frontal sinus

Special Considerations
1. Associated central nervous system injury
2. Cerebrospinal fluid (CSF) leak
3. Status of the posterior table
4. Associated ethmoid complex fracture
5. Medial canthal tendon integrity

Preoperative Preparation
1. Computed tomographic (CT) evaluation utilizing bony windows without contrast
2. CT scan of brain with contrast if cerebral injury is suspected

Special Instruments, Position, and Anesthesia
1. Headlight
2. Maxillofacial miniplate system
3. Sinus endoscopes
4. Access to entire head if a coronal flap repair is contemplated

Tips and Pearls
1. Adequate reduction of the fracture segments before applying fixation
2. Determine the integrity of the frontal sinus mucosa.
3. Maintain the patency of the frontoethmoid recess and tract.

Pitfalls and Complications
1. Continued external deformity
2. Missing segments
3. Associated soft tissue injury
4. Late mucocele formation
5. CSF leak

Postoperative Care Issues
1. Avoid any further trauma to the repaired sinus
2. Restoration of normal sinus physiology and mucociliary flow
3. Management of associated soft tissue injuries or injuries below the neck
4. Careful follow-up assessment to diagnose and treat mucocele formation

References
Shockley WW, Stucker FF, Gage-White L, Anthony SO. Frontal sinus fractures: some problems—some solutions. Laryngoscope 1988;98:18.
Wallis A, Donald PJ. Frontal sinus fractures: a review of 72 cases. Laryngoscope 1988;98:593–598.

Operative Procedure
With the patient in the supine position, the entire face is prepped and draped in a sterile fashion. Cocaine pledgets or other topical nasal decongestants are placed within the nasal cavity to provide vasoconstriction, allowing adequate examination of the lateral nasal wall and frontal ethmoid recess to be undertaken.

For mildly displaced or greenstick-type fractures with intact skin and no other associated significant mucosal injuries, open reduction without internal fixation can be undertaken through a frontal sinus trephine approach (Fig. 211-1). An incision is made just beneath the eyebrow through the skin and soft tissue overlying the floor of the frontal sinus. The soft tissue is dissected with care to avoid injury to the supraorbital and supratrochlear nerves. Injuries to these nerves result in ipsilateral anesthesia of that portion of the forehead and scalp. The floor of the frontal sinus is then opened with a medium cutting bur. This should be performed anterior to the plane of the pupillary line to avoid injury to the posterior table of the frontal sinus or cribriform plate. After the frontal sinus is entered, the trephine can be enlarged with a biting Kerrison rongeur. A 30° or 70° endoscope is placed through the trephine and the frontal sinus cavity inspected. It is irrigated to clean any blood or loose mucosal debris. A small Joseph elevator or other appropriately sized and shaped instrument is placed within the frontal sinus cavity, and gentle pressure is placed on the fracture segments to reduce these. Often, the integrity of the frontal sinus can be restored and maintained in excellent reduction for minimally or noncomminuted frontal sinus fractures. The cavity is suctioned free of all irrigant and blood, and the external incision is closed with interrupted synthetic sutures.

For more extensively comminuted anterior table fractures, exposure of the entire frontal sinus must be obtained (Fig. 211-2). Depending on the degree of associated soft tissue injury and the patient's natural hairline, this can be performed through a bicoronal incision placed high behind the patient's hairline or through a butterfly incision going beneath the eyebrows and crossing over the bridge of the nose. Both are cosmetically excellent incisions and provide good access to the frontal sinus.

The bicoronal or butterfly flap is elevated in a plane deep to the galea aponeurotica and superficial to the periosteum of the frontal bones. Using small nerve and bone hooks, the segments of the frontal sinus fracture are reduced and held in fixation using one of many available low-profile miniplate systems with appropriate sizes of plates and screws (Fig. 211-3). The use of dynamic compression on these fractures is unnecessary. Care should be taken to try to restore the external contour as completely as possible.

For fractures that involve extensive disruption of the mucosa and disruption of the frontal ethmoid recess, obliteration of the frontal sinus can be considered (Fig. 211-4). The necessity for this is usually rare, and the procedure should be reserved for extensively comminuted fractures with significant mucosal disruption. The surgeon should remove all of the mucosa with a diamond bur. To obliterate the sinus, cortical bone that is harvested from the parietal skull is preferred. This can be obtained through the same bicoronal incision that was used to provide exposure for the frontal sinus or through a separate incision posterior and superior to the top of the ear. Temporalis fascia can be used to stuff the nasal frontal recess and block off the communication between the nose and the frontal sinus. Abdominal fat is another source of material to obliterate the sinus and may be used if the surgeon is unable or unwilling to obtain the cortical bone from the parietal area. After the sinus has been filled with the bone paté, the anterior table can then be reconstructed and held in fixation with miniplates. After the frontal sinus anterior table has been reconstructed, the skin is closed in a layered fashion. If a butterfly incision has been made, careful approximation over the brow and bridge of the nose is made to obtain the most cosmetically acceptable closure.

Postoperatively, the patient's head is kept elevated, and the patient is told to avoid straining, nose blowing, heavy lifting, and bending over for 2 weeks. Sutures are usually removed at about 1 week.

GERALD S. GUSSACK

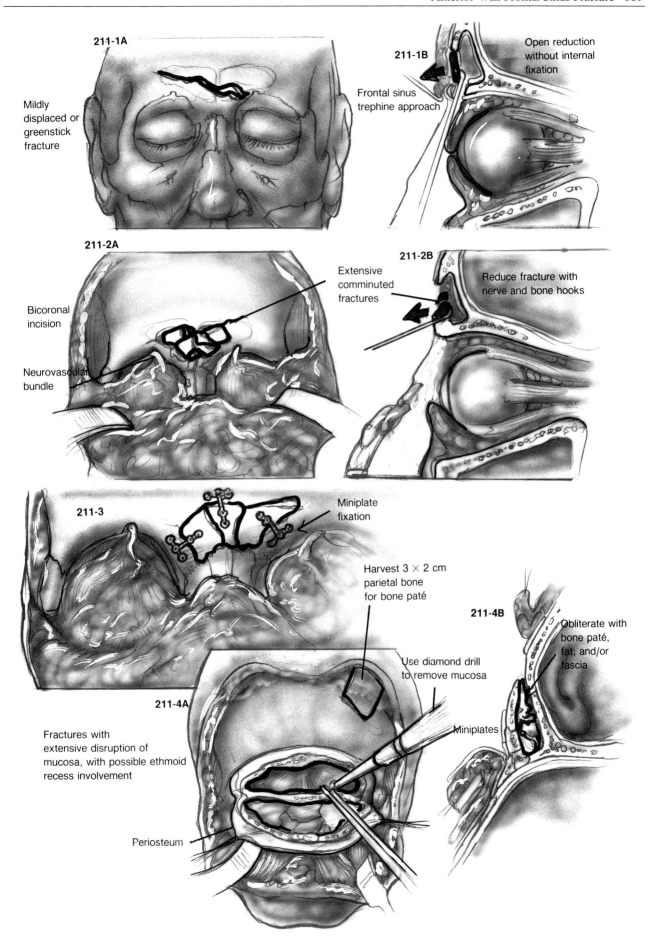

211-1A

Mildly
displaced or
greenstick
fracture

211-1B

Open reduction
without internal
fixation

Frontal sinus
trephine approach

211-2A

Bicoronal
incision

Neurovascular
bundle

Extensive
comminuted
fractures

211-2B

Reduce fracture with
nerve and bone hooks

211-3

Miniplate
fixation

Harvest 3 × 2 cm
parietal bone
for bone paté

Use diamond drill
to remove mucosa

211-4B

Obliterate with
bone paté,
fat, and/or
fascia

Miniplates

211-4A

Fractures with
extensive disruption of
mucosa, with possible ethmoid
recess involvement

Periosteum

■ *212.* POSTERIOR WALL FRONTAL SINUS

FRACTURE— A disruption of the integrity of the posterior table of the frontal sinus from blunt or penetrating trauma

Indications

1. Any displaced fracture of the posterior table of the frontal sinus

Special Considerations

1. Associated central nervous system trauma
2. Status of the dura overlying the frontal lobe
3. Status of the anterior table of the frontal sinus
4. Cerebrospinal fluid leak
5. Associated injuries of the neck and C-spine

Preoperative Preparations

1. Axial and coronal computed tomography (CT) scans of the sinuses without contrast
2. Axial CT scan of the brain with contrast

Special Instruments, Position, and Anesthesia

1. Headlight
2. Miniplate fixation system
3. Drill with diamond and cutting burs
4. Bone-cutting Kerrison rongeurs

Tips and Pearls

1. Consider obliteration or cranialization for all but the most limited posterior table injuries.
2. Determine the patency of the frontoethmoid recess drainage pathways.
3. Labeling any or all of the anterior table fragments that are removed and will be used for repair
4. Complete obliteration of the nasofrontal ducts for those undergoing obliteration or cranialization

Pitfalls and Complications

1. Determine the integrity of the frontal lobe dura, and rule out an associated epidural or subdural hematoma.
2. Complete removal of all frontal sinus mucosa
3. High incidence of cerebral and anterior cranial fossa injuries

Postoperative Care Issues

1. Avoid further trauma to the forehead
2. Counsel the patient to avoid lifting, straining, and bending over.
3. Annual follow-up examination with a CT scan to detect late mucocele formation

References

Donald PJ. Frontal sinus ablation by cranialization. Arch Otolaryngology 1982;108:142.

Grus JJ. Frontal naso-orbit trauma. Clin Plast Surg 1982;9:577.

Operative Procedure

With the patient under adequate general anesthesia, the face, head, and scalp are prepped and draped in a sterile fashion. Cocaine pledgets or other topical nasal decongestants are placed in the nasal cavity to provide vasoconstriction, which enables examination of the lateral nasal wall and frontoethmoid recess. The CT scans are kept in the operating room and referred to during the operative procedure. The choice of three approaches depends on the severity of the fracture, the status of the soft tissue and frontal nasal duct, and the degree of mucosal disruption.

For minimally displaced posterior frontal sinus table fractures, reconstruction of the sinus can be undertaken if the nasofrontal duct is patent. The procedure is similar to that for the anterior table fracture (see Procedure 211). Access to the frontal sinus is obtained through a frontal sinus trephination or by removal of the fractured anterior table segments. The posterior table is carefully inspected (Fig. 212-1*A*). The posterior table fractures can be reduced if no significant mucosal disruption is found and particularly if no mucosa is trapped between the fracture segments extending into the intracranial cavity (Fig. 212-1*B*). The integrity of the posterior wall and mucosa is confirmed, and the patency of the frontal nasal recess (duct) is determined by following the passage of saline irrigant from the frontal sinus into the nasal cavity. The anterior table is then reconstructed. All fractures are reduced. The soft tissues are closed in a standard fashion.

For fractures that are more severe, obliteration of the frontal sinus should be considered. In addition to the steps taken for the management of severe anterior table fractures of the frontal sinus, the entire mucosa and any displaced fragments on the posterior table are removed (Fig. 212-2). If only a small amount of disruption of the posterior table has occurred and the dura overlying the frontal lobe is intact, the small fracture segments can be removed after all of the mucosa has been drilled away from the frontal sinus (Fig. 212-3). After the nasal frontal ducts and nasal frontal ethmoid recesses are denuded of all mucosa, this area is plugged with some temporalis fascia. The frontal sinus then is obliterated in the standard fashion, preferably with cancellous bone from the parietal area or with abdominal fat (Fig. 213-4). The anterior table is then replaced and secured with low-profile miniplates and screws. The soft tissue is closed in a standard fashion (Fig. 213-5).

The preferred technique for extensively comminuted or severe fractures of the posterior table of the frontal sinuses is cranialization. The entire posterior table of the frontal sinus and all of the mucosa of the anterior table are removed, preferably through a frontal craniotomy approach, although the contents can be removed through an osteoplastic sinusotomy. After good exposure of the posterior table is obtained, the posterior wall is totally removed with bone-cutting Kerrison rongeurs and cutting and diamond burs. All of the rough edges of the posterior table are smoothed until they are even with the frontal bone and taken down to the floor and lateral walls of the frontal sinus. The nasal frontal ducts are then packed with temporalis fascia. The frontal lobe dura is carefully inspected, and any tears are repaired. The surgeon carefully inspects for spinal fluid leaks. The brain is allowed to expand to obliterate the entire frontal sinus cavity. The anterior table of the frontal sinus is replaced and secured with low-profile miniplates in the standard fashion, as would be used for reduction of anterior table fractures.

Postoperatively, the patient's head is kept elevated, and the patient is instructed to avoid straining, nose blowing, heavy lifting, and bending over. Sutures are usually removed within about 1 week. Careful follow-up examinations during the next several years ensure the completeness of the obliteration and assess any mucocele formations resulting from retained mucosa. A screening CT scan is usually obtained annually.

GERALD S. GUSSACK

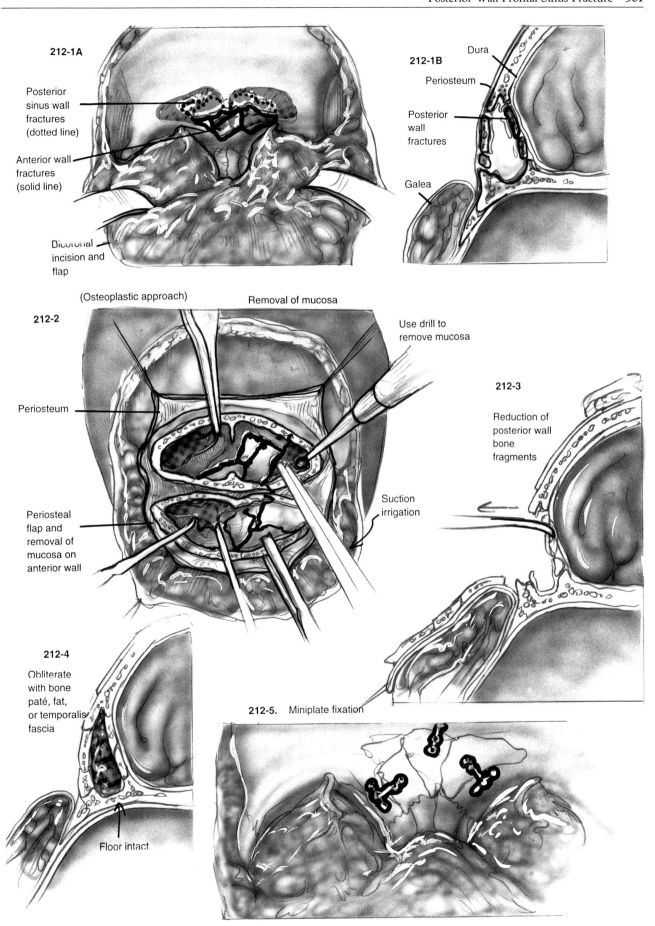

212-1A

Posterior sinus wall fractures (dotted line)

Anterior wall fractures (solid line)

Dicoronal incision and flap

212-1B

Dura

Periosteum

Posterior wall fractures

Galea

(Osteoplastic approach)

Removal of mucosa

212-2

Use drill to remove mucosa

Periosteum

Periosteal flap and removal of mucosa on anterior wall

Suction irrigation

212-3

Reduction of posterior wall bone fragments

212-4

Obliterate with bone paté, fat, or temporalis fascia

Floor intact

212-5. Miniplate fixation

■ *213.* FRONTONASAL DUCT INJURY

Disruption of the inferior frontal and anterior superior ethmoid cells that connect the frontal sinus to the nasal cavity

Indications

1. Blunt or penetrating trauma to the frontonasal duct that results in disruption of the anatomic integrity of the mucosa or bone

Special Considerations

1. Status of the anterior and posterior tables of the frontal sinus
2. Careful endoscopic nasal examination
3. Associated nasoethmoid complex fracture and medial canthal ligament injury
4. Indwelling Silastic or latex stent for an extended period

Preoperative Preparation

1. Computed tomography (CT) scan of the paranasal sinuses
2. Careful documentation of all associated injuries

Special Instruments, Position, and Anesthesia

1. Headlight
2. Sinus endoscopes (30° and 70°)
3. Silastic or latex T-tubes
4. Kuhn-Bolger frontal sinus instrumentation sets, including curets, giraffe forceps, and seekers

Tips and Pearls

1. Careful determination of the integrity of the ethmoid cells along the frontonasal drainage tract
2. Preservation and redraping of the mucosa of the frontoethmoid recess
3. Stenting for 8 to 12 weeks
4. Frequent cleaning, irrigation, and suctioning of the reestablished drainage tract
5. Consider frontal sinus obliteration or cranialization for extensive fractures or those that include the posterior table.
6. Three-dimensional computer reconstructions for help in determining anatomic disruptions

Pitfalls and Complications

1. Restenosis of the reconstructed frontonasal duct
2. Mucocele formation
3. Chronic ethmoid and frontal sinusitis

Postoperative Care Issues

1. Irrigation and patency of the stent
2. Frequent cleaning and removal of granulations from the frontoethmoid recess
3. Follow-up CT at 1 year to assess the status of the sinuses

References

Heller EM, Jacobs JB, Holliday RH. Evaluation of the frontonasal duct in frontal sinus fractures. Head Neck 1989;11:46.

Levine SB, Rowe LD, Keame WH, Arkins JP. Evaluation and treatment of frontal sinus fractures. Otolaryngol Head Neck 1986;95:19.

Stanley RB, Becker TS. Injuries of the nasofrontal orifices in frontal sinus fractures. Laryngoscope 1989;99:1011.

Operative Procedure

With the patient under general anesthesia, the nose is instilled with a cocaine solution or other appropriate topical decongestant, and the lateral nasal wall and the frontal nasal recess are anesthetized with a solution of Xylocaine with epinephrine. Exploration of the frontal sinus is undertaken through a Lynch approach or an osteoplastic frontal sinusotomy.

The type of reconstruction depends on the degree of injury to the frontal nasal duct. The long-term patency of any reconstruction of the frontal ethmoid recess or frontal nasal duct depends on maintaining the integrity of the bony supporting structures of the frontal ethmoid recess, including the lamina papyracea, the posterior table of the frontal sinus, the lacrimal bone, the nasal process of the frontal bone, and the remaining ethmoid sinus. For patients with severe telescoping frontoethmoidal injuries combined with a frontal sinus fracture, I recommend against reconstruction of the frontoethmoid tract and instead suggest cranialization or obliteration of the frontal sinus and duct along with management of the telescoping nasal ethmoid fracture.

The indications for frontal and nasal duct reconstruction after trauma are limited to linear-type fractures through the posterior table of the frontal sinus and extending down into the ethmoid, with minimal disruption of the overlying mucosa and only a small degree of separation (Fig. 213-1). The techniques described for endoscopic drainage of the frontoethmoid recess are applicable to the management of frontonasal duct injuries.

The initial portion of the procedure is begun by removing the uncinate process through an endoscopic approach with a combination of a sickle knife and straight binding Blakesley forceps. The bulla ethmoidalis is identified and entered through its inferior lateral aspect. The entire bulla is removed, taking care to avoid injury to the superior medial aspect of the middle turbinate attachment adjacent to the cribriform plate (Fig. 213-2). The agger nasi cells are identified in the lateral nasal wall in the direction of the frontal ethmoidal recess. Careful endoscopic evaluation of this area helps to determine the route for drainage of the supraorbital ethmoid cells and the route toward the frontal sinus. The agger nasi cells are removed with 45° and 90° frontal sinus curets, carefully removing the bony partitions in a posteromedial to anterolateral direction. This protects the integrity of the vertical lamina of the cribriform plate. All bone fragments are removed. Care is taken to preserve as much of the frontal ethmoid mucosa as possible; this mucosa is redraped over the overlying bone.

If status of the area permits, the frontal sinus injury is reconstructed in a standard fashion (Fig. 213-3). Reconstruction of the frontonasal duct of the frontal sinus should be undertaken only in patients in whom normal physiology can be restored.

Most of the reconstructed ducts require stenting, usually with a small indwelling tube that is self-retaining. A 14- or 16-Fr cholangiogram T-tube works well (Fig. 213-4). The horizontal portion of the T is placed within the frontal sinus, and the vertical portion of the T traverses the area of the frontal nasal recess into the nasal cavity. After all the mucosa has been removed from the frontal ethmoid recess, nasal flaps can be developed from the nasal mucosa to reline the tract. Two parallel incisions are made approximately 2 cm apart along the superior aspect of the upper nasal vault and along the anterior lateral surface of the nasal mucosa. The incisions are extended inferiorly approximately to the area between the upper lateral and lower lateral cartilages. The incisions are then connected, and the tissue is cut horizontally. A superiorly based flap is elevated and rotated back on itself, extending into the frontal sinus (Fig. 213-5). The tube is placed such that it can stent the reconstructed flap in good apposition to the surrounding soft tissue and drainage can be maintained.

The patients are usually kept on antibiotics perioperatively, and a moderate amount of attention is required to maintain the patency of the tube or stent that was left in place and to clean any crust or granulation that collects around the lateral aspect of the stent as it traverses the frontal ethmoid recess. The catheters can be irrigated and suctioned free of all mucus, blood, and collected debris. Stents are removed in 8 to 12 weeks.

GERALD S. GUSSACK

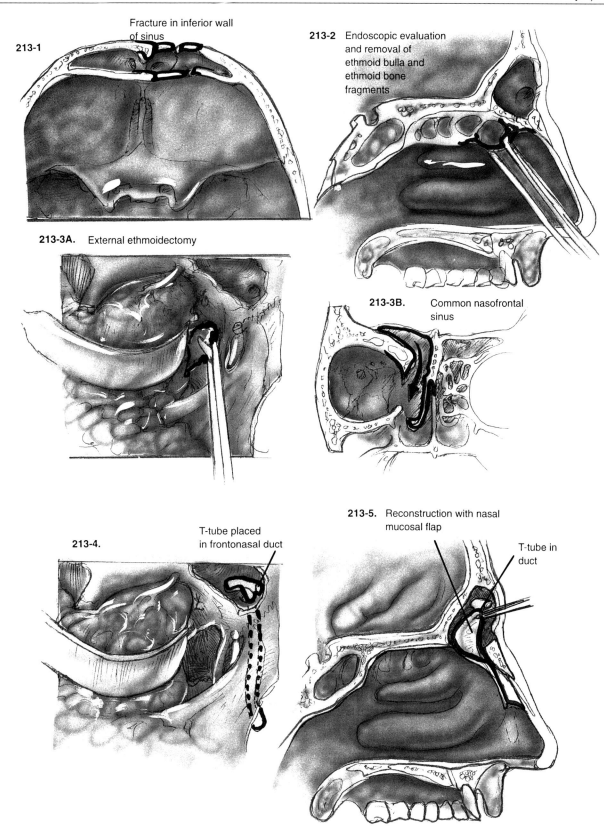

213-1

Fracture in inferior wall of sinus

213-2 Endoscopic evaluation and removal of ethmoid bulla and ethmoid bone fragments

213-3A.   External ethmoidectomy

213-3B.   Common nasofrontal sinus

213-4.

T-tube placed in frontonasal duct

213-5.   Reconstruction with nasal mucosal flap

T-tube in duct

■ *214.* LATE REPAIR OF TRAUMATIC EN-OPHTHALMOS—Open repair of a malpositioned globe after orbital trauma. Although usually caused by traumatic displacement of the orbital floor, wall, or roof, it may be associated with a malpositioned zygoma.

Indications
1. Enophthalmos greater than 3 mm
2. Hypophthalmos greater than 3 mm
3. Enophthalmos or hypophthalmos with associated zygoma malposition

Contraindications
1. Only seeing eye
2. Unstable visual acuity secondary to previous surgery (relative contraindication)

Preoperative Preparation
1. Coronal and axial computed tomography (CT) scans
2. Full ophthalmologic evaluation, including visual acuity, globe position measurements, and globe restriction measurements

Special Instruments, Position, and Anesthesia
1. Headlight
2. Oculoplastic instrumentation
3. Bone graft harvesting equipment
4. Alloplastic materials (if bone not used)
5. Osteotomes and saw for zygomatic repositioning

Tips and Pearls
1. Precise preoperative planning is essential.
2. Malar malposition commonly is associated with enophthalmos.
3. Meticulous, deep orbital dissection is required.
4. Isolation of solid posterior bone is required.
5. Bone grafts or alloplastic materials are carefully placed over solid bony ledges.
6. Reproduction of the normal, cone-shaped orbital cavity is essential.
7. Forced duction examination preoperatively and at the end of the operation

Pitfalls and Complications
1. Inadequate preoperative evaluation
2. Improper repositioning of the zygomatic and orbital rim segments
3. Inadequate orbital dissection
4. Inadequate volume constriction with implants
5. Inadequate soft tissue restoration

Postoperative Care Issues
1. Frequent postoperative visual acuity examinations
2. Lubrication of the cornea

References
Mathog RH. Orbital wall fractures. In: Mathog RH, ed. Atlas of craniofacial trauma. Philadelphia: WB Saunders, 1992:303.
Pearl RM. Treatment of enophthalmos. Clin Plast Surg 1992;19:99.

Operative Procedure
Critical to the reconstruction of the posttraumatic enophthalmic globe is the proper diagnosis of the deformity. Enophthalmos usually is caused by traumatic displacement of the orbital floor, walls, or roof. Displacement of the zygomatic segment further exacerbates the enophthalmos. The surgical plan should incorporate the diagnosis of all components of the orbit and zygoma. This discussion assumes normal zygomatic positioning with pure orbital enophthalmos. A coronal CT scan can demonstrate areas of volume expansion secondary to fractures of the various components of the orbital cavity. These most commonly involve the floor, medial wall, and lateral wall.

A lower eyelid incision (ie, subciliary, transconjunctival, with or without lateral canthotomy) or a middle eyelid crease incision may be used (Fig. 214-1*A*). Through this incision, the orbital rim is approached, and the periosteum incised throughout the extent of the infraorbital rim (Fig. 214-1*B*). Careful subperiosteal dissection is carried inferiorly, medially, and laterally through this incision (Fig. 214-1*C*). The most difficult aspect of the dissection commonly is in the region of the inferior orbital fissure (Fig. 214-2). This area is often comminuted, with bone resorption and herniation of scarred orbital contents into the superior aspect of the maxillary sinus. It is essential to dissect in all directions of the bony orbital cone such that solid bony ledges are located posteriorly (Fig. 214-3). Without adequate dissection and location of these bony landmarks, the proper restoration of the superiorly, posteriorly, and medially based apex of the orbital cone is extremely difficult. Similarly, without adequate dissection, proper reduction of the orbital contents within this orbital cone cannot occur.

Medial wall, lateral wall, and orbital roof displacements must be addressed. These may be approached through small incisions in the medial orbit (ie, partial Lynch) and eyebrow region, or they may be approached with greater exposure through the transcoronal incision (Fig. 214-4). The latter allows complete visualization of all components of the orbit. Dissection through these approaches enables a 360° elevation of the orbital periosteum and soft tissues, as is required. Preoperative CT evaluation dictates the dissection required.

After periosteal elevation and retraction of the orbital contents with a flat orbital retractor, reconstruction may ensue. The choice of materials may include autologous materials, including bone (eg, calvarial, rib, iliac), autogenous cartilage (eg, costal, septal, conchal), or alloplastic materials. With all bony ledges isolated, implant materials are positioned to overlay these bony ledges (Fig. 214-5). In cases of substantial volumetric expansion, a significant amount of material may be required in the posttraumatic setting. However, overzealous implantation may lead to the postoperative sequelae of increased intraocular pressure and visual disturbance, although this is extremely unusual.

It is important to always visualize the posterior extent of all implants to avoid any pressure of the orbital apex. In most cases, the implants are designed such that they lie in a stable fashion within the dissection pockets. However, they occasionally need to be secured by screw fixation to the underlying stable bony fragments or by suture fixation in a similar fashion. A variety of titanium and Vitallium implants can be used for very large subtotal orbital deformities.

After bony implantation, the globe position is evaluated (Figs. 214-5 and 214-6). The position at the end of orbital implantation should not be solely relied on. This evaluation is only useful if there is obviously inadequate repositioning of the globe and further augmentation is required. However, if the globe appears to be in a relatively normal position, the surgeon should remember that there is some degree of edema within the orbital contents that may provide a false representation of eventual globe position. Accordingly, a slight overcorrection is often indicated. After orbital reconstruction, it is important to secure the orbital cavity by resuturing of all periosteal incisions at the various locations around the orbital rim. Similarly, if complete orbital dissection has taken place, it is extremely important to resecure the canthi to limit postreconstructive soft tissue deformities.

JOHN L. FRODEL

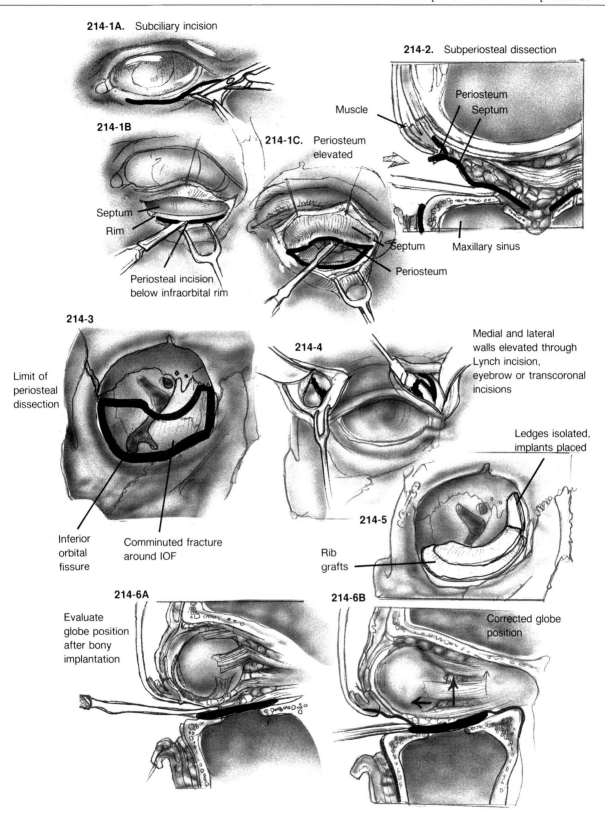

214-1A. Subciliary incision

214-1B

Septum

Rim

Periosteal incision below infraorbital rim

214-1C. Periosteum elevated

Septum

Periosteum

214-2. Subperiosteal dissection

Muscle

Periosteum

Septum

Maxillary sinus

214-3

Limit of periosteal dissection

Inferior orbital fissure

Comminuted fracture around IOF

214-4

Medial and lateral walls elevated through Lynch incision, eyebrow or transcoronal incisions

Ledges isolated, implants placed

214-5

Rib grafts

214-6A

Evaluate globe position after bony implantation

214-6B

Corrected globe position

215. PEDIATRIC FACIAL FRACTURE

Disruption of the integrity of the bones of the face by blunt or penetrating trauma in patients 13 years of age and younger

Indications

1. Displaced fractures of the bones of the face

Special Considerations

1. High incidence of associated chest and extremity injuries in motor vehicular trauma
2. Associated cranial trauma
3. Lower circulating blood volume than adults
4. Growth centers of the nose, face, and mandible
5. Rapid healing of the pediatric skeleton and decreased need for prolonged immobilization and fixation

Preoperative Preparation

1. Complete assessment of child for associated injuries
2. Laboratory evaluation
3. Volume replacement, if indicated
4. Airway management
5. Facial and neck radiographs and computed tomography (CT) scan

Special Instrumentation, Position, and Anesthesia

1. Miniplates and screws
2. Uncuffed endotracheal tubes

Tips and Pearls

1. Treat most nondisplaced fractures nonoperatively
2. Intermaxillary fixation times of 2 to 3 weeks are usually sufficient
3. The blood loss and hemodynamic status of pediatric patients should be monitored closely.
4. High incidence of associated intracranial injuries
5. Postoperative nutrition requires attention.
6. Be aware of evolving and mixed dentition status.
7. Lingual splints

Pitfalls and Complications

1. Missed injury
2. Fractures affecting the growth centers of the condyle, nasal septum, and maxilla
3. Dental caries
4. Hypovolemic shock

Postoperative Care Issues

1. Airway control
2. Physical therapy to restore occlusion
3. Remove intermaxillary fixation in 2 to 3 weeks.
4. Nutritional support

References

Angelillo JC. Fractures of the mandible in children. In: Serafin D, Georgiade N, eds. Pediatric plastic surgery. St. Louis: CV Mosby, 1984: 531.

Gussack GS, Luterman A, Powell RW, Rodgers K, Ramenofsky ML. Pediatric maxillofacial trauma: unique features in diagnosis and treatment. Laryngoscope 1987;97:925.

James D. Maxillofacial injuries in children. In: Rowe NL, Williams JL, eds. Maxillofacial trauma. Edinburgh: Churchill Livingstone, 1985: 538.

Operative Procedure

The patient is carefully evaluated for the degree of facial injury and for associated injuries. There is a very high incidence of associated thoracoabdominal and extremity injuries in children who have sustained facial fractures, particularly those involved in motor vehicle or motor vehicle–pedestrian injuries. The degree of blood loss is evaluated, and and careful monitoring of the patient's hematocrit, blood pressure, and pulse should be maintained. Blood loss from scalp wounds can be significant. There is often associated cranial trauma, and a complete neurologic examination should be undertaken for suspected cases. Pediatric airway management is also essential, and laryngospasm may be associated with blood in the oral and hypopharynx.

A CT scan of the head and neck can document the degree and severity of the maxillofacial and mandibular injuries and the status of the cervical spine. The cervical spine should be maintained in an appropriate collar until its status is documented. The growth centers of the face should be considered in patients who have displaced fractures of the condyle, nasal septum, or midface. These fractures should be reduced, and the parents should be informed of the possible long-term consequences of this degree of injury.

Most mandibular fractures can be managed with short periods of intermaxillary fixation. Nondisplaced condylar fractures can be managed with a soft diet if the occlusion is intact. Open reduction and internal fixation for mandibular fractures is usually reserved for severely comminuted or displaced fractures. Intermaxillary fixation between the upper and lower jaws can be undertaken with Ivy loops, as demonstrated in the accompanying figure (Fig. 215-1). Fixation should be maintained for approximately 2 to 3 weeks. Adequate nutrition is a source of concern, and the physician must consider the use of liquid caloric and oral vitamin supplements. Follow-up radiographs are usually obtained before removal of the intermaxillary fixation.

Early intervention should be considered for facial and mandibular fractures in the pediatric population, because rapid healing can start within 3 or 4 days after injury. Reduction and fixation of the fracture should be undertaken within the first 72 hours. A nasal fracture should be reduced in the standard fashion, and the nasal septum should be examined carefully. Repositioning of the nasal septum and bone should be undertaken instead of performing a formal septoplasty for children with nasal and septal fractures (Fig. 215-2). The junction of the quadrangular cartilage and perpendicular plate of the ethmoid is where the growth center of the nose is located. Hematomas or fractures in this area can be associated with subsequent shortening of the nose if these are not recognized and addressed. For displaced mandible fractures in a patient younger than 5 years of age, an occlusal splint can be fabricated (Fig. 215-3). This usually requires the services of a dental laboratory, which can be fashioned after appropriate impressions of the mandible are made. The occlusal splint allows good reduction of the mandibular segments and lets the patient eat during the perioperative period.

Midface injuries in the pediatric population are rare because of the lack of pneumatization of the ethmoid and maxillary sinuses. These injuries should be evaluated with a CT scan. For LeFort I and LeFort II fractures, internal fixation after open reduction can be maintained with the use of low-profile miniplates without requiring intermaxillary fixation (Fig. 215-4). The patient should be instructed by a physical therapist how to establish occlusion and should be maintained a full liquid or soft diet during the initial 2 to 3 weeks. Postoperative physical therapy should also be considered.

Midface fractures are associated with a high incidence of intracranial injuries. Consultation with the appropriate pediatric general surgical and neurosurgical colleagues should be made early in the patient's course.

GERALD S. GUSSACK

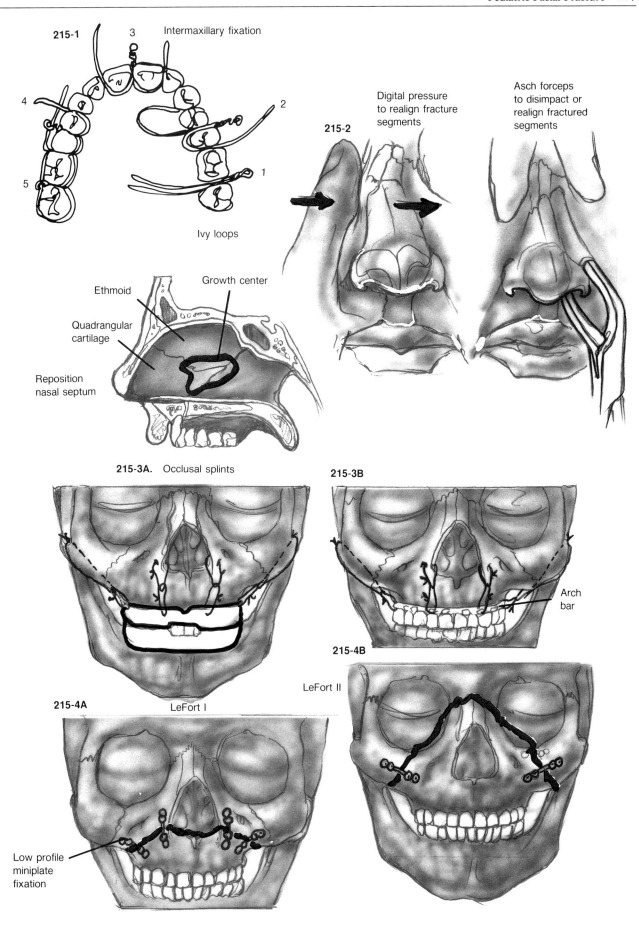

215-1 Intermaxillary fixation

Ivy loops

215-2 Digital pressure to realign fracture segments

Asch forceps to disimpact or realign fractured segments

Ethmoid

Growth center

Quadrangular cartilage

Reposition nasal septum

215-3A. Occlusal splints

215-3B

Arch bar

215-4A

LeFort I

215-4B

LeFort II

Low profile miniplate fixation

■ 216. INTERMAXILLARY FIXATION

Mechanism for holding the mandible in a normal position relative to the maxilla

Indications

1. Temporary reduction of mandibular fractures while placing rigid internal fixation
2. Fractures of the condyle area
3. Fractures of the body
4. Fractures of the angle or symphyseal areas; usually combined with open reduction and internal fixation
5. Multiple fractures; often combined with open reduction and internal fixation

Special Considerations

1. Protection of the operating team from glove penetration while handling hardware

Preoperative Preparations

1. Appropriate imaging studies
2. Appropriate laboratory tests

Special Instruments, Positions, and Anesthesia

1. Head light
2. Wire twisting instrument (ie, Hagar needle holder)
3. Instrument to hold wire ligature in the gingival sulcus while tightening (eg, Freer elevator, "pickle fork")
4. Tongue and cheek retractor
5. Nasotracheal intubation

Tips and Pearls

1. Accurate contouring of arch bars
2. Prestretching of wire ligatures
3. Proper technique for tightening of wire ligatures

Postoperative Care Issues

1. Prevention of vomiting
2. Accurate instructions to nursing personnel, patient, and family in case vomiting becomes imminent
3. Maintenance of oral hygiene
4. Maintenance of nutrition
5. Antibiotics to reduce incidence of infection
6. Weekly examinations and others as needed

References

Clark WD, Bailey BJ. Management of fractures of the mandible. In: Mathog , ed. Maxillofacial trauma. Baltimore: Williams & Wilkins, 1984:148.

Clark WD. Management of mandibular fractures. Am J Otolaryngol 1992;13:125.

Shelton DW. Fractures of the mandible. In: Miller RH, ed. The surgical atlas of airway and facial trauma. New York: Grune & Stratton, 1983:23.

Operative Procedure

Intermaxillary fixation (IMF) may be achieved through several techniques. This discussion is limited to the use of stock arch bars. The arch bar material is cut to approximate the length of the dental arch. The bar is then bent into a curve and placed against the dental arch to access its length (Fig. 216-1). Any excess material is trimmed.

The importance of properly contouring the arch bar to conform to the dental arch cannot be overemphasized. Without proper contouring, an arch bar lacks optimal stability and acts as an orthodontic appliance. Teeth ligated to a poorly contoured arch bar become subjected to forces that may move, loosen, or even extract them.

As viewed from the side, the occlusal plane curves superiorly, usually beginning with the first molar (Fig. 216-2). This is called the curve of Spee, and it should be reproduced in the maxillary and mandibular arch bars.

Incisor and molar teeth have faciolingual inclinations up to 28° from the vertical plane. The maxillary anterior teeth and molars are inclined to the facial plane, and the premolars of both arches are almost perpendicular to the occlusal plane. Mandibular incisors are inclined facially, and mandibular molars are inclined to the lingual (Fig. 216-3). With a little effort, an arch bar can be contoured to match the inclinations of these different zones and the curve of Spee.

The arch bar is then ligated to the canine, premolar, and molar teeth using 24- to 26-gauge stainless steel wire that has been prestretched. It is convenient to ligate one tooth on each side of the arch to hold the arch bar in position for placing the remainder of the wires (Fig. 216-4); the first premolar is a good choice.

The wire ligatures are passed through the gingival embrasure (ie, potential space on the gingival side of the contact areas of each tooth, normally filled with the papillary gingiva) on each side of the tooth to be ligated, taking care that it passes above the arch bar on one side and below on the other. A Freer elevator or similar instrument should be used to hold the wire ligature in the gingival sulcus while it is tightened (Fig. 216-5). Proper tightening of the ligature is done by applying traction on the wire and then twisting to take up the slack as the tension is lessened. This is repeated until the ligature is tight against the arch bar.

The ligatures are left at full length until all have been placed. This reduces soft tissue trauma and the danger of glove puncture. After testing each one for tightness, the wires are cut to a length of 1 to 1.5 cm and twisted on themselves to bury their sharp ends.

Any fracture that an arch bar crosses must be reduced before the arch bar is secured. Otherwise, the arch bar acts to resist fracture reduction. In some cases, it may be advantageous to apply the arch bar loosely, reduce the fracture, and then tighten the ligatures. An alternative is to place the arch bars in segments, with the breaks at the fracture lines. This is less desirable, because a continuous arch bar offers more stability.

After arch bars are securely in place, IMF may be obtained by elastics or wires (Fig. 216-6). Each has advantages and disadvantages, but a good compromise is the placement of a few elastics initially, replacing them with wires after the high-risk period for nausea has passed and any anticipated dynamic improvement has been realized.

WILLIAM D. CLARK

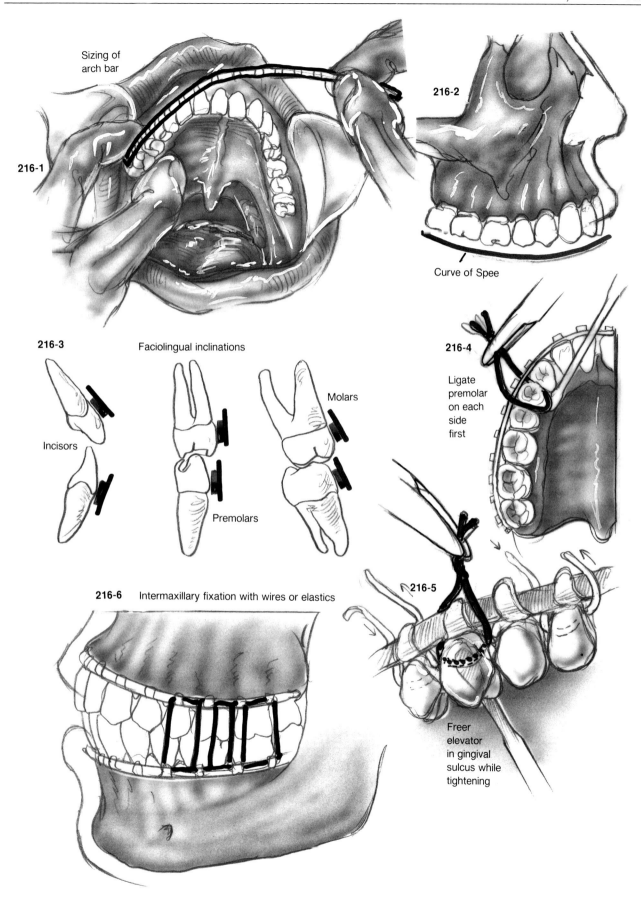

216-1

Sizing of arch bar

216-2

Curve of Spee

216-3   Faciolingual inclinations

Incisors

Premolars

Molars

216-4

Ligate premolar on each side first

216-5

Freer elevator in gingival sulcus while tightening

216-6   Intermaxillary fixation with wires or elastics

■ 217. MANDIBULAR FRACTURES: OPEN REDUCTION AND INTERNAL FIXATION WITH COMPRESSION PLATING—Repair of a through-and-through fracture of the mandible from the dental arch through the lower border with a compression plate, which is designed so a planned interaction between the plate and the screws results in predictable compression of the bones across the fracture site

Indications

1. Repair of nonoverlapping mandible fractures in which there is adequate bone-to-bone contact for compression

Contraindications

1. Overlapping fragments will slide and overlap more under compression.
2. A straight compression plate should not be used without a tension band along the tension portion of the fracture.

Special Considerations

1. Reestablishment of the proper occlusal relation is a primary concern.
2. Tension banding (eg, arch bar, wire, miniplate) is necessary along alveolar portion of fracture.
3. The compression plate is placed along the basal border of the mandible.

Preoperative Considerations

1. If dentition is not sufficient to reestablish occlusion, dentures or splints are required.

Special Instruments, Position, and Anesthesia

1. Anesthesia is administered by a nasal tube so it does not interfere with intermaxillary fixation.
2. The patient is supine.
3. Headlights
4. Arch bars
5. Plating sets and instruments, including appropriate bone-reduction forceps

Tips and Pearls

1. A proper occlusal relation is a primary concern, and if it cannot be accomplished, consider not plating.
2. Proper bending and positioning of the plate are keys to a correct outcome.
3. When no tension band is possible, an eccentric dynamic compression plate can be used.

Pitfalls and Complications

1. Malocclusion equals malunion.
2. Tooth root injury
3. Inferior alveolar nerve injury
4. Injury to the marginal mandibular branch of the facial nerve
5. Infection
6. Osteomyelitis
7. Nonunion

Postoperative Care Issues

1. Keep the oral mucosa clean.
2. Drain wounds to avoid hematoma.

References

Kellman RM, Marentette LJ. Atlas of cranio-maxillofacial fixation. New York: Raven Press, 1995.
Spiessl B. Internal fixation of the mandible. Berlin: Springer-Verlag, 1989.

Operative Procedure

The successful use of compression plating for the repair of mandibular fractures depends on attention to two principles. First, correctly using a compression plate requires proper positioning of the screws in the compression holes to produce tightening that forces the bone fragments together across the fracture line. Second, compression of mandibular fractures requires the use of bicortical screws, which necessitates placement of the compression plate along the biomechanically unfavorable compression side of the mandible, the basal border. Except in a few cases of screw placement in an edentulous mandibular body and at the symphysis, bicortical screws in the midportion of the bone or at the biomechanically favorable tension side result in injury to the tooth roots and the inferior alveolar nerve. To use compression plating along the inferior border of the mandible, a tension band must be applied along the tension side. This can be an arch bar across the teeth or a wire or miniplate on the bone. A tension band miniplate is applied between the tooth roots and inferior alveolar nerve using monocortical screws.

The arch bars are applied, and occlusion is reestablished using intermaxillary fixation. The fracture is then exposed intraorally or extraorally. When an intraoral incision is used, it is made perpendicular to the mucosa, 5 to 10 mm below the gingival margin. Posteriorly, it extends along the oblique line of the mandible onto the ramus. If an extraoral incision is made, it is placed in an appropriate line of relaxed skin tension to minimize scar formation. Care is taken to avoid injury to the marginal mandibular branch of the facial nerve.

If an arch bar tension band is in place, the surgeon can proceed directly to compression plate application. Precompression of the fracture helps position the fragments and hold them during plate application. A modified towel clip can be used by drilling a small notch in the bone on either side of the fracture (Fig. 217-1). Mandibular reduction-compression pliers can be used by screwing the holders to the inferior border of the mandible temporarily with screws. The forceps is then screwed onto the holders, which can be used to reduce and compress the fracture (Fig. 217-2). Except for the symphysis, this device can only be used through an extraoral approach. If no arch bar has been placed, a tension band miniplate should be applied (Fig. 217-3).

After the fracture is reduced and precompressed, an appropriate plate is selected. A pliant template is placed across the fracture and bent to shape. The selected plate is bent to match the template. The plate is positioned across the fracture and held in position. The first compression hole is drilled such that the shaft of the screw is positioned in the plate hole away from the fracture, with the head of the screw overlapping the metal of the plate (Fig. 217-4). The hole is measured with a depth gauge, making sure to catch both cortices, because bicortical screw purchase is necessary to prevent shifting under compressive forces. The hole is tapped if a non–self-tapping system is used, and the screw is placed but not tightened. The second compression screw is similarly placed on the opposite side of the fracture (Fig. 217-4A). Tightening this screw compresses the fragments together. The first screw is tightened also, completing compression (Fig. 217-4B).

Additional screws are positioned centrally in their plate holes such that they are neutral and add no further compression. At least two screws on each side of the fracture are required, although three or four per side are preferable. Behind the midbody, transoral plate application requires transbuccal screw placement.

Reduction forceps are removed. The wound is drained, and closure is completed in layers, according to the surgeon's preference.

In the absence of a tension band, an eccentric dynamic compression plate may be used. Proper application of this plate closes the alveolar (ie, tension) side of the fracture from its position along the basal border. Precompression is necessary, using a modified towel clip or a reduction-compression pliers with side rollers for superior compression. The horizontal compression screws are applied and tightened as described previously. Vertical compression forces are then applied by placing screws in the inferior portion of the diagonal compression holes (Fig. 217-5).

ROBERT M. KELLMAN

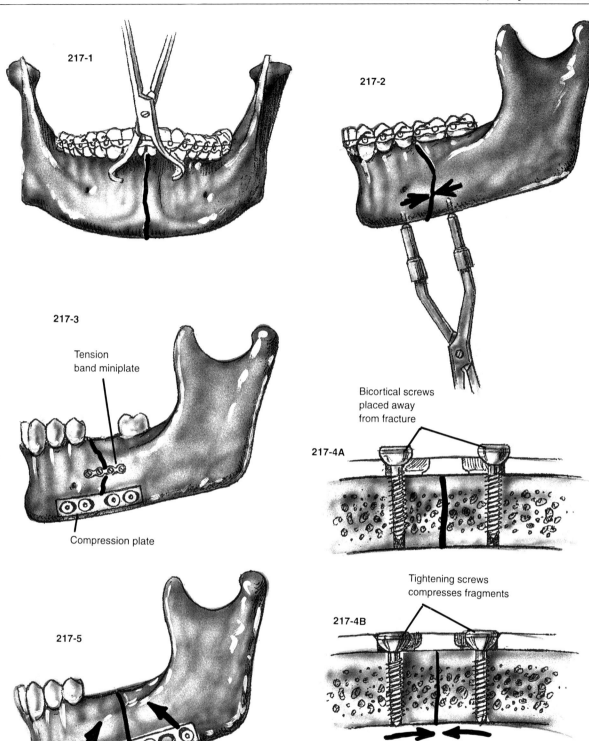

217-1

217-2

217-3

Tension
band miniplate

Compression plate

Bicortical screws
placed away
from fracture

217-4A

Tightening screws
compresses fragments

217-4B

217-5

Eccentric
compression plate

■ 218A. MANDIBULAR FRACTURE: OPEN REDUCTION AND INTERNAL FIXATION WITH NONCOMPRESSION PLATING—Repair of a through-and-through fracture of the mandible from the dental arch through the lower border with a noncompression plate, which is designed so a plate screwed to the bone on either side of a fracture supplies support for the fragments and rigidly fixes them without compression, allowing healing to occur

Indications
1. Repair of mandible fractures that are not overlapping

Contraindications
1. Overlapping fragments, for which a lag screw technique should be used
2. Neutral miniplates should not be used for comminuted fractures. Larger reconstruction plates should be used for these.

Special Considerations
1. Reestablishment of a proper occlusal relation is a primary concern.
2. Miniplating along the ideal line of osteosynthesis requires monocortical screws to avoid injury to tooth roots and the inferior alveolar nerve.
3. The surgeons must use mandibular miniplates that are 1 to 1.2 mm thick, because thinner plates may result in failure.

Preoperative Considerations
1. If dentition is not sufficient to reestablish occlusion, dentures or splints are required.

Special Instruments, Position, and Anesthesia
1. Anesthesia is administered by a nasal tube so it does not interfere with intermaxillary fixation.
2. The patient is supine.
3. Headlights
4. Arch bars
5. Plating sets and instruments, including towel clip bone-holding forceps and transbuccal instrumentation.

Tips and Pearls
1. A proper occlusal relation is a primary concern, and if it cannot be accomplished, consider not plating.
2. Proper bending and positioning of the plate are keys to a correct outcome.
3. The plating usually is applied transorally.

Pitfalls and Complications
1. Malocclusion equals malunion.
2. Tooth root injury
3. Inferior alveolar nerve injury
4. Infection
5. Osteomyelitis
6. Nonunion

Postoperative Care Issues
1. Keep the oral mucosa clean.
2. Drain wounds to avoid hematoma.

References
Champy M, Pape H-D, Gerlach KL, Lodde JP. Mandibular fractures: the Strasbourg miniplate osteosynthesis. In: Kruger E, Schilli W, Worthington P, eds. Oral and maxillofacial traumatology, vol 2. Chicago: Quintessence Publishing, 1986:19–43.
Kellman RM, Marentette LJ. Atlas of cranio-maxillofacial fixation. New York: Raven Press, 1995.
Worthington P, Champy M. Monocortical miniplate osteosynthesis. Otolaryngol Clin North Am 1987;20:607–620.

Operative Procedure
Noncompression plating of mandible fractures includes two types of repair. The main form is miniplate fixation, which refers to the placement of monocortical miniplates along the ideal lines of osteosynthesis, as described by Champy (Fig. 218-1). For the symphysis, parasymphysis, and angle regions, two miniplates should be applied. For the body region, one miniplate along the ideal line is sufficient, although two are more stable and therefore safer.

Occlusion is reestablished using intermaxillary fixation by whatever means is appropriate. Miniplate fixation usually is carried out through an intraoral incision. The incision is made perpendicular to the mucosa, 5 to 10 mm below the gingival margin. Posteriorly, it extends along the oblique line of the mandible onto the ramus. The incision is taken to bone, and an elevator is used to expose the bone on either side of the fracture. Care is used to avoid injury to the inferior alveolar nerve.

In the symphyseal and parasymphyseal regions, a modified towel clip can be used to hold the fragments in reduction. At the angle, a Kocher clamp on the posterior fragment allows it to be pulled forward to abut the body. Body fractures usually must be reduced manually.

Attention is turned to placement of the miniplates. An upper miniplate is positioned over the area between the tooth roots and the inferior alveolar nerve, which is 1.5 to 2 crown heights below the gingival margin. The plate is bent to shape. Each hole is drilled, and a monocortical self-tapping screw is placed. The process is repeated sequentially until all screws have been placed. A minimum of two screws on each side of the fracture are required. At the angle, the first plate is positioned along the oblique line.

A second plate is placed along the inferior (ie, basal) border of the mandible (Fig. 218-2); the exception is the angle region, where the second plate is placed above the inferior alveolar nerve (Fig. 218-3). At the basal border, monocortical or bicortical screws can be used, because there are no structures at risk. Drilling and screw placement into the lateral mandible behind the parasymphysis or anterior body generally requires use of the transbuccal trocar.

Wounds are irrigated, drained, and closed, using suture according to the surgeon's preference. The intermaxillary fixation may then be released.

Another noncompression technique involves the use of the mandibular reconstruction plate. This involves the use of a long, strong plate to replace areas of the mandible that are absent or functionally defective due to severe comminution. The use of a long, rigid device with multiple fixation points provides enough stability to replace such defective areas. This type of fixation requires the use of bicortical screws along the basal border of the mandible. At least four screws placed into the solid bone on either side of a defective area are recommended, although the use of more fixation points increases the stability of the fixation (Fig. 218-4).

Another noncompression technique is the three-dimensional miniplate. Although experience has been limited in the United States thus far, early results suggest that the technique is effective and safe. It is actually a variation on the miniplate technique.

ROBERT B. KELLMAN

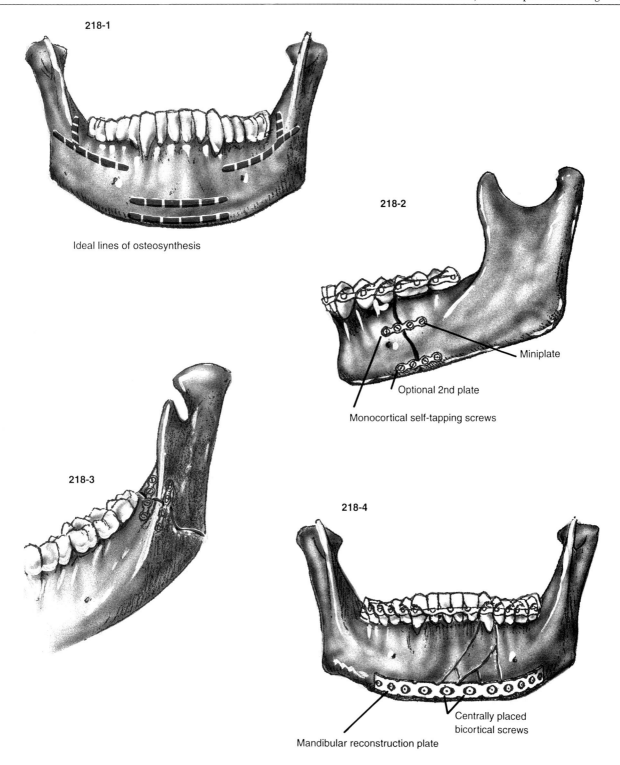

218-1

Ideal lines of osteosynthesis

218-2

Miniplate

Optional 2nd plate

Monocortical self-tapping screws

218-3

218-4

Centrally placed
bicortical screws

Mandibular reconstruction plate

■ *218B.* MANDIBULAR FRACTURES: OPEN REDUCTION AND INTERNAL FIXATION WITH LAG SCREWS—A fracture of the mandible in which the fragments overlap each other is repaired using lag screws. Lag screws placed through both overlapping fragments pull them together in compression.

Indications
1. Repair of overlapping bone fragments

Contraindications
1. Inadequate bone through which to fix the screws

Special Considerations
1. Reestablishment of a proper occlusal relation is a primary concern.
2. Reduce the fracture with a modified towel clip first, if possible.

Preoperative Considerations
1. If dentition is not sufficient to reestablish occlusion, dentures or splints are required.

Special Instruments, Position, and Anesthesia
1. Anesthesia is administered by a nasal tube so it does not interfere with intermaxillary fixation.
2. The patient is supine.
3. Headlights
4. Arch bars
5. Plating sets and instruments, including towel clip bone-holding forceps, drill bits for gliding (nonthreaded) and threaded holes, drill sleeve for threaded holes (if available)

Tips and Pearls
1. A gliding hole should be the size of the thread to minimize play around the screw.
2. Countersink the first hole.
3. Two lag screws are typically the minimum; three are safer.
4. Lag screw fixation of mandibular angle fractures is difficult.
5. A proper occlusal relation is a primary concern, and if cannot be accomplished, consider a less rigid fixation technique.

Pitfalls and Complications
1. Malocclusion equals malunion.
2. Tooth root injury
3. Inferior alveolar nerve injury
4. Infection
5. Osteomyelitis
6. Nonunion

Postoperative Care Issues
1. Keep the oral mucosa clean.
2. Drain wounds to avoid hematoma.

References
Ellis E, Galli GE. Lag screw fixation of mandibular angle fractures. J Oral Maxillofac Surg 1991;49:234–243.

Kellman RM, Marentette LJ. Atlas of cranio-maxillofacial fixation. New York: Raven Press, 1995.

Niederdellmann H, Shetty V. Solitary lag screw osteosynthesis in the treatment of fractures in the angle of the mandible: a retrospective study. Plast Reconstr Surg 1987;80:68–74.

Operative Procedure
Lag screw fixation is applied when bone fragments overlap (Fig. 218-5). A lag screw does not thread or catch in the first fragment, called the gliding hole, but does catch in the second, called the threaded hole. When the screw is tightened, the first cortex behaves as a washer and the second as a nut, and the first cortex is compressed between the head of the screw and the second cortex, compressing the bone surfaces together. Lag screw fixation is ideal for overlapping (ie, oblique) fractures, and it can also be used effectively for abutting fractures of the mandibular symphysis and angle, because the curvature of the bone in these areas leads to overlapping cortices despite the lack of obliquity of the fractures.

Occlusion is reestablished using intermaxillary fixation by whatever means is appropriate. Exposure of the fracture is accomplished according to the surgeon's preference. Intraoral incisions are made perpendicular to the mucosa, 5 to 10 mm below the gingival margin. Extraoral incisions are made in appropriate relaxed skin tension lines. The bone is exposed and reduced, using a modified towel clip to stabilize the fractured fragments (Fig. 218-6).

The lag screws must penetrate both cortices, approximately perpendicular to the fracture. Ideal angles have been calculated, but they are rarely a concern. The outer cortex is drilled using a drill bit that is the size of the thread of the screw to be used, creating a gliding hole in which the thread does not catch (Fig. 218-7). If available, a drill sleeve that fits into the gliding hole is used to stabilize the drill bit and direct the drilling of the smaller-diameter hole in the second cortex. Because this hole is the size of the shaft of the screw, the thread catches. A countersink is used to widen the surface of the outer hole for better metal to bone contact and less screw head protrusion. The depth of the hole is measured with a depth gauge, being sure to catch both cortices. When necessary, the threaded hole is tapped. The appropriate-length screw is then placed and tightened (Fig. 218-8). The process is repeated for a second and, when possible, additional lag screws.

At the symphysis, lag screws are passed across the fracture so that the solid cortical bone on either side of the fracture is compressed. The first hole is overdrilled (to form a gliding hole), and the second is threaded. Tightening the screw compresses the fragments together (Fig. 218-9). Two lag screws are preferred in this area for adequate stabilization.

When the fracture is beyond the anterior body or midbody, the approach requires transbuccal placement of the drill holes and screws. Lag screw fixation of the mandibular angle fracture is a technically tricky procedure. Great care must be used to direct the drill hole to penetrate both cortices and avoid the inferior alveolar nerve. The drill must be directed posteromedially and slightly superiorly, and drilling must be performed through the cheek using the transbuccal trochar.

ROBERT M. KELLMAN

218-5

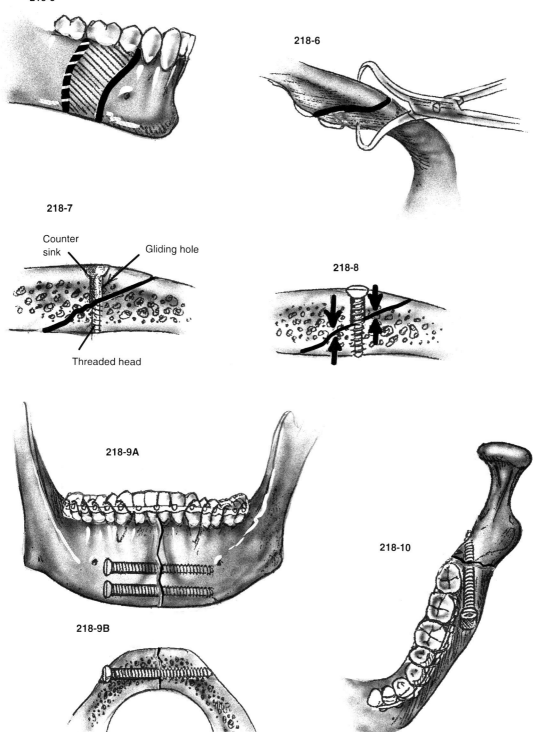

218-6

218-7

Counter
sink   Gliding hole

Threaded head

218-8

218-9A

218-10

218-9B

■ 219. MANDIBULAR FRACTURES: EXTERNAL FIXATION WITH A BIPHASE APPARATUS

—Mandible fractures involving through-and-through fractures, bone loss, infection, and multiple fragments may be treated with a biphase apparatus, which is a solid bar of methylmethacrylate attached percutaneously with pins to the mandibular fragments.

Indications
1. Unstable fractures
2. Comminuted fractures
3. Bone loss
4. Infection
5. Medically unstable patient

Contraindications
1. Patient too unstable for even minor surgery
2. No uninfected or vascularized bone for pin placement
3. Severe damage to or infection of the overlying skin (relative contraindication)

Special Considerations
1. External fixation can be a temporizing maneuver in treating the medically unstable patient.
2. As definitive treatment, external treatment requires great skill to reposition bones precisely and maintain position.

Preoperative Considerations
1. If the dentition is not sufficient to reestablish occlusion, dentures or splints are required.

Special Instruments, Position, and Anesthesia
1. Pins
2. Methylmethacrylate
3. Mold or endotracheal tube

Tips and Pearls
1. External fixation is a fall-back technique that can be used when other techniques fail.
2. External fixation may be interchangeable with using a mandibular reconstruction plate in many situations.

Pitfalls and Complications
1. Skin injury from heat as the methylmethacrylate sets
2. Infection of soft tissues
3. Osteomyelitis
4. Malocclusion creating malunion

Postoperative Care Issues
1. Preventing infection around the pins
2. Maintaining health of the skin

References
Mathog RH. Atlas of craniofacial trauma. Philadelphia: WB Saunders, 1992.

Morris JH. Biphase connector: external skeletal splint for reduction and fixation of mandibular fractures. J Oral Surg 1949;2:1382.

Operative Procedure

The successful use of external pin fixation requires proper reduction of the fractures, followed by stable placement of an adequate number of transosseous pins. These must be fixed to a solid bar, which provides the continuity and stability. The rigidity of the bar is transmitted to the bone by means of the pins. The fixation pins are placed percutaneously through stab holes, and a separate incision is used to reduce the bone fragments (Fig. 219-1).

When a patient is medically unstable, closed reduction can be combined with percutaneous pin fixation placed under local anesthesia, although this method is considered suboptimal (Fig. 219-2).

Occlusion is reestablished using intermaxillary fixation by whatever means is appropriate. The area of the fracture or fractures is exposed through an appropriate incision, although the periosteum is usually left intact. The bone fragments are manually reduced. When multiple small fragments intervene between larger ones, the smaller ones usually are kept in position by manipulating them and, if possible, compressing them between the larger fragments. Pins should be placed only into fragments that can be properly stabilized with two pins or tightly fixed in position between other fragments; otherwise, rotation around a single pin leads to movement and probable malposition and infection.

The locations of the pins are planned and marked. A small stab hole is made over each intended pin site, keeping the blade parallel to the direction of the facial nerve, and dissection is carried down to the bone. A transbuccal trocar from a plating set helps. A small area of periosteum is elevated for pin placement.

The pins that are commonly used are threaded at both ends, one end for insertion into the bone and the other for a nut that screws down to the fixation acrylic, which rests on a fixed nut. If a Kirschner wire is used, it is cut flush with the acrylic. A drill the size of the screw shaft is used, and a bicortical hole is drilled. The pin is screwed into the hole, penetrating both cortices for pin stability, but there should be minimal protrusion through the lingual cortex to avoid mucosal irritation and infection. This process is repeated until all the pins have been placed.

Fittings that tighten onto each pin are placed such that a bendable rigid bar can be fixed across all of the pins (Fig. 219-3). The fittings and the bend of the bar are adjusted until the fracture fragments have been properly reduced. These attachments are close to the mandible, leaving room for placement of the acrylic over the ends of the pins onto the fixed nuts. When this technique is used for simpler fractures, this step can be skipped, and the fragments can be held manually in reduction while the acrylic bar is applied.

The remainder of the fixation involves replacing the metal bar fixation with an acrylic bar, which is the second phase of the biphase fixation. A rod of acrylic must be created. This can be accomplished by mixing the acrylic and pouring it into a greased bar-shaped mold (Fig. 219-4). When it is firm, but not solid, it is removed from the mold and placed over the screws so they pass through the material. As this bar hardens, it holds all of the pins rigidly in position. Nuts can be placed onto the screws down to the acrylic (Fig. 219-5).

As an alternative to the mold, an endotracheal tube can be passed over the pins by making through-and-through holes in the tube walls. Liquid acrylic is then squirted into the tube using a syringe.

In either case, it is important to cool the pins near the skin while the acrylic sets, because the pins transmit heat that could burn the tissues. The metal bar fixation, if present, is then removed.

The wounds are irrigated and closed. The pin sites must be kept meticulously clean and coated with antibiotics.

The main alternative to external pin fixation is the use of the mandibular reconstruction plate. When appropriate, this plate provides even greater stability, and it is possible to use more fixation points. However, the technique is more technically demanding, and it requires wider exposure.

ROBERT M. KELLMAN

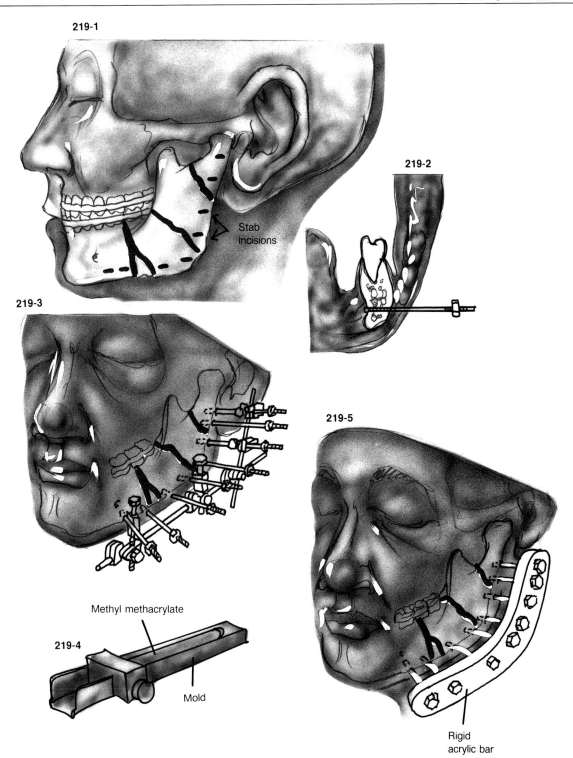

219-1

Stab incisions

219-2

219-3

219-5

Methyl methacrylate

219-4

Mold

Rigid acrylic bar

■ 220. MANDIBULAR FRACTURES: USE OF DENTURES AND SPLINTS

—Splints and dentures that function as splints can be used to prevent fractured mandibular segments from splaying, to stabilize periodontally involved teeth, to replace missing teeth temporarily, and to provide for intermaxillary fixation.

Indications

DENTURES AS SPLINTS
1. To provide for intermaxillary fixation (IMF) in the edentulous patient
2. To treat a body of mandible fracture in the edentulous patient with a severely atrophic mandible or medical contraindications to an open procedure

SPLINTS
1. As an occlusiolingual splint and sole treatment for an isolated body of mandible fracture in child 8 to 9 years of age
2. Bilateral body fracture (ie, bucket handle fracture) with inferior rotation of anterior segment
3. Symphyseal and parasymphyseal fractures combined with bilateral posterior fractures
4. Multiple fractures with poor stability
5. Numerous loose or missing teeth

Special Considerations
1. Preoperative study models (eg, plaster casts) to evaluate the occlusion and plan the splint are not needed for edentulous patients with serviceable dentures.
2. Fabricating the splint by producing the fractures in plaster, reducing the fractures by occluding the fragments of the sectioned cast with the cast of the maxilla, stabilizing the study model in its anatomic position, and using the repaired cast to form the template for the splint

Preoperative Preparation
1. Having all dental laboratory work completed and soaked in antiseptic solution before anesthesia
2. Laboratory studies as appropriate for the patient

Special Instruments, Positions, and Anesthetics
1. Nasotracheal intubation
2. Head light
3. Equipment to pass wires around the mandible and zygomatic arches
4. Drill for ligature holes

Tips and Pearls
1. Fractured dentures are easily repaired by a dental laboratory
2. Remove mandibular central incisors from the denture to provide for alimentation and egress of secretions and vomitus.
3. Counsel an edentulous patient that dentures may not be serviceable, even with repair, after their use as splints.

Pitfalls and Complications
1. Failure to have the splints or dentures completely prepared preoperatively
2. Failure to employ adequate fixation of the splint or denture to the patient

Postoperative Care Issues
1. Avoidance of and provisions for nausea and vomiting
2. Maintenance of oral hygiene
3. Maintenance of nutrition
4. Weekly examinations to verify the status of hardware, maintenance of occlusion, state of nutrition, and freedom from infection

References
Clark WD. Management of mandibular fractures. Am J Otolaryngol 1992;13:125.
Shelton DW. Fractures of the mandible. In: Miller RH, ed. The surgical atlas of airway and facial trauma. New York: Grune & Stratton, 1983:23.

Operative Procedure

Splints can be of several designs. A lingual splint is the classic and works well to hold the mandibular segments from splaying. An occlusal splint can stabilize periodontally involved teeth or "lock in" the occlusion when the surfaces of the teeth are worn flat. An occlusiolingual splint is an excellent combination of the first two. It is physically stronger and more stable, and it provides a mechanism to temporarily replace missing teeth. Because the intermeshing of opposing teeth tends to reduce and stabilize fractures, this splint offers great benefit.

Dentures function as facio-occlusiolingual splints. They may be fixed to the mandible and maxilla and used to furnish a base for IMF. Needed repairs may be easily provided by a dental laboratory. A simple and aesthetic way to apply hardware for IMF is shown in Figure 220-1, although there are several acceptable alternatives.

Some dental laboratories are familiar with the fabrication of splints suitable for use in the treatment of mandibular fractures. Such a facility may require only impressions of the two arches to carry the task to completion. When provided design instructions and repaired casts, most dental laboratories should be able to make an acceptable splint.

Several steps are necessary for designing and making a splint. Impressions are taken of both dental arches; a general anesthetic may be required. Plaster casts are made. As seen in Figure 220-2A, a malocclusion becomes obvious when occluding the casts. The mandibular cast is sectioned along the lines of the fractures. The segments of the mandibular cast are brought into tight occlusion with the cast of the maxillary arch (see Fig. 220-2B). While holding the fragments in occlusion, they are joined together in a temporary fashion (dental "sticky wax" works well) first and then permanently joined with plaster. The repaired mandibular cast then becomes the foundation for making the splint.

If a dental laboratory cannot complete the splint, the cast is coated with a separating medium (eg, thin layer of petrolatum ointment), and self-curing polymethylmethacryate is used in the "sprinkle on" method to form then desired appliance.

The lingual portion of an occlusiolingual splint should cover the attached gingiva of the alveolar ridge and the lingual surface of the teeth. The occlusal portion should, at a minimum, replace any missing posterior teeth. If desirable (eg, pediatric body fractures, adults who need locking of occlusion or stabilization of individual teeth) the splint may be designed to extend over the occlusal and incisal surfaces of all mandibular teeth. This opens the bite a few millimeters and requires that the models be mounted on a dental articulator for accurate fabrication.

The external surface of the splint should be smoothed and polished for the patient's comfort.

WILLIAM D. CLARK

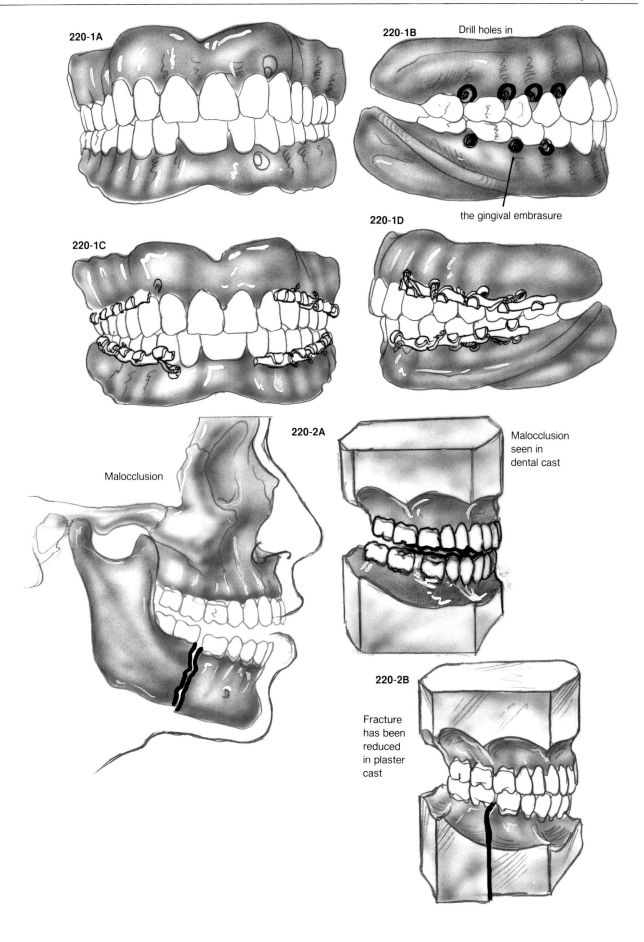

220-1A

220-1B Drill holes in

the gingival embrasure

220-1C

220-1D

Malocclusion

220-2A Malocclusion seen in dental cast

220-2B

Fracture has been reduced in plaster cast

■ *221.* MANDIBULAR FRACTURES: SPECIAL PROBLEMS IN CHILDREN—There are difficulties in treating mandibular fractures that are peculiar to children.

Special Considerations

1. Fewer, smaller, and less favorably shaped teeth
2. Teeth less stable within the alveolus because of smaller roots, roots incompletely formed, or partially resorbed by permanent tooth buds
3. Mandible smaller with less dense bone and less room to accommodate drill holes and hardware
4. Temporomandibular joint more prone to loss of mobility, even ankylosis
5. Potentially less cooperation or tolerance from patient

Tips and Pearls

1. Accurate contouring of arch bars with careful ligation using fine wire (26–28-gauge)
2. Use of circumferential wiring to support intermaxillary fixation (IMF)
3. Use of occlusiolingual splints to supplement or, in selected cases, replace IMF
4. Careful use of open reduction with interosseus wiring
5. Shortened periods of IMF
6. Careful examination of imaging studies to determine safe areas for drill holes

References

Clark WD, Bailey BJ. Management of fractures of the mandible. In: Mathog RH, ed. Maxillofacial trauma. Baltimore: Williams & Wilkins; 1983.

Clark WD. Management of mandibular fractures. Am J Otolaryngol 1992;13:125.

Operative Procedure

Fractures of the mandible are uncommon in children but present special challenges when they do occur.

Deciduous teeth are few (20 versus 32 teeth in adults), small, poorly shaped for wire ligation, and often have incomplete root systems (Fig. 221-1). They also tend to be spaced so as to have poor or open contact areas between them. The mixed dentition years are further complicated by spaces and loose teeth. All of this contributes to difficulties in obtaining stable IMF.

The rapid healing of fractures in children necessitates early treatment and shorter periods of fixation. The temporomandibular joints of children seem more prone to become limited in range of motion after IMF. Periods of IMF need to be shorter than in adults, typically 2 to 3 weeks. Nighttime elastics are useful for 1 to 2 weeks after releasing brief periods of IMF.

On the positive side are the better healing capabilities and more forgiving nature of the developing dental apparatus in children.

Fine wire (26- to 28-gauge) and meticulous techniques are recommended for the application of IMF in children. Circumferential wiring is an excellent way to stabilize IMF in children. Three-point circummandibular wires are used for mandible, and bilateral circumzygomatic plus anterior nasal spine (versus piriform aperture) wiring are used for maxillary arch bars (Fig. 221-2).

Splints are useful for improving mandibular stability. Occlusiolingual splints can fill in spaces left by missing teeth, providing the stops and locks normally associated with occluding dental arches.

Body of mandible fractures seem relatively more common in children than adults, probably because of weakening by numerous, large tooth buds. This case has the potential for a less complex treatment. Occlusiolingual splints wired to the mandible with three-point circumferential wiring for 4 weeks is an alternative to IMF for treating these fractures.

Open reduction with internal fixation of fractures of the child's mandible is limited by the small size of the bone and presence of tooth buds. In the young child, drill holes for interosseus wiring should be placed no more than a few millimeters from the inferior border of the mandible and a like distance from the fracture line. Imaging studies should always be consulted before drilling any holes in the pediatric mandible. Rigid internal fixation is out of the question for the young child. The older child may have sufficient room to permit placement of miniplate fixation devices. Careful study of radiographs is essential to make such judgments.

WILLIAM D. CLARK

221-1A

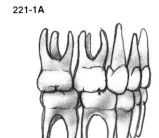

221-1B

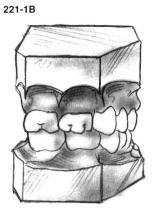

Mixed dentition

221-1C

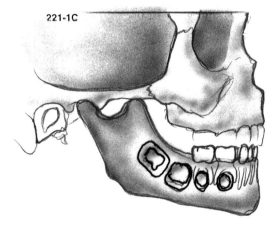

221-1D

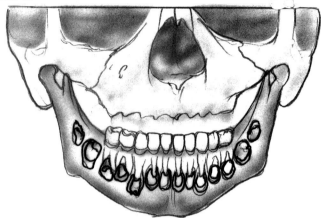

221-2

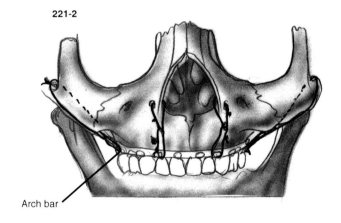

Arch bar

■ *222.* ANTERIOR LARYNGOTRACHEAL DECOMPRESSION (ANTERIOR CRICOID SPLIT)—
Anterior midline division of the cricoid ring, with or without division of upper tracheal cartilages, to enlarge the subglottic airway

Indications
1. As an alternative to tracheotomy or chronic nonfibrotic subglottic pathology (eg, edema)
2. Mild to moderate acquired subglottic stenosis
3. Mild congenital subglottic stenosis
4. Anterior glottic web

Special Considerations
1. Extubation failure on at least two occasions secondary to pathologic laryngeal process
2. Infant weight greater than 1500 g
3. No assisted ventilation for 10 days before the procedure
4. Supplemental O_2 less than 30%.
5. No evidence of congestive heart failure
6. No evidence of acute upper or lower respiratory tract infection
7. No antihypertensive medication for 10 days before evaluation

Preoperative Preparation
1. Complete endoscopic evaluation of the airway
2. Anteroposterior and lateral soft tissue views of the subglottic space and trachea
3. Careful evaluation of vocal cord mobility

Special Instruments, Position, and Anesthesia
1. Headlight
2. Tracheotomy position, with the shoulders elevated and the head hyperextended and stabilized
3. Patient intubated with endotracheal tube or bronchoscope
4. General anesthesia
5. Postprocedure intubation: for infant body weight of 1500 to 2000 g, 3.0-mm endotracheal tube; for 2000 to 2500 g, 3.5-mm endotracheal tube; for 2500 to 3000g, 4.0-mm endotracheal tube
6. Adequate drainage
7. Stay sutures

Tips and Pearls
1. Minimal dissection
2. Insertion of augmentation graft of auricular cartilage or midportion of hyoid
3. Hemostasis

Pitfalls and Complications
1. Excessive dissection may lead to pneumomediastinum or pneumothorax.
2. Accidental extubation

Postoperative Care
1. Sedation; short-term paralysis in some cases
2. Duration of intubation: body weight less than 2500 g, 10 to 14 days; more than 2500 g, 7 to 10 days.
3. Antibiotics
4. Careful monitoring in intensive care unit for accidental extubation
5. Corticosteroids, administered 6 to 12 hours before extubation (dexamethasone, 1.0 mg/kg to a maximum dose of 10 mg).

References
Cotton RT, Myer CM, et al. Anterior cricoid split, 1977–1987. Arch Otolaryngol Head Neck Surg 1988;114:1300.
Cotton FT, Seid AB. Management of the extubation problem in the premature child: anterior cricoid split as an alternative to tracheotomy. Ann Otol Rhinol Laryngol 1980:89:508.
Holinger LD, Stankiewicz JA, Livingston GL. Anterior cricoid split: the Chicago experience with an alternative to tracheotomy. Laryngoscope 1987;97:19.

Operative Procedure
Flexible laryngoscopy is performed to evaluate vocal cord motion. General anesthesia is induced using a mask to prepare the patient for the endoscopic portion of procedure. Spontaneous respiration is required. The larynx is sprayed with topical Xylocaine (lidocaine), the endotracheal tube, if present, is withdrawn into the hypopharynx, and anesthesia is maintained using an insufflation technique. This allows an unimpaired view of the larynx using the 0° Hopkins rod telescope. A careful evaluation of the subglottic pathology is undertaken and photographic documentation employed if possible. The trachea and bronchi are examined to rule out other abnormalities. The patient is then carefully reintubated and prepared for anterior decompression.

Positioning as for tracheotomy is accomplished with the shoulders elevated and the head hyperextended. A horizontal skin incision is made over the cricoid to expose the cricoid and the upper tracheal rings (Fig. 222-1). The lower half of the thyroid cartilage is also exposed. A vertical incision is made through the anterior cartilaginous ring of cricoid and through the mucosa to expose the endotracheal tube. The incision may be extended inferiorly to the tracheal rings (Fig. 222-2). Superior extension may be necessary, depending on the degree of pathology. It is necessary if the procedure is undertaken for a glottic web (Fig. 222-3).

After making the incision, the cricoid should spring open, and the endotracheal tube should be readily visible. Stay sutures of 3-0 silk are placed on each side of the incised cricoid (Fig. 222-4). A small cartilage or hyoid graft may be interposed at this point for further expansion (Fig. 222-5). The graft can be used as retractors in the event of accidental extubation. The skin is then loosely approximated around a small rubber band drain (Fig. 222-6).

GERALD B. HEALY

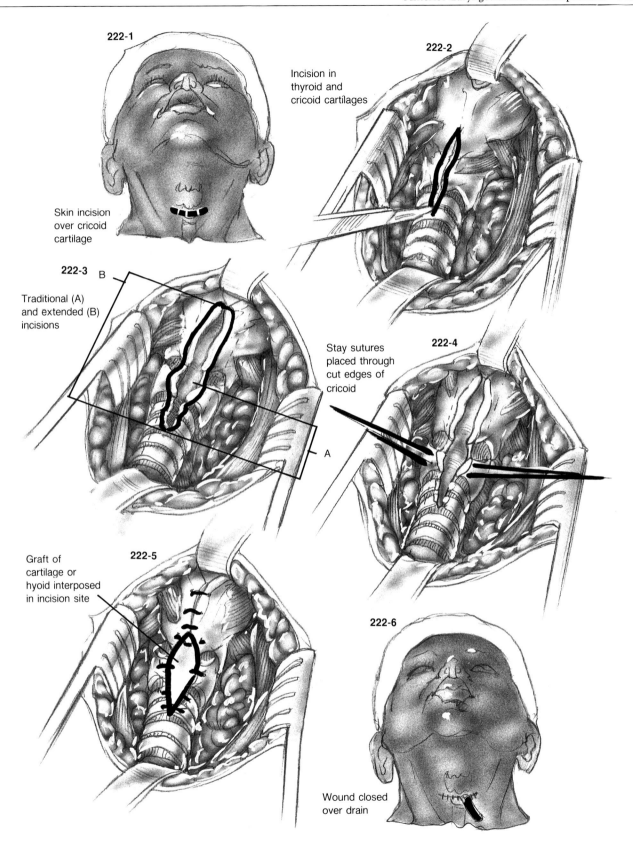

222-1

Skin incision over cricoid cartilage

222-2

Incision in thyroid and cricoid cartilages

222-3

Traditional (A) and extended (B) incisions

B

A

222-4

Stay sutures placed through cut edges of cricoid

222-5

Graft of cartilage or hyoid interposed in incision site

222-6

Wound closed over drain

■ *223.* POSTERIOR GLOTTIC SPLIT WITH CARTILAGE GRAFT—Restoration of laryngotracheal patency with normal oronasal respiration, preventing damage to the laryngeal structures essential for normal vocalization

Indications

1. Cotton's grade 3 or 4 subglottic stenosis
2. Impaired vocal fold mobility
3. In conjunction with an anterior glottic graft (see Procedure 222)

Special Considerations

1. Upper respiratory infection or asthma
2. Gastroesophageal reflux
3. Preoperative vocal fold function

Preoperative Preparation

1. Routine laboratory studies
2. Bleeding and clotting studies
3. Significant subglottic stenosis (see Procedure 222)
4. Vocal fold dynamics
5. Laryngeal electromyogram (optional)

Special Instruments, Position, and Anesthesia

1. Headlight
2. Supine position with shoulder roll
3. Potts scissors
4. Second instrument set to harvest costal cartilage
5. Sterile endotracheal tube (ie, Reye tube), with extension tubing on the back table

Tips and Pearls

1. Minimal dissection
2. Insertion of an anterior augmentation graft (ie, costal cartilage)
3. Hemostasis
4. Do not excise scar tissue.
5. Divide the posterior cricoid plate completely.
6. Divide interarytenoid scar tissue submucosally with Potts scissors.
7. Fit a cartilage graft in position between the distracted halves of the cricoid plate, and secure it with 5-0 Vicryl sutures.
8. The graft should be less wide than the space created between the cricoid halves. If the graft is larger, the lateral pressure exerted by the cricoid halves pushes the graft out of position.
9. Suture the laterally based mucosal flap down. The flap acts as a tarpaulin to hold the cartilage graft in position.

Pitfalls and Complications

1. Graft extrusion
2. Esophageal injury
3. Pneumothorax
4. Pneumomediastinum
5. Poor voice

Postoperative Care Issues

1. Sedation; short-term paralysis in some cases
2. Duration of intubation: body weight less than 2500 g, 10 to 14 days; more than 2500 g, 7 to 10 days.
3. Antibiotics
4. Careful monitoring in the intensive care unit for accidental extubation
5. Corticosteroids, administered 24 hours before extubation (dexamethasone, 0.25 mg/kg/dose q6h).

References

Cotton R. The problem of pediatric laryngotracheal stenosis: a clinical and experimental study on the efficacy of autogenous cartilage grafts placed between the vertically divided halves of the posterior lamina of the cricoid cartilage. Laryngoscope 1991;101:1.

Cotton R, Myer C. Innovations in pediatric laryngotracheal reconstruction. J Pediatr Surg 1992;27:196.

Operative Procedures

The patient is placed in the supine position, using a shoulder roll to flex the neck and extend the head. The neck and chest are prepared and draped. A posterior glottic split with a cartilage graft is used in conjunction with an anterior cartilage graft as part of a laryngotracheoplasty. The operative description is similar to that of Procedure 222, and only the points pertinent to the exposure and placement of the posterior glottic graft are discussed here.

After the larynx and trachea are opened, the stenosis is inspected (Fig. 223-1). Redundant scar tissue is not excised. If placement of an anterior graft does not provide an adequate airway, the posterior plate of the cricoid is divided. Division is usually necessary for severe stenosis (ie, Cotton's grade 3 or 4) or in cases of marked interarytenoid scarring with limited vocal fold motion.

A vertical incision is made through the overlying cricoid mucosa approximately 5 mm to the right or to the left of the midline to expose part of the posterior cricoid plate (Fig. 223-2). The incision is carried through the perichondrium overlying the cricoid plate. Using a Cottle elevator, a subperichondral pocket is created medially. The vertical incision is extended medially at the superior and inferior edge of the cricoid plate to a point 1 mm across the midline on the opposite side. This results in a laterally based subperichondral flap that exposes the midline of the cricoid plate. The posterior cricoid plate is divided in the midline from the superior to inferior aspects. Halves of the cricoid are distracted using a Freer elevator to expose the underlying fibers of the esophagus (Fig. 223-3). The size of the posterior cricoid defect is measured (about 2 mm) and an adequate piece of costal cartilage harvested.

The harvested cartilage is cut into a rectangle to bridge the posterior cricoid defect. The width of the posterior cricoid graft is cut slightly smaller than the size of the defect, and the length of the graft is cut equal to the height of the cricoid plate. The graft should not be forced into position, because lateral pressure from the cricoid halves will push the too-tight graft into the airway.

After the graft is in position, it is sutured at its corners. This is extremely difficult. Usually, two sutures can be secured. The laterally based mucosal flap is sutured over the graft. The flap acts like a tarpaulin and eliminates any potential for graft movement. Firmly anchor the graft with 5-0 Vicryl sutures (Fig. 223-4).

A posterior graft is usually done in conjunction with an anterior graft as part of a two-stage laryngotracheal procedure. It is also possible to use a posterior graft in a one-stage procedure. Details of these operations are described in Procedure 222. If a one-stage procedure is performed, the patient should be extubated in the operating room so that the posterior glottis can be carefully inspected. A small amount of granulation tissue may be seen over the area of the laterally exposed cricoid cartilage (Fig. 223-5).

RICHARD J.H. SMITH

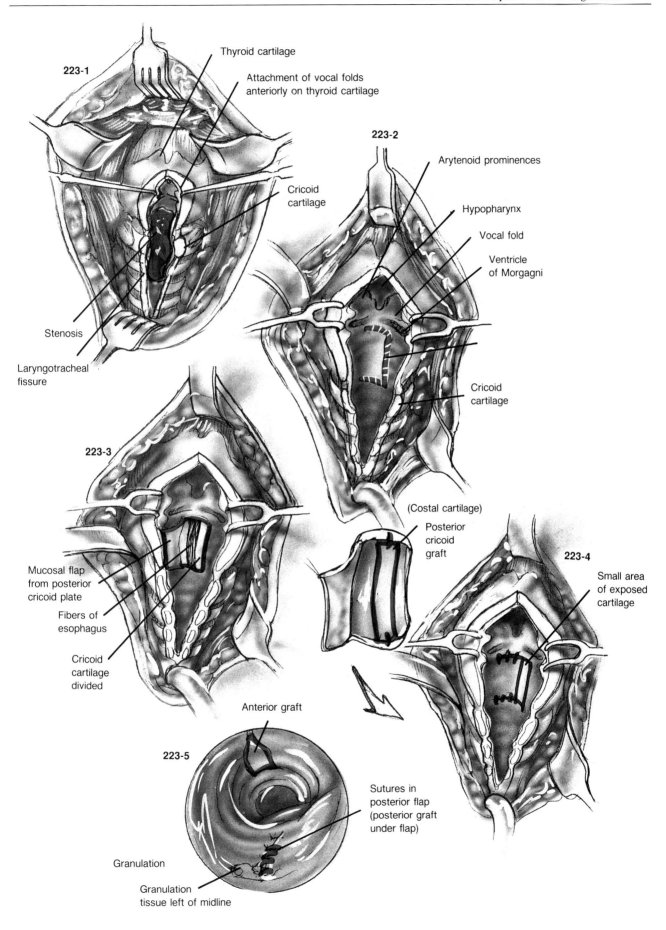

223-1

Thyroid cartilage

Attachment of vocal folds
anteriorly on thyroid cartilage

Cricoid
cartilage

Stenosis

Laryngotracheal
fissure

223-2

Arytenoid prominences

Hypopharynx

Vocal fold

Ventricle
of Morgagni

Cricoid
cartilage

223-3

Mucosal flap
from posterior
cricoid plate

Fibers of
esophagus

Cricoid
cartilage
divided

(Costal cartilage)

Posterior
cricoid
graft

223-4

Small area
of exposed
cartilage

Anterior graft

223-5

Sutures in
posterior flap
(posterior graft
under flap)

Granulation

Granulation
tissue left of midline

224. ANTERIOR AND POSTERIOR LARYNGO-
TRACHEAL RECONSTRUCTION—Repair to restore laryngotracheal patency with normal oronasal respiration and to prevent damage to laryngeal structures essential for normal vocalization

Indications
1. Cotton's grade 2 to 4 stenosis
2. Impaired vocal fold mobility

Special Considerations
1. Upper respiratory infection or asthma
2. Gastroesophageal reflux
3. Preoperative vocal fold evaluation
4. Location, length, consistency, and degree of stenosis
5. Potential problems in other areas of the airway, such as choanal atresia or stenosis, tracheomalacia, and bronchopulmonary dysplasia

Preoperative Preparation
1. Routine laboratory studies
2. Bleeding, clotting studies
3. Recognition of associated problems
4. Soft tissue films or xeroradiographs of the airway
5. Computed tomography (CT) scan or cine CT scan of the airway (optional)
6. Flexible fiberoptic laryngoscopy
7. Microsuspension laryngoscopy and bronchoscopy
8. A 24-hour pH probe (optional)
9. Chest radiograph

Special Instruments, Position, and Anesthesia
1. Pott's scissors
2. Second instrument set to harvest costal cartilage
3. Sterile endotracheal tube (ie, Reye tube) with extension tubing on the back table
4. Supine position, using a shoulder roll

Tips and Pearls
1. Obtain a tracheal aspirate for Gram stain, and culture the sample at the beginning of treatment.
2. Expose stenosis before harvesting costal cartilage.
3. If possible, avoid dividing the anterior commissure.
4. If the anterior commissure is divided, immediately tag the anterior ligament on either side with colored Vicryl. The anterior ligament must be reapproximated exactly for optimal vocalization postoperatively.
5. Do not excise scar tissue.
6. Preserve perichondrium on one side of the cartilage graft.
7. Pack the laryngotracheal fissure with cocaine-wetted cottonoids while harvesting cartilage.
8. Close the donor site before continuing with the laryngotracheoplasty.
9. For one-stage procedures, reintubate orally with an appropriately sized endotracheal tube; for two-stage procedures, select the appropriate Aboulker stent.
10. Secure the anterior graft in position; the tracheal mucosal surface must be flush with the costal cartilage perichondrium.
11. If an Aboulker stent is used, anchor with a transtracheal suture.

(continued)

Operative Procedure
The patient is placed in the supine position, using a shoulder roll to flex the neck and extend the head. The neck and chest are prepared and draped. A transverse incision is made across the midline of the neck at the level of the midpoint of the stenosis. In cases of subglottic stenosis, this usually corresponds to a point 5 to 10 mm below the inferior edge of the cricoid cartilage. The incision is extended through the platysma, and superiorly and inferiorly based subplatysmal flaps are elevated to expose the underlying strap muscles. Retraction is provided by stay sutures.

The underlying strap muscles are divided in the midline and reflected laterally to expose the trachea and larynx (Fig. 224-1). Stay sutures are used to retract the strap muscles. If the patient has a tracheotomy and a one-stage procedure is being done, dissection should be carried inferiorly to expose the tracheotomy site. If a two-stage procedure is being performed and the stenosis does not extend to the tracheotomy site, the tracheotomy site does not need to be exposed during the dissection. However, for long segmental stenosis, the tracheotomy site frequently must be included in the dissection.

After obtaining adequate tracheal and laryngeal exposure, a laryngotracheal fissure is performed. If the stenosis is Cotton's grade 2 or 3 and the tracheal lumen can be easily entered inferior to the stenosis, the trachea is opened at that point. Using a Cottle elevator, the tracheal lumen is probed. A #12 blade is placed into the tracheal lumen, and the trachea is opened in the midline from the mucosal surface outward, progressing slowly superiorly. As the subglottic area is approached, it is important to stay in the midline. If the stenosis does not extend to the level of the vocal folds, the anterior commissure should not be divided. However, if the stenosis extends to the vocal folds and the thyroid cartilage and anterior commissure are divided, immediately reattach the vocal folds to the edges of the thyroid cartilage. It is important to oppose the vocal folds exactly when closing the laryngofissure to obtain a good postoperative voice result. The mucosal edges along the laryngotracheal fissure are sewn to the free edges of cartilage to provide hemostasis and prevent mucosal tearing.

By gently retracting on the edges of the laryngotracheal fissure, the stenosis can be inspected. Redundant scar tissue is not excised. If placement of an anterior graft can provide an adequate airway, division of the posterior plate of the cricoid is unnecessary. However, in cases of severe stenosis (ie, Cotton's grade 3 or 4) or marked interarytenoid scarring with limited vocal fold motion, a posterior graft is necessary. Measure the laryngotracheal defects so that an adequate piece of costal cartilage is harvested. Place cocaine-soaked cottonoids in the airway for hemostasis, cover the operative site, and change gown and gloves.

Use a second instrument set to harvest the costal cartilage. Make an incision parallel to and 1 cm above the right or left costal margin, approximately 3 cm from the midline. The incision should be approximately 5 cm long. Extend the incision through the rectus abdominis to expose the underlying costal cartilage. Mark an appropriately sized piece of cartilage to harvest, preserving the perichondrium on the exposed surface. Obtain meticulous hemostasis, and gently incise around the marked perimeter. Use a Freer elevator carefully to extend the incision through the cartilage, taking full-thickness cartilage but leaving the perichondrium on the inner surface down. Dissect from lateral to medial aspects, gently retracting on the free lateral edge as the cartilage is mobilized.

After the donor cartilage has been removed, fill the wound with saline, and apply positive-pressure ventilation to establish whether the pleural cavity has been entered. The wound bed should be carefully inspected for a consistent air leak, which would signify the presence of a pneumothorax. Verify the pneumothorax on an intraoperative chest x-ray film, and if significant, insert a chest tube.

The laryngofissure then is reinspected. Secure a posterior cricoid graft in position if one is required. If a one-stage laryngotracheoplasty is being performed, the Reye tube should be removed and the patient should be intubated with an appropriately sized endotracheal tube. Help the anesthesiologist by directing the tip of the endotracheal

(continued)

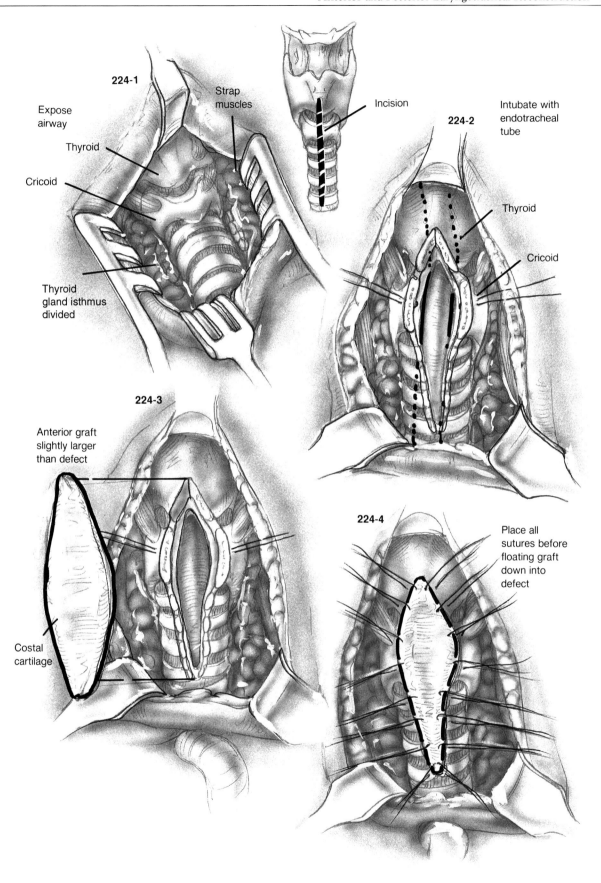

224-1

Expose
airway

Thyroid

Cricoid

Thyroid
gland isthmus
divided

Strap
muscles

Incision

224-2

Intubate with
endotracheal
tube

Thyroid

Cricoid

224-3

Anterior graft
slightly larger
than defect

Costal
cartilage

224-4

Place all
sutures before
floating graft
down into
defect

224. ANTERIOR AND POSTERIOR LARYN-GOTRACHEAL RECONSTRUCTION *(continued)*

Pitfalls and Complications

1. Restenosis
2. Poor voice
3. Pneumothorax
4. Pneumomediastinum
5. Graft extrusion

Postoperative Care Issues

One-Stage Repair

1. Paralysis
2. Broad-spectrum antibiotic coverage
3. Reflux precautions (i.e., Ranitidine, 0.5 mg/kg, given intravenously every 8 hours)
4. Daily chest x-ray films and daily record of the patient's weight
5. Chest physical therapy with log-rolling every 4 hours
6. Perform a leak test beginning on postoperative day 4. To perform this test, remove the patient from the ventilator; place the head in a neutral position; ventilate with Ambu bag; and auscultate over the cervical trachea for an air leak. An air leak at a pressure of 20 cm H_2O or less is a good prognostic sign for successful extubation.

Two-Stage Procedure

1. Broad-spectrum antibiotic coverage
2. Reflux precautions (i.e., Ranitidine, 0.5 mg/kg, given intravenously every 8 hours)
3. Chest radiograph
4. Remove Aboulker stent in operating room 3 months after the procedure.
5. Bronchoscopy 2 weeks after Aboulker stent removal
6. Decannulate

References

Cotton R. Pediatric laryngotracheal stenosis. J Pediatr Surg 1984;19:699.
Smith RJH. Laryngotracheal stenosis. Head Neck 1987;10:38.

tube into the distal trachea after suctioning blood and secretions from the right and left main bronchi (Fig. 224-2).

After the endotracheal tube is in position, the size of the anterior defect is readily apparent (see Fig. 224-2). The anterior graft must be slightly larger than the observed defect to minimize mucosal compression by the endotracheal tube after the anterior graft is sewn in position (Fig. 224-3). Use 5-0 Vicryl sutures passed through the tracheal cartilage and costal graft, placing all sutures in position before floating the graft carefully down into the defect (Fig. 224-4). The graft should be secured carefully, and the sutures should exactly approximate the perichondrial surface of the graft to the mucosal surface of the trachea. Because the cartilage graft is thicker than the tracheal rings, the outer tracheal surface and graft will not be flush. The closure should be airtight; after the graft is sewn in position, positive pressure should be used to test for leaks. Close any leaks with additional sutures (Fig. 224-5). The wound is drained and closed in layers, reapproximating strap muscles and platysma.

If a two-stage laryngotracheoplasty is performed, an appropriately sized Aboulker stent should be selected to maintain the lumen. The length of the stenosis must be measured, and the Aboulker stent must be slightly longer to extend above and below the stenotic segment. Aboulker stents have removable plugs. The plug should be removed and the stent trimmed to the appropriate length. The plug is refitted so that both ends of the Aboulker stent are smooth. If the stent does not extend above the vocal folds, the ends of the plug, which are normally sealed, can be opened; however, if the Aboulker stent extends above the vocal folds, the ends of the plug should not be opened to avoid aspiration.

After the stent has been appropriately fitted, it is soaked in normal saline until it is needed. A posterior graft is secured in position at this time. The anterior graft then is carved from the harvested costal cartilage. Usually the graft is boat shaped, coming to a point at the "bow" and "stern" (see Fig. 224-3). The width of the graft should be slightly larger than the width of the stenotic segment. Using 5-0 Vicryl suture, the tracheal rings are approximated to corresponding points in the cartilage graft. When the graft is sewn in position, the perichondrial surface of the graft should be flush with the mucosal surface of the trachea. Place all sutures before floating the graft into position.

After all sutures have been placed in the costal graft, the Aboulker stent should be slipped into the airway. Using a 2-0 nylon transtracheal suture, the stent is secured by passing a suture through one side of the trachea, through the stent, and through the opposite side of the trachea. When this suture is pulled taut, the stent should be properly positioned and extend from slightly above to slightly below the stenotic segment. The anterior graft is floated down into the tracheal defect, and the 5-0 Vicryl sutures are tied. Because the distal aspect of the graft often is more difficult to secure, these sutures should be tied first (Fig. 224-6).

After the graft has been secured, the strap muscles are approximated. The stay suture anchoring the stent is tied with a small piece of feeding tube over the right arm of the stay suture to prevent overtightening and cutting the airway. The suture is tied on the left side (Fig. 224-7). It is a good idea to be consistent and to tie the stay suture on the same side in each case. This makes it easier to find the knot several months later. The remainder of the incision is drained and closed in layers (Fig. 224-8).

An essential aspect of a laryngotracheoplasty is postoperative patient care. For a one-stage procedure, this necessitates 7 to 10 days in the intensive care unit with the patient under heavy sedation and paralysis. Beginning on the fourth postoperative day, the patient should be tested for an air leak. An audible air leak at a pressure of 20 cm H_2O or less is a valuable sign for a successful extubation. Two days before the time of anticipated extubation, Decadron is started. Twenty-four hours before extubation, furosemide is used to remove excess body water, and narcotics and paralytics are tapered. For complicated repairs or if an audible leak is not detected, extubation in the operating room is advisable. However, for simple one-stage repairs with an audible leak before extubation, this is unnecessary (Fig. 224-9).

RICHARD J. H. SMITH

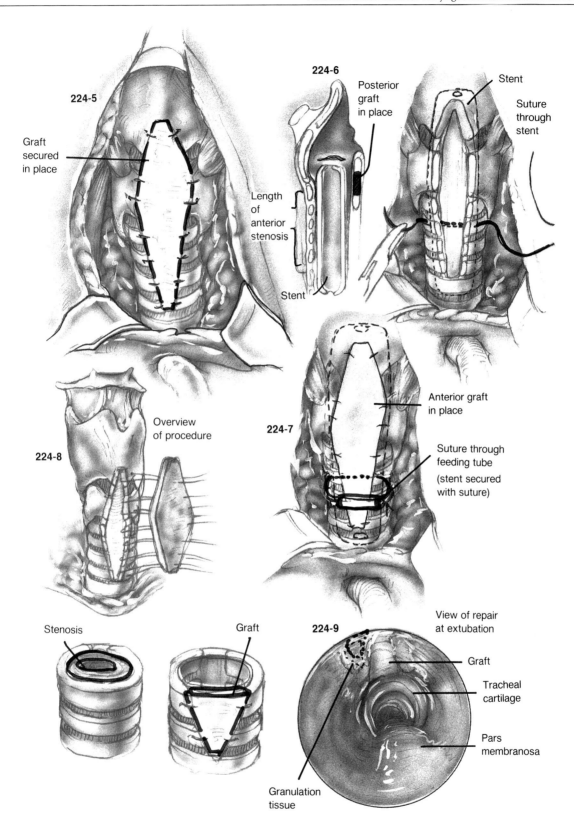

224-5

Graft
secured
in place

224-6

Posterior
graft
in place

Length
of
anterior
stenosis

Stent

Stent

Suture
through
stent

Anterior graft
in place

224-7

Suture through
feeding tube
(stent secured
with suture)

224-8

Overview
of procedure

Stenosis

Graft

224-9

View of repair
at extubation

Graft

Tracheal
cartilage

Pars
membranosa

Granulation
tissue

■ *225.* LARYNGEAL WEBS

Web lysis by microlaryngeal surgery with subsequent serial dilatation until healed or by tissue lysis with the endoscopic insertion of a keel

Indications

1. For microlaryngeal surgery and dilatation, an anterior glottic web that is 50% of the area or less and confined to the vocal cords
2. For the endoscopic keel approach, an anterior web of the larynx tethering both vocal cords in the midline

Special Considerations

1. For microlaryngeal surgery and dilatation
   a. Cooperative patient with minimal gag reflex
   b. Anatomy must be such that the patient is easy to examine indirectly.
   c. Bleeding and clotting abnormalities
   d. Airway maintenance
2. For the endoscopic keel approach
   a. Airway maintenance
   b. Bleeding or clotting abnormalities
   c. Ability to visualize the larynx by endoscopic technique

Preoperative Preparation

1. Routine laboratory studies
2. Bleeding and clotting studies
3. Definition of the extent of the web, possibly using magnetic resonance imaging (MRI) or computed tomography (CT)

Special Instruments

1. For microlaryngeal surgery and dilatation
   a. Microlaryngeal set
   b. Curved blunt local anesthetic laryngeal cannula
   c. Fiberoptic laryngoscope (preferred, but optional)
2. For the endoscopic keel approach
   a. A microlaryngeal set, including microlaryngeal scissors, microlaryngeal alligators, and 0-gauge nylon thread
   b. Silastic (Exmoor Plastics Taunton, England) with a flat posterior keel or one made out of Teflon

Tips and Pearls

1. Proper patient selection
2. Adequate visualization of the anterior commissure
3. The web must be no greater than 60% of the area.
4. The web must not extend subglottically.

Pitfalls and Complications

1. For microlaryngeal surgery and dilatation
   a. Improper patient selection (eg, hand grabber, bad gag reflex)
   b. Airway compromise
   c. Postoperative bleeding
2. For the endoscopic keel approach
   a. Airway obstruction
   b. The sutures may break, and the stent may be lost in the airway.

Postoperative Care Issues

1. For microlaryngeal surgery and dilatation, office visits twice weekly for approximately 4 weeks during the healing process.
2. For the endoscopic keel approach, careful observation for the healing period, which usually is less than 4 weeks, to detect granulation tissue, mucous, or other problems that may complicate the postoperative period.

References

Dedo HH. Endoscopic Teflon keel for anterior glottic web. Ann Otol 1979;88:467.

Jackson C. The nose, throat and ear and their diseases. Philadelphia: WB Saunders, 1930;755.

Parker DA, Das Gupta AR. An endoscopic Silastic keel for anterior glottic webs. J Laryngol Otol 1987;101:1055.

Operative Procedures

Microlaryngeal Web Lysis

The patient is taken to the operating room, where standard microlaryngeal surgery is performed. The larynx is exposed with a microlaryngeal set, and using scissors or a laryngeal knife, a midline cut is made through the web, dividing it to the anterior commissure. If the web was extensive, approximately a 0.1 mL of Kenalog 40 is injected in the incised margins of the newly lysed cord, and the patient is awakened.

The patient is counseled to take a very deep breath at least eight or ten times each day to keep the cords apart during the healing process. The patient comes to the office twice weekly for approximately the next 4 weeks, during which time the larynx is dilated to allow posterior to anterior epithelialization. Recurring webs are broken until epithelialization is complete. During these visits, 4 mL of a 4% solution of Xylocaine, a local anesthetic, is dripped on to the vocal cords using a curved, blunt cannula. After sufficient anesthesia is obtained, the cannula is inserted between the vocal cords with mirror visualization or with fiberoptic visualization and brought quickly anteriorly and superiorly, breaking the reforming web during the healing process. This allows posterior to anterior epithelialization to occur and diminishes the likelihood of the recurrence of a significant web. Using this approach, the web should be minimal and the voice good after healing has occurred (approximately 4 weeks).

Endoscopic Keel Approach

In the operating room, with the patient in the supine position, under general endotracheal anesthesia (or Venturi jet), and prepped and draped in a routine fashion, an anterior commissure laryngoscope is inserted (Fig. 225-1). It is important to visualize the anterior commissure of the cords. After the web is inspected, its depth is estimated. If it is suitable for the procedure, the web is divided precisely in the midline to the thyroid cartilage. A laryngeal knife or up-biting microlaryngeal scissors are preferred for this procedure (Fig. 225-2); I think using the laser to divide the cords results in a more complicated healing process, but this is an alternative for those so inclined.

If the divided web is sufficiently thick, less than 0.1 mL Kenalog is injected on either side, near the anterior commissure, which diminishes on granulation tissue during the healing process (Fig. 225-3).

Two 20-gauge intravenous cannulas (usually obtained from the anesthesiology service) are placed, with one through the cricothyroid membrane and one above the anterior commissure. Zero-gauge nylon suture is inserted through this into the lumen of the larynx. It is grasped with an alligator forceps and brought out through the mouth in both locations. The nylon is secured to the appropriate Silastic or the Teflon keel to prevent raw surfaces from coapting. The keel does not extend near the posterior commissure to prevent a problem in this area. The nylon is fixed to the anterosuperior and anteroinferior aspects of the keel (Fig. 225-4). The keel is then brought down endoscopically toward the anterior commissure and anchored there with buttons tied over anterior neck skin (Fig. 225-5).

The patient is awakened, and the airway is monitored. After discharge, the patient is examined in the office twice weekly and is taken back to the operating room in 3 to 4 weeks for endoscopic removal of the keel, performed under general endotracheal anesthesia. The suture is cut, and the keel is pulled out through the mouth. At this time, any residual web and granulation tissue can be removed with cautery or by injection of another small amount of Kenalog 40 (less than 0.1 mL).

C. RICHARD STASNEY

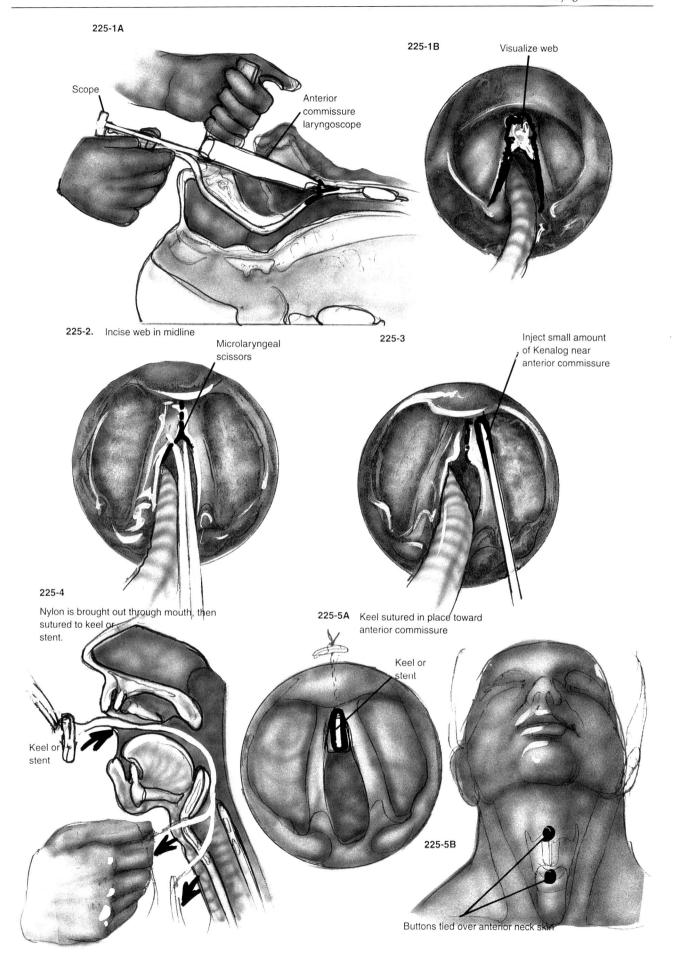

225-1A

Scope

Anterior commissure laryngoscope

225-1B   Visualize web

225-2.   Incise web in midline

Microlaryngeal scissors

225-3

Inject small amount of Kenalog near anterior commissure

225-4

Nylon is brought out through mouth, then sutured to keel or stent.

Keel or stent

225-5A   Keel sutured in place toward anterior commissure

Keel or stent

225-5B

Buttons tied over anterior neck skin

■ 226. STROBOSCOPY

Detailed study of the vibratory characteristics of the vocal cords during phonation to analyze symmetry, amplitude, periodicity, mucosal wave, and glottal closure

Indications

1. Dysphonia with a lesion
2. Dysphonia without a lesion
3. Dysphonia with paralysis or paresis

Special Considerations

1. Preoperative and postoperative examinations
2. Total aphonia

Special Instrumentation, Position, and Anesthesia

1. Stroboscope
2. A 90° endoscope with zoom capabilities
3. Flexible fiberoptic scope
4. Machida 70° endoscope
5. 23- and 38-mm lenses
6. Video cassette recorder (VCR) and television (TV) monitor
7. Camera
8. Glass bead sterilizer or other means of warming the lens to prevent fogging
9. Large-millimeter lens for close up views
10. Smaller-millimeter lens for brighter light
11. Flexible fiberoptic scope for hyperpharyngeal sensitivity
12. Patient positioned with the tilted forward from the waist

Tips and Pearls

1. Speech pathologist, with a specialty in voice, to facilitate behavioral modification for best study
2. Sustained "E" vowel to facilitate viewing of true vocal cords
3. Videotaping enables slow-motion observation of phonation and allows comparison, review, and consultation.

Operative Procedure

Videostroboscopic examination is used to view the vibratory characteristics of the vocal cords during phonation (Fig. 226-1). It provides a detailed investigation of the integrity of the vocal cords. The endoscopic light source allows examination of abduction and adduction and superior surface, medium to large lesions. The stroboscopic light source presents a slow-motion view of the cords, permitting examination of the infraglottic surface, glottal closure, integrity of the mucosal wave, adynamic segments, symmetry, periodicity, and amplitude. Stroboscopy clearly defines lesion borders, stiffness, and infringement not visible under endoscopic light. The procedure helps to avoid missed diagnoses and misdiagnoses, differentiates lesions, differentiates between mucus and a lesion, and detects lesions hidden on infraglottic surface. The more comprehensive diagnosis refines the prognosis and helps in the choice of behavioral modification, surgical remediation, or a combination of these options for treatment.

Indications include paralysis or paresis or dysphonia with or without an identifiable lesion on examination. Because the strobe light triggers only with phonation, an aphonic patient cannot be strobed. Stroboscopic evaluation is often used in preoperative and postoperative examinations for specific definition of the operative sight and for reviewing the healing process when approaching rehabilitation.

The patient provides an acoustic sample by reading a standard passage. This allows perceptual analysis and documentation of the voice. The patient is seated, tilted forward from the waist, in an examination chair with his or her mouth at approximately the clinician's eye level (Fig. 226-2). The scope is attached to a lens and camera to allow VCR input and viewing on a TV monitor (Fig. 226-3). The patient provides sustained "E" vowel trials for endoscopic and stroboscopic examination. The examiner is able to guide the patient through tasks to facilitate viewing the cords in different aspects of the vibratory cycle for examination of the stroboscopic parameters. The pedal is held in the first position for endoscopic light, second position for "running strobe," and feathered to hold an open or closed phase, inspect the vertical phase difference, and view surfaces of the cord visible only with strobe.

Each of the following parameters refers to the cords during motion under stroboscopy; all parameters depend on lesion size and composition. *Symmetry* is the degree to which the cords provide a mirror image of each other. They should proceed into lateral excursion and return to median position at the same time. Classic asymmetry, which appears as the cords chasing each other, can be seen in unilateral vocal cord paralysis. *Amplitude* is the extent that each cord moves into lateral excursion from the midline of the glottis. The degree of amplitude can be influenced by intensity, pitch, unilateral lesions, or broad-based bilateral lesions. *Periodicity* refers to the regularity of the glottal cycle. This should be evaluated over successive cycles. Aperiodicity appears as a fluttering of the cords and usually obliterates any reliable judgment of the other parameters.

Mucosal wave is the wave like motion that is observed as a result of the Bernoulli effect, alternately bringing the cords together and apart. A normal wave usually extends from the medial edge of each cord laterally to about 50% of the superior surface. A stiffened or unequal wave can indicate stiffness of the cover. An adynamic segment in the wave can indicate a very stiff, mature lesion or cystic mass. A full, extended wave can represent full cord edema that is invisible on endoscopic examination.

Glottal closure is the degree to which the vocal cords approximate each other in the closed phase of the cycle. The alternating closure of the inferior and superior lip can be referred to as vertical *phase* difference. Many lesions are hidden on the infraglottic edge of the cords and can be discovered through observing this parameter. True closure cannot be evaluated under endoscopic light.

ELIZABETH S. LUKEN
JAMES L. NETTERVILLE

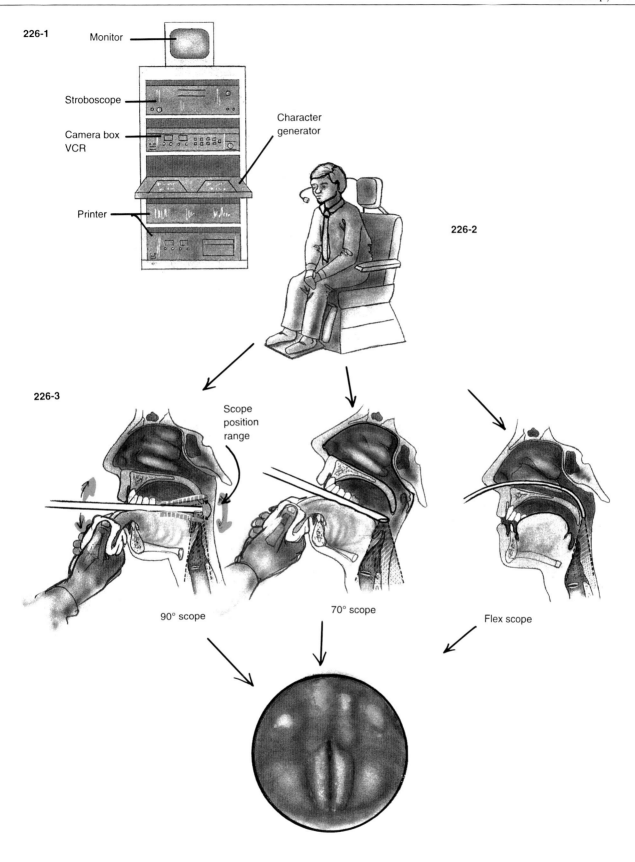

226-1

Monitor

Stroboscope

Camera box
VCR

Printer

Character
generator

226-2

226-3

Scope
position
range

90° scope

70° scope

Flex scope

■ *227.* THYROPLASTY (PHONOSURGERY)

TYPE I—Surgical medialization of a vocal cord

Indications

1. Paralyzed vocal cord with inadequate closure for acceptable voice
2. Incompetent glottis and inadequate closure of the vocal cords

Special Considerations

1. Airway management
2. Bleeding or clotting abnormalities
3. Adequate time must elapse to ensure the vocal cords cannot regain mobility after temporary paralysis or the opposite cord cannot compensate for the immobile cord; this requires at least 1 year in most cases and an adequate trial of speech therapy.

Preoperative Preparation

1. Bleeding and clotting studies
2. Evaluation of the airway and lung function

Special Instruments, Position, and Anesthesia

1. Thyroidectomy set, angled Weitlaner retractors (eg, X-298, X-300, X-300), and Storz instruments as follows: N-2348 Freer elevator, N-2248 Rosen cartilage knife, N-2252 Freer septum knife, N-5420 Brown-Adson tissue forceps, E-2404 calipers (essential), and a Silastic block at least 2 cm^3
2. Patient in the supine position

(continued)

Operative Procedure

With the patient in the supine position, prepped and draped as for a thyroidectomy, and under local monitored anesthesia, the procedure is begun. A 7-cm incision is made over the midportion of the thyroid cartilage eccentrically located to the side of laryngeal paralysis or incompetence (Fig. 227-1). Strap muscles are divided in the midline and retracted using the Weitlaner retractors. Care is taken to skeletonize the anterolateral portion of the thyroid cartilage, leaving the perichondrium intact but moving the cricothyroid muscle on the paralyzed side posteriorly enough so an adequate window can be created.

With the calipers, the anterior thyroid cartilage is measured from the notch superiorly to its inferior margin (Fig. 227-2). This distance is divided by one half, and a Bovie needle is used to mark this halfway point. This marks the projection of the anterior commissure within 1 to 2 mm. At this point, the size of the thyroid cartilage is evaluated subjectively. In a large male larynx with a heavy thyroid cartilage, a window is outlined, starting anterosuperiorly at a point approximately 5 to 6 mm directly back from the anterior commissure and then outlining a rectangular window of approximately 6 × 12 mm. In a smaller female larynx, this window would be correspondingly smaller, approximately 4 × 9 mm. Four corners of the rectangular window are marked using a Bovie needle point with a very light cautery touch to permanently mark the cartilage on the undersurface of the perichondrium. A #15 blade is used to outline a posteriorly based U-shaped perichondral flap, which is elevated carefully with a Cottle or Freer elevator with the curve anterior and overlapping the previously marked rectangle by several millimeters superiorly, anteriorly, and inferiorly (Figs. 227-3 and 227-4). The window should not be parallel to the superior or inferior edges of the thyroid cartilage, because these are quite irregular. It should be perpendicular to the plane of the patient, although it is better to err more inferiorly than superiorly.

The rectangle is again identified, remeasuring if necessary. In noncalcified cartilage, the surgeon can cut through the outer 50% of the thyroid cartilage with a #11 blade and finish the cut with a combination of a Rosen cartilage knife or a weapon (Fig. 227-5).

(continued)

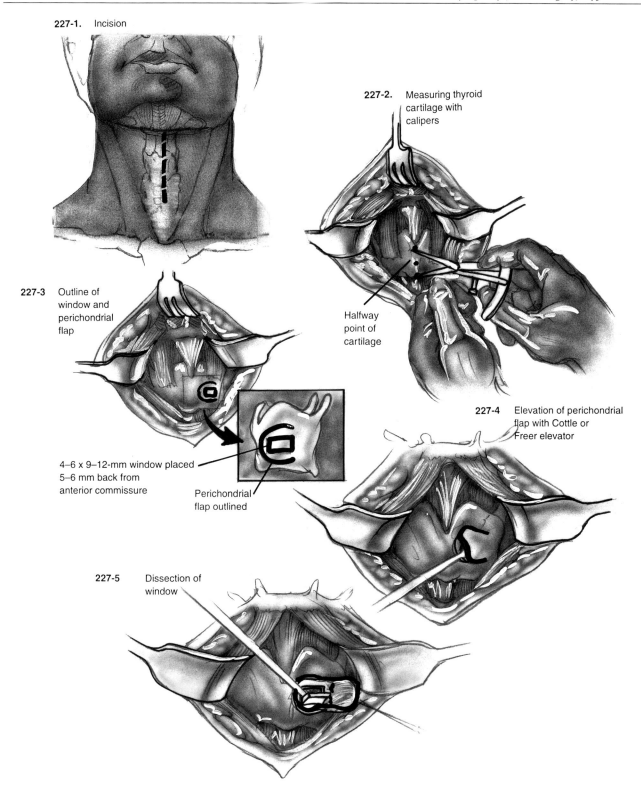

227-1.   Incision

227-2.   Measuring thyroid cartilage with calipers

Halfway point of cartilage

227-3   Outline of window and perichondrial flap

4–6 x 9–12-mm window placed 5–6 mm back from anterior commissure

Perichondrial flap outlined

227-4   Elevation of perichondrial flap with Cottle or Freer elevator

227-5   Dissection of window

■ 227. THYROPLASTY (PHONOSURGERY)
TYPE I (continued)

Tips and Pearls

1. Adequate exposure
2. Adequate dissection around the cartilage window, with an adequate elevation of the inner perichondrium to allow mobility of the cartilage fragment
3. Meticulous measuring of the window for construction of the stent
4. Meticulous suturing of the Silastic stent so it does not move in the postoperative period

Pitfalls and Complications

1. Bleeding
2. Inadequate exposure
3. Making the window too high in the ventricle or too low, causing mobility to be limited by the cricoid

Postoperative Care Issues

1. At least 1 night of hospitalization to monitor the airway and to remove the drain the morning after surgery

References

Ford CN, Bless D. Phonosurgery, assessment and surgical management of voice disorders. New York: Raven Press, 1991.

Isshiki N. Phonosurgery, theory and practice. Tokyo: Springer-Verlag, 1989.

Isshiki N. Phonosurgery videotapes. Philadelphia: The Voice Foundation, 1993.

The weapon is then used to remove the cartilage and elevate around the inner perichondrium for approximately 3 mm on all sides to allow insertion of the implant and adequate medialization of the vocal fold (Fig. 227-6). The surgeon should not to invade the inner perichondrium more than is absolutely necessary.

This technique must be modified in patients with calcified cartilage, as in most males older than 20 years of age and in the posterior aspect of the window in most females. In these cases, a small, fast-cutting microdrill is used to outline the window, and the same caveats apply to the inner perichondrium as stated before. If troublesome bleeding occurs, a small pledget of cotton moistened with epinephrine is placed in the window for a few minutes, and the bleeding usually subsides.

If it is difficult to medialize the window by depressing the inner perichondrium with the blunt posterior surface of the weapon, the window is too low and bound by the cricoid, or there has not been sufficient elevation of the perichondrium. The problem should be corrected before proceeding to the next step.

At this point, the patient's nose is anesthetized, and after modifying the drapes, an assistant or cooperative anesthesiologist inserts a flexible laryngoscope to visualize the vocal folds and display them on a monitor easily seen by the surgeon. By manipulating the inner perichondrium, the surgeon can identify where the implant must go to achieve optimal results and ensure that she or he is not in the ventricle or bound by the cricoid posteroinferiorly. If the medialization is satisfactory, a Silastic implant is prepared as in the illustration (Fig. 227-7, A–C).

Many implant shapes are used, depending on the particular patient and whether more is needed anteriorly, posteriorly, superiorly, or inferiorly (Fig. 227-7). If the vocal process is very lateral, the surgeon can fashion a tail for the Silastic implant to extend under the vocal process and force it medially. The implant is then inserted into the window, and the position and voice are checked before the flexible laryngoscope is removed.

If everything is satisfactory, the implant is removed, and four holes are drilled (Fig. 227-8). Four sutures of 4-0 nylon are used, bringing the needles out as in Figure 227-9, ensuring that the needles exit inside the window such that the implant can be sewn in as a mitral valve is implanted (Fig. 227-10). This prevents the implant from migrating, especially medially.

Hemostasis is ensured, and the wound is irrigated. A mini-Hemovac drain is used. The wound is closed in layers. A thyroidectomy-type dressing is applied. In most cases, the drain is removed the next morning, and the patient is sent home. The voice usually requires several weeks to return to normal, because the cord invariably becomes swollen during the postoperative period. Postoperatively, the surgeon must be certain that there is no compromise of the airway and that the neck heals satisfactorily.

C. RICHARD STASNEY

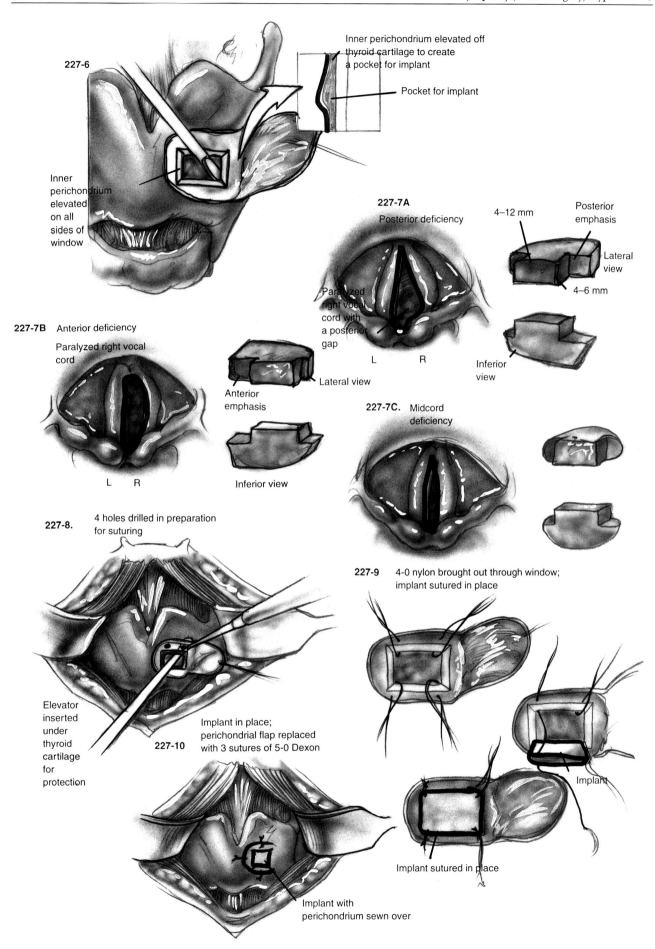

227-6

Inner perichondrium elevated on all sides of window

Inner perichondrium elevated off thyroid cartilage to create a pocket for implant

Pocket for implant

227-7A
Posterior deficiency

Paralyzed right vocal cord with a posterior gap

L   R

4–12 mm

Posterior emphasis

Lateral view

4–6 mm

Inferior view

227-7B Anterior deficiency

Paralyzed right vocal cord

L   R

Lateral view

Anterior emphasis

Inferior view

227-7C. Midcord deficiency

227-8.

4 holes drilled in preparation for suturing

Elevator inserted under thyroid cartilage for protection

227-9   4-0 nylon brought out through window; implant sutured in place

Implant

Implant sutured in place

Implant in place; perichondrial flap replaced with 3 sutures of 5-0 Dexon

227-10

Implant with perichondrium sewn over

■ *228.* THYROPLASTY (PHONOSURGERY)

TYPE II—Thyroplasty is a classic example of surgery done to improve the voice. In thyroplasty, voice change is accomplished by altering the laryngeal cartilaginous framework. Vocal fold lateralization and decreased force of glottic closure are accomplished with type II thyroplasty as described by Isshiki.

Indications
1. Adductor spasmodic dysphonia
2. Mixed dysphonias with hyperadduction
3. Fails or refuses nonsurgical treatment

Contraindications
1. Responsive to chemolysis, voice therapy, or other nonsurgical management
2. Patient does not accept risk of failure or secondary breathy dysphonia.
3. Chronic lung disease or impaired pulmonary function

Special Considerations
1. Procedure is adjustable and technically reversible
2. Intraoperative voice not as useful a predictor of outcome, as in medialization thyroplasty
3. Experience with this procedure is limited, and long-term results are unknown.

Preoperative Preparation
1. Complete voice evaluation and recording
2. Adequate trial voice therapy
3. Explain the options and limitations of the procedure.

Special Instruments, Position, and Anesthesia
1. A #11 BP scalpel, angled elevator (eg, Penfield #4, Woodson), fine (0.5-mm) side-end cutting bur (eg, Microaire Surgical #ZB100)
2. Supine position, with the neck slightly extended
3. Anesthesia screen
4. Local anesthesia with 1% lidocaine plus monitored intravenous sedation
5. Flexible fiberoptic laryngoscope and video monitor

Tips and Pearls
1. Meticulous hemostasis
2. Perichondrium should be preserved, and elevation should be just sufficient to achieve thyroid cartilage overlap.
3. Silastic or miniplate bolster to tie over if cartilage fragile
4. Use miniplate fixation if the larynx is unstable.

Pitfalls and Complications
1. Inner perichondrium disruption favors bleeding and edema.
2. Bleeding and edema mask the result and may obstruct the airway.
3. Patients may be less responsive to Botox chemolysis postoperatively.
4. Mild glottic insufficiency can result in aspiration and breathiness.

Postoperative Care Issues
1. Hospitalization overnight with relative voice rest, monitored vital signs with attention to the airway, head elevated, mist, and analgesics
2. Follow-up voice assessment and voice therapy in 2 to 4 weeks

References
Isshiki N. Phonosurgery theory and practice. Tokyo: Springer-Verlag, 1989.

Woo P. Laryngeal framework reconstruction with miniplates. Ann Otol Rhinol Laryngol 1990;99:772.

Operative Procedure

The patient is premedicated and monitored by an anesthesiologist throughout the procedure. Cottonoids soaked with a 4% solution of cocaine are inserted into the nose on the most patent side, and the neck is prepped with Betadine. A malleable screen (Allen Malleable Anesthesia Screen) is used to support the drapes and create a non-sterile space for the endoscopist to interact with the patient. Sterile drapes are applied, and a 5-cm horizontal incision is marked over the midthyroid cartilage. The soft tissues are infiltrated using a solution of 1% lidocaine with a 1:100,000 concentration of epinephrine. General anesthesia delivered with a small endotracheal tube is a possible alternative.

The skin incision is carried down through platysma muscle, and superior and inferior flaps are developed. The strap muscles are separated with a scissors in the midline, and dissection carried down to the thyroid cartilage perichondrium. Exposure is accomplished from the superior margin of the thyroid cartilage to the cricoid inferiorly and completed posteriorly approximately two thirds of the distance to the posterior cartilaginous edge. Avoidance of trauma to the cricothyroid muscle helps ensure a dry operative field.

A vertical incision is made in the thyroid cartilage at the junction of the anterior one fourth and posterior three fourths using the #11 BP scalpel (Fig. 228-1). Calcified cartilage requires the use of a fine (0.5-mm) side-end cutting bur. Cuts should be placed just short of the inner perichondrium and carefully completed to avoid a perichondrial tear (Fig. 228-2). Approximately 5 mm of inner perichondrium is carefully elevated from the anterior free edge of posterior thyroid cartilage segment with an angled elevator. Elevation of inner perichondrium should be limited to preserve the stability of the cartilaginous framework. After the posterior cartilage is easily displaced lateral to the anterior segment, elevation is terminated.

The endoscopist then inserts and positions a flexible endoscope and observes while the segments are overlapped and the patient is asked to phonate. If there is any bleeding, this is the best time to achieve hemostasis with topical epinephrine or low-voltage thermal cautery. The segments of thyroid cartilage are secured in position with 3-0 nylon sutures (Figs. 228-3 and 228-4). Additional relaxation can be achieved by interposing a wedge of thyroid cartilage harvested from the superior thyroid cartilage rim (Figs. 228-5 and 228-6). If the larynx appears unstable, miniplate fixation can be used to secure the segments.

The wound is closed in layers with 3-0 polyglycolic acid and 5-0 monofilament nylon sutures. A 0.25-in (0.6-cm) Penrose drain is left in place for 12 hours, and the patient is kept on relative voice rest overnight. A mist mask is provided. Perioperative antibiotics or steroids are not used routinely. The patient is discharged the day after surgery and returns in 1 week for suture removal and evaluation by the speech pathologist. Optimal voice results may require adjunctive voice therapy, and these patients need continued follow-up to address their needs and evaluate recurrent symptoms.

CHARLES N. FORD

Thyroplasty Type II

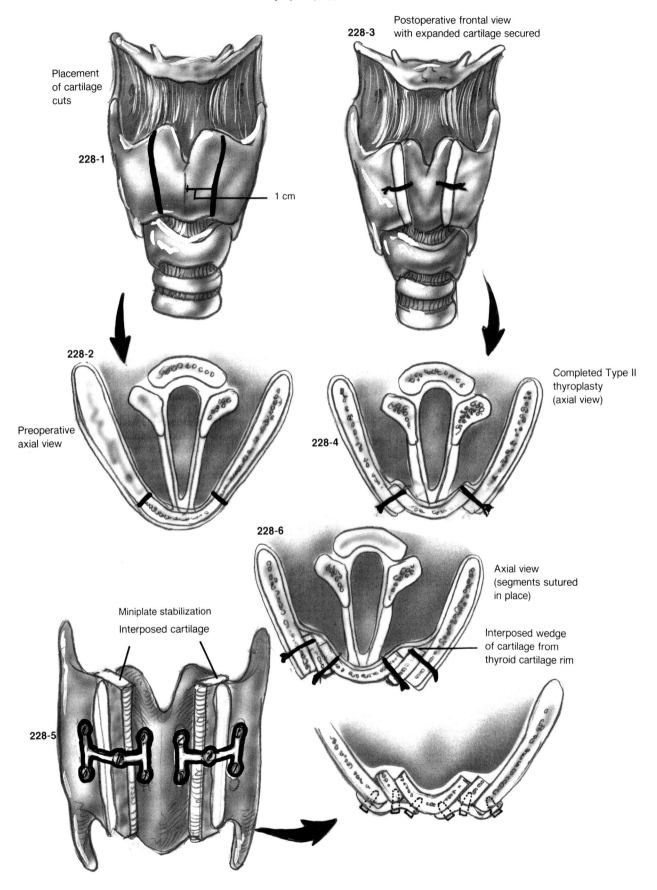

Placement of cartilage cuts

228-1

1 cm

228-3 Postoperative frontal view with expanded cartilage secured

228-2

Preoperative axial view

Completed Type II thyroplasty (axial view)

228-4

228-6

Axial view (segments sutured in place)

Miniplate stabilization

Interposed cartilage

Interposed wedge of cartilage from thyroid cartilage rim

228-5

■ *229.* THYROPLASTY (PHONOSURGERY)

TYPE III—Surgery done to improve the voice by altering the laryngeal cartilaginous framework. Isshiki described a technique in which vertical strips of thyroid cartilage are excised to shorten and relax the tension of vocal folds, thereby lowering the pitch.

Indications

1. Adductor spasmodic dysphonia
2. Refractory mutational falsetto and inappropriately high-pitched male voice
3. High-pitched breathy dysphonia with narrow glottic chink and reduced amplitude of vibration, suggesting an underlying vocal fold stiffness (expect limited results)

Contraindications

1. Responsive to voice therapy or other noninvasive management
2. Sulcus vocalis or other conditions associated with vocal fold scarring and glottic insufficiency
3. Vocal fold paralysis, prior recurrent laryngeal nerve section, Teflon injection, or diminished glottic airway
4. Chronic lung disease or impaired pulmonary function

Special Considerations

1. The procedure is adjustable and technically reversible.
2. Intraoperative voice assessment is more useful in predicting pitch change than control of spasmodic dysphonia.
3. The effect on spasmodic dysphonia may be delayed.
4. Management of subsequent recurrent spasmodic dysphonia symptoms with Botox injections may be more difficult.

Preoperative Preparation

1. Complete voice evaluation and recording
2. Adequate voice therapy trial
3. Manual testing by anterior to posterior thyroid cartilage compression
4. Explain management options and limitations of this procedure to the patient.

Special Instruments, Position, and Anesthesia

1. Bard-Parker #11 scalpel, angled elevator (Penfield #4 or Woodson), fine bur (eg, 0.5-mm side-end cut tapered: Microaire surgical #ZB100)
2. Supine position, with the neck slightly extended; anesthesia screen in place
3. Local anesthesia consists of 1% lidocaine plus intravenous monitored sedation.
4. Flexible fiberoptic laryngoscope and video monitor

Tips and Pearls

1. Meticulous hemostasis
2. Preserve the inner perichondrium.
3. Use a Silastic block or two-hole miniplate bolster to tie over if the cartilage is fragile.
4. Use miniplate fixation if the larynx is unstable.

Pitfalls and Complications

1. Inner perichondrium disruption favors bleeding and edema.
2. Bleeding and edema mask the result and may obstruct the airway.
3. Patients are less responsive to Botox chemolysis postoperatively.

Postoperative Care Issues

1. Hospitalization overnight with relative voice rest, airway observation, head elevation, mist mask, and analgesics
2. The patient should avoid straining, lifting, and attempting to speak at extremes of pitch or loudness for 2 weeks.
3. Follow-up voice assessment and voice therapy in 2 to 4 weeks
4. Refractory recurrent spasmodic dysphonia can subsequently be treated by unilateral surgical neurolysis.

References

Isshiki N. Phonosurgery theory and practice. Tokyo: Springer-Verlag, 1989.

Operative Procedure

The patient is premedicated and monitored by an anesthesiologist throughout the procedure. Cottonoids soaked with a 4% cocaine solution are inserted into the nose on the most patent side, and the neck is prepped with Betadine. A malleable screen (ie, Allen Malleable Anesthesia Screen) is used to support the drapes and create a nonsterile space for the endoscopist to interact with the patient. Sterile drapes are applied, a 5-cm midthyroid cartilage horizontal incision marked, and the soft tissues are infiltrated using a solution of 1% lidocaine with 1:100,000 epinephrine. General anesthesia with a small endotracheal tube is a less desirable alternative and should not be used if pitch change is the primary surgical goal.

The skin incision is carried down through the platysma muscle, and superior and inferior flaps are developed. The strap muscles are separated in the midline, and dissection is carried down to the thyroid cartilage perichondrium. The anterior thyroid cartilage is bluntly exposed in a plane superficial to the perichondrium. Exposure is accomplished from the superior margin of the thyroid cartilage to the cricoid inferiorly and posteriorly, approximately two thirds of the distance to the posterior edge. Avoidance of trauma to the cricothyroid muscle facilitates a dry operative field.

Vertical incisions are placed 0.5 cm posterior to the midline and extended from the superior to inferior rim of the thyroid cartilage (Fig. 229-1). Calcified cartilage requires the use of a fine (0.5-mm) side-end cutting bur. Cuts should extend through the outer perichondrium and the thyroid cartilage but remain just short of the inner perichondrium to avoid inner perichondrial injury (Fig. 229-2). The anterior 1 cm of inner perichondrium is carefully elevated from the posterior thyroid cartilage segment with an angled elevator. The anterior cartilage segment with attached Broyle's ligament is then retrodisplaced into the larynx, allowing the posterior segments to override laterally.

The endoscopist then positions the flexible endoscope and observes while the degree of retrusion is adjusted to achieve an optimal voice. If there is any bleeding, this is the best time to achieve hemostasis with topical epinephrine or low-voltage thermal cautery. The segments of thyroid cartilage are secured in position with 3-0 Nylon sutures (Figs. 229-3 and 229-4) or miniplates.

The wound is closed in layers with 3-0 polyglycolic acid and 5-0 monofilament nylon sutures. A Penrose 0.25-in (6-mm) drain is left in place for 12 hours, and the patient kept on relative voice rest overnight. A mist mask is provided. Perioperative antibiotics or steroids are not used routinely. The patient is discharged the day after surgery and returns in 1 week for suture removal and evaluation by the speech pathologist. Optimal voice results may require adjunctive voice therapy, and these patients need continued follow-up examinations to address their needs and detect recurrent symptoms.

CHARLES N. FORD

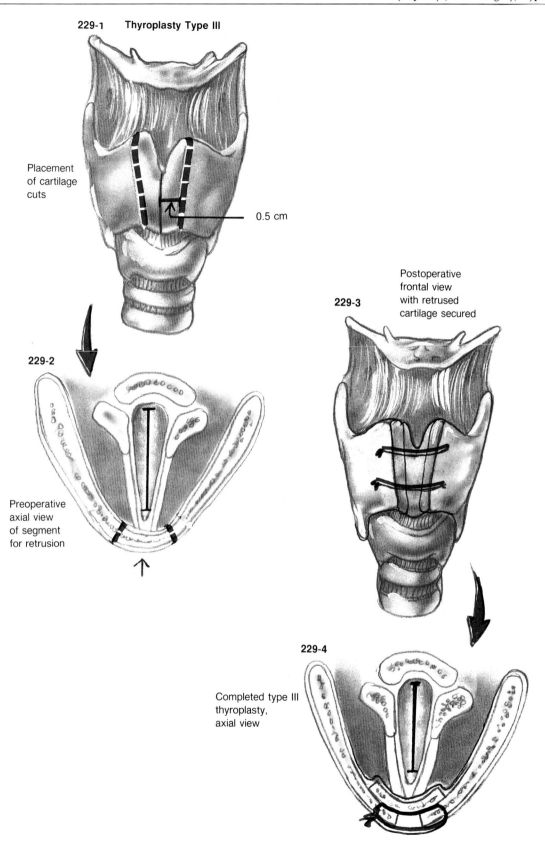

229-1   Thyroplasty Type III

Placement of cartilage cuts

0.5 cm

229-2

Preoperative axial view of segment for retrusion

229-3

Postoperative frontal view with retrused cartilage secured

229-4

Completed type III thyroplasty, axial view

230. THYROPLASTY (PHONOSURGERY)

TYPE IV—Vocal pitch can be raised by approximating the cricoid and thyroid cartilages anteriorly, expanding the thyroid cartilage anteroposterior dimension, intracordal injection of steroids, or altering mass and stiffness by vocal fold incisions or CO_2 laser vaporization. The simplest technique is cricothyroid approximation (thyroplasty type IV), which does not preclude concurrent or subsequent use of the other techniques.

Indications

1. Androphonia
2. Gender-reassigned (transsexual) female
3. Cricothyroid muscle paralysis
4. Acceptable rise in pitch produced by manual cricothyroid approximation (Fig. 230-1)

Contraindications

1. Emotionally unstable individual with unrealistic expectations
2. Presence of other treatable vocal fold pathology, such as Reinke's edema
3. Singer or someone unwilling to accept possible loss of pitch range

Special Considerations

1. If vocal fold mass is the primary problem, it should be addressed by adjunctive measures to secure the best result.
2. Voice therapy and counseling play important roles in the perioperative period.
3. Although the voice is tunable at surgery, fluctuations and deterioration require continued assessment and management by a competent speech pathologist.
4. Additional stability can be gained by the use of an H-shaped miniplate, which is particularly useful in soft cartilage where sutures tend to pull through.

Preoperative Preparation

1. Complete voice evaluation and recording
2. Adequate trial voice therapy
3. Manual testing by cricothyroid approximation (see Fig. 230-1)
4. Explain the options and limitations of the procedure to the patient, and consider psychiatric consultation.

Special Instruments, Position, and Anesthesia

1. Miniplate (two holes) or Silastic block for tie-over bolster
2. Supine poistion, with the neck slightly extended; anesthesia screen in place
3. Local anesthesia with 1% lidocaine plus monitored intravenous sedation

Tips and Pearls

1. Attempt maximum correction because some loosening will occur over time.
2. Try to avoid passing a suture through the inner mucosal lining.
3. The voice may seem unnatural, strained, or almost aphonic immediately after tightening but will achieve the desired quality and pitch within weeks.

Pitfalls and Complications

1. Undercorrection is the most common long-term problem.
2. The thyroid cartilage may be fragile, and sutures under tension can pull through without the use of a tie-over bolster.

Postoperative Care Issues

1. Hospitalization overnight with relative voice rest, airway observation, head elevation, mist mask, and analgesics
2. Patient should avoid straining, lifting, and attempting to speak at extremes of pitch or loudness for 2 weeks.
3. Voice therapy should begin within 2 weeks.
4. Alternative adjunctive measures should be considered if results are judged inadequate.

References

Isshiki N. Phonosurgery theory and practice. Tokyo: Springer-Verlag, 1989.

Isshiki N. Surgical alteration of the vocal pitch. J Otolaryngol 1983;12: 335.

Operative Procedure

The patient is premedicated and monitored by an anesthesiologist throughout the procedure. With the patient in the supine position and with the neck slightly extended, the neck is prepped with Betadine, and sterile drapes are applied. A malleable screen (ie, Allen Malleable Anesthesia Screen) is used to support the drapes and create a nonsterile space for the anesthesiologist to interact with the patient. A 4-cm horizontal incision is marked at the inferior margin of the thyroid cartilage, and the soft tissues are infiltrated with a solution of 1% lidocaine and 1:100,000 epinephrine.

The skin incision is carried down through the platysma muscle, and superior and inferior flaps are developed. The strap muscles are separated with a scissors in the midline, and dissection is carried down to expose the anterior surface of the thyroid and cricoid cartilages (Fig. 230-2). A 3-0 nylon suture or fine-gauge swedged-on wire suture is passed through the midthyroid cartilage just off midline and brought out through the cricothyroid membrane. The same suture is then reinserted through the cricothyroid membrane, hugging the cricoid cartilage to emerge just inferior to the cricoid. The cricoid is circumscribed by then placing the suture back through the cricothyroid membrane and bringing it out through the thyroid cartilage within 3 to 5 mm of where the needle was originally inserted (Figs. 230-3 through 230-5). Care should be taken to hug the cartilage on inner surface passes to avoid intraluminal penetration. One or two such sutures are then placed on either side of midline.

The thyroid cartilage ends are then passed over bolsters, and a single throw of a tie is tightened on either side of the midline while the patient is asked to phonate. When pitch elevation is demonstrated, the first suture is secured while the assistant relieves suture tension by approximating the suture on the opposite side and a second assistant pushes the cricoid cartilage superiorly. The remaining sutures are then tied on alternate sides. Some overcorrection is always desirable. Surgical trauma to the plexus of vessels associated with the cricothyroid muscle is inevitable, but bleeding is easily controlled. The wound is closed in layers with 3-0 polyglycolic acid and 5-0 monofilament nylon sutures. A Penrose 0.25-in (6-mm) drain is left in place for 12 hours, and the patient is kept on relative voice rest overnight. A mist mask is provided. Perioperative antibiotics or steroids are not used routinely. The patient is discharged the day after surgery and returns in 1 week for suture removal and evaluation by a speech pathologist. Patients benefit from close supportive follow-up and treatment by a speech pathologist. Patients who undergo surgery during sexual transition periods need careful psychologic management through their gender-reassignment surgery.

CHARLES N. FORD

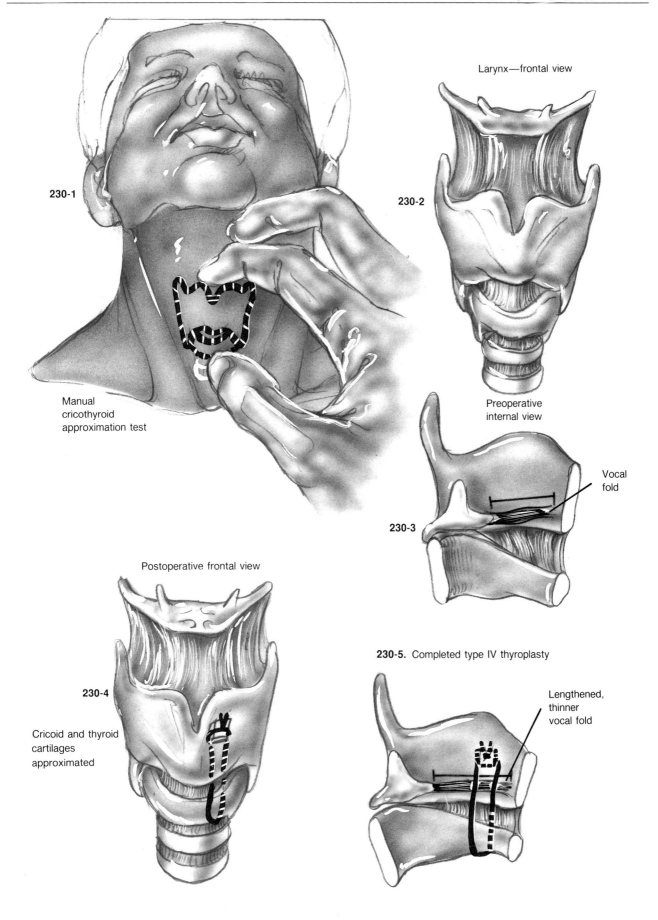

230-1

Manual
cricothyroid
approximation test

Larynx—frontal view

230-2

Preoperative
internal view

Vocal
fold

230-3

Postoperative frontal view

230-4

Cricoid and thyroid
cartilages
approximated

230-5. Completed type IV thyroplasty

Lengthened,
thinner
vocal fold

■ 231. VOCAL CORD INJECTION FOR PARALYSIS

RALYSIS—Glottic insufficiency resulting from vocal cord paralysis can be treated by injecting a filler substance to displace the medial edge of the paralyzed fold toward the midline.

Indications

1. Unilateral vocal fold paralysis with known disruption of nerve, electromyographic evidence of denervation, or persistent immobile vocal fold after 1 year
2. Symptomatic glottic insufficiency with breathy dysphonia, dysphagia, or aspiration
3. Failure to achieve satisfactory improvement with voice therapy

Contraindications

1. Possible laryngeal malignancy or known treatable laryngeal disease causing impaired vocal fold mobility
2. Contralateral vocal fold paresis or glottic airway impairment from any other cause

Special Considerations

1. Alloplastics (eg, Teflon) should be considered first when immediate rehabilitation is needed, especially in the older patient with a known malignancy.
2. Bioimplants are advantageous when some resorption is tolerable.

Preoperative Preparation

1. Laryngoscopy and a complete workup to determine cause of paralysis (an immobile vocal cord does not mean paralysis)
2. A laryngeal electromyogram is useful in determining the prognosis.
3. Minimal voice evaluation should include a voice recording and maximum phonation time.
4. Videostroboscopy can help in assessing effect of paralysis on vocal fold function and in detecting reinnervation.

Special Instruments, Position, and Anesthesia

1. Injections are preferably done using indirect laryngoscopy with the patient under local anesthesia and in the sitting position.
2. When general anesthesia is used, large endotracheal tubes should be avoided, and the laryngoscope should be carefully inserted to avoid glottic distortion.

Tips and Pearls

1. Overinjection must be avoided, and if the vocal fold edge is not medializing with injection, reposition the needle but do not continue to inject.
2. Redistribution of injectate is possible by rubbing the medial edge of the vocal fold with the hub of the injector.
3. The initial placement of the Teflon injection should be lateral to the vocal process to facilitate arytenoid rotation and closure of the posterior commissure.

Pitfalls and Complications

1. Failure to monitor displacement during injection can result in airway obstruction, requiring tracheotomy.
2. Injection of the anterior one third of the vocal fold disturbs vibration of the contralateral vocal fold and prevents posterior glottic closure.
3. Superficial (medial) injection of Teflon results in symptomatic granuloma formation.
4. Subglottic injection produces a strained brassy voice that may be worse than the presenting breathy dysphonia.
5. Injection should be guided by tactile, visual, and auditory senses, even when using a guarded needle.

Postoperative Care Issues

1. Overnight hospitalization for airway observation is appropriate.
2. Voice therapy can enhance the vocal result.

References

Ford CN. Laryngeal injection techniques. In: Ford CN, Fless DM, eds. Phonosurgery—assessment and management of voice disorders. New York: Raven Press, 1991.

Ford CN, Bless DM, Loftus JM. Role of injectable collagen in the treatment of glottic insufficiency: a study of 119 patients. Ann Otol Rhinol Laryngol 1992;101:237.

Operative Procedure

It is important to consider the properties of the specific material being injected. In general, alloplastics must be buried deep in the thyroarytenoid muscle to prevent distortion, increased stiffness, and possible extrusion. Collagen must be injected superficially to produce optimum results and to prevent rapid resorption. Regardless of the material or technique used, it is necessary to visually monitor the morphologic changes during the injection procedure. Ideally, the procedure should be done with the patient awake so that morphologic alterations can be correlated with changes in the patient's voice. Using indirect laryngoscopy and topical anesthesia (Fig. 231-1), the surgeon can monitor the voice result while performing the procedure quickly and with minimal intraoperative risk.

Polytef Paste is provided in 7-mL tubes suitable for instillation into a Bruening intracordal injector (Storz). The 18- and 19-gauge needles are available for direct (straight) or indirect (curved) laryngoscopy. After the paste is squeezed into the barrel of the injector, the ratchet handle is pumped several times until the material appears at the needle tip. The device is designed to deliver 0.2 mL with each click of the ratchet, but the actual volume delivered varies somewhat because of the delay caused by the dissipation of the compression throughout the chamber and needle. It is advisable to wait about 1 minute while the material continues to run out of the needle before beginning injection.

The needle is initially inserted at a point just lateral to the tip of the vocal process of the arytenoid. The tip is aimed a bit laterally so that the bolus of material is lateral to the vocalis (Fig. 231-2) and is in the most lateral aspect of the thyroarytenoid muscle; when the arytenoid is passively mobile, it is possible to medialize the vocal process by placing the bolus at this lateral location. Proper placement may require retracting the posterior false vocal fold with the side of the needle. Typically, 0.6 to 0.8 mL of material is injected at this point (Fig. 231-3), but the actual volume is determined by the degree of medialization achieved and the change in phonation. If the voice is still breathy or if a concavity persists in the midmembranous vocal fold, a second site is injected at the middle of the membranous vocal fold (see Fig. 231-3). This is done incrementally until the medialization is satisfactory. To avoid complications at this site, it is particularly important to place the needle deep (laterally) in the thyroarytenoid muscles.

It is not advisable to inject alloplastics superficially because of the risk of distortion, stiffness, extrusion, and granuloma formation. Injection in the anterior one third of the vocal fold may further compromise glottic closure. If the material is not distributed appropriately, the contour can be modified by rubbing the edge of the needle against the medial edge of the vocal fold; this type of manipulation is only successful at the time of initial injection before the implant is encapsulated. The surgeon should strive for optimal results the first time, because it is difficult to make modifications later. It is also important to avoid overinjection. The injection of too much material—often associated with injection in the subglottic plane—results in reduced vocal function and a noisy, brassy voice quality.

Autologous collagen is being evaluated. The injection device is inserted transorally and directed to the posterior one third of the membranous vocal fold, where the needle is carefully inserted (Fig. 231-4). After the initial resistance of the epithelium is overcome, the next point of resistance is the vocal ligament. The injection is started at this point, and incremental displacement occurs as the collagen is introduced. Generally, 0.3 to 0.8 mL of collagen is sufficient for an atrophic paralyzed vocal fold. In the absence of scar tissue, the collagen spreads forward and fills out the vocal fold in the midmembranous and anterior portion. Additional collagen can be injected if there is insufficient dispersion, and this is best done at the midpoint of maximal residual concavity or defect.

CHARLES N. FORD

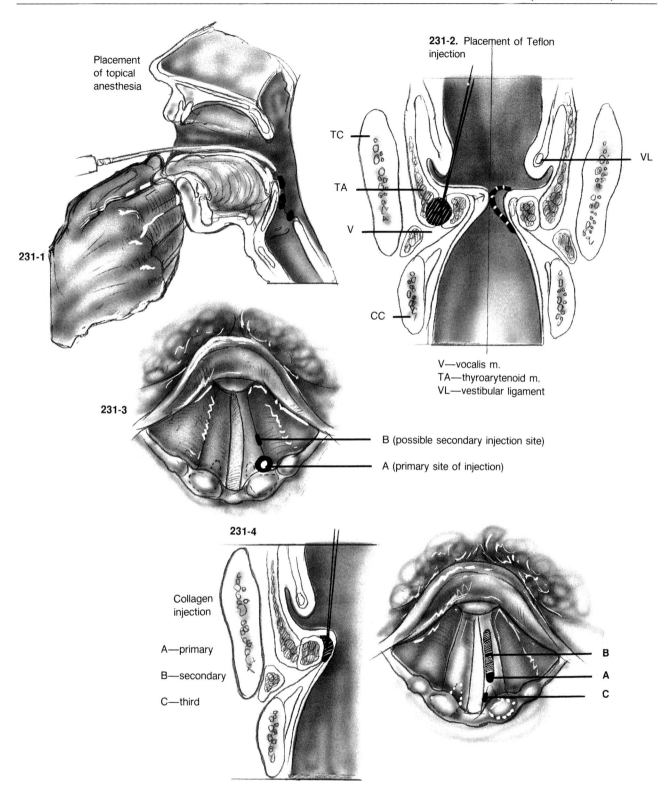

Placement of topical anesthesia

231-1

231-2. Placement of Teflon injection

TC

TA

V

CC

VL

V—vocalis m.
TA—thyroarytenoid m.
VL—vestibular ligament

231-3

B (possible secondary injection site)

A (primary site of injection)

231-4

Collagen injection

A—primary

B—secondary

C—third

B

A

C

232. LARYNGEAL FRACTURE REPAIR

Laryngeal fracture implies damage to the osseocartilaginous framework of the larynx with mucosal disruption. Surgical intervention is necessary to preserve the functional integrity of the larynx, prevent stenosis, and preserve the airway.

Indications

1. History of neck trauma resulting in dyspnea, stridor, dysphonia, difficulty swallowing, and aspiration
2. Physical signs of cervical subcutaneous emphysema with tenderness and loss of detail of the anterior laryngeal landmarks
3. Flexible or indirect laryngoscopic findings of mucosal lacerations, bleeding, or exposed cartilage
4. Indirect findings,such as edema, ecchymosis, hematoma, asymmetric glottis, displaced arytenoids, impaired arytenoid motion, glottic shortening secondary to epiglottic displacement.

Contraindications

1. History of cervical trauma in a stable or improving patient with normal laryngoscopic or minimal findings.
2. Comatose patient or other life-threatening problems needing immediate attention

Special Considerations

1. Rule out associated mandibular or other facial fractures.
2. Consider the possibility of associated cervical spine injury until cervical spine radiographs are evaluated.
3. Tracheotomy under local anesthesia is the proper way to secure the airway in cases of laryngeal trauma.

Preoperative Preparation

1. Physical examination must include indirect laryngoscopy or flexible fiberoptic laryngeal examination.
2. Neck CT scans and cervical spine and chest x-ray films are useful.
3. Steroids should be limited to cases for which surgery is deferred.

Special Instruments, Position, and Anesthesia

1. Stryker saw, hand drill, elevators, and soft tissue instruments
2. Stent pan with preformed stents, Silastic sheeting, Portex tubing.
3. Positioning of the patient varies.
   a. Semisitting position may be necessary for a dyspneic patient during local tracheotomy.
4. After tracheotomy is performed under local anesthesia, general anesthesia is administered.

Tips and Pearls

1. Look for associated aerodigestive tract injuries, such as esophageal tears, cricotracheal separation, and hyoid fractures.
2. An abnormally high hyoid and disrupted tracheal air column may indicate laryngotracheal separation.
3. Place holes for reapproximation of the thyroid cartilage before performing a thyrotomy.
4. Preserve all available mucosa.
5. If primary closure is not possible, use local mucosal flaps (eg, epiglottis, piriform sinus) or grafts.

Pitfalls and Complications

1. Nonrecognition of severe laryngeal injury results in a permanently dysfunctional larynx. Do not underestimate the injury.
2. Do not injure the superior and recurrent laryngeal nerves.
3. Unnecessary stenting increases morbidity. Stent only if needed for skeletal stability or in cases of extensive soft tissue injury.

Postoperative Care Issues

1. Nasogastric suction followed by nasogastric feedings in 24 to 48 hours, as tolerated.
2. Antibiotics are continued in the perioperative period.
3. Defer oral feedings if the stent is poorly tolerated.
4. Use H_2 blockers postoperatively for 2 to 4 weeks.

References

Olsen NR. Acute injuries and chronic stenosis of the larynx, pharynx, and trachea. In: Johnson J, Derkay C, Mandell-Brown MK, Newman RK, eds. Instructional courses of the AAO-HNS. St. Louis: Mosby Year Book, 1991.

Schaefer SD, Close LG. Acute management of laryngeal trauma—update. Ann Otol Rhinol Laryngol 1989;98:98.

Operative Procedures

The patient is placed in a semirecumbent to supine position, with the neck in a neutral to slightly extended position, as tolerated. A horizontal incision is marked 2 to 3 cm above the sternal notch. A tracheotomy is performed and an endotracheal tube is inserted and sutured to the chest. General anesthesia is administered, and the head is repositioned. Direct laryngoscopy and esophagoscopy are performed to assess internal injuries.

A second horizontal incision is made at the midinferior margin of the thyroid cartilage and the subplatysmal flaps are elevated (Fig. 232-1). The strap muscles are separated up to the hyoid bone. The laryngeal exoskeleton and the associated joints, ligaments, and muscles are inspected. If the laryngeal interior can be visualized through an existing defect, it should be used. If thyrotomy is necessary for further diagnosis or management, the periosteum is incised at the midline (Fig. 232-2) and reflected 2 to 3 mm. On either side, two holes are drilled to facilitate reapproximation, and the Stryker saw is used to make a shallow cut through the thyroid cartilage in the midline. The cricothyroid membrane is cut horizontally to allow entrance into the subglottic lumen.

Using direct visualization with a headlight, the inner perichondrium and remaining soft tissues are incrementally sectioned with a #11 blade until the undersurface of the anterior commissure is seen. The commissure is precisely divided and the incision carried up to the thyrohyoid membrane. At this level, a sharp scissors is used to continue the cut superiorly and obliquely off midline to avoid the petiole of the epiglottis and section the aryepiglottic fold on one side if necessary for adequate exposure. The epiglottic cartilage is preserved, and the mucosa is left intact for possible use in grafting.

Soft tissue damage can be assessed and repaired directly. Dislocations of the cricoarytenoid and cricothyroid joints should be repositioned if possible. All mucosal surfaces should be approximated primarily with 4-0 chromic catgut sutures. Denuded cartilage must be covered with soft tissue. If there is insufficient mucosa for primary closure, adjacent mucosa should be recruited or a mucosal graft placed. The lingual surface of the epiglottis and piriform sinus are excellent sources for rotation flaps, and buccal mucosal is a good alternative source for free grafts. If there is extensive mucosal injury or tissue loss, a thin split-thickness skin graft (0.012 in [0.3 mm]) is helpful. The graft can be wrapped around a soft stent constructed from a sponge covered with a double-layered finger cot and secured with 4-0 absorbable suture with the dermal side out (Fig. 232-3).

If a skin graft is not required, a more rigid internal stent that is preformed or constructed from Portex tubing can be used effectively. The preformed stents are particularly useful if there is extensive damage to the cricoid and the larynx is unstable. Stents are used for three purposes: support of grafts and flaps, maintaining the stability of disrupted cartilaginous framework, and prevention of scar contracture and loss of laryngeal lumen. In the absence of these needs, stenting is unnecessary.

Before initiating closure, a small feeding tube is inserted. Closure is started by suturing foreshortened true and false vocal folds to the anterior ends of the thyroid cartilage. The stent is positioned to extend up through the true and false vocal folds and secured with 2-0 nylon sutures that traverse the stent superiorly at the thyrohyoid membrane or upper thyroid lamina and inferiorly through the cricothyroid membrane. The sutures are passed through the strap muscles laterally and then through a button on either side and left to be cinched down later (Fig. 232-4). The larynx is folded together over the stent, and the cartilaginous fragments are aligned and joined together with fine-gauge stainless steel wires. Skip areas and unstable areas can be bridged with miniplate fixation. The stent is then secured by cinching down the buttons over the strap muscles.

The wound is closed, approximating the perichondrium, platysmal, and subcutaneous layers with 3-0 polyglycolic acid suture. The drains are secured and staples used for skin closure. A tracheotomy tube is then inserted to replace the endotracheal tube. In 2 to 3 weeks, the stent is removed.

CHARLES N. FORD

232-1. Incisions for repair of laryngeal fracture

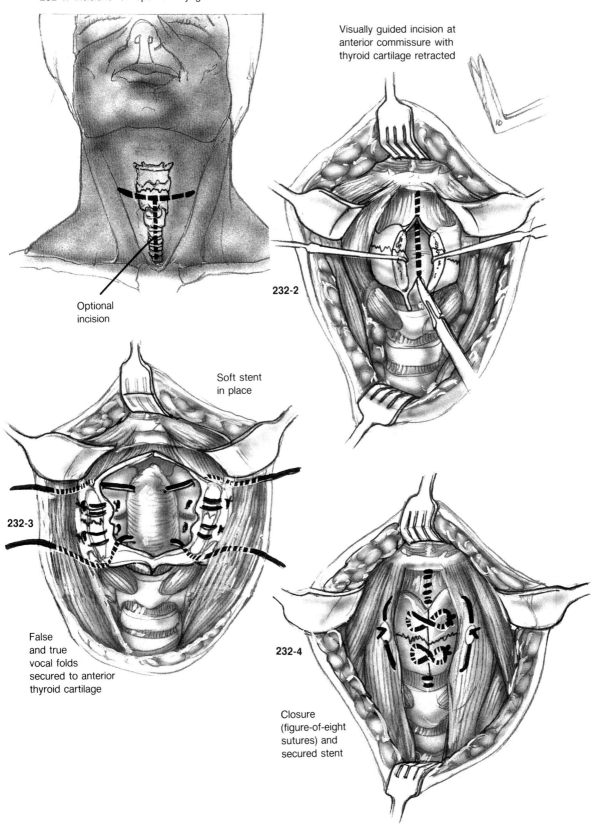

Optional
incision

Visually guided incision at
anterior commissure with
thyroid cartilage retracted

232-2

Soft stent
in place

232-3

False
and true
vocal folds
secured to anterior
thyroid cartilage

232-4

Closure
(figure-of-eight
sutures) and
secured stent

■ *233.* NASOLABIAL FLAP

A random-pattern skin flap with axially oriented blood supply composed of skin and subcutaneous tissue of cheek adjacent to nasolabial and nasofacial groove

Indications

1. Reconstruction of lateral, dorsal, alar, tip, and columellar nasal defects
2. Reconstruction of defects of the upper and lower lip
3. Reconstruction of floor of the mouth and oral cavity defects

Contraindications

1. Excessive scarring due to previous surgery or radiation therapy in the nasolabial region
2. Larger defects of nose exceeding the coverage capability of the nasolabial flap
3. Younger patients with inadequate skin redundancy in the nasolabial region
4. Skin with significant actinic changes secondary to sun exposure

Special Considerations

1. The flap is a random-pattern flap receiving blood supply directly through the axially oriented subdermal plexus (septocutaneous system) fed by branches of the angular and infraorbital vessels.
2. Longitudinal orientation of subdermal plexus confers a "degree of axiality" to the flap.[1]
3. Provides good color and texture match and good contour for nasal reconstruction
4. Donor site scar hidden in the nasolabial fold

Preoperative Preparation

1. Analysis of the defect with consideration of reconstructive alternatives, such as split-thickness and full-thickness skin grafts, other rotation, and advancement flaps
2. Evaluation of the condition of facial skin, with attention to actinic damage, which may preclude the use of the nasolabial flap

Special Instruments, Position, and Anesthesia

1. Routine plastic surgical tray
2. Local anesthesia achieved with 1% Xylocaine with 1:100,000 epinephrine or general anesthesia

Tips and Pearls

1. Dissection in subdermal plane beneath subdermal plexus, preserving underlying facial musculature and facial nerve branches
2. Thinning of subcutaneous fat to accommodate thickness of defect
3. Wide undermining around surgical defect to minimize "trap door" or "pincushion" deformity in nasal reconstruction
4. The flap can be used even after previous sacrifice of ipsilateral facial artery (ie, previous neck dissection).

Pitfalls and Complications

1. "Dog ear" at the base of flap rotation
2. Elevation and bulging of flap postoperatively, secondary to scar contracture, known as pincushioning or trap door effect
3. Potential with larger flaps for transfer of hair-bearing tissue to non–hair-bearing regions in males
4. Potential distortion of nasolabial groove and ala
5. Hypertrophic scarring in the nasolabial area in younger patients

Postoperative Care Issues

1. Sutures removed by 1 week
2. Injection of triamcinolone (40 mg) 3 to 6 weeks postoperatively if pincushioning deformity occurs
3. Various revisions of the pedicle, including inlaying of flap and revision of pincushioning or dog ear, at the base of the flap may be required.

References

1. Hynes B, Boyd B. The nasolabial flap—axial or random? Arch Otolaryngol Head Neck Surg 1988;114:1389.
2. Levine PA. Reconstruction of large nasal defects with a subcutaneous pedicle nasolabial flap: an underutilized technique. Arch Otolaryngol 1985;111:628.
3. Cameron RR. Nasal reconstruction with nasolabial cheek flaps. In: Grabb W, Myers M, eds. Skin flaps. Boston: Little, Brown, 1975: 323.

Operative Procedure

Superiorly, inferiorly, laterally, or medially based flaps can be designed, depending on the size, shape, and location of the defect to be reconstructed. The superiorly based nasolabial flap is most commonly employed to reconstruct lateral, dorsal, and alar nasal defects.

The lesion plus an appropriate margin to be excised is outlined. After attaining local anesthesia with a solution of 1% lidocaine with 1:100,000 epinephrine, the lesion is excised with frozen-section control of the margins. An exact template of the surgical defect is constructed by placing a surgical glove or aluminum suture material wrapper over the defect and cutting out a segment precisely matching the defect. The template is then transposed to the nasolabial skin, providing the exact dimension of the defect (Fig. 233-1). The approximate width of the flap is then determined, and the lateral outline of the flap is drawn superiorly toward the orbit. The line is then carried inferiorly across the cheek into the nasolabial fold. The medial aspect of the flap is outlined from the inferolateral aspect of the proposed defect inferiorly in the nasolabial groove to join the previously designed lateral margin (see Fig. 233-1). The flap is sharply incised as outlined through skin, dermis, and into the subcutaneous tissue.

The flap is then elevated, beginning inferiorly in the subdermal plane with a scalpel, thermal knife, or scissors, and using skin hooks for retraction (Fig. 233-2). If the dissection is kept within the subcutaneous fat, the underlying facial musculature and facial nerve branches are not damaged. The flap is then rotated into the defect. A gentle arc of rotation of the flap is desirable, because too sharp an angulation of the pedicle onto the nose may lead to flap engorgement and dog ear formation. To avoid this acute angulation, base the flap more superiorly, ensuring a better arc of rotation. The cheek skin lateral to the flap donor defect is then widely undermined in the subdermal plane to facilitate closure of the donor site.

The donor site defect is closed in standard two-layer fashion, placing the scar in the nasolabial groove. The recipient site is also undermined to facilitate closure, and the underside of the flap is thinned of subdermal fat to accommodate the thickness of the recipient defect. Suturing of the flap is begun proximally and continued distally. The distal triangular tail of the flap is left in place until the coverage of the recipient site is ensured; only then is the terminal triangle resected and the distal flap inset (Fig. 233-3).

One variation of the nasolabial flap, the subcutaneous pedicle nasolabial flap, has been used by the senior author for reconstruction of larger defects of the lower nasal bridge.[2] The donor skin and underlying fat is rotated from the nasolabial region, based on a subcutaneous pedicle from the infraorbital region as wide as the length of the flap. The subcutaneous pedicle is released from the dermis and from the underlying deep muscles of the face to allow the flap to be rotated into position (Fig. 233-4). The donor flap is tunneled under an intact skin bridge and sutured into the recipient defect, and the donor site is closed primarily (Fig. 233-5). When a large flap with a wide-based pedicle is used, a second stage may be necessary to defat the pedicle in the region deep to the skin bridge.

When full-thickness defects of the alar and lateral nose are present after resection, a nasolabial flap can be constructed of sufficient length to create the inner nasal lining and the outer skin lining of the defect.

Superiorly or inferiorly based nasolabial flaps may be employed to resurface intraoral and floor of mouth defects. Inferiorly based nasolabial flaps can be used to resurface floor of mouth defects, and superiorly based flaps can be used to resurface palatal defects. To resurface floor of mouth defects, an inferiorly based nasolabial flap is tunneled into the oral cavity through a buccal opening of appropriate size to prevent constriction of the flap pedicle. The flap is inset in a single step by de-epithelialization of the base of the pedicle with primary closure of the donor defect or as a two-step procedure with secondary division and insetting of the pedicle completed at 2 to 3 weeks. If the patient has teeth, a temporary bite block may be necessary to avoid dental trauma to the flap or amputation. Other uses of nasolabial flaps include reconstruction of defects of the upper and lower lip, nasal floor, ala, and columella.[3]

PAUL A. LEVINE
SCOTT D. MEREDITH

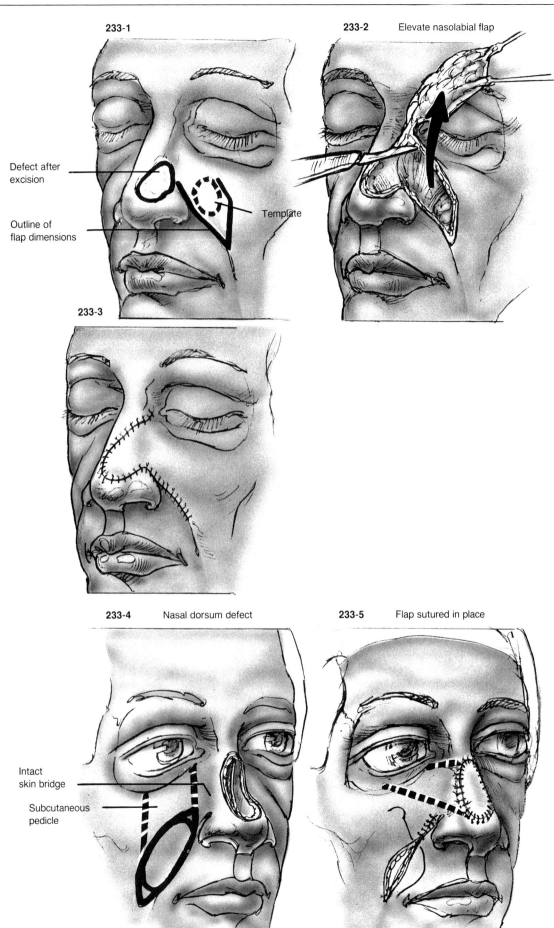

233-1

Defect after excision

Outline of flap dimensions

Template

233-2   Elevate nasolabial flap

233-3

233-4   Nasal dorsum defect

Intact skin bridge

Subcutaneous pedicle

233-5   Flap sutured in place

■ 234. BILOBED FLAP

Two flaps based on a common pedicle and rotated to cover a skin defect. The primary flap rotates into the defect, and the secondary flap is used to close the defect resulting from the primary flap. The defect left by the secondary flap is closed primarily. The flaps capitalize on the laxity of adjacent skin to produce a closure with minimum distortion.

Indications
1. Skin defects less than 1.5 cm on the lower one third of the nose
2. Defects on the cheek or temple when adjacent skin is lax

Contraindications
1. Large defects
2. Poor laxity of adjacent skin

Special Considerations
1. Lesions that cross anatomic boundaries
2. Full-thickness lesions of the nose

Preoperative Preparation
1. Routine preoperative laboratory tests

Special Instruments, Position, and Anesthesia
1. Fine plastic surgery instruments
2. Local anesthetic with or without general anesthesia

Tips and Pearls
1. Wide undermining of the flaps and the surrounding skin
2. The donor site must have adequate skin mobility.
3. The total angle of rotation may range from 45° to 180°.
4. The flaps may be the same size as the defect; more commonly, each flap is progressively smaller (up to 20%) than the defect it fills.
5. The defect created by the second flap is more readily closed if this flap is tapered.

Pitfalls and Complications
1. Flaps should not cross boundaries of facial units.
2. Pincushoning can develop, usually with a greater angle of rotation.
3. Excess tissue may be present at the point of rotation and may require excision later.

Postoperative Care Issues
1. Routine wound care
2. Dermabrasion may be required later.

References

McGregor JC, Soutar DS. A critical assessment of the bilobed flap. Br J Plast Surg 1981;34:197.
Zitelli JA. The bilobed flap for nasal reconstruction. Arch Dermatol 1989;125:957.

Operative Procedure

The patient is positioned appropriately for excision of the primary lesion. Local anesthetic is injected in the area of the lesion and the donor site. The lesion is excised to an appropriate level, often to the perichondrium on the lower nose.

Flaps are designed to rotate into the defect. Both flaps must come from an adjacent area with greater skin mobility than the lesion site. The flap immediately adjacent to the defect is the primary flap (A) and covers the original defect. Mobilization of this flap creates a second defect, which is filled by the second flap (B). The defect that remains after rotation of the second flap is closed primarily (Figs. 234-1 through 234-4).

The anatomic site plays an important role in flap design. Reconstruction of a defect near the nasal tip is often best accomplished by a laterally based flap, and medially based flaps may be used for defects on the ala (Figs. 234-5 and 234-6). When a bilobed flap is used on the cheek or temple, some of the incisions should be aligned, if possible, with the relaxed skin tension lines. The flaps should not lie across the boundaries of anatomic units, because this may lead to distortion.

When the flaps are designed, it is useful to envision a semicircle that encompasses the outer edge of the defect and the distal ends of both flaps. The point of rotation is the center of this arc (see Fig. 234-1). The rotation of each element of the bilobed flap can be between 45° and 90°. The total arc of rotation is measured from the long axis of the original defect to the long axis of the second flap. As this arc increases, the risk of developing a "dog ear" at the point of rotation increases. This excess skin can be excised, although this may compromise the blood supply to the flap.

The first flap is typically rounded. It may be the same size or slightly smaller (20%) than the defect. The secondary flap may be tapered and somewhat smaller (20%) than the primary flap. The tapering of the second flap facilitates closure of this donor site.

After the design is complete, the flap incisions are made. The flaps and the skin surrounding the donor sites are widely undermined in the subcutaneous plane with sharp scissors. The pedicle of the flaps should be undermined sufficiently to allow transposition of both flaps (see Figs. 234-2 and 234-3).

Hemostasis is obtained, and the wound is closed. The secondary flap donor site is closed primarily with interrupted buried absorbable sutures. The flaps are trimmed as needed and set into the defects. If needed, back cuts may be made at the base of the flaps and dog ears may be excised, but in doing so, the blood supply to the flaps should not be compromised. The primary flap and the secondary flap are secured in place with buried sutures. The skin is closed with 6-0 nylon suture (see Fig. 234-4).

JACQUELINE F. MOSTERT

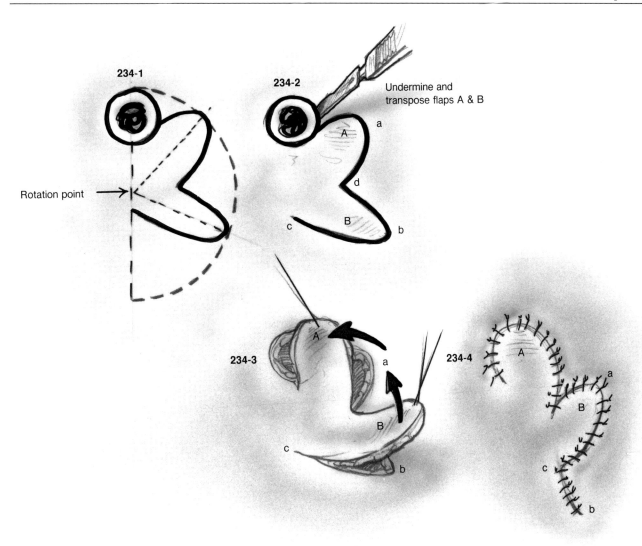

234-1

Rotation point

234-2

Undermine and
transpose flaps A & B

234-3

234-4

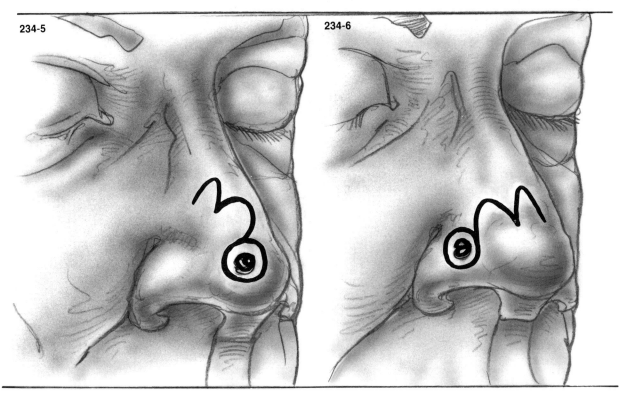

234-5

234-6

■ *235.* MEDIAN FOREHEAD FLAP

Axial pattern flap based on the supratrochlear artery and vein.[1]

Indications

1. Reconstruction of soft tissue defects, primarily of the nose.
2. Reconstruction of brow and other facial defects, in some cases.

Special Considerations

1. One must attain clear margins of resection prior to reconstruction.
2. A previous incision on the forehead may have compromised the supratrochlear vascular bundle and preclude use.

Preoperative Preparation

1. Routine lab tests, including coagulation studies
2. Comprehensive discussion with the patient to point out that this type of reconstruction will require at least three operations.

Special Instruments, Position, and Anesthesia

1. Sterile hand-held Doppler probe to locate the vascular pedicle
2. Bipolar cautery
3. Small, delicate plastic surgery instruments

Tips and Pearls

1. Use a Doppler probe to outline the supratrochlear vascular pedicle as it exits the medial orbit.
2. Use the subunit principle of Burget. Complete excision of tissue within involved nasal subunits.
3. Always provide intranasal lining to close full-thickness nasal defects (eg, turnover flaps, septal flaps, nasolabial flaps)
4. Reconstitute cartilage deficits of the upper and lower lateral cartilages with septal or auricular cartilage grafts.
5. Do not hesitate to extend the flap into hair-bearing scalp to provide additional flap length.
6. Use a precise template to mark out the pattern of the forehead flap to match the outline of the defect.
7. Create a narrow (1 to 1.5 cm) pedicle to allow maximal rotation of the flap without compression of the vascular pedicle.
8. Thin out the distal 1 to 2 cm of forehead flap to match the depth of the defect by excising subcutaneous tissue.
9. Perform precise skin eversion closure of the distal 1 to 2 cm.
10. Leave the forehead defect open to heal by secondary intention if the donor site defect does not close primarily.
11. Apply a split-thickness skin graft to the undersurface of the forehead flap pedicle to minimize postoperative drainage.
12. When the pedicle is divided, do not replace remaining skin into forehead defect. Inset if the base of the pedicle will reconstitute the contour of the glabellar region.

Pitfalls and Complications

1. Flap compromise may occur if there is excessive torque or kinking of the pedicle of the flap.
2. Significant scar contracture and deformity may occur if one fails to reconstitute nasal lining or reconstruct structural defects of the upper or lower lateral cartilages.

Postoperative Care Issues

1. Flap viability can be monitored by examining flap color and capillary refill.
2. If healing by secondary intention is necessary for closure of the donor site defect, the wound should be kept moist under an occlusive dressing until complete epithelialization has taken place.
3. Patients should be instructed on wound care.

References

1. Shumrick KA, Smith TL. The anatomic basis for the design of forehead flaps in nasal reconstruction. Arch Otolaryngol Head Neck Surg 1992;118:373.
2. Burget GC, Menick FJ. The subunit principle in nasal reconstruction. 1985;76:239.
3. Burget GC. Aesthetic reconstruction of the nose. Clin Plast Surg 1985;12:463.
4. Burget GC, Menick FJ. Nasal reconstruction: seeking a fourth dimension. Plast Reconstr Surg 1986;78:722.
5. Burget GC, Menick FJ. Nasal support and lining: the marriage of beauty and blood supply. Plast Reconstr Surg 1989;84:189.

Operative Procedure

With the patient in the supine position, general anesthesia is induced and endotracheal intubation is performed. The borders of the involved subunits of the nose are outlined with a marking pen. If more than 50% of a nasal subunit is involved, the remaining skin of that subunit can be excised (Fig. 235-1). All deficits in intranasal lining or cartilage support should be reconstituted. Intranasal lining can be transferred from the nasal septum, local turnover flaps or nasolabial flap. Septal or auricular cartilage can be used to reconstruct the upper or lower lateral cartilages. If the ala is reconstructed, supporting alar grafts should be fixed with mattress sutures as close to the alar margin as possible to prevent postoperative alar retraction.

A malleable template can be cut from the foil suture package to precisely match the shape of the nasal defect. The template is positioned on the upper extent of the forehead to outline the tissue transfer. A folded gauze can be used to simulate the transfer of the tissue to determine if the flap will reach the defect. If necessary, the flap can be designed to extend into the frontal hairline to gain additional flap length. If the nasal defect is situated on the left side of the midline, a left sided paramedian forehead flap should be used to allow maximal rotation into the defect.

A sterile Doppler probe can be used to locate and trace the course of the supratrochlear vascular bundle for the proposed flap. The vascular pedicle is usually located just above the medial aspect of the brow. The vessels exit the superior medial orbit approximately 1.7 to 2.2 cm lateral to the midline and continue about 2 cm from the midline.[1] The pedicle of the flap can be narrowed to 1 cm to 1.5 cm to allow maximal rotation of the flap. The distal third of the flap is elevated in the subcutaneous plane above the frontalis muscle (Fig. 235-2). The proximal two thirds of the flap is elevated below the frontalis muscle down to the orbital rim. The proximal third of the flap can be elevated off the periosteum down to a level just below the orbital rim. The supratrochlear vessels can be followed with the Doppler throughout the dissection to insure preservation of the vascular supply of the flap. The distal 1.5 to 2 cm of the flap can be thinned down to the dermis to allow a precise match in skin thickness with the edges of the defect.

The flap is oriented into the defect by twisting it 180° and transposing it 180° (Fig. 235-3). Care is taken to be sure there is no tension or kinking of the pedicle. The flap is sutured into position using deep everting skin sutures and vertical mattress sutures for skin closure (Fig. 235-4).

After the flap is inset, the undersurface of the pedicle of the forehead flap is covered with a split-thickness skin graft to minimize drainage of serous fluid. The forehead defect is closed in two layers using everting subcutaneous and vertical mattress sutures. If the defect cannot be closed primarily, it can be left open to granulate and heal by secondary intention.

After waiting 3 to 4 weeks, the pedicle is divided and the proximal segment of the flap is debulked prior to closure (Fig. 235-5). The distal third of the flap must be left intact because the blood supply to the flap is from this distal segment. When closing the incision, skin eversion techniques should be used in preparation for followup dermabrasion. The base of the pedicle of the skin flap is trimmed and inset into the region of the glabella as an inverted "V" (Fig. 235-6).

In patients with possible small vessel disease (eg, smokers, diabetics), we prefer to debulk the middle third of the flap 3 to 4 weeks after reconstruction, with the pedicle of the flap divided 6 to 8 weeks after inset of the flap. This method leaves the pedicle in place for an additional period of time and the dual blood supply allows more aggressive debulking.

Dermabrasion of the margins of the reconstructed region can be performed as early as 8 weeks after division of the pedicle. Additionally, scar revision or dermabrasion of the donor site incision (forehead) can be performed.

DEAN M. TORIUMI

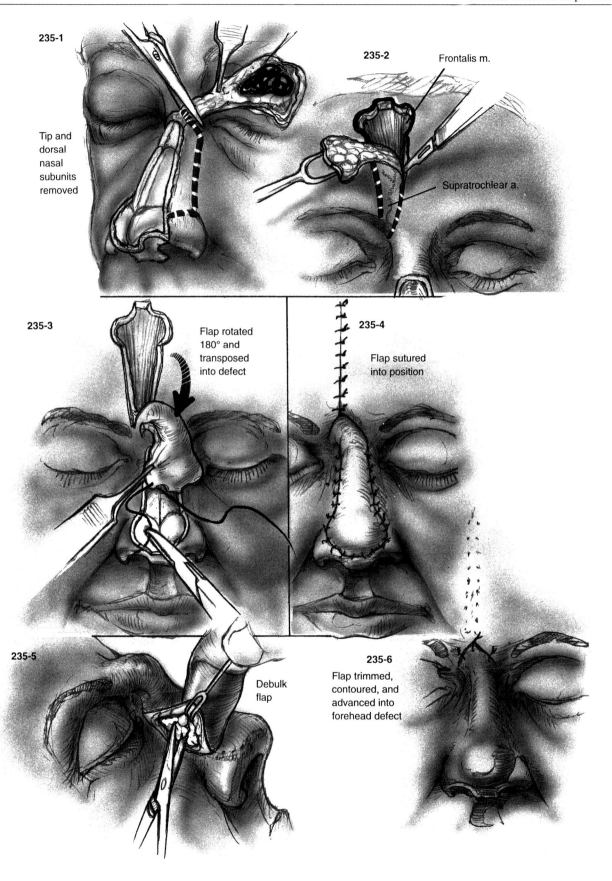

235-1

Tip and dorsal nasal subunits removed

235-2

Frontalis m.

Supratrochlear a.

235-3

Flap rotated 180° and transposed into defect

235-4

Flap sutured into position

235-5

Debulk flap

235-6

Flap trimmed, contoured, and advanced into forehead defect

■ 236. GLABELLAR FLAPS

Midline flap of nasal glabellar tissue

Indications

1. Defects of medial canthus (≤15 mm)
2. Dorsal lateral nasal defects
3. For covering a raw bone defect, for which a skin graft is less suitable

Contraindications

1. Horizontal scarring, which could decrease blood supply

Special Considerations

1. Good tumor margins (if defect is from tumor); flap may mask recurrence.
2. May be combined with other flaps for larger lesions
3. Single-stage reconstruction without requirement to take down a pedicle

Preoperative Preparation

1. Careful measurement
2. No aspirin or anticoagulants

Special Instruments, Position, and Anesthesia

1. Delicate plastic surgery instruments (eg, hooks)
2. Bipolar cautery
3. Head slightly elevated
4. Local or general anesthesia

Tips and Pearls

1. May be midline or paramedian incision
2. Avoid heaped-up appearance close to the eye by carefully thinning the flap tip.

Pitfalls and Complications

1. Avoid hair-bearing skin next to the eye.
2. Watch for vascular congestion (may need "milking").
3. Brows may be medialized; be sure the patient has consented.

Postoperative Care Issues

1. Daily cleaning with hydrogen peroxide
2. Twice-daily application of antibiotic ointment
3. May be revised after 4 to 6 weeks

References

Field LM. The glabellar transposition "banner" flap. J Dermatol Surg Oncol 1988;14:376.

Mustarde JC. V-Y glabellar skin flap to the medial canthal region. In: Strauch B, Vasconez LO, Hall-Findlay EJ, eds. Grabb's encyclopedia of flaps. Boston: Little, Brown, 1990:107.

Operative Procedure

After definitive resection of the area to be reconstructed, the patient is placed with the head elevated in a semi-Fowler position if under local anesthesia. The appropriate flap is marked on the patient. The pedicle may be based on either of the supratrochlear arteries or may be a random flap. The vertical dimension may be up to three times the breadth of the flap; the rich anastomotic network of vasculature of this area makes this possible (Fig. 236-1). One side ends near the lesion, with the pedicled base ending more superiorly on the opposite side (Fig. 236-2A).

The incision lines are injected with a solution of 1% lidocaine with 1:100,000 epinephrine for local anesthesia and hemostasis. The incision is made with a #15 blade to just below the subdermal plexus or to the galea aponeurotica for a thicker flap. The thicker flap is used for a full-thickness loss of nasal tissue, and the thinner flap is used for a partial loss or loss immediately next to the eye. The flap can be lifted using knife or scissors dissection. Bipolar cautery is used for hemostasis as needed. If the primary lesion excision extends into either eyelid from the medial canthus, the tarsal plate should be sutured to the periosteum of the medial canthal tendon before relocating the flap. The flap is then moved into position and sutured with 5-0 and 6-0 nylon suture in a V-Y closure (Fig. 236-2B).

Surgical Variations

The glabellar flap can be used as a sliding flap or as a rotation flap. For a rotation flap, the technique for elevating the flap is largely the same as previously described. The flap is elevated just below the subdermal plexus. The pedicle should end in a glabellar furrow to allow maximum aesthetic closure (Fig. 236-3A). After rotating the flap, closure is begun at the base of the flap and extended to the tip. The tip is trimmed as necessary. The vertical defect is closed primarily, undermining as necessary, with care not to undermine beyond the medial brow edge (Fig. 236-3B).

The glabellar flap may also be developed in a paramedian position, with closure still in a glabellar furrow (Fig. 236-4) and rotated or used to cover a midline nasal defect.

LINDA GAGE-WHITE

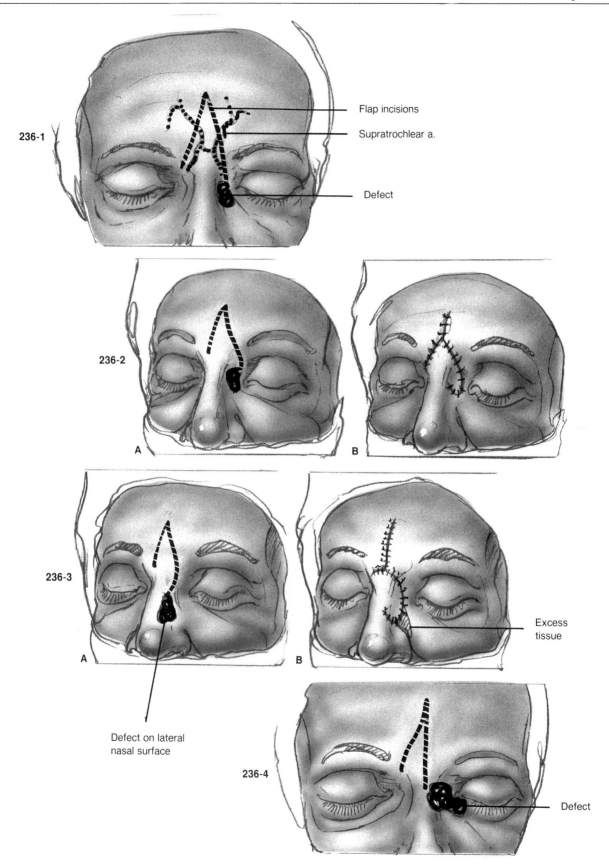

236-1

Flap incisions

Supratrochlear a.

Defect

236-2

A

B

236-3

A

B

Excess tissue

Defect on lateral nasal surface

236-4

Defect

■ 237. CHEEK-NECK ROTATION FLAP

A mixed axial-pattern and random-pattern cutaneous rotation flap supplied by the contralateral external carotid vasculature or the first through third intercostal perforators from the internal mammary artery.

Indications

1. Reconstruction of large cutaneous defects of the cheek, temple, and lateral face

Contraindications

1. Previous irradiation to the cheek and neck skin is a relative contraindication.

Special Considerations

1. Smaller cheek and temple defects can be closed by a random-pattern cervicofacial rotation flap.
2. Large lateral face defects are closed with an axial-pattern cervicofacial flap.
3. The flap provides an excellent color and thickness match.
4. Oncologic resection of the skin is not compromised.
5. Exposure after flap elevation is adequate for neck dissection.
6. A split-thickness skin graft, if needed, is hidden inferior to clavicle.

Preoperative Preparation

1. Sterile preparation of the face, neck, shoulder, and chest inferior to costal margin
2. Prepare a separate donor site to provide the split-thickness skin graft.

Special Instruments, Position, and Anesthesia

1. The patient is supine, with the neck in the neutral position, with minimal flexion or extension when the flap is rotated for closure.

Tips and Pearls

1. Design the excision so the superior margin is horizontal and above the level of the lateral canthus to minimize lower lid ectropion.
2. Preserve the ipsilateral facial artery when oncologically sound.
3. Cervicopectoral flap design should incorporate the entire length of the deltopectoral flap for later use, if necessary.
4. The plane of dissection is deep to the superficial musculoaponeurotic system in the face, deep to the platysma in the neck, and deep to the pectoralis major fascia inferior to the clavicle.
5. A bolster can be used along the suture line to relieve tension.

Pitfalls and Complications

1. Preserve the marginal mandibular nerve during flap elevation.
2. Preserve the spinal accessory nerve.
3. Closure of the superior aspect of the flap in the facial defect should have minimal tension.
4. Preserve the first through third intercostal perforating arteries when using a cervicopectoral flap.

Postoperative Care Issues

1. Closed suction drainage under flap

References

Patterson HC, Anonsen CA, Weymuller EA, Webster RC. The cheek-neck rotation flap for closure of temporozygomatic cheek wounds. Arch Otolaryngol 1984;110:388.

Wallis A, Donald PJ. Lateral face reconstruction with the medial-based cervicopectoral flap. Arch Otolaryngol Head Neck Surg 1988;114:729.

Operative Procedure

The area of skin excision is outlined around the tumor to provide adequate margins. This area can be incorporated in a triangular defect with an M-plasty. If a cervicofacial flap is planned, the superior horizontal incision should be placed above the zygomatic arch level to prevent tension on the anterosuperior aspect of the repair from resulting in inferior displacement of the eyelid. The superior incision is carried into a standard parotidectomy incision, except that the inferior limb is carried lower into the midline neck, usually at the level of the cricoid cartilage (Fig. 237-1).

For larger defects, the flap is designed in a wide, broad, gently curved line incorporating the preauricular skin crease to extend behind the whole of the ear and inferiorly along the anterior border of the trapezius. This is carried to the acromion and then into the lower limb of a standard deltopectoral flap (Fig. 237-2). The flap is carried deep to the superficial musculoaponeurotic system layer in the face, deep to the platysma muscle in the neck, and deep to the pectoralis major fascia over the chest. The marginal mandibular branch of the facial nerve and the spinal accessory nerve, when tumor free, are spared. The flap is elevated to the midline in the neck and to within 2 cm of the sternal border in the chest to preserve the intercostal perforating vessels and to maximize the arc of rotation. After flap elevation, the oncologic resection is performed, which may include parotidectomy, neck dissection, and maxillectomy.

Reconstruction begins by placing the head in the neutral position and then rotating the flap into position to ensure a tension-free closure (Fig. 237-3). Bolster sutures with dental rolls can be used on the superior and posterior closure to alleviate tension, if needed, particularly if the cervical skin has been previously irradiated.

Dog-ear defects are judiciously excised with Burow's triangles, and the wound usually can be closed primarily. Closed suction drainage is used. Occasionally, a split-thickness skin graft is required to close a donor site defect over the pectoralis muscle.

RAMON M. ESCLAMADO

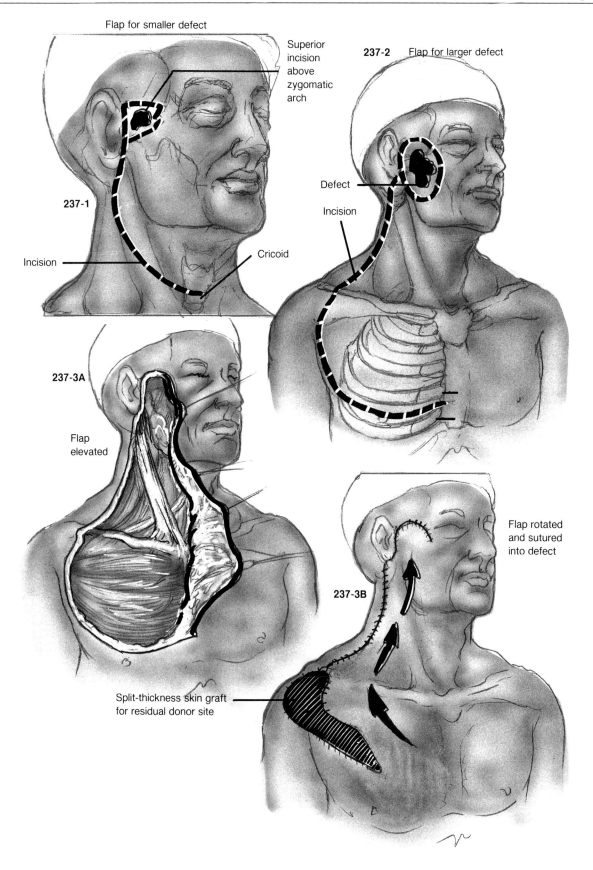

Flap for smaller defect

Superior incision above zygomatic arch

237-2 Flap for larger defect

237-1

Defect

Incision

Incision

Cricoid

237-3A

Flap elevated

Split-thickness skin graft for residual donor site

Flap rotated and sutured into defect

237-3B

■ *238.* RHOMBOID FLAP

A transposition flap for the repair of local skin defects. The rhomboid flap by definition contains two 120° angles and two 60° angles, with four sides of equal length. Variations of this design that use modified rhomboids do exist. This flap was originally described by Limberg.[1]

Indications

1. Repair of skin cancer defects
2. Repair of traumatic avulsion injuries

Special Considerations

1. This flap is useful throughout the face, but especially in the cheek and temple regions.
2. When a classic rhomboid flap is employed, tailoring the defect into the desired configuration may require excision of significant normal skin. Modifications of the rhomboid flap or other method should be considered if this is the case.
3. Placement of the flap to take advantage of the resting skin tension lines (RSTLs) will enhance the final result.

Preoperative Preparation

1. In the design and placement of rhomboid flaps on the face the effect of transposition and wound tension on the donor site must be considered. This is especially important around the eyelids and oral commissure.
2. It is useful to draw the rhomboid on the face and visualize the potential donor sites before making incisions.
3. Patients should be asked to refrain from smoking and any platelet-inhibiting drugs for as long as possible before surgery.

Special Instruments, Position, and Anesthesia

1. Most facial rhomboid flaps can be performed under local anesthesia in an ambulatory setting.
2. Fine instruments such as skin hooks and non-crushing forceps should be used to avoid trauma to the skin flaps.

Tips and Pearls

1. Consider axial blood flow and the RSTLs in the design of all flaps to decrease complications.
2. Wide undermining and meticulous hemostasis will make closure easier.

Pitfalls and Complications

1. Poor flap design with inadequate consideration of closing tension and incision placement is the most common source of complications. With a rhomboid flap the majority of tension is at the closure of the donor site[2] (Fig. 238-1).
2. Skin necrosis may result with high flap-closing tension or subcutaneous hematoma (or both) if not addressed immediately.
3. Hypertrophic or keloid scars may result in some lateral facial defects.

Postoperative Care Issues

1. Prophylactic antibiotics are frequently used, but the infection rate for facial flaps is extremely low.
2. Routine incision care is provided with peroxide and antibiotic ointment applied twice per day.
3. Suture removal is done at 5 to 7 days, with routine taping for 1 week.
4. Dermabrasion may be considered later if healing is not desirable.

References

1. Larrabee WF, Trachy R, Sutton D, et al. Rhomboid flap dynamics. Arch Otolaryngol 1981;107:755.
2. Limberg AA. The planning of local plastic operations on the body surface: theory and practice. Toronto: Cullamore Press, 1984.
3. Webster RC, Davidson TM, Smith RC. The 30 degree transposition flap. Laryngoscope 1978;88:85.

Operative Procedure

After it is determined that a rhomboid flap is appropriate for facial reconstruction the design can be drawn on the skin. The rhomboid is constructed with four equal sides containing two 120° angles and two 60° angles. The rhomboid is drawn to take advantage of the RSTLs, with placement of the donor defect closure along this plane (Fig. 238-2)

The four possible rhomboid flaps are then considered, and the most advantageous flap is selected. The subcutaneous tissues are then infiltrated with local anesthetic and the flap incisions are made. Wide undermining is performed and the flap is transposed into position. The donor site is closed first with subcutaneous suture, and the flap will usually rest with minimal tension in the recipient site. A careful two-layer closure can then be performed with little trauma to the flap itself. Meticulous hemostasis must be maintained.

Variations of the rhomboid flap include the Dufourmentel flap and the 30° transposition flap in combination with the rhomboid. The Dufourmentel flap is useful in situations where the surgeon utilizes rhombic defects with acute angles of 60° to 90°, allowing the preservation of skin normally excised to execute a rhomboid flap (Fig. 238-3). The flap is designed by bisecting the angle between an extension of the short axis and one of the rhomboid sides. This line is extended the length of a rhomboid side, and a second line is drawn parallel to the long axis of the rhomboid. The line of tension at closure is as shown, and should be placed as close to the RSTLs as possible.

Also useful is the 30° transposition flap transferred into a rhomboid defect shortened by an M-plasty. This variation of a rhomboid will help to decrease dog-ear formation and spread closing tension more evenly throughout the wound (Fig. 238-4). This flap is more difficult to design,[3] but does offer the advantages mentioned above.

IRA D. PAPEL

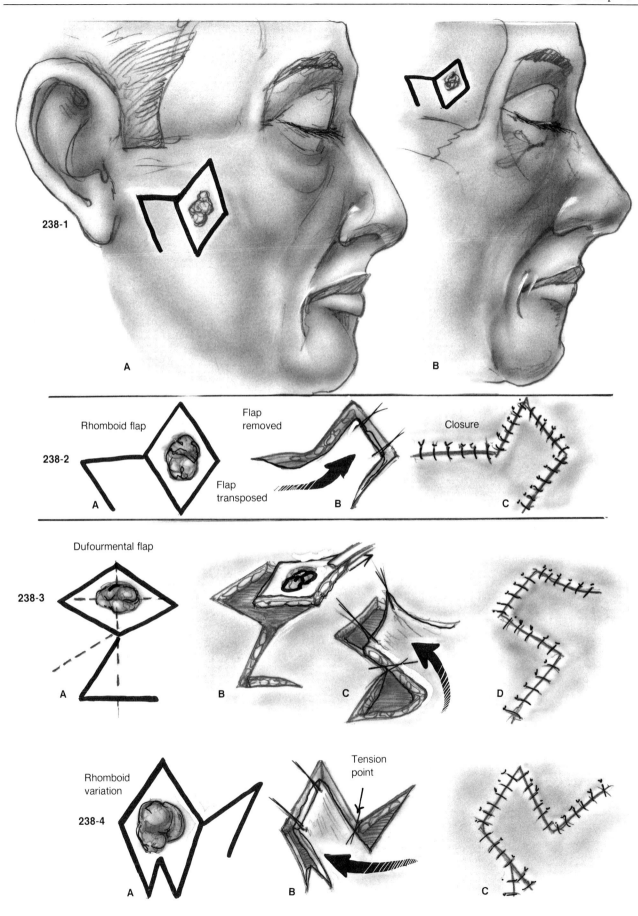

238-1

238-2   Rhomboid flap   Flap removed   Closure
A   Flap transposed   B   C

238-3   Dufourmental flap
A   B   C   D

238-4   Rhomboid variation   Tension point
A   B   C

◼ 239. DELTOPECTORAL FLAP

Axial skin flap of the upper chest that is medially based and horizontally oriented. The flap is supplied by the first three or four perforating intercostal branches of the internal mammary artery.

Indications

1. External defects of the neck or face
2. Oral defect reconstruction
3. Partial or circumferential pharyngeal or cervical esophageal reconstruction
4. Options include a rotational transfer, subcutaneous transfer with a portion of the flap pedicle de-epithelialized, transfer with a tubed pedicle bridge, transfer with the distal flap split longitudinally, and flap "waltzing" after time elapsed for neovascularization at the recipient site.

Contraindications

1. Prior surgery that has interrupted the perforating intercostal vessels
2. Prior thoracic surgery using the internal mammary artery (eg, coronary artery bypass graft)
3. Nonacceptance of donor site deformity

Special Considerations

1. Flap delay is necessary if an extended flap is planned.
2. Consider flap delay if the patient is a smoker or is elderly or for associated diabetes mellitus, arteriosclerosis, nutritional deficiency, or prior radiation therapy to the donor site.
3. The donor site is usually out of the field of prior radiation therapy.
4. The deltoid segment of the flap is usually not hair bearing.
5. May be used in conjunction with other flaps

Preoperative Preparation

1. With flap delay, flap length can be extended as far as the posterolateral deltoid area or superiorly to the scapular spine.
2. A skin graft may be applied to the distal fascial surface of the flap for use in through-and-through defects.

Tips and Pearls

1. Elevate the flap in a plane deep to the pectoralis and deltoid fascia.
2. Avoid excessive medial dissection of the flap base, which may disrupt perforating vessels.
3. Handle the flap gently, and avoid pinching of the flap or flap pedicle.
4. Avoid tension or torsion of the flap pedicle.
5. Avoid pressure on the flap pedicle (eg, tracheotomy, gown ties).
6. Do not drape the flap over the reconstruction plate.
7. Adequate hemostasis and wound drainage are important.

Pitfalls and Complications

1. Partial flap necrosis (5% to 20%)
2. Protect the donor site from possible tumor implantation.
3. The flap is prone to stenosis when used for circumferential pharyngeal reconstruction.
4. Hematoma under the flap may contribute to flap necrosis. The early identification and evacuation of a hematoma is important.
5. Infection is unusual but may occur in setting of salivary contamination of the donor site.

Postoperative Care Issues

1. Careful monitoring of flap viability and factors that may contribute to vascular compromise of the flap
2. Immobilize the split-thickness skin graft on the donor site with nonadherent dressing for approximately 5 days.
3. Minimize shoulder movement postoperatively.

References

Bakamjian VY. A two-stage method for pharyngoesophageal reconstruction with a primary pectoral skin flap. Plast Reconstr Surg 1965;36:173.

Bakamjian VY. The deltopectoral flap. In: Stark RB, ed. Plastic surgery of the head and neck. New York: Churchill Livingstone, 1987;926.

McGregor IA, Jackson IT. The extended role of the deltopectoral flap. Br J Surg 1970;23:173.

Operative Procedures

With the patient in the supine position, the anterior chest and shoulder are prepped and draped in the usual sterile fashion. The flap is designed according to the reconstructive requirements, and the length of the flap required is determined (Fig. 239-1). Abduction of the arm allows visualization of the inferior flap border's elongation potential.

After the flap has been outlined, a superior horizontal incision is made along the inferior aspect of the clavicle, extending laterally from the sternoclavicular joint region. An inferior horizontal incision is also made parallel to the superior incision, beginning at the third or fourth intercostal space and crossing onto the shoulder at the level of the apex of the anterior axillary fold. A lateral curvilinear vertical incision over the deltoid connects the previously made horizontal incisions. The incisions are carried down through the pectoralis and deltoid fascia. The flap is elevated by sharp dissection from the lateral to medial aspects in a plane deep to the muscular fascia (Fig. 239-2). After the flap length is sufficient to reach the recipient site adequately, medial dissection and elevation are terminated to prevent injuring the intercostal perforating vessels.

After it is elevated, the flap is transferred to the recipient site by using one of the transfer options previously listed in the Indications section. If the flap is transferred with the flap pedicle bridging over intact skin, the pedicle is tubed on itself using absorbable sutures for subcutaneous closure and nylon sutures for cutaneous closure. Exercise care to avoid vascular compromise of the flap when tubing the pedicle, particularly in an obese patient. The recipient site defect is closed with the flap using absorbable sutures for mucosal and subcutaneous closure and nylon sutures or staples for cutaneous closure (Fig. 239-3).

After hemostasis is ensured at the donor site, a split-thickness skin graft is harvested from the thigh or other donor site with a dermatome at a thickness of 0.0015 in (0.04 mm). It should be of sufficient width and length that, when meshed, the skin graft adequately covers the donor site (Fig. 239-3). The skin graft is secured at the donor site with sutures or staples, and a nonadherent gauze compression dressing (eg, Xeroform) is applied over the skin graft and secured with Montgomery straps.

If flap delay is warranted for the purpose of extending the length of the flap or for other factors listed in the Special Considerations section, 1 to 2 weeks before elevation of the flap, the cutaneous deltoid branch from the thoracoacromial artery is divided, and the skin along the outline of the planned flap is incised. As an alternative to a continuous skin incision around the distal flap, the skin over the deltoid extension of the flap can be divided segmentally, leaving intact segments of skin that are divided at the time of flap elevation. The flap-delay skin incisions are closed with staples or nylon sutures, and routine postoperative wound care is instituted.

Allow 4 weeks after the flap transfer for adequate neovascularization of the distal flap. The flap pedicle may then be divided, the resultant wound closed, and the flap pedicle remnant returned to the chest donor site if the pedicle remnant is large enough to improve chest cosmesis (Fig. 239-4). Umbilical tape can be applied as a tourniquet to the pedicle base before division of the pedicle to confirm adequate distal flap neovascularization from the recipient site.

DAVID W. EISELE

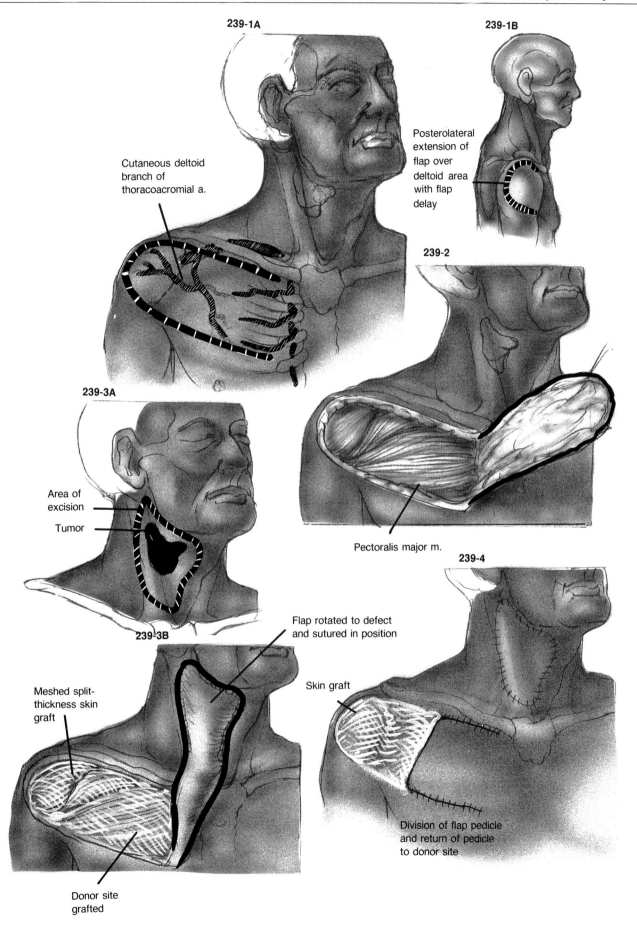

239-1A

Cutaneous deltoid branch of thoracoacromial a.

239-1B

Posterolateral extension of flap over deltoid area with flap delay

239-2

Pectoralis major m.

239-3A

Area of excision

Tumor

239-3B

Meshed split-thickness skin graft

Donor site grafted

Flap rotated to defect and sutured in position

239-4

Skin graft

Division of flap pedicle and return of pedicle to donor site

■ 240. A TO T FLAP

A complex of two local flaps for coverage of a skin defect

Indications

1. Triangular (ie, A-shaped) or round skin defect
2. Movable skin (ie, no landmarks such as eyelid or nasal ala) on two of its three sides
3. Excellent for 1- to 2-cm defects on the face and neck; can also be used for 3- to 4-cm defects, especially on the forehead and temple

Special Considerations

1. Used with care in heavy smokers

Preoperative Preparation

1. Patient should not take any aspirin or nonsteroidal antiinflammatory drug–containing medications for 2 weeks before surgery, if possible.
2. Patients are encouraged to quit or reduce smoking.

Special Instruments, Position, and Anesthesia

1. Fine instrument tray, including Bishop-Harmon forceps, Beaver knife handle and a #64 blade, small sharp iris scissors, and Castroviejo needle holders
2. Surgical loupes
3. Local or general anesthesia, depending on the patient's medical conditions and preference

Tips and Pearls

1. Use of a half-buried suture for the trifurcation decreases the chance of necrosis of flap tips.
2. Skin closure with absorbable suture such as 6-0 Fastsorb chromic obviates the need for suture removal with its potential for disturbance of the skin alignment.
3. If nonabsorbable sutures are used, use loupes or the microscope for excellent visualization during removal.
4. Addition of one part sodium bicarbonate to five parts local anesthetic brings the pH closer to neutral and diminishes the burning sensation associated with injection.

Pitfalls and Complications

1. The chance of flap necrosis is diminished if adequate hemostasis is obtained and drainage is allowed with a rubber band drain or by using interrupted sutures so that drainage can occur between sutures.

Postoperative Care Issues

1. Suture lines are kept continuously moist with antibiotic ointment until cutaneous healing is complete.
2. Use of Steri-strips to decrease tension on the healing wound may decrease the chance of scar spreading.
3. Consider dermabrasion 6 to 8 weeks after surgery.

Operative Procedure

With the patient in a supine position, the skin is infiltrated with local anesthesia (Fig. 240-1). The wound is widely undermined in a subcutaneous plane, leaving a thin layer of subcutaneous fat on the skin flap. A decision is made about the location of the base of the flap, which becomes the arms of the T shape. Two arms equal in length are drawn on the skin. The length of the arms is roughly two to three times the height of the defect (Fig. 240-2). The #64 Beaver blade is used to incise along these lines.

A buried horizontal stitch of 4-0 or 5-0 Vicryl is placed at the trifurcation. If significant tension is needed to bring the three flaps together, slightly lengthening the arms sometimes allows additional movement of the flaps. Creation of small Burow's triangles at the ends of the T arms, on the side opposite the defect, is usually required for low-tension closure (Fig. 240-3).

After this key trifurcation stitch is placed, the three lines of the T are closed with subcutaneous horizontal sutures (ie, 4-0 or 5-0 Vicryl). Skin closure is begun with the trifurcation, where a half-buried horizontal suture is used. A separate running suture (ie, 6-0 Fastsorb chromic) is used for each arm of the T, or interrupted simple sutures can be used (Fig. 240-4). If a running stitch is used, more equal tension on the skin wound and a more pleasing appearance are produced by diagonally traveling under the skin and by perpendicular crossings over the skin.

Antibiotic ointment is applied, and Steri-strips can be used if desired.

KAREN H. CALHOUN

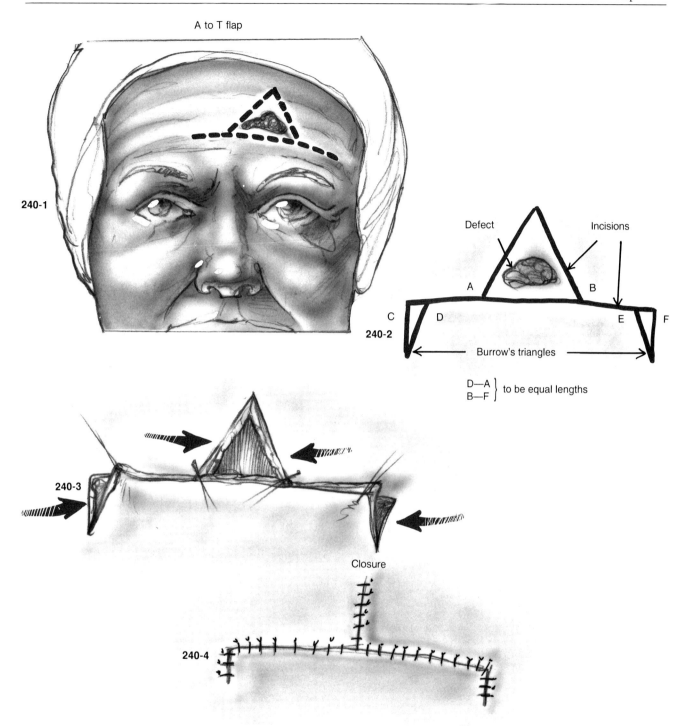

A to T flap

240-1

Defect

Incisions

A   B

C   D   E   F

240-2

Burrow's triangles

$\left.\begin{array}{c} D—A \\ B—F \end{array}\right\}$ to be equal lengths

240-3

Closure

240-4

■ 241. Z-PLASTY

A transposition flap in which two equal-sized triangular flaps are transposed

Indications

1. To rotate the dominant axis of a scar to a more favorable orientation with the relaxed skin tension lines (RSTLs)
2. To lengthen a scar contraction or avoid a contracture in an incision across a concavity
3. To align anatomic lines that are in an unfavorable position

Special Considerations

1. Z-plasty is the procedure of choice for lengthening scars or altering their direction. For other indications, techniques such as W-plasty and geometric line closure may be indicated.
2. The degree of lengthening can be controlled by the angles at the apices of the two flaps. The larger the angle, the greater is the degree of lengthening:

   A 30° angle produces 25% lengthening
   A 45° angle produces 50% lengthening
   A 60° angle produces 75% lengthening

3. Z-plasties designed with angle outside the 30° to 60° range tend to have significant protrusion when rotated, compromising the aesthetic result.
4. When planning a Z-plasty scar revision, the surgeon must accept that the new scar will be three times the length of the original lesion.
5. Multiple Z-plasty techniques may be helpful in long scar contractures in a concavity or for lengthy scar oriented perpendicular to the RSTLs.

Preoperative Preparation

1. Evaluate the RSTLs and orientation of the scar. In general, the limbs of the Z-plasty should be placed in the surrounding RSTLs to obtain a scar in the desired direction (Fig. 241-1).
2. Assessment of skin elasticity and mobility
3. Careful marking of planned incisions and excisions on the skin before injection of local anesthetic
4. Inspect previous facial scars to predict healing traits.

Special Instruments, Position, and Anesthesia

1. Most head and neck Z-plasties can be performed under local anesthesia or under sedation. A solution of lidocaine with a 1:100,000 dilution of epinephrine is infiltrated with a 27- or 30-gauge needle. General anesthesia may be necessary in pediatric cases and special situations.
2. Instrumentation should include fine skin hooks, dissecting scissors, gentle tissue forceps, and a fine caliper to measure the limbs of the Z-plasty accurately.

Tips and Pearls

1. Careful planning is the key to good results.
2. Z-plasty limbs less than 0.5 cm long may cause pincushion deformities.
3. Wide undermining helps to approximate wound edges with less tension.
4. Careful closure without compromising the blood supply to the flap tips is essential.
5. Delayed dermabrasion may enhance the results.

Pitfalls and Complications

1. Poor flap design is the major cause of flap necrosis and poor aesthetic results.
2. These delicate flaps must be handled with care. Avoid crushing forceps, and use fine skin hooks if possible.

References

Borges AF. Principles of scar camouflage. Facial Plast Surg 1984;1:226.
Thomas JR, Holt GR, eds. Facial scars: incision, revision, and camouflage. St. Louis: Mosby-Year Book, 1989.

Operative Procedure

Only after proper planning and skin marking is the surgical area infiltrated with local anesthetic and the area prepped for surgery. If appropriate, the scar is then excised, and the limbs of the Z-plasty are incised. The flaps are mobilized by subcutaneous dissection, and wide undermining of the surrounding tissues is performed as necessary. Hemostasis is meticulously obtained using bipolar cautery.

The flaps are then transposed (Fig. 241-2) and fixed into position by using fine nylon-tip sutures at the apex of each flap. The free sides of the triangular flaps are sutured into position. Care is taken not to crush the flaps with forceps, and the sutures are not tightened excessively. Antibiotic ointment is applied to the wound. Sutures are removed in 5 days from the face and 7 days from the neck. On thin facial skin a single layer closure is usually sufficient. With the thicker neck skin, a subcutaneous closure is usually employed in addition to fine skin closure.

Multiple Z-plasties must be planned and executed in a similar manner. Multiple small Z-plasties may be preferable to one or two large flaps in treating an elongated scar. In multiple Z-plasties, there may be some overlapping of flaps, requiring trimming to achieve a flat final scar (Fig. 214-3).

IRA D. PAPEL

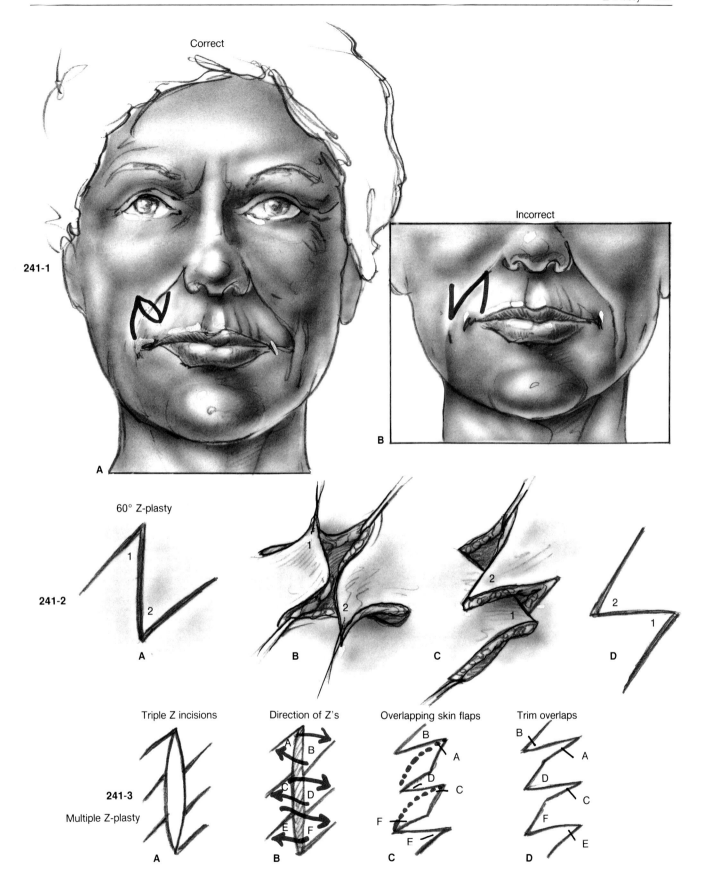

Correct

Incorrect

241-1

A

B

60° Z-plasty

241-2

A

B

C

D

Triple Z incisions

Direction of Z's

Overlapping skin flaps

Trim overlaps

241-3

Multiple Z-plasty

A

B

C

D

■ *242.* ADVANCEMENT FLAPS

Movement of skin into an adjacent area or defect without rotation or lateral movement

Indications

1. Primary closure of an elliptical excision
2. Closure of wound with adjacent redundant skin
3. Trauma

Contraindications

1. A dirty wound may close better by secondary intention.

Special Considerations

1. Use the simplest closure.
2. Design an ellipse if possible so that the closure is along relaxed skin tension lines.

Preoperative Preparation

1. Thorough cleaning, if needed
2. Standard clotting studies

Special Instruments, Position, and Anesthesia

1. Delicate plastic surgery instruments
2. Local anesthesia with a solution of 1% lidocaine with 1:100,000 epinephrine

Tips and Pearls

1. Meticulous hemostasis
2. Undermine equally in both directions

Pitfalls and Complications

1. Too much tension
2. Uneven closure by starting at one end

Postoperative Care Issues

1. Daily cleaning with hydrogen peroxide
2. Daily application of antibiotic ointment

Reference

Grabb WC. Classification of skin flaps. In: Grabb WC, Myers MB, eds. Skin flaps. Boston: Little, Brown, 1975:145.

Operative Procedure

After positioning the patient to optimally expose the area to be addressed, the area is prepped with Betadine or other antibacterial solution, and local anesthesia injected.

For a simple advancement flap, the edges are freshened and made perpendicular if necessary, and the advancement areas are undermined with a #15 blade or scissors dissection. In all cases, the plane of dissection should be just below the subdermal plexus. Initially, the midportion of the flaps are approximated. The wound is then closed, dividing the remaining open area by one half with each stitch to spread the tension and any unevenness between sides (Figs. 242-1 and 242-2). Continue until the entire length is closed. Absorbable subcuticular suture may be used to take tension off of a wide ellipse before skin closure.

For a single pedicle advancement flap, the flap is developed to advance into the defect area by using the skin's natural elasticity (Fig. 242-3) or by excision of Burow's triangles (Fig. 242-4). Undermining the receiving end allows it to advance as well, and balances the scar contracture. The flap is sutured into place, beginning with the corner stitches after meticulous hemostasis is achieved.

Variation

A bipedicle advancement flap may be used to close a visible area and move the defect to a less obvious site. Figure 242-5 illustrates use of a bipedicle flap near the scalp, with the new wound covered by a skin graft in a area easily covered by hair.

LINDA GAGE-WHITE

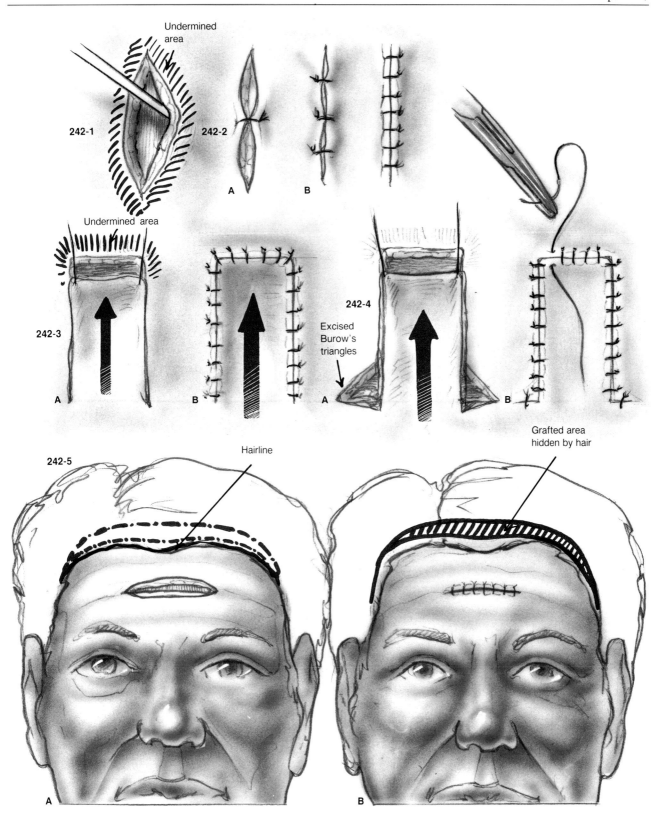

Undermined area

242-1

242-2

A   B

Undermined area

242-3

A   B

242-4

Excised Burow's triangles

A   B

242-5

Hairline

Grafted area hidden by hair

A   B

■ 243. TRIPLE RHOMBOID FLAPS

A complex of three local rhomboid-shaped skin flaps used to cover a skin defect

Indications

1. A circular defect, usually 3 to 8 cm in diameter (Fig. 243-1)
2. Movable skin (ie, no landmarks such as eyelid or nasal ala) on three equal sides of the defect

Special Considerations

1. Used with care in heavy smokers

Preoperative Preparation

1. The patient should avoid aspirin-containing compounds for 2 weeks before surgery, if possible.
2. Patients are encouraged to quit or reduce smoking.

Special Instruments, Position, and Anesthesia

1. Fine instrument tray with Bishop-Harmon forceps, Beaver knife handle with #64 blade, small sharp iris scissors, and Castroviejo needle holders
2. Surgical loupes
3. Performed under local or general anesthesia, depending on the patient's medical condition and preference

Tips and Pearls

1. Skin closure with absorbable suture, such as 6-0 Fastsorb chromic, obviates the need for suture removal with its potential for disturbance of the skin alignment.
2. If nonabsorbable sutures are used, use loupes or the microscope for meticulous visualization during removal.
3. Addition of one part sodium bicarbonate to five parts local anesthetic brings the pH closer to neutral and diminishes the burning sensation associated with injection.

Pitfalls and Complications

1. Chance of flap necrosis is diminished if adequate hemostasis is obtained and drainage is allowed with a rubber band drain or by using interrupted sutures so that drainage can occur between sutures.

Postoperative Care Issues

1. Suture lines are kept continuously moist with antibiotic ointment until healing is complete.
2. Use of Steri-strips to decrease tension on the healing wound may decrease the chance of the scar spreading.
3. Consider dermabrasion 6 to 8 weeks after surgery.

Reference

Larrabee WF, Trachy R, Sutton D, Cox K. Rhomboid flap dynamics. Arch Otolaryngol 1981;107:755.

Operative Procedure

With the patient in a supine position, the skin is infiltrated with local anesthesia. The skin is widely undermined in a subcutaneous plane, leaving a thin layer of subcutaneous fat on the skin flap. The circular defect is then divided into three equal sections. A best-fit rhomboid is drawn into each section. The central axis of each rhomboid is extended onto the surrounding skin, and rhomboid flaps are drawn (Fig. 243-2). Careful planning in this step is crucial to a successful outcome. The lines dividing the circle into thirds may be placed anywhere around the circumference, as long as they are equidistant. Each rhomboid may be drawn in one of two directions, but it is essential that all are drawn in a similar direction.

Points B1, B2, and B3 are brought together, and a horizontal subcutaneous 4-0 or 5-0 Vicryl suture is used to join them (Fig. 243-3). The opposite edges of the rhomboid flaps are sutured into position (eg, A1 to C1). Additional subcutaneous sutures are placed as needed to close the wounds. Fine skin stitches are placed, usually as three separate running sutures (Fig. 243-4).

Antibiotic ointment is applied to the wound.

KAREN H. CALHOUN

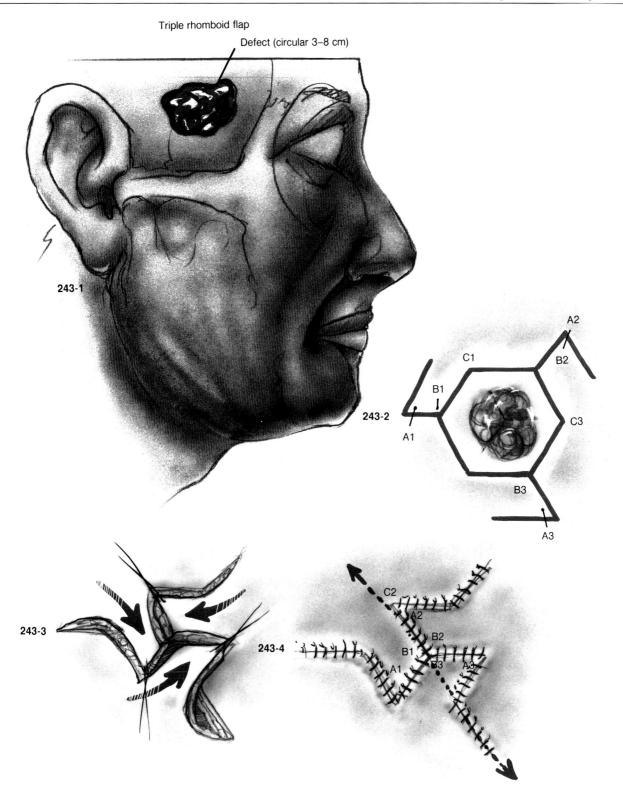

Triple rhomboid flap
Defect (circular 3–8 cm)

243-1

243-2

C1
A2
B2
B1
A1
C3
B3
A3

243-3

243-4
C2
A2
B2
B1
B3
A1
A3

■ *244.* PERICRANIAL FLAP

Flap consisting of loose areolar tissue (connective tissue) and cranial periosteum, together defined as the pericranium

Indications

1. Reconstruction of small to medium-sized defects of the floor of the anterior cranial fossa[1,2]
2. Combined with laterally based temporalis fascia and muscle for reconstruction of lateral defects in the anterior skull base
3. Coverage for cartilage grafts in reconstruction of the ear
4. Augmentation of facial soft tissue defects
5. Combined with temporalis muscle and fascia, tunneled beneath the zygoma for closure of lateral oropharyngeal wall and oral cavity defects after tumor resection[3]

Special Considerations

1. Rich vascular supply
   a. Axial pattern: deep division of the supraorbital artery
   b. Random pattern: supratrochlear and perforating branches through the galea aponeurotica of the superficial division of the supraorbital and superficial temporal arteries
2. Contiguity of pericranium with temporalis fascia allows its inclusion with temporalis muscle to increase the amount of transferred tissue
3. Can be combined with overlying galea aponeurotica, skin, or underlying bone to create composite flaps for head and neck reconstruction

Special Instruments, Position, and Anesthesia

1. Periosteal elevator
2. Thermal or cold knife

Tips and Pearls

1. Dissection between the subgaleal plane and subperiosteal plane to create the pericranial flap
2. Flap must be planned and elevated during the initial exposure to the anterior cranial fossa to prevent damage to flap tissue.
3. The flap can be based inferiorly (ie, supraorbital and supratrochlear arteries), laterally (ie, superficial temporal artery), or bilaterally on the superficial temporal arteries as a visor flap.

Pitfalls and Complications

1. When used alone, the pericranial flap is limited to small to medium-sized defects of the anterior skull base; larger defects require the use of regional myofascial flaps or distant vascularized tissue, such as myocutaneous flaps or revascularized free flaps that may contain bone.
2. Although the flap is extremely durable, potential exists for flap breakdown, resulting in cerebrospinal fluid leaks, pneumocephalus, and retrograde infection producing meningitis and other intracranial infections.

References

1. Stiernberg CM, Bailey BJ, et al. Reconstruction of the anterior skull base following craniofacial resection. Arch Otolaryngol Head Neck Surg 1987;113:710.
2. Johns ME, Winn RH, McLean WC, Cantrell RW. Pericranial flap for the closure of defects of craniofacial resections. Laryngoscope 1981;91:952.
3. Hüttenbrink KB. Temporalis muscle flap: an alternative in oropharyngeal reconstruction. Laryngoscope 1986;96:1034.

Operative Procedure

The combined approach of craniofacial resection for lesions of the anterior skull base, nasal cavity, and paranasal sinuses has been well described elsewhere, and only details pertinent to the pericranial flap reconstruction are discussed here. From above, access is gained to the anterior cranial fossa using a bicoronal incision elevated in the subgaleal plane down to the supraorbital rim, followed by any of a variety of frontal craniotomies. From below, transfacial exposure is attained using a lateral rhinotomy or facial degloving approach. The exposure allows en block resection of the involved structures, including the cribriform plate, the involved paranasal sinuses, nasal cavity, orbit, orbital contents, and dura.

The pericranial flap used to reconstruct the resulting defect is elevated in conjunction with the creation of the bicoronal flap early in the procedure. The layers contributing to the pericranium are illustrated in (Fig. 244-1). The bicoronal flap is initially elevated in the subgaleal plane, leaving the pericranial layers intact. An inferiorly based U-shaped or apron flap based on the supraorbital and supratrochlear arteries is then sharply outlined (Fig. 244-2). A periosteal elevator is used to raise the flap from the cranium to the level of the supraorbital rims. It is then retracted using silk sutures and carefully laid over the previously created bicoronal flap and protected with a moistened sponge until the time of reconstruction (Fig. 244-3).

After tumor resection, reconstruction of the defect is begun by repairing any dural tears; larger dural defects are closed using fascial grafts such as fascia lata. The pericranial flap is then rotated posteriorly through the craniotomy site to cover the anterior cranial fossa defect (Fig. 244-4). It is secured in place by suturing it to the deepest portion of exposed dura, to the bony margins of anterior fossa defect, reinforcing areas of dural tears. The flap provides structural support for the anterior cranial fossa contents, a watertight closure preventing cerebrospinal fluid leaks, and a barrier preventing retrograde infection from the contaminated nose and paranasal sinuses. The anterior cranial fossa contents are returned to their original position, and the bone flap is replaced. As an additional layer of closure, a skin graft or an abdominal fat graft (Scarpa's fascia-free graft) may be placed against the nasal side of the pericranial flap and held in place by antibiotic-impregnated gauze nasal packing. The remaining surgical incisions are closed. The nasal packing is left in place for 7 days.

A laterally based pericranial flap with axial blood supply provided by the superficial temporal vessels, incorporating galea, temporalis fascia, and muscle, can be elevated and used to reconstruct larger and more laterally based anterior cranial fossa defects (Fig. 244-5). A similar flap using pericranium, temporalis fascia, and muscle can be tunneled beneath the zygoma via the infratemporal fossa for closure of defects in the maxilla or lateral pharynx.[3] Other uses for the pericranial flap are coverage of cartilaginous structures in ear reconstruction and augmentation of facial defects.

Because of its rich vascularity, proximity to the defect, and technical ease of elevation, the pericranial flap is ideal for reconstruction of small to medium-sized anterior skull base defects. When combined with contiguous fascia and muscle, the pericranial flap provides a versatile method of head and neck reconstruction.

PAUL A. LEVINE
SCOTT D. MEREDITH

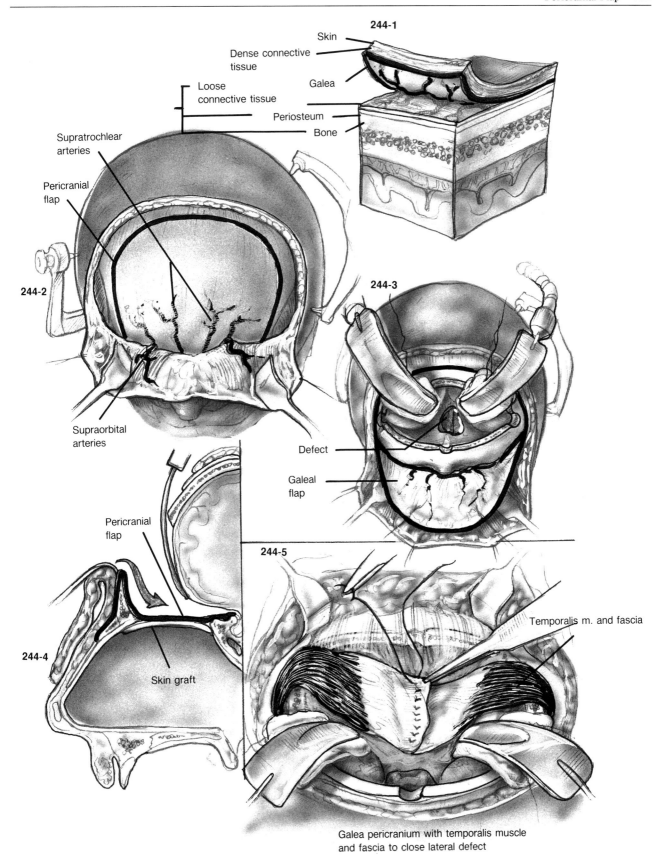

244-1

Skin

Dense connective tissue

Galea

Loose connective tissue

Periosteum

Bone

Supratrochlear arteries

Pericranial flap

244-2

Supraorbital arteries

244-3

Defect

Galeal flap

Pericranial flap

244-4

Skin graft

244-5

Temporalis m. and fascia

Galea pericranium with temporalis muscle and fascia to close lateral defect

■ 245. TISSUE EXPANSION

Repeated inflation of an implanted Silastic balloon, resulting in the expansion of overlying soft tissue and skin

Indications

1. Creation of extra skin for local flaps in the head and neck
2. Provision of skin flaps of similar color, texture, and hair-bearing qualities as required by local defects
3. Treatment of localized baldness or alopecia
4. Cranioplasty

Special Considerations

1. Discussions with patient regarding head and neck deformity during expansion process
2. Placement of incisions for inserting expanders
3. Proposed flap to be used after expansion
4. Blood supply of surrounding tissues
5. Previous irradiation of the area of intended expansion
6. Size and contour of expander to be used
7. Contingency plans in case of expander infection or extrusion

Preoperative Preparation

1. Routine laboratory studies
2. Bleeding and clotting studies
3. Detailed informed consent
4. Preplanning of proposed expander placement and proposed flap creation
5. Procurement of appropriately sized expander
6. Appropriate amount of expansion before expander removal

Special Instruments, Position, and Anesthesia

1. Headlight
2. A 1% solution of Xylocaine with 1:100,000 epinephrine
3. Adequate retractors (eg, Richardson, Deaver, facelift)
4. Bipolar cautery

(continued)

Operative Procedure

The preoperative workup is critical to the success of this surgery. Assessment of the skin quality, scarring, previous radiation therapy, blood supply, and hair-bearing characteristics of the defect and the adjacent tissues to be used for the reconstruction is required. A careful psychological assessment of the patient is needed, with extensive counseling about the expected head and neck changes associated with chronic tissue expansion. Preoperative planning should yield a surgical strategy regarding the most appropriate flap coverage of the defect, including the incisions and lines of tension for closure of such a flap. The size and shape of the expander is dictated by the location of these incisions and by the amount of tissue expansion required to produce the flap (Figs. 245-1 through 245-3 and 245-5). This expander, together with a spare in case of a defective product, should be available at the time of surgery.

With the patient in a supine position and suitably prepped and draped, the intended expander pocket, the placement incision, and an adjacent pocket for placement of the remote injection reservoir are marked on the patient (Figs. 245-4 and 245-7). The area is injected with a 1% solution of Xylocaine with a 1:100,000 concentration of epinephrine. Injection provides anesthesia and vasoconstriction for improved hemostasis. If the placement incision is going to be within hair-bearing scalp, a 1-cm strip of hair is shaved, and the area is carefully reprepped. Adhesive transparent dressings are used to keep adjacent hair out the wound.

An incision is made through the skin and subcutaneous tissue to the level intended for expander placement. On the scalp, this is usually subgaleal; on the face, it is subdermal; and in the neck, it is subplatysmal or subdermal. Sharp and blunt dissection are used to create a tunnel from the placement incision to the proposed pocket for the tissue expander. This pocket should be at least 2 cm away from the placement incision. Ideally, the placement incision and tunnel should be narrower than the width of the expander pocket. The expander pocket should be just large enough to accept the expander in its flattened, unfolded state. By placing the expander through a tunnel of smaller dimensions at a distance from the incision, migration of the inflatable tissue expander before and during expansion can be minimized.

Careful hemostasis is secured within the elevated pocket. This can usually be accomplished with the use of a headlight and various retractors, depending on the size and location of the expander pocket. Flat-bladed retractors with fiberoptic light sources attached, as used in facelift and breast augmentation surgery, are often helpful in identifying bleeding points in the distal pocket. Bipolar cauterization is used.

If a tissue expander with an integrated injection port is to be used, the expander pocket needs to be slightly larger than the base dimensions of the expander. This allows tension-free draping of the overlying soft tissues, because the integrated expander port is relatively thick and increases the vertical profile of the deflated expander when in place. If a remote injection port connected to the expander by Silastic tubing is to be used, a second pocket for this injection reservoir should be created. This reservoir should be placed far enough away from the expander to prevent an inadvertent puncture of a partially inflated expander during transcutaneous needle puncture of the reservoir. The tubing connecting the reservoir to the expander should be oriented to avoid overlap with the injection reservoir and inadvertent puncture during inflation. This usually can be achieved by placing the reservoir on the opposite side of the placement incision from the expander. If the placement incision is adjacent to a defect (Figs. 245-3 through 245-6), this is not possible,

(continued)

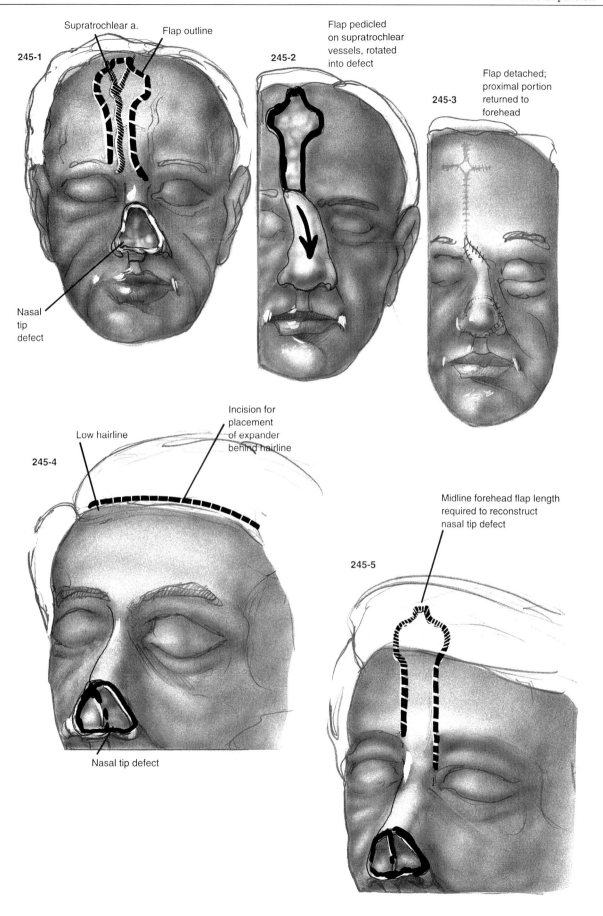

245-1 Supratrochlear a. Flap outline

Nasal tip defect

245-2 Flap pedicled on supratrochlear vessels, rotated into defect

245-3 Flap detached; proximal portion returned to forehead

245-4 Low hairline Incision for placement of expander behind hairline

Nasal tip defect

245-5 Midline forehead flap length required to reconstruct nasal tip defect

■ *245.* TISSUE EXPANSION *(continued)*

Tips and Pearls

1. Create a pocket of appropriate size for the expander.
2. Place the expander away from the incision line.
3. Locate the remote infusion port far enough from the expander to avoid needle injury to the expander during inflation.
4. Use previous scars when available for placement of the expander.
5. Always overexpand, because tissues naturally contract.
6. Obtain good hemostasis.
7. Place a drain, if necessary.
8. Expect higher complication rates when expanding irradiated tissues.
9. Avoid scalp expansion in children before closure of the cranial suture lines.
10. Expect the fibrous capsule around the expander, including the fibrous "bowl" between the expander and skull, to resorb over time.
11. The amount of expansion over a rigid base such as the cranium is easy to estimate, but expansion in the neck frequently deceives surgeon. Overexpand the neck skin.
12. If a knuckle of the Silastic expander is palpable through the skin, deflate the expander by 50 mL, massage the expander to remove the pressure point, and reinflate.
13. Telangiectasia of the expanded skin resolves spontaneously after the expander removed.

Pitfalls and Complications

1. Improper planning may result in an incision for expander placement that severs the blood supply of the proposed flap to be used after expansion.
2. Infection leading to premature removal of the expander
3. Expander placement too close to fresh suture lines, leading to extrusion during expansion
4. Overzealous expansion, leading to tissue thinning, striae formation, alopecia, or extrusion
5. Inadvertent puncture of the expander during placement or during inflation
6. Hematoma formation
7. Pocket size too large, leading to expander migration and inadvertent expansion of soft tissues not intended for expansion, such as eyebrows or the junction with hair-bearing skin
8. Inadequate expansion, expanders removed too soon, or flaps inadequate to cover the defect

Postoperative Care Issues

1. Care of the expander placement incision to avoid local infection
2. Early detection of hematoma formation, with evacuation under sterile conditions without puncturing the expander
3. Two-week delay between expander placement and inflation
4. Continued patient counseling about the enlarging expander in the head or neck region
5. Careful observation and patient counseling about the potential for infection around the expander
6. Accurately conceived surgical strategy to avoid underexpansion

and the reservoir needs to be placed on the same side of the placement incision as the expander but in a separate location.

After the appropriate surgical pockets have been created, the expander is fully inflated with air and immersed in saline to detect potential leaks, as evidenced by bubble formation. If the expander is intact, the air is evacuated, and it is reinflated to 10% of its proposed volume with sterile saline. After copious irrigation of the wound, the expander and the remote reservoir are placed in sterile fashion into their respective pockets. Careful attention is required to avoid folding the expander and to ensure that neither it nor the connecting tubing overlaps the reservoir port.

After proper orientation of expander, tubing, and reservoir has been attained, the wound can be closed in layers. Deep layer closure usually is carried out with interrupted sutures of 30 Maxon, and skin closure is achieved with a subcuticular monofilament. If there is any question of inadequate hemostasis, a small suction drain can be placed in the pocket with the expander and brought out through a separate stab wound; the drain is removed on the second postoperative day. A light pressure dressing is applied to help obliterate any dead space within the tunnel connecting the placement incision with the expander pocket. Antibiotic ointment is applied to the placement incision.

Careful postoperative assessment on the first, third, and seventh postoperative days reveals any evidence of hematoma or seroma formation. Sterile evacuation of such accumulations should avoid puncturing the buried expander. In the absence of hematoma, seroma, or infection, graduated expansion is usually begun after 2 weeks.

At each expander inflation the injection port is localized, and the overlying skin is prepped with Betadine (Figs. 245-6 and 245-8). Transcutaneous injection of sterile saline through a 23-gauge needle is continued until the skin over the expander shows decreased capillary filling or until the patient complains of discomfort. At this point, the injection needle is withdrawn, and pressure is applied to the injection site with a sterile pad until bleeding has stopped. In most cases, 10% of the expander volume can be administered on a weekly basis. More frequent expansions can be carried out, usually on a biweekly basis.

At each office visit for graduated expansion, patient counseling is continued about the negative aesthetic results of increasing expansion within the head or neck region. The expander site is also checked for evidence of inflammation, infection, or tissue thinning that could lead to premature expander exposure and extrusion.

After appropriate expansion has been accomplished, usually after 6 to 8 weeks, the patient is returned to the operating room for removal of the expander, creation of the intended flap, and reconstruction of the defect. With the expander fully inflated, the flap is outlined over the expanded skin. The maximal length of the skin flap will be attained by designing it over the convexity of the expander rather than along the perimeter of the expander. The patient is prepped and draped in routine fashion, and the area injected with a 1% solution of Xylocaine with 1:100,000 epinephrine. The expander can be deflated with a large-bore needle and a 50-mL syringe through the injection port. Flap incisions are carried through the skin, subcutaneous tissue, and fibrous capsule surrounding the expander. The expander is visualized and removed. Remote ports can be removed through separate incisions after division of the connecting tube.

The edges of the defect to be repaired are freshly incised. The skin graft or scar is removed, and the flap is transferred to the defect. Donor and recipient wounds are closed in routine fashion after hemostasis is secured (Fig. 245-9).

RICHARD E. HAYDEN

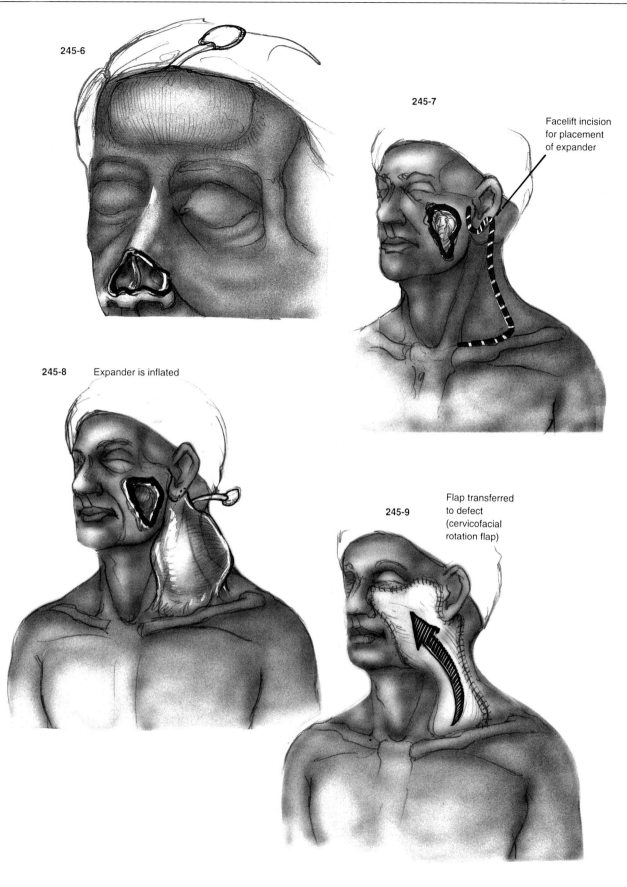

245-6

245-7

Facelift incision for placement of expander

245-8   Expander is inflated

245-9   Flap transferred to defect (cervicofacial rotation flap)

■ 246. PECTORALIS MAJOR MYOCUTA-NEOUS FLAP—A flap of pectoralis major muscle and the overlying skin that is pedicled on the thoracoacromial vessels

Indications

1. Bulky soft tissue defects of the neck and lower face, especially the oral cavity and oropharynx
2. Need for a flap that reaches as high as the zygomatic arch
3. Use of this flap in the face or neck in conjunction with a neck dissection also provides carotid artery coverage.

Contraindications

1. There are no absolute contraindications.
2. Primary closure of the flap donor site creates a restrictive pulmonary defect. This usually causes minimal morbidity but may be clinically troublesome in a patient with very poor pulmonary reserves.
3. The flap is more likely to fail in a patient with severe systemic vascular disease, diabetes, or obesity.

(continued)

Operative Procedure

The skin is prepped from the midaxillary line to the across the midline and from the neck across the chest wall to below the coastal margin.

A bipedicled deltopectoral flap should be outlined first to allow preservation of the vascular supply to this flap (Fig. 246-1). The pectoralis skin paddle is outlined inferior to this overlying muscle. The arc of rotation is increased by placing the skin paddle at the inferior margin of the pectoralis muscle. A crescent-shaped skin paddle in the inframammary crease in women provides a more cosmetic result (Fig. 246-2).

After incising the skin and muscle, temporary sutures are used between the skin and muscle to prevent inadvertent shearing of the skin from the muscle during the rest of the harvest (Figs. 246-3 and 246-4). The pectoralis muscle fascia is elevated under the outlined deltopectoral flap to preserve its vascularity (Figs. 246-5 through 246-7). The skin is widely undermined, allowing easier identification of the lateral border of the pectoralis muscle and facilitating later closure.

The vascular pedicle is identified before the muscle cuts, particularly on the lateral portion of the pectoralis muscle. The vessel is most readily identified laterally, where the pectoralis minor muscle and fascial planes are more easily found. The pedicle can also be identified from medial and inferior approaches, although the multiple muscle insertions onto the ribs makes establishing the correct fascial plane more difficult. The flap is then elevated, and with the vessels in direct view, the pedicle is trimmed.

(continued)

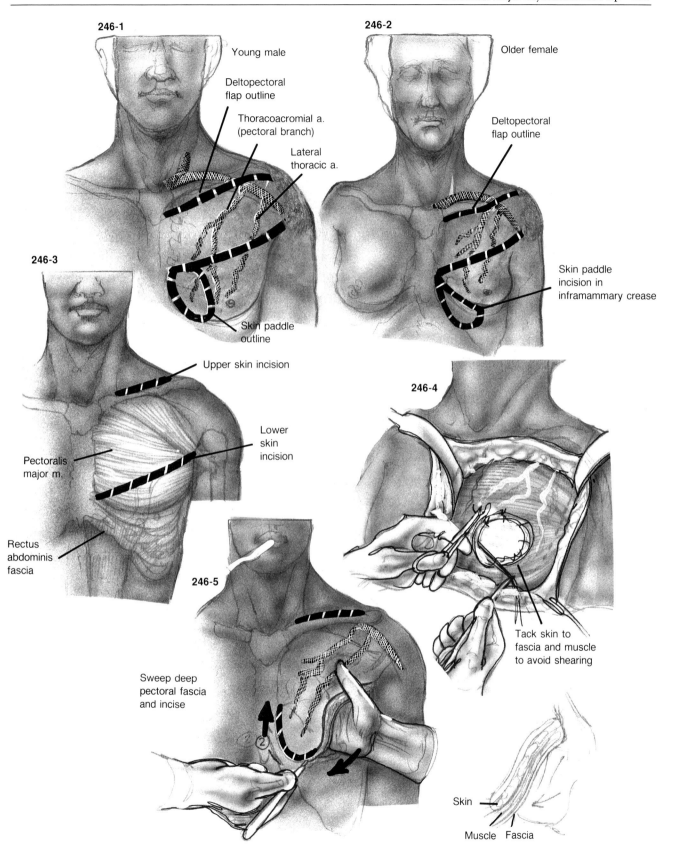

246-1

Young male

Deltopectoral flap outline

Thoracoacromial a. (pectoral branch)

Lateral thoracic a.

Skin paddle outline

246-2

Older female

Deltopectoral flap outline

Skin paddle incision in inframammary crease

246-3

Upper skin incision

Lower skin incision

Pectoralis major m.

Rectus abdominis fascia

246-4

Tack skin to fascia and muscle to avoid shearing

246-5

Sweep deep pectoral fascia and incise

Skin

Muscle   Fascia

■ 246. PECTORALIS MAJOR MYOCUTA-
NEOUS FLAP (continued)

Special Considerations
1. Harvesting this flap does not require a position change during most head and neck cases.
2. Allows repair using nonirradiated tissue in most head and neck cases
3. Donor site morbidity is minimal, and the site usually can be closed primarily.
4. The cutaneous paddle is very thick in some patients, especially obese patients, and this may limit its use.
5. In hirsute individuals, hair can continue to grow after flap transfer, which can be problematic in the OC/OP.
6. The flap creates breast distortion in women; this can be minimized by designing the skin paddle in the inframammary crease.

Preoperative Preparation
1. Routine laboratory studies

Special Instruments, Position, and Anesthesia
1. Prep the chest before beginning head and neck surgery.
2. Place central lines on the opposite side of the chest.

The use of back lighting and transillumination may help, and a Doppler probe may be useful, especially for thick muscle. A cervical tunnel broad enough to prevent compression is developed beneath the deltopectoral flap over the clavicle. Easy passage of four fingers through the tunnel indicates an appropriate size. A McFee neck incision for tumor removal adapts well for the passage of a pectoralis flap, because it is often performed with a neck dissection. Adequate undermining of the cervical skin usually permits. Rarely, a skin graft is necessary to cover over the pectoralis pedicle.

The flap is passed superiorly through the prepared tunnel (Fig. 246-8). The tunnel and flap placement are checked to ensure there is no tension that could cause spasm or occlusion of the artery.

For flap insetting, a single-layer watertight closure is sufficient. It is important to provide tacking sutures on the muscle, especially superiorly, to prevent the muscle from shearing away from the cutaneous portion of the flap (Fig. 246-9).

The chest wall is closed after meticulous hemostasis is achieved. With wide undermining, defects as wide as 8 to 10 cm may be closed primarily. Suction drains are placed and left until the drainage becomes minimal, usually in 3 to 4 days.

Postoperatively, the capillary refill time is assessed frequently. The skin color is often somewhat paler than surrounding skin, but it should be pale pink and not congested or mottled. Venous congestion causes excessive bleeding around the edges of the flap after insetting. Explicit orders should be left to prevent anything from compressing the vascular pedicle, including the tracheostomy ties, hospital gowns, or oxygen masks.

ERNEST A. WEYMULLER, JR.
MICHAEL G. GLENN

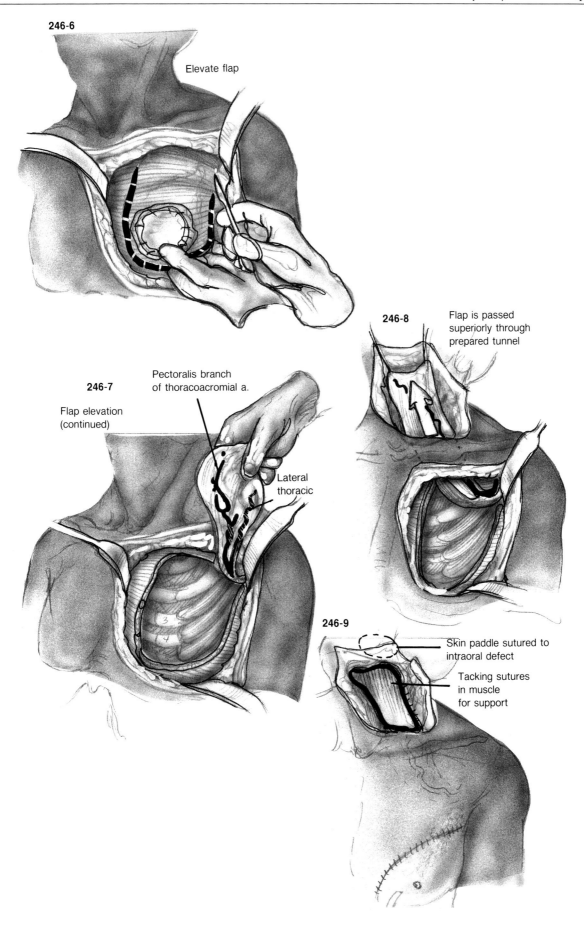

246-6

Elevate flap

246-7

Flap elevation
(continued)

Pectoralis branch
of thoracoacromial a.

Lateral
thoracic

246-8

Flap is passed
superiorly through
prepared tunnel

246-9

Skin paddle sutured to
intraoral defect

Tacking sutures
in muscle
for support

■ 247. SUPERIOR TRAPEZIUS FLAP

An axial-pattern myocutaneous flap developed from the upper two thirds of the trapezius muscle along with its overlying skin. The attached pedicle is proximal, near the midline.

Indications

1. Cutaneous cover loss over the lower face and the ipsilateral cervical region
2. Coverage of exposed carotid after wound breakdown
3. Creation of an orocutaneous fistula after wound breakdown
4. Ipsilateral oropharyngeal defects
5. Ipsilateral hypopharyngeal defects

Special Considerations

1. Previous surgery in the region
2. State of innervation to the trapezius muscle

Preoperative Preparation

1. Routine laboratory studies
2. Inspection of the trapezius area for previous surgery or traumatic injury
3. Inspection of the contralateral trapezius for normal function

Special Instruments, Position, and Anesthesia

1. Routine major surgical tray
2. Patient's head positioned on horseshoe headrest, with the entire shoulder exposed

Tips and Pearls

1. The anterior incision follows the anterior border of the trapezius muscle.
2. The posterior incision follows the spine of the scapula and then runs parallel to the anterior incision.
3. The maximum random extension is 10 cm.
4. If the transverse cervical artery does not tether the rotation, do not ligate it.
5. If the harvest defect is less than 10 cm, close primarily.
6. Although the flap may be used to reconstruct the pharynx, it requires a controlled fistula with a second-stage takedown of the flap base, and it therefore is not the first choice for this region.

Pitfalls and Complications

1. Random extension beyond 10 cm may lead to distal flap loss.
2. A skin graft over the harvest site is prone to abrasion and breakdown.

Postoperative Care Issues

1. Position a pillow under the ipsilateral shoulder to prevent pressure on the proximal portion of the flap.
2. Remove the bolster on the skin graft in 5 to 7 days.
3. After waiting 6 months to 1 year, flap revision may be necessary to debulk the dog-ear defect at the base or to defat thick areas of the flap.

References

Donald PJ, Chole RA. Superiorly based trapezius flap. 1984;94:969.
Maves MD, Netterville JL, Boozan JA, Keenan MJ. Superiorly based trapezius flap for emergency carotid artery coverage. 1992;13:342.
Netterville JL, Panje WR, Maves MD. The trapezius myocutaneous flaps. Arch Otolaryngol 1987;113:271.

Operative Procedure

With the patient in the supine position after adequate general anesthesia has been obtained, the head is stabilized as the horseshoe headrest is attached to the bed. For extra padding the firm surface of the headrest is wrapped with felt rolls. The rest is extended out from the table until the shoulders overhang the edge of the bed; this position provides access to the region of the scapular spine.

When outlining incisions for a resection of a primary site, it is wise to align the cervical incisions along the anterior border of the trapezius flap to prevent a small strip of elevated skin between the resection incisions and the incisions needed to outline the trapezius flap. The superior trapezius flap is composed of the superior two thirds of the trapezius muscle along with its overlying skin and a distal segment of random skin extension. The axial-pattern flap has its base oriented toward the midline of the back. Its major vascular supply is from the ipsilateral intercostal perforating arteries (Fig. 247-1). The occipital and the transverse cervical arteries provide supplementary blood supply.

The use of this flap necessitates the loss of function of the trapezius muscle. If resection has not resulted in the loss of the spinal accessory nerve, I am hesitant to use this flap. If the trapezius function is still intact, I exhaust all other reconstructive options before employing this flap, because the loss of trapezius function results in significant morbidity after head and neck surgery.

The flap is outlined with its anterior border along the anterior edge of the trapezius muscle. The posterior edge roughly parallels the anterior edge, incorporating all of the trapezius muscle above the spine of the scapula. The distal extent of the muscle is identified by the junction of the acromion process with the clavicle. As necessary for length, a distal random segment is outlined beyond this point, but it should not exceed 10 cm.

The initial incision is created a the distal aspect of the flap and down to the deltoid muscle, and the deltoid fascia is raised with the distal flap. As the clavicle is exposed, finger dissection is used to tunnel deep to the trapezius muscle where it attaches to the clavicle and the acromion process (Fig. 247-2). The anterior and posterior incisions are extended as the flap is raised, and the muscle is incised from front to back off the clavicle, the acromion process, and then the spine of the scapula. In most situations employing this flap, a previous radical neck dissection has been performed. If the transverse cervical artery is still intact, the surgeon can usually leave it inserting into the flap. The rotation toward the cervical region is not hindered by this vessel.

The trapezius muscle is raised up off the supraspinatus and the levator scapulae muscles. As the rhomboid minor muscle is visualized, the perforating dorsal scapular artery is also seen. The dorsal scapular must be ligated for flap mobilization. At this point, the flap is rotated into position to test for adequate length. If the length needed for rotation is insufficient, the posterior incision is extended until the rotation is complete (Fig. 247-3). Care is taken as the trapezius muscle is elevated toward the midline to prevent injury to the intercostal perforating arteries, which provide the major blood supply to the flap.

The flap is rotated into position and sutured in place with strong sutures, such a 2-0 Vicryl, in a subcutaneous fashion (Fig. 247-4). If the rotation is forward to the cervicofacial region, a large, superior dog-ear is produced. A Penrose drain is brought out through this region, which is dependent when the patient is supine. If all edges of the closure can be sealed, I prefer closed suction drainage, but if the upper edge at the dog-ear cannot be closed well, the Penrose is used.

The harvest site is closed primarily, if possible, or a split-thickness skin graft is placed immediately or transferred in a delayed fashion after an adequate granulation bed has been produced by secondary healing (see Fig. 247-4). If primary grafting is used, the bolster is removed 5 to 7 days later.

The patient is positioned in the postoperative period with a pillow under the ipsilateral back to prevent any pressure on the proximal portion of the flap.

JAMES L. NETTERVILLE

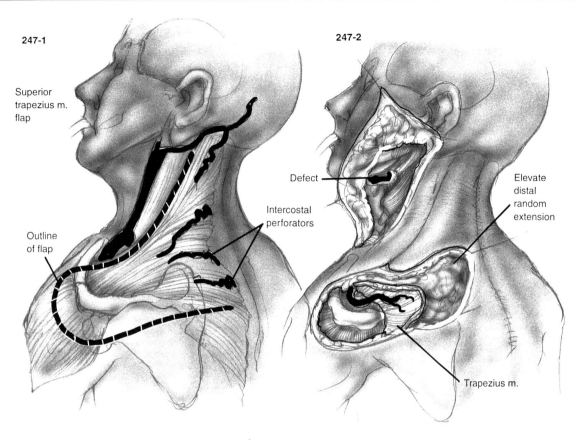

247-1

Superior trapezius m. flap

Outline of flap

Intercostal perforators

247-2

Defect

Elevate distal random extension

Trapezius m.

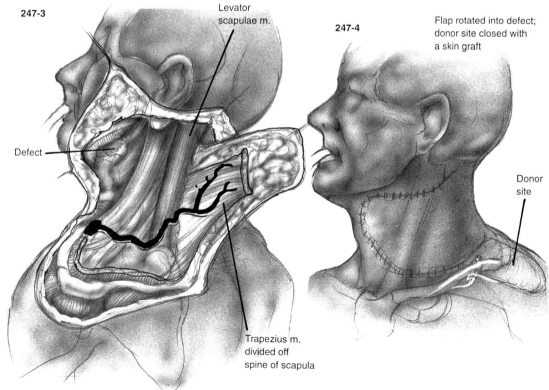

247-3

Levator scapulae m.

Defect

Trapezius m. divided off spine of scapula

247-4

Flap rotated into defect; donor site closed with a skin graft

Donor site

■ *248.* LATERAL ISLAND TRAPEZIUS FLAP

An island-pattern myocutaneous flap developed from the upper lateral trapezius muscle along with its overlying skin and a lateral random extension.

Indications

1. Ipsilateral oropharyngeal defects
2. Ipsilateral hypopharyngeal and cervical esophageal defects
3. Cutaneous cover loss over the ipsilateral face, temporal, and cervical regions

Special Considerations

1. Previous surgery in the region
2. Integrity of the transverse cervical artery and vein
3. State of innervation to the trapezius muscle

Preoperative Preparation

1. Routine laboratory studies
2. Inspection of the trapezius area for previous surgery or traumatic injury
3. A preoperative angiogram is necessary to establish the vascular supply to the flap if the patient has had radical neck dissection.
4. Inspection of the contralateral trapezius for normal function

Special Instruments, Position, and Anesthesia

1. Routine major surgical tray
2. Patient's head positioned on horseshoe headrest, with the entire shoulder exposed

Tips and Pearls

1. The anterior incision follows the anterior border of the trapezius muscle.
2. The posterior incision follows the spine of the scapula and then runs parallel to the anterior incision.
3. The maximum random extension is 10 cm.
4. If the harvest defect is less than 10 cm, close primarily.
5. If trapezius function is still normal, avoid the use of this flap if another flap is equally useful.
6. Always have an alternate plan when planning reconstruction with this flap.

Pitfalls and Complications

1. Random extension beyond 10 cm may lead to distal flap loss.
2. The transverse cervical artery may be injured during concurrent neck dissection.
3. The transverse cervical artery may arise laterally off the dorsal scapular artery, limiting the arch of rotation of the flap into pharyngeal defects.

Postoperative Care Issues

1. Prevent cervical ties on the tracheotomy tube or the oxygen mask from encircling the neck, resulting in pressure on the flap pedicle.
2. If the flap develops vascular compromise, it should be debrided and replaced before necrosis and infection occur.

References

Demergasso F, Piazza MV. Trapezius myocutaneous flaps in reconstructive surgery for head and neck cancer: an original technique. J Surg 1979;138:533.
Guillamondegui OM, Larson DL. The lateral trapezius musculocutaneous flap: its use in head and neck reconstruction. Plast Reconstr Surg 1981;67:143.
Panje WR. Myocutaneous trapezius flap. Head Neck Surg 1980;2:206.

Operative Procedure

With the patient in the supine position the head is stabilized in the Mayfield horseshoe headrest attached to the bed (Fig. 247-2). It is wrapped with orthopedic felt rolls to pad the surface of the headrest. The rest is extended out from the table until the shoulders overhang the edge of the bed to provide access to the region of the scapular spine.

It is wise to align the cervical incisions along the anterior border of the trapezius flap to prevent a small strip of elevated skin between the resection incisions and the incisions needed to outline the trapezius flap. The lateral island trapezius flap is composed of the superior lateral trapezius fibers and the overlying skin. The major blood supply to the flap comes from the transverse cervical artery and vein (Fig. 248-1). The origin of this artery is not consistent, limiting the use of this flap. Most commonly, the artery arises from the thyrocervical trunk and runs superior to the deep cervical fascia and over the levator muscle to insert onto the undersurface of the trapezius muscle near the insertion of the spinal accessory nerve.

The course of the transverse cervical also varies. Most commonly, it lies parallel to the artery. The external jugular vein is dissected after the skin flaps have been elevated and after protecting any veins draining into the vein in the lower lateral neck. The external jugular vein is ligated above these veins as the dissection progresses. If metastatic nodes are found in the lateral triangle, the use of the flap is aborted.

The skin paddle is drawn out over the superior lateral trapezius fibers (Fig. 248-3). To acquire the greatest arc of rotation, the paddle may be centered over the acromion process. The thin, supple skin of the distal random extension overlying the deltoid muscle is one of its main attributes. The paddle may be 25 to 250 cm^2, with an average size of 8 × 12 cm. In laying out the paddle, the surgeon must be sure that the transverse cervical artery inserts into the muscle beneath the skin paddle to ensure maximum viability. With the previously described anatomic variations in mind, the transverse cervical vein and artery are isolated in a systematic fashion, using the Doppler probe as needed to substantiate vascular flow early in the course of a neck dissection or through a limited incision over the clavicle. The outline of the skin paddle is incised down to the trapezius and deltoid fascia, and the skin paddle is stabilized to this fascia with temporary sutures.

The dissection starts at the lateral edge by raising the deltoid fascia with the flap (Fig. 248-4). As the edge of the clavicle is approached, blunt dissection is used to develop a plane between the supraspinatus and the fat on the undersurface of the trapezius. The transverse vessels lie within this fatty tissue. The insertion of the trapezius muscle is divided off the clavicle, the acromion, and the spine of the scapula (Fig. 248-5). The elevation continues deep to the trapezius muscle, separating it from the levator scapulae and the rhomboid minor muscles. During this elevation, the ascending branch of the dorsal scapular artery may be encountered just medial to the spine of the scapula inferior to the rhomboid muscle. Before division of this branch, the surgeon must be certain of the continuity and insertion of the transverse cervical artery and vein into the myocutaneous paddle. Doppler confirmation of the integrity of the transverse cervical artery is useful. It is prudent to divide the perforating dorsal scapular vessels low, leaving a 1-cm cuff of vessel on the undersurface of the flap. This provides the surgeon with the option of reanastomosis of the artery into the carotid system.

If the transverse cervical artery enters the trapezius lateral to the insertion of the accessory nerve, a small island flap may be raised lateral to the accessory insertion point. Occasionally, the spinal accessory nerve bifurcates into superior and inferior branches, allowing harvesting of a lateral island flap that may only partially denervate the trapezius muscle.

With the flap completely elevated on the deep surface, the trapezius fibers are divided medial to the skin paddle, freeing the flap for rotation into the defect (Fig. 248-6). The donor defect is usually closed primarily, but for larger flaps, it may be necessary to cover the site with a split-thickness skin graft.

JAMES L. NETTERVILLE

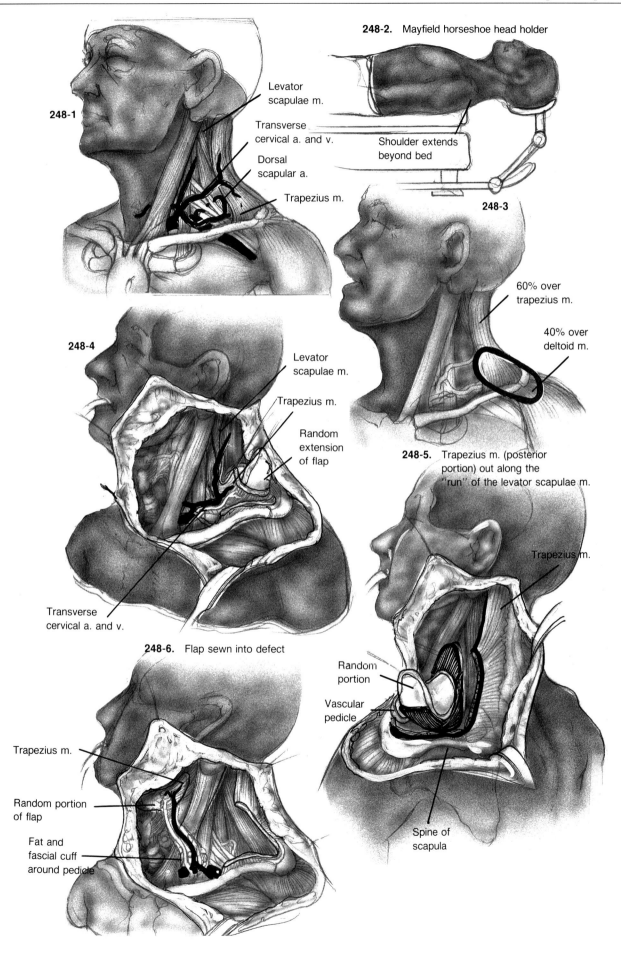

248-1

Levator scapulae m.

Transverse cervical a. and v.

Dorsal scapular a.

Trapezius m.

248-2. Mayfield horseshoe head holder

Shoulder extends beyond bed

248-3

60% over trapezius m.

40% over deltoid m.

248-4

Levator scapulae m.

Trapezius m.

Random extension of flap

Transverse cervical a. and v.

248-5. Trapezius m. (posterior portion) out along the "run" of the levator scapulae m.

Trapezius m.

Random portion

Vascular pedicle

Spine of scapula

248-6. Flap sewn into defect

Trapezius m.

Random portion of flap

Fat and fascial cuff around pedicle

■ 249. LOWER ISLAND TRAPEZIUS FLAP

An island-pattern myocutaneous flap developed from the lower medial trapezius muscle fibers along with its overlying skin and an inferolateral random skin extension.

Indications

1. Temporal-cutaneous defects
2. Lateral and occipital skull base defects
3. Ipsilateral oropharyngeal defects
4. Ipsilateral hypopharyngeal and cervical esophageal defects

Special Considerations

1. Previous surgery in the region
2. Integrity of the transverse cervical artery and vein
3. Integrity of the dorsal scapular artery and vein

Preoperative Preparation

1. Routine laboratory studies
2. Inspection of trapezius area for previous surgical or traumatic injury
3. A preoperative angiogram is necessary to establish the vascular supply to the flap if the patient has had radical neck dissection.
4. Special preoperative orders to prevent use of the ipsilateral arm by the anesthesia service for arterial monitoring or venous access

Special Instruments, Position, and Anesthesia

1. Routine major surgical tray
2. Patient in the lateral decubitus position, with a bean bag placed under patient for stability
3. Axillary roll to prevent injury to the brachial plexus

Tips and Pearls

1. Inclusion of the dorsal scapular artery allows a lower skin paddle position.
2. A lower skin paddle position allows an extended arch of rotation without injury to the upper trapezius fibers.
3. The proximal skin paddle is de-epithelialized to allow a greater muscle-fat interface.

(continued)

Operative Procedure

The skin overlying the trapezius muscle receives its blood supply from four sources: the transverse cervical artery, the dorsal scapular artery, the intercostal perforators lying just off the midline, and branches from the occipital artery. The transverse cervical and dorsal scapular arteries contribute blood supply to the lower trapezius muscle and its overlying skin, from which the lower trapezius flap is harvested. To be comfortable with the use of this flap, the surgeon must be familiar with the anatomy of these two vessels. The transverse cervical artery originates from the thyrocervical trunk. It then passes over the brachial plexus, and the levator muscle descends in the investing fascia on the deep surface of the trapezius muscle (Figs. 249-1 and 249-2). The dorsal scapular artery takes its origin from the subclavian artery, just lateral to the anterior scalene insertion. This branch is approximately 2 cm lateral to the origin of the thyrocervical trunk. The dorsal scapular artery then travels between the branches of the brachial plexus and takes a serpentine course as it dives deep to the levator muscle and the superior angle of the scapula (see Fig. 249-1). It divides at the level of the scapular spine. The major branch penetrates between the rhomboid major and minor muscles, and it then descends along the deep surface of the trapezius to supply the inferior trapezius region (see Fig. 249-2). The smaller branch or branches travel deep to the rhomboid major, yielding several small muscular perforators that may pass laterally through the rhomboid major into the trapezius in a more inferior position.

The previous description summarizes the more commonly described anatomic path of each of the arteries. However, equal-caliber arteries are found in a minority of dissections. In most dissections, the dorsal scapular or the transverse cervical artery is usually the larger, dominant vessel. The the proximal portion of the nondominant vessel often does not exist or is less than 1 mm in diameter and has no distal connection to the trapezius. If a proximal dominant artery occurs, the distal portions of the dorsal scapular and the transverse cervical arteries arise from that dominant vessel. If the transverse cervical artery is dominant, as it was in 9 of 30 cadaver dissections, the dorsal scapular artery branches off of it just proximal to the levator muscle and passes deep to the levator in its customary course. If the dorsal scapular artery is the dominant vessel, as it was in 15 of 30 dissections, the transverse cervical artery branches off of it just proximal to the levator and passes over the levator in its customary course.

Although there are variations in the proximal arterial anatomy, the vascular anatomy distal to the levator muscle is more consistent, with the transverse cervical artery following its usual pattern over the levator muscle and the dorsal scapular artery traveling in its usual path deep to the levator muscle and the upper border of the scapula. The importance of understanding these vascular variations is that, in cases of previous ipsilateral neck surgery, a preoperative angiogram is necessary to ensure an intact dorsal scapular arterial system supplying the lower trapezius region.

Based on these findings, a surgical technique is outlined for isolating and using the dorsal scapular artery during the harvest of the lower trapezius flap. The patient is positioned in the lateral decubitus position and prepped and draped so that the back is visible down to the lilac crest and past the midline, as identified by the spinal processes (Fig. 249-3). The ipsilateral arm is kept free of arterial or

(continued)

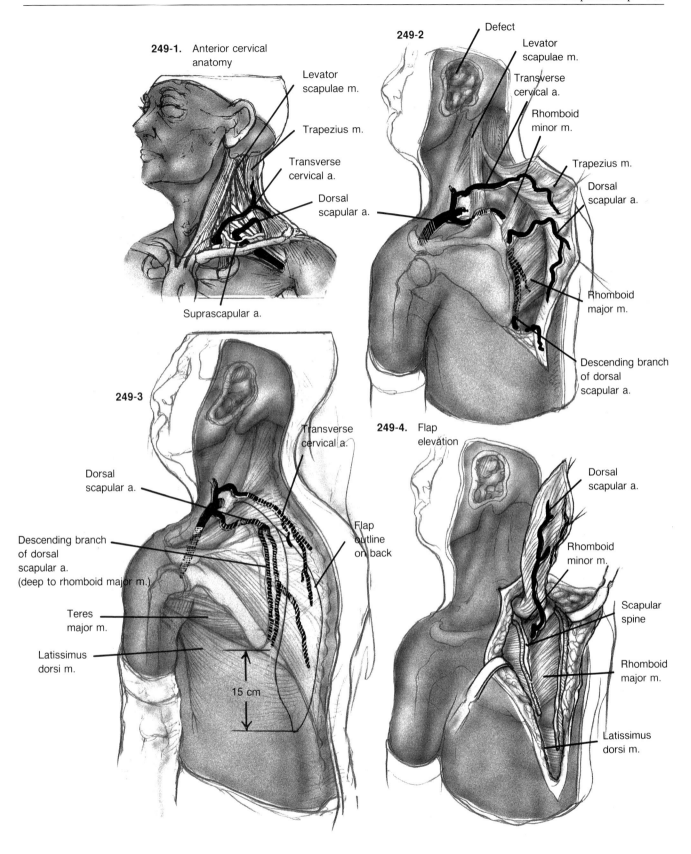

249-1. Anterior cervical anatomy

Levator scapulae m.

Trapezius m.

Transverse cervical a.

Dorsal scapular a.

Suprascapular a.

249-2

Defect

Levator scapulae m.

Transverse cervical a.

Rhomboid minor m.

Trapezius m.

Dorsal scapular a.

Rhomboid major m.

Descending branch of dorsal scapular a.

249-3

Dorsal scapular a.

Descending branch of dorsal scapular a. (deep to rhomboid major m.)

Teres major m.

Latissimus dorsi m.

Transverse cervical a.

Flap outline on back

15 cm

249-4. Flap elevation

Dorsal scapular a.

Rhomboid minor m.

Scapular spine

Rhomboid major m.

Latissimus dorsi m.

■ *249.* LOWER ISLAND TRAPEZIUS FLAP
(continued)

Pitfalls and Complications

1. Division of the dorsal scapular artery may necessitate moving the skin paddle into a more superior position and amputation of the distal portion of the paddle.
2. Previous cervical surgery with injury to the transverse cervical artery may produce a poorly vascularized flap.
3. Pressure on the upper back at the site of trapezius muscle rotation in the early postoperative period may result in flap necrosis.

Postoperative Care Issues

1. The patient is positioned with a pillow supporting the middle to lower back to prevent pressure on the upper back.
2. A caution sign is created with tape on the upper back over the site of muscle rotation to prevent pressure on this area in the early postoperative period.
3. Prevent cervical ties on the tracheotomy tube or the oxygen mask from encircling the neck, resulting in pressure on the flap pedicle.
4. If the flap develops vascular compromise, it should be debrided and replaced before necrosis and infection occur.

References

Netterville JL, Panje WR, Maves MD. The trapezius myocutaneous flaps. Arch Otolaryngol 1987;113:271.

Netterville JL, Wood DE. The lower trapezius flap: vascular anatomy and surgical technique. Arch Otolaryngol 1991;117:73.

Urken ML, Naidu RK, Lawson W, Biller HF. The lower trapezius island musculocutaneous flap revisited. Arch Otolaryngol Head Neck Surg 1991;117:502.

venous access lines and is draped sterilely into the field. This allows its mobility during the procedure. From this position, the surgeon can easily perform ablative procedures, including neck dissection, pharyngeal resection, temporal bone–skull base resection, or cutaneous resection. This prevents an intraoperative change of position, which always risks breaks in surgical techniques and sterility.

After the arm is placed in an anteriorly rotated position, the flap is outlined over the lower medial trapezius fibers. The medial edge of the flap is placed as close to the midline as possible, which allows a greater distal extension of the flap still overlying the inferior aspect of the trapezius muscle. The flap is purposely outlined longer than necessary and later tailored to fit the size of the surgical defect. This increase in paddle length allows a more cosmetic closure of the back incision with less dog-ear formation at each end and allows the inclusion of more potential perforators into the subcutaneous aspect of the flap. The distal aspect of the flap may extend 15 cm below the tip of the scapula, which creates a significant random extension on the inferior lateral aspect of the skin paddle.

The outlined skin paddle is incised and elevated over the latissimus dorsi, starting on the inferior lateral border. Following this plane medially, the surgeon can readily identify the lower trapezius fibers. The flap is further elevated deep to the trapezius until the lower border of the rhomboid major is identified. In most situations, this muscle is left in place, which prevents postoperative winging of the scapula. At this point, the distal arcade of the dorsal scapula artery is usually identified lying in the deep fascia on the undersurface of the trapezius muscle (Fig. 249-4). It is followed until it departs from the muscle at the interface between the rhomboid minor and the rhomboid major muscles adjacent to the medial portion of the scapular spine. Rarely, when the major branch of the dorsal scapular artery perforates more inferiorly through the body of the rhomboid major, the muscle is divided to free the vessel.

In most cases, additional pedicle length is needed. The descending branches of the dorsal scapular artery that pass deep to the rhomboid major are ligated with fine vascular clips and divided (Fig. 249-5). Usually, two or three sets of descending vessels must be divided. After this division, gentle dissection along the dorsal scapular artery allows the surgeon to uncoil it from its serpentine path under the scapula, which provides an additional 2 to 3 cm of pedicle length. If further rotation is needed, the rhomboid minor is divided on either side of the vascular pedicle (see Fig. 249-5, *dotted lines*), which supplies several more centimeters of rotation with no venous tension.

The upper trapezius fibers are divided superiorly just enough to rotate the distal portion of the skin paddle into the defect, protecting the superior portion of the muscle. This allows normal shoulder elevation postoperatively. The flap can then be passed through a subcutaneous tunnel over the remaining superior trapezius fibers into a pharyngeal defect or rotated onto a temporal-cutaneous defect. With the flap in position, the skin paddle is outlined and tailored to fit the defect (Fig. 249-6). If the proximal portion of the cutaneous paddle is too long, the necessary amount of skin is de-epithelialized, leaving the subcutaneous tissues on the muscle (Fig. 249-7), allowing a greater subcutaneous tissue–muscle interface that ensures more perforators into the cutaneous tissue. The distal end of the flap can be divided or de-epithelialized using the distal subcutaneous tissue for bulk.

The back is closed primarily. Postoperatively, the patient is positioned on a pillow that contacts the back inferior to the scapular spine, with a second pillow under the head (Fig. 249-8). This prevents pressures on the vessels as they rotate over the superior trapezius fibers.

If necessary, the surgeon can cut the dorsal scapular artery and continue the superior muscle division, allowing the flap to be vascularized only by the more superiorly placed transverse cervical artery. This works well for flaps positioned above the level of the scapula tip, but skin paddles positioned inferior to the scapula tip may suffer from arterial insufficiency without input from the dorsal scapular artery. This superior division also results in a complete loss of trapezius function.

JAMES L. NETTERVILLE

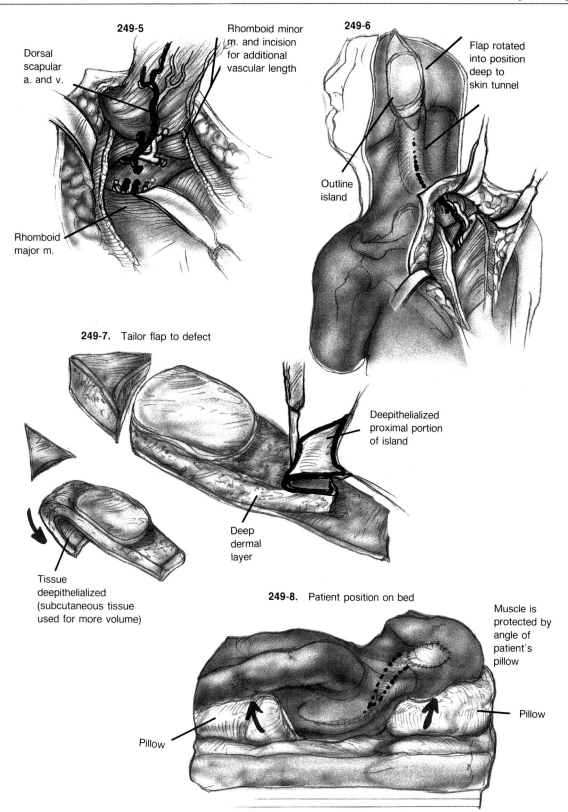

249-5

Dorsal scapular a. and v.

Rhomboid minor m. and incision for additional vascular length

Rhomboid major m.

249-6

Flap rotated into position deep to skin tunnel

Outline island

249-7. Tailor flap to defect

Deepithelialized proximal portion of island

Deep dermal layer

Tissue deepithelialized (subcutaneous tissue used for more volume)

249-8. Patient position on bed

Muscle is protected by angle of patient's pillow

Pillow

Pillow

■ *250.* LATISSIMUS DORSI MYOCUTANEOUS
FLAP—An island-pattern myocutaneous flap developed from the latissimus dorsi muscle along with its overlying skin

Indications
1. Cutaneous cover loss over the ipsilateral head and neck
2. Ipsilateral oropharyngeal defects
3. Ipsilateral hypopharyngeal defects
4. Cutaneous loss over the ipsilateral chest and shoulder region

Special Considerations
1. Previous surgery in the region
2. The thickness of the subcutaneous fat in the region may exclude use as a myocutaneous flap in obese patients; a myofascial flap may substitute in this group.
3. Functional deficit from loss of latissimus function

Preoperative Preparation
1. Routine laboratory studies
2. Inspection of the latissimus area for previous surgical or traumatic injury
3. Patient education about postoperative physical therapy for rehabilitation

Special Instruments, Position, and Anesthesia
1. Routine major surgical tray
2. Patient positioned in the lateral decubitus position, with the use of a bean bag
3. Careful padding of the contralateral axilla
4. Ipsilateral arm prepped into the field

(continued)

Operative Procedure
The patient is positioned in the lateral decubitus position, using a bean-bag support. The contralateral axilla is carefully padded with a wrapped bag of intravenous fluids, and the contralateral arm is supported on an arm rest. No intravenous or intraarterial access is allowed in the ipsilateral arm so it can be prepped into the field. This enables easy intraoperative positioning of the arm during flap dissection and closure of the donor defect. During resection of the head and neck primary tumor, the bean bag may be deflated, allowing the patient to settle into the 45° position. After the completion of the resection, the patient is shifted back into the lateral decubitus position, and the air is withdrawn from the bag.

The latissimus muscle has a dual blood supply, with the dominant vascular source formed by the thoracodorsal artery and veins (Fig. 250-1). The secondary blood supply is from the posterior paraspinous perforators. Both of these systems are diffusely interconnected. The myocutaneous flap is based on the thoracodorsal pedicle, necessitating sacrifice of the paraspinous perforators.

The subscapular artery, which is a branch off the third portion of the axillary artery (Fig. 250-2), gives rise to the thoracodorsal artery, which enters the latissimus muscle on its anterior lateral margin, yielding a vascular pedicle that is 10 to 12 cm long. The first branch of the subscapular is the circumflex scapular artery, which rarely restricts the rotation of the flap and is not usually sacrificed during flap rotation. Several centimeters distal to its takeoff, the branch to the teres major is seen passing laterally. This vessel is usually sacrificed during flap harvest. Distal to this, one or two branches to the serratus anterior are encountered just before the entry of the thoracodorsal artery into the latissimus muscle. These vessels are divided unless the serratus muscle is harvested with the flap for unusually large defects.

The thoracodorsal artery divides into two major intramuscular divisions. The superior branch travels parallel to the upper border of the muscle, about 3 cm inferior to the upper edge. The lateral branch travels parallel to the lateral margin of the muscle, approximately 2 to 3 cm from the lateral edge. This intramuscular division allows a bipedicled flap to be developed, which is helpful for simultaneous coverage of the intraoral lining and cutaneous coverage in cases of large pharyngocutaneous defects.

After the conclusion of the resection, the anterior border of the latissimus muscle is palpated and outlined on the skin. The cutaneous paddle is outlined over the lateral inferior aspect of the muscle, allowing for the added length needed to reach the head and neck defect (Fig. 250-3). The skin paddle is created larger than necessary to allow for later tailoring into the defect. An initial incision, which is created along the anterior lateral border of the flap, is extended up to but not into the axillary region (Fig. 250-4). The anterior

(continued)

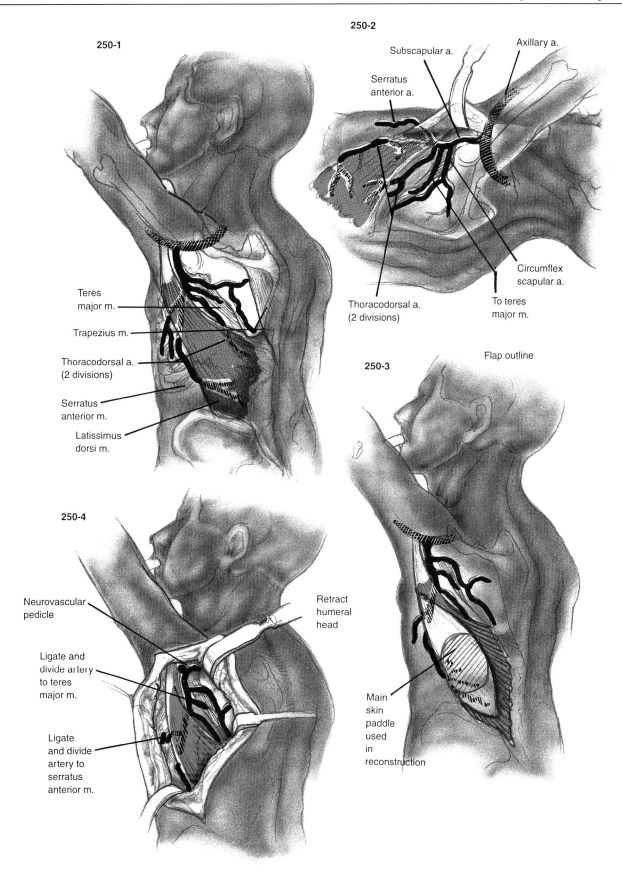

250-1

Teres
major m.

Trapezius m.

Thoracodorsal a.
(2 divisions)

Serratus
anterior m.

Latissimus
dorsi m.

250-2

Subscapular a.

Axillary a.

Serratus
anterior a.

Circumflex
scapular a.

Thoracodorsal a.
(2 divisions)

To teres
major m.

250-3

Flap outline

Main
skin
paddle
used
in
reconstruction

250-4

Neurovascular
pedicle

Ligate and
divide artery
to teres
major m.

Ligate
and divide
artery to
serratus
anterior m.

Retract
humeral
head

250. LATISSIMUS DORSI MYOCUTANEOUS FLAP (continued)

Tips and Pearls

1. The anterior incision follows the anterior border of the latissimus muscle.
2. Do not take the incision into the hair-bearing axillary region.
3. Maintain a relaxed position of the arm during surgery to prevent hyperabduction and a stretch injury of the brachial plexus.

Pitfalls and Complications

1. Venous compression within the anterior tunnel commonly causes of flap loss.
2. Skin grafts over the harvest site often fail because of the increased mobility of the region.
3. Seromas frequently form at the donor site.

Postoperative Care Issues

1. A pillow is positioned under the ipsilateral arm to hold it in a neutral position to prevent compression of the venous outflow.
2. Initiate a physical therapy program before the patient's discharge.
3. After waiting 6 months to 1 year, flap revision may be necessary to debulk or defat thick areas of the flap. If the thoracodorsal nerve is divided, the muscle may take as long as 1 year to atrophy.

References

Chowdhury CR, Mclean NR, Harrop-Griffiths K, Breach NM. The repair of defects in the head and neck region with the latissimus dorsi flap. J Laryngol Otol 1988;102:1127.

Maves MD, Panje WR, Shagets F. Extended latissimus dorsi myocutaneous flap reconstruction of major head and neck defects. Otolaryngol Head Neck Surg 1984;92:551.

Sabatier RE, Bakamjian VY. Transaxillary latissimus dorsi flap reconstruction in head and neck cancer. Am J Surg 1985;150:427.

border of the muscle is isolated and followed up to the tendinous insertion onto the humerus. With careful dissection into the axillary fat pad, the thoracodorsal vessel is identified with the associated vein and nerve. The neurovascular pedicle is developed proximally, ligating the vessels supplying the teres major and the serratus. The circumflex scapular vessels are identified but left intake. After flap rotation, they can be divided if further pedicle length is needed.

The skin island is incised down to the muscle, and the surrounding skin is elevated to expose the muscle (Fig. 250-5). The latissimus is separated from the serratus in a superior to inferior direction, where the plane between the two muscle becomes less distinct. After the remaining distal attachments of the muscle are separated, the humeral head is divided (Fig. 250-6). The flap, which is only attached by the neurovascular pedicle, is passed through the axilla through a tunnel created between the heads of the pectoralis major and minor (Fig. 250-7). If more room is needed within the tunnel, the head of the pectoralis minor can be divided. The surgeon can create a path through the pectoralis major for passage of the pedicle by spreading apart the muscle fibers or dividing some of the central fibers. Care is taken to prevent injury to the thoracoacromial vascular pedicle during this dissection in case the pectoralis flap is needed for future use.

The flap then passes over the clavicle into the defect. After initially insetting the flap into position, the pedicle is examined within the tunnel to check for compression. The arm is abducted and adducted to see if the tunnel needs enlargement to prevent vascular compression. The thoracodorsal nerve is divided only if atrophy of the muscle is desired, or if it results in venous compression during the rotation of the flap.

The flap is tailored into the defect, and the back is closed primarily over several closed suctioned drains. If needed, the tendinous humoral portion of the muscle is attached to the chest wall or the pectoralis minor tendon to prevent further pull on the pedicle (Fig. 250-8). Rarely, after harvesting an extensive flap, the defect must be resurfaced with a split-thickness skin graft. Because of the constant movement in this area of the chest wall, the result of skin-graft healing is often frustrating. Postoperatively, the ipsilateral arm is positioned in a neutral position, resting on a pillow, for several days to prevent venous compression.

JAMES L. NETTERVILLE

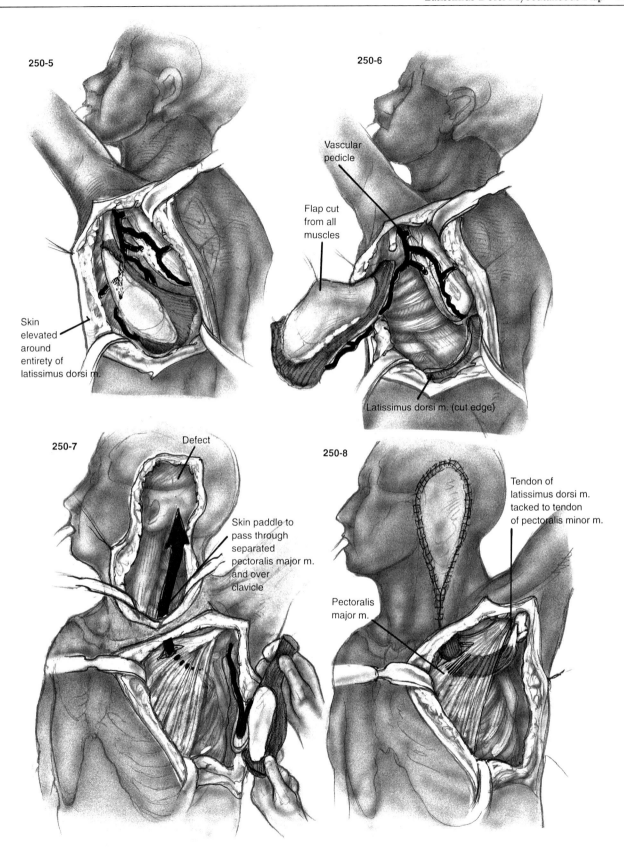

250-5

Skin elevated around entirety of latissimus dorsi m.

250-6

Vascular pedicle

Flap cut from all muscles

Latissimus dorsi m. (cut edge)

250-7

Defect

Skin paddle to pass through separated pectoralis major m. and over clavicle

250-8

Tendon of latissimus dorsi m. tacked to tendon of pectoralis minor m.

Pectoralis major m.

■ *251.* TEMPOROPARIETAL FASCIA FLAP

Richly vascularized fascia from the temporoparietal scalp can be transferred as a pedicled transposition flap or as a microvascular free tissue transfer.

Indications

1. The need for vascularized soft tissue coverage of auricle, orbit, face, oral cavity, and mastoid can be met by a pedicled transposition flap.
2. The need for a vascularized sheet of tissue anywhere in the body can be supplied by a microvascular free tissue transfer.

Contraindications

1. Defects requiring bulk or large surface area coverage
2. Compromised axial blood supply

Special Considerations

1. A detailed knowledge of scalp anatomy is mandatory.
2. The skin's vascular supply is provided by the external carotid (ie, superficial temporal artery, occipital, postauricular) and internal carotid (ie, supraorbital, supratrochlear) systems. Multiple anastomotic connections occur with the temporoparietal fascia flap and galea vessels.
3. A temporoparietal fascia flap is primarily supplied by the superficial temporal artery, but anastomoses also occur with vessels supplying skin. The fascia is contiguous with the superficial musculoaponeurotic system, galea, and epicranius musculature.
4. Deep temporal fascia is supplied by the middle temporal artery off the superficial temporal artery (deep aspect of fascia). Anastomoses occur through temporalis muscle with deep temporal artery. The fascia is contiguous with the periosteum.
5. The temporalis muscle is supplied by deep temporal vessels off the internal maxillary artery, with anastomoses to the middle temporal artery supply of the deep temporal fascia.

Preoperative Preparation

1. Routine head and face preparation
2. External auditory canal protection
3. Minimal hair removal

Special Instruments, Position, and Anesthesia

1. Supine position
2. Head of bed elevation
3. Doppler probe
4. Bipolar electrocautery

Tips and Pearls

1. Cautious use of flaps greater than 12 × 12 cm
2. Begin flap elevation inferiorly and proceed superiorly
3. Avoid hair follicle injury.
4. Avoid facial nerve injury in the temporal area.

Postoperative Care Issues

1. Closed suction drainage of flap and donor sites
2. Head of bed elevation
3. Prolonged flap edema

References

Brent B, Bryd HS. Secondary ear reconstruction with cartilage grafts covered by axial, random, and free flaps of temporoparietal fascia. Plast Reconstr Surg 1983;72:141.

East CA, Brough MD, Grant HR. Mastoid obliteration with the temporoparietal fascia flap. J Laryngol Otol 1991;105:417.

Abul-Hassan HS, von Drasek Ascher G, et al. Surgical anatomy and blood supply of the fascial layers of the temporal region. Plast Reconstr Surg 1986;77:17.

Operative Procedure

Figure 251-1 shows an auricle with no vessels available for microvascular replantation (Fig. 251-2). The patient is positioned supine and prepped in the standard fashion. The external auditory canal is occluded with sterile cotton or otic ointment. The amputated auricle is also prepped, wrapped in sterile saline sponges, and placed on ice. Antibiotics are administered.

Palpation and a Doppler probe are used to mark the course of the superficial temporal artery and its anterior and posterior branches from the preauricular crease to the parietal region. The course of the facial nerve's frontal branch from the inferior tragus to 1 cm lateral to the eyebrow is marked and protected during dissection. Subcutaneous epinephrine is safe for pedicled flaps but should be avoided in the preauricular region for free flaps.

The skin incision is begun at the anterior attachment of the superior helix and continued up in the preauricular crease toward the temporal area hairline. The scalp incision is continued coronally to the parietal region. A posterior limb and Y-shaped incision can be used for large flaps. In scalps with low hair follicle density, a zigzag coronal skin incision reduces visible scar-related alopecia.

The skin is incised to the immediately subfollicular level. Flap elevation is initiated inferiorly over the superficial temporal artery trunk. Superiorly, the temporoparietal fascia flap becomes more adherent to the dermis. Veins are carefully preserved. Bipolar electrocautery and sharp dissection preserve flap vessels and the subdermal hair follicles. Flaps are elevated, avoiding facial nerve branches. The superficial temporal artery and its branches are seen within the red, filmy temporoparietal fascia.

After the anterior, posterior, and superior flap border cuts are made, the temporoparietal fascia flap is reflected off the deep temporal fascia (Fig. 251-3). There are minimal vascular interconnections between these two layers. The skin is dissected off the perichondrium of the amputated segment and stored (Fig. 251-4). The cartilage is sutured into anatomic position with clear monofilament sutures. The temporoparietal fascia flap is reflected over the replaced cartilage and sutured to the peripheral subcutaneous soft tissues while being tucked under surrounding skin (Fig. 251-5). A small-gauge suction catheter is placed under the flap to assist flap coaptation to the cartilage and is brought out through a postauricular puncture. If viable, the amputated skin is replaced over the temporoparietal fascia flap–covered auricle (Fig. 251-6). Otherwise, a split-thickness skin graft is harvested. Plain gut sutures secure the skin graft to surrounding skin, and the auricle's convolutions are packed with petroleum gauze.

The scalp donor site is closed over a suction drain with absorbable dermal sutures and cutaneous chromic sutures. A well-padded otomastoid head dressing is placed. The scalp drain can be removed the next day. The auricle drain remains until output is scant for a 24-hour period. The petroleum gauze is removed at 5 days, and a protective shield is worn over the reconstruction for 2 to 4 weeks, depending on skin graft healing. Flap edema continues to subside over a 1-year period.

STEVEN L. GARNER
S. ANTHONY WOLFE

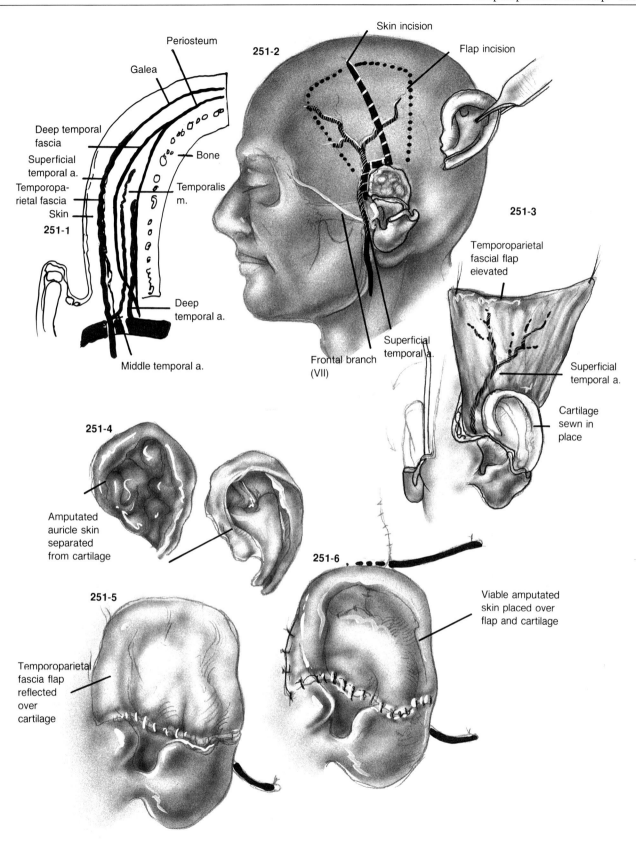

251-1
Periosteum
Galea
Deep temporal fascia
Superficial temporal a.
Temporoparietal fascia
Skin
Bone
Temporalis m.
Deep temporal a.
Middle temporal a.

251-2
Skin incision
Flap incision
Frontal branch (VII)
Superficial temporal a.

251-3
Temporoparietal fascial flap elevated
Superficial temporal a.
Cartilage sewn in place

251-4
Amputated auricle skin separated from cartilage

251-5
Temporoparietal fascia flap reflected over cartilage

251-6
Viable amputated skin placed over flap and cartilage

■ *252.* TEMPORALIS MUSCLE FLAP

A regional muscle flap available for vascularized tissue cover, for soft tissue augmentation, or as a motorized functional unit

Indications

1. Facial reanimation
2. Skull base defects
3. Oral defects
4. Facial defects
5. Temporomandibular joint ankylosis
6. Orbital reconstruction

Contraindications

1. Prior surgical injury to muscle or blood supply

Preoperative Preparations

1. Preoperative surgical soap shampoo
2. Perioperative antibiotics for contaminated cases

Special Instruments, Position, and Anesthesia

1. Patient supine, with the head of the bed elevated
2. External auditory canal occlusion
3. Minimal hair removal

Tips and Pearls

1. The blood supply to the temporalis muscle is from the anterior and posterior deep temporal arterial branches of the internal maxillary artery.
2. Vessels lie between muscle and periosteum.
3. V_3 motor nerve supply
4. The flap can include contiguous periosteum extended to sagittal midline and can carry vascularized cranial bone.
5. May require zygomatic arch osteotomies and coronoid process resection

Pitfalls and Complications

1. Facial nerve injury (frontal branch)
2. Temporal fossa hollow
3. Zygomatic bulge
4. Scar alopecia

Postoperative Care Issues

1. Elevation of the head of the bed
2. Suction drainage
3. Perioperative antibiotics in contaminated cases
4. Physical therapy rehabilitation for functional flaps

References

May M, Drucker C. Temporalis muscle for facial reanimation: A 13-year experience with 224 procedures. Arch Otolaryngol Head Neck Surg 1993;119:378.

Shagets FW, Panje WR, Shore JW. Use of temporalis muscle flaps in complicated defects of the head and face. Arch Otolaryngol 1986;112:60.

Van der Wal KGH, Mulder JW. The temporal muscle flap for closure of large palatal defects in CLP patients. Int J Oral Maxillofac Surg 1992;21:3.

Operative Procedure

The temporalis muscle can be used be alone or as a composite flap with periosteum, fascia, cranial bone, or some combination of these (Fig. 252-1). Each use dictates specific technical details (see references). These include orbital, maxillary, zygomatic, mandibular, and calvarial osteotomies as well as technical aspects of insetting the flap in specific regions (eg, orbit, skull base, palate defects). In this case, the patient had a partial maxillectomy performed through Weber-Fergusson and buccal sulcus incisions with preservation of the orbital floor, orbital contents, and soft palate (Fig. 252-2).

The scalp is injected with dilute epinephrine solution 15 minutes before dissection. Minimal hair removal is necessary, and the external auditory canal is occluded with sterile cotton or otic ointment. A coronal flap is incised from auricle to auricle, with care to avoid straying anteriorly. Zigzag incisions or more posterior incision placement may be useful for patients with a receding hairline or sparse hair. Although smaller incisions are technically possible, they require greater traction on the anterior flap and risk injury to the frontal branch of the facial nerve. The skin flaps are elevated in a subgaleal plane from above and downward toward the superior aspect of the temporalis muscle. Judicious use of electrocautery reduces the risk of scar alopecia, and scalp clips reduce blood loss. The temporoparietal (ie, superficial temporal) fascia is elevated with the scalp off the deep temporal fascia (DTF); respecting these planes protects the facial nerve branches. When the temporal fat pad becomes visible at the level of the supraorbital rims, the deep temporal fascia is incised transversely, and dissection continues just deep to this fascia and superficial to the adipose tissue. This soon connects with the prior ablative subperiosteal maxillary dissection field.

Electrocautery is used to incise the temporalis muscle and DTF 1 cm posterior to the anterior lip of the temporal fossa, leaving a soft tissue cuff on this bony rim. Posteriorly and superiorly, the incisions include several centimeters of periosteum, which is elevated with the muscle and the DTF (Fig. 252-3). The soft tissues of the flap are elevated in a subperiosteal plane toward the arch and are reflected down through the medial arch defect left by the ablative procedure. The coronoid process can be transected, but this usually is unnecessary. Care must be taken during all ablative and reconstructive surgical dissection around the internal maxillary artery and its deep temporal artery branches to the flap. The middle temporal artery branch of the superficial temporal artery should be preserved because it supplies the DTF and forms anastomoses with the muscle's vascular supply.

The entire flap is reflected into the oral cavity (Fig. 252-4). The flap can be split longitudinally to return excess posterior muscle to the temporal fossa. The intraoral flap is secured with Vicryl sutures to drill holes in the free edge of the cut hard palate and to the surrounding muscle and mucosa. The fascia and periosteum attached to the muscle help to hold these sutures securely. A split-thickness skin graft can be applied to both surfaces of the muscle, but these vascularized surfaces will mucosalize if left bare (Fig. 252-5).

The flap excess from the posterior muscle, which was returned to the temporal fossa, is advanced anteriorly and sewn to the soft tissue cuff left on the bony lip of the fossa with Vicryl sutures. This usually prevents the temporal depression in the non–hair-bearing part of the region. I prefer not to use alloplastic materials. The scalp is closed over a suction drain with galea-subcutaneous Vicryl sutures and cutaneous chromic sutures. The Weber-Fergusson incision is closed in a standard fashion (Fig. 252-6). The bulk of the transposed muscle is such that a maxillary alveolar ridge bone graft capable of holding osseointegrated implants may be placed later.

Postoperatively, the head remains elevated, and the drains are removed when output has diminished. Perioperative antibiotics are administered. The physician should avoid dressing or positioning pressure on the flap at its zygomaticomalar prominence.

STEVEN L. GARNER
S. ANTHONY WOLFE

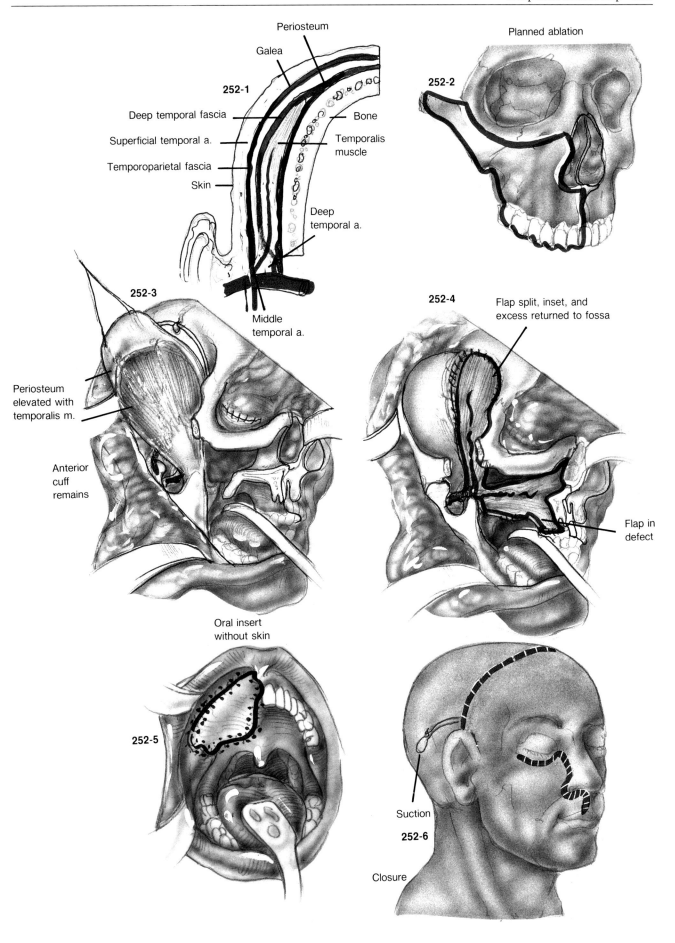

252-1

Periosteum

Galea

Deep temporal fascia

Superficial temporal a.

Temporoparietal fascia

Skin

Bone

Temporalis muscle

Deep temporal a.

Middle temporal a.

252-2

Planned ablation

252-3

Periosteum elevated with temporalis m.

Anterior cuff remains

252-4

Flap split, inset, and excess returned to fossa

Flap in defect

Oral insert without skin

252-5

252-6

Suction

Closure

■ *253.* PLATYSMA FLAP

A regional muscle or musculocutaneous flap based on the platysma muscle that is available for head and neck reconstruction

Indications

1. A skin or skin-muscle defect in the oral cavity, lower face, or neck

Contraindications

1. Contraindicated in cases of prior facial artery ligation, prior neck dissection, established facial paralysis, or prior irradiation

Preoperative Preparation

1. Wide cervicofacial preparation, including the chest
2. Preparation for alternative reconstructive options if the flap does not appear viable

Special Instruments, Position, and Anesthesia

1. The patient is supine, with the neck extended and the head supported.
2. The patient is kept warm, well hydrated, and normotensive.

Tips and Pearls

1. The platysma receives its primary blood supply from the submental branch of the facial artery.
2. Motor innervation through the cervical branches of the facial nerve may be preserved for functional lip reconstruction.
3. Cervical plexus branches supply sensation to the overlying skin.
4. The skin paddle is designed to fit the defect in a 1:1 ratio.
5. The skin paddle is at least 5 cm wide.
6. Consider the male beard pattern in flap design.

Pitfalls and Complications

1. Skin paddle losses of 20% are common. The platysma flap is rarely the best reconstructive choice.

References

Coleman JJ III, Jurkiewicz MJ, Nahai F, Mathes SJ. The platysma musculocutaneous flap: experience with 24 cases. Discussion by JW Futrell and JA Rabson. Plast Reconstr Surg 1983;72:315.

McGuirt WF, Matthews BL, Brody JA, May JS. Platysma myocutaneous flap: caveats reexamined. Laryngoscope 1991;101:1238.

Talmant JC. Emploi du peaucier cervical dans la correction des asymétries faciales—le lambeau de Barron-Tessier. Rev Stomatol Chir Maxillofac 1983;84:283.

Operative Procedure

A superiorly based platysma flap can be used for reconstruction of a defect of the floor of the mouth (Fig. 253-1). The platysma receives its primary blood supply from the submental branch of the facial artery (Fig. 253-2).

A template of the defect is made of sterile aluminum foil. The skin paddle is oriented so that down-site closure will be a transverse linear scar in or parallel to natural skin creases (Fig. 253-3). Rotation of the planned flap is simulated with an unfolded sponge to assess the design.

Subcutaneous epinephrine injections are not used in the preparation. After incising the borders of the flap skin paddle down to the fascia overlying the platysma muscle, all other surrounding skin is elevated widely in a subcutaneous plane. Inferiorly, the platysma muscle is divided along with perforating supraclavicular sensory branches of the cervical plexus. The muscle is divided at least 1 cm below the inferior border of the skin paddle. The platysma is separated and elevated off the inferior portion of the sternocleidomastoid muscle along with the deep cervical fascia investing it. This fascia helps to protect the platysma muscle and its inferior vascular pedicle. The external jugular vein and any major tributaries under the platysma muscle portion of the flap are ligated inferiorly and elevated with the flap.

If necessary, a transverse skin counterincision can be made below the border of the mandible to facilitate flap dissection and preparation of the tunnel through which the flap is passed superiorly. Flap elevation continues superiorly along the posterior border of the sternocleidomastoid muscle, where cervical plexus sensory nerves usually must be transected to allow flap rotation.

Care is taken not to injure the spinal accessory nerve or marginal mandibular branches of the facial nerve during flap elevation. Preservation of motor innervation to the platysma from cervical branches of the facial nerve is possible and may be useful in lip reconstruction. The facial artery is preserved or divided distal to the submental branch.

The flap is passed under the mandible and folded to place the skin paddle into the floor of the mouth defect (Fig. 253-4). The skin paddle is sutured to the floor of the mouth mucosa with absorbable sutures for a spit-tight closure, and the flap muscle edges are secured to surrounding muscle and periosteum (Fig. 253-5). The surgeon continuously assesses and maintains flap circulation and tension-free insetting.

The wounds are irrigated copiously with warm saline. Suction drains are used for the defect site and the donor site. The donor site is closed primarily (Fig. 253-6).

Perioperative antibiotics, head elevation, and suction drainage are continued as needed.

STEVEN L. GARNER
S. ANTHONY WOLFE

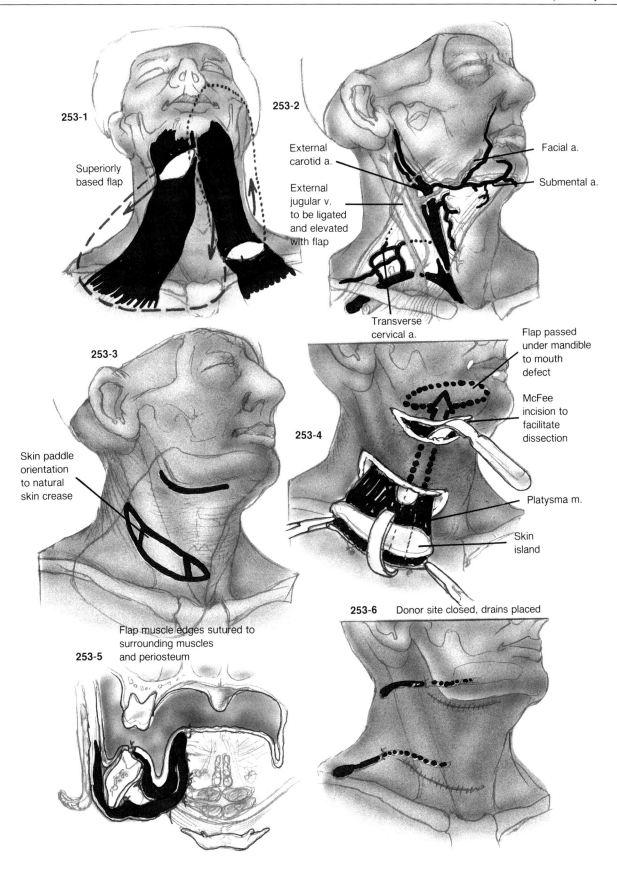

253-1

Superiorly based flap

253-2

External carotid a.

External jugular v. to be ligated and elevated with flap

Transverse cervical a.

Facial a.

Submental a.

253-3

Skin paddle orientation to natural skin crease

253-4

Flap passed under mandible to mouth defect

McFee incision to facilitate dissection

Platysma m.

Skin island

Flap muscle edges sutured to surrounding muscles and periosteum

253-5

253-6   Donor site closed, drains placed

■ *254.* STERNOCLEIDOMASTOID FLAP

A regional muscle, musculocutaneous, or composite flap based on either of the sternocleidomastoid muscles and its multiaxial blood supply, used for head and neck reconstruction

Indications

1. Augmentation of soft tissue defects
2. Orocutaneous fistula closure
3. Vascular coverage
4. Composite skin and bone oral defect
5. Laryngotracheal-esophageal stenosis
6. Frey's syndrome

Contraindications

1. Extracapsular lymph node metastatic cancer
2. Sternocleidomastoid muscle (SCM) muscle inclusion with neck dissection

Preoperative Preparation

1. Wide field cervicofacial preparation including chest, preparation for alternative reconstructive options (ie, flap, graft)

Special Instruments, Position, and Anesthesia

1. Supine, with the head elevated
2. No local epinephrine injection

Tips and Pearls

1. SCM has a three-level blood supply: occipital artery, superior or inferior thyroid artery, and thyrocervical trunk.
2. Preservation of the thyroid pedicle augments flap circulation whether superiorly or inferiorly based. This may, however limit flap rotation, as may the spinal access nerve.
3. Skip paddles should be less than 36 cm².
4. Minimize random extension beyond the muscle.

Pitfalls and Complications

1. The skin paddle is tenuous with partial necrosis rates of almost 50%.
2. Large defects, prior radiation, and carotid coverage may warrant consideration of reconstructive alternatives.
3. Short and fat necks add to flap rotation limitations.
4. Donor site deformities are relative to the skin paddle size, ability for primary closure, and neck flatness from muscle rotation.

Postoperative Care Issues

1. Closed suction drainage of donor and recipient sites
2. No tape or straps across flap
3. Head of bed elevation

References

Ariyan S. One-stage reconstruction for defects of the mouth using a sternomastoid myocutaneous flap. Plast Reconstruct Surg 1979:63: 518.

Friedman M, Mayer AD. Laryngotracheal reconstruction in adults with the sternocleidomastoid myoperiosteal flap. Ann Otol Rhinol Laryngol 1992;101:897.

Larson DL, Goepfert H. Limitations of the sternocleidomastoid musculocutaneous flap in head and neck cancer reconstruction—discussion by Stephan Ariyan, M.D. Plast Reconstruct Surg 1982;70:328.

Operative Procedure

The SCM flap can be used as a muscle flap alone or with any combination of skin, clavicular bone, or clavicular periosteum. The choice of a superiorly or inferiorly based flap depends on the available arc of rotation, the tissue requirements, and the muscle's mutiaxial vascular status (Fig. 254-1). The SCM flap is available for immediate or delayed reconstruction.

The patient is positioned supine, with wide preparation of the head and neck. Head of the bed elevation reduces venous engorgement and improves hemostasis. Maintaining the ability to rotate the head and neck during the procedure allows the surgeon to test flap tension in all possible head positions to ensure that adequate design and mobilization are executed. I prefer not to use subcutaneous epinephrine injections for hemostasis if a skin paddle is included with the flap. Maintenance of core temperature, blood and fluid repletion, and systolic blood pressure at physiologic levels is critical for flap survival, especially if a skin paddle is included.

Before neck dissection, the planned skin paddle is oriented over the superior portion of the SCM muscle (Fig. 254-2), and the arc of rotation to the intraoral defect is tested with a sterile towel. An assessment of the defect area is made, and a 1:1 flap is planned. Underestimation of the defect and subsequent inadequate flap harvesting can produce a tense and tenuous closure.

The skin paddle is incised to a subdermal level, and the cervical skin surrounding the paddle is undermined an additional 2 cm. This allows an augmented capture of vascular perforators to the skin paddle. The skin paddle incisions are then carried down to the investing fascia of the SCM muscle, and the skin paddle dermis is tacked down to the fascia with interrupted sutures. This can prevent shearing injuries to vascular perforators during dissection. Any additional incisions that provide adequate exposure without compromising cervical skin circulation are acceptable (eg, MacFee, hockey stick). The SCM fascia is incised longitudinally over the muscle and reflected into the anterior and posterior triangles, respectively. The muscle is divided at the mastoid level at least 2 cm above the superior border of the skin paddle and reflected inferiorly out of its fascial envelope. This requires ligation of the superior vascular pedicle from the occipital artery. The muscle is elevated only as far as is necessary to allow tension-free rotation to the intraoral defect.

The neck dissection can proceed around the flap, and removal of the submandibular gland facilitates delivery of the flap into the mouth (Fig. 254-3). If it is possible to preserve central vascular contributions from the superior thyroid artery without compromising tension-free flap rotation, this approach augments circulation. However, the flap can be carried on the inferior thyrocervical vascular contributions alone. The least amount of dissection necessary generates the least risk to the flap.

Before insetting the flap, I remove the sutures tacking the skin paddle to the muscle. These sutures are no longer necessary, and they can prevent ideal wound closure and edge eversion at the suture lines. The muscle and fascia first are secured to deep soft tissue (ie, mandible periosteum, floor of the mouth musculature) with Vicryl sutures (Fig. 254-4). The skin paddle then is sutured to surrounding oral mucosa for a spit-tight closure. Adequate skin flap perfusion is assessed by color and dermal bleeding during suturing. If compromised, the surgeon should evaluate pedicle tension and revise as needed. This is a vital point in the operation, because the surgeon must not assume that the flap circulation will improve beyond the intraoperative status.

The wounds are irrigated copiously. Closed suction drains are placed in the donor and recipient sites. The cervical skin flaps have been elevated and undermined in a subplatysmal plane and are advanced and trimmed to close the neck primarily in layers.

Postoperatively, the head remains elevated, the general physiologic status of the patient (eg, temperature, fluid volume, blood replacement) is maintained, and perioperative prophylactic antibiotics are administered. Drains are removed when output is below 30 to 50 mL/day.

STEVEN L. GARNER
S. ANTHONY WOLFE

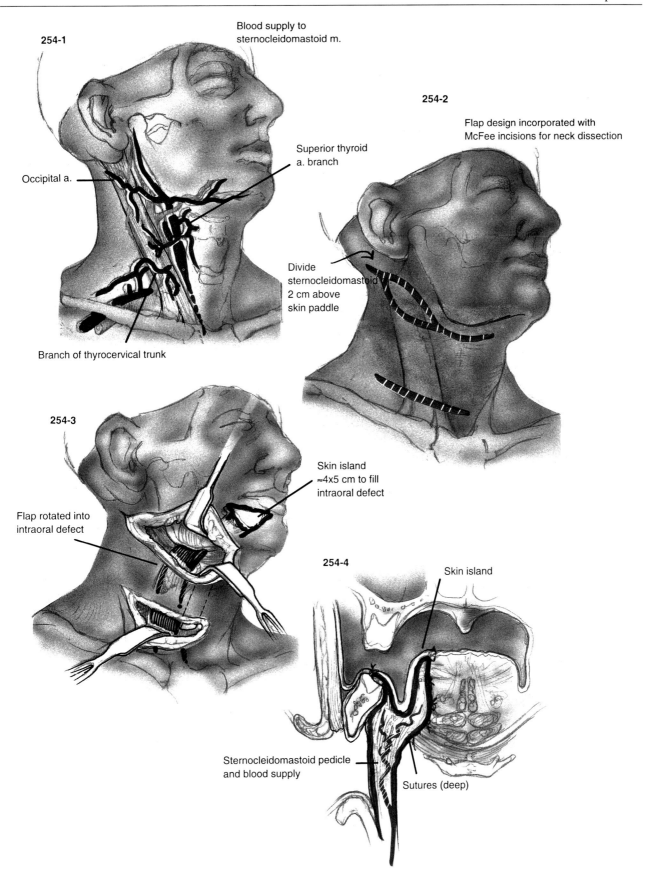

254-1

Blood supply to
sternocleidomastoid m.

254-2

Flap design incorporated with
McFee incisions for neck dissection

Occipital a.

Superior thyroid
a. branch

Branch of thyrocervical trunk

Divide
sternocleidomastoid
2 cm above
skin paddle

254-3

Flap rotated into
intraoral defect

Skin island
≈4x5 cm to fill
intraoral defect

254-4

Skin island

Sternocleidomastoid pedicle
and blood supply

Sutures (deep)

■ *255.* SKIN GRAFTS, DERMAL GRAFTS, AND MUCOSAL GRAFTS—

Avascular grafts, usually autogenous from the donor site, are transferred to a recipient site for soft tissue coverage. Variations include a full-thickness skin-dermal graft with the epidermal skin layer; split-thickness skin-epidermis graft with a partial dermal layer; dermal-subepithelial grafts of dermis; and mucosal–secretory mucous epithelium grafts.

Indications

1. Soft tissue coverage (eg, burns, head and neck defects)
2. Reconstruction of extirpated cancer defect (eg, surveillance for recurrence)
3. Line cavities (eg, maxilla, orbital)
4. Regional flap and donor site coverage
5. Aerodigestive tract coverage
6. For dermal grafts
   a. Carotid artery and vein graft protection
   b. Pharyngeal suture line protection
   c. Primary enucleation implant
   d. Mucous membrane reconstruction of nasal or oral cavity
7. For mucosal grafts
   a. Surface coverage of the nasal cavity, conjunctiva of the eye, and aerodigestive tract

Contraindications

1. Recipient site infection or granulation
2. Donor site lesions
3. Bone without periosteum or cancellous bed
4. Cartilage without perichondrium

Special Considerations

1. Skin elastosis
2. Nutritional status
3. Consider aesthetic units of the face in graft selection.
4. Donor site quality, such as color, texture, and other characteristics
5. Full-thickness graft selection (eg, preauricular, postauricular, supraclavicular nasolabial groove, upper eyelid)
6. Primary contracture of 40% for full-thickness skin graft (FTSG) and 10% to 20% for a split-thickness skin graft (STSG)
7. Direct, rapid, proven reconstructive alternative with a low morbidity rate, high survival rate, and wide application

Preoperative Preparation

1. Clean, viable recipient bed
2. Preoperative donor site selection
3. Routine laboratory and clotting studies

Special Instruments, Position, and Anesthesia

1. For skin and dermis grafts
   a. Mineral oil
   b. Modern dermatome
   c. Epinephrine (1:200,000)
   d. Graft mesher with 1:15 dermacarrier
   e. Reston, Adaptic, and occlusal dressing
2. For mucosal grafts
   a. Mouth gag retractor
   b. 1% Solution of lidocaine with 1:100,000 epinephrine
   c. Fine surgical instrument set

(continued)

Operative Procedure

Split-Thickness and Dermal Skin Grafts

The patient is positioned on the operating table to allow preparation of the recipient graft site and harvesting of the skin graft. The recipient and donor sites are prepped and draped in the usual sterile fashion. The lesion is extirpated, or the recipient site is prepared. The recipient site must be free of all infection, eschar, or granulation tissue. Preparation may be performed using a standard scrub brush. Hemostasis of the recipient site is obtained using gauze soaked with 1:200,000 epinephrine. Dimensions of the recipient site are measured, and these are transferred to the proposed donor site, which is preferably the lateral thigh of the leg. A template may be cut from sterile paper (eg, glove package) and used to map the graft needed onto the donor site.

The donor site is then infiltrated in a subdermal plane with a 1% solution of Xylocaine with a 1:100,000 concentration of epinephrine. Mineral oil lubricant is applied to the donor site. A gas-powered dermatome is set at a thickness of 0.013 to 0.015 in (0.33 to 0.38 mm), and a guard of appropriate width is chosen. Maintaining of constant pressure on the skin with the use of a tongue blade, the dermatome is placed against the epidermis and activated (Fig. 255-1). The epidermal flap is elevated with the assistant maintaining constant pressure in front of the dermatome and holding the graft taught with forceps. The flap is left attached at one end.

If an STSG is to be harvested, the epidermal flap is transected at its base and transferred to the appropriate recipient site (Fig. 255-2). The decision for using meshed or unmeshed STSG depends on the donor site. For aesthetic reasons, most facial grafts are not meshed or meshed at the lowest ratio possible. For large surface area defects, a graft mesher with a 1:1.5 dermacarrier is used. The skin graft is spread over the ridges of the dermacarrier and passed through the graft mesher. The graft is then transferred to the recipient site, where it is sutured in place with 4-0 interrupted chromic sutures or stapled with 35-mm-wide staples. If a relatively small surface area is to be covered, the intact, nonmeshed graft is placed over the recipient site and sutured with 4-0 interrupted chromic sutures. Excess graft material is excised with small Stevens scissors.

Before suturing the graft in place, it should be pie-crusted to release fluid collections with a series of longitudinal cuts through the flap over a firm surface with a #15 blade. Adaptic gauze is placed over the recipient site. Reston is covered with dry gauze, placed over the adaptic, stapled in place using 35-mm-wide staples. When meshed grafts are used, the Reston gauze is soaked with an antibiotic solution. When grafts are placed intraorally, a Xeroform or emollient-coated gauze bolster is placed over the graft and secured with overlapping 3-0 chromic sutures placed around the periphery of the graft.

If a dermal graft is to be harvested, the split-thickness skin flap is reflected and remains attached at one end. The dermatome is reset at a thickness of 0.013 to 0.020 in (0.33 to 0.5 mm), typically with a narrower guard in place. The dermal graft is harvested with a second pass of the dermatome in a manner similar to that for the epidermal graft. Dermis or subcutaneous fat is seen below the level of the dermal graft (Fig. 255-3). The dermal graft is transected at its base with a #15 blade and placed in saline solution. The elevated skin flap is then pie-crusted. After appropriate hemostasis has been obtained, the elevated epidermal flap is returned to its original site and secured with interrupted 4-0 nylon sutures.

(continued)

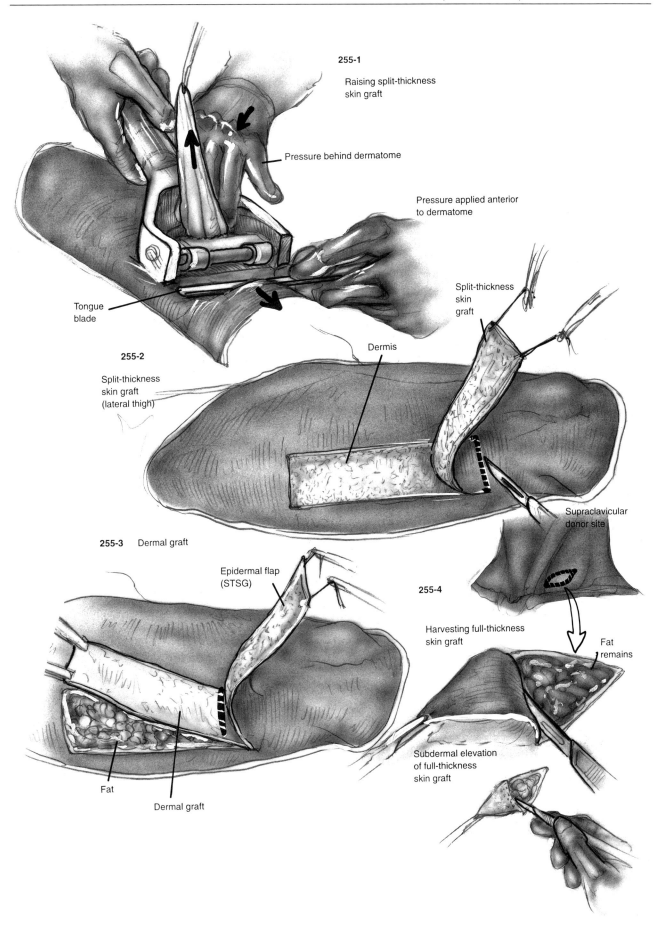

255-1

Raising split-thickness skin graft

Pressure behind dermatome

Pressure applied anterior to dermatome

Tongue blade

Split-thickness skin graft

255-2

Split-thickness skin graft (lateral thigh)

Dermis

Supraclavicular donor site

255-3   Dermal graft

Epidermal flap (STSG)

255-4

Harvesting full-thickness skin graft

Fat remains

Fat

Dermal graft

Subdermal elevation of full-thickness skin graft

■ *255.* SKIN GRAFTS, DERMAL GRAFTS, AND MUCOSAL GRAFTS *(continued)*

Tips and Pearls

1. Bevel of a #15 knife blade between the blade and dermatome of approximately 0.013 in (0.3 mm)
2. STSG thickness of 0.013 to 0.015 in (0.33 to 0.38 mm)
3. Assistant to maintain firm pressure in front of the dermatome
4. Pie-crusting prevents hematoma and seroma
5. Size and thickness of FTSG limited by metabolic demands
6. For dermal grafts
   a. Dermal graft thickness of 0.013 to 0.020 in (0.33 to 0.5 mm)
   b. Use in cases with high probability of fistula formation
   c. High reliability in irradiated field
   d. Exposure results in re-epithelization of the dermal graft, which may take days to weeks.
7. For mucosal grafts
   a. Size of the graft is limited by closure of the donor site (approximately 2 to 3 cm without the use of local flap closure)

Pitfalls and Complications

1. Hematoma or seroma
2. Graft failure secondary to lack of immobilization, infection, or poorly vascularized recipient beds
3. Scarring at recipient or donor site

Postoperative Care Issues

1. For skin and dermal grafts
   a. Monitor for infection
   b. Bolster dressing: meshed grafts (5 to 7 days), unmeshed (7 to 14 days)
   c. Occlusal dressing (eg, Tegaderm, Op-Site) to donor site (10 to 14 days)
   d. Emollient dressing (eg, antibiotic ointment, mineral oil) to donor and recipient sites after primary healing is complete
   e. Sunscreens used over donor and recipient sites
   f. Dermabrasion and camouflage of recipient area, as needed
2. For mucosal grafts
   a. Intraoral irrigation with one-half strength hydrogen peroxide four times daily
   b. Soft diet

References

Branham GH, Thomas JR. Skin grafts. Otolaryngol Clin North Am 1990;23:889.

Reed GF. The use of dermal grafts in the head and neck. In: Conley J, et al, eds. Plastic and reconstructive surgery of the face and neck. New York: Grune & Stratton, 1972:177.

Donor site hemostasis is obtained with 1:200,000 epinephrine-soaked gauze. Benzoin or Mastisol is applied along the periphery of the donor site, and Tegaderm or Op-Site is applied, followed by a light compression wrap.

Full-Thickness Skin Grafts

The patient is placed in the supine position. After appropriate general or local anesthesia, the donor and recipient sites are prepped and draped in the usual sterile fashion. After meticulous hemostasis, debridement, and cleaning, the recipient site is measured, and the dimensions are transferred to donor site, allowing for contracture of the FTSG. The donor site is designed for closure along relaxed skin tension lines and includes consideration of local flap closure when necessary. The area is infiltrated with a 1% solution of Xylocaine with a 1:100,000 concentration of epinephrine in a subcutaneous plane, and a skin incision of appropriate dimensions is then performed with a #15 blade. Hemostasis is obtained with electrocautery. The end of the graft is grasped with fine-toothed forceps or skin hooks for retraction (Fig. 255-4). The remainder of the graft is elevated in a subdermal plane with the #15 blade or sharp scissors. The graft is trimmed with Stevens scissors and sutured into the recipient site using 5-0 nylon sutures in an interrupted fashion (Fig. 255-5). Stay sutures are tied over a bolster of Xeroform or emollient gauze (Fig. 255-5*A*). After undermining circumferentially or performing local flaps, if necessary, the donor site is closed primarily in two layers. Antibiotic ointment is applied to the donor site.

Mucosal Grafts

Buccal mucosal grafts are the most common type of mucosal graft. Donor graft size is limited to approximately 2 × 3 cm because of scarring and potential problems with mouth opening. After appropriate anesthesia is instituted, a bite block or mouth gag is placed to gain adequate exposure. The buccal mucosa is infiltrated with a 1% solution Xylocaine with a 1:100,000 concentration of epinephrine. An anterior incision through the mucosa is created with a #15 blade (Fig. 255-6). Meticulous dissection with Metzenbaum scissors in the superficial submucosal plane is used to widely undermine a mucosal flap (Fig. 255-6*A*). Care must be taken to avoid damage to the deeper vasculature or entry into the buccal fat pad. Closure is simplified by extending the mucosal flap elevation beyond the planned graft edges, completing undermining before making the final graft incisions. The area of the parotid duct must be left undisturbed. An appropriately sized graft is harvested, typically in an elliptical fashion, and placed into saline solution. Hemostasis is obtained using electrocautery. The oral cavity is irrigated, and the intraoral defect is closed primarily with interrupted 3-0 chromic gut suture.

The mucosal graft is sutured into the recipient site, and an appropriate bolster or splint is applied for immobilization and protection.

BRUCE A. SCOTT
THOMAS V. CONLEY

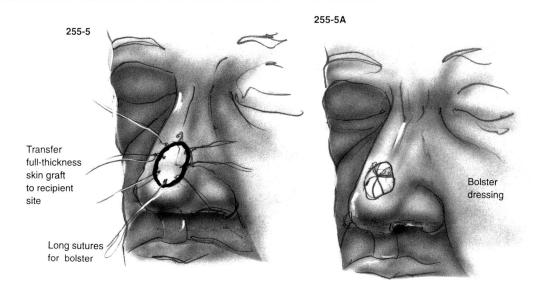

255-5

Transfer
full-thickness
skin graft
to recipient
site

Long sutures
for bolster

255-5A

Bolster
dressing

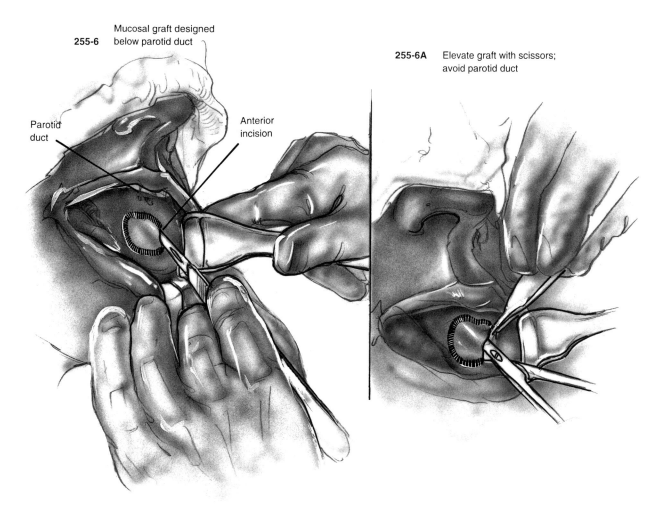

255-6   Mucosal graft designed
below parotid duct

Parotid
duct

Anterior
incision

255-6A   Elevate graft with scissors;
avoid parotid duct

■ *256.* CARTILAGE GRAFTS FROM THE SEP-
TUM—Surgical harvest of autologous cartilage

Indications
1. Cosmetic and reconstructive nasal surgery
2. Eyelid reconstruction
3. Repair of orbital floor defect
4. Repair of other cartilaginous or bony facial defect

Contraindications
1. Preexisting septal perforation
2. Midline granulomatous disease

Special Considerations
1. Bleeding and clotting abnormalities
2. Previous nasal surgery, septoplasty, or submucous resection
3. Poor nasal-tip support, columellar retraction, or dorsal saddle deformity (all suggesting a lack of adequate septal cartilage)

Preoperative Preparation
1. Routine laboratory and bleeding studies
2. Complete nasal examination

Special Instruments, Position, and Anesthesia
1. Headlight and nasal specula
2. Standard nasal instrument set with Freer or Cottle elevator
3. Topical vasoconstrictor-anaesthetic (4% cocaine)
4. Injectable solution of 1% lidocaine with a 1:100,000 dilution of epinephrine
5. Intravenous sedation or general anesthesia

Tips and Pearls
1. Careful injection for hemostasis and hydrodissection
2. Careful elevation in the submucoperichondrial plane and great care at junction of mucoperichondrium and mucoperiosteum along floor
3. Maintain undisturbed dorsal and caudal struts for nasal support.
4. Improved visualization with progressively longer nasal specula
5. Cartilage near the dorsum tends to be thicker and straighter.

Pitfalls and Complications
1. Cocaine toxicity (4 mg/kg)
2. Bleeding or septal hematoma
3. Septal perforation
4. Cosmetic deformity: columella retraction, loss of tip support, dorsal saddle
5. Nasal obstruction: loss of support, septal deviation, compensatory turbinate hypertrophy

Postoperative Care Issues
1. Minimize nasal packing. All packing is saturated with antibiotic ointment or cream and removed at 24 hours or sooner. A nasal drip pad is used.
2. Head elevation decreases nasal congestion and edema. Ice is used to decrease swelling in the nasal area.
3. The patient should avoid heavy lifting, straining, and nose blowing for 2 weeks.
4. Begin saline nasal drops after the packing is removed.

References
Burget GC. Nasal restoration with flaps and grafts. In: Bailey BJ, ed. Head and neck surgery—otolaryngology. Philadelphia: JB Lippincott, 1993:2034.

Wood R-P, Jafek BW, Eberhard R. Nasal obstruction. In: Bailey BJ. ed. Head and neck surgery—otolaryngology. Philadelphia: JB Lippincott, 1993:302.

Operative Procedure
The patient is placed in the supine position, with the neck gently flexed, the head secured on a foam doughnut, and the head of the bed elevated. A focused beam headlight is used by the surgeon for visualization throughout the procedure. If endotracheal anesthesia is elected, a moistened throat pack should be placed. Cotton pledgets or thin strips of gauze saturated with a 4% cocaine solution (total, 4 mL) are carefully placed along each side of the nasal septum, maximizing mucosal contact for vasoconstrictive and anesthetic effect. An injection of 1% lidocaine with 1:100,000 epinephrine (total, 5 to 10 mL) is performed using a long 27-gauge needle into the submucosal perichondrial plane on each side of the septum. It is important to wait at least 10 minutes for maximal vasoconstrictive and anesthetic effect. The patient is sterilely prepped and draped during this time.

The left side of the nasal septum is exposed with a nasal speculum, and a Killian incision is created through the mucosa and perichondrium down to the level of the septal cartilage (Fig. 256-1). It is placed approximately 1 cm posterior and parallel to the caudal end of the cartilaginous septum, with a gradual curve near the nasal floor. The incision should allow exposure of the entire vertical height of the cartilaginous septum. Initially, sharp dissection may be required to find the anatomic plane between the mucoperichondrium and cartilage. Exposure is maximized with a nasal speculum and retraction by an assistant using an Adson forceps. Extra effort initially to ensure dissection into the correct submucoperichondrial plane is rewarded by almost effortless blunt elevation of an intact sheet of mucosa posteriorly (Fig. 256-2). Careful dissection is necessary along the floor of the nose at the junction between the perichondrium of the cartilaginous septum and periosteum of the vomer (a discontinuous plane). Sharp dissection may also be necessary at areas of previous septal surgery, preexisting fracture sites, and the posterior cartilaginous-bony junction. Wide elevation provides improved visualization and access.

After the available septal cartilage is exposed, the portion to be harvested is determined, leaving at least 1 cm of cartilage undisturbed along the dorsal and caudal borders to maintain nasal support. A cartilage-only incision (sparing the contralateral mucoperichondrium) is created approximately 2 mm offset from the initial Killian mucosal incision with the Cottle elevator or cartilage knife. The contralateral mucoperichondrial flap elevation is then performed again in the submucoperichondrial plane under direct visualization by placing a medium speculum with one tine on each side of the incised cartilage. The mucosa is elevated only over the portion of cartilage to be harvested (Fig. 256-3). After the cartilage graft is completely free of the perichondrium on both sides, it is bluntly released from the bony septum posteriorly and the vomer inferiorly with the Cottle elevator, and it is removed with polyp forceps (Fig. 256-4). The graft must be kept moist in normal saline until it is implanted. Any excess harvested portions should be crushed and replaced between the mucoperichondrial flaps.

Closure of the Killian incision is performed using 5-0 plain gut suture in an interrupted fashion. The mucoperichondrial layers are reapproximated using a 4-0 chromic suture in a running through-and-through quilting fashion (Fig. 256-5). Alternatively, a septal splint may be created from a 0.02-in (0.5-mm) thickness of Silastic sheeting placed on each side of the septum and held in place with at least two through-and-through 3-0 silk sutures. Any mucosal tears, particularly if bilateral, should be closed with 5-0 plain gut suture. At the conclusion of the nasal portion of the procedure, a small amount of soft nasal packing (ie, rolled Telfa pad or commercially available soft packing) saturated with antibiotic ointment or cream is placed into each nostril and secured anteriorly with a silk suture taped to the malar area. A nasal drip pad is created from cotton gauze and placed under the nose.

BRUCE A. SCOTT

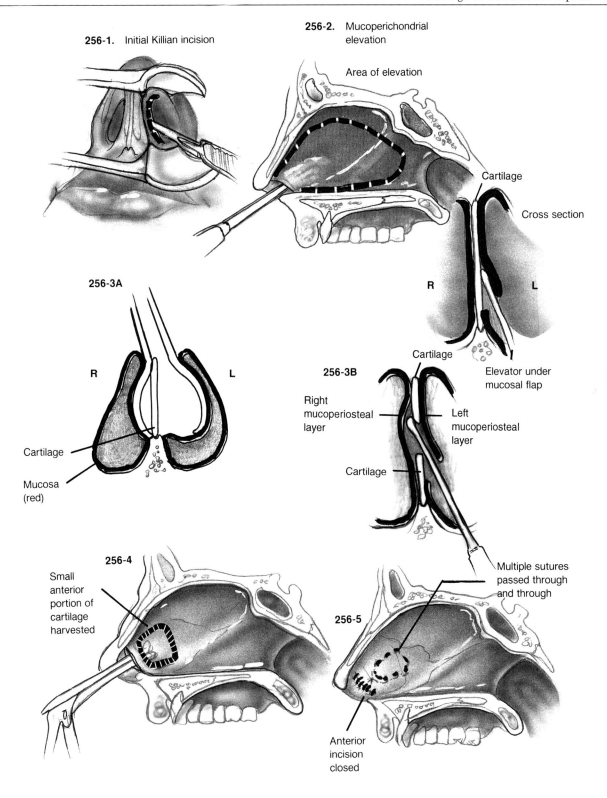

256-1.   Initial Killian incision

256-2.   Mucoperichondrial elevation

Area of elevation

Cartilage

Cross section

R   L

Cartilage

Elevator under mucosal flap

256-3A

R   L

Cartilage

Mucosa (red)

256-3B

Cartilage

Right mucoperiosteal layer

Left mucoperiosteal layer

Cartilage

Multiple sutures passed through and through

256-4

Small anterior portion of cartilage harvested

256-5

Anterior incision closed

■ 257. EAR CARTILAGE GRAFTS

The external ear has as much as 7.0 cm² of cartilage available for harvest without violating its structural integrity. Composite grafts with a skin-cartilage interface are also available for soft tissue augmentation and nasal defect reconstitution.

Indications

1. Structural and contour defects of the nose.
2. Partial defects of the trachea.
3. eyelid facial deficits.

Contraindications

1. Patients with relapsing polychondritis.
2. Bleeding or clotting disorders.

Special Considerations

1. The antihelical fold must not violated with cartilage incisions or excisions.

Preoperative Preparation

1. Broad-spectrum antibiotics are begun the day of surgery and continued for 5 days.

Special Instruments, Position, and Anesthesia

1. Standard delicate soft tissue instruments suffice for cartilage harvest.
2. Infiltration local anesthesia of 1% Lidocaine with 1:100,000 epinephrine.

Tips and Pearls

1. Hydraulic dissection with the local anesthetic injection beneath the perichondrium anterolaterally.
2. Thick cartilage posterior to the ear canal makes an excellent tip graft.

Pitfalls and Complications

1. Cartilage more friable in older patients handle gently to prevent fragmentation.
2. Incisions/excisions violating the antihelical fold can change external ear appearance.
3. Meticulous hemostasis essential since hematoma may result in postoperative infection with permanent changes in ear appearance.

Postoperative Care Issues

1. Antibiotic coverage maintained for five days.
2. Bolster compression dressing prevents hematoma, facilitates healing; is removed by cutting the single stitch at 4–6 days.

References

Tardy ME. The versatile cartilage autograft in reconstruction of the nose and face. Laryngoscope 1985;95:810.

Operative Procedure

Reconstruction of the nose often requires cartilage autografts or composite grafts from the external auricle (Fig. 257-1). The various concave and convex contours of the ear cartilage allow great versatility for dorsal profile onlay grafts, columellar struts, alar sidewall battens, nasofrontal and nasolabial region augmentation grafts, spreader grafts, tip contour grafts, and composite grafts for soft tissue and structural repair.

After local anesthetic infiltration of the overlying anterior and posterior ear cartilage and skin, the skin deep (medial) to the crest of the antihelical fold is incised for a distance sufficient to harvest a portion or all of the cavum-cymba-concha complex (Fig. 257-2). The antihelical fold is preserved. A significant amount of cartilage exists in the cephalic aspect of the concha, beneath the inferior crus.

With blunt scissors dissection in the hydraulically infiltrated subperichondrial plane, the anterior skin slap is elevated, usually bloodlessly. The cartilage is incised, and the posterior surface of the cartilage is freed by sharp dissection. A small amount of soft tissue is preserved on the posterior surface of the cartilage graft or grafts for more rapid adherence at the donor site.

Alternately, access for harvesting the ear cartilage may be gained through a posterior incision (Fig. 257-3). Meticulous microcautery of the soft tissue bed is critical to ensure absolute hemostasis (Fig. 257-4). Postoperative hematoma must be prevented.

Closure of the incision is achieved with a running 5-0 fast-absorbing catgut suture. The incision is further sealed with Histoacryl blue tissue adhesive.

A double layer of Telfa is placed on either surface of the ear and secured with a single, firmly tied, through-and-through 4-0 white Tevdek suture, which provides firm compression of the wound for further prevention of hematoma. The suture is removed after 4 to 6 days.

M. EUGENE TARDY, JR.
ERIC O. LINDBECK
JAMES A. HEINRICH

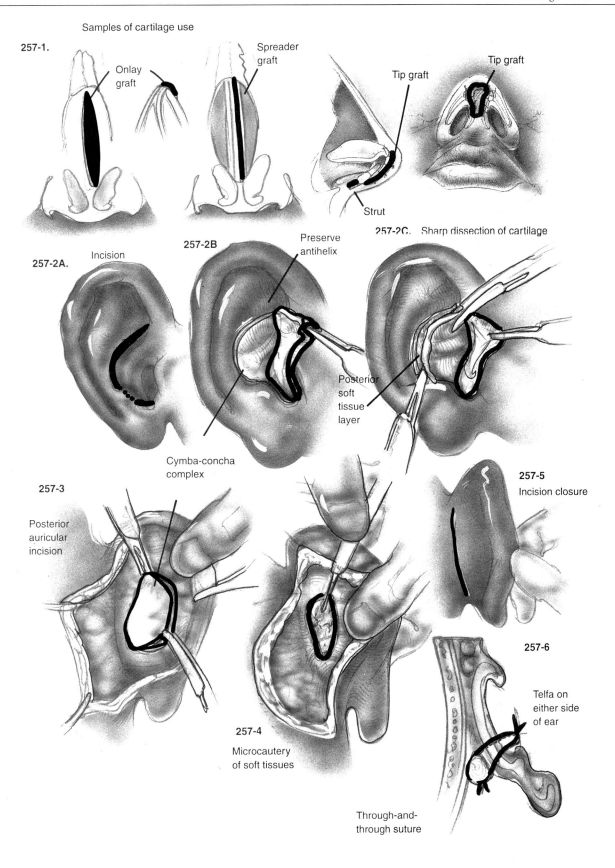

Samples of cartilage use

257-1.

Onlay graft

Spreader graft

Tip graft

Tip graft

Strut

257-2A. Incision

257-2B Preserve antihelix

257-2C. Sharp dissection of cartilage

Posterior soft tissue layer

Cymba-concha complex

257-3

Posterior auricular incision

257-4

Microcautery of soft tissues

257-5

Incision closure

257-6

Telfa on either side of ear

Through-and-through suture

■ *258.* COMPOSITE GRAFTS FROM THE EAR

Use of a two- or three-layer free auricular graft for reconstructing tissue defects involving cartilage and overlying soft tissue, which is particularly useful to reduce risk of contracture or retraction of soft tissue grafts. The cartilage graft is harvested with intact perichondrium and overlying skin (one or both surfaces).

Indications

1. Nasal defects: alar rim, soft triangle, columella, nasolabial fold
2. Contralateral auricular defects
3. Eyelid defects or retraction

Contraindications

1. Infection of the auricular harvest site or recipient site
2. Defect size greater than limit of available auricular graft

Special Considerations

1. The center of the graft should not be farther than 2.0 cm from any wound edge.
2. Increased graft survival compared with cartilage graft alone or separate cartilage and soft tissue grafts
3. Preserve or restore integrity of antihelical fold to minimize the donor ear deformity.

Preoperative Preparation

1. Preoperative photography and documentation of the defect
2. Select the most appropriate donor site, such as postauricular skin with a helical rim, fossa triangularis, cavum concha, crus of the helix, tragus, or inner aspect of the helical rim.
3. After the anesthetic injection, allow time for anesthetic and vasoconstrictive effect.
4. Sterile preparation of the donor and recipient site

Special Instruments, Positions, and Anesthesia

1. Minimize handling of the graft and shearing forces.
2. Inject local anesthetic, even when using general anesthesia, for vasoconstriction and hydraulic dissection.
3. Minimize the use of ligatures and electrocautery on the graft and recipient sites.
4. Position the patient to allow access to the donor and recipient sites while maintaining a sterile field.

Tips and Pearls

1. Use an intraoperative template to help delineate the extent of the graft.
2. Harvest a graft larger than the defect site to allow for later tissue shrinkage. Grafts get smaller, and defects get bigger.
3. May use 5-0 or 6-0 chromic suture in a mattress fashion in order to help stabilize the graft
4. Plan incisions to minimize visible scars by using anatomic folds and shadows.

Pitfalls and Complications

1. Partial or complete graft loss
2. Contracture or scarring of donor or recipient site
3. Hematoma of donor or recipient site
4. Infection of the donor or recipient site, including chondritis or perichondritis
5. External auditory canal meatal collapse or obstruction

Postoperative Care Issues

1. Donor site compression dressing with a thin strip of gauze or cotton saturated with antibiotic (eg, gentamicin) ointment and placed into the folds of the ear and postauricular sulcus with a mastoid dressing or through-and-through sutures
2. Immobilization of the graft at the recipient site, covering with antibiotic ointment

References

Adams JS. Grafts in the head and neck. In: Bailey BJ, ed. Head and neck surgery—otolaryngology. Philadelphia: JB Lippincott, 1993: 1895.

Walter C. Aspects of facial correction and reconstruction by using transplants (composite grafts and implants) with special reference to surgical membrane implants. Otolaryngol Head Neck Surg 1994;19:524.

Operative Procedure

Position the patient with the head elevated above the operating table on a foam doughnut to expose the entire auricular area. The surrounding hair is covered with adhesive tape, and a cotton ball is placed into the meatus before the sterile prep. The recipient site should be debrided, if necessary, and then prepped and draped as well. Excision and debridement must be carried to an edge of well-vascularized tissue. To harvest a more exact composite graft, a template of the defect may be created from the suture pack foil wrapper or paper. After considering the available auricular composite donor sites (Fig. 258-1), the surgeon maps the template (slightly larger to allow for tissue shrinkage) onto the ear. Thoughtful planning is required to design the graft because of the variety of contours, curvatures, and potential layers (eg, cartilage with one or two layers of overlying soft tissue) available. Acceptable closure of the donor defect must also be considered.

After the designed graft is drawn, the lateral and medial surfaces of the ear should be injected with a solution of 1% lidocaine with 1:100,000 epinephrine. Time must be allowed for the anesthetic and vasoconstrictive effects. Three-layer composite grafts, requiring through-and-through incisions, are best harvested with a #11 blade, being careful not to inadvertently bevel the cut (Fig. 258-2). A #15 blade is best for cutting grafts from the crus of the helix and most two-layer grafts. Gentle technique with fine-toothed forceps should be used to limit tissue damage and minimize the shearing forces. Temporary through-and-through mattress sutures may be placed to prevent separation of the composite layers; these should be released after the graft is in place. The graft should be kept moist and sterile until transplanted.

Auricular composite grafts are particularly well suited for reconstruction of nasal alar rim defects, because primary closure or soft tissue grafts invariably contract with healing, resulting in unacceptable alar rim retraction or notching. The alar tissue loss is configured to a wedge shape, and a corresponding wedge is harvested from the helical rim. At the recipient site, layers of tissue corresponding to the composite graft layers must be identified and exposed. After final trimming of the graft is complete, like tissue elements are sutured together (Fig. 258-3). The skin on the concave (ie, lateral surface before harvest) side of the graft is sutured to the skin and mucosa of the nasal vestibule with absorbable sutures. Precise approximation of the rim margin and external closure line is completed next. The number of sutures should be kept to a minimum, and knots should be secure but not strangulating. Tails of suture may be kept long to hold a bolster dressing over the graft. The underside of the graft may be supported with antibiotic-saturated gauze placed within the nostril.

Smaller defects of the alar rim and soft triangle can be reconstructed with a composite graft from the crus of the helix. Simple primary closure of the donor site results in an inapparent scar. Composite grafts are also useful to repair contralateral auricular tissue loss (Fig. 258-4). A graft approximately one-half the size of the deficit may be used to allow acceptable closure of both ears.

Absolute hemostasis must be obtained before closure. Closure of the donor site may require extension of the graft incisions, advancement flaps, or rotational flaps (Fig. 258-5). It is best to undermine slightly at the subperichondrial plane and trim the cartilage edge to allow tension-free closure of the perichondrium and skin. Topical antibiotic ointment (ie, gentamicin) is placed over the closure line and used to saturate cotton pulled into thin strips and packed along the folds of the ear. Saturated cotton is also placed into the meatus and posterior sulcus. A mastoid dressing is applied to maintain compression and protect the ear for 48 hours. Alternately, a compression dressing may be created by positioning dental rolls or gauze pads onto the lateral and medial surfaces of the ear. These are held in place by through and through 4-0 silk sutures.

BRUCE A. SCOTT
TAPAN A. PADHYA

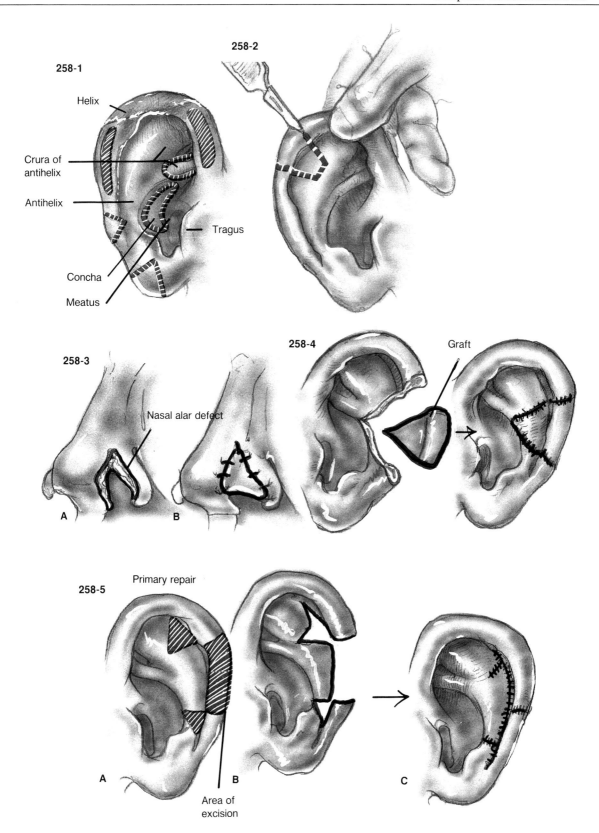

258-1

Helix

Crura of antihelix

Antihelix

Tragus

Concha

Meatus

258-2

258-3

Nasal alar defect

A

B

258-4

Graft

258-5

Primary repair

Area of excision

A

B

C

■ *259.* HARVESTING RIB GRAFTS

Surgical removal of one or more ribs containing bone or cartilage

Indications

1. Reconstruction of craniomaxillofacial osseous defects or depressions
2. Nasal reconstruction
3. Auricular reconstruction (ie, costal cartilage)
4. Temporomandibular joint reconstruction (ie, costochondral graft)

Contraindications

1. History of restrictive lung disease or recent pulmonary infection

Preoperative Preparation

1. Routine laboratory studies, including bleeding and clotting studies
2. Chest radiograph
3. Discussion with patient regarding postoperative scar position and potential contour deformity

Special Instruments, Position, and Anesthesia

1. Curved periosteal elevators, wide retractors, Doyen rib stripper, and rib cutter
2. Bipolar cautery, partial left lateral decubitus position, and general anesthesia with paralysis

Tips and Pearls

1. Use right chest, which avoids confusion with postoperative cardiac pain
2. Meticulous hemostasis
3. Check for postresection plural tear
4. Place incision in inframammary crease over the sixth or seventh rib

Pitfalls and Complications

1. Plural tear with pneumothorax
2. Thorax depression when contiguous ribs harvested (harvest every other rib, when necessary)
3. Postoperative pleuritic pain
4. Pneumonia
5. Postoperative scar and contour deformity

Postoperative Care Issues

1. Incentive spirometry
2. Chest tube, if persistent pneumothorax after plural tear
3. Pressure dressing with or without a Penrose drain

Reference

Frodel JL. Complications of bone grafting. In: Eisele DW, ed. Complications in head and neck surgery. St. Louis: CV Mosby, 1993:773.

Operative Procedure

The patient is positioned on the operating table with the right thorax elevated. The right arm can be included in the surgical preparation or rotated anteriorly and draped. The former approach is recommended, because it allows more flexibility in the donor and recipient head and neck sites. An incision is marked in the right inframammary crease over approximately the sixth or seventh rib. The procedure should be performed through an incision of approximately 5 to 6 cm, although extension may be necessary if an extremely long length of rib is required.

The incision is made through the skin and subcutaneous tissues to the level of the periosteum over the selected rib, followed by a further incision through the periosteum over the anterior surface of the rib for a length several centimeters longer than the desired rib graft length (Figs. 259-1 and 259-2). Careful subperiosteal dissection ensues medially, laterally, and superiorly. This is facilitated by the use of a wide, curved osteotome that allows subperiosteal dissection over the superior surface of the rib. Similar dissection is undertaken inferiorly, taking into account the presence of the intercostal neurovascular bundle, which lies in a concavity along the inferior aspect of each rim. After elevation in a subperiosteal plane anteriorly, superiorly, and inferiorly, dissection then ensues along the posterior aspect of the rib. Extreme caution must be used to stay within the subperiosteal plane to prevent tearing the periosteum and potentially injuring the tightly adherent parietal pleura. A large, wide, curved elevator then may be used to further elevate on the posterior surface of the rib, or a Doyen rib elevator may be used to perform the same maneuver (Fig. 259-3). The latter provides quick and efficient subperiosteal elevation if the elevator is in the proper plane.

The completed subperiosteal elevation includes elevation in a subperichondrial plane medially over the costal cartilage and laterally to approximate the anteriorly axillary line. A bone-grasping clamp is used to stabilize the bone proximally, followed by separation of the proximal and the distal segments of the rib segment with a rib cutter or large bone-cutting instrument (Fig. 259-4). If cartilage is required for a costochondral graft, it is excised sharply in a subperichondrial plane with similar care not to injure the underlying pleura.

After removal of the rib segment, hemostasis is obtained using bipolar cautery. The donor site is then examined for pleural tears. This is best undertaken after filling the donor site area with physiologic saline solution and having the anesthesiologist provide intermittent positive pressure while observing for air bubbles. If no air escape is noticed, the wound is closed in layers. The interosseous musculature that had been dissected superiorly and inferiorly in the subperiosteal dissection is closed with its attached periosteum (Fig. 259-5). Subcutaneous tissue is closed, followed by subcuticular closure of the skin. If there is a problem with complete hemostasis, a suction or Penrose drain is placed through the outer aspect of the wound (Fig. 259-6). A pressure dressing is then applied.

If positive-pressure ventilation reveals air escape through the pleura, the surgeon should assume that a pleura tear and pneumothorax exist. The initial management of this problem includes placement of a small, red rubber catheter through a pleura tear into the pleural space. This is placed on suction while a pursestring suture is placed around the tear and catheter. The wound is closed in layers as previously described around the catheter. After complete closure, the anesthesiologist is asked to again provide positive pressure to allow maximal inflation of the lungs, and the red rubber catheter is removed. Ventilation sounds are auscultated, and if normal sounding breath sounds are heard on the involved side, the procedure is completed. If the air sounds are diminished in the involved side, a portable chest radiograph should be ordered immediately to check for the presence of a pneumothorax, for which a chest tube is necessary.

After completion of the procedure, a chest radiograph is routinely obtained to observe for pneumothorax.

JOHN L. FRODEL

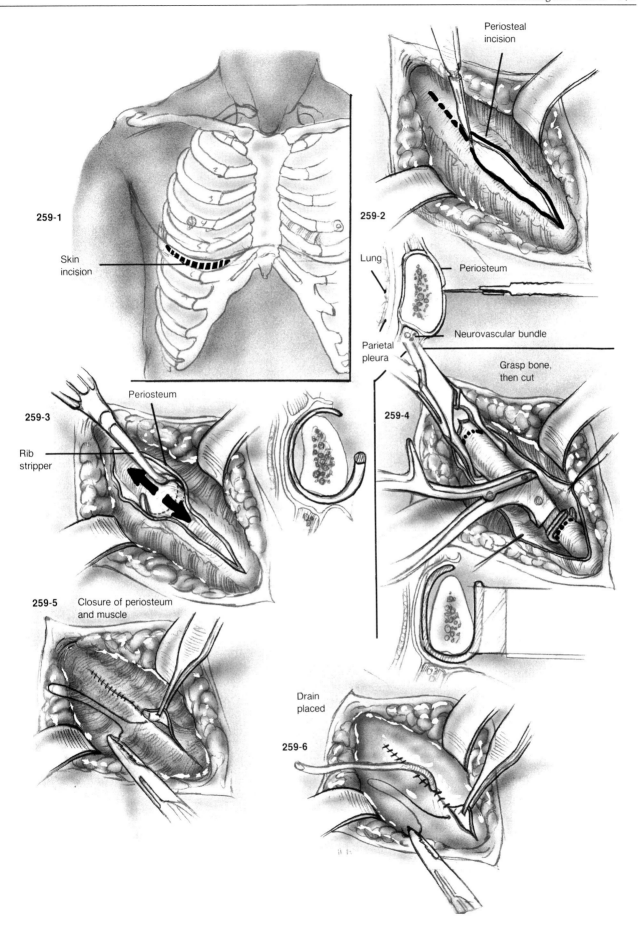

259-1

Skin incision

259-2

Periosteal incision

Lung

Periosteum

Parietal pleura

Neurovascular bundle

259-3

Periosteum

Rib stripper

259-4

Grasp bone, then cut

259-5   Closure of periosteum and muscle

259-6

Drain placed

■ 260. HARVESTING CALVARIAL BONE
GRAFTS—Surgical removal of a portion of the cranial inner or outer cortex or both

Indications
1. Craniomaxillofacial defects or depressions
2. Nasal reconstruction

Special Considerations
1. History of prior cranial trauma with or without intracerebral injury
2. Known thin calvarium
3. Young patient age (<5 years)

Preoperative Preparation
1. Routine laboratory studies
2. Computed tomography scan if the history is questionable for intracerebral injury

Special Instruments, Position, and Anesthesia
1. Surgical drill with sharp cutting burs
2. Sharp, curved osteotomes or sagittal saw
3. Bipolar cautery, reciprocating saw (if inner cortex graft to be harvested from craniotomy bone flap)
4. Mayfield head holder or elevated, circular head holder

Tips and Pearls
1. Coronal incision, as appropriate
2. Anteroposterior incision within hair-bearing region, as necessary
3. Bone harvested in parietal region, posterior to the coronal suture
4. Avoid the midline (ie, sagittal sinus)
5. Avoid bone dissection inferior to the squamosal suture.
6. In general, harvest grafts no wider than 1.5 to 2 cm.
7. Bur edges to prevent contour deformity.
8. All osteotomies should be within the diploic plane or in a direction parallel to the inner and outer cortices.

Postoperative Care Issues
1. Pressure dressing or drainage of wound

References
Frodel JL. Complications of bone grafting. In: Eisele DW, eds. Complications in head and neck surgery. St. Louis: CV Mosby, 1993:773.

Frodel JL, Marenttete LJ, Quatela VC, et al. Calvarial bone graft harvest: techniques, considerations, and morbidity. Arch Otolaryngol Head Neck Surg 1993;119:17.

Powell NB, Riley RW. Calvarial bone grafting in facial anesthetic and reconstructive contouring. Arch Otolaryngol Head Neck Surg 1987;113:713.

Operative Procedure
With the patient in a Mayfield head holder or on an elevated head-holding cushion, the surgical approach to the calvarium is begun. Ideally, a coronal incision is made over the vertex of the skull for use in craniofacial reconstruction. If this incision is not required, an incision is placed within the hair-bearing scalp over the parietal region. This incision is down to and through the galea and periosteum, and elevation ensues using a periosteal elevator to widely undermine the parietal region, which is the donor area. Self-retaining retractors facilitate this dissection if a coronal incision is not used. Before graft design, the "danger" areas of the parietal skull must be recognized (Fig. 260-1). These include the area of the sagittal sinus in the midline, the temporal line laterally, and the coronal suture anteriorly. Depending on the bone graft needs, the graft is then outlined such that the curvature of the skull is optimally used for the reconstructive needs. Generally, a graft 1.5 to 2 cm wide by 5 to 6 cm long is designed.

A drill with a large cutting bur is used to create a "trough" along one of the long edges of the proposed graft (Fig. 260-2). This trough enables later placement of an osteotome or right-angled sagittal saw. If this trough is not made wide enough, the osteotome or saw may be misdirected. It is best to place the trough at the edge of the bone, which is least suitable for bone harvest (eg, along the temporal line or the coronal suture). The trough's inner limit is the diploic layer of the skull between the outer and inner cortex. Sometimes this layer is quite thin, and the surgeon should be aware of approaching dura that does not appear to have a diploic space. After creation of the trough, a smaller cutting bur is used to outline the graft around the remaining three sides. The depth of drilling is to the diploic layer.

The outer cortical bone graft is then elevated in the diploic plane. I recommend the use of a sharp osteotome if an adequate diploic space exists. If an inadequate diploic space exists, a right-angled sagittal saw may allow for more precise cutting of the bone (Fig. 260-3). However, the use of the saw "wastes" 1 to 2 mm of bone thickness during the elevation process. After elevation of the bone graft, the inner cortex is checked for dural exposure. If the latter exists, it is imperative to check for dural tears. If a tear and cerebrospinal fluid are found, neurosurgical consultation may be advised. The bone edges surrounding the exposed dura and tear are carefully elevated in a supradural plane, followed by the use of a Kerrison rongeur to remove bone until the entirety of the drill tear is well visualized. The dural tear is oversewn with 4-0 Neurolon. Occasionally, a small fascial graft from the temporal region is necessary to close the dural defect.

In the usual scenario in which no dural exposure or tears are present, further grafts may be harvested by outlining them with a small cutting bur to the diploic layer, followed by elevation of subsequent grafts with an osteotome or sagittal saw. After elevation of the remaining grafts, the large cutting bur is again used to smooth down the edges to minimize the palpability of the deformity. Some surgeons recommend placing alloplastic material into this donor defect to minimize the deformity. I have not found this to be necessary.

In patients who have undergone craniotomy or have had a full-thickness bone flap elevated because of cranial trauma, an inner cortex bone graft may be harvested from this full-thickness calvarium (Fig. 260-4). This may also be indicated in children younger than 5 years of age because of the thin nature of their skulls. After the bone flap has been elevated, an osteotome is used to separate the two cortices within the diploic space. This should be done circumferentially around the bone flap. Care must be taken to minimize fracturing of the outer cortex of the skull, because this will be repositioned to approximate normal contour. A reciprocating or oscillating saw may facilitate separation of the cortices. After separation has been performed, the bone grafts may be further cut and contoured as necessary for the reconstructive needs, and the outer cortex is eventually replaced to allow a normal contour of the skull.

JOHN L. FRODEL

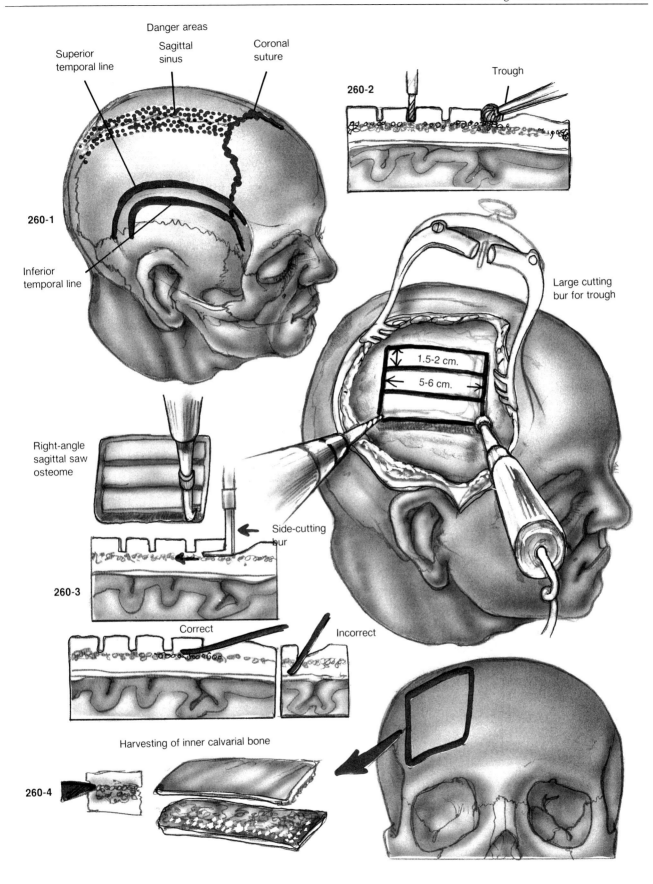

Danger areas

Superior
temporal line

Sagittal
sinus

Coronal
suture

260-1

Inferior
temporal line

Trough

260-2

Large cutting
bur for trough

1.5-2 cm.

5-6 cm.

Right-angle
sagittal saw
osteome

Side-cutting
bur

260-3

Correct

Incorrect

Harvesting of inner calvarial bone

260-4

■ *261.* NERVE GRAFTS USING THE GREATER AURICULAR AND SURAL NERVES—Using a technique for neural anastomosis, the greater auricular nerve and sural nerve can be used for nerve grafts. The greater auricular nerve supplies the sensory innervation of the pinna and postauricular area. The sural nerve provides sensory innervation for the lateral portion of the distal extremity. The technique of anastomosis provides end-to-end approximation of two nerve segments for primary repair or with a nerve graft, which is used especially for repairing the facial nerve.

Indications

1. For harvesting the greater auricular nerve
   a. Intact sensory function to the pinna and postauricular area
   b. Facial nerve defect of 3 to 12 cm
2. For harvesting the sural nerve
   a. Intact sensory function to the distal extremity
   b. Facial nerve defect greater than 12 cm
   c. Cross-facial nerve graft
3. For using the neural anastomosis technique
   a. Patient with complete facial paralysis
   b. Duration of paralysis of less than 1 year

Contraindications

1. For harvesting the greater auricular nerve
   a. Inability to locate nerve endings, as in cases of massive trauma
   b. Extensive defect
2. For using the neural anastomosis technique
   a. Inability to locate facial nerve endings
   b. Atrophied motor end plates
   c. Extensive massive facial trauma

Special Considerations

1. For using the neural anastomosis technique
   a. Preoperative assessment of facial function to determine absolute total facial paralysis
   b. Primary repair is done preferably within 48 hours to take advantage of the persistent stimulatory capabilities of the distal segment to facilitate nerve location.
   c. Epineural repair (nerve sheath) is preferable and technically easier than fascicular coaptation.

Special Instruments, Position, and Anesthesia

1. For harvesting the greater auricular nerve
   a. Operating binocular microscope or spectacle loupes (2.5×)
   b. Headlight
   c. Curved Castroviejo needle holders
   d. Curved and straight Westcott scissors
   e. Bishop-Harman forceps, with and without teeth
   f. Castroviejo calipers
   g. Kelman tying forceps
   h. Weck-cel sponges
   i. McCabe dissector
   j. Marking pen
   k. Tongue blade
   l. Standard ear, nose, and throat plastics set

(continued)

Operative Procedures

Greater Auricular Nerve

Two types of incision may be used. In the classic Blair incision, the incision is marked with marking pen, starting in the preauricular crease and making a lazy S along the angle of the mandible down to two fingerbreadths below and parallel to the mandible for about 4 cm (Fig. 261-8). As an alternative, a rhytidectomy may be used. The incision starts in the preauricular crease and extends around the earlobe and into the postauricular area. The incision is then extended posteriorly and notched to prevent contracture. It is then extended into the hairline, which has been previously shaved, and travels down into the neck area. The incision is then carried down into the appropriate plane below the skin and subcutaneous tissue until the surgeon identifies the parotid fascia superiorly and the sternocleidomastoid inferiorly (Fig. 261-9). Double-pronged skin hooks are applied to the skin edge to produce traction posteriorly and anteriorly as countertraction is applied (Fig. 261-10). With the use of electrocautery or scissors, the flap is raised mostly anteriorly, and the surgeon identifies the parotid gland and the sternocleidomastoid muscle (Fig. 261-11).

A posterior flap is created to allow further identification of the sternocleidomastoid muscle. Care must be taken to avoid transecting the greater auricular nerve.

Using the landmarks of the angle of the mandible and the mastoid tip, the surgeon should delineate the sensory cervical plexus nerve, which originates between C2 and C3 and innervates the pinna and postauricular area. The surgeon can obtain additional length of the great auricular nerve by continuing to trace it around the sternocleidomastoid muscle. After adequate length is obtained, with appropriate visualization, the nerve is gently grasped, and with a fine dissecting scissors, the nerve is transected and carefully lifted out of its position from the sternocleidomastoid muscle, tracing it to the other end and again sharply transecting it. It is immersed in physiologic saline for later use.

Sural Nerve

The patient is in the supine position, with the table slightly rotated away and the patient's leg elevated. A longitudinal incision is marked 1 to 2 cm posterior to the lateral malleolus (Fig. 261-6). The incision curves around and extends up to the middle portion of the calf. An alternative is to use step-wise incisions that require multiple wounds and a fascia stripper (Fig. 261-7).

Small flaps can be raised on either side of the incision using double-pronged skin hooks and countertraction (Fig. 261-7*B*). With adequate exposure and using the lateral malleolus as a landmark, the nerve should be 1 to 2 cm posterior to this, intimately associated with the short saphenous vein. The sural nerve is identified and cleared of overlying tissue. After adequate nerve length is obtained, the surgeon can then transect one end of the nerve, grasping it gently adjacent to its epineurium. With sharp dissection, the surgeon can continue to harvest the nerve to the other end, where a sharp scissors cut is made to remove the nerve.

After the nerve is harvested, the wounds are closed in a layered fashion with 3-0 chromic buried stitches and 4-0 continuous or interrupted nylon. As an alternative, a subcuticular closure can be achieved with 4-0 polyvinyl. A pressure dressing must be applied, and the leg must be kept elevated postoperatively for 24 hours.

Nerve Technique of Anastomosis

To identify the facial nerve, the patient is placed in the supine position, with the head slightly extended with the use of a shoulder roll and doughnut head holder and with the patient's head turned slightly away from the surgeon. The incisions employed are those described for harvesting the greater auricular nerve.

After the flaps have been raised and the parotid gland and sternocleidomastoid muscle have been identified, the parotid gland is dissected away from the anterior border of the sternocleidomastoid muscle, reflecting it anteriorly and superiorly (Fig. 261-1). The surgeon should not proceed too deeply to avoid trauma to the facial nerve. This can be accomplished by hugging the cartilaginous ear

(continued)

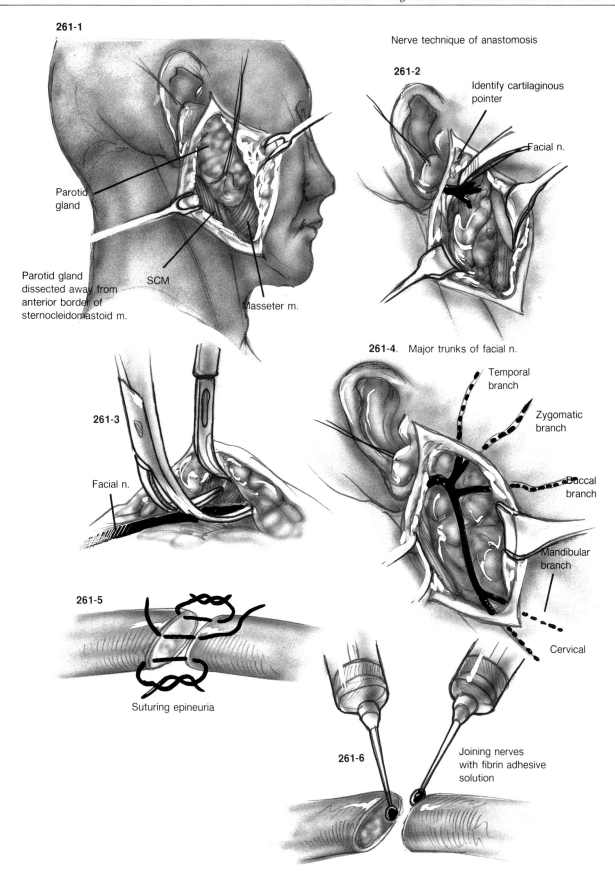

261-1

Parotid gland

Parotid gland dissected away from anterior border of sternocleidomastoid m.

SCM

Masseter m.

Nerve technique of anastomosis

261-2

Identify cartilaginous pointer

Facial n.

261-3

Facial n.

261-4. Major trunks of facial n.

Temporal branch

Zygomatic branch

Buccal branch

Mandibular branch

Cervical

261-5

Suturing epineuria

261-6

Joining nerves with fibrin adhesive solution

■ 261. NERVE GRAFTS USING THE GREATER AURICULAR AND SURAL NERVES (continued)

2. For harvesting the sural nerve
   a. All items listed for using the greater auricular nerve
   b. Fascia stripper
3. For using the neural anastomosis technique
   a. All items listed for using the greater auricular nerve
   b. 8-0 Nylon suture with GS-8 needles
   c. Fibrin tissue adhesive

Tips and Pearls

1. For harvesting the greater auricular nerve
   a. Nerve consistently runs perpendicular to an imaginary line drawn from the mastoid tip to the angle of the mandible
   b. Nerve repair to be done without tension
2. For harvesting the sural nerve
   a. The nerve lies just posterior to the lateral malleolus and is intimately associated with the short saphenous vein.
3. For using the neural anastomosis technique
   a. Because the anastomosis must be done without tension, the surgeon must mobilize the proximal and distal nerve segments in primary repair, or if tension is apparent, a greater auricular or sural nerve graft must be employed.

Pitfalls and Complications

1. Meticulous hemostasis to prevent hematoma
2. Wound closure without tension

Postoperative Care Issues

1. For harvesting the greater auricular nerve
   a. Patient to be informed of sensory deprivation to the pinna
   b. Return of function is not expected before 6 to 12 months, depending on the defect's location. Weakness and possible synkinesis should be anticipated.
2. For harvesting the sural nerve
   a. The patient is informed about the resulting numbness of the lateral portion of the distal leg.
   b. Ace bandage wrapping and elevation are necessary to reduce postoperative edema.
3. For using the neural anastomosis technique
   a. Absolute hemostasis must be obtained to avoid wound hematoma.
   b. The patient should be told about the delayed return of sensation (at least 6 months) and about the resultant weakness and probable synkinesis.

References

Baker, Connolly. Facial nerve grafting: a thirty year retrospective review. Clin Plast Surg 1979;6:343.

Bento, Miniti. Anastomosis of the intratemporal facial nerve using fibrin tissue adhesive. ENT J 1993;72:663.

Johns, Crumley. Facial nerve injury, repair and rehabilitation. SIPAC 1984;31.

canal until the pointer is identified (Fig. 261-2). The pointer represents the distal end of the cartilaginous canal and 2 to 3 mm above the point of exit of the facial nerve from the stylomastoid foramen. After wide exposure is obtained, the surgeon palpates the area to locate the mastoid tip and the styloid process, which provide bony reference points for the exit of the facial nerve (Fig. 261-3).

The surgeon must use some type of magnification at this point, either a microscope or, preferably, magnification loupes, and use excellent illumination. The tissues overlying the facial nerve are teased away gently, using anterior to posterior strokes parallel to the nerve. Because the surgeon usually is dealing with some type of trauma or transection, facial nerve stimulation may not be applicable. Hemostasis must be achieved before identification of the nerve to avoid working in a wet, obscured field.

After the facial nerve is identified, the surgeon carefully traces the nerve distally. The McCabe dissector, an excellent instrument for this purpose, is placed very close to the nerve, and lifting the tissue above, cutting is achieved with a #12 blade or electrocautery to reduce bleeding. As the surgeon dissects down to the pointer, the digastric muscle can also be identified. The fibers of this muscle are somewhat oblique or perpendicular to the sternocleidomastoid, allowing differentiation of the two muscles. The posterior belly of the digastric is identified; it can be traced superiorly to assist identification of the facial nerve because the muscle lies just under and posterior to the point of the facial nerve from the stylomastoid foramen. This continues until the main division (ie, pes anserinus) is identified, ensuring positive identification of the facial nerve. The major trunks (Fig. 261-4), the cervical fascia and the zygomatic temporal, can be traced out as is necessary, depending on the extent of the trauma and whether there is one or multiple transections. If this exploration occurs within 48 hours of the injury (ie, at a primary resection), the surgeon can use a nerve stimulator to help dissect out the distal segments.

The nerve segments must then be mobilized for a tension-free anastomosis. This is accomplished by gently picking up the nerve, and with sharp dissection, cutting the tissue attachments on the undersurface. If there is a small defect, the proximal segment can be further mobilized by tracing the nerve to the stylomastoid foramen and then removing the bone and tissue at the distal end of the mastoid. The digastric muscle fascia is extremely thick, and this process can be quite tedious. Further proximal exposure can be obtained by removing the tissue over the mastoid bone and drilling down to identify the facial nerve in the fallopian canal.

After the segments are fully mobilized and can be approximated without tension, the two ends are sutured together. It is helpful to use some type of hard surface underneath, such as a portion of a tongue blade, for support of the nerve structures.

The nerves are then gently grasped with a Bishop forceps. With an 8-0 nylon suture on a GS-8 needle, the epineurium is grasped on one end and then sutured to the other, avoiding deep cuts into the perineurium. Three square knots are applied. Three sutures are usually adequate to maintain the anastomosis (Fig. 261-5). As an alternative to sutures, the surgeon may employ fibrin tissue adhesive (Fig. 261-6). This is particularly helpful in the intratemporal segment, where it is difficult to use sutures because the bony fallopian canal limits exposure. In this case, the ends of the nerve segments are coapted and stabilized with two drops of two fibrin adhesive solutions, dropped by the needle of each syringe.

If adequate nerve length cannot be obtained because of a persistent defect, a nerve graft, usually employing the greater auricular nerve, can be applied using the previously described anastomosis technique. However, the graft produces two anastomotic points. It is preferable to use two suture sites without tension than to apply one with significant tension on the suture line.

Meticulous hemostasis is achieved, and the wound is closed with buried 3-0 chromic suture, followed by continuous 5-0 nylon or subcuticular polyvinyl sutures. A Penrose drain with a pressure dressing is applied. Alternatively, suction drainage may be used, but it the suction must avoid any contact with the nerve structures.

STEVEN M. PARNES

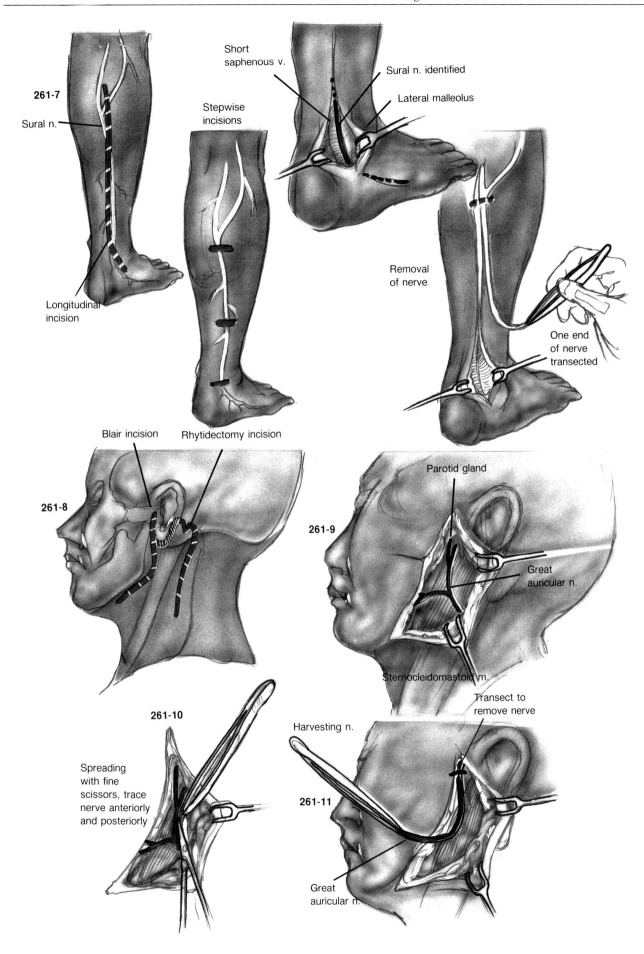

261-7

Sural n.

Longitudinal incision

Stepwise incisions

Short saphenous v.

Sural n. identified

Lateral malleolus

Removal of nerve

One end of nerve transected

Blair incision

Rhytidectomy incision

261-8

Parotid gland

261-9

Great auricular n.

Sternocleidomastoid m.

Transect to remove nerve

261-10

Spreading with fine scissors, trace nerve anteriorly and posteriorly

Harvesting n.

261-11

Great auricular n.

■ *262.* MICROVASCULAR SURGERY

The transfer of tissue from a donor site to a distant recipient site by division of the dominant arterial and venous blood supply, followed by reconstruction of arterial inflow and venous outflow

Indications

1. Absolute: anterior mandible defects, circumferential pharyngeal defects, and large, complex soft tissue losses not suitable for pedicled flap reconstruction.
2. Relative: prior high-dose irradiation and recurrent tumors. Consider a free flap first.

Contraindications

1. Inadequate recipient vessels or donor tissue
2. Medically compromised patients

Special Considerations

1. Available recipient blood vessels
2. Available specialized equipment, nursing services, physicians, and surgeons to provide adequate care

Special Instruments, Position, and Anesthesia

1. Double-head binocular operating microscope with magnifications of 3 to 20× and focal lengths of 200 to 250 mm
2. Sutures: 8-0, 9-0, and 10-0 suture on tapered vascular needles
3. Basic microvascular set
   a. Straight and curved jewelers forceps (2 each)
   b. Curved blunt-tip dissection scissors without clamp, straight adventitia scissors without clamp
   c. Curved-tip needle holder without clamp
   d. Vessel dilator, microbipolar forceps
   e. Tenotomy scissors (4.5 in), 30° microknife
4. Basic microvascular clamp set
   a. 4v Straight single clamps (4), DeBakey bulldog vein clamps (4), 4-in DeBakey 45° vascular clamps (2), Silastic vascular loops (4)
5. Flap harvest set
   a. Major head and neck tumor resection set
   b. Long DeBakey vascular forceps (2), DeBakey bulldog vein clamps (4), 45° DeBakey peripheral vascular clamps (2), straight and curved Satinsky clamps (2)
6. Microsurgery pharmacologic solutions
   a. Vein solution for irrigation: 1 L of Ringer lactate with 4000 units of heparin added
   b. Plain lidocaine solution (2% or 4%)

Tips and Pearls

1. Laboratory practice requires the use of high-quality instruments.
2. Coordinate recipient site preparation with simultaneous free flap harvest.
3. Place intravenous lines so that they do not interfere with flap harvest or inset
4. Harvest vein grafts if necessary.
5. Pharmacologic vasopressor agents should be avoided.
6. No ties around the patient's neck

Pitfalls and Complications

1. Place drains and position patient carefully to prevent compression of the free flap pedicle.

Postoperative Care Issues

1. Round-the-clock monitoring of the free flap vascular status is essential for the first 72 hours.
2. Maintenance of adequate patient fluid volume status and a hematocrit between 27 and 32.

References

Sullivan MJ. Microvascular surgical technique. In: Baker SR, ed. Microsurgical reconstruction of the head and neck. New York: Churchill Livingstone, 1989:1.

Operative Procedure

The donor and recipient vessels are individually clamped with appropriate-sized microvascular clamps, with approximately 2 to 4 mm of vessel protruding from the tips (Fig. 262-1). The adventitia of the vessel, is gently lifted and the vessel lumen fully visualized. The lumen is irrigated with vein solution and 4% plain lidocaine solution, each in a 3-mL Luer-Lok syringe with a 22-gauge blunt needle (Fig. 262-2).

The adventitia is grasped with straight or curved jeweler's forceps and pulled along the long axis of the blood vessel toward its cut end. A small cut is made in the adventitia. One blade of the straight adventitia scissors is placed inside this cut, another blade is placed outside, and the adventitia is removed from the full circumference of the vessel (Fig. 262-3).

The vessels are dilated to separate the cut edges while stretching the smooth muscle lining to prevent vasospasm. The closed vessel dilator is inserted 1 to 2 mm into the lumen. The vessel dilator is then gently opened until the vessel wall is stretched to 1.5 times its natural size (Fig. 262-4). Divide the vessel into thirds.

Gently insert the tips of straight forceps into the vessel lumen. Do not grasp the vessel edges with the forceps; simply support and elevate the vessel wall (Fig. 262-5*A*). The microvascular needle should enter the outer circumference of the vessel between the forceps tips and approximately 0.5 to 1 mm back from the cut edge of the vessel. Briskly pass the needle through the vessel wall, and stabilize it with the tips of the straight forceps in the vessel lumen (Fig. 262-5*B*). Regrasp the needle with the needle holder, and following the curve of the needle, gently pull it through the vessel wall. Repeat this step at the opposite vessel edge with the microvascular needle first entering through the lumen side and exiting through the outer wall (Fig. 262-5*C*). Gently pull the suture through the vessel wall until 5 to 10 mm of suture remains on the opposite side.

Holding the long end of the suture in the needle holder, gently create a double loop around the tips of the straight forceps, and grasp the short end of the suture (Fig. 262-6*A*). While holding the short end of the suture with the needle holder and the long end with the forceps, gently pull the suture in opposite directions to tighten the knot (see Fig. 262-6*B*). Repeat this step twice more with single loops to create a flat square knot. The surgeon should leave a 20- to 30-mm length of suture on the knot to secure the anastomosis to the microvascular clamp (see Fig. 262-6*C*).

Select a second site approximately 120° around the circumference of the vessel from the first stay suture, and using the same technique, place the second stay suture. Single interrupted sutures are then placed between the two stay sutures to complete that section of the microvascular anastomosis (Fig. 262-7).

The vessel is then rotated 180°, and a third stay suture is placed approximately 120° from each of the previous two stay sutures. Using the same technique of interrupted suture, the "backwall anastomosis" is completed.

After the microvascular anastomosis is complete, it is again copiously irrigated with vein solution and 4% plain lidocaine solution. The distal clamp is released first, and any bleeding sites along the anastomosis are identified and repaired. The proximal clamp is then released. Brisk flow through the anastomosis should be seen, and pulsation should extend into the vessel distal to the microvascular anastomosis.

The patency of the anastomosis is assessed using the strip test (Fig. 262-8). The artery or vein distal to the anastomosis is occluded. A second forceps is placed just distal to the first, and the vessel is stripped or milked for several millimeters in the direction of blood flow away from the anastomosis. The proximal clamp is then released, and prompt filling of the vessels should be seen. If prompt filling does not occur, the anastomosis should be investigated for thrombosis or an error in suturing.

EUGENE L. ALFORD

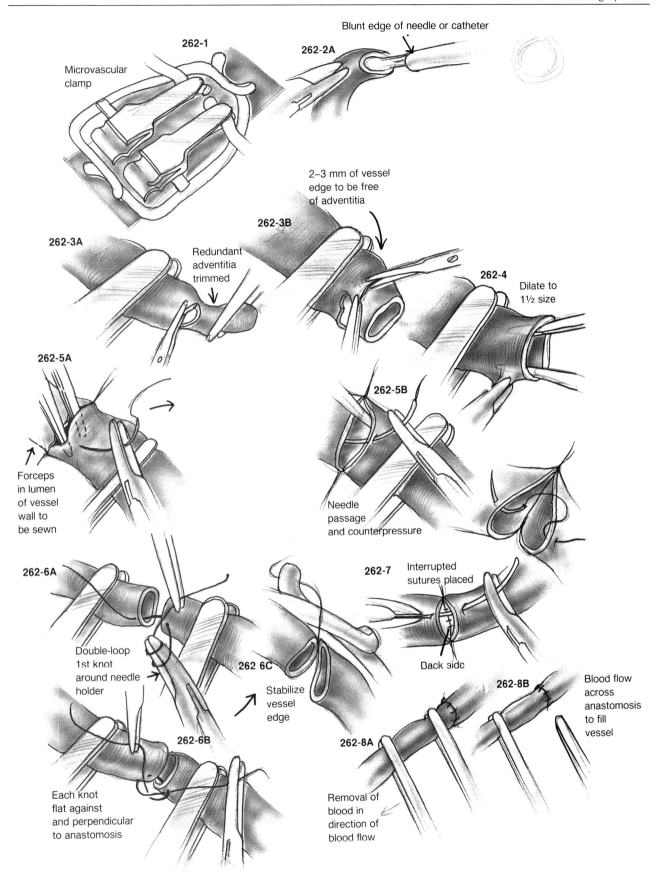

262-1
Microvascular clamp

262-2A
Blunt edge of needle or catheter

262-3A
Redundant adventitia trimmed

262-3B
2–3 mm of vessel edge to be free of adventitia

262-4
Dilate to 1½ size

262-5A
Forceps in lumen of vessel wall to be sewn

262-5B
Needle passage and counterpressure

262-6A
Double-loop 1st knot around needle holder

262-6B
Each knot flat against and perpendicular to anastomosis

262 6C
Stabilize vessel edge

262-7
Interrupted sutures placed

Back side

262-8A
Removal of blood in direction of blood flow

262-8B
Blood flow across anastomosis to fill vessel

■ *263.* SCAPULAR FREE FLAP, WITH AND WITHOUT BONE—A free composite flap consisting of vascularized skin and subcutaneous tissue of the scapular region that can incorporate vascularized segments of the lateral scapular border. The osseous and cutaneous portions of the flap receive nutrients from branches of the circumflex scapular artery and vein.

Indications

1. Reconstruction of selected oromandibular defects, including bone-only deficits or composite defects of bone, mucosa, or skin
2. Midfacial maxillary reconstruction, including the hard palate or orbital floor
3. Resurfacing of cutaneous defects of the scalp, face, or neck

Special Considerations

1. Previous axillary surgery may have resulted in ligation of the vascular pedicle, mandating selection of the contralateral scapula.
2. Scapula flap harvest disrupts various muscles that contribute to shoulder girdle function. Select the scapula opposite previous or synchronously performed radial neck dissection to avoid potentiating shoulder disability.

Preoperative Preparation

1. Routine serum chemistries and hematologic studies
2. Donor site examination to ascertain scars indicative of previous axillary surgery

Special Instruments, Position, and Anesthesia

1. Lateral decubitus position, if possible
2. Vacuum bean bag
3. Reciprocating saw
4. Bipolar cautery
5. Magnifying loupes

Tips and Pearls

1. Expose recipient vessels before flap harvest.
2. An assistant lifts and rotates the shoulder during flap harvest to facilitate dissection and improve exposure of the vascular pedicle.
3. The lateral or superior extent of the scapular or parascapular skin paddles, respectively, should overlap the muscular triangle to avoid inadvertent injury to the circumflex scapular vessels when making the skin incisions.
4. An optimal way of isolating vascular pedicle during flap elevation is to maintain sharp dissection close to the muscles bounding the triangular space as the latter is approached.

(continued)

Operative Procedure

Flap elevation is easiest with the patient supported by a vacuum bean bag in the lateral decubitus position. This allows access to the entire back, shoulder, upper chest, and arm, all of which are included in the sterile preparation. An assistant situated across the patient supports the upper arm and maintains the shoulder joint positioned properly throughout the procedure.

The blood supply of the scapular region is based on osseous and cutaneous branches of the circumflex scapular artery. This vessel is the posterior continuation of the subscapular artery after the latter gives off the thoracodorsal artery. The subscapular artery originates from the third portion of the axillary artery (Fig. 263-1). The circumflex scapular artery supplies the skin of the scapular region after passing through a triangular space bounded by the long head of the triceps laterally and the divergence of the teres major and minor muscles inferiorly and superiorly, respectively. Before emerging from this space, several branches provide nutrient flow to the periosteum of the lateral border of the scapula. After emerging from the triangular space, the circumflex scapular artery divides into horizontal and descending fasciocutaneous branches that supply the skin of the back (Figs. 263-1 and 263-2).

Before flap elevation, it is helpful to mark the location of the triangular space, which is usually palpable 2 cm cephalad to the posterior axillary fold. Alternatively, a Doppler probe may be used to pinpoint the location of the vascular pedicle at the muscular triangle.

Elliptical cutaneous paddles are designed to simplify donor site closure after flap harvest. The long axis of the horizontally oriented scapular paddle is centered over the scapular fasciocutaneous branch of the circumflex scapular artery. This branch originates at the triangular space laterally and extends medially parallel to the scapular spine. The lateral end of the elliptical skin paddle is placed over the previously identified muscular triangle. Medially, the skin paddle can extend to the midline of the back. The superior limit of the scapular flap is the scapular spine. The inferior limit is the tip of the scapula. Alternatively, a vertically oriented parascapular cutaneous paddle may be designed along the lateral border of the scapula, centered over the descending fasciocutaneous branch of the circumflex scapular artery. The superior end of the ellipse is placed just over the muscular triangle. Its inferior limit extends just below the tip of the scapula. Width is limited to approximately 14 to 18 cm to allow primary closure of the donor defect (Fig. 263-3).

Medial incisions are made and deepened to the deep fascia of the infraspinatus muscle. Flap elevation proceeds from the medial to lateral aspects in the avascular plane just superficial to this muscular fascia. The teres major and minor muscles are identified inferiorly and medially. The long head of the triceps is identified superiorly and laterally as the flap is reflected off the deltoid muscle. Elevation of the skin paddle continues with sharp dissection that is kept close to the muscles bounding the muscular triangle (Fig. 263-4). The circumflex artery and its fasciocutaneous branches are identified in the fibrofatty tissue contained within the triangular space. With right-angle retractors separating the teres major and minor muscles in their respective directions, the circumflex scapular vessels are carefully skeletonized. The multiple branches encountered supply the adjacent musculature and the periosteum of the lateral scapular border. Muscular branches are ligated individually with small vascular clips. If a purely cutaneous flap is being harvested, the periosteal branches must be similarly ligated. Proximal dissection

(continued)

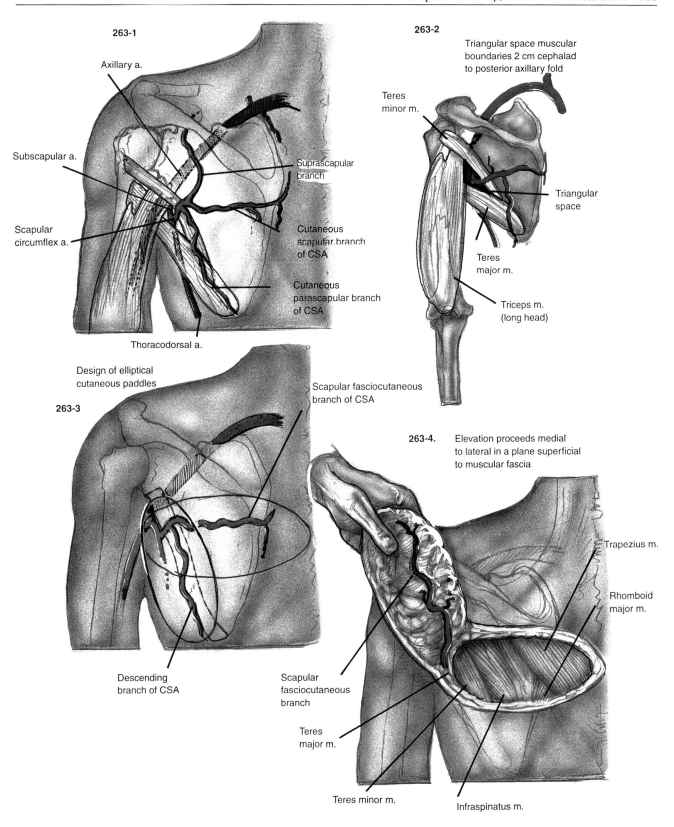

263-1

Axillary a.

Subscapular a.

Scapular circumflex a.

Suprascapular branch

Cutaneous scapular branch of CSA

Cutaneous parascapular branch of CSA

Thoracodorsal a.

263-2

Triangular space muscular boundaries 2 cm cephalad to posterior axillary fold

Teres minor m.

Triangular space

Teres major m.

Triceps m. (long head)

263-3

Design of elliptical cutaneous paddles

Scapular fasciocutaneous branch of CSA

Descending branch of CSA

263-4. Elevation proceeds medial to lateral in a plane superficial to muscular fascia

Trapezius m.

Rhomboid major m.

Scapular fasciocutaneous branch

Teres major m.

Teres minor m.

Infraspinatus m.

■ 263. SCAPULAR FREE FLAP, WITH AND WITHOUT BONE (continued)

5. When contouring of the scapular border is necessary, ostectomies allow better fitting of the bone segments than what can be achieved with osteotomies alone.

6. Elevate the periosteum at the ostectomy site with a Freer elevator to allow tunneling of the saw and avoid possible injury to periosteal feeders downstream from the ostectomy site.

7. Separate, independently mobile osseous segments of the lateral scapular border can be harvested based on the branches of the subscapular vessels. A proximal one, near the glenoid fossa, may be raised based on branches of the circumflex scapular artery. A distal segment, near the inferior angle, is supplied by the angular branch of the thoracodorsal artery.

8. Closure of the osteocutaneous donor site requires approximately 60 minutes and must be performed before flap insetting and revascularization. As much contouring as possible should be performed in situ before transecting the nutrient pedicle.

Pitfalls and Complications

1. Patient positioning makes simultaneous flap harvest and tumor ablation difficult.
2. Donor site seroma
3. Flap failure

Postoperative Care Issues

1. The ipsilateral upper extremity is placed in a sling for the initial 3 to 5 postoperative days.
2. Antithrombotic therapy with low-molecular-weight dextran is employed during first 5 postoperative days. Low-dose aspirin is administered for 2 weeks.
3. Maintain the head position arrived at during surgery, which prevents excessive tension or redundancy of the vascular pedicle.
4. Meticulous wound surveillance to detect early vascular compromise or salivary fistulization
5. Range of motion and shoulder strengthening exercises begin on postoperative day 5 under the supervision of a physical therapist.

References

Baker SR, Sullivan M. The osteocutaneous scapular flap for one stage reconstruction of the mandible. Arch Otolaryngol Head Neck Surg 1988;114:267.

Swartz WM, Banis JC, Newton ED, et al. The osteocutaneous scapular flap for mandibular and maxillary reconstruction. Plast Reconstr Surg 1986;77:530.

of the vascular pedicle then proceeds toward the axilla (Fig. 263-5).

If a composite osteocutaneous flap is being raised, the periosteal branches must be carefully preserved. In this case, the dissection is simplified, and exposure is improved by detaching the insertion of the teres major muscle to the inferior and lateral aspect of the scapula. A tunnel is created with blunt dissection around the teres major, and electrocautery is used to transect the muscle. A 2- to 3-cm cuff of muscle is left attached to the lateral border of the scapula to protect the underlying periosteal feeders. The nutrient pedicle is then easily skeletonized proximal to its origin from the axillary artery and vein. This requires identification and ligation of the thoracodorsal artery and vein (Fig. 263-6). However, if a segment of inferolateral scapular border is being harvested based on the angular branch of the thoracodorsal artery, both vessels must be skeletonized and preserved. The angular branch is identified on the chest wall, deep to the teres major muscle, when this muscle is detached from the lateral scapular border. The vessel originates directly from the thoracodorsal artery or from its crossing branch to the serratus anterior muscle in equal numbers of cases.

With the vascular pedicle isolated, a vertical incision is made through the teres minor and infraspinatus muscles down to scapular bone, staying 3 cm medial to the lateral border of the scapula. A periosteal elevator is used to strip the scapular periosteum medially before performing osteotomies. A vertical bone cut is made with a reciprocating saw approximately 2.5 cm medial to and parallel to the lateral scapular border. A short, transverse cut is made superiorly, just below the glenoid fossa. Care must be taken in making this cut to preserve the joint structures and the circumflex scapular vessels in the triangular space. Muscular remnants attached to the osteotomized lateral scapular border can be transected with Metzenbaum scissors. On the ventral aspect of the scapular border, these muscles include the serratus anterior and subscapularis muscles. A small portion of these are left attached to bone to prevent the disruption of the periosteal blood supply. Further dissection of the vascular pedicle toward the axilla may proceed, if necessary. The length of the harvested scapular border varies from 10 to 14 cm, depending on the patient's sex and build (Fig. 263-7).

When the recipient site is ready for insetting, the subscapular artery and vein are ligated in that order, and the flap is transferred. Flap insetting usually is performed before completion of the microvascular anastomoses. If an osteocutaneous flap has been harvested for maxillary or mandibular reconstruction, ostectomies are preferred over osteotomies for bony contouring. These may be safely performed with a small reciprocating saw after first elevating periosteum and muscle over the ostectomy site with a Freer elevator. The saw can then be inserted into the created tunnel to perform the bone cuts. The resultant bony segments are stabilized to one another and to the mandibular or maxillary remnants with interosseous wiring or miniplates. The skin paddles are used to resurface external or intraoral soft tissue defects and to cover the scapular bone and hardware (Fig. 263-8).

After carefully securing hemostasis, closure of the cutaneous defect is performed over suction drains. Primary closure can be achieved in most cases with wide undermining of the surrounding skin of the back and axilla. Closure of the osteocutaneous scapular flap defect requires restitution of disrupted muscle groups. Multiple drill holes are made along the remaining lateral border of the scapula. Nonabsorbable sutures are then passed through these holes and used to approximate the teres muscles, the long head of triceps, and subscapularis muscles to the lateral border of the scapula. Closure of the cutaneous defect is performed as described previously.

Antithrombotic therapy is routinely administered postoperatively and consists of low-molecular-weight dextran (500 mL) infused over 12 hours once daily for the first 5 days after surgery. In addition, the patient is placed on aspirin (81 mg, once daily) for 2 weeks. The ipsilateral upper extremity is immobilized in a sling until the third to fifth postoperative day. At that time, physical therapy is initiated to increase shoulder range of motion and increase the strength of the shoulder girdle.

JUAN F. MOSCOSO

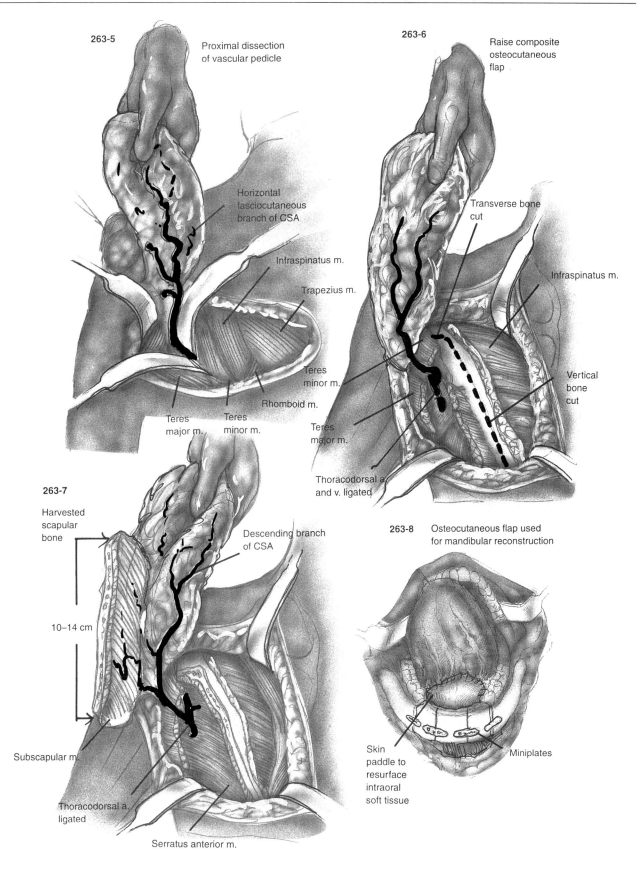

263-5

Proximal dissection
of vascular pedicle

Horizontal
fasciocutaneous
branch of CSA

Infraspinatus m.

Trapezius m.

Teres
minor m.

Rhomboid m.

Teres
major m.

Teres
minor m.

263-6

Raise composite
osteocutaneous
flap

Transverse bone
cut

Infraspinatus m.

Vertical
bone
cut

Teres
major m.

Thoracodorsal a.
and v. ligated

263-7

Harvested
scapular
bone

Descending branch
of CSA

10–14 cm

Subscapular m.

Thoracodorsal a.
ligated

Serratus anterior m.

263-8   Osteocutaneous flap used
for mandibular reconstruction

Skin
paddle to
resurface
intraoral
soft tissue

Miniplates

■ 264. ILIAC CREST INTERNAL OBLIQUE

FREE FLAP—A free tissue flap consisting of a segment of vascularized, bicortical ilium and overlying skin and subcutaneous tissue based on osseous and musculocutaneous perforators of the deep circumflex iliac artery and vein, which includes the internal oblique muscle based on the ascending branch of the same artery and vein

Indications

1. Reconstruction of selected segmental oromandibular defects, particularly composite defects including mucosa, bone, and skin and especially where osteointegrated implants are to be used to restore a functional dental arch
2. Reconstruction of combined total or near-total glossectomy defects with segmental defects of the anterior mandibular arch

Special Considerations

1. Morbid obesity complicates placement of the skin paddle over the zone of cutaneous perforators and makes abdominal dissection difficult.
2. Previous groin or inguinal surgery may have resulted in ligation of or injury to the deep circumflex iliac vessels.
3. Preoperative selection of the left or right ilium is based on the expected ablative defect and availability of recipient vessels.

Preoperative Preparation

1. Routine serum chemistries and hematologic studies

Special Instruments, Position, and Anesthesia

1. Magnifying loupes
2. Reciprocating saw
3. Bipolar cautery
4. Donor site elevation with a roll placed underneath the hip to improve access to the posterior ilium

Tips and Pearls

1. The skin paddle design may be shifted 2.0 cm cephalad to the axis joining the anterior-superior iliac spine to the inferior angle of ipsilateral scapula to ensure capturing the musculocutaneous perforators and improving the mobility of the skin paddle relative to bone.
2. Avoid excessive tension or twisting of the mesentery transmitting musculocutaneous perforators and connecting cutaneous paddle with a bicortical segment of iliac crest.
3. The cutaneous defect to be resurfaced should not extend above level of the zygomatic arch. Insetting the skin paddle above this level can result in excessive stretching of the mesentery.

(continued)

Operative Procedure

With the patient in the supine position, a soft roll is placed underneath the hip to improve access to the posterior portions of the iliac crest. An elliptical skin paddle is drawn centered on a line joining the ASIS to the inferior angle of the ipsilateral scapula. The skin paddle must be large enough to ensure incorporation of musculocutaneous perforators of the DCIA and DCIV, which exit through the three layers of abdominal wall musculature along the inner aspect of the iliac crest.

The superior incision is made first and extends inferiorly and medially, parallel to the inguinal ligament, to the palpable pulse of the femoral vessels, and superiorly and laterally toward the inferior angle of the scapula (Fig. 264-1). This incision is deepened to the external oblique muscle and aponeurosis (Fig. 264-2). The external oblique muscle is incised inferiorly and medially down to, but not through, the internal oblique muscle, which is preserved (Fig. 264-3). Finger dissection separates the two muscles, and Metzenbaum scissors are used to extend the incision cephalad through the external oblique along the entire length of the previously described skin incision, maintaining a 3-cm cuff of muscle attached to the inner table of the iliac crest. Using rake retractors, the external oblique muscle and overlying abdominal wall are sharply elevated as a unit in a plane superficial to the internal oblique, exposing the full extent of this muscle from its costal attachments to the inguinal ligament, and from the midaxillary line to the rectus sheath.

The internal oblique muscle is harvested by incising the muscle along its cephalad, lateral, and medial boundaries. The initial incision through the internal oblique muscle is made superiorly and laterally and extends medially, following the outline of the lower rib cage. Medially, the internal oblique muscle is incised 1 cm lateral to the linea semilunaris (Fig. 264-4). The plane between the internal oblique and transversus abdominis is identified superiorly and laterally, and this broad sheet of muscle is elevated to within 3 cm of the iliac crest. This maneuver is facilitated by an assistant gently lifting the cut edge of the internal oblique muscle with Babcock clamps. The operating surgeon applies countertraction against the transversus abdominis muscle with one hand while sharply developing the plane between the two sheets of muscle with the other hand.

As the internal oblique muscle is elevated, the ascending branch of the DCIA is identified on its undersurface and is preserved. The ascending branch is then carefully traced back through the transversus abdominis muscle to its origin from the DCIA and DCIV. These vessels are isolated to the external iliac artery and vein. Before joining the external iliac vein, paired DCIVs join to form a common venous trunk that gives off a pelvic branch that requires ligation. This common venous trunk (ie, DCIV) continues its course to the external iliac vein, passing superficial or deep to the external iliac artery.

The transversus abdominis and transversalis fascia are incised parallel to the iliac crest, preserving a 3-cm cuff of these layers to protect the musculocutaneous perforators. Exposed preperitoneal fat is retracted medially with malleable retractors to expose the iliacus muscle on the inner surface of the iliac crest. The iliacus is then incised down to periosteum, preserving a 2-cm cuff of muscle attached superiorly to the inner table of the iliac crest to protect the deep circumflex iliac vessels. As the iliacus is being incised, the lateral femoral cutaneous nerve is encountered and may be harvested to use as a nerve graft if one is needed. The iliacus fibers are reflected inferiorly with a periosteal elevator to expose the necessary depth of iliac crest.

Lateral exposure is obtained by incising the caudad aspect of the skin paddle down to the lateral lip of the iliac crest. Care must be taken not to carry this incision medially over the iliac crest, because this would result in transection of the mesentery transmitting the musculocutaneous perforators to the skin paddle. The tensor fascia lata and gluteus medius muscles are detached from the lateral aspect of the iliac crest with the cautery and are reflected inferiorly with a periosteal elevator to expose the necessary depth of iliac crest. Anterior exposure is obtained by detaching the sartorius muscle from the ASIS and transecting the iliopsoas as it courses under the ASIS.

(continued)

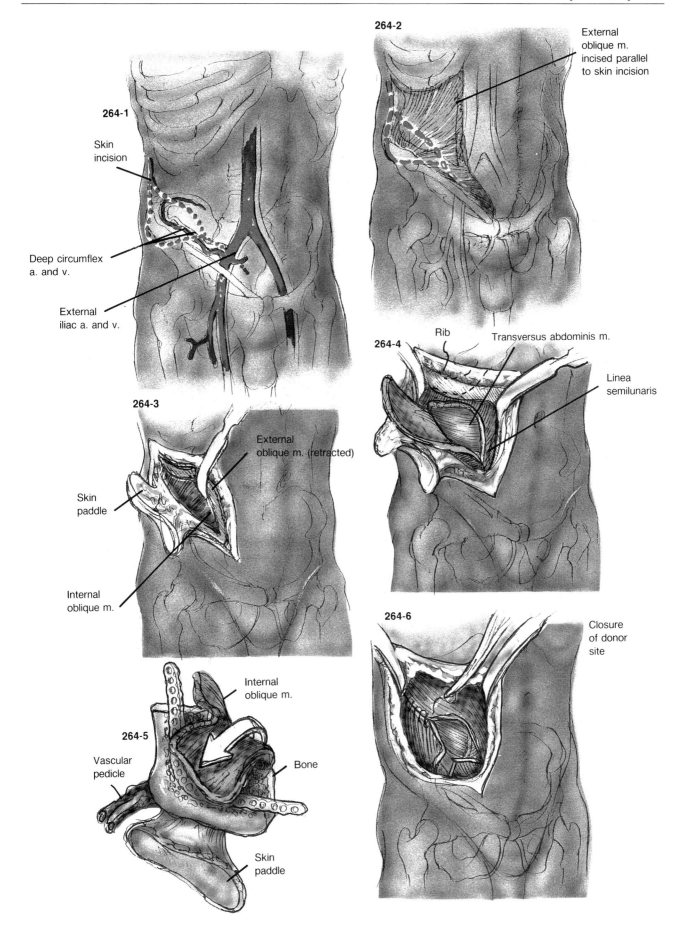

264-1

Skin incision

Deep circumflex a. and v.

External iliac a. and v.

264-2

External oblique m. incised parallel to skin incision

264-3

External oblique m. (retracted)

Skin paddle

Internal oblique m.

264-4

Rib

Transversus abdominis m.

Linea semilunaris

264-5

Internal oblique m.

Vascular pedicle

Bone

Skin paddle

264-6

Closure of donor site

■ 264. ILIAC CREST INTERNAL OBLIQUE FREE FLAP *(continued)*

4. After flap harvest, back cuts can be made in the internal oblique muscle toward the ascending branch. This improves the maneuverability of the muscle relative to the other components of the flap.
5. Hip flexion facilitates closure of the donor defect.

Pitfalls and Complications

1. Total flap loss
2. Necrosis of the skin paddle due to tension or pressure on the mesentery transmitting musculocutaneous perforators
3. Abdominal hernia formation
4. Femoral nerve injury

Postoperative Care Issues

1. Slight hip flexion, with a pillow underneath the ipsilateral knee
2. Antithrombotic therapy with low-molecular-weight dextran is employed during first 5 postoperative days. Low-dose aspirin is administered for 2 weeks.
3. Maintain the head position arrived at during surgery, which prevents excessive tension or redundancy of the vascular pedicle.
4. Assisted ambulation and physical therapy commence on postoperative days 5 to 7.
5. Meticulous wound surveillance to detect early vascular compromise or evidence of salivary fistulization

References

Moscoso JF, Urken ML. The internal oblique–iliac crest osseomyocutaneous free-flap for the reconstruction of composite oromandibular defects. Oper Techn Otolaryngol Head Neck Surg 1993;4:132.

Urken ML, Buchbinder D, Weinberg H, et al. Primary placement of osseointergrated implants in microvascular mandibular reconstruction. Otolaryngol Head Neck Surg 1989;101:56.

Urken ML, Weinberg H, Vickery C, et al. The internal oblique–iliac crest free flap in composite defects of the oral cavity involving bone, skin, and mucosa. Laryngoscope 1991;101:257.

This maneuver can be performed with the cautery after first isolating and protecting the deep circumflex iliac vessels just medial to the ASIS.

A bicortical segment of iliac crest is harvested based on the dimensions of the resected mandibular segment. The bone cuts are made with a reciprocating saw from the lateral aspect of the iliac bone using malleable retractors to protect the abdominal contents. The osteomyocutaneous flap will be turned 180° such that the crest forms the inferior border of the neomandible. Harvesting the flap from the same side as the segmental mandibular defect positions the vascular pedicle at the angle of the neomandible and allows anastomoses to recipient vessels in the ipsilateral neck. Osseous reconstruction of the ramus and condyle can be achieved by incorporation of the ASIS as part of the bone graft. Otherwise, the depth of the osteotomy through iliac bone remains constant at 2.5 cm from the iliac crest throughout the length of the segment to be harvested. Harvest of the flap from the hip opposite the side of the segmental mandibular defect positions the vascular pedicle anteriorly, closer to recipient vessels in the contralateral neck. Osseous reconstruction of the ramus and condyle can be achieved in this instance by harvesting a greater depth of bone from the posterior aspect of the iliac crest.

Final contouring to the shape of the resected mandibular segment can be performed with osteotomies through the outer cortex of the iliac crest. The reciprocating saw is used to make these osteotomies, which can be performed with the flap isolated on its vascular pedicle or after transfer to the head and neck. When the recipient bed is ready for insetting, the DCIA and DCIV are transected in that order, and the flap is transferred.

Mandibular reconstruction is typically performed with the flap inverted by 180°. In this configuration, the iliac crest forms the inferior border of the neomandible. The internal oblique muscle attaches to the lingual surface of the bone graft and can be used to resurface mucosal defects of the pharynx or oral cavity. A portion of the muscle may also be used to cover the bone graft and the reconstruction plate used to procure rigid fixation to the residual mandibular segments (Fig. 264-5). It is not always necessary to cover the internal oblique muscle with split-thickness skin grafts. If there is sufficient mucosa available in the cheek, floor of the mouth, or ventral tongue, direct approximation of mucosa to muscle results in adequate healing and preserved mobility of these structures. The skin paddle remains attached to the inferior and lingual aspect of the neomandible and can be used to resurface external cutaneous defects. When no external cutaneous defect exists, the skin paddle is incorporated into a cervical suture line to serve as a monitor of flap viability in the postoperative period.

After obtaining hemostasis, a meticulous closure of the donor site is performed in three layers (Fig. 264-6). This is facilitated by removing the roll placed under the donor hip and gently flexing the ipsilateral knee. Multiple drill holes are made through the remnants of the osteotomized iliac crest. The transversalis fascia and transversus abdominis muscles are approximated to iliacus muscle and directly to bone with interrupted, mattressed, permanent sutures passed through the drill holes. A portion of the gluteus medius and tensor fascia lata muscles may be incorporated with each suture. Inferior and medial to the ASIS, the transversus abdominis muscle and transversalis fascia are approximated to the inguinal ligament, with care taken to avoid injury to the femoral nerve. The second layer in the closure consists of the external oblique muscle and aponeurosis, which are sutured to the gluteus medius and tensor fascia lata muscles and fascia. Nonabsorbable, interrupted, mattress sutures are also used in this layer. In the final layer, the cutaneous defect is closed over a suction drain after sufficient undermining is performed to allow coaptation of the skin edges.

Postoperatively, a pillow is placed under the ipsilateral knee to maintain the donor site hip in slight flexion. Antithrombotic therapy is routinely administered and consists of low-molecular-weight dextran (500 mL) infused once daily over 12 hours for the first 5 days after surgery. In addition, the patient is placed on aspirin (81 mg, once daily) for 2 weeks.

JUAN F. MOSCOSO

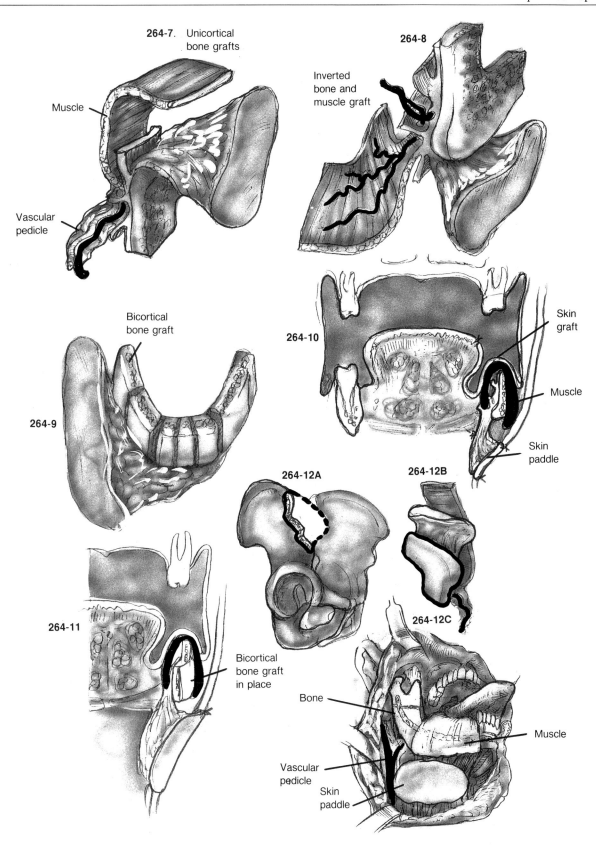

264-7. Unicortical bone grafts

Muscle

Vascular pedicle

264-8

Inverted bone and muscle graft

Bicortical bone graft

264-9

264-10

Skin graft

Muscle

Skin paddle

264-11

264-12A

264-12B

Bicortical bone graft in place

264-12C

Bone

Muscle

Vascular pedicle

Skin paddle

265. RADIAL FOREARM FLAP

Free tissue flap consisting of vascularized skin and subcutaneous tissue of the forearm based on cutaneous perforators of the radial artery. Venous drainage occurs through paired vena comitantes of the radial artery and superficial forearm veins. Sensory neurotization is possible through the antebrachial cutaneous nerves of the forearm.

Indications

1. Correction of cervical skin contractures in burn patients.
2. Resurfacing of mucosal defects of oral cavity and pharynx after limited or near-total glossectomy and after partial or circumferential pharyngectomy
3. Total lower lip reconstruction
4. Reconstruction after hemilaryngopharyngectomy

Contraindications

1. Osteocutaneous radial flaps are no longer favored in oromandibular reconstruction.

Special Considerations

1. Inadequate ulnar circulation to the hand (ie, incomplete palmar arch)
2. Recent use of indwelling catheters or recent venipuncture of superficial veins of the forearm
3. Selection of the nondominant arm for flap harvest

Preoperative Preparation

1. Routine serum chemistries and hematologic studies
2. Allen's test to document the adequacy of palmar circulation
3. Avoidance of trauma to the superficial veins of the forearm

Special Instruments, Position, and Anesthesia

1. Pneumatic tourniquet
2. Magnifying loupes
3. Bipolar cautery

Tips and Pearls

1. Design the skin paddle to maximize residual tongue mobility.
2. Incorporate at least one superficial vein (cephalic or basilic) in the flap design.
3. Preserve the superficial radial nerve and its branches.
4. Preserve the paratenon of the wrist flexor tendons.
5. Incorporate a portion of the flap into the cervical suture line for postoperative monitoring of the tissue.

Pitfalls and Complications

1. Vascular insufficiency of the hand (rare)
2. Radial fracture after harvest of osteocutaneous flaps (20% incidence)
3. Delayed donor site wound healing due to flexor tendon exposure
4. Superficial radial nerve injury and neuroma formation
5. Donor site hematoma
6. Flap failure

Postoperative Care Issues

1. Skin grafted donor site is immobilized with an ulnar splint and kept elevated for the first 7 postoperative days.
2. Clinical evaluation of the hand's circulation
3. Antithrombotic therapy with low-molecular-weight dextran is employed during the first 5 postoperative days. Low-dose aspirin is administered for 2 weeks.
4. Meticulous wound surveillance to detect early flap compromise or evidence of salivary fistulization
5. Maintain the head position arrived at during surgery, which prevents excessive tension or redundancy of the vascular pedicle.

References

Timmons MJ. The vascular basis of the radial forearm flap. Plast Reconstr Surg 1986;77:80.
Urken ML, Moscoso JF. A new bilobed design for the sensate radial forearm flap to preserve tongue mobility following significant glossectomy. Arch Otolaryngol Head Neck Surg 1994;120:26.
Urken ML, Moscoso JF, Lawson W, Biller HF. A systematic approach to functional reconstruction of the oral cavity following partial and total glossectomy. Arch Otolaryngol Head Neck Surg 1994;120:589.

Operative Procedure

After elevation and exsanguination of the extremity, a previously placed pneumatic tourniquet is inflated to 250 mm Hg. Flap elevation therefore proceeds in a dry field. The skin paddle design is based on the size of the ablative defect and is projected over the course of the radial artery and one subcutaneous forearm vein (Fig. 265-1). The skin paddle should be placed over the distal forearm to maximize the length of the vascular pedicle. There are no limitations to the shape of the skin island, a portion of which may be incorporated into a cervical suture line to serve as a postoperative monitor of flap viability. Alternatively, the flap may be designed with a second, proximal skin island that is exteriorized in the lower neck.

Skin incisions are made about the periphery of the flap and carried through the subcutaneous tissue and deep muscle fascia, except at the proximal portion of the skin paddle, where the incision extends through skin only. Distally, the radial vessels are identified just lateral to the flexor carpi radialis tendon and ligated. Flap elevation proceeds in the plane deep to the muscular fascia from the radial and ulnar aspects of the flap toward the intermuscular septum of the forearm (Fig. 265-2). The superficial branch of the radial nerve runs in the cubital fossa after emerging from deep to the brachioradialis muscle in its distal third. This nerve and its variable number of branches, supplying sensation to the thumb and first two digits, should be carefully isolated and preserved during flap elevation. Septocutaneous perforators are easily seen as the intermuscular septum is identified between the bellies of the brachioradialis and flexor carpi radialis muscles. Care is taken to preserve the paratenon overlying the wrist flexor tendons, which provides a vascularized bed for healing of the skin graft to be used for closure of the donor defect. Branches of the cephalic or basilic veins are ligated in the distal aspect of the flap but are protected as the dissection proceeds toward the antecubital fossa. A curvilinear incision extends from the proximal portion of the flap toward the antecubital fossa and facilitates exposure of the vascular pedicle.

With the intermuscular septum widely exposed, the radial vessels are elevated from the groove between the flexor carpi radialis and brachioradialis muscles in a distal to proximal direction. Tenotomy scissors are ideal for this step. Individual muscular and periosteal branches of the radial vessels are ligated or electrocoagulated with bipolar cautery as they are encountered. Proximal dissection of the vascular pedicle to the bifurcation of the brachial artery requires careful separation of the bellies of the flexor carpi radialis and brachioradialis muscles. At the proximal portion of the flap, the antebrachial cutaneous nerves of the forearm are identified (Fig. 265-3) next to the cephalic and basilic veins and are harvested to reinnervate the flap by performing microneural repairs between them and appropriate sensory nerves in the head and neck.

With the flap attached only to the nourishing pedicle, the pneumatic tourniquet is released, and the flap is perfused until ready for transfer (Fig. 265-4). The adequacy of the circulation to the skin paddle is easily ascertained at this time.

At the time of harvest, the radial artery is ligated just distal to the bifurcation of the brachial artery. The vena comitantes and the preserved branches of the cephalic or basilic veins are then ligated. The flap is then transferred to the head and neck for insetting and revascularization (Fig. 265-5). The donor defect usually is too large to allow closure with local transposition flaps unless tissue expansion of the donor site has been accomplished preoperatively. A split-thickness skin graft is used in most cases to resurface the donor defect. At the end of the procedure, the wound is dressed in a sterile fashion and the forearm is placed in an ulnar splint.

The forearm is maintained elevated, and the wound is examined 7 days later, when the splint is removed. Antithrombotic therapy is routinely administered and consists of low-molecular-weight dextran (500 mL) infused over 12 hours each day for the first 5 days after surgery. In addition, the patient is placed on aspirin (81 mg, once daily) for 2 weeks.

JUAN F. MOSCOSO

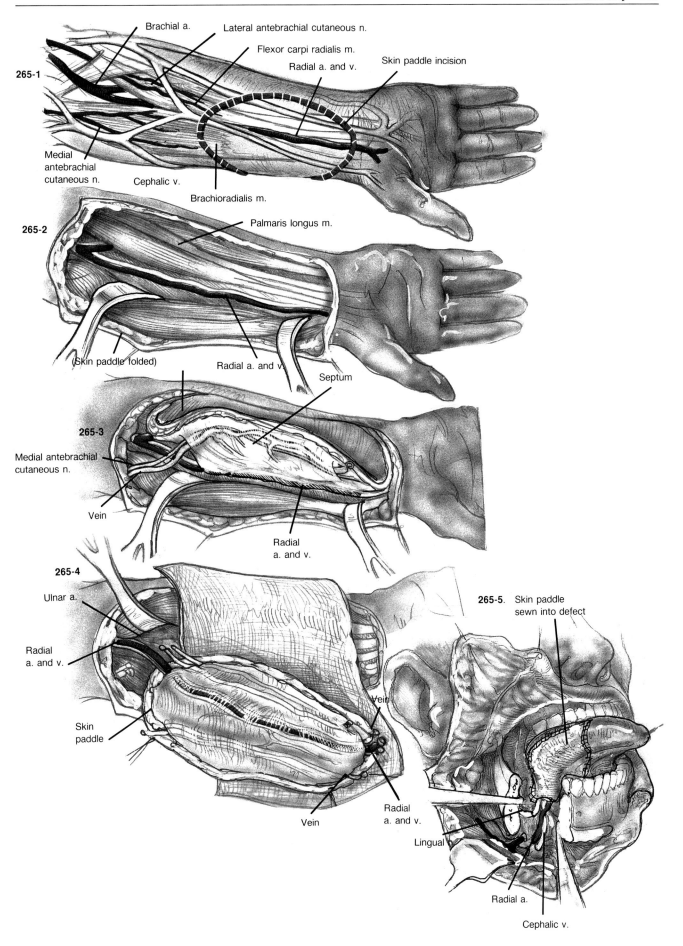

265-1

Brachial a.

Lateral antebrachial cutaneous n.

Flexor carpi radialis m.

Radial a. and v.

Skin paddle incision

Medial antebrachial cutaneous n.

Cephalic v.

Brachioradialis m.

265-2

Palmaris longus m.

(Skin paddle folded)

Radial a. and v.

Septum

265-3

Medial antebrachial cutaneous n.

Vein

Radial a. and v.

265-4

Ulnar a.

Radial a. and v.

Skin paddle

Vein

Vein

Radial a. and v.

265-5. Skin paddle sewn into defect

Lingual

Radial a.

Cephalic v.

■ 266. LATERAL ARM FREE FLAP

A fasciocutaneous flap based on the intermuscular septum of the arm that receives its blood supply from the posterior radial collateral artery

Indications

1. Reconstruction of head and neck defects requiring thin, pliable soft tissue with potential for sensory reinnervation
2. Soft tissue augmentation of head and neck defects
3. Vascularized nerve graft, with or without soft tissue

Contraindications

1. Large soft tissue defects (<8 × 10 cm)
2. Inability to close the donor site primarily when cosmesis is important
3. Previous trauma to skin of posterolateral arm

Special Considerations

1. Flap harvest results in a permanent sensory deficit of the volar aspect of the upper forearm.
2. Primary closure can be achieved by harvesting up to one third of the the the circumference of the arm skin.
3. The flap can be harvested with a 10 × 1 cm segment of humerus, but this method is infrequently used.

Preoperative Preparation

1. Flap harvest from the arm opposite the side of tumor resection facilitates a two-team approach.
2. Sterile preparation of the entire arm to the axilla
3. Use of a tourniquet is optional; it limits superior exposure.

Special Instruments, Position, and Anesthesia

1. Supine position, with the arm flexed and internally rotated
2. Headlight
3. Surgical loupes enhance visualization of the 1- to 2-mm vascular pedicle

Tips and Pearls

1. The lateral intermuscular septum is parallel and 1 cm posterior to a line drawn from the deltoid insertion to the lateral epicondyle.
2. The vascular pedicle is more easily visualized with a posterior approach, because the triceps muscle fibers do not insert into the intermuscular septum.
3. Identification of the radial nerve distally between the brachialis and brachioradialis muscles facilitates its preservation.

Pitfalls and Complications

1. The radial nerve must be identified, separated from the vascular pedicle, and preserved.
2. The lower lateral cutaneous nerve of the arm, not the posterior cutaneous nerve of the forearm, should be anastomosed to a sensory nerve at the recipient site to restore sensation of the flap.
3. The entire length of the vascular pedicle should be identified before detaching the intermuscular septum from the humerus.
4. The vessels of the lateral arm free flap are among the smallest of the free flaps commonly used for head and neck reconstruction.

Postoperative Care Issues

1. Closed suction drainage of the donor site
2. Watch for radial nerve compression syndrome.

References

Katsoros J, Schusterman M, Beppu M, Banis JC, Acland RD. The lateral upper arm flap: anatomy and clinical applications. Ann Plast Surg 1984;12:489.

Sullivan MJ, Carroll WR, Kuriloff DB. Lateral arm free flap in head and neck reconstruction. Arch Otolaryngol Head Neck Surg 1992;118: 1095.

Operative Procedure

The posterior radial collateral artery (PRCA) is the terminal branch of the profunda brachial artery and is the vessel supplying the lateral arm flap. From its origin in the spiral groove of the humerus, it follows the lateral intermuscular septum, and three or four dominant perforating branches ascend in the septum to supply the deep investing fascia of the upper arm and the subdermal plexus. The lateral intermuscular septum, containing the PRCA, lies parallel and 1 cm posterior to a line drawn from the deltoid insertion on the humerus to the lateral epicondyle. The location of the septal perforating branches can be confirmed with a Doppler ultrasound probe.

The skin paddle is designed with its central axis over the septal perforating branches in the lateral intermuscular septum (Fig. 266-1). The cutaneous territory of the PRCA varies from 8 × 10 to 14 × 15 cm, and it extends from the lateral epicondyle to 12 cm proximally. Distally, skin can be harvested to 3 to 4 cm below the epicondyle, although we typically do not extend below the epicondyle. The width of skin available is estimated by pinching enough skin together on each side of the central axis that allows primary closure.

Identification of the vascular pedicle is facilitated by a posterior approach to the intermuscular septum. The skin, subcutaneous fat, and deep investing fascia of the triceps muscle are incised and elevated. Dissection between the triceps and its investing fascia allows identification and preservation of the intermuscular septum and the perforating branches of the PRCA. As dissection is carried down to the humerus, the PRCA is visualized. The intermuscular septum is then exposed and approached in similar fashion anteriorly. Dissection is carried out in the plane deep to the investing fascia of the brachialis and brachioradialis muscles. Some brachioradialis muscle fibers attach directly on the intermuscular septum and require sharp division (Fig. 266-2).

Identification and preservation of the radial nerve is essential at this point in the dissection. The radial nerve follows the intermuscular septum from the deltoid insertion to the superior border of the brachioradialis muscle, where it turns anteromedially to course between the brachialis and brachioradialis muscles. The nerve is easily identified between these two muscles and then followed proximally to determine its relation to the PRCA and vena comitantes. The radial nerve in the septum should not be confused with the posterior cutaneous nerve of the forearm, which lies deep within the septum and just below the vascular pedicle. With the vascular pedicle in full view, the radial nerve is separated from the intermuscular septum and preserved (Fig. 266-3).

A superior extension of the skin incision following the posterior border of the deltoid facilitates dissection of the vascular pedicle and radial nerve in the spiral groove of the humerus. Exposure is improved by partially detaching the origin of the lateral head of the triceps from the humerus. Dissection of the vascular pedicle into the spiral groove adds 2 to 3 cm to the pedicle length and provides an arterial diameter of 1 to 2.4 mm, with venous diameters averaging 2 mm. At this point, the posterior cutaneous nerve of the forearm and lower lateral cutaneous nerve of the arm arise from the radial nerve and enter the septum. The maximal length of these nerves should be obtained if neurorrhaphy is anticipated to create a sensate flap.

The flap is ready to detach from the humerus after the vascular pedicle has been dissected throughout its course and the radial nerve has been separated from the pedicle and preserved. The septum is divided distally, with ligation of the distal extension of the PRCA and distal transection of the posterior cutaneous nerve of the forearm. With the vascular pedicle in full view, the intermuscular septum is detached from the humerus. The vascular pedicle is separated from muscle and soft tissue proximally into the spiral groove, where it is ligated and divided to provide maximum pedicle length (Fig. 266-4).

Closure begins with reattachment of the proximal head of the triceps to the deltoid muscle near its humeral insertion. The wound is irrigated, and hemostasis is achieved. A soft suction drain is placed, and the skin is undermined to allow primary closure in two layers.

RAMON ESCLAMADO
WILLIAM R. CARROLL

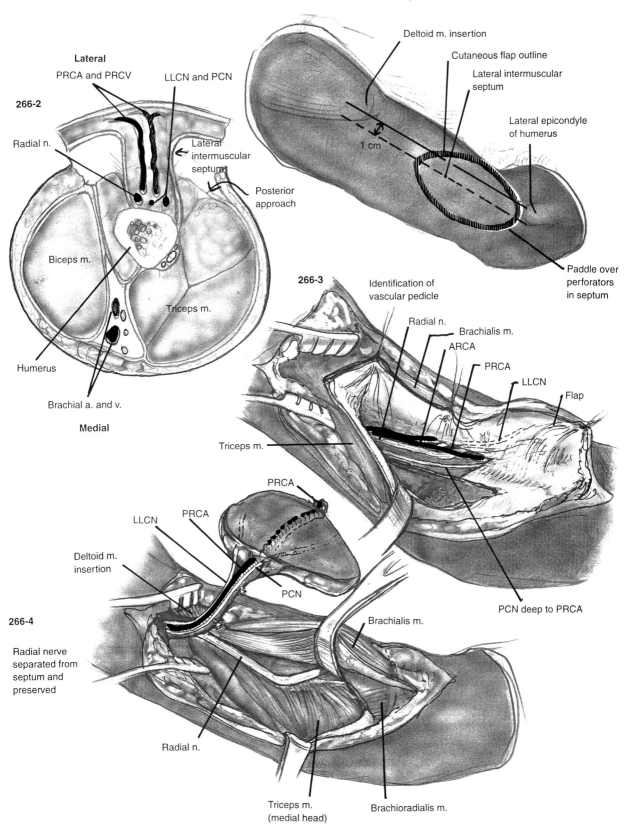

266-1. Location of lateral intermuscular septum

266-2

Lateral

PRCA and PRCV

LLCN and PCN

Radial n.

Lateral intermuscular septum

Posterior approach

Biceps m.

Triceps m.

Humerus

Brachial a. and v.

Medial

Deltoid m. insertion

Cutaneous flap outline

Lateral intermuscular septum

Lateral epicondyle of humerus

1 cm

Paddle over perforators in septum

266-3

Identification of vascular pedicle

Radial n.

Brachialis m.

ARCA

PRCA

LLCN

Flap

Triceps m.

PCN deep to PRCA

LLCN

PRCA

PRCA

Deltoid m. insertion

PCN

Brachialis m.

266-4

Radial nerve separated from septum and preserved

Radial n.

Triceps m. (medial head)

Brachioradialis m.

■ 267. FIBULA OSSEOCUTANEOUS FREE

FLAP— An osteocutaneous flap providing a long segment of cortical bone for reconstruction of mandibular and other head and neck defects with minimal donor site morbidity

Indications

1. Primary or secondary reconstruction of mandibular defects and associated moderate-sized skin and mucosal defects
2. Maxillary or orbital reconstruction requiring vascularized bone

Contraindications

1. Significant peripheral vascular occlusive disease of the lower extremities
2. Venous stasis of the lower extremities
3. Arterial anomalies in which the peroneal artery is a major supplier of blood flow to the foot, as occurs in 5% to 7% of the population
4. Previous fractures of the fibula

Special Considerations

1. The soft tissue obtained with the fibular osteocutaneous flap is insufficient for reconstructing large mucosal defects (eg, near-total glossectomy) or combined skin and mucosal defects.
2. A skin graft often is necessary for donor site closure.

Preoperative Preparation

1. Estimate the position of the posterior intermuscular septum preoperatively.
2. Bump the ipsilateral hip to improve access to the lateral surface of the lower leg.

Special Instruments, Position, and Anesthesia

1. A second set of surgical instruments to allow simultaneous and sterile harvest of the fibular flap by a second team
2. Doppler flow meter
3. Hemostatic tourniquet (optional)

Tips and Pearls

1. Approach the posterior intermuscular septum from the anterior aspect initially. If no septocutaneous vessels are identified in the intermuscular septum, a cuff of soleus and flexor hallucis longus muscle must be preserved to protect musculocutaneous perforators.
2. Model the fibula to fit the recipient defect before transecting the blood supply to minimize the duration of ischemia.
3. If cutaneous portion is to be used intraorally, harvest the fibula contralateral to the side of the recipient vessels, if possible.

Pitfalls and Complications

1. Harvest of the peroneal artery if it is a major source of blood supply to the foot
2. Ligation of the posterior tibial artery
3. Ankle instability if 8 to 10 cm of fibula above the lateral malleolus is not preserved

References

Hidalgo DA. Fibula free flap: a new method of mandible reconstruction. Plast Reconstr Surg 1989;84:71.

Kadir S. Arterial anatomy of the trunk and extremities. In: Atlas of normal and variant audiographic anatomy. Philadelphia: WB Saunders, 1991:124.

Shusterman MA, Reece GP, Miller MJ, Harris S. The osteocutaneous free fibula flap: is the skin paddle reliable? Plast Reconstr Surg 1992;90:787.

Operative Procedure

If a skin island is to be included in the flap, it should be centered over the posterior intermuscular septum. The location of the septum is approximated by a line drawn between the fibular head and the lateral malleolus. Identification of the posterior intermuscular septum is begun preoperatively when the patient can flex the lateral and posterior compartment muscles to delineate the septum. A Doppler flow meter may help to identify perforating cutaneous vessels adjacent to the line and located 15 to 25 cm distal to the fibular head. The skin paddle should be drawn to match the recipient defect and is positioned to include the maximal number of skin perforators (Fig. 267-1).

Dissection begins at the anterior edge of the skin paddle. Skin, subcutaneous tissue, and investing fascia of the peroneus muscles are incised. The investing fascia is elevated sharply toward the intermuscular septum, and the septum subsequently is followed down to its attachment on the fibula. Frequently, septocutaneous perforators can be identified in the intermuscular septum at this point. The posterior border of the flap is incised, and then the fascia overlying the soleus muscle is incised. The investing fascia is elevated sharply, and the intermuscular septum is approached from the posterior side (Fig. 267-2). If no perforating vessels have been previously identified in the posterior intermuscular septum, a 1.0-cm cuff of soleus muscle adjacent to the intermuscular septum should be included in the flap to protect essential musculocutaneous branches.

Bone cuts are made 8 to 10 cm below the fibular head and above the lateral malleus. These cuts allow rotation of the fibula to facilitate the remaining dissection (Fig. 267-3). The mobile segment of bone is rotated posteriorly to expose the attachments of the lateral compartment muscles (ie, peroneus longus and brevis muscles). These muscles are separated from the fibula, leaving a 1- to 2-mm cuff on the bone to protect the periosteum. As the lateral compartment muscles are elevated, the anterior intermuscular septum begins to come into view (Fig. 267-4). The anterior septum is divided sharply adjacent to the fibula, and the anterior compartment muscles (ie, extensors digitorum and hallucis longus and tibialis anterior muscles) must be separated from the fibula in a similar fashion.

The next structure encountered is the interosseous membrane. The membrane is divided sharply, approximately 2 to 3 mm from the fibular periosteum. After the interosseous membrane has been sectioned, the fibula becomes quite mobile and much easier to distract from the leg. The muscle immediately deep to the interosseous membrane is the tibialis posterior. This muscle overlies the peroneal artery and vein. The vessels are identified distally on the posterior medial surface of the fibula, adjacent to the distal osteotomy site. The pedicle is traced from its distal to proximal aspects as the overlying tibialis posterior muscle is sharply divided (Fig. 267-5). The posterior tibial vessels should be palpated and protected. The proximal limit of dissection is the bifurcation of the posterior tibial and the peroneal vessels.

The final muscles to be detached from the fibula are the flexor hallucis longus and brevis. If musculocutaneous perforators are to be preserved to improve perfusion of the skin, a 1-cm cuff of the flexor hallucis longus should be maintained as the muscle is separated from the fibula. The vascular pedicle is directly visualized to avoid injury during this portion of the dissection. After this dissection, the fibular flap is attached only by its vascular pedicle (Fig. 267-6).

A significant portion of bony contouring can be performed before detaching the fibular flap from its vascular supply to minimize the duration of ischemia. Using a template of the bony defect, osteotomies are made in the fibular bone and plated with miniplates to approximate the contour of the resected mandible. Too much bone is typically available if the flap is harvested as described. Using the more distal portions of the donor bone maximizes pedicle length for subsequent microvascular anastomosis.

Closure of the donor defect is uncomplicated. A suction drain is left in the space vacated by the fibula. There is no need to reapproximate the muscle groups. Skin grafts are usually needed to close the skin defect.

WILLIAM R. CARROLL
RAMON ESCLAMADO

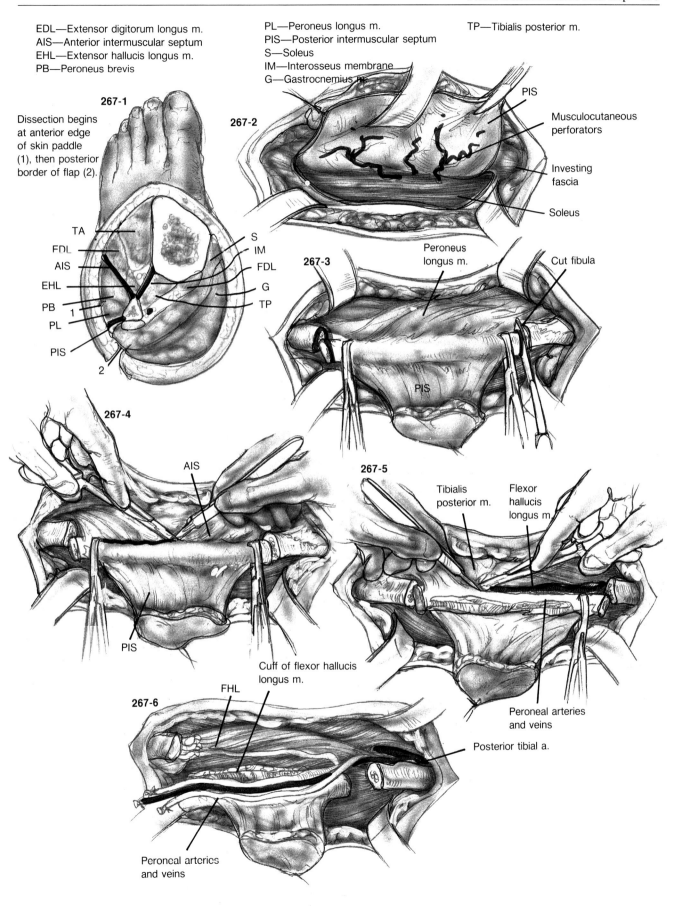

EDL—Extensor digitorum longus m.
AIS—Anterior intermuscular septum
EHL—Extensor hallucis longus m.
PB—Peroneus brevis

PL—Peroneus longus m.
PIS—Posterior intermuscular septum
S—Soleus
IM—Interosseus membrane
G—Gastrocnemius m.

TP—Tibialis posterior m.

267-1

Dissection begins at anterior edge of skin paddle (1), then posterior border of flap (2).

TA
FDL
AIS
EHL
PB
PL
PIS
1
2

S
IM
FDL
G
TP

267-2

PIS
Musculocutaneous perforators
Investing fascia
Soleus

267-3

Peroneus longus m.
Cut fibula
PIS

267-4

AIS
PIS

267-5

Tibialis posterior m.
Flexor hallucis longus m.
Peroneal arteries and veins
Posterior tibial a.

Cuff of flexor hallucis longus m.

267-6

FHL

Peroneal arteries and veins

◼ 268. INFERIOR RECTUS ABDOMINIS FREE

FLAP—Microvascular transfer of the rectus abdominis muscle based on the deep inferior epigastric artery and vein

Indications

1. Reconstruction of a variety of small and large soft tissue defects

Special Considerations

1. Status of abdominal wall fascia
2. Previous chevron incision, which may limit the amount of rectus muscle available for transfer or predispose to development of direct ventral hernia
3. Intact inferior epigastric artery and vein
4. Flap anatomy (Fig. 268-1)
   a. The deep inferior epigastric artery originates from the medial surface of external iliac artery.
   b. Paired venae comitantes.
   c. Musculocutaneous perforators are concentrated in the paraumbilical region, oriented parallel to a line from the umbilicus to the scapular tip.
   d. The muscle component may include the entire length of the rectus muscle or only the paraumbilical portion to capture the musculocutaneous perforators.
   e. The cutaneous and subcutaneous component may be harvested from the ipsilateral midaxillary line to the contralateral linea semilunaris, oriented parallel to paraumbilical perforators.

Contraindications

1. Previous injury to inferior epigastric artery or vein
2. History of direct ventral hernia

Preoperative Preparation

1. Preoperative mechanical bowel preparation
2. Routine laboratory studies

Special Instruments, Position, and Anesthesia

1. Microvascular set
2. Marlex mesh available
3. Supine position
4. Anesthesia equipment at the head or foot of the patient

Tips and Pearls

1. Always suture the anterior rectus sheath to the posterior rectus fascia at the arcuate line (Fig. 268-2).
2. Preserve when possible a medial and lateral cuff of anterior rectus sheath.
3. Reinforce the anterior rectus sheath closure with Marlex to prevent ventral hernia development.
4. Rectus abdominis free flap variations (Fig. 268-3).
   a. Muscle-only flap
   b. Musculosubcutaneous flap
   c. Musculocutaneous flap
   d. Reduced muscle flap—harvesting only that portion of the muscle that contains the musculocutaneous perforators
5. Ligate the superior epigastric artery to prevent late bleeding and hematoma.
6. Avoid injury to the contents of the inguinal ring.

Pitfalls and Complications

1. Development of a ventral hernia
2. Bleeding at the donor site from failure to ligate the superior epigastric artery

Postoperative Care Issues

1. Bowel ileus common for 48 to 72 hours
2. Abdominal support while coughing after surgery

References

Boyd J, Taylor GI, Corlett R. The vascular territories of the superior epigastric and deep inferior epigastric systems. Plast Reconstr Surg 1984;73:1–14.

Shindo ML, Sullivan MJ. Soft tissue microvascular free flaps. Otolaryngol Clin North Am 1992;27:173.

Urken ML, Turk JB, Weinberg H, Vickery C, Biller HF. The rectus abdominis free flap in head and neck reconstruction. Arch Otolaryngol Head Neck Surg 1991;117:857.

Operative Procedure

With the patient in the supine position, the abdomen and chest are prepped and draped from 4 cm above the xiphoid to the pubis and laterally to the midaxillary line. Important superficial landmarks of the rectus abdominis free flap donor site are marked on the patient (see Fig. 268-1). The linea alba defines the medial border of the paired rectus abdominis muscles. The anterior superior iliac crest is marked, because it approximates the location of the arcuate line. The linea semilunaris marks the lateral border of the rectus abdominis muscle.

Outlines of the skin incisions for harvesting the rectus abdominis free flap are determined by the recipient site needs with regard to tissue thickness, bulk, and cutaneous coverage. If no cutaneous coverage is needed and a muscle-only flap is to be harvested, a paramedian vertical skin incision can be made from the costal margin to the arcuate line down to the anterior rectus fascia. If a skin or subcutaneous component is necessary, this area should be marked, centered over the paraumbilical region to capture the greatest concentration of musculocutaneous perforators (Fig. 268-4). These musculocutaneous perforators ascend in a subcutaneous and cutaneous arcade, paralleling a line drawn from the umbilicus to the scapular tip. Orientation of the skin paddle along this axis allows the surgeon to harvest the largest skin and subcutaneous paddle possible while facilitating primary closure of the donor defect.

The first incisions are made along the outline of the skin paddle down to the level of the anterior rectus sheath and external oblique fascia. Inferiorly, the skin incision is extended along the lateral border of the rectus muscle. At the arcuate line, the incisions turn 45° to the ipsilateral inguinal ring. Skin and subcutaneous tissue are elevated superficial to the anterior rectus sheath and external oblique fascia to fully expose the amount of rectus muscle needed for reconstruction.

The anterior rectus sheath above the arcuate line is opened in the median portion of the muscle, except in the paraumbilical region, where it is left intact to preserve the musculocutaneous perforators. This cuff of anterior rectus sheath is secured to the underlying muscle with several interrupted sutures of 3-0 chromic gut suture to prevent a shearing injury to the musculocutaneous perforators. Proper harvesting technique should leave a 1- to 2-cm cuff of medial and lateral anterior rectus sheath for later closure of the abdominal donor site.

The rectus abdominis muscle is divided at its appropriate location superiorly with Bovie electrocautery. Care should be taken to identify and suture ligate the superior epigastric artery. The dissection of the flap proceeds from superior to inferior, with care taken not to penetrate the posterior rectus fascia. Small branches of intercostal arteries, veins, and nerves encountered laterally along the border of the rectus muscle should be ligated and divided.

Just above the arcuate line, the deep inferior epigastric artery enters the deep surface of the rectus abdominis muscle. This vascular pedicle is carefully dissected inferiorly and laterally, to its origin from the medial surface of the external iliac vessels. The inguinal ring is identified and care is taken not to injure it or its contents by dissection or retraction. The inferior portion of the muscle is elevated with a Kelly clamp below the arcuate line and divided with Bovie electrocautery. The deep inferior epigastric artery and vein are separately clamped, divided, and double suture ligated at their origin.

Donor site closure technique uses 2-0 Prolene sutures to approximate the anterior rectus fascia to the posterior rectus fascia at the level of the arcuate line, followed by reconstruction of the anterior rectus fascia using Marlex mesh. The mesh is cut to exactly match the defect found in the anterior rectus fascia and is secured with multiple interrupted 2-0 Prolene sutures placed every 0.5 to 1 cm along the medial and lateral borders of the anterior rectus fascia.

A large suction drain is placed, Scarpa's fascia and the subcutaneous tissue are individually closed in layers with 3-0 Vicryl suture, the skin is closed with staples, and an abdominal binder is applied and kept in place for 2 weeks. The patient is also instructed to place pressure and abdominal support on the abdomen when coughing.

EUGENE L. ALFORD

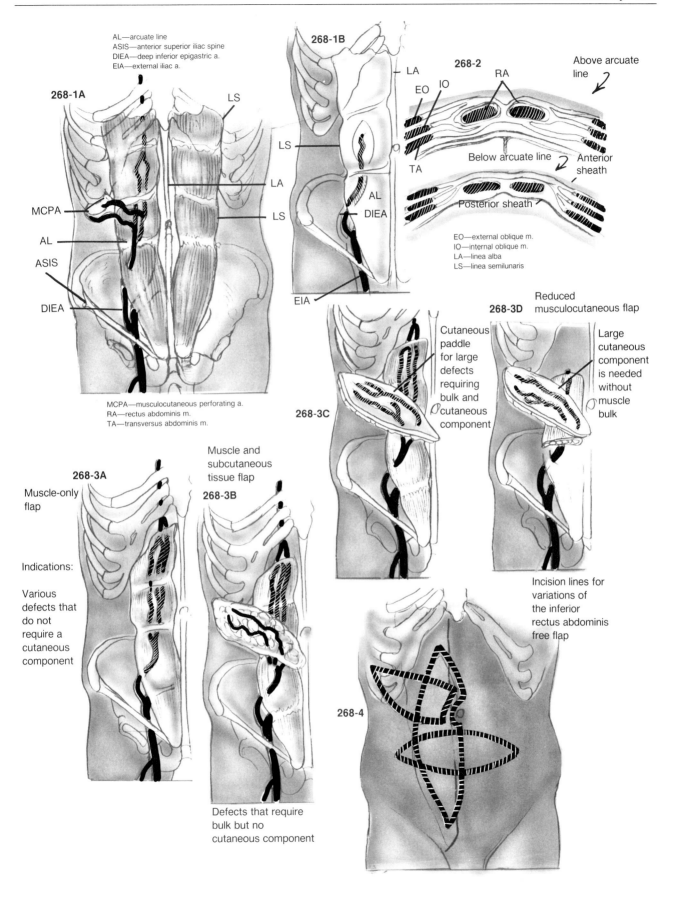

268-1A

AL—arcuate line
ASIS—anterior superior iliac spine
DIEA—deep inferior epigastric a.
EIA—external iliac a.

LS
LS
LA
LS

MCPA
AL
ASIS
DIEA

MCPA—musculocutaneous perforating a.
RA—rectus abdominis m.
TA—transversus abdominis m.

268-1B

LA
EO
IO
TA
AL
DIEA
EIA

268-2

RA

Above arcuate line

Below arcuate line

Anterior sheath

Posterior sheath

EO—external oblique m.
IO—internal oblique m.
LA—linea alba
LS—linea semilunaris

268-3A

Muscle-only flap

Indications:

Various defects that do not require a cutaneous component

Muscle and subcutaneous tissue flap

268-3B

Defects that require bulk but no cutaneous component

268-3C

Cutaneous paddle for large defects requiring bulk and cutaneous component

Reduced musculocutaneous flap

268-3D

Large cutaneous component is needed without muscle bulk

Incision lines for variations of the inferior rectus abdominis free flap

268-4

■ 269. FREE JEJUNAL TRANSFER

Reconstruction of the pharynx and cervical esophagus with a jejunal segment of small bowel using techniques of microvascular free tissue transfer

Indications

1. Cancer of the larynx or pharynx if resection does not allow primary (ie, removal of 60% or more of the surface of the hypopharynx)
2. Primary carcinoma of the cervical esophagus
3. Cervical esophageal strictures that cannot be corrected with more conservative measures, such as dilatation
4. Treatment of pharyngocutaneous fistulas

Contraindications

1. History of duodenal ulcers
2. Cancer invading the prevertebral space, deep neck structures, or tumor extension below the thoracic inlet of the esophagus
3. Previous laparotomy, small bowel resection, and abdominal trauma or pathology.

Special Considerations

1. Availability of recipient arteries and veins
2. General surgeon to harvest bowel segment
3. Placement of gastrostomy and feeding jejunostomy

Preoperative Preparation

1. Clear liquid diet for 48 to 72 hours preoperatively or mechanical bowel preparation 24 hours before surgery

Special Instruments, Position, and Anesthesia

1. Microvascular instrument set (see Procedure 262)
2. Arteriovenous access graft set and vascular clamp set

Tips and Pearls

1. To avoid unnecessary laparotomy, separation of the pharynx from the deep neck structures and prevertebral space should be determined early in the operation.
2. Placement of the jejunal autograft in an isoperistaltic orientation
3. Double-layer pharyngojejunal anastomosis followed by venous anastomosis, arterial revascularization, and then double-layer esophagojejunal bowel anastomosis
4. Avoid the use of auto staplers for pharyngojejunal and esophagojejunal anastomosis
5. Avoid redundancy or kinking of the jejunal segment in the neck
6. The reconstructive surgeon assists the general surgeon in selection of the proper jejunal sement for transfer
7. Dissect the vascular pedicle well proximal to the hilum of the selected branch of the superior mesenteric artery.
8. An externalized segment of jejunum is the best method by which to monitor the vascular status of the autograft.

Pitfalls and Complications

1. Dissection of the jejunal autograft may lead to vascular compromise of nearby small bowel segments.
2. Mild dysphagia due to continued jejunal peristalsis in the neck.

Postoperative Care Issues

1. Use of postoperative anticoagulants, antiplatelet agents, or volume expanders is determined by the microsurgeon.
2. Visual and Doppler monitoring of an externalized segment of the jejunum is the best way to check the graft's vascular status.
3. Isotonic jejunostomy tube feedings may begin immediately postoperatively.

References

Bradford C, Esclamado RM, Carroll WR. Monitoring of revascularized jejunal autografts. Arch Otolaryngol Head Neck Surg 1992;118:1042.

Salamovin W. Swartz WM, Johnson JT, et al. Free jejunal transfer for reconstruction of the laryngopharynx. Otolaryngol Head Neck Surg 1987;96:149.

Operative Procedure

Skin prep extends from the nose to the pubis and from the mastoid tip to midaxillary line laterally. The abdomen is prepped and draped separately for an upper midline laparotomy (Fig. 269-1).

Harvest of the jejunal segment and placement of a feeding jejunostomy and gastrostomy tube is carried out by the general surgeon simultaneously with the laryngopharyngectomy. An upper midline laparotomy is performed. Abdominal exploration is performed, searching for disease such as gallstones or malignancy. The complete small bowel is explored, and the ligament of Treitz is localized. A 20- to 25-cm-long segment of jejunum is selected 20 to 60 cm distal to the ligament of Treitz. A single branch of the superior mesenteric artery supplying an adequate length of jejunum for reconstruction is located by transillumination of the mesentery (Fig. 269-2).

The reconstructive surgeon assists the general surgeon in selection of the appropriate jejunal segment for reconstruction. The proximal and distal ends of the jejunal segment are divided with a stapling device. The proximal end of the jejunum is marked with a suture for later identification and isoperistaltic orientation to the native esophagus. The jejunal segment remains perfused on its pedicle, and the mesentery on either side of the selected superior mesenteric artery and vein is divided. The selected branch of the superior mesenteric artery is dissected proximally to the hilum to ensure adequate vascular pedicle length (Fig. 269-3). After the ablative procedure is completed, the recipient arteries and veins in the neck are dissected and cleaned of their adventitia along a 3- to 5-cm length. The jejunal segment vascular pedicle is then divided. To prevent venous congestion, the mesenteric artery is clamped first, divided, and tied.

The proximal and distal ends of the donor of jejunum are re-anastomosed, and feeding gastrostomy and jejunostomy tubes are placed for bowel decompression and long-term enteral feeding. Careful examination of the jejunal segments proximal and distal to the harvested free graft is carried out, and any portion of the jejunum showing signs of arterial insufficiency or venous congestion should be resected.

The free jejunal segment is placed isoperistaltically, and the proximal pharyngojejunal anastomosis is performed. Bovie electrocautery is used to open the antimesenteric border of the jejunal autograft longitudinally. This filets the proximal jejunal segment to increase the diameter of the pharyngojejunal anastomosis (Fig. 269-4). A double-layer anastomosis is carried out using running interrupted Connell stitches of 3-0 Vicryl on an intestinal needle. The outer layer anastomosis is completed using 3-0 silk pop-off sutures on an intestinal needle (Fig. 269-5). The mesenteric artery and vein are cleaned of surrounding fat and adventitia. Microvascular anastomoses are carried out to the appropriate venous and arterial recipient vessels. The venous anastomosis should be performed first, followed by the arterial. After the arterial and venous anastomoses are completed, the length of bowel needed is determined.

Using Bovie electrocautery, a distal segment of jejunum of adequate length to eliminate redundancy in the neopharynx is separated from the antimesenteric border of the graft, with careful attention paid to the vascular supply to the distal segment. This segment of jejunum is sutured to the skin of the neck so that it may be observed (Fig. 269-6). This monitor is supplied by the same arterial and venous system that supplies the jejunal autograft in the neck and reflects the vascular status of the flap. An 18-Fr (6-mm) nasogastric tube is placed through the proximal and distal pharyngeal anastomosis and acts as a short-term stent. The distal anastomosis is carried out, using interrupted Connell stitches of 3-0 Vicryl on an intestinal needle. The 3-0 silk intestinal sutures are used as a reinforcing serosal layer to achieve the final distal closure. The wound is copiously irrigated with warm saline. Large suction drains are placed and secured so that the vascular pedicle is not harmed.

The viability of the jejunal free graft is determined using the externalized monitoring segment of jejunum.

Five to seven days after completion of the microvascular free tissue transfer, the externalized segment of jejunal free graft may be divided from its arterial and venous blood supply.

EUGENE L. ALFORD

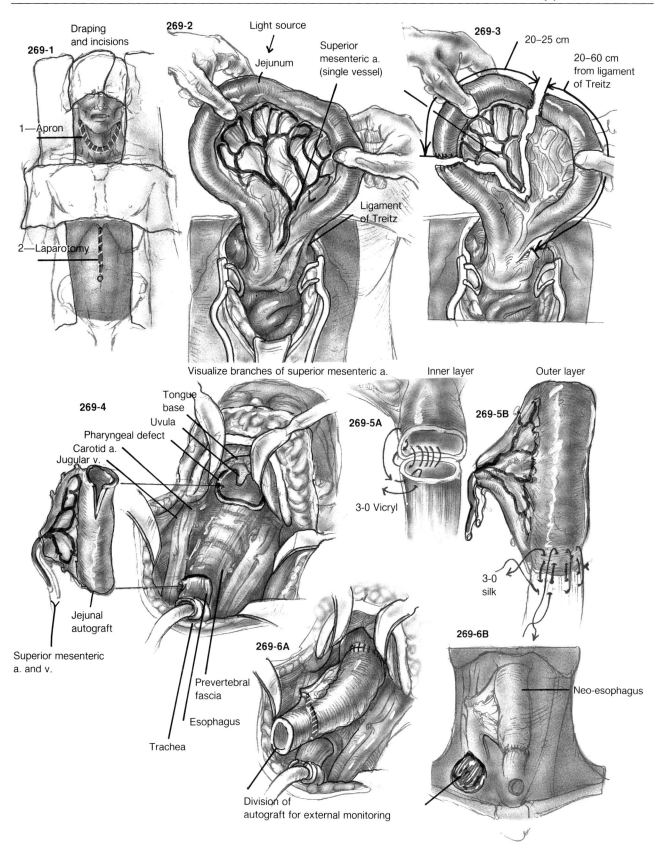

269-1 Draping and incisions

1—Apron

2—Laparotomy

269-2 Light source

Jejunum

Superior mesenteric a. (single vessel)

Ligament of Treitz

269-3 20–25 cm

20–60 cm from ligament of Treitz

Visualize branches of superior mesenteric a.

269-4 Tongue base

Uvula

Pharyngeal defect

Carotid a.

Jugular v.

Jejunal autograft

Superior mesenteric a. and v.

Prevertebral fascia

Esophagus

Trachea

269-5A Inner layer

3-0 Vicryl

269-5B Outer layer

3-0 silk

269-6A Division of autograft for external monitoring

269-6B Neo-esophagus

■ 270. CROSS FACIAL NERVE GRAFT

Dynamic facial nerve reanimation by attaching a branch of the contralateral functioning facial nerve to the ipsilateral facial nerve

Indications

1. Complete facial nerve paralysis
2. Motor end plates intact
3. Contralateral facial nerve function intact
4. Proximal facial nerve unavailable
5. Ipsilateral 12th nerve unavailable

Contraindications

1. Facial paralysis for longer than 1 year
2. Functioning proximal facial nerve on the ipsilateral side
3. Possible dysfunction of contralateral facial nerve

Special Considerations

1. The surgeon must harvest a large nerve graft, preferably the sural nerve, to obtain adequate length.

Preoperative Preparation

1. Routine laboratory studies
2. Facial nerve testing to determine normal contralateral response and response to electromyographic testing on the ipsilateral side

Special Instruments, Position, and Anesthesia

1. Operating binocular microscope or spectacle loupes (2.5×)
2. Headlight
3. Curved Castroviejo needle holders
4. Curved and straight Westcott scissors
5. Bishop-Harman forceps, with and without teeth
6. Castroviejo caliper
7. Kelman tying forceps
8. Weck-cel sponges
9. McCabe dissector
10. Marking pen
11. 8-0 Nylon suture with GS-8 needles
12. Nerve stimulator
13. Standard ear, nose, and throat plastics set

Tips and Pearls

1. The simplest technique is to identify the contralateral marginal branch of the facial nerve. This is the best-suited donor site with the least morbidity.

Postoperative Care Issues

1. Meticulous hemostasis to avoid hematoma
2. Patients should be made aware that they will have some loss of function on the normal contralateral side, particularly a lack of function of the depressor anguli muscle and a resultant asymmetric smile.
3. Function returns not sooner than 6 months, and the final result demonstrates some weakness and synkinesis.

References

Anderle H. Cross-face nerve transplant. Clin Plast Surg 1979;6:433.
Conley J. Perspectives in facial reanimation. In: May M, ed. The facial nerve. New York: Thieme, 1986:646.
Gary-Bobo A, Fuentes J. Long term follow-up report on cross-facial nerve grafting in the treatment of facial paralysis. Br J Plast Surg 1983;36:48.

Operative Procedure

The patient is placed in the supine position, with the head extended, which is facilitated by the use of a shoulder roll and doughnut head holder. With a marking pen, the surgeon outlines a Blair incision or bilateral rhytidectomy incisions, as described in Procedure 261 (Fig. 270-1). The surgeon should start on the ipsilateral side and be certain that the distal end of the facial nerve can be identified (Fig. 270-2). This incision is carried down through the subcutaneous tissue, and a flap is elevated to expose the parotid gland. This can be done with a scissors or electrocautery to minimize some of the bleeding. The facial nerve is identified by exposing the cartilaginous canal down to the pointer; the nerve usually is 2 to 3 mm inferior to this. Palpating the mastoid tip and styloid process greatly enhance the ability to locate the facial nerve.

The facial nerve is carefully exposed by further removing parotid tissue anteriorly. The extent of exposure of the nerve depends on the extent of the injury and the particular technique employed. Scarmella's technique identifies the buccal branch on the normal side to be reanastomosed to the main trunk of the paralyzed side. Fisher's technique uses several distal branches, connecting the normal to the paralyzed side and passing the nerve grafts over the lip. Anderle's modification uses three or four separate grafts, with each one applied at the appropriate distal branch. However, all of these approaches are technically difficult, with unpredictable results and with increased potential injury to the normal contralateral side. A simpler technique is to locate the marginal branch on the normal side and attach this to the main trunk on the paralyzed side, as proposed by Conley.

The normal marginal mandibular nerve is exposed by tracing the facial nerve to the pes anserinus and continuing along the inferiorly located cervical facial trunk. An alternative to finding the marginal mandibular nerve is to identify it as it crosses over the angle of the mandible and then trace it proximally back to the pes anserinus. The facial nerve stimulator can greatly facilitate this maneuver.

With both facial nerves identified, the surgeon may harvest a sural nerve graft, as described in Procedure 261 (Fig. 270-3). A tunnel must be created under the lip by using a Cryostat or by finger dissection. A long suture is attached to the graft. The graft is introduced through the tunnel by grasping the long sutures and gently pulling the graft through. With the sural nerve graft in place, adequate length is determined to avoid tension at either anastomotic site. On the normal side, the marginal mandibular nerve is sharply transected and sutured to the sural nerve (see Procedure 261). On the paralyzed, ipsilateral side, the surgeon performs anastomosis to the main trunk or alternately to the upper facial nerve branches, depending on the extent of the injury (Fig. 270-4).

Hemostasis is meticulously obtained, and a Penrose drain is placed on either side. The wounds are closed with 3-0 chromic buried stitches, followed by a 5-0 nylon continuous running stitch (Fig. 270-5), and pressure dressings are applied. Taking care not to place the suction over the nerves, suction drainage can be applied, obviating the need for pressure dressings.

STEVEN M. PARNES

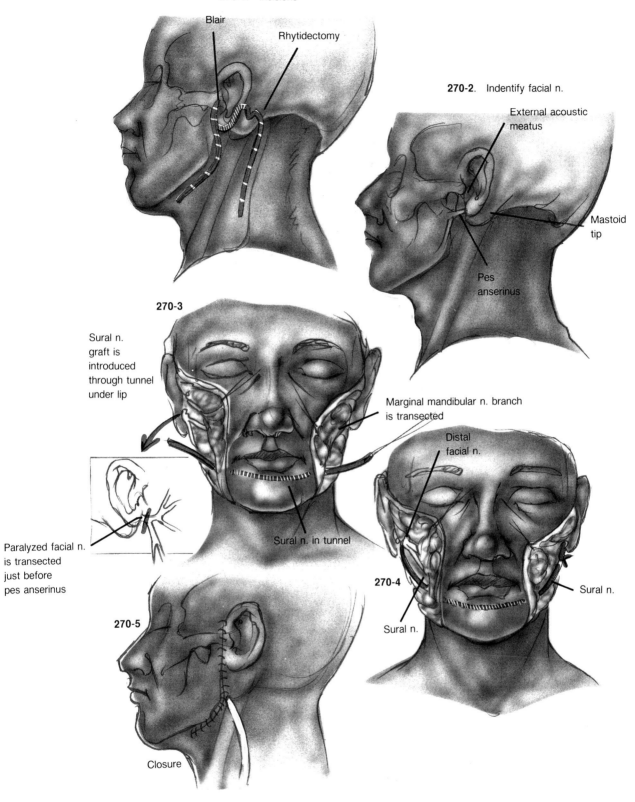

270-1. Incisions

Blair

Rhytidectomy

270-2. Indentify facial n.

External acoustic meatus

Mastoid tip

Pes anserinus

270-3

Sural n. graft is introduced through tunnel under lip

Marginal mandibular n. branch is transected

Distal facial n.

Paralyzed facial n. is transected just before pes anserinus

Sural n. in tunnel

270-4

Sural n.

Sural n.

270-5

Closure

■ *271.* NERVE-MUSCLE PEDICLE

Transfer of a nerve with its intact motor end plate, specifically ansa hypoglossal and strap muscle end plates rotated and attached to the facial muscles

Indications

1. Facial paralysis for less than 1 year
2. Integrity of facial nerve is uncertain, as in cases of acoustic neuroma resection in which the facial nerve is preserved, but recovery is uncertain
3. Intact cranial nerves X and XII

Special Considerations

1. No sacrifice of any other major cranial nerve
2. Facial nerve recovery is uncertain

Preoperative Preparation

1. Routine laboratory studies
2. Facial nerve electromyogram

Special Instruments, Position, and Anesthesia

1. Operating binocular microscope or spectacle loupes (2.5×)
2. Headlight
3. Curved Castroviejo needle holders
4. Curved and straight Westcott scissors
5. Bishop-Harman forceps, with and without teeth
6. Castroviejo caliper
7. Kelman tying forceps
8. Weck-cel sponges
9. McCabe dissector
10. Tongue blade
11. Marking pen
12. 6-0 nylon sutures with GS-8 needle
13. Nerve stimulation
14. Standard ear, nose, and throat plastics set

Tips and Pearls

1. Identification of the posterior belly of the digastric muscle to facilitate location of the hypoglossal and cervicalis nerves
2. Ligating the posterior segment of the cervicalis branch for lengthening the pedicle

Pitfalls and Complications

1. Atrophy of facial musculature due to a lack of reinnervation for more than 12 months
2. Counsel the patient that, because only the lower division will be innervated, full normal function will not be restored.
3. Patients need to be retrained for facial movement by tensing the strap muscles.

References

Anonsen CK, Duckert LG, Cummings CW. Preliminary observations after facial rehabilitation with the ansa hypoglossal pedicle transfer. Otolaryngol Head Neck Surg 1986;94:302.

Johnson J, Tucker H. Selective experimental reinnervation of paralyzed facial muscles. Arch Otolaryngol 1977;103:22.

Operative Procedure

The patient is in the supine position, with a shoulder roll placed with a doughnut head holder for slight extension of the head. The patient is turned slightly away from the surgeon. Two parallel incisions are made in the neck; one is 2 to 3 cm below the mandible, and the second is made over the cricoid area (Fig. 271-1). The incisions are carried down through the skin, subcutaneous tissue, and platysma. The flaps are raised by traction and countertraction, establishing a tunnel between the two flaps and then extending the lower flap down to the level of the sternocleidomastoid muscle and identifying the anterior border of the muscle (Fig. 271-2). The sternocleidomastoid muscle is isolated and retracted laterally until the posterior belly of the digastric muscle and the internal jugular vein can be identified. If the middle thyroid vein is encountered, it should be transected and ligated.

At this point, the surgeon should be able to locate the ansa hypoglossal nerve's anterior and posterior segments (Fig. 271-3). The anterior segment lies along the jugular vein until the point where anterior and posterior ramifications are identified. The nerves are then traced anteriorly to their respective strap muscles. To identify the nerves, the nerve stimulator may be used to observe movement of the strap muscles. With a fine forceps, the anterior ramification is grasped and then sharply dissected off the jugular vein superiorly up to its attachment to the hypoglossal nerve. The branches of the ansa hypoglossal nerves are then traced into the respective muscles. The surgeon must dissect further into the muscle to ensure that the motor end plates are not sacrificed. Several segments, each with 2 to 3 mm of surrounding muscle, are then sharply dissected from the belly of the straps (Fig. 271-4). The nerve-muscle pedicle is then gently retracted upward. Further lengthening may be achieved by tracing the posterior ramification and transecting it if necessary.

Attention is then turned to the upper skin incision, where a plane is established under the platysma. The flap is raised over the mandible until the lower facial muscles are identified. The marginal mandibular nerve must be preserved. This can be easily accomplished by identifying the submandibular gland, where the nerve courses over and is incorporated into the submandibular gland fascia. Sharp dissection under this area can reflect it out of harm's way. The ansa hypoglossal nerve–strap muscle pedicles are then rotated and transferred under the previously created flaps and placed onto the various lower facial muscles, particularly the depressor and elevator anguli and the orbicularis oris (Fig. 271-5). It is important to abrade the fascial muscles and to incorporate the nerve-muscle pedicle within the bellies of the muscles for maximum contact. The muscles are then sutured into place with 6-0 nylon.

Excellent illumination with magnification is necessary during these maneuvers. After the nerve-muscle pedicles are secured, the wounds can be closed with 3-0 chromic buried interrupted stitches and 4-0 nylon continuous suture. A Penrose drain and a pressure dressing are applied.

STEVEN M. PARNES

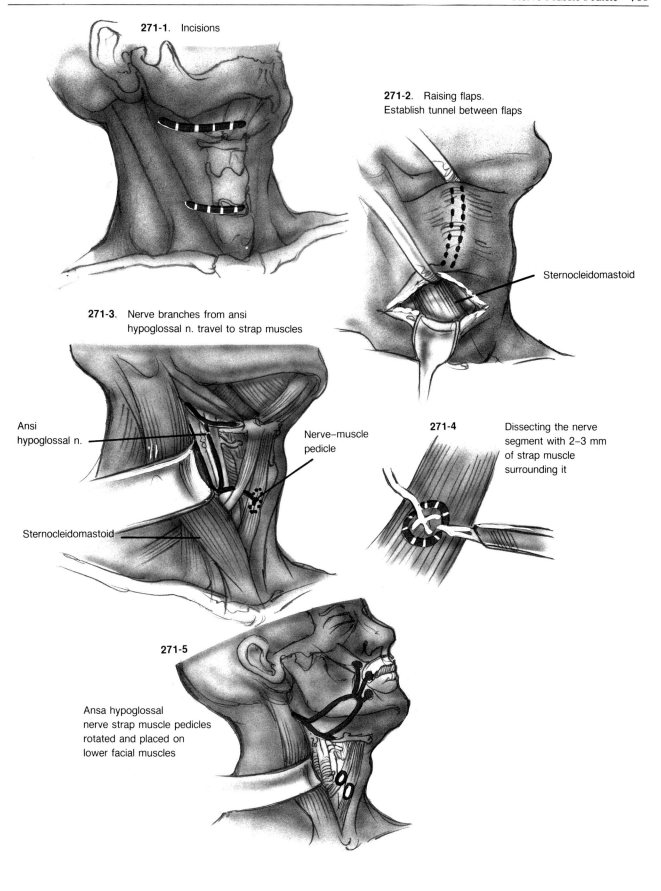

271-1.   Incisions

271-2.   Raising flaps.
Establish tunnel between flaps

Sternocleidomastoid

271-3.   Nerve branches from ansi
hypoglossal n. travel to strap muscles

Ansi
hypoglossal n.

Nerve–muscle
pedicle

Sternocleidomastoid

271-4   Dissecting the nerve
segment with 2–3 mm
of strap muscle
surrounding it

271-5

Ansa hypoglossal
nerve strap muscle pedicles
rotated and placed on
lower facial muscles

■ *272.* STATIC SLINGS

Fibrous connective tissue used to resuspend the facial muscles from the lateral facial skeleton after facial nerve resection or paralysis when other procedures, such as facial nerve grafting or dynamic muscle transposition, are not indicated

Indications

1. Permanent facial paralysis after multiple cranial neuropathy
2. After cancer ablation of parotid if the temporalis or masseter muscles are not available
3. In older patients if a dynamic muscle transposition is not desired or contraindicated because of prolonged anesthetic risk
4. When the lateral face should not be covered by large muscle bulk to rule out tumor recurrence
5. When a simple, fast, and effective support of the face is needed

Special Considerations

1. Possibility of obtaining long fascia strips from lateral thigh or temporal-parietal skull region
2. Will an additional procedure, such as a gold weight, be required for the eyelids to promote closure?
3. Is the lateral facial skin sufficiently supple to allow for elevation or tunneling?
4. Is there still a possibility for return of facial function or the use of a more dynamic procedure?

Preoperative Preparation

1. Complete ophthalmologic evaluation
2. Close-up and full facial photographs
3. Routine laboratory tests as appropriate for general anesthesia
4. Inspection of legs to see if donor site is satisfactory
5. Perioperative intravenous antibiotics

Special Instruments, Position, and Anesthesia

1. Fascia stripper
2. Preparation of ipsilateral leg with patient in the semi-oblique position
3. General anesthesia with injection of facial incisions to decrease bleeding

(continued)

Operative Procedure

The procedure is normally performed under general anesthesia because of the extensive undermining or exposure required for obtaining the fascia lata grafts. The facial site can be prepared concomitantly with obtaining of the donor fascia to save operating time. With the patient in a supine, semi-oblique position, the lateral thigh is exposed. Although it is possible to obtain the fascia by undermining between two parallel incisions on the thigh and obtaining the fascia by using the fascia stripper subcutaneously, for those who are not experienced in that technique, the direct approach is simpler (Figs. 272-1 and 272-2).

A long incision at the lateral thigh is made parallel to the axis of the leg, extending for approximately 15 cm. The sides of the incision are undermined and elevated in the subcutaneous plane, exposing the fascia overlying the quadriceps muscle and extending posterior to the hamstring muscles. Multiple, long rectangular strips, approximately 1.5 × 12 cm may be excised from the exposed fascia, similar to obtaining a temporalis fascial graft for tympanoplasty (Fig. 272-3A). If the strips are cut like the stripes on a flag, so there is a strip of fascia remaining between defects, large herniation of the muscle is not as likely. The fascial strips may be placed in a saline-soaked gauze until needed.

A running 4-0 chromic catgut or Vicryl suture can be placed in a running fashion along each defect to form a "net," which tends to reduce the risk of muscle herniations (see Fig. 272-3B). The skin can then be closed over a small Penrose or suction drain with 4-0 Vicryl and 4-0 Prolene sutures (Fig. 272-4). A Bactroban-coated Telfa pad, ABD dressings, and a gauze wrap complete the isolation and dressing of the leg wound.

(continued)

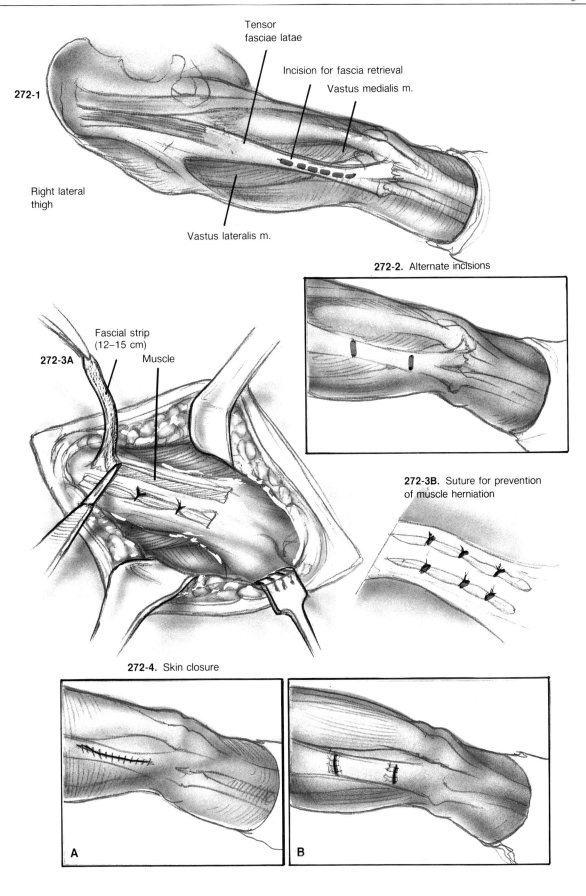

272-1

Tensor
fasciae latae

Incision for fascia retrieval

Vastus medialis m.

Right lateral
thigh

Vastus lateralis m.

272-2. Alternate incisions

Fascial strip
(12–15 cm)

Muscle

272-3A

272-3B. Suture for prevention
of muscle herniation

272-4. Skin closure

A

B

■ 272. STATIC SLINGS (continued)

Tips and Pearls

1. The fascial strips should be at least 12 cm long in most patients. Gore-Tex soft tissue strips may also be used.
2. A modified Blair or facelift incision is used for exposure of the zygoma and temporal fascia, and small perioral and periorbital incisions are made to facilitate proper attachment distally of the strips.
3. The fascial strips should be secured at both ends with permanent suture, such as clear nylon.

Pitfalls and Complications

1. Facial hematoma
2. Herniation of quadriceps muscle
3. Undercorrection or overcorrection of the facial resuspension
4. Slippage of fascia over time if not well secured in position

Postoperative Care Issues

1. Use compression dressings on the face and a leg for 48 hours to prevent a hematoma.
2. Perioperative antibiotics
3. Cool compresses around eyes and lips during the first 48 hours to reduce edema.
4. Eye lubricant and artificial tears should be continued as long as advised by the ophthalmologist.
5. Vitamin E gel may be used daily on the wound after suture removal.

References

Berson MI. Procurement of fascia for facial paralysis. In: Atlas of plastic surgery. New York: Grune & Stratt, 1963:82.

Freeman BS. Correction of facial nerve paralysis. In: Long-term results in plastic and reconstructive surgery, vol 1. Boston: Little, Brown & Co, 1980:408.

The facial skin may be elevated through a modified Blair parotidectomy incision or a standard facelift incision, depending on whether a previous incision exists (Fig. 272-5). The skin is elevated in the subdermal facelift plane all the way to the peripheral attachment of the facial muscles. If a previous parotidectomy had been performed, it is wise to leave some scar tissue on the unelevated tissue to protect against salivary leaks from any residual glandular elements. The flap should be elevated sufficiently to visualize the temporalis fascia, zygoma, lateral orbit, nasolabial fold, and corner of the mouth. Hemostasis can be achieved with monopolar cautery, because nerve injury is not problematic.

Using long Cushing forceps in the wound, the lateral portion of the eyelids, alar crease, nasolabial fold, and oral commissure are grasped and pulled superiorly and laterally to gain an appreciation of the location and vector of pull that will be required to achieve a satisfactory facial suspension. Small incisions are made in these areas (in relaxed skin tension folds) at just about the site where the best location of attachment of the fascial strips has been determined.

The fascial strips are then placed in the facial wound and tunneled slightly into the distal facial muscle to the peripheral incisions. Horizontal mattress sutures of clear 4-0 nylon are placed through the small incisions through the distal end of the fascial strip and back out the incision again, sewing the strip to the underlying muscle and dermis. These are tied firmly in place; multiple sutures at each site may be necessary for a secure connection of fascia to muscle and dermis. Fascial strips should be located, at a minimum, at the lateral boundary of each of the upper and lower eyelids, the lateral nasal ala, the nasolabial fold, and the lateral commissure of the lips; usually four or five strips suffice.

After the distal ends of the strips have been secured, each strip is pulled in the desired vector and attached to the zygomatic arch periosteum with a single securing suture (Fig. 272-6). As each strip is vectored, pulled, and secured, the previous ones may need to be repositioned slightly, until all of the strips are in the proper position. They may be finally secured to the periosteum with 3-0 or 4-0 clear nylon sutures. Excessive proximal ends of the fascial strips may be trimmed.

On the operating table, the affected side of the face should be suspended in a pleasant "half-smile" position, with the eyelids slightly closed. If the eyelids remain open, a gold weight can be placed in the upper eyelid beneath the pretarsal skin and secured to the tarsus with interrupted 4-0 Vicryl sutures. The proper weight is determined in the office by taping increasingly heavy weights to the upper eyelid skin until the upper lid just covers the top of the pupil. This same weight can be sterilized and placed in the eyelid if needed.

The facial wound can be drained with a Penrose drain or closed suction drainage. The flap is sutured back into place with 4-0 chromic catgut and 6-0 Prolene (Fig. 272-7). A facelift-type pressure dressing is applied. The drain may be removed in 24 to 48 hours, depending on the extent of drainage, and the sutures may be removed in 7 to 10 days.

G. RICHARD HOLT

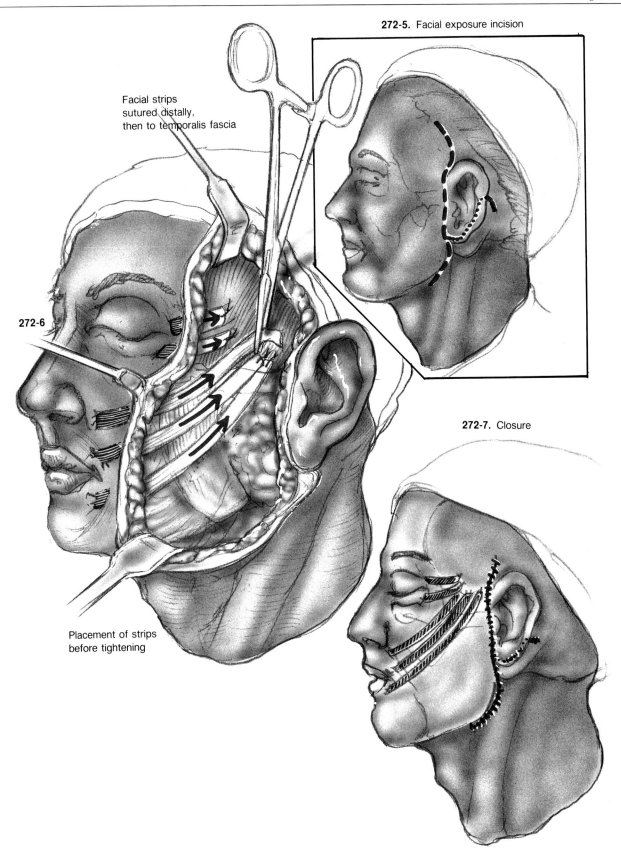

272-5. Facial exposure incision

Facial strips
sutured distally,
then to temporalis fascia

272-6

Placement of strips
before tightening

272-7. Closure

■ 273. DYNAMIC TEMPORALIS AND MASSE-TER MUSCLE TRANSPOSITION—Use of the muscles of mastication to provide an innervated musculofascial support for facial expression and movement

Indications

1. Congenital facial paralysis
2. Permanent paralysis after removal of an intracranial, intratemporal, or parotid tumor
3. Permanent and complete idiopathic facial paralysis
4. Traumatic paralysis due to injury to the brain, temporal bone, or face in which nerve reanastomosis or grafting has not been possible or successful

Special Considerations

1. What is the integrity of facial skin on the side of injury?
2. Has the trigeminal nerve supply to the muscles of mastication been damaged?
3. Has there been a history of temporomandibular joint dysfunction or surgery on the affected or normal side?
4. Would a dynamic muscle transposition prevent early detection of a possible recurrence?
5. Is the patient capable of learning to use jaw tension to control facial motion?

Preoperative Preparation

1. Complete ophthalmologic examination
2. Schirmer's test
3. Jaw tension test
4. Mandibular radiographs, with close attention to the temporomandibular joint and condyle
5. Routine laboratory tests appropriate for age and general anesthesia

Special Instruments, Position, and Anesthesia

1. General anesthesia
2. Facelift or parotidectomy positioning
3. Prepare for hemicoronal scalp incision
4. Straight Keith needle for passing of anchoring suture
5. Fiberoptic headlight
6. Abdominal preparation if fat graft is necessary
7. Curved retractors for face and double, sharp skin hooks for muscle translocation

(continued)

Operative Procedure

The approach to exposing the facial structures with dynamic muscle transpositions is similar to that used for static facial slings except for one factor. If a temporalis muscle transfer is planned, the entire temporal fossa and parietal fascia must be exposed through a hemicoronal extension of the modified Blair or facelift incisions (Fig. 273-1). The entire facial skin is elevated subdermally, leaving a small amount of fat on the undersurface of the flap and some fascia or scar tissue on the deep layers. It is necessary to expose the entire masseter muscle if that type of transposition is selected. This may necessitate the removal of any parotid remnants or an entire superficial parotidectomy if that structure is intact.

The flap elevation and exposure should be extended to include the lateral position of the orbicularis oculi muscle, nasolabial fold, and the lateral portion of the orbicularis oris muscle. The reason for this extensive exposure is to allow the onlay or interposition of the transferred muscle flap directly to the recipient muscle bed. It is possible, at least in theory, that some neuronal "budding" could occur from the transposed muscle to the paralyzed muscle, but such neoneuronization would be physiologically effective only if neuromotor endplates remained in the recipient muscle.

After total exposure has been achieved, the surgeon must observe the anatomy and linear associations between the potential donor and recipient muscles and decide what type or combination of muscle transfer would be best for the patient. With the masseter transfer, only the eye or the corner of the mouth and lips can be selected as a recipient site, because the muscle is too short and narrow. The support of the eyelids usually is preferred, although in the rare case, the eyelid closure is satisfactorily remediable with just a gold weight, and the mouth can be the sole recipient of the masseter transposition. The temporalis muscle is large and expansive enough that it can be translocated to all areas of the face, from the eyelids to the lower lip and corner of the mouth.

If the masseter has been selected, its attachment to the inferior border of the mandible is identified (Fig. 273-2). Using a scalpel, the tendinous insertion is sharply excised from the bony cortex. A Freer elevator or a Joseph periosteal elevator can be used to elevate the muscle from its attachments to the underlying mandibular ramus. It is somewhat alarming at this point to see the muscle contract and shorten, but it can be stretched again almost to its former length when inserted into its new distal recipient site or sites. The neurovascular bundle enters the inner or medial surface of the muscle just below its attachment to the zygomatic arch. Its integrity must be preserved for proper dynamic functioning; otherwise, the transposed muscle becomes a static sling. The distal muscle can be separated into two bundles, stopping the split just short of the neurovascular bundle. Using double skin hooks passed through the small incisions at the corners of the eyelids or of the mouth, the split ends of the muscle can be pulled into position at their new location. After the proper tension is decided to tighten the eyelids or raise the lips and corner of the mouth, these ends may be sutured into the recipient muscle beds (ie, orbicularis oculi or oris) using the Keith needle threaded with 4-0 clear nylon (Figs. 273-3 and 273-4).

(continued)

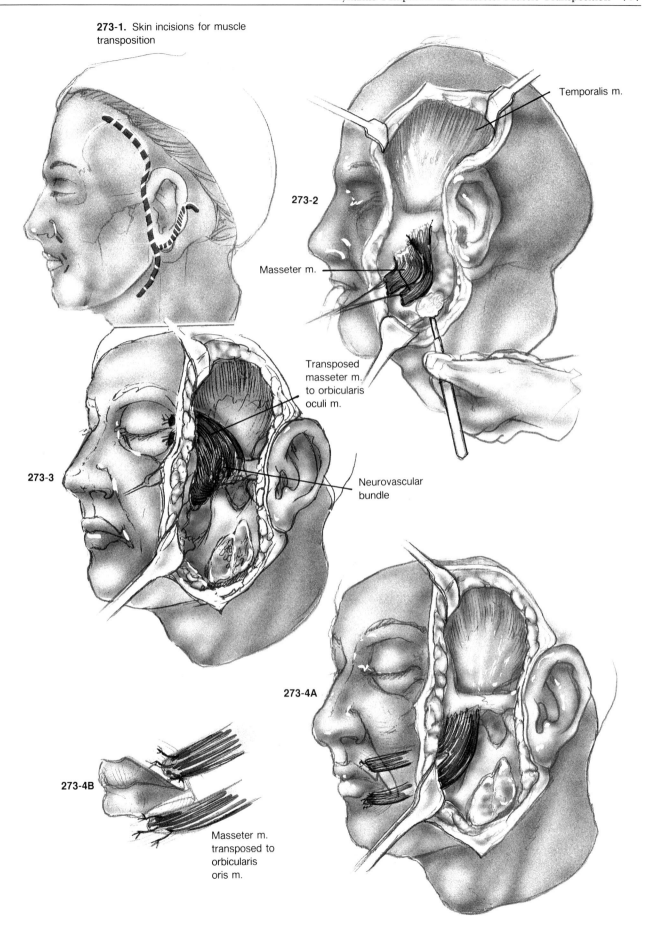

273-1. Skin incisions for muscle transposition

273-2

Temporalis m.

Masseter m.

Transposed masseter m. to orbicularis oculi m.

Neurovascular bundle

273-3

273-4A

273-4B

Masseter m. transposed to orbicularis oris m.

■ *273.* DYNAMIC TEMPORALIS AND MASSE- TER MUSCLE TRANSPOSITION *(continued)*

Tips and Pearls

1. The zygomatic arch may be resected in part with a saw to provide greater length of transposition for the temporalis muscle and to reduce the unsightly muscle bulge.
2. In lieu of resecting the arch, an abdominal fat graft may be used to fill out the temporal fossa and improve the postoperative appearance.
3. The distal ends of the transposed muscle must be securely attached to the specific facial landmark with mattress nonabsorbable su- tures to avoid late slippage.

Pitfalls and Complications

1. Chewing dysfunction and temporomandibular joint syndrome due to altered and asymmetric mastication efforts
2. Hematoma or seroma beneath facial flap or in temporal fossa
3. Injury to neurovascular supply to muscle
4. Undercorrection or overcorrection of the face

Postoperative Care Issues

1. Wound drainage should continue for at least 48 hours or until drainage has subsided.
2. Cool compresses to face, mouth, and eye may help reduce edema and bruising.
3. Early mobilization of the face with exercises may begin within 2 weeks after surgery.
4. Ophthalmic lubricant and artificial tears should be continued indefinitely.

References

Dentlinger M, Freilinger G. Transfer of the temporal muscle for lagoph- thalmos according to Gillies. Scand J Plastic Reconstr Hand Surg 1991;25:151.

May M. Muscle transposition for facial reanimation. Facial Plast Surg 1992;8:115.

Rubin LR. Reanimation of the paralyzed face by continuous muscle transfers. In: Current therapy in plastic and reconstructive surgery. Philadelphia: BC Decker, 1989:151.

Multiple mattress sutures are used to secure the new attachment. The facial flap is closed over a Penrose drain or closed suction drain with 4-0 chromic catgut sutures and 4-0 and 6-0 Prolene sutures for the skin. The eyelid or lip and corner of the mouth incisions are closed in a similar fashion.

If the temporalis muscle transposition is selected, a very wide exposure is necessary. The temporoparietal fascia is incised approx- imately 1 cm beyond the muscle itself to provide a strong fascial attachment to the new facial sites. Using a Freer elevator and blunt dissection, the entire temporalis muscle is elevated out of its fossa down to the level of the zygoma. If the muscle is quite thick when folded down over the zygoma, the arch may be removed with an oscillating saw to provide a "channel" for the muscle to lie more flush against its insertion into the condylar neck. The main drawback to resecting the arch is that the origin of the masseter muscle is taken away, and mechanical dysfunction of some degree results. A good alternative is to leave the arch intact and fill the vacant temporal fossa with a large abdominal fat graft; this decreases the disparity of soft tissue fullness when the muscle is "flipped" or transposed in- feriorly and medially to the face.

In the same manner as the masseter transfer, the temporalis muscle and fascia (which is fan shaped) are split and divided into five separate slips or "fingers" (Fig. 273-5). The neurovascular bundle of the temporalis muscle enters deep to the belly and just at the level of the zygomatic arch, and careful blunt dissection at this level can preserve the bundle. The five slips of muscle and fascia (still attached together behind the zygoma) are transposed into the five recipient sites: the lateral upper eyelid, lateral lower eyelid, upper nasolabial fold, lateral upper lip and lateral lower lip. The strips are brought out the small incisions in each of these areas and the eyelids and lower face tightened or elevated until a pleasant appearance is achieved on the table (Fig. 273-6). The head should be turned to the midline to do this. The excessive ends of the muscle strips are trimmed, and the remaining ends are sutured into or onto the distal muscles (ie, orbicularis oris and oculi and zygomaticus) with 4-0 clear nylon. If used, the fat graft is trimmed to the volume of the temporalis fossa and secured into position with a few 4-0 chromic catgut sutures. The facial wound is closed over one or more drains, as described previously (Fig. 273-7).

Rarely are gold weights also necessary for the upper eyelid when a dynamic muscle transposition to the orbicularis oculi muscle has been performed. A bulky facelift-type dressing is placed for compression and to serve the drains. Eyelid lubrication is mandatory.

After adequate wound healing, the patient is begun on a course of educational therapy to learn how to use varied pressures of mas- tication to achieve graded elevation of the lower face and closure of the eyelids. A pleasant neutral position of the affected face in repose is a worthy goal. As the temporalis muscle undergoes some atrophy (due to reduced strength of contraction), its bulk over the zygomatic arch decreases, and the appearance in that area improves.

G. RICHARD HOLT

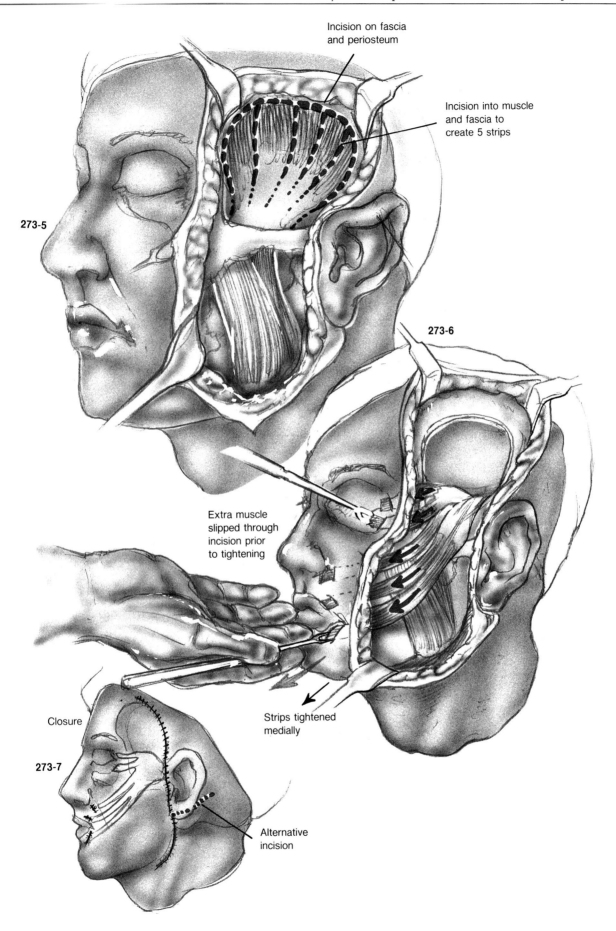

Incision on fascia
and periosteum

Incision into muscle
and fascia to
create 5 strips

273-5

273-6

Extra muscle
slipped through
incision prior
to tightening

Closure

273-7

Strips tightened
medially

Alternative
incision

■ *274.* SAGITTAL OSTEOTOMY OF THE MANDIBULAR RAMUS—A sagittal osteotomy of the mandibular ramus produces an osseous split in the sagittal plane, preserving the inferior alveolar neurovascular bundle, which allows anteroposterior and limited rotational correction of mandibular deformities.

Indications

1. Mandibular prognathism (ie, class III malocclusion and associated jaw malrelation)
2. Retrognathia (ie, class II malocclusion and associated jaw malrelation)
3. Mild to moderate asymmetry can also be corrected by sagittal osteotomy

Contraindications

1. Correction of an anterior open bite as an isolated procedure
2. Inadequate size of the ascending ramus, as in some severe cases of hemifacial microsomia

Special Considerations

1. The operation usually is done in conjunction with orthodontic treatment.
2. Sagittal osteotomy is frequently combined with LeFort I osteotomy or genioplasty.

Preoperative Preparation

1. Clinical evaluation of facial esthetics and the occlusion
2. Cephalometric analysis is performed.
3. Dental models are placed on an articulator.
4. Mock surgery is performed to determine the optimal procedure.
5. Final occlusion of the articulated models is used to create an acrylic occlusal splint that is used to transfer the occlusion to the patient during surgery.

Special Instruments, Position, and Anesthesia

1. Channel retractors
2. Rotary drill with Lindemann and #703 burs
3. Series of osteotomes, including one thin 6- to 8-mm osteotome
4. Rigid fixation screws

Tips and Pearls

1. The cortical cut through the inferior mandibular border must be complete to achieve a proper split.

Pitfalls and Complications

1. A variety of "bad splits" can occur, most of which can be corrected.
2. The inferior alveolar bundle often requires dissection out of the mandibular canal remnant in the proximal fragment.
3. The condyles must be properly seated posteriorly and superiorly within the glenoid fossa to avoid immediate "relapse" after release of intermaxillary fixation.
4. Temporary sensory impairment of the inferior alveolar and mental nerve distribution is to be expected.

Postoperative Care Issues

1. Secure rigid fixation allows early release of intermaxillary fixation; many surgeons prefer to leave the jaws wired for 1 week.
2. Patients who also undergo a LeFort I maxillary osteotomy benefit from 1 to 2 weeks of intermaxillary fixation.

References

Epker BN. Modifications in the sagittal osteotomy of the mandible. J Oral Surg 1977;35:157.

Wolford LM, Bennett MA, Rafferty CG. Modifications of the mandibular ramus sagittal split osteotomy. Oral Surg Oral Med Oral Pathol 1987;64:146.

Operative Procedure

The sagittal split osteotomy is used for advancement of a horizontally deficient mandible, retraction of a horizontally excessive mandible, or correction of mandibular asymmetry. It is not used alone for the closure of an anterior open bite. The operation is almost always done in conjunction with orthodontic therapy and as part of a combined orthodontic and surgical treatment plan. The surgical plan is determined by preoperative clinical and cephalometric analysis and mock surgery on articulated dental models. Before surgery, the orthodontist will have applied orthodontic arch wires with lugs suitable for intermaxillary fixation.

The operation is performed under general nasal endotracheal anesthesia. Epinephrine containing local anesthesia aids in hemostasis, as does hypotensive general anesthesia. The incision is placed in the posterior buccal mucosa, slightly lateral to the mandibular ascending ramus, extending from the mucobuccal fold superiorly. The superior end of the incision extends no farther than the midpoint of the ascending ramus to avoid herniation of the buccal fat pad into the wound. The anterior border of the mandible is exposed, and the temporalis muscle insertion is stripped up to the coronoid process, which is clamped with a curved Kocher clamp to aid in retraction. Masseter muscle attachments to the lateral cortex of the mandible are preserved, and subperiosteal exposure of the lateral mandibular body is limited to the area of the first and second molar. The subperiosteal dissection is extended to fully expose the inferior mandibular border. Medially, a subperiosteal dissection is performed superior to the mandibular foramen and is extended posteriorly to the posterior border of the ascending ramus. The inferior alveolar neurovascular bundle is retracted medially as a channel retractor is placed so that it engages the posterior ramus border.

After placement of a second channel retractor beneath the inferior border, a series of cuts are made through the cortical bone of the mandible to prepare for the sagittal split. A #703 fissure bur is generally used with a Stryker or similar rotary instrument. The first is a vertical cut through the lateral cortex of the mandibular body in the area of the first molar (Fig. 274-1). The cortical bone at the inferior border must be completely transected to ensure a successful split. The second is a horizontal cut through the medial cortex of the ascending ramus, just above the mandibular foramen (Fig. 274-2). This cut is best performed with a Lindemann bur and is often preceded by slight reduction of the internal oblique ridge with a pineapple bur to improve visualization in this area. The third cortical cut connects the previous two, passing just medial to the external oblique ridge and well lateral to the molar teeth (Fig. 274-3). After all cortical cuts are checked again for completeness, the split is begun.

A very thin osteotome is driven to an initial depth of 1 cm along the superior aspect of the external oblique ridge cut, closely approximating the medial surface of the lateral cortex. A Smith separator or a similar instrument is positioned within the inferior border cut to apply lateral splitting pressure as thicker osteotomes are used to carefully pry apart the bone superiorly, creating the split (Fig. 274-4). During the split, the inferior alveolar neurovascular bundle is often exposed and may require careful dissection out of the proximal fragment. After completion of the split, the periosteal envelope is transected with a Freer elevator to allow passive repositioning of the fragments. The teeth are then wired together into the new occlusion, using a previously made acrylic splint. The proximal segment is passively repositioned posteriorly, so that the condyle is optimally positioned within the glenoid fossa. Rigid fixation is then applied with transosseous stabilization screws (Fig. 274-5).

The wound is closed with running, locking 3-0 chromic gut suture. Release of the intermaxillary fixation is optional, depending on the stability of the rigid fixation and the surgeon's preference.

On the first or second postoperative day, a lateral cephalogram is obtained to ensure that the mandibular condyles are properly seated posteriorly within the glenoid fossae. If the radiograph demonstrates that one or both condyles have shifted anteriorly, the patient is returned to surgery for revision of the rigid fixation to allow correction of the condylar position.

ERIC J. DIERKS

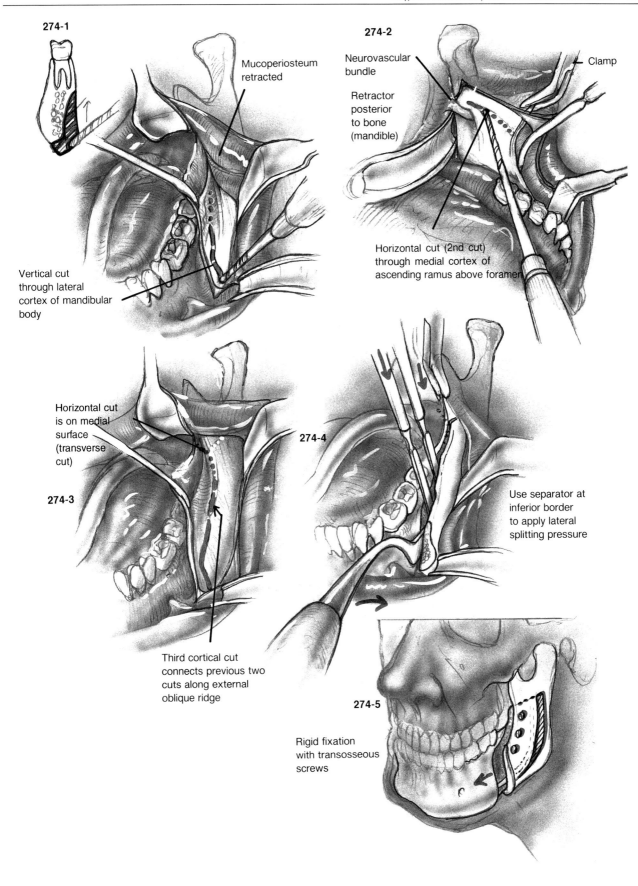

274-1

Mucoperiosteum retracted

Vertical cut through lateral cortex of mandibular body

274-2

Neurovascular bundle

Clamp

Retractor posterior to bone (mandible)

Horizontal cut (2nd cut) through medial cortex of ascending ramus above foramen

Horizontal cut is on medial surface (transverse cut)

274-3

274-4

Use separator at inferior border to apply lateral splitting pressure

Third cortical cut connects previous two cuts along external oblique ridge

274-5

Rigid fixation with transosseous screws

■ *275.* LEFORT I OSTEOTOMY AND ADVANCEMENT

The LeFort I osteotomy horizontally separates the alveolar process of the maxilla and the palate from the midface, preserving blood supply through the posterior soft tissue attachments. This allows repositioning of the upper jaw to correct a variety of occlusal and facial deformities.

Indications
1. Maxillary excess or deficiency in any plane
2. Anterior open bite

Contraindications
1. Not performed before the maxillary teeth have completely erupted

Special Considerations
1. Usually done in conjunction with orthodontic treatment
2. Frequently combined with sagittal osteotomy or genioplasty
3. Cleft palate patients require special planning.

Preoperative Preparation
1. Clinical evaluation of facial aesthetics and the occlusion
2. Cephalometric analysis is performed.
3. Dental models and mock surgery to determine the optimal procedure
4. The final occlusion of the articulated models used to create an acrylic occlusal splint that is used to transfer the occlusion to the patient during surgery.

Special Instruments, Position, and Anesthesia
1. Hypotensive general nasal endotracheal anesthesia
2. Vasoconstrictor containing local anesthesia
3. Obwegeser retractors
4. Osteotomes, including a curved pterygomaxillary osteotome
5. Reciprocating saw or rotary bur

Tips and Pearls
1. Careful attention to complete bone removal in the posterior aspects of the maxilla
2. Preservation of the descending palatine arteries is not essential.

Pitfalls and Complications
1. Careful occlusal and aesthetic planning is essential.
2. The maxilla can be segmented, although it may increase the risk of devascularizing part of the maxilla.

Postoperative Care Issues
1. Solid rigid fixation allows early release of intermaxillary fixation.
2. Patients who undergo concomitant sagittal osteotomy of the mandible benefit from 1 to 2 weeks of intermaxillary fixation.

References
Bell WH. LeFort I osteotomy for correction of maxillary deformities. J Oral Surg 1975;33:412.
Posnick JC, Tompson B. Modification of the maxillary LeFort I osteotomy in cleft-orthognathic surgery: the unilateral cleft lip and palate deformity. J Oral Maxillofac Surg 1992;50:666.

Operative Procedure

The LeFort I osteotomy allows the surgeon to advance the maxilla in cases of horizontal maxillary deficiency and to correct malposition of the upper jaw in all three dimensions. Closure of an anterior open bite is achieved by LeFort I osteotomy with intrusion of the posterior aspect of the maxilla. The LeFort I osteotomy allows the maxilla to be divided into as many as four segments to correct complex multidimensional facial and occlusal problems. The operation usually is done in conjunction with orthodontic therapy and as part of a combined orthodontic and surgical treatment plan.

The operation is performed under general hypotensive nasal endotracheal anesthesia. The addition of epinephrine containing local anesthesia aids in hemostasis. The incision is placed in the maxillary mucobuccal fold, extending from first molar to first molar. A subperiosteal dissection exposes the anterior wall of the maxillary sinus up to the infraorbital foramen. Laterally, the zygomaticomaxillary buttress is exposed, allowing access to the junction of the posterior maxilla with the pterygoid plates. Medially, the piriform aperture is identified and intranasal elevation of the mucoperiosteum from the lateral wall of the nose is performed. Vertical reference marks are scribed into the anterior maxillary wall with a rotary bur before the osteotomy.

A rotary bur or reciprocating saw is used to make the horizontal osteotomy, preserving at least a 3-mm margin of bone above the roots of the maxillary teeth (Fig. 275-1). Medially, a thin osteotome is used to divide the lateral nasal wall. This same thin osteotome is used to create a corresponding horizontal osteotomy across the thin bone of the posterior wall of the maxillary sinus. A U-shaped osteotome is employed to separate the nasal crest of the maxilla from the nasal floor, while preserving the anterior nasal spine. A curved osteotome is then placed vertically between the maxillary tuberosity and the pterygoid plates and is struck with a mallet to separate these structures (Fig. 275-2).

The maxilla is firmly grasped and manually down-fractured as the mucoperiosteum of the nasal floor is elevated and preserved. The descending palatine arteries are preserved, if possible. A pedicle of the posterior soft tissue attachments of the maxilla is created. Removal of bone is then dictated by the direction of the planned movement. The frequently encountered condition of vertical maxillary excess requires removal of a planned amount of bone from the anterior, posterior, medial, and lateral walls of the maxillary sinus (Fig. 275-3). In this situation, a double horizontal osteotomy is created on the anterior maxillary wall before the down-fracture, corresponding to the predetermined amount of bone to be removed. Removal of the nasal crest of the maxilla and resection of some of the caudal aspect of the nasal septum is usually needed, regardless of the direction of maxillary movement. A septoplasty can be performed from this approach, if needed. Advancement of the maxilla requires gentle and repeated stretching of the soft tissues, allowing the maxilla to lie passively in its new position. The final position of the maxilla is checked after the teeth are wired together into their new occlusal association, which is established by a prefabricated interdental acrylic splint. The maxillomandibular complex is then gently pushed posteriorly to seat the mandibular condyles and then rotated upward as the surgeon and assistant check for bony interferences (Fig. 275-4).

After removal of any bony projections and the establishment of good osseous interface at the osteotomy site, rigid fixation is applied. Typically, four L-shaped miniplates are used, one at each piriform rim and one at each zygomaticomaxillary buttress (Fig. 275-5). The mucobuccal fold incision is closed in one layer with 3-0 chromic gut. Incorporation of a small V- or Y-plasty in the midline of the mucosal closure often helps to restore upper lip contour.

Immediate postoperative release of the intermaxillary fixation is optional and depends on the degree of comfort the surgeon has with the stability of the repositioned maxilla. Maxillary and mandibular osteotomies are often combined, and despite the use of rigid fixation in each jaw, 1 week of intermaxillary fixation helps to ensure stability after the postoperative edema resolves.

ERIC J. DIERKS

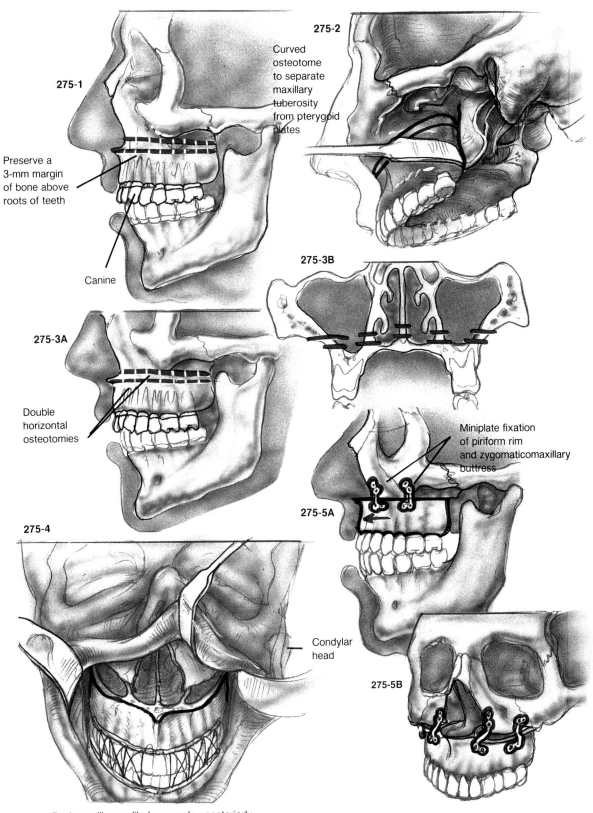

275-1

Preserve a
3-mm margin
of bone above
roots of teeth

Canine

275-2
Curved
osteotome
to separate
maxillary
tuberosity
from pterygoid
plates

275-3A

Double
horizontal
osteotomies

275-3B

Miniplate fixation
of piriform rim
and zygomaticomaxillary
buttress

275-5A

Condylar
head

275-5B

275-4

Push maxillomandibular complex posteriorly
to seat mandibular condyles

■ 276. TRANSNASAL REPAIR OF CHOANAL ATRESIA—To restore nasal patency and to prevent damage to any structures important in facial development

Indications
1. Bilateral choanal atresia
2. Unilateral choanal atresia

Special Considerations
1. Repair bilateral choanal atresia as soon as possible.
2. Repair unilateral choanal atresia early if symptomatic; otherwise, repair can be delayed, usually until preschool age.
3. Associated abnormalities include the CHARGE syndrome, trisomy 21, and Treacher Collins syndrome.
4. Transnasal approach in infants and young children

Preoperative Preparations
1. Routine laboratory studies
2. Bleeding and clotting studies
3. For thin-cut axial computed tomography, use topical decongestants and suction mucus from the nares before scanning.
4. Evaluation of associated abnormalities

Special Instruments, Position, and Anesthesia
1. CO_2 laser and microscope with 400-mm lens
2. Aural specula
3. Dingman mouth gag
4. Nasal endoscopes (0° and 120°)
5. Stammberger-Lusk backbiting antral punch
6. Mastoid curettes
7. Sphenoid punch
8. Van Buren dilators
9. Argyle chest tubes
10. Afrin
11. Supine position, using a shoulder roll (ie, sniffing position)

Tips and Pearls
1. Vasoconstrict nasal mucosa.
2. Out-fracture the inferior turbinates.
3. Vaporize the atretic plate just above the floor of the nose.
4. Consider pressure-equalizing tubes.
5. Check the operative site frequently with a 120° nasal endoscope (operate under visual control).
6. Stent for 6 months.

Pitfalls and Complications
1. Restenosis after stent removal
2. Persistent sinusitis during stenting
3. Otitis media during stenting

Postoperative Care Issues
1. Careful suctioning and cleaning of stents to ensure patency
2. Prophylactic antibiotics to prevent sinusitis and otitis

References
Jones KM, Bauer BS, Pensler JM. Maintenance of airway patency following treatment of choanal atresia. Plast Reconstr Surg 1989;84: 669.
Pirsig W. Surgery of choanal atresia in infants and children: historical notes and updated review. Int J Pediatr Otorhinolaryngol 1986;11: 153.

Operative Procedure

The patient is positioned supine, with a shoulder roll to flex the neck and extend the head. The surgeon is seated at the head of the table. Both nares are packed with 0.25 × 0.25 inch Afrin-soaked neurosurgical cottonoids, and the pharynx is exposed with a Dingman mouth gag. A stay suture is placed through the uvula, and by retracting gently on this suture, the soft palate is elevated. A 120° nasal endoscope is passed into the oral cavity to examine the nasopharynx. The posterior choanal atresia is carefully assessed (Fig. 276-1).

The cottonoids are removed from the nares. A 5-Fr (1.6-mm) Frazier suction catheter is used to clear the nasal cavity of mucus, and with a 0° nasal endoscope, the atretic plate is examined. An appropriately sized aural speculum is placed in the anterior nares, and the nasal cavity is inspected through the operating microscope using the 400-mm objective lens. The inferior turbinate is fractured laterally to better expose the atretic plate.

The patient is draped so that the CO_2 laser can be used safely. At a setting of 10 watts and 0.1 seconds, the laser is used in the pulse mode to vaporize the atretic plate. It is important to vaporize the atretic plate just above the floor of the nose; if the atretic plate is vaporized superiorly, the alae of the vomer or the sphenoid rostrum can be inadvertently damaged. After opening the atretic plate, the choanae should be inspected from the nasopharynx using the 120° nasal endoscope (Fig. 276-2). Usually, the choanae are compromised medially by the thickened posterior aspect of the vomer and laterally by medial encroachment of the medial wall of the maxilla.

Using mastoid curettes or rongeurs, the choanal opening can be enlarged. The endoscopic backbiting antral punch (Stammberger-Lusk) is passed down the naris (the contralateral naris in cases of unilateral atresia), and the size of the vomer is reduced. It is important to reduce the vomer in an inferior-to-superior manner, not in a posterior-to-anterior direction (Fig. 276-3). After the vomer has been reduced, the choanal opening should be reinspected using the 120° endoscope. The medial aspect of the maxilla then can be reduced using a sphenoid punch under direct visual control with the 120° endoscope (Fig. 276-4).

Van Buren dilators are used to dilate the posterior choanae before placement of Argyle polyethylene chest tube stents. Slip the dilators along the floor of the nose using the 120° nasal endoscope for observation (Fig. 276-5). Continue to dilate the choanae with serially larger dilators until a larger-than-normal opening is obtained. The choanae then should be stented.

To position the Argyle chest tubes properly, red rubber catheters are passed through the nose and into the nasopharynx, where they are retrieved and delivered through the mouth. A suture is used to secure an appropriately sized Argyle polyethylene chest tube to the red rubber catheter. The chest tube is positioned in the naris in retrograde fashion, with the flared end of the tube stenting the posterior choana and extending a short distance into the nasopharynx. The tube should be trimmed posteriorly so that the eustachian tube is not obstructed (Fig. 276-6). The tube also must be shortened anteriorly so that it neither protrudes from the nostril nor abuts the nasal rim. A single 2-0 nylon suture secures the tube to the cartilaginous septum next to the floor of the nose. Tubes are removed under general anesthesia after 6 months.

Postoperative care requires irrigation with normal saline and frequent suctioning to prevent crusting. In dry environments, bedside humidification is advisable. Prophylactic antibiotics should be used to prevent sinusitis and otitis media. Children with a history of otitis media should have pressure-equalizing tubes placed in their tympanic membranes.

RICHARD J. H. SMITH

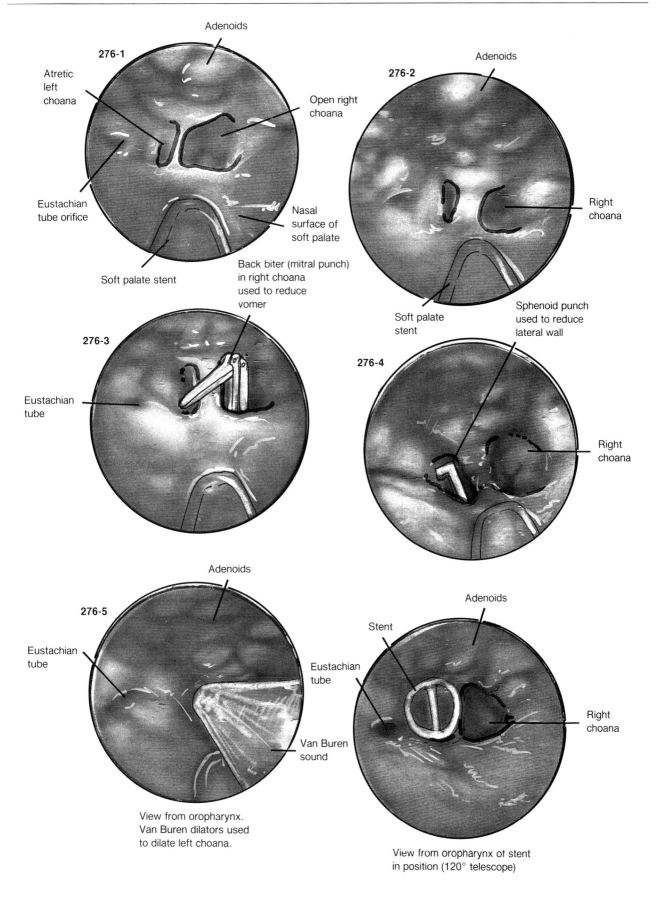

276-1

Adenoids

Atretic left choana

Open right choana

Eustachian tube orifice

Nasal surface of soft palate

Soft palate stent

Back biter (mitral punch) in right choana used to reduce vomer

276-2

Adenoids

Right choana

Soft palate stent

Sphenoid punch used to reduce lateral wall

276-3

Eustachian tube

276-4

Right choana

276-5

Adenoids

Eustachian tube

Eustachian tube

Van Buren sound

View from oropharynx. Van Buren dilators used to dilate left choana.

Stent

Adenoids

Eustachian tube

Right choana

View from oropharynx of stent in position (120° telescope)

■ *277.* TRANSPALATAL REPAIR OF CHOANAL ATRESIA—To restore nasal patency and prevent damage to any structures important in facial development

Indications
1. Bilateral choanal atresia
2. Unilateral choanal atresia
3. Failed prior repairs

Special Indications
1. Visualization of the atretic area is better than with the transnasal approach.
2. Blood loss, operative time, and convalescence are longer than with the transnasal approach.
3. Mucosal flaps can be sutured into position.
4. This procedure should be considered only after puberty.

Preoperative Preparations
1. Routine laboratory studies
2. Bleeding and clotting studies
3. For thin-cut axial computed tomography, use topical decongestants and suction mucus from the nares before scanning.
4. Evaluate the dentition.

Special Instruments, Position, and Anesthesia
1. Microscope with 400-mm lens
2. Dingman mouth gag
3. Drill
4. Kerrison rongeurs
5. Beaver #6910 miniblade
6. Argyle chest tubes
7. Cocaine
8. Supine position, using a shoulder roll (ie, sniffing position)

(continued)

Operative Procedure

The patient is positioned supine, with a shoulder roll to flex the neck and extend the head. The surgeon is seated at the head of the table. Both nares are packed with 0.25 × 0.25 inch cocaine-soaked neurosurgical cottonoids. Exposure to the oral cavity and pharynx is obtained with a Dingman mouth gag. A mucosal flap is outlined on the hard palate, beginning just inside the second molar on one side and following the dental arch to the second molar on the opposite side. Adequate mucosa is preserved along the dental arch to permit easy flap closure at the conclusion of the procedure (Fig. 277-1).

The mucosal incision is carried down to bone using a Beaver #6910 miniblade to facilitate making the incision perpendicular to the bony palate. The flap is elevated with a periosteal elevator to the posterior border of the hard palate. The greater palatine vessels should be lifted from their groove in the hard palate and seen in relief on the under surface of the flap (Fig. 277-2). Inclusion of these vessels in the flap ensures a good blood supply to the elevated tissue.

A Woodson elevator is used to elevate the mucosa lining the posterior aspect of the atretic plate without entering the nasopharynx. After tissue elevation is adequate enough to place a small cottonoid or a malleable retractor between the mucosa and bone, the drill is used to remove the posterior edge of the palate and expose the atretic plate (Fig. 277-3). The atretic plate is carefully thinned, progressing in a posterior-to-anterior manner until the anterior extent of the atresia is visualized. The bone over the anterior edge of the atretic plate is removed without entering the nose. A Woodson or Cottle elevator is used to further elevate the mucosa lining the anterior aspect of the atretic plate (Fig. 277-4).

(continued)

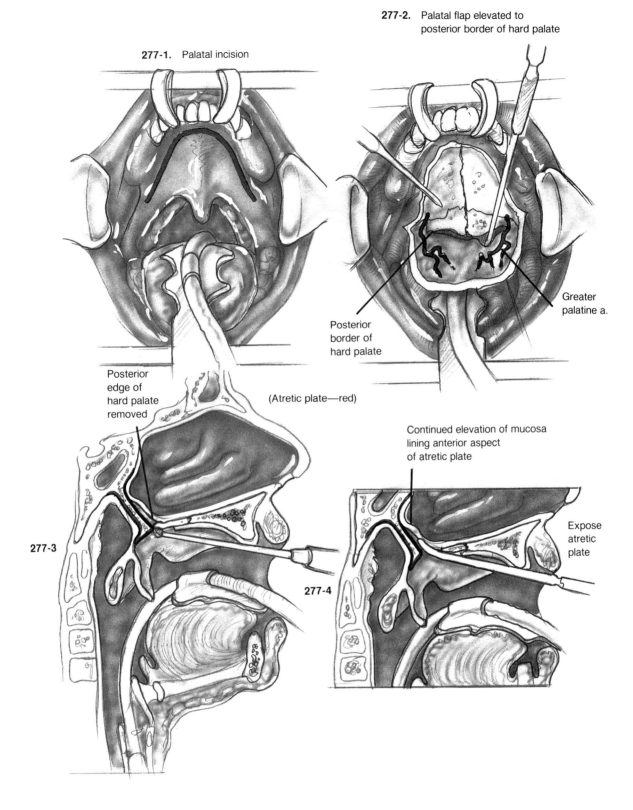

277-1. Palatal incision

277-2. Palatal flap elevated to posterior border of hard palate

Greater palatine a.

Posterior border of hard palate

Posterior edge of hard palate removed

(Atretic plate—red)

277-3

Continued elevation of mucosa lining anterior aspect of atretic plate

Expose atretic plate

277-4

■ *277.* TRANSPALATAL REPAIR OF CHOANAL ATRESIA *(continued)*

Tips and Pearls

1. Vasoconstrict nasal mucosa using cocaine-soaked pledgets.
2. At the junction of the hard and soft palate, do not enter the nasopharynx.
3. Preserve the mucosa on the posterior and anterior surfaces of the atretic plate.
4. Use preserved mucosa to line the newly created choana.
5. Use stents.

Pitfalls and Complications

1. Restenosis
2. Palatal fistulization
3. Development of a cross bite
4. Otitis media during stenting

Postoperative Care Issues

1. Careful suctioning and cleaning of stents to ensure patency
2. Prophylactic antibiotics to prevent sinusitis and otitis

References

Owens H. Observations in treating twenty-five cases of choanal atresia by the transpalatal approach. Laryngoscope 1965;75:84.

Persig W. Surgery of choanal atresia in infants and children: historical notes and updated review. Int J Pediatr Otorhinolaryngol 1986;11: 153.

The remainder of the bony atresia is removed with the drill (Fig. 277-5). Laterally, bony removal is limited by the greater palatine vessels. Medially, enough bony septum is removed to ensure that an adequate opening is created.

To minimize the likelihood of restenosis, mucous membrane continuity is reestablished in the posterior choana. The anterior flap is hinged to fit the roof of the choana by making an incision along the floor of the nose (Fig. 277-6). The posterior flap is hinged to meet the mucosa of the floor of the nose by making an incision near the superior extent of the choana (see Fig. 277-4). Both flaps are sutured in position using 4-0 Vicryl. The raw surface over the posterior aspect of the nasal septum is covered by reapproximating the mucosa on either side of the nasal septum. If necessary, additional septum is removed posteriorly to facilitate this closure (Fig. 277-7).

An Argyle chest tube is positioned in the nares, with the flared end of the tube stenting the posterior choana. Check tube placement in relation to the eustachian tube orifice to determine whether a pressure-equalizing tube may be required. In cases of unilateral stenosis, the chest tube can be secured to the nasal septum; in cases of bilateral stenosis, a wire passed posteriorly through one chest tube, around the posterior aspect of the nasal septum, and anteriorly through the contralateral chest tube can be secured to the anterior nasal spine. A small gingival buccal incision is required to tie the wire in place (Fig. 277-8).

The palatal flap is reapplied to the hard palate. To eliminate dead space and improve palate-to-flap opposition, the midportion of the flap is sutured to the hard palate (Fig. 277-9). The mucosa incision is closed tightly with 4-0 Vicryl. A palatal stent can be used for a few days but is not essential.

RICHARD J. H. SMITH

277-5. Remaining atretic plate drilled

Retractor
on mucosa

277-6

Incise anterior flap to
line roof

Posterior flap lines
floor of nose

PF

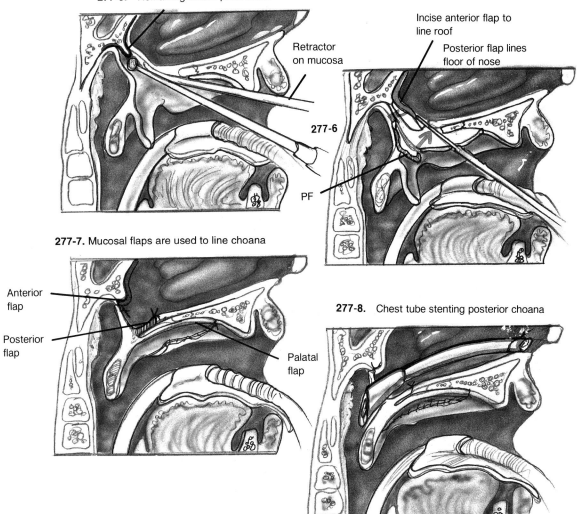

277-7. Mucosal flaps are used to line choana

Anterior
flap

Posterior
flap

Palatal
flap

277-8. Chest tube stenting posterior choana

277-9. Closure of palatal flap

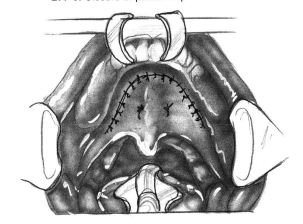

■ *278.* UNILATERAL CLEFT LIP REPAIR USING A ROTATION-ADVANCEMENT TECHNIQUE— Flap rotation and advancement for the repair of a unilateral cleft lip deformity

Indications
1. Incomplete or complete unilateral cleft lip, with or without cleft palate

Contraindications
1. Medically unstable patient
2. Rule of tens: 10 weeks of age, 10 lb of weight, and 10 g of hemoglobin

Special Considerations
1. In patients with extremely wide clefts, consider using a preoperative prosthetic appliance to improve alignment of the maxillary arches and to decrease the cleft size.
2. Perform a preliminary lip adhesion procedure at 6 weeks of age to convert a wide complete cleft to an incomplete cleft.

Preoperative Preparation
1. Routine laboratory studies
2. Bleeding and clotting studies (if history warrants)

Special Instruments, Position, and Anesthesia
1. Fine, sharp plastic instruments to minimize tissue trauma; measuring calipers and sterile, malleable wire
2. The patient is supine, with the surgeon seated at the head of the table with the patient's head in the surgeon's lap.
3. General anesthesia with an endotracheal tube

Tips and Pearls
1. The goal of surgical repair is establishment of normal form and function.
2. Identify and preserve normal lip architecture and landmarks.
3. Muscle closure to reconstitute an intact oral sphincter.
4. This is a surgery of judgment instead of measurement, with the ultimate goal of achieving symmetry while restoring form and function.
5. Adequate rotation of the medial lip segment and adequate lateral lip length should be achieved on completion.
6. Adjust the back cut on the medial segment to increase rotation, but do not cross the opposite philtral ridge.
7. The length of lateral lip segment may be increased by extending the releasing incision around nasal ala to "borrow" lateral lip tissue.
8. A collapsed lower lateral cartilage may be repositioned and supported with bolster sutures during the primary repair. This helps with nasal symmetry, but definitive nasal reconstruction is required, except in extremely mild cases.
9. Minimize wound edge tension on closure.
10. Minimize the degree of undermining.
11. Anticipate a minor touch-up procedure after the primary repair.

(continued)

Operative Procedure
The operation is begun with the patient in the supine position under general anesthesia with oral endotracheal intubation. The oral endotracheal tube is bent 90° onto the lower lip and positioned out of the operative field. The tube should be taped in the midline such that it does not affect the resting position of the upper or lower lips. The normal side is measured to provide a template for the closure of the cleft side. Several points are marked as shown in the illustration (Fig. 278-1):
1. Center of cupid's bow on the mucocutaneous vermilion
2. Peak of cupid's bow on the noncleft side
3. Peak of cupid's bow on the cleft side; the distance between 1 and 2 is usually about 4 mm and should equal the distance between 1 and 3.
4. The position of the alar base on normal side
5. Extent of the rotation curve on the medial cleft side before placement of the back cut; small letter x indicates the extent of the back cut from point 5 to achieve adequate downward rotation of central segment
6. Lateral commissure on normal side
7. Lateral commissure on cleft side
8. Lateral cupid's bow peak on the cleft side, which must be matched to point 3
9. Medial-most point of the lateral cleft segment, which is needed to achieve a satisfactory philtral length
10. Alar base on the cleft side
11. Extension of the alatomy incision on the cleft side

Key points 1, 2, 3, 5, 8, and 9 may be tattooed with a 27-gauge needle and tincture of violet directly into the skin to minimize being erased during the remainder of the procedure. The points may be established by precise caliper measurements based on the normal side. The usual distance between points 1 and 2 is approximately 4 mm. The vertical distance between points 2 and 4, which should be matched by the distance between points 8 and 10 on the cleft side, is about 10 mm. The distance from the cupid's bow peak to the commissure is generally about 20 mm, and this should be marked on the cleft side and the normal side. Occasionally, the vermilion on the lateral lip segment is atrophic and foreshortened, and point 8 may need to be lateralized to find satisfactory tissue for philtral ridge closure. In that case, point 8 may be shifted laterally, toward point 7, to achieve satisfactory vertical lip height at the expense of lateral lip length.

The rotation incision may be marked with a malleable wire extending from point 3 to point 5. This distance should approximate the cupid's peak through the columella base distance along the noncleft side and should also approximate the distance between points 8 and 9 on the lateral segment of the cleft side. The back cut from point 5 may be necessary to achieve satisfactory rotation. This back cut may be extended toward the normal philtrum, but it should never cross it. The back cut usually is 1 to 2 mm.

(continued)

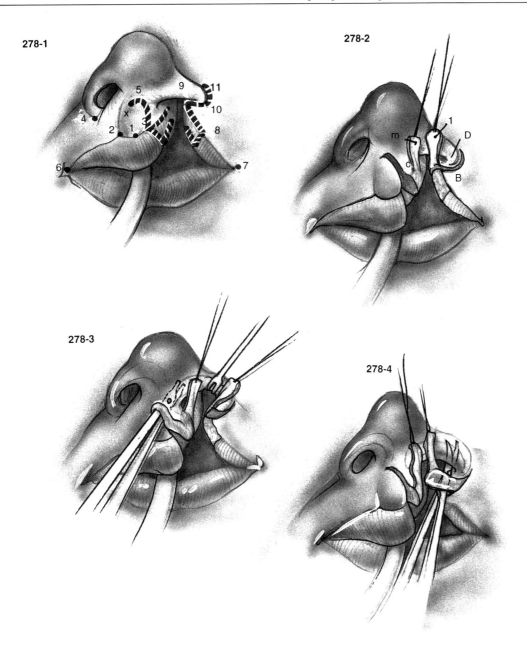

278-1

278-2

278-3

278-4

■ 278. UNILATERAL CLEFT LIP REPAIR US-ING A ROTATION-ADVANCEMENT TECH-NIQUE *(continued)*

Pitfalls and Complications

1. Wide clefts may result in excess tension and an unfavorable scar; consider preliminary lip adhesion.
2. Secondary lip and nasal deformities may persist. They may be mild to severe, depending on the cleft and surgical technique.
3. Rotation or lip length may be inadequate or excessive.
4. The vermilion may be notched or asymmetric.
5. The columella may be short or deviated
6. An abnormal nostril or alar base may result from intranasal incisions.
7. Vestibular stenosis resulting from extensive intranasal scarring
8. Lip scar contracture or hypertrophy
9. Maxillary arch collapse
10. Dehiscence of closure
11. Soft tissue infection after closure

Postoperative Care Issues

1. The incision should be kept clean. Antibiotic ointment should be applied 1 week after surgery to prevent scabs and crusting.
2. Oral antibiotics are administered for 1 week after surgery.
3. Arm restraints are used for 2 weeks after surgery.

References

Bumsted RM. Management of unilateral cleft lip In: Smith JD, Bumsted RM, eds. Pediatric facial plastic and reconstructive surgery. New York: Raven Press, 1993.

Millard RJ Jr. Cleft craft. Vol 1. Unilateral deformity. Boston: Little Brown, 1977.

After the points and incisions have been marked, the surgeon should inspect the markings to ascertain the appropriate relationship of all the units. The marking should be corrected or changed at this point to improve symmetry. After satisfactory marking is achieved, the lip may be sparsely infiltrated with local anesthetic containing epinephrine, particularly near the incision lines to aid in hemostasis.

The rotation flap is cut perpendicular to the skin surface, with the incision extended up to point 5 (Fig. 278-2). Satisfactory rotation is achieved when points 2 and 3 line up in a horizontal, symmetric position. If necessary, the back cut can be extended from point 5 to point x to help achieve this horizontal symmetry. The medial lip segment is undermined from the maxilla sharply to help with the rotation. The lip should sit freely in the symmetric position without any external retraction. The advancement is next incised along the previously marked incision lines. The lateral lip segment and alar base may be undermined from the anterior maxilla in limited fashion to facilitate the advancement. The mucosal flaps *m* and *l* in Figure 278-3 should have their superior attachments preserved so the flaps may be used to line the intranasal incisions or help create upper labial sulcus. Flap *c* is also released from its underlying attachments to allow its incorporation into the columella on the cleft side (Fig. 278-3).

The lower lateral cartilage on the cleft side may be freed from its skin and mucosal attachments with scissors dissection to facilitate its repositioning in a superior medial direction (Fig. 278-4). Closure is begun by attaching the tip of the alar flap D in Figure 278-5 to the nasal spine to medialize the nasal base (Fig. 278-5). The *c* flap is advanced into the columella for lengthening (Fig. 278-6). Advancement flap B is sutured to the nasal spine, taking care to obtain a substantial bite of the muscle to securely anchor this flap medially (Fig. 278-7). This advancement helps to push the rotation flap and maintain the appropriate relation of the reconstructed work. The skin edges along the new philtral borders may be undermined for a distance of 1 to 2 mm to facilitate eversion on closure.

The lip is closed in three layers, with the muscle layer closed in tight approximation using 4-0 polydioxanone sutures. It is important to achieve tight approximation, particularly along the inferior border, to minimize notching or surface irregularities. The mucosal layer and the vermilion may be closed with 4-0 Vicryl interrupted sutures. The skin is closed first with a stitch aligning the mucocutaneous vermilion precisely. All incisions are closed with 6-0 fast-absorbing gut sutures. With a skin hook supporting the nostril rim, two through-and-through bolsters sutures are placed through the lower lateral cartilage to anchor it in a superior medial direction to approximate a more normal architecture (Fig. 278-8). Antibiotic ointment may be placed along the incision lines and the procedure terminated. The bolster sutures may be removed in 5 to 7 days. The lip scar tends to shorten in the course of the first 3 to 4 months. It thereafter softens and lengthens to its more normal position (Fig. 278-9).

TOM D. WANG

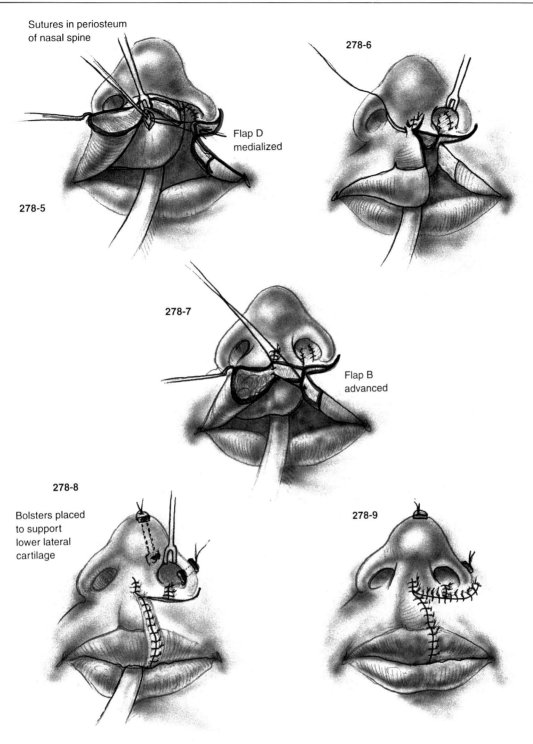

Sutures in periosteum
of nasal spine

278-6

Flap D
medialized

278-5

278-7

Flap B
advanced

278-8

Bolsters placed
to support
lower lateral
cartilage

278-9

■ *279.* BILATERAL CLEFT LIP REPAIR
Surgical repair for bilateral cleft lip deformity

Indications
1. Incomplete or complete bilateral cleft lip, with or without a cleft palate

Contraindications
1. Medically unstable patient
2. Excessively wide clefts with thin, atrophic tissue, preventing one-stage closure

Special Considerations
1. Excessively protuberant premaxilla may require unilateral or bilateral lip adhesion before definitive closure.

Preoperative Preparation
1. Routine laboratory studies
2. Bleeding and clotting studies (if history warrants)

Special Instruments, Position, and Anesthesia
1. Fine, sharp plastic instruments to minimize tissue trauma; measuring calipers and sterile, malleable wire
2. The patient is supine, with the surgeon seated at the head of the table with the patient's head in the surgeon's lap.
3. General anesthesia with an endotracheal tube

Tips and Pearls
1. Goal of repair is to establish and maintain symmetry while restoring form and function.
2. Lateral prolabial tissue may be banked for secondary columella elongation.
3. The lip height is determined by prolabial tissue medially, not by lateral lip segments, and the lip length tends to elongate over time as child grows.
4. Minimize trauma to the premaxilla. Do not resect the premaxilla, no matter how protuberant.
5. Do not use the prolabial vermilion in anterior vermilion closure, because this tissue will never match the surrounding vermilion.

Pitfalls and Complications
1. Rarely, prolabial ischemia occurs in bilateral incomplete cleft lip cases.
2. Dehiscence of the closure secondary to protuberant premaxilla
3. A foreshortened and tethered columella with minimal tip projection is an expected outcome after primary lip repair.
4. Maxillary arch collapse after lip repair requires orthodontia.
5. Secondary lip and nasal deformities vary from mild to severe, depending on the cleft presentation and surgical technique.
6. Vermilion notching or asymmetry
7. An abnormal nostril or alar base is to be expected because of columella tethering.
8. Scar contracture or hypertrophy
9. Soft tissue infection after surgery

Postoperative Care Issues
1. The incision should be kept clean. Antibiotic ointment should be applied for 1 week after surgery to prevent scabs and crusting.
2. Oral antibiotics are administered for 1 week after surgery.
3. Arm restraints are used for 2 weeks after surgery.

References
Millard RJ Jr. Cleft craft. Vol 2. Bilateral deformities. Boston: Little Brown, 1977.

Seibert RW. Bilateral cleft lip repair. In: Smith JD, Bumsted RN, eds. Pediatric facial plastic and reconstructive surgery. New York: Raven Press, 1993.

Operative Procedure
The patient is placed supine on the operating table. The procedure is performed under general anesthesia with oral endotracheal intubation. The tube is secured inferiorly, taped to the center of the lower lip to minimize any distortions of the lip architecture. Calipers are used to measure the normal cupid's bow peak from the center of the prolabium; this is usually 2 mm on each side. This distance is marked along the lateral segment vermilion in a slightly longer fashion to help produce the central lip tubercle. The distance between the lateral commissure and the cupid's bow peak is determined bilaterally; this is usually between 18 and 22 mm. The lateral vertical height of the prolabium is determined next. This is matched along the mucocutaneous junction of the lateral segment and usually measures between 8 to 13 mm. It is imperative to find satisfactory vermilion thickness to establish the new central tubercle. The measure points may be tattooed with a fine-gauge needle and tincture of violet to minimize inadvertent erasure. A small portion of the central inferior vermilion designated as the *e* flaps is marked for incorporation into the central tubercle behind the lateral vermilion segments (Fig. 279-1).

After the markings have been completed, the lip is infiltrated with a small amount of local anesthetic containing epinephrine for hemostasis, and all incisions are made (Fig. 279-2). The prolabial and lateral lip segments are undermined to facilitate mobilization. The tips of the alar flaps are de-epithelialized and sutured with 4-0 polydioxanone suture to the nasal spine (Fig. 279-3). The segments may be sutured together with one suture or individually with two sutures, one at a time. The suture is placed beneath the elevated prolabium. The undermined mucosa covering the premaxilla and prolabium is elevated and positioned down onto the premaxilla to serve as the posterior mucosal lining of the new labial sulcus. The tips of the lateral lip segments are also sutured to each other and the nasal spine just below the alar flap junction (Fig. 279-4). It is important to obtain a deep muscle suture in this region for satisfactory union. The previously elevated prolabial elements—the bilateral banked fork flap along the alar rim and the central philtral segment—are then sutured down.

Flap *e* is inserted behind the vermilion tubercle to add bulk to the vermilion (Fig. 279-5). This type of closure typically results in a short, tethered columella that requires secondary columellar lengthening using the banked fork flaps (Fig. 279-6). At this point, antibiotic ointment is placed over the closed incisions, and the procedure is completed.

TOM D. WANG

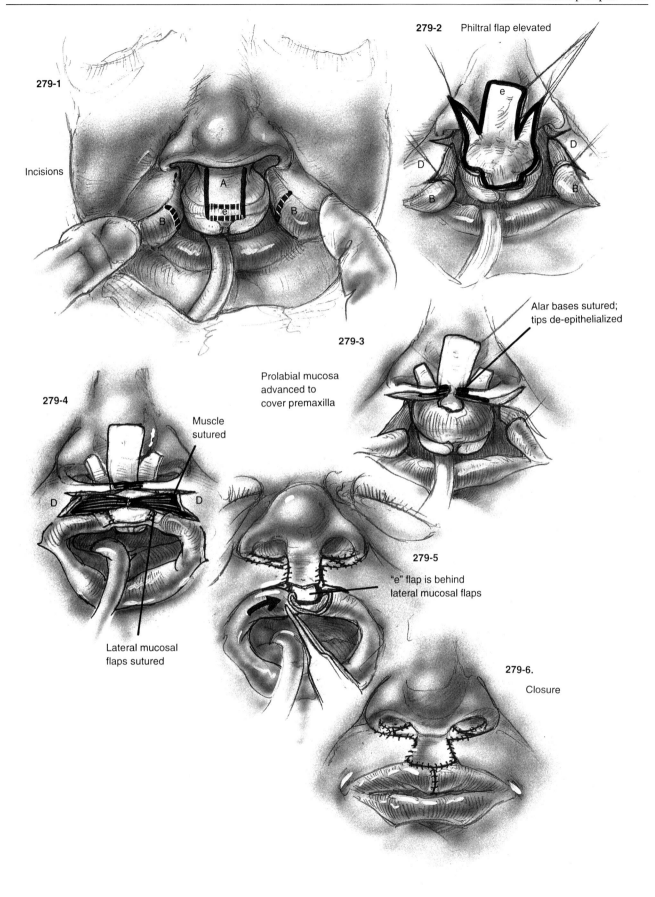

279-1

Incisions

279-2   Philtral flap elevated

Alar bases sutured;
tips de-epithelialized

279-3

Prolabial mucosa
advanced to
cover premaxilla

279-4

Muscle
sutured

Lateral mucosal
flaps sutured

279-5

"e" flap is behind
lateral mucosal flaps

279-6.

Closure

■ 280. COMPLETE SECONDARY PALATAL CLEFT REPAIR (TWO-FLAP PALATOPLASTY WITH INTRAVELAR VELOPLASTY)

—The secondary palatal defect involves the entire soft palate and hard palate to the incisive foramen. The surgical goal of repair is to accomplish closure of the defect while reconstructing a competent velopharyngeal sphincter for adequate speech development. The repair involves closure of the oral mucoperiosteal layer, the nasal layer using a vomerine flap, and reconstruction of the velar muscular sling. Various surgical procedures and their modifications have been used. The two-flap palatoplasty with intravelar veloplasty, incorporating a midline vomerine flap, is discussed.

Indications

1. Unrepaired cleft of the secondary palate
2. Symptoms of velopharyngeal insufficiency

Special Considerations

1. Closure ideally completed before speech development begins, usually between 6 and 18 months
2. Potential maxillofacial growth disturbances and occlusal abnormalities related to surgery
3. Concomitant middle ear disease, affecting hearing and speech
4. Nutrition and feeding
5. Team management involving speech pathology, orthodontists, and cleft surgeons
6. Psychosocial concerns

Preoperative Preparation

1. Routine laboratory studies
2. Evaluate patient for cleft width, palatal shelf position, and presence of vomer in the cleft midline.

Special Instruments, Position, and Anesthesia

1. Headlight
2. Trendelenburg position, with the head in a foam doughnut
3. Dingmann mouth gag
4. Injection of palate with 0.5% solution of lidocaine with 1:100,000 epinephrine
5. Woodson elevator, nerve hook, and Dean scissors
6. Oxidized cellulose (Surgicel)

Tips and Pearls

1. Judicious dissection of neurovascular pedicle from flap to increase mobility and reduce tension
2. Infracture of the hamulus as needed if further mobilization required
3. Three-layered closure of soft palate with reconstruction of palatal muscle sling
4. Two-layered closure of hard palate, followed by approximation of the oral and nasal layers to eliminate dead space

Pitfalls and Complications

1. Postoperative bleeding
2. Mucoperiosteal flap necrosis
3. Oronasal fistula formation
4. Infection
5. Persistent velopharyngeal incompetence

Postoperative Care Issues

1. Postoperative monitoring for airway obstruction, adequate fluid balance, and hemostasis
2. Counsel parents about pain management, fever, diet restrictions, and fluid intake.
3. Feed with spoon or bulb syringe; avoid pacifiers or sucking on nipples for 2 weeks postoperatively.

References

Bardach J, Salyer KE. Surgical techniques in cleft lip and palate. St. Louis: Mosby-Year Book, 1991:224.

Dado DV. Early cleft palate repair with intravelar veloplasty. In: Kernahan DA, Rosenstein SW, eds. Cleft lip and palate: a system of management. Baltimore: Williams & Wilkins, 1990:189.

Operative Procedure

With the patient supine in the Trendelenburg position, the Dingmann mouth gag is positioned to expose the palate. The proposed mucoperiosteal flaps are marked posteriorly on the descending palatine artery and are designed so that the anterior tip of each flap is adjacent to the lateral incisor (Fig. 280-1).

A #15 blade scalpel is used to incise the medial aspect of the flap, starting at the uvula and continuing to the anterior extent of the cleft, while holding traction on the uvula tip with a Cushing forceps. Along the soft palate, the incision is placed at the junction of the oral and nasal mucosa. Along the hard palate, the incision is placed 1 to 2 mm lateral to the cleft edge. This strip of oral mucoperiosteum is rotated medially with the nasal mucosa to facilitate tension-free closure of the nasal layer. From the anterior aspect of the cleft, the medial incision is carried toward the lateral incisor. Laterally, the incision is begun about 1 cm posterior to the maxillary tuberosity, curving around the tuberosity and anteriorly along the base of the alveolus to meet the medial incision.

The mucoperiosteal flaps are elevated from the hard palate, using a Freer or Woodson elevator. The anterior V-shaped mucoperiosteum covering the primary hard palate is left intact. Posteriorly, it is important to identify and preserve the neurovascular bundle exiting from the greater palatine foramen. The nerve is gently stretched and dissected from the posterior flap using a nerve hook. The flap elevation should continue to the posterior edge of the hard palate both medial and lateral to the neurovascular bundle.

Beginning at the posteromedial edge of the cleft, the mucosa is elevated from the nasal surface of the hard palate to allow mobilization of the nasal mucoperiosteum. A Woodson elevator or right-angle palatal elevator is particularly helpful for elevating around the curve of the cleft edge. When the vomer is found in the midline, vomerine flaps are created by incising along the lower edge of the vomer. Mucoperiosteal flaps are elevated on each side of the vomer (Fig. 280-2). When it is absent, widely undermine the nasal mucoperiosteum for closure to itself.

Using the sharp edge of the Woodson elevator, dissect the velar muscles from the attachment to the posterior border of the hard palate. Continue the dissection of the nasal mucosa from the nasal side of the hard palate along its posterior edge. Complete detachment of the soft tissues from the posterior edge of the hard palate helps lengthen the soft palate. The velar muscles are then sharply dissected from the oral and nasal mucosal layers for 2 to 3 mm from the medial cleft edge, permitting reorientation of the muscle fibers into a transverse palatal sling.

Grasp the medial edges of the oral and nasal mucosa and gently pull toward the midline. Approximation of the edges should be possible without tension. If further mobilization is needed to allow tension-free closure dissection in the space of Ernst between the superior constrictor muscles and pterygoids may be carried out. The neurovascular bundle can also be further mobilized by dissecting it free from the mucoperiosteal flap for approximately 1 cm. In cases of severe clefting, the hamulus may be infractured, or the attachment of the tensor veli palatini muscle may be dissected free to maximize medial mobility of the flap.

The nasal mucosa, velar musculature, and oral mucoperiosteal flaps are closed in three separate layers. The vomerine flaps are sutured to the nasal mucoperiosteal layer in the region of the hard palate (Fig. 280-3). Interrupted sutures are placed with the knot on the nasal side, using 4-0 chromic suture. The nasal layer closure is continued posteriorly to the uvula. The velar muscles are approximated in the midline using 4-0 Vicryl suture. Starting at the uvula, the oral layer is then closed. Vertical mattress sutures are used in the region of the hard palate for stabilization of the mucoperiosteal flaps to the underlying nasal mucosa. This reduces the risk of hematoma formation and flap detachment postoperatively.

After medial closure, the anterior and lateral incisions are loosely approximated. If the lateral incisions cannot be closed without tension, partial closure is accomplished, and oxidized cellulose is inserted between the wound edges to cover the exposed bare bone (Fig. 280-4).

BECKY MCGRAW-WALL

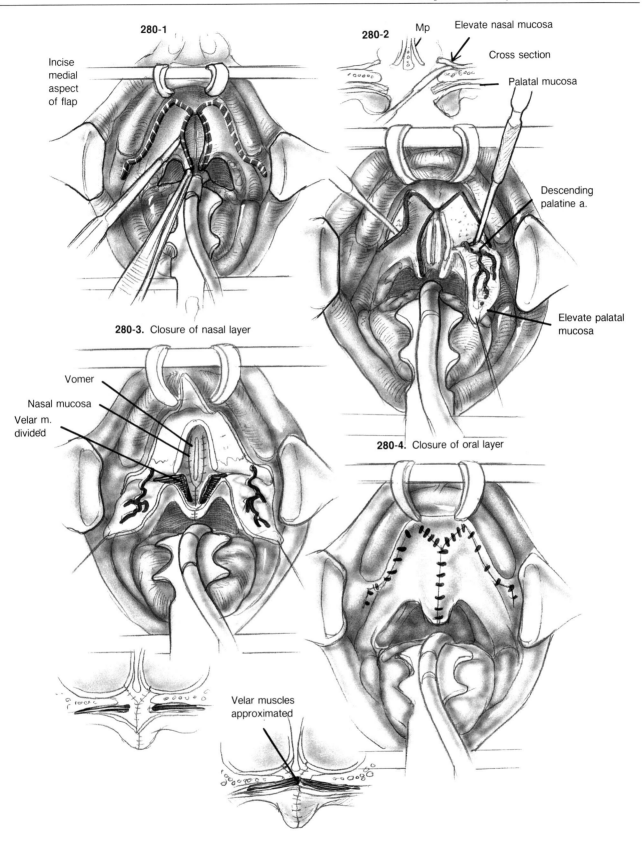

280-1

Incise medial aspect of flap

280-2   Mp   Elevate nasal mucosa

Cross section

Palatal mucosa

Descending palatine a.

Elevate palatal mucosa

280-3. Closure of nasal layer

Vomer

Nasal mucosa

Velar m. divided

280-4. Closure of oral layer

Velar muscles approximated

■ *281.* INCOMPLETE SECONDARY PALATAL CLEFT REPAIR—Two-flap palatoplasty with intravelar veloplasty is used for closure of the defect and for reconstructing a competent velopharyngeal sphincter for adequate speech development. The repair involves closure of the oral and nasal mucosal layers and renovation of the soft palate musculature. Incomplete secondary palatal defects may involve only the soft palate or may involve the entire soft palate and a portion of the posterior hard palate.

Indications
1. Unrepaired incomplete cleft of the secondary palate
2. Symptoms of velopharyngeal insufficiency

Special Considerations
1. Closure ideally is completed before speech development, usually between 6 and 18 months of age.
2. Potential maxillofacial growth disturbances and occlusal abnormalities related to surgery
3. Concomitant middle ear disease and its impact on hearing and speech
4. Nutrition and feeding issues
5. Management team involving speech pathologists, orthodontists, and cleft surgeons
6. Psychosocial concerns

Preoperative Preparation
1. Routine laboratory studies
2. Evaluate the cleft width and presence or absence of the vomer in the cleft midline.

Special Instruments, Position, and Anesthesia
1. Headlight
2. Trendelenburg position, foam doughnut
3. Dingmann mouth gag
4. Injection of the palate with a 0.5% solution of lidocaine with 1: 100,000 epinephrine
5. Woodson elevator, nerve hook, and Dean scissors
6. Oxidized cellulose (Surgicel)

Tips and Pearls
1. Judicious dissection of the neurovascular pedicle from the flap to increase mobility and reduce tension
2. Infracture of the hamulus if further mobilization is required
3. Three-layer closure of the soft palate, with reconstruction of the palatal muscle sling
4. Two-layer closure of the hard palate, followed by approximation of the these layers to eliminate dead space

Pitfalls and Complications
1. Postoperative bleeding
2. Mucoperiosteal flap necrosis
3. Oronasal fistula formation
4. Infection
5. Persistent velopharyngeal incompetence

Postoperative Care Issues
1. Postoperative monitoring for airway obstruction, adequate fluid balance, and hemostasis
2. Counsel the parents about pain management, fever, diet restrictions, and fluid intake.
3. Feed the patient with a spoon or bulb syringe; the child must avoid pacifiers or sucking on nipples 2 weeks postoperatively.

References
Bardach J, Salyer KE. Surgical techniques in cleft lip and palate. St. Louis: Mosby-Year Book, 1991:224.
Dado DV. Early cleft palate repair with intravelar veloplasty. In: Kernahan DA, Rosenstein SW, eds. Cleft lip and palate: a system of management. Baltimore: Williams & Wilkins, 1990:189.

Operative Procedure
With the patient supine in the Trendelenburg position, the Dingmann mouth gag is positioned to expose the palate. The proposed mucoperiosteal flaps are marked with gentian violet before infiltrating with a 0.5% solution of lidocaine with a 1:100,000 concentration of epinephrine.

The flaps are based posteriorly on the descending palatine artery and are designed such that the anterior tip of each flap is adjacent to the canine tooth (Fig. 281-1). A #15 blade scalpel is used to incise the medial aspect of the flap, starting at the uvula and extending the incision to the anterior extent of the cleft, while holding traction on the uvula tip with a Cushing forceps. The scalpel or Dean scissors can be used to continue this incision posteriorly to the tip of the uvula. Along the soft palate, the incision is placed at the junction of the oral and nasal mucosa. Along the hard palate, the incision is placed 1 to 2 mm lateral to the cleft edge, leaving a strip of oral mucosa attached to the nasal mucosa. This strip of oral mucoperiosteum is rotated medially with the nasal mucosa to facilitate tension-free closure of the nasal layer. From the anterior aspect of the cleft, the medial incision is carried anterolaterally toward the canine tooth. Laterally, the incision is begun about 1 cm posterior to the maxillary tuberosity, curving around the tuberosity and anteriorly along the base of the alveolus to meet the medial incision.

The incisions are carried to the subperiosteal plane, after which the mucoperiosteal flaps are elevated from the hard palate, starting laterally and using a Freer or Woodson elevator. The anterior V-shaped mucoperiosteum covering the uncleft portion of the hard palate is left intact. Posteriorly, it is important to identify and preserve the neurovascular bundle exiting from the greater palatine foramen. The nerve is gently stretched and dissected from the posterior flap using a nerve hook. The flap elevation should continue to the posterior edge of the hard palate medial and lateral to the neurovascular bundle (Fig. 281-2). Beginning at the posteromedial edge of the cleft, the mucosa is elevated from the nasal surface of the hard palate to allow mobilization of the nasal mucosa. A Woodson elevator or right-angle elevator is particularly helpful for elevating around the curve of the cleft edge.

The sharp edge of the Woodson elevator is used to dissect the velar muscles from the attachment to the posterior border of the hard palate. The dissection of the nasal mucosa is continued from the nasal side of the hard palate along its posterior edge. The velar muscles are then sharply dissected from the oral and nasal mucosal layers for 2 to 3 mm from the medial cleft edge, permitting reorientation of the muscle fibers into a transverse palatal sling (see Fig. 281-2).

The medial edges of the oral and nasal mucosa are grasped and gently pulled toward the midline. Approximation of the edges should be possible without tension. If further mobilization is needed to allow tension-free closure in the midline, three additional maneuvers may be performed (lateral dissection in the space of Ernst between the superior constrictor muscles and pterygoids, further mobilization of the neurovascular bundle by sharply dissecting it free from the mucoperiosteal flap, or infracturing the hamulus).

After achieving adequate medial mobilization, the nasal mucosa, the velar musculature, and the oral mucoperiosteal flaps are closed in three separate layers. Closure of the nasal layer begins anteriorly and proceeds toward the uvula using 4-0 chromic suture with a small G-2 or PS-4-CP needle. Interrupted, inverted sutures are placed with the knot on the nasal surface (Fig. 281-3). The velar muscles are approximated in the midline using 4-0 Vicryl suture (Fig. 281-4). The oral layer is then closed with 4-0 chromic suture, starting at the uvula and advancing anteriorly toward the hard palate. Vertical mattress sutures are used in the region of the hard palate for approximation of the wound edges and for stabilization of the mucoperiosteal flaps to the underlying nasal mucosa. This reduces the risk of hematoma formation and flap detachment postoperatively.

After medial closure, the lateral incisions are loosely approximated using chromic suture. If the lateral incisions cannot be closed without tension, partial closure is accomplished, and oxidized cellulose is inserted between the wound edges to cover the exposed bare bone (Fig. 281-5).

BECKY MCGRAW-WALL

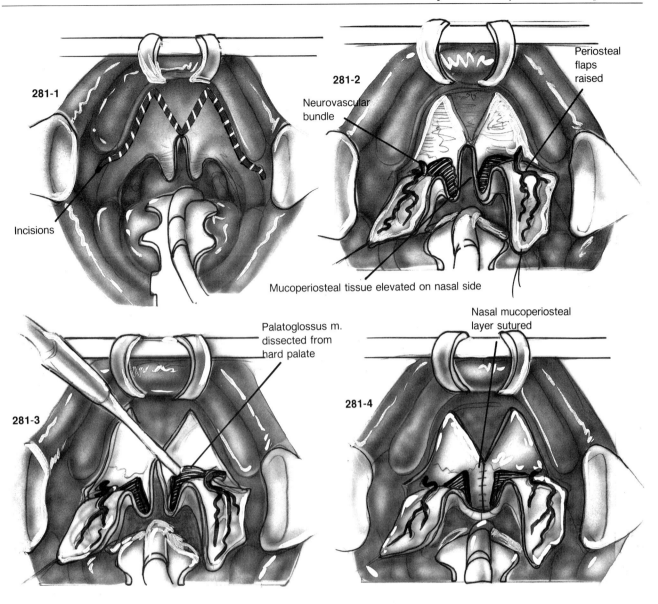

281-1

Incisions

281-2

Periosteal
flaps
raised

Neurovascular
bundle

Mucoperiosteal tissue elevated on nasal side

281-3

Palatoglossus m.
dissected from
hard palate

Nasal mucoperiosteal
layer sutured

281-4

281-5. Palatoglossus m. and oral mucosa sutured

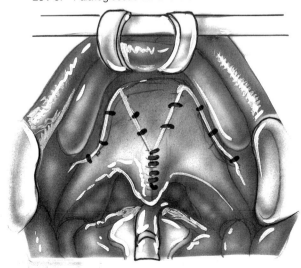

282. COMPLETE UNILATERAL CLEFT PALATE REPAIR (TWO-FLAP PALATOPLASTY WITH INTRAVELAR VELOPLASTY)—Complete

unilateral cleft palate defects involve the soft palate, secondary and primary hard palate, and extend to the alveolus, which is usually clefted. The surgical goal of palatoplasty is to accomplish closure of the defect, while reconstructing a competent velopharyngeal sphincter to prevent nasal emission of air during speech. The repair involves closure of the oral and nasal mucosal layers in addition to the repair of the soft palate musculature.

Indications
1. Unrepaired unilateral cleft of the palate
2. Symptoms of velopharyngeal insufficiency

Special Considerations
1. Closure ideally completed before speech development, usually between 6 and 18 months
2. Potential maxillofacial growth disturbances and occlusal abnormalities related to surgery
3. Concomitant middle ear disease, affecting hearing and speech
4. Nutrition and feeding
5. Team management involving speech pathology, orthodontists, and cleft surgeons

Preoperative Preparation
1. Evaluation of cleft width, inclination of palatal shelves, and attachment of vomer to noncleft side
2. Bleeding and coagulation studies

Special Instruments, Position, and Anesthesia
1. Headlight
2. Trendelenburg position, foam doughnut
3. Dingmann mouth gag
4. Injection of palate with a solution of 0.5% lidocaine with 1:100,000 epinephrine
5. Woodson elevator, nerve hook, and Dean scissors
6. Oxidized cellulose (Surgicel)

Tips and Pearls
1. Judicious dissection of neurovascular pedicle from flap to increase mobility and reduce tension
2. Infracture of the hamulus as needed if further mobilization required
3. Three-layered closure of soft palate with reconstruction of palatal muscle sling
4. Two-layered closure of hard palate, followed by approximation of these layers to eliminate dead space

Pitfalls and Complications
1. Postoperative bleeding
2. Mucoperiosteal flap necrosis
3. Oronasal fistula formation
4. Infection
5. Persistent velopharyngeal incompetence

Postoperative Care Issues
1. Postoperative monitoring for airway obstruction, adequate fluid balance, and hemostasis
2. Counsel parents about pain management, fever, diet restrictions, and fluid intake.
3. Feed with spoon or bulb syringe postoperatively; avoid pacifiers or sucking on nipples.

References
Bardach J, Salyer KE. Surgical techniques in cleft lip and palate. St. Louis: Mosby-Year Book, 1991:224.

Dado DV. Early cleft palate repair with intravelar veloplasty. In: Kernahan DA, Rosenstein SW, eds. Cleft lip and palate: a system of management. Baltimore: Williams & Wilkins, 1990:189.

Operative Procedure

With the patient supine in the Trendelenburg position, the Dingmann mouth gag is positioned to expose the palate. The proposed mucoperiosteal flaps are marked with gentian violet before infiltrating with local anesthetic. The flaps are based posteriorly on the descending palatine artery (Fig. 282-1).

A #15 blade scalpel is used to incise the medial aspect of the flap, starting at the base of the uvula and extending the incision to the alveolus, while holding traction on the uvula. The incision is then continued posteriorly to the tip of the uvula. Along the soft palate, the incision is placed at the junction of the oral and nasal mucosa. Along the hard palate, notice whether the vomer is attached to the palatal shelf on the noncleft side. If the vomer is not attached to the palate, the incision is placed 1 to 3 mm lateral to the cleft edge (see Fig. 282-1). This leaves a strip of oral mucosa attached to the nasal mucosa that can be rotated medially to facilitate tension-free closure of the nasal layer. If the vomer is attached to the palatal shelf, the incision is placed at the medial edge of the cleft and a flap of mucoperiosteum from the vomer is developed to facilitate closure of the nasal layer.

Laterally, the incision is begun about 1 cm posterior to the maxillary tuberosity, curving around the tuberosity along the base of the alveolus to meet the medial incision. The mucoperiosteal flaps are elevated from the hard palate using a Freer or Woodson elevator. Posteriorly, it is important to identify and preserve the neurovascular bundle exiting from the greater palatine foramen. The nerve is gently stretched and dissected from the posterior flap using a nerve hook to mobilize the flap (Fig. 282-2). The flap elevation should continue to the posterior edge of the hard palate medial and lateral to the neurovascular bundle.

Beginning at the posteromedial edge of the cleft, the mucosa is elevated from the nasal surface of the hard palate to allow medialization of the nasal mucosa. A Woodson elevator or right-angled palatal elevator is helpful for elevating around the curve of the cleft edge. Using the Woodson elevator, dissect the velar muscles from their attachment to the posterior border of the hard palate. Continue the dissection of the mucosa from the nasal side of the hard palate along its posterior edge. The velar muscles are then sharply dissected from the oral and nasal mucosa for 2 to 3 mm from the medial cleft edge (Fig. 282-3). Mobilizing the nasal mucosa and detaching the muscles permit lengthening of the palate and reorientation of the muscle fibers into a functional palatal muscle sling.

Grasp the medial edges of the oral and nasal mucoperichondrial flaps, and gently pull them toward the midline. If further mobilization is needed to allow tension-free closure, lateral dissection in the space of Ernst may be carried out. The neurovascular bundle can also be further mobilized by sharply dissecting it free from the mucoperiosteal flap posteriorly for approximately 1 cm. In cases of severe clefting, the hamulus may be identified laterally and infractured, or the attachment of the tensor veli palatini muscle tendon may be dissected free to maximize medial mobility of the flap.

The nasal mucosa, velar musculature, and oral mucoperichondrial flaps are closed in three separate layers. Closure of the nasal layer starts anteriorly and proceeds toward the uvula using interrupted, inverted sutures placed with the knots on the nasal side (Fig. 282-4). If the vomer is attached to the noncleft side, a vomerine flap is developed and rotated medially, and is then approximated to the nasal mucoperiosteum on the cleft side. The velar muscles are approximated in the midline using 4-0 Vicryl suture (Fig. 282-5). Starting at the uvula tip, the oral mucoperiosteum is closed using 4-0 chromic. Vertical mattress sutures are used in the region of the hard palate for stabilization of the oral flaps to the underlying nasal mucosa, reducing the risk of hematoma formation and flap detachment postoperatively.

After medial closure, the lateral incisions are loosely approximated. If the lateral incisions cannot be closed without tension, partial closure is accomplished, and oxidized cellulose is inserted between the wound edges to cover the exposed bare bone laterally (Fig. 282-6).

BECKY MCGRAW-WALL

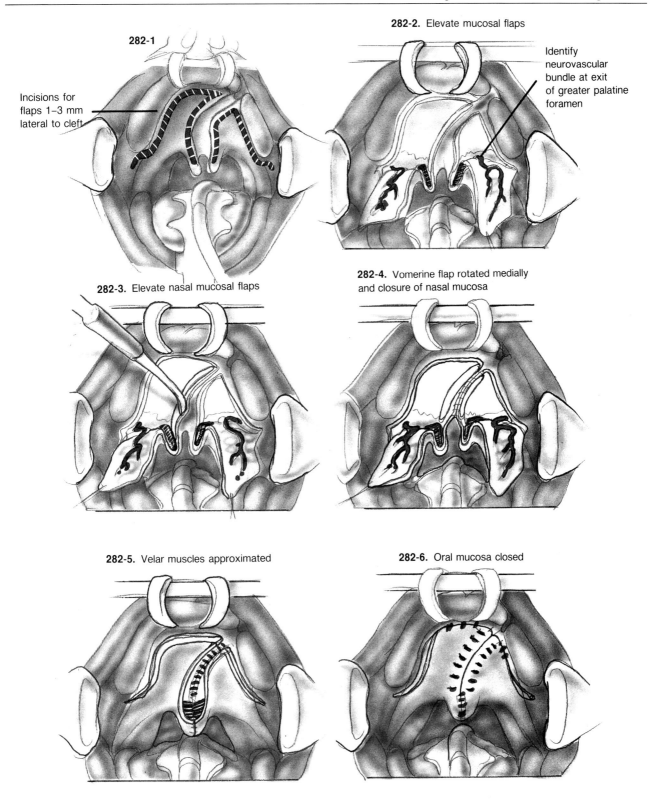

282-1

Incisions for
flaps 1–3 mm
lateral to cleft

282-2. Elevate mucosal flaps

Identify
neurovascular
bundle at exit
of greater palatine
foramen

282-3. Elevate nasal mucosal flaps

282-4. Vomerine flap rotated medially
and closure of nasal mucosa

282-5. Velar muscles approximated

282-6. Oral mucosa closed

■ *283.* ORONASAL AND OROANTRAL FISTULA REPAIR

ORONASAL AND OROANTRAL FISTULA REPAIR—Closure of a communication between the oral and nasal cavity (ie, oronasal fistula) or between the oral cavity and maxillary antrum (ie, oroantral fistula). Most commonly, such communications develop as a complication after cleft palate repair, but they may result from accidental or iatrogenic trauma, neoplasm, dental extractions, or infection. Symptoms may include the passage of air, fluids, or food through the fistula and may interfere with speech production or cause maxillary sinusitis, depending on the location of the fistula. Ideally, the repair involves closure of the oral and nasal mucosal layers, using mucoperiosteal rotation-advancement flaps.

Indications

1. Presence of symptomatic oronasal or oroantral fistula

Special Considerations

1. The size, shape, and location of the fistula are important when considering the approach to repair.
2. Complete revision of the palatoplasty procedure is indicated for large fistulas resulting from cleft palate repair.
3. Presence or absence of teeth adjacent to the fistula affects the repair technique.
4. Sinus infection requires treatment before the repair of oroantral fistula.

Preoperative Preparation

1. Routine laboratory studies
2. Bleeding and coagulation studies as indicated

Special Instruments, Position, and Anesthesia

1. Headlight
2. Trendelenburg position, with the head in a foam doughnut
3. Dingmann mouth gag
4. Injection of the fistula and proposed flap with a solution of 1% lidocaine with 1:100,000 epinephrine

Tips and Pearls

1. Two-layered closure of nasal and oral layers ensures complete repair of fistula.
2. Wide elevation and mobilization of the palatal flaps for tension-free closure of repair
3. Preservation of the greater palatine artery pedicle is important for flap survival.
4. Placement of the oral suture line 3 to 5 mm away from fistula edge improves the success of repair.
5. Large oronasal fistulas may require elevation of bilateral mucoperiosteal flaps for closure.

Pitfalls and Complications

1. Postoperative bleeding or infection
2. Mucoperiosteal flap necrosis with reformation of oronasal fistula

Postoperative Care Issues

1. Postoperative antibiotics for 7 to 10 days to cover oral flora
2. Avoid nose blowing for 2 weeks after surgery
3. Soft diet for adults; spoon or bulb syringe feedings for children
4. No pacifiers or sucking on nipples for 2 weeks postoperatively
5. Dental appliances may not be worn for 6 weeks after repair.

References

Bardach J, Salyer KE. Surgical techniques in cleft lip and palate. St. Louis: Mosby Year Book, 1991:224.

Del Junco R, Rappaport I, Allison GR. Persistent oral antral fistulas. Arch Otolaryngol Head Neck Surg 1988;114:1315.

Operative Procedure

With the patient supine in the Trendelenburg position, the Dingmann mouth gag is positioned to expose the palate and fistula. The proposed mucoperiosteal flaps are marked with gentian violet before infiltrating a solution of 1% lidocaine with 1:100,000 epinephrine. Oronasal and oroantral fistulas may be closed using a combination of a turnover flap to close the inner layer and a rotation-advancement flap to close the oral layer (Fig. 283-1).

A turnover flap is created from the oral mucosa adjacent to the fistula, equal to the diameter of the fistula. The turnover flap is incised with a #15 blade scalpel through the periosteum. The flap is then elevated based on the edge of the fistula and rotated inward with the mucosa facing the nasal or antral cavity. The incision around the fistula opposite the turnover flap is placed 1 to 2 mm lateral to the fistula edge, leaving a strip of oral mucosa adjacent to the fistula. This strip of oral mucosa is rotated inward to allow tension-free closure of the inner layer. Undermining of the nasal or antral mucosa adjacent to the fistula is carried out using a Woodson or cleft palate elevator. The turnover flap is sutured to the opposite mucosa, closing the inner layer of the fistula (Fig. 283-2). Interrupted, inverted sutures are placed with the knot on the nasal surface. A small G-2 or PS-4-CP needle is useful for approximation of the nasal layer.

The oral rotation-advancement flap is designed on the side of the fistula opposite the turnover flap and is based posteriorly on the greater palatine artery. The flap needs to be appropriately sized to completely cover the fistula and the donor site for the turnover flap. Laterally, the flap is usually extended to the junction of the alveolus and hard palate, and posteriorly, it is extended to the maxillary tuberosity. If the fistula is centrally located in the palate, the medial incision follows the midline. If the fistula is laterally located or oroantral, the incision away from the fistula may be placed in the midline or, depending on the size of the fistula to be repaired, may extend around the opposite alveolar-palatine junction to incorporate the entire palatal mucosa.

The rotation-advancement flap incision is carried to the subperiosteal plane, after which the flap is elevated from the hard palate using a Freer or Woodson elevator. Care is taken to preserve the integrity of the neurovascular pedicle. The oral mucoperiosteal flap is then rotated to cover the fistula completely. Approximation of the mucosal edges should be possible without tension. If further mobilization is needed to allow tension-free closure, the neurovascular bundle can be gently stretched, and lateral dissection in the space of Ernst between the superior constrictor muscles and pterygoids may be bluntly carried out. The oral layer is then sutured and secured to the nasal layer using 4-0 chromic vertical mattress sutures (Fig. 283-3). The flap donor site is left to granulate, usually healing within 6 weeks.

Anterior fistulas of the hard palate often require elevation of bilateral mucoperiosteal flaps, similar to the flaps used in the repair of a unilateral cleft palate (Fig. 283-4). Adequate mobilization of the rotation-advancement flaps and careful approximation of the nasal layer are essential to the success of the repair. Larger fistulas following cleft palate repair generally require total reoperation of the palatoplasty, with mobilization of bilateral mucoperiosteal flaps and two-layered repair of the hard palate fistula (see Procedure 282). Fistulas located or extending into the soft palate demand three-layered repair to reconstruct the velopharyngeal musculature.

When dealing with nasoantral fistulas, all necrotic tissue and infected bone must be debrided before closure. If periapical or periodontal disease is present in adjacent teeth, extraction may be indicated before repair. The rotation flap can not be adequately anchored to diseased mucosa adjacent to the fistula, and extraction can facilitate advancement of the mucoperiosteal flap. It may be necessary to tailor the rotation-advancement flap to conform to the neighboring teeth without buckling or tension. Occasionally, a buccal advancement flap may be required in combination with the palatal rotation-advancement flap for closure of large oroantral fistulas.

BECKY L. MCGRAW-WALL
JENNIFER KEIR-GARZA

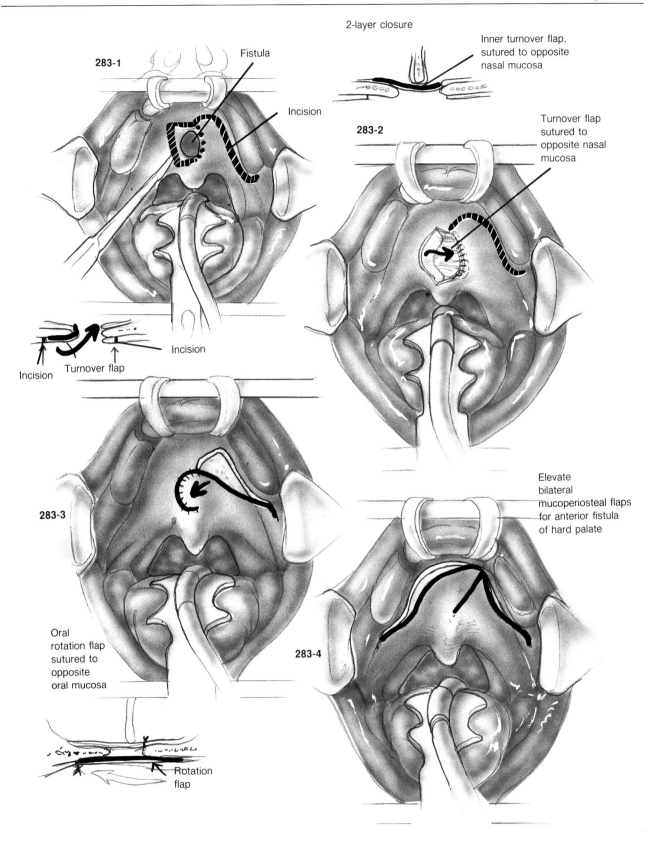

2-layer closure

Inner turnover flap, sutured to opposite nasal mucosa

283-1

Fistula

Incision

283-2

Turnover flap sutured to opposite nasal mucosa

Incision

Incision   Turnover flap

283-3

Elevate bilateral mucoperiosteal flaps for anterior fistula of hard palate

283-4

Oral rotation flap sutured to opposite oral mucosa

Rotation flap

■ 284. SUPERIORLY BASED PHARYNGEAL
FLAP—Surgical correction of velopharyngeal insufficiency with a superiorly based musculomucosal flap from the pharynx

Indications
1. Correction of velopharyngeal insufficiency with central movement defect but good lateral wall motion

Contraindications
1. The procedure is relatively contraindicated in patients with velopharyngeal insufficiency with poor or absent lateral wall motion. Sphincter pharyngoplasty may yield better results.

Special Considerations
1. The surgical decision is made with input from the speech therapy evaluation.
2. Appropriate evaluations, including nasopharyngoscopy, must be performed to confirm a correct diagnosis.

Preoperative Preparation
1. Routine laboratory studies
2. Bleeding and clotting studies, if the history warrants

Special Instruments, Position, and Anesthesia
1. Dingman mouth gag, palatal elevators, cleft palate instruments
2. Surgeon seated at the head of the table, with the patient's head in the surgeon's lap
3. General anesthesia with oral endotracheal intubation

Tips and Pearls
1. The surgical goal is to allow velopharyngeal competency without nasal obstruction.
2. The flap, level of the flap base, and the lateral port size are determined by preoperative evaluations.
3. Pediatric endotracheal tube sizes 3 to 3.5 are used in patients with poor lateral wall motion.
4. Endotracheal tube sizes 4 to 4.5 are used in patients with modest lateral wall motion.
5. Endotracheal tube sizes 5 to 5.5 are used in patients with good lateral wall motion.
6. Patients with minimal lateral wall movement have a higher risk of developing hyponasality and airway obstruction.
7. Flap base level should be placed at the level of maximal lateral wall movement. This can be determined by preoperative nasal endoscopy. The prominence of the first cervical vertebra is a helpful landmark in making this determination.

Pitfalls and Complications
1. Hyponasality and airway obstruction may result from excess flap width and from scar tissue formation, leading to obliteration of the lateral ports.
2. Persistent velopharyngeal insufficiency can result if the flap is too narrow.
3. The soft palate may become immobilized secondary to surgical manipulation and scarring, increasing reliance on lateral wall movement for closure.

Postoperative Care Issues
1. Patients are typically hospitalized for overnight observation and dismissed the next day. It is important to have room mist to enhance humidification. Antibiotics are given for 1 week postoperatively. The airway needs to be monitored for 1 night after surgery.
2. Port-controlled tubes are removed the morning after surgery.

References
Crockett DM. Velopharyngeal incompetence. In: Healy GB, ed. Common problems in pediatric otolaryngology. Chicago: Year Book Medical Publishers, 1990.

Shprintzen RJ. Surgery for speech: the planning of operations for velopharyngeal insufficiency with emphasis on the preoperative assessment of both pharyngeal physiology and articulation. In: Huddart AJ, Ferguson MWJ, eds. Cleft lip and palate: long term results and future prospects, vol I. New York: Manchester University Press, 1990: 430–447.

Operative Procedure
The procedure is performed with the patient placed supine and under general anesthesia with oral endotracheal intubation. The surgeon is seated at the head of the table with the patient's head in the surgeon's lap. The mouth is held open with a Dingman mouth gag. Local anesthetic containing epinephrine may be infiltrated into the midline of the soft palate and the posterior pharyngeal wall.

The soft palate is split in the midline in full-thickness fashion (Fig. 284-1). Two retaining sutures may be placed, one on each side of the split uvula to offer countertraction. At this point, more anesthetic solution may be deposited under the nasal mucosal side of the soft palate. The posterior pharyngeal wall is then marked for the pharyngeal flap. The width of the flap is determined by the amount of velopharyngeal insufficiency. The superior base of the flap should be positioned at a level high enough into the nasopharynx that the entire flap is not visible postoperatively on direct inspection with the patient's mouth open. This ensures positioning the pharyngeal flap at the appropriate level of velopharyngeal closure.

The pharyngeal flap is incised with a #15 scalpel down to the loose areolar layer, superficial to the prevertebral fascia (Fig. 284-2). Elevation is accomplished up to the superior base of the flap. The nasal mucosa of the soft palate is incised in a horizontal fashion, extending from the lateral soft palate borders across to the apex of the palatal split incision. The nasal mucosa is reflected, based on the posterior palatal borders bilaterally (Fig. 284-3). The pharyngeal flap is sutured to the nonreflected nasal mucosal edge using 4-0 Vicryl simple interrupted sutures (Fig. 284-4). It is helpful to place a substantial mattress suture in the center of this closure to help minimize tension. The previous nasal mucosal layers are redraped down along the raw undersurface of the elevated pharyngeal flap (Fig. 284-5). A few tacking sutures may be placed to anchor the mucosa in position. The palatal split is closed in layers, and the pharyngeal flap donor site may be closed or left open, depending on the amount of lateral port aperture required (Fig. 284-6). If endotracheal tubes are to be used for port control, they should be inserted before suturing the pharyngeal flap to the posterior nasal surface of the soft palate. These control tubes are usually removed the day after surgery.

TOM D. WANG

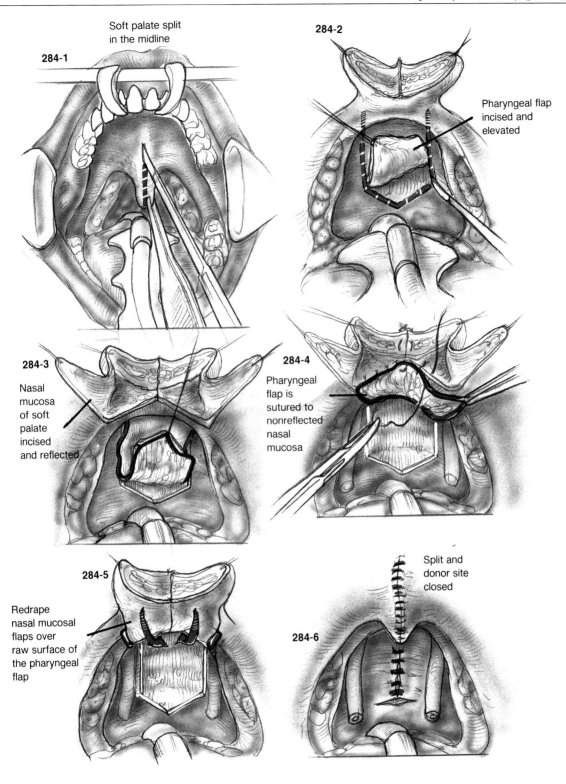

284-1

Soft palate split in the midline

284-2

Pharyngeal flap incised and elevated

284-3

Nasal mucosa of soft palate incised and reflected

284-4

Pharyngeal flap is sutured to nonreflected nasal mucosa

284-5

Redrape nasal mucosal flaps over raw surface of the pharyngeal flap

284-6

Split and donor site closed

■ *285.* SURGICAL APPROACHES TO THE TEMPOROMANDIBULAR JOINT—Several approaches

are used to treat diseased temporomandibular joints:

Preauricular: 2.5- to 3.5-cm vertical incision in the preauricular fold

Endaural (modified): 2.0- to 3.0-cm vertical incision along the posterior tragal cartilage (tragus is not split)

Postauricular: 5-cm incision, 3 to 5 mm posterior to the auriculocephalic sulcus, extending from the superior auricle to the mastoid tip; the external auditory canal is transected.

Hemicoronal: curvilinear temporal incision; can be an extension of any of the previous incisions

Submandibular: 2.5- to 5-cm incision 1 cm inferior to the inferior border of the mandible in the angle region

Indications

1. Preauricular: traditional approach; may encounter superficial temporal vessels
2. Endaural (modified): cosmetic, quick and easy dissection, and excellent access; best approach
3. Postauricular: cosmetic, increased bleeding (eg, postauricular artery), and auditory canal stenosis (rare); rarely indicated
4. Hemicoronal: exposure of the zygomatic arch or temporalis muscle-fascia flap
5. Submandibular: access to the ramus

Preoperative Preparation

1. Antibiotic prophylaxis for *Staphylococcus*
2. Preparation of the ear canal

Special Instruments, Position, and Anesthesia

1. Nasal endotracheal tube
2. Hypotensive anesthesia provides increased visibility.

Tips and Pearls

1. Inject the superior joint space with 1 to 2 mL of local anesthetic with a vasoconstrictor before making the incisions.

Pitfalls and Complications

1. Medial bleeding
2. Facial nerve injury (eg, frontal, zygomatic)
3. Frey's syndrome
4. External auditory canal perforation

Postoperative Care Issues

1. Pressure dressing for 24 hours
2. Cotton ear plug for 24 hours to prevent blood in the canal
3. Adequate pain control; use a PCA pump
4. Liquid diet; advance as tolerated to soft foods

References

Howerton DW, Zysset M. Anatomy of the temporomandibular joint and related structures with surgical anatomic considerations. Oral Maxillofac Clin North Am 1989;1:229.

Ide Y, Nakazawa K. Anatomical atlas of the temporomandibular joint. Tokyo: Quintessence, 1991.

Operative Procedures

Endaural Approach

The endaural approach to the temporomandibular joint (TMJ) is preferred because the auriculotemporal nerve and superficial temporal vessels are avoided, surgical access is excellent, potential complications are minimized, and aesthetic results are superior (Figs. 285-1 and 285-2). After prepping, 1 to 2 mL of local anesthetic with a vasoconstrictor is injected into the superior joint space.

The incision is started superiorly in the crease above the tragal cartilage. It is 2.5 to 3.5 cm long and follows the posterior margin of the tragal cartilage, ending just superior and anterior to the lobe. Supraperichondrial dissection along the anterior tragal cartilage is performed with a small tenotomy scissors (Fig. 285-3).

After exposure of 0.5 to 1 cm of tragal cartilage, blunt dissection over the temporal arch with a hemostat exposes the deeper temporalis fascia. After the temporalis fascia is identified, a hemostat is slid inferiorly, along the anterior tragal margin, between the deep and superficial temporalis fascia layers for the full length of the incision. This defines the temporal fascia plane, which continues inferiorly as the parotidomasseteric fascia. The tissue over the hemostat is incised with electrocautery. A Dean scissors incises the temporal fascia over the posterior temporal arch, and a flap is elevated anteriorly just below the temporal fascia to the articular eminence. The auriculotemporal nerve, temporal vessels, and facial nerve are retracted superiorly and anteriorly within the flap (Fig. 285-4).

With electrocautery, the lateral ligament of the TMJ and periosteum over the glenoid fossa are incised horizontally along the inferior margin of the temporal arch. The lateral ligament is reflected inferiorly, exposing the superior extent of the TMJ capsule and its attachment to the lateral fossa. A #15 scalpel blade is directed superiorly and anteriorly, and the superior joint space is entered through the lateral capsule (Fig. 285-5A). By previously distending the superior joint space and by angling the blade superiorly, damage to the disc is avoided (Fig. 285-5B). A Freer elevator is gently placed into the space, taking care not to damage the lining of the fossa, which can lead to scarring and adhesions (Fig. 285-6). The remainder of the surgery is then completed.

Incision closure is uncomplicated. The lateral capsule and ligament are clinically indistinguishable, and as a unit, they are repaired with several resorbable sutures to the lateral temporal arch.

Preauricular Approach

The preauricular approach, with or without temporal extension, is the more traditional approach (see Figs. 285-1 and 285-2). Recently described techniques involve an incision in the pretragal fold. The disadvantage of this approach includes a more evident scar and a greater chance of damage to the auriculotemporal nerve and superficial temporal vessels. The surgical dissection is similar to the endaural approach.

Postauricular Approach

The postauricular approach requires a large postauricular incision and transection of the external auditory canal (see Figs. 285-1 and 285-2). A 3- to 5-cm incision posterior to the auriculocephalic sulcus is extended from the superior extent of the auricle down to the mastoid tip. A superficial dissection is carried above the superficial fascia and through the auricularis muscle. The posterior auricular artery may be encountered. The external auditory canal is transected, and the tragal cartilage is exposed anteriorly. The remaining dissection proceeds as described previously. If conchal cartilage is to be harvested, this approach provides excellent access.

Hemicoronal Approach

Any of the previously described approaches can be extended into a hemicoronal flap for access to the temporalis muscle and fascia (see Figs. 285-1 and 285-2). A curvilinear incision extends superiorly into the temporal region. Branches of the superficial temporal artery are often palpable and can be avoided in the incision. Dissection proceeds down to the deep temporalis fascia, directly overlying the muscle, and a free temporalis fascia graft can be harvested from the muscle surface. If an axial-based muscle-fascia flap is desired, incision should be parallel to the direction of the muscle fibers.

DAVID A. COTTRELL

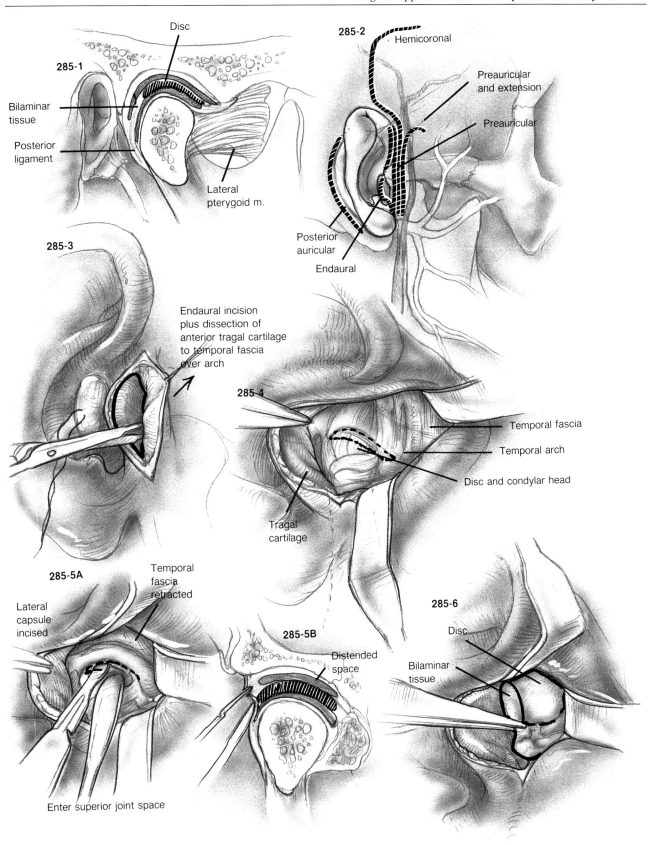

285-1

Disc

Bilaminar tissue

Posterior ligament

Lateral pterygoid m.

285-2

Hemicoronal

Preauricular and extension

Preauricular

Posterior auricular

Endaural

285-3

Endaural incision plus dissection of anterior tragal cartilage to temporal fascia over arch

285-4

Temporal fascia

Temporal arch

Disc and condylar head

Tragal cartilage

285-5A

Temporal fascia retracted

Lateral capsule incised

Enter superior joint space

285-5B

Distended space

285-6

Disc

Bilaminar tissue

■ 286. TEMPOROMANDIBULAR JOINT AR- TICULAR DISC REPOSITIONING—Procedure to reposition and stabilize a displaced temporomandibular joint articular disc

Indications
1. Failed conservative therapy
2. Internal derangement with pain or dysfunction
3. Pathology (eg, pannus in rheumatoid arthritis)

Special Considerations
1. Diagnostic blocks

Preoperative Preparation
1. Magnetic resonance imaging and tomograms
2. Routine laboratory studies

Special Instruments, Position, and Anesthesia
1. Microneedle holder
2. Polydioxanone (PDS) or Vicryl suture on a P-2 needle
3. A 1.5-mm twist drill, 28-gauge wire, #0 braided nylon, and French-eye needle (optional)

Tips and Pearls
1. Anterior disc release
2. Meniscoplasty
3. Posterior and lateral ligament repair
4. Smooth osteophytes

Pitfalls and Complications
1. Damage to fibrocartilage lining the fossa and condyle
2. Disc repair to elastic portion of bilaminar tissues only
3. Failure to release the disc anteriorly

Postoperative Care Issues
1. Alteration of parafunctional habits
2. Physical therapy
3. Altered diet (ie, full liquid; advance to dental soft as tolerated)
4. Pain Control (patient-controlled analgesia pump)

References
Zetz MR, Ash DC. Double-layered closure for temporomandibular joint discoplasty. J Oral Maxillofac Surg 1986;44:965.

Operative Procedure

A standard endaural incision and dissection to the superior joint space is performed (see Procedure 285), and the disc is identified. The lateral ligament and capsular attachments to the temporal arch should be released to ensure proper access and mobility of the disc. A horizontal incision is made over the lateral pole of the condyle, and a small Freer elevator is passed into the inferior joint space. Additional disc attachments to the lateral condylar head are released with a Dean scissors. Care is taken not to scratch or damage the fibrocartilage covering the fossa or condyle. The disc is then mobilized and pulled over the condyle by releasing the anterior, lateral, and if needed, medial capsule and disc attachments with a Freer elevator. This is performed by passing a Freer elevator anterior to the arch, with the curve of the elevator tip aimed superiorly (Figs. 286-1 and 286-2). Resistance is encountered, and with firm but controlled pressure, the Freer "pops" through the anterior capsule. This approach is performed incrementally, from a medial to lateral direction until the Freer can be passed without resistance. Greater mobility of the disc should be achieved, but often, anterior and lateral capsular and ligament attachments to the temporal arch and condyle require further releasing. By applying a posterior pull on the disc with a toothed forceps, the point of the restriction can often be identified. If the disc can not be adequately repositioned laterally, medial releasing may be required. This must be done with extreme caution because of potential damage to medial vessels.

Significant venous bleeding is often encountered when the anterior capsule is freed because of the pericapsular venous network. This bleeding is usually self-limited, but it can be stopped by pushing the mandible and condyle up into the fossa and by injecting local anesthesia with vasoconstrictor.

The retrodiscal bilaminar tissue is identified and grasped just behind the posterior band of the disc with an Adson forceps (Fig. 286-3A). Using a Dean scissors, the bilaminar tissue is transected along the forceps, which leaves small bilaminar attachment to the disc (see Fig. 286-3B). Transection is carried to the medial wall of the fossa. Posteriorly, the bilaminar tissue is also transected in a similar fashion, and the wedge of bilaminar tissue is removed. The volume resected varies with the degree of displacement of the articular disc, but a small amount of bilaminar tissue usually remains attached to the posterior disc.

The bilaminar zone is plicated to the posterior band of the disc with several individual sets of running 4-0 PDS sutures on a P-2 needle (Fig. 286-4A). Suturing begins medially and can be tedious; magnifying loupes can help with suturing. Care is taken to ensure that the needle passes not only through the elastic portion of bilaminar tissue but also through the posterior ligament (ie, fibrous layer of the bilaminar zone). The posterior ligament rests against the condylar head, contains no elastic fibers, is stable enough to suture to, and resists stretching. To accomplish this, the needle is angled inferiorly into the bilaminar tissue and driven toward the condylar neck. The needle is then directed superiorly, out of the tissue (see Fig. 286-4B). If the fibrous layer is properly engaged, there is minimal play in the suture. The suture then passes through the posterior disc, engaging approximately 2 mm of the posterior band. Suturing continues laterally to the lateral pole, closing the inferior joint space (Fig. 286-5). The mandible is mobilized to ensure good disc position and function. The incision is then closed in a layered fashion. At the completion of surgery, the occlusion is examined, and if significant shifting has occurred or further correction of an existing jaw deformity is indicated, appropriate orthognathic procedures are performed.

Additional support to the repositioned disc can be provided by passing a #0 braided nylon suture through a prepared tunnel in the posterior condylar head. The suture is first passed through the posterior band of the disc in a horizontal mattress fashion. The needle is removed, and the suture is pulled through the prepared hole in the condyle with a 28-gauge pull-through wire. The suture is then passed through the lateral disc with a French-eye needle, and the suture is tied (Fig. 286-6). This technique provides posterior and lateral support to the disc.

DAVID A. COTTRELL

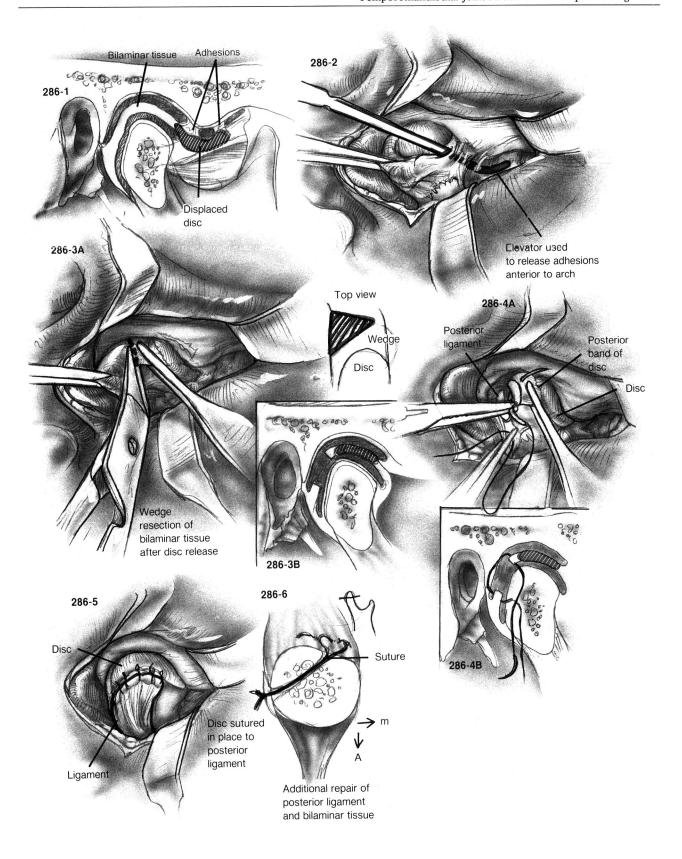

286-1

Bilaminar tissue   Adhesions

Displaced
disc

286-2

Elevator used
to release adhesions
anterior to arch

286-3A

Top view

Wedge

Disc

Wedge
resection of
bilaminar tissue
after disc release

286-3B

286-4A

Posterior
ligament

Posterior
band of
disc

Disc

286-4B

286-5

Disc

Ligament

286-6

Suture

m

A

Disc sutured
in place to
posterior
ligament

Additional repair of
posterior ligament
and bilaminar tissue

■ *287.* BONE GRAFT RECONSTRUCTION OF THE TEMPOROMANDIBULAR JOINT—Procedure

to replace the condyle or ramus with a free bone graft. For a costochondral graft, the contralateral fifth or sixth rib with a cartilaginous cap replaces the mandibular condyle. For a sternoclavicular graft, a split clavicular graft with fibrocartilaginous cap and disc replaces the mandibular condyle.

Indications
1. Congenital defects
2. Traumatic avulsion
3. Ankylosis
4. Pathology
5. Congenital and acquired condyle growth center deformities

Contraindications
1. Previous Proplast/Teflon implants
2. Sternoclavicular graft in a patient younger than 5 years of age

Special Considerations
1. A sternoclavicular graft can be harvested with its own fibrocartilage disc. A costochondral graft requires an interpositional graft.
2. A sternoclavicular graft contains a greater volume of cortical and cancellous bone, is stronger, and histologically more closely resembles the temporomandibular joint (TMJ).
3. For a sternoclavicular graft, the ipsilateral donor site is harvested for lateral placement of the graft, and contralateral harvest is indicated for posterior or medial placement of the graft.
4. The rib on the contralateral side is harvested for lateral placement.

Preoperative Preparation
1. Computed tomography scan
2. Dental model workup
3. Splint construction

Special Instruments, Position, and Anesthesia
1. Rigid fixation
2. Arch bars and intermaxillary fixation (IMF)

Tips and Pearls
1. Delay donor graft harvest until the recipient site is prepared.
2. IMF during graft placement

Pitfalls and Complications
1. Malocclusion
2. Tinnitus, vertigo, and middle ear effusion
3. Injury to cranial nerves V and VII
4. Clavicle fracture (donor site) postoperatively
5. Pneumothorax

Postoperative Care Issues
1. Figure-of-eight clavicle harness and no heavy lifting for 3 months with sternoclavicular harvest
2. Physical therapy for jaw
3. Liquid diet for 6 weeks and soft diet for 3 months

Reference
Wolford LM, Cottrell DA, Henry CH. Sternoclavicular grafts for TMJ reconstruction. J Oral Maxillofac Surg 1994;52:119.

Operative Procedure

Arch bars are first applied to the upper and lower teeth. A standard preauricular or endaural dissection is performed to expose the TMJ. The condyle and condylar neck are isolated, and medial protection is provided with a Dautray retractor. Using a reciprocating saw, a condylectomy is performed, and the joint area is debrided. In ankylosis cases, the fossa commonly needs reshaping with a large, round bur. A coronoidectomy is sometimes necessary.

An autogenous interpositional material usually is placed between the bone graft and the fossa. If a sternoclavicular graft is used, the disc is harvested with the clavicular head (Fig. 287-4). If a costochondral graft is used, dermis, temporalis fascia, or a temporalis muscle-fascia flap are probably the best options. These are placed to line the fossa and can be fixed medially, anteriorly, and posteriorly with sutures to soft tissue and laterally to the temporal arch with sutures through prepared bone holes.

After the preparation of the recipient site, the appropriate donor site is approached, and the graft is harvested. Multiple holes are placed in the graft with a round bur to improve revascularization. The graft is positioned into the surgical site with the cartilaginous portion seated into the depth of the fossa (Fig. 287-5). Manual pressure is maintained on the graft during fixation in a superior direction to ensure it is fully seated. The graft can be placed medially, laterally, or posteriorly against the ramus. The position of the ramus relative to the glenoid fossa determines the best graft placement. Fixation of the graft to the ramus requires bone screws if placed medially or laterally, and they should be placed to avoid the inferior alveolar nerve (usually posterior to the nerve). A minimum of four screws is recommended. Occasionally, the graft needs to be placed along the posterior border of the ramus. It can be applied with bone plates, adapted and applied to the graft outside the surgical site, and then positioned on the ramus and fixed (Figs. 287-4 and 287-6). Lag screws can also be used.

After graft placement, the maxillomandibular fixation is released, and the occlusion is checked. To evaluate the occlusion, superior pressure is applied at the mandibular angles, and the mandible is rotated closed. This ensures full seating of the condyles (grafts) into the fossa. If the bite is incorrect, maxillomandibular fixation is reapplied, and the graft is repositioned.

Maxillomandibular fixation may be continued postoperatively.

Sternoclavicular Graft Harvest

The graft is harvested from the ipsilateral side if it is to be placed laterally; otherwise, the contralateral donor site is chosen for the best fit. Only the superior one half of the clavicle is harvested (Fig. 287-1). An 8- to 10-cm incision, 1 cm above and parallel to the clavicle, is made from the clavicular head and carried laterally. The incision is pulled over the clavicle, and electrocautery completes the dissection down to the periosteum (Fig. 287-2). The periosteum is incised, and subperiosteal dissection is completed over the superior aspect of the clavicle and is carried medially. Dissection around the clavicular head is supraperiosteal to maintain the ligamentous attachment to the articular disc. Great care must be exercised medially to avoid perforating into the plural cavity. The planned osteotomy cut is outlined with a small fissure bur (#701), and a reciprocating saw completes the osteotomy cut (Fig. 287-3). Laterally, the cut is tapered, rather than squared off, to avoid a weak point in the clavicle. Medially, the cut is continued through the clavicular head and is incised with a #15 blade. Medial protection during the osteotomy is imperative to prevent pleural or vascular injury. The periosteum is sutured, and the wound is closed in a layered fashion.

A figure-of-eight clavicular support is worn by the patient for 3 months to prevent clavicular fracture. Aesthetically, no clinical defect is noticeable at the donor site, because the superior portion of the clavicle regenerates to a large degree.

Costochondral Graft

Normally, the contralateral donor site is chosen for laterally positioned grafts. A standard approach to the fifth or sixth rib is used. The rib is harvested with a 1-cm cartilage cap and with the periosteum and perichondrium maintained at the costochondral junction. The wound is closed in a layered fashion.

DAVID A. COTTRELL

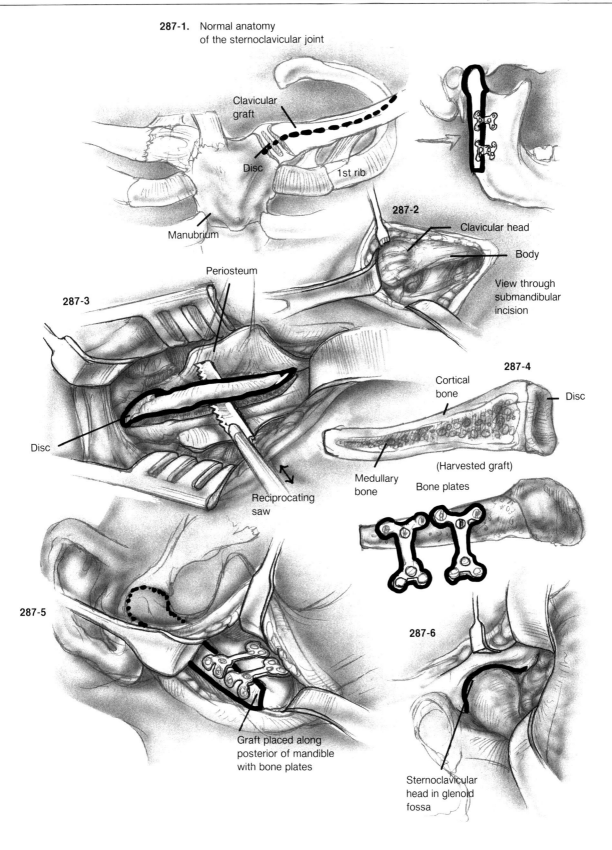

287-1. Normal anatomy of the sternoclavicular joint

Clavicular graft

Disc

1st rib

Manubrium

287-2

Clavicular head

Body

View through submandibular incision

Periosteum

287-3

Disc

Reciprocating saw

287-4

Cortical bone

Disc

Medullary bone

(Harvested graft)

Bone plates

287-5

Graft placed along posterior of mandible with bone plates

287-6

Sternoclavicular head in glenoid fossa

288. SKELETAL CORRECTION OF HEMIFACIAL MICROSOMIA—Surgical correction of the skeletal asymmetry secondary to deficient midface and mandibular growth

Indications

1. Congenital hypoplastic facial skeleton and normal occlusion (Munro Ia)
2. Congenital hemifacial flattening with a hypoplastic condyle, occlusal and labial cant and malocclusion (Munro Ib)
3. Congenital hemifacial flattening with malocclusion and absent ascending ramus, condyle, and glenoid fossa (Munro II through V)

Special Considerations

1. Timing of surgery may need to coincide with onset of school if psychosocial problems are associated with the facial deformity
2. Secondary surgery may be required when skeletal growth is completed in the teenage years.

Preoperative Preparation

1. Anteroposterior and lateral cephalograms
2. Panorex view
3. Dental impressions
4. Orthodontic consultation
5. Occlusal splint
6. Three-dimensional computed tomography scanning, particularly for severe cases (Munro III through V)

Special Instruments, Position, and Anesthesia

1. Headlight
2. Instruments for LeFort I, sagittal-split osteotomies (see Procedures 274 and 275) and rib and cranial bone graft harvests (see Procedures 259 and 260)

Tips and Pearls

1. Scars should be minimized, and a neck scar is almost never necessary.
2. Cranial bone should be used if possible for onlay grafting.
3. Costochondral grafts are necessary for ascending ramus and zygomatic arch reconstruction.

Pitfalls and Complications

1. Abnormal facial nerve position predisposes it to injury.
2. Inadequate skeletal fixation

Postoperative Care Issues

1. Careful airway monitoring is essential.
2. Intensive care unit observation is frequently necessary.

References

Munro IR. One-stage reconstruction of the temporomandibular joint in hemifacial microsomia. Plastic Reconstr Surg 1980;66:699.

Murray JE, Kaban LB, Mulliken JB. Analysis and treatment of hemifacial microsomia. Plast Reconstr Surg 1984;74:186.

Operative Procedure

A lower buccal sulcus incision is made on the affected side, and subperiosteal exposure of the mandible and vestigial ascending ramus and condylar remnant is performed. Dissection is carried anteriorly to the mental foramen. A temporal incision with a preauricular extension is made, and dissection is carried through the subcutaneous tissue and temporoparietal (ie, superficial temporal) fascia to the level of the innominate fascia. The dissection is developed in a cephalad to caudad direction on top of the superficial layer of the deep temporal fascia. This fascia is transected approximately 1 cm above the zygomatic arch, and subperiosteal dissection is used to expose the arch and the glenoid fossa. A tunnel is made to connect the temporal and oral exposures. The facial nerve, which is medially displaced, must be avoided; a nerve stimulator is an invaluable aid.

For a patient with a complete but hypoplastic skeleton, onlay cranial bone grafts are placed to augment the facial skeleton (see Fig. 288-1). Rib offers the advantage of easy contourability but is more prone to resorption and leaves a more conspicuous and painful donor site than cranial bone grafts. Split cranial grafts are harvested (see Procedure 260) and fixed using miniplate lag screws of appropriate length.

A patient with an intact skeleton but a labial and occlusal tilt requires two jaw osteotomies for correction of the deformity. Through an upper buccal sulcus incision, a LeFort I osteotomy is made (see Procedure 275). The normal side is shortened by removing a predetermined wedge of bone, and the contralateral side is lengthened and advanced (see Fig. 288-2A). The osteotomy fulcrum must be planned around the facial midline rather than the zygomatic buttress of the normal side to prevent excessive incisor show. Removal of a wedge of bone from the normal side and insertion of a graft on the affected side allow maxillary leveling without excessive vertical lengthening (see Fig. 288-2A). Bilateral sagittal-split osteotomies are performed, and occlusion is established with a premade occlusal splint (see Procedure 274). In the patient with deciduous dentition, circummandibular, circumzygomatic, and piriform aperture wires are essential to allow splint fixation. With rigid plating of the osteotomies, intermaxillary fixation is unnecessary. A leveling and advancement genioplasty completes the correction of the hypoplastic skeleton (see Fig. 288-2 and Procedures 180 and 181).

The more severe types of hemifacial microsomia (types II through V) require condylar and often zygomatic arch and glenoid fossa reconstruction. After LeFort I and sagittal-split osteotomies have been performed as described previously, a new ascending ramus and condyle can be constructed using an autogenous rib graft (see Figs. 288-3 and 288-4). While harvesting the graft (see Procedure 259), the periosteal-perichondral junction must be left intact to prevent separation of the cartilage from the bone. The cartilage cap is made convex to simulate a condylar head and should not be longer that 5 to 7 mm, because a longer segment may predispose to later overgrowth of the new ascending ramus. The graft is passed into the mouth through the preauricular incision and secured to the residual mandibular body with miniplate lag screws. The graft may extend to the pogonion if necessary to allow increased skeletal projection (see Fig. 288-4B). Additional onlay grafts can be used if necessary to augment the reconstruction and increase skeletal bulk on the affected side (see Fig. 288-4A).

A coronal incision is necessary if the zygomatic arch is absent (types III and IV). After exposure of the lateral orbital wall and residual anterior arch, a full-thickness rib graft, beveled anteriorly, is attached to the zygoma and curved backward in a convex manner to the temporal bone to form a zygomatic arch (see Fig. 288-4). Fixation of the graft is accomplished with miniplates or lag screws. A concave indentation is made in the graft to cancellous bone to create a glenoid fossa. This cavity is lined by chondral cartilage wired to the rib (Fig. 288-5). LeFort I and sagittal-split osteotomies and ramus reconstruction are then performed as described previously. Additional onlay grafts can be used around the orbit and the new zygomatic arch to increase projection.

The timing of surgery depends on the patient's age, the severity of the condition, and psychosocial considerations. Children rarely are teased by their peers until they begin school.

MICHAEL WHEATLEY

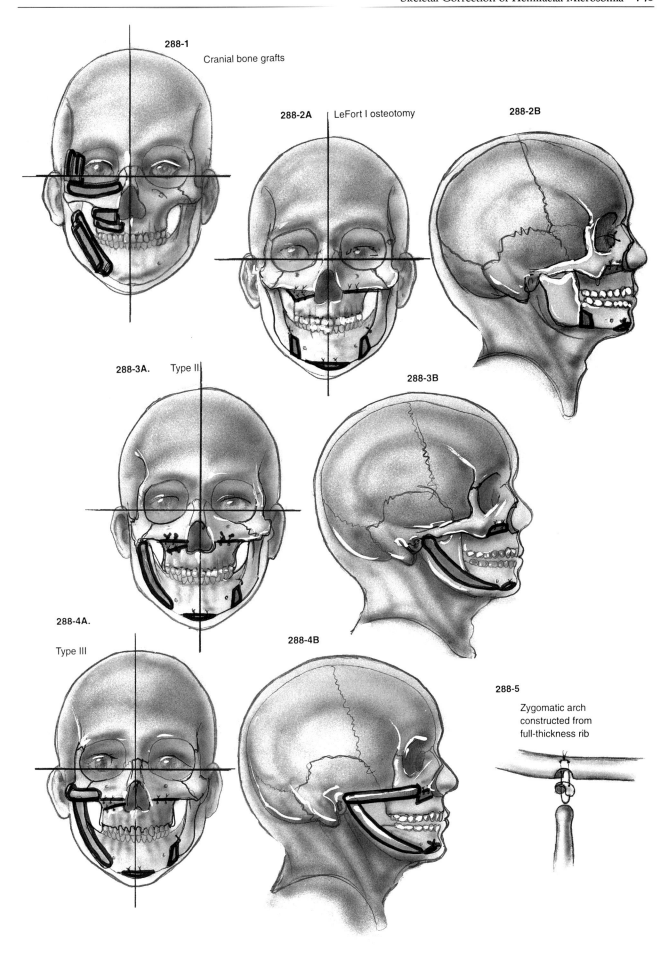

288-1

Cranial bone grafts

288-2A   LeFort I osteotomy

288-2B

288-3A.   Type II

288-3B

288-4A.

Type III

288-4B

288-5

Zygomatic arch
constructed from
full-thickness rib

■ 289. AESTHETIC FACIAL SUBUNITS

The subunit principle divides the face into several aesthetic units and subunits that are demarcated by ridges, shadows, and creases. The anatomic relations of the subunits are employed to obtain optimal cosmetic results in reconstructing facial defects.

Facial Subunits

1. The *forehead* unit extends from the eyebrows to the hairline. Horizontal creases and glabellar lines subdivide this area.
2. The *brow* is composed of hair-bearing tissue that must be properly positioned and aligned during reconstruction.
3. The *periorbit* is subdivided into the supraorbital, infraorbital, upper lid, and lower lid subunits, all of which have extremely thin skin.
4. The *cheek* unit extends from the zygomatic arch to the mandibular margin and from the melolabial fold to the preauricular crease. The cheek consists of anterior and posterior subunits.
5. The *nose* unit extends from the brow to the columellar base and between the lateral edges of the nasal sidewalls. Subunits of the nose include the dorsum, sidewall, alar lobule, soft triangle, and tip.
6. In the *lip and perioral area*, mucosal and cutaneous tissue meet at the vermilion border. This area may be divided into upper lip, lower lip philtrum, and five lip subunits.
7. The *chin* describes the area enclosed between the labiomental fold and the mandibular margin.
8. The *ear* has four subunits: helix, triangular fossa, conch, and lobule.

References

Burget GC, Menick FJ. The subunit principle in nasal reconstruction. Plast Reconstr Surg 1985;76:239.

Thomas JR. Local skin flaps. In: Thomas JR, ed. Cutaneous facial surgery. St Louis: Mosby-Year Book, 1991.

Zitelli JA. Secondary intention healing: an alternative to surgical repair. Clin Dermatol 1984;2:92.

The Subunit Principle

The face can be divided into several aesthetic or anatomic units (Fig. 289-1). Certain areas, particularly the nose, can be further divided into smaller subunits.

Excess tissue may exist along the junctions of units. This excess may be incorporated into grafts or flaps with minimal cosmetic deformity as the junction is restored (Fig. 289-2).

Observations of wounds healing by secondary intention have led to an additional grouping of the various facial subunits. The favorable sites, where wounds heal with good cosmetic results, have been categorized as the concave surfaces of the nose, ear, eye and temple (ie, NEET areas). Wounds located on the convex surfaces heal less favorably (Fig. 289-3). These convex surfaces include portions of the nose, oral lips, cheeks and chin, and helix of the ear (ie, NOCH areas). This classification aids the surgeon in determining the cosmetic result of a wound allowed to heal secondarily.

The surgeon can use various aesthetic units and subunits of the face to advantage in facial reconstruction.

Forehead

The forehead extends from the eyebrows to the hairline. It consists of relatively thick skin and is influenced by the frontalis muscle, which causes horizontal lines, and the procerus and corrugator supercilii muscles, which cause horizontal and vertically oriented creases, respectively, in the glabellar region. These glabellar lines help to create an additional subdivision of the forehead in the midline. The temple may be considered an additional subunit.

Brow

The brow or supraorbital region is aesthetically important because of its hair-bearing tissue. Any reconstruction must be concerned with potential hair loss and proper orientation of hairs in free grafts or flaps.

Periorbit

The periorbital area may be subdivided into the supraorbital, infraorbital, upper, and lower lid areas. All have extremely thin skin. The infraorbital subunit may be grouped with the zygomatic or cheek region. This principle accounts for the success of the cheek advancement flap in nasal and cheek reconstruction (Fig. 289-4).

Cheek

The cheek describes the area from the zygomatic arch to the mandibular edge and the melolabial fold to the preauricular crease. The cheek skin varies from thin in the preauricular region to thickest at the melolabial fold. This skin differentiation allows a further subdivision into an anterior or buccal subunit, which is soft and mobile, and a posterior or masseteric subunit, which is firm and less mobile. An additional zygomatic unit lying over the malar eminence of the zygomatic bone has been described.

Nose

The nose extends from the brow to the columellar base and between the lateral edge of the sidewalls (Fig. 289-5). This lateral edge is demarcated by a margin of light and shadow that sets off the cheek from the nose. The subdivision of the nose into smaller units is extremely important in planning reconstruction. If scars can be positioned so they resemble the ridges and depressions of previously existing subunits, they will be less apparent. When a reconstructive flap is planned appropriately and contraction occurs, the resulting bulge may resemble a normal topographic subunit. If a defect includes a significant portion of a subunit, excising the uninvolved healthy skin and making a defect larger to conform to a regional subunit may be necessary.

The lateral borders of the dorsum are defined by ridges that reflect a line of light separating the dorsal subunit from the sidewall. The dorsum begins at the supratip depression and extends to the nasion, where a horizontal crease perpendicular to the procerus muscle may mark its limit. The alar groove separates the alar lobule from the sidewall, tip, cheek, and lip. The soft triangle is a flat or slightly depressed area between the arched caudal border of the medial and lateral crus of the lower lateral cartilage. This area is an excellent recipient of a skin graft. The tip area is separated from the sidewall and alar lobule by a slight drop off in the level of the skin surface. In the bifid nose, the tip may be divided into two hemitip subunits by a crease that extends to the base of the columella. The columella has a wide base that narrows as it meets the tip at the columellar-lobular angle.

Lip and Perioral Area

The lip area provides many subunits and borders that can be used in reconstruction. In this area, mucosal and cutaneous surfaces abut. The vermilion border provides an excellent place to camouflage incisions. The region is limited by the nasolabial folds and secondary lines of expression situated lateral to the angle of the mouth and the labiomental fold. It can be further subdivided into upper lip, philtrum, lower lip, and five lip segments, including the prolabia and two lateral segments superiorly and two segments inferiorly (Fig. 289-6).

Chin

The chin extends from the labiomental fold to the mandibular margin. Preserving the labiomental fold is an important consideration in planning reconstruction. The increased thickness of subcutaneous tissue in this unit must also be considered.

Ear

The ear may be divided into four subunits: helix, triangular fossa, concha, and lobule. The relatively thin skin and cartilaginous support in all subunits except the lobule and the increased subcutaneous soft tissue in the lobule must be considered in reconstructive planning.

AARON SHAPIRO
J. REGAN THOMAS

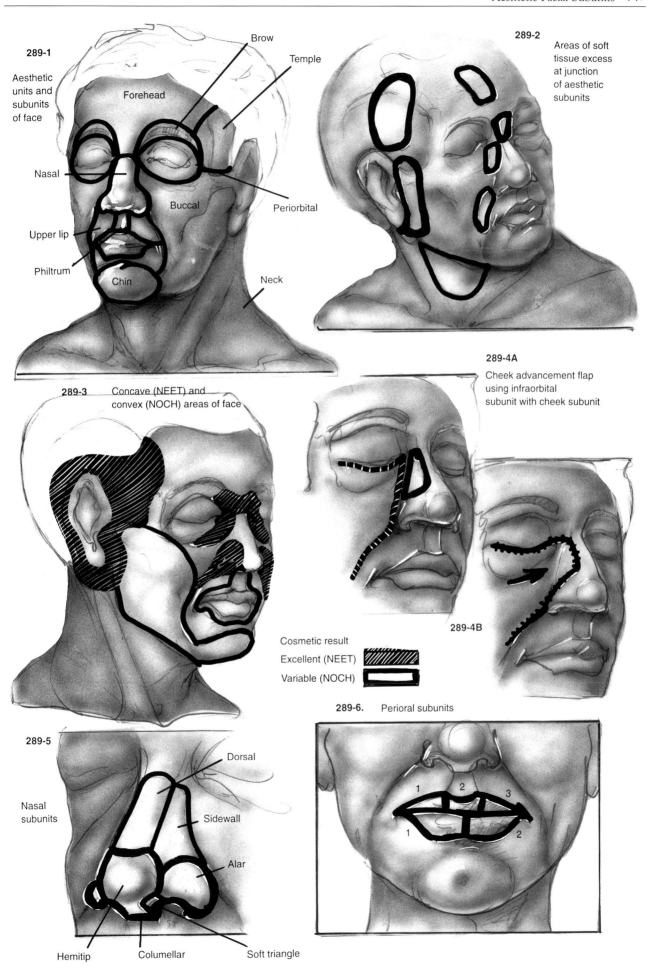

289-1 Aesthetic units and subunits of face

Brow
Temple
Forehead
Nasal
Buccal
Periorbital
Upper lip
Philtrum
Chin
Neck

289-2 Areas of soft tissue excess at junction of aesthetic subunits

289-3 Concave (NEET) and convex (NOCH) areas of face

289-4A Cheek advancement flap using infraorbital subunit with cheek subunit

289-4B

Cosmetic result
Excellent (NEET)
Variable (NOCH)

289-5 Nasal subunits

Dorsal
Sidewall
Alar
Hemitip
Columellar
Soft triangle

289-6. Perioral subunits

■ 290. LOCAL EXCISION AND PRIMARY

CLOSURE— Local excision and primary closure is used for small skin lesions (usually smaller than 2 cm in diameter). Primary closure is closure of small skin defects accomplished without the use of flaps or grafts.

Indications

1. Small skin defects

Contraindications

1. Primary closure resulting in excess tension as shown by puckering or extreme skin pallor

Special Considerations

1. Primary closure
   a. Adequate undermining is crucial.
   b. Interrupted absorbable dermal sutures with buried knots
   c. Ensure that inversion of the skin edges does not occur.
   d. Dog ear deformities are corrected with standing cone excision.
   e. Antibiotic ointment keeps the wound moist and eschar free, and it minimizes depressed scar formation.
   f. Taping minimizes wound tension during healing.
2. Local excision
   a. Excision performed so resultant scar parallels resting skin tension lines (RSTLs)
   b. Scar camouflage is enhanced by incision in a natural skin crease or rhytid, inside an orifice, within a hair-bearing area, or at the junction of anatomic subunits.
   c. Best performed with fusiform incision with 3:1 length to width ratio
   d. Incisions in hair-bearing areas are beveled to prevent hair loss from root transection.
   e. Running W-plasty closure is sometimes helpful for scar camouflage.

Preoperative Preparation

1. Routine laboratory studies
2. Marking of relaxed skin tension lines

Special Instruments, Position, and Anesthesia

1. Fine surgical instruments, including Castroviejo needle holder and Bishop-Harmon forceps

References

Freeman MS. Incision planning and basic soft tissue surgery. Otolaryngol Clin North Am 1990;23:865.
Thomas JR. Incision techniques in cutaneous surgery. In: Thomas JR, Roller J, eds. Cutaneous facial surgery. New York: Thieme Medical, 1992.
Thomas JR. Scar revision and camouflage. In: Thomas JR, Roller J, eds. Cutaneous facial surgery. New York: Thieme Medical, 1992.

Operative Procedure

Local excision begins with incision planning. A favorable incision enhances repair and is best made so the resultant scar falls in the RSTLs (Fig. 290-1). RSTLs are formed by anatomic and gravitational pull acting on relaxed skin and can be reliably determined by pinching the skin. Incisions can also be camouflaged by placing them in natural skin creases or wrinkles. These are referred to as favorable skin tension lines or lines of minimal tension. In many areas of the head and neck, these lines parallel the RSTLs, but in the glabella and temple, these lines are different (Fig. 290-2). The surgeon chooses, based on the patient's unique facial characteristics, which incision placement is best. Other techniques for incision camouflage include placing the incision inside an orifice, within a hair-bearing area, or at the junction of anatomic subunits.

A fusiform incision with approximately a 3:1 length to width ratio provides the easiest closure, and ending the fusiform in a 30° or smaller angle avoids creating a dog ear deformity. The incision should not cross a normal anatomic border. A #11 or #15 scalpel blade is used, and the skin in incised at a 90° angle or beveled slightly away from the lesion (Figs. 290-3 and 290-4). An M-plasty can shorten the length of the incision (Fig. 290-5). Incisions in hair-bearing areas are beveled parallel to the hair root, preventing hair loss from root transection. Incisions near a hairline can be beveled to cut through the follicles, allowing hair to grow through the incision and aid in scar camouflage.

If an incision must be made perpendicular to the RSTL and no other camouflage technique is available, a running W-plasty incision and closure yields the best results (Fig. 290-6).

After the excision is performed, undermining is carried out in a subdermal plane for 1 to 2 cm in all directions (Fig. 290-7). This usually allows wound closure with minimal tension. Tissue expansion can be used in specific circumstances to aid in decreasing wound closing tension. Hemostasis before wound closure prevents hematoma formation. Gentle tissue handling with a single hook or a small single-toothed forceps minimizes tissue damage.

After undermining, interrupted dermal sutures (absorbable, usually 4-0 or 5-0 Vicryl) are placed with the knot buried. These align the skin for surface closure and take additional tension off the wound edges. Everting the skin edges is crucial to producing a level scar. This is performed by placing the dermal sutures so that more tissue is grasped in the horizontal than in the vertical plane or by placing the stitch slightly beyond the wound edge (Fig. 290-8).

If epidermal closure is performed with simple or running sutures, the needle at skin entry is perpendicular or slightly greater than perpendicular. This suture encompasses more subcutaneous than epithelial tissue, which everts the skin. Running subcuticular or vertical mattress sutures can also be used for skin closure. In all suture techniques, care is taken to ensure that skin inversion does not occur. Typically a 5-0 or 6-0 nonabsorbable suture is used for epidermal closure, but 6-0 rapidly absorbing catgut yields similar results.

When a dog ear deformity occurs during closure, it is corrected with a standing cone excision. An M-plasty can be used with the standing cone excision if the dog ear abuts an anatomic landmark (Fig. 290-9).

After closure, the wound is kept moist and free of eschar with an antibiotic ointment. Reepithelialization occurs more quickly in the moist wound and takes place in the same plane as the surrounding epidermis, avoiding a depressed scar surface.

Taping the wound after suturing may help relieve wound tension during healing. Skin adhesives such as Mastisol or tincture of benzoin aid tape adherence. The ideal tape is flesh colored and microporous.

AARON L. SHAPIRO
J. REGAN THOMAS

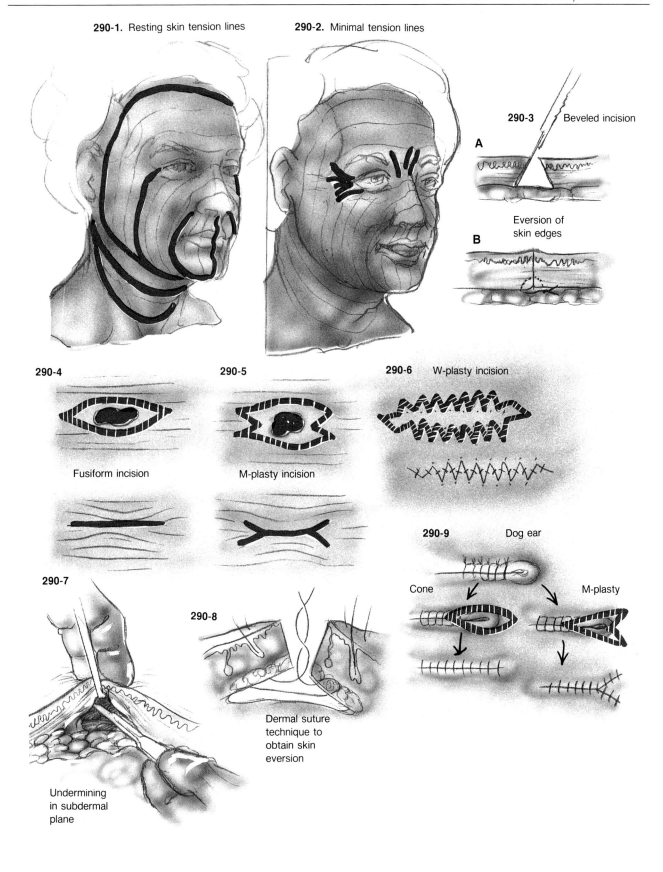

290-1. Resting skin tension lines

290-2. Minimal tension lines

290-3 Beveled incision

A

Eversion of skin edges

B

290-4

Fusiform incision

290-5

M-plasty incision

290-6 W-plasty incision

290-7

Undermining in subdermal plane

290-8 Dermal suture technique to obtain skin eversion

290-9 Dog ear

Cone

M-plasty

■ *291.* SCAR EXCISION

Surgical removal of a visible scar, with closure employing any of several techniques that camouflage the scar

Indications

1. Depressed scar
2. Widened scar
3. Malpositioned scar (ie, perpendicular to relaxed skin tension lines or those crossing junctions between facial units)
4. Contracted scar
5. Discolored scar

Contraindications

1. Scars located over regions of high tension, such as over the sternum, deltoid, or knee are contraindicated. Scar revision in these areas may result in worsening of the scar.
2. Keloids should be excised and closed using the simplest method possible. The surgeon should avoid complex closures (eg, geometric broken line closure) in patients undergoing excision of keloids.

Special Considerations

1. Relaxed skin tension lines (RSTLs) run perpendicular to the underlying muscle fibers. Scars can be placed parallel to RSTLs or reoriented using Z-plasty to follow the RSTLs.
2. Scars of the thin neck skin are oriented to follow the RSTLs and should not be dermabraded.
3. The standard simple closure of the incision in a RSTL uses skin eversion techniques; the incision is everted to prevent a depressed scar.[1]
4. In Z-plasty, two equal-sized triangular flaps are transposed along the axis (central limb) of the scar.[1] The two lines at either end intersect the central limb at 30°, 45°, or 60°. The Z-plasty lengthens the scar, changes the direction of the scar, and breaks up a straight-line scar.
5. W-plasty uses a repeating saw-tooth pattern along the axis of the scar. The W-plasty breaks up a straight-line scar, aiding scar camouflage.
6. Geometric broken line closure uses a random pattern of different geometric shapes (eg, squares, triangles, rectangles) along the axis of the scar.[1] The multiple geometric patterns break up the scar and aid in scar camouflage.
7. To maximize scar camouflage, all techniques can be followed with dermabrasion 8 to 16 weeks after scar revision.

(continued)

Operative Procedure

Simple Closure

A fusiform excision of the scar is marked out on the skin with a marking pen. To decrease the length of the excision, M-plasties can be placed at each end of the excision (Fig. 291-1). The excision is positioned along the RSTLs. A solution of 1% lidocaine with 1:1,000,000 epinephrine is injected just deep to the scar and around the periphery of the scar. Overinjection distorts the tissues and makes precise scar excision difficult. After waiting at least 10 minutes, a #15 blade is used to excise the scar. The scar is excised, leaving a thin layer of scar at the base of the wound.

The wound edges are undermined 3 to 10 mm around the edges of the wound. Wider undermining is performed in larger scar excisions. Then a 5-0 polydioxanone (PDS, Ethicon, Sommerville, NJ) Webster-type subcutaneous everting suture is used to create pronounced skin edge eversion (Fig. 291-2). The degree of skin edge eversion depends on the location of the incision and the tension at the operative site. Pronounced skin edge eversion can be used above the brow because of the degree of mimetic activity of the frontalis muscle and the thickness of the skin. However, the relatively thin skin of the neck does not tolerate pronounced skin eversion. After the wound edges are approximated with everting sutures, 6-0 or 7-0 nylon vertical mattress sutures can be used to close the epidermis. Gilles's corner stitches can be used to close the bilateral M-plasties.

Z-Plasty

In the Z-plasty technique, two equal-sized triangular flaps are transposed along the central line or limb of the scar (Fig. 291-3). The central limb is oriented along the axis of the scar or line of scar contracture. The two lines at either end are equal in length and intersect the central limb at identical angles of 30°, 45°, or 60°. These intersecting lines are placed parallel to the RSTLs. The incisions are of equal length to the central limb. After making the incisions, the flaps are undermined up to 1 cm around the surgical site and transposed (see Fig. 291-3). Transposition of the flaps results in lengthening of the central limb of the pattern and reorientation of the central limb by 90° (see Fig. 291-3).

The degree of lengthening attained in Z-plasty depends on the angles between the central limb and the intersecting lines (angle at apices of transposed flaps). Proposed Z-plasties of 30°, 45°, and 60° result in increases in the length of the central limb by 25%, 50%, and 75%, respectively.

(continued)

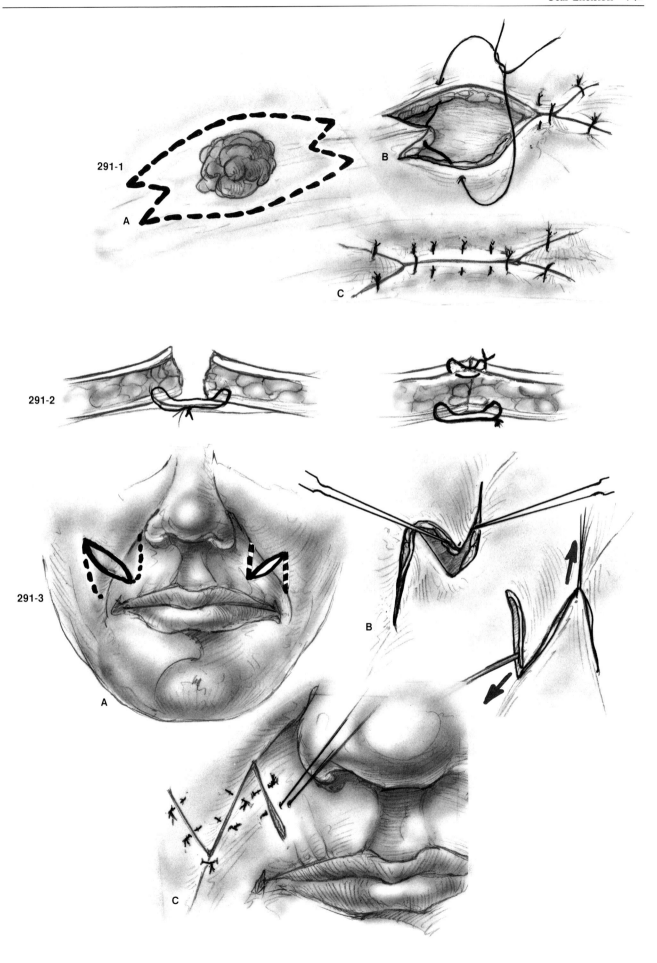

291-1

A

B

C

291-2

291-3

A

B

C

■ 291. SCAR EXCISION (continued)

Preoperative Preparation

1. Photographically document the scar using conventional and tangential lighting.[2] Tangential lighting casts a shadow in the depth of the scar and allows easier identification.
2. Inform the patient that the scar may look worse before it looks better. In the short term, extreme eversion of the skin edges makes the scars look more prominent. Everted scars will efface over several months. Discuss the possibility of a secondary dermabrasion to maximize scar camouflage.

Special Instruments, Position, and Anesthesia

1. Small delicate plastic surgery instruments
2. Bipolar cautery
3. Anesthesia with a solution of 1% lidocaine with 1:1,000,000 epinephrine

Tips and Pearls

1. Allow the epinephrine in the local anesthetic to take effect for at least 10 minutes before making the incision.
2. Leave a layer of scar at the base of the dissection to act as a foundation for the scar excision. This helps support the wound and decreases the degree of scar contracture postoperatively.
3. Use Webster-type subcutaneous everting sutures to create pronounced eversion of the skin edges.[3] This pronounced skin edge eversion will efface over several months and leave a slightly everted wound that can be easily dermabraded. Webster-type subcutaneous eversion sutures are most important in areas where the underlying muscle is very active (eg, forehead or frontalis muscle, upper lip or orbicularis oris muscle).

Pitfalls and Complications

1. Poor planning resulting in unfavorable scar orientation
2. Failure to evert skin edges, resulting in a widened or depressed scar

Postoperative Care Issues

1. Remove the skin sutures early (5 days) to prevent suture marks or related scarring.
2. Use antitension taping for at least 4 weeks postoperatively to minimize tension on the wound edges and help prevent a widened or depressed scar.

References

1. Borges AF. Principles of scar camouflage. Facial Plast Surg 1984;1: 226.
2. Thomas JR, Holt GR. Facial scars: incisions, revision and camouflage. St. Louis: CV Mosby, 1989.
3. Davidson TM, Webster RC. Scar revision. American Academy of Facial Plastic and Reconstructive Surgery, Self-Instructional Package, 1977.

Multiple or serial Z-plasties are designed in a repeating fashion and transposed with the contralateral flap (Fig. 291-4). Multiple Z-plasties can be used to camouflage longer scars requiring more than one Z-plasty flap to correct the deformity. Multiple Z-plasty can also be used to correct trap door, pincushioned, and circumferential scars.

W-Plasty

In the W-plasty technique, a repeating saw-tooth pattern is marked around the scar. The pattern is created so that the edges of the incision will meet in a tongue-in-groove fashion (Fig. 291-5). This technique breaks up the line of the scar and replaces it with a repeating W-shaped pattern. After excising the scar and undermining the skin edges, Webster-type subcutaneous sutures are used to evert the skin edges. Fine 6-0 nylon suture is used to align the epidermal closure.

Geometric Broken Line Closure

A random pattern of squares, rectangles, and triangles are marked along the line of the scar excision (Fig. 291-6). The pattern is planned so that the pattern of one side of the incision fits into the other side in a tongue-in-groove fashion. All the geometric shapes should be at least 4 to 5 mm in diameter, because the skin retracts after the incisions are made. If the incision is curvilinear, the size of the geometric shapes should increase on the longer limb and be reduced on the shorter limb. After the pattern is carefully incised with a #11 blade, the wound edges should be undermined for about 5 to 10 mm.

Webster-type subcutaneous everting 5-0 PDS sutures can be used to create pronounced eversion of the skin edges. If skin eversion is not attained, tension on the wound edges causes a widened, depressed scar. After the wound edges are approximated, fine 6-0 or 7-0 nylon suture can be used to complete the epidermal closure. While aligning the skin edges, the geometric shapes should be sutured into an everted orientation to prevent depression of the scar. Any elevated portions of the pattern can be dermabraded later. However, any depressed segment of the scar may require reexcision. In some cases, a running interlocking mattress suture that aligns the corners of the geometric shapes can be used to complete the epidermal closure.

DEAN M. TORIUMI

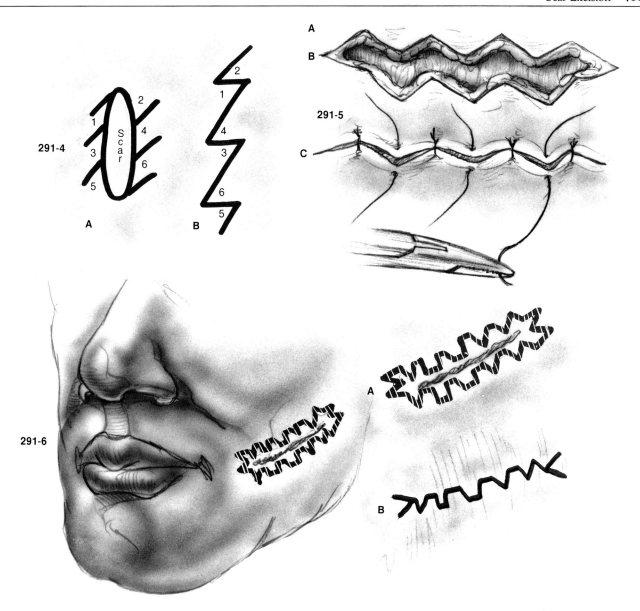

291-4

291-5

291-6

A

B

C

A

B

■ *292.* COMPLEX FACIAL LACERATION RE-PAIR—Surgical repair of soft tissue defects limited to the facial skin. The techniques used to repair complex defects include subcutaneous skin eversion sutures (Webster-type sutures), Gilles corner stitch, repair of a trap door defect, and stellate laceration repair.

Indications
1. Complex facial lacerations requiring specialized suture repair techniques

Special Considerations
1. Patients with a history of hypertrophic scar or keloid formation have a greater chance of unsightly scar formation.
2. Darker-pigmented (non-Caucasian) skin may undergo pigmentary changes.

Preoperative Preparation
1. Meticulous cleaning of the wound
2. Incisions may demonstrate pronounced skin edge eversion that efface over several months.

Special Instruments, Position, and Anesthesia
1. Fine facial plastic instruments
2. Monofilament suture material (ie, 4-0 or 5-0 polydioxanone [PDS] and 6-0 or 7-0 nylon) helps to avoid infection.

Tips and Pearls
1. In acute wounds, preserve as much viable tissue as possible.[1]
2. To maximize the result, close the incision using subcutaneous skin edge eversion sutures (Webster-type sutures).[2] If slight skin eversion persists at 3 months, dermabrasion can be performed.
3. Tension on incisions may result in widening and inversion of the scar.

Pitfalls and Complications
1. Asymmetric alignment of skin edges
2. Hypertrophic scar formation
3. Wound infection due to inadequate wound debridement

Postoperative Care Issues
1. Early suture removal: 5 days after surgery
2. Use antitension taping for 2 to 4 weeks after surgery. My colleagues and I prefer to use flesh-colored Steri-Strips (Cat. #1551, 3M Medical Surgical Division, St. Paul, MN).

References
1. Thomas JR, Holt GR. Facial scars: incisions, revision, and camouflage. St. Louis: CV Mosby, 1989.
2. Davidson TM, Webster RC. Scar revision. Self-instructional package. American Academy of Otolaryngology. 1977.

Operative Procedure
The wound and surrounding skin are injected with a 1% solution of lidocaine with a 1:100,000 concentration of epinephrine.

The skin edges of the wound are trimmed if there is damaged or macerated tissue along the margins of the wound. Only conservative tissue excision is performed to avoid a large defect with excessive tension on the closure.

Subcutaneous Skin Eversion Sutures
Before closure, the edges of the wound are undermined 5 to 10 mm to allow application of deep Webster-type subcutaneous sutures (Fig. 292-1). These sutures are inserted into the dermis away from the wound and exit the dermis before reaching the edge of the skin incision. Special care should be taken to ensure symmetric suture placement; otherwise, the suture will produce improper skin edge alignment. To avoid skin puckering, exceedingly deep suture bites should not be taken, and these sutures should not be used in thin skin. If used properly, the deep sutures can evert the skin edges and take all tension off the wound closure. The degree of skin edge eversion should be greater in areas of high mimetic activity (eg, forehead, cheek). A 4-0 or 5-0 PDS suture can be used for these subcutaneous sutures and are applied at 1- to 1.5-cm intervals along the length of the wound. After these sutures are applied, fine 6-0 or 7-0 nylon vertical mattress sutures can be used to approximate the epidermal skin edges. If these sutures are tied too tightly, skin suture marks may develop.

Before using the sutures that create pronounced eversion of skin edges, the surgeon should explain to the patient that the everted scar will efface over several months. If scar eversion persists, secondary dermabrasion may be necessary.

Gilles Corner Stitch
In some cases, a corner stitch is necessary to inset the corner of an angulated wound edge precisely into the apex of the defect. In such cases, a Gilles corner stitch can approximate the skin edges and encourage eversion. If there is significant tension on the closure, a deep subcutaneous suture can be used to take tension off the skin edges. The Gilles corner stitch is a modified (half buried) horizontal mattress suture that traverses the apex of the skin edge. The suture advances the point of the flap into the apex of the incision (Fig. 292-2). The point of the flap should not carry an angle less than 30° to avoid necrosis of the distal point of the flap.

Repair of a Trap Door Defect
"Trap door" defect and "pincushioning" refer to the inverted scar effect of contractual wound healing that can occur with small flaps of skin. This problem occurs most commonly with circular flaps, such as bilobed transposition flaps. Trap door defects can be corrected by debulking the flap by resecting excessive fibrofatty subcutaneous tissue, wide undermining of the skin edges around the scar to create more uniform draping and healing, recruiting subdermal tissue into the junctional zone between flap and skin edges, and performing multiple Z-plasties along the circumference of the circular flap.

The flap can be debulked through the old scar, followed by wide undermining (1 to 1.5 cm) around the margins of the scar (Fig. 292-3). After undermining, deep subcutaneous sutures can be applied to recruit subdermal tissue under the scar to prevent scar inversion (Fig. 292-4). In more severe deformities, multiple Z-plasties can be performed around the circumference of larger flaps to break up the circular scar (Fig. 292-5). The multiple Z-plasties act to make scar formation irregular and decrease deformity due to scar contracture.

Stellate Laceration Repair
Stellate lacerations frequently require specialized closure to avoid unsatisfactory scarring. In many cases, the underlying problem is a subdermal soft tissue deficit resulting in a depressed scar. To prevent necrosis of skin flaps, the distal points of flaps should be rounded off if the angle of the distal end of the flap is less than 30°. Before closing the skin, the subdermal tissue is approximated with 4-0 or 5-0 PDS suture to minimize the subdermal soft tissue deficit (Fig. 292-6). The lacerations are closed under no tension.

DEAN M. TORIUMI

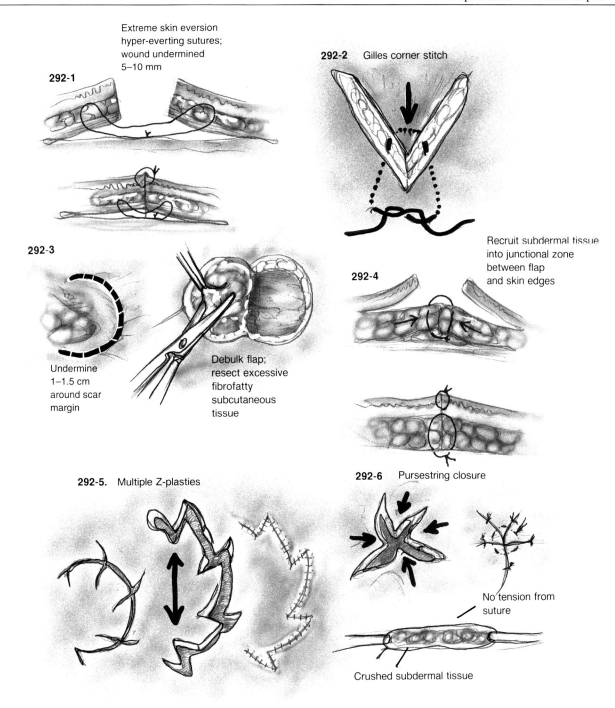

292-1

Extreme skin eversion
hyper-everting sutures;
wound undermined
5–10 mm

292-2   Gilles corner stitch

292-3

Undermine
1–1.5 cm
around scar
margin

Debulk flap;
resect excessive
fibrofatty
subcutaneous
tissue

Recruit subdermal tissue
into junctional zone
between flap
and skin edges

292-4

292-5.   Multiple Z-plasties

292-6   Pursestring closure

No tension from
suture

Crushed subdermal tissue

293. GRAFTS FOR HAIR TRANSPLANTA-
TION— Relocation of hair-bearing scalp to a bald area using various sizes of grafts.

Indications
1. Patient's age
2. Sizes of future bald area and recipient area
3. Hair color, texture, and density
4. Punch grafts or minigrafts if bald skin is removed
5. Slit grafts or micrografts if no bald skin is removed

Special Considerations
1. Number of sessions
2. Graft placement
3. Sizes of donor site and recipient area

Preoperative Preparation
1. Graft harvesting
2. Local factors

(continued)

Operative Procedure
Punch Grafts

For punch grafts, I use the power-driven carbon steel punch developed by Robbins Instruments, Inc. (Chatham, NJ). The punches are always sharpened after each procedure. When dull punches are used, the skin is compressed, which causes splaying of the hair shafts and cuts the follicles at the margin of the graft (Fig. 293-1). If sharp punches are not used, the results of hair transplantation are unsatisfactory.

The scalp is prepared with a 3% solution of hexachlorophene. Hair in the donor site is then cut short, leaving stubble that is 1 to 2 mm long. Local anesthesia is used. After anesthesia is achieved, the individual graft recipient sites are marked by scratching the skin with a hand-held punch.

The recipient holes are cut at the angle appropriate for each part of the scalp. The hair on top of the head normally grows anteriorly and anterolaterally toward the forehead. The direction of graft placement in the crown varies as grafting progresses around the swirl. Bald skin is left in place until the donor grafts are harvested.

With the patient in a lateral or prone position, the donor area is locally infiltrated with anesthetic solution and then injected with normal saline solution to add turgor. The grafts are cut with the power punch parallel to the hair shafts, as demonstrated in Figure 293-1. I remove every third or fourth graft and inspect it to ensure that the punches are being cut at the proper angle. An alternative method is to cut an entire block with a #10 blade into 4-mm grafts with the edges (ie, minigrafts or micrografts).

The grafts are removed by cutting through the fatty layer just deep to the follicles. The grafts are kept moist, and the holes at the donor site are then closed. If more than one row has been harvested, a running-locking suture of 4-0 polypropylene is placed. If an area has been totally harvested or a single row taken, the Pierce interdigitating closure technique is performed using the staple gun (Fig. 293-2).

The bald skin is removed from the previously cut recipient holes. The full thickness of the skin and galea is removed to prevent a cobblestone effect. Placement of the grafts with the proper orientation of hair growth is essential. A Telfa and gauze dressing is placed.

Crusts that form on the grafts usually fall off in 2 to 3 weeks. The hair in the grafts falls out 4 to 6 weeks after surgery, when the follicle develops telogen effluvium secondary to the shock of surgery. New hair growth starts about 3 months after the procedure. Four sessions are necessary to fill any area. All transplantations at each session are separated by the width of one graft (Fig. 293-3).

Minigrafts

Minigrafting is actually an old technique with a new name. In 1970, Ayres described the use of small grafts in 1.5-mm holes for "fill-ins" but did not call them minigrafts.

Minigrafts contain three to six hairs. Grafts that are 4.5 to 4.75 mm in diameter are harvested and then bisected or quadrisected using sharp iris scissors or a #10 blade. In this case, the bald skin is excised from the recipient area before placement of the grafts.

(continued)

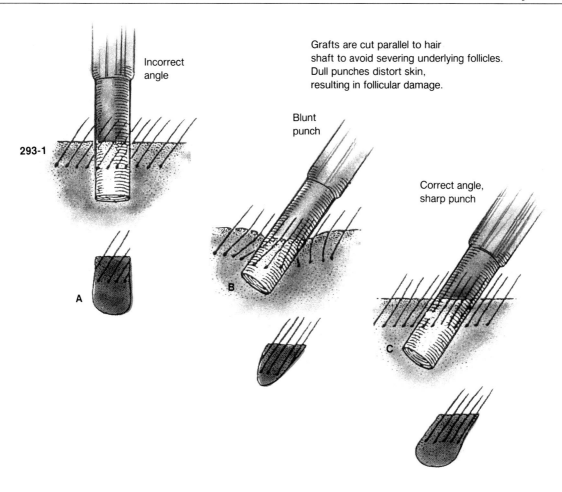

293-1

Incorrect angle

Grafts are cut parallel to hair shaft to avoid severing underlying follicles. Dull punches distort skin, resulting in follicular damage.

Blunt punch

A

B

Correct angle, sharp punch

C

293-2. Primary closure of donor punch defects with interdigitating suture placement minimizes scarring.

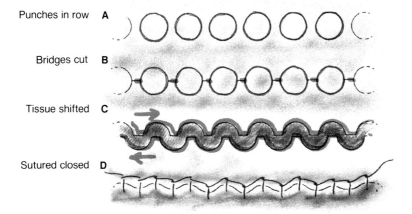

Punches in row A

Bridges cut B

Tissue shifted C

Sutured closed D

■ 293. GRAFTS FOR HAIR TRANSPLANTATION (continued)

Tips and Pearls

1. Sharp punches for optimal result
2. Saline infiltration before cutting donor grafts
3. Cutting donor grafts by hand

Pitfalls and Complications

1. Too many grafts during one procedure can decrease circulation.
2. Cutting grafts with a dull punch
3. Aggressive trimming of fat on the deep surface of the transplant
4. A cobblestone effect is created if the grafts are not "seated" well.

References

Mayer TG, Fleming RW. Aesthetic and reconstructive surgery of the scalp. St. Louis: Mosby Year Book, 1992.

Norwood OT, Shiell R, eds: Hair transplant surgery, 2nd ed. Springfield, IL: Charles C Thomas, 1984.

Unger WP, Nordstrom RE, eds. Hair transplantation, 2nd ed. New York: Marcel Dekker, 1988.

Slit Grafts

Slit grafting is a type of minigrafting, except that no bald skin is removed. Instead, a slit is created, and the de-epithelialized donor graft of three or four hairs is placed.

We first draw the proposed grafts in ink with the patient prone or on his side. Local anesthesia consisting of a 0.5% solution of lidocaine hydrochloride with a 1:200,000 concentration of epinephrine is administered. At the donor site, one or two rectangles of 3.0 mm × 15 cm are cut to yield 100 to 125 or 200 to 250 grafts, respectively. The galea of the donor site is closed with 0 polydioxanone (PDS), and staples are used for cutaneous closure.

With the patient in a supine position, a 1% solution of lidocaine hydrochloride with a 1:100,000 concentration of epinephrine is injected in a field block and to the recipient area. The #15 Bard-Parker blade incisions are initiated at the most posterior recipient area and are continued anteriorly.

The first procedure involves a fully staggered pattern with each graft being separated by 6.0 mm. A staggered pattern must be used, or the result appears artificial (Fig. 293-4). The staggered pattern terminates approximately 1 cm before the hairline. At this point, a partially staggered pattern of #15 blade incisions is placed 4 mm apart circumferentially. This establishes the natural hairline. Micrografts of three or four hairs are then placed in front to further soften the hairline.

Four months are allowed between sessions. All procedures are performed as for the first session, except that the incisions are placed 2.0 mm from those of the previous session (see Fig. 293-4). The anterior hairline is softened with one- or two-hair micrografts using dilators.

After another 4 months, the third procedure is performed. This session's slits are made between those of the first and second sessions. Further softening can be done with several more sessions of micrografts. This slit grafting procedure gives a thinning look and does not produce the density of conventional grafting.

Micrografts

Micrografts, which by definition contain one or two hair follicles, are most frequently used to refine the hairline after punch grafting and soften the cornrow appearance and abruptness within the first row of standard-sized grafts at the hairline. Micrografts are taken from donor hairs of smaller caliber. Micrografts are also used to reconstruct hairline scars, to fill in small areas of alopecia in eyebrow and mustache reconstruction, and to soften a "flap" hairline.

These grafts are harvested by taking a linear strip of hair-bearing scalp approximately 2 mm wide. The donor strip is de-epithelialized, and small one- or two-hair grafts are cut from the strip of donor skin. An 18-gauge needle is used to puncture holes within the recipient site. When used at the hairline, these holes are made within 2 mm of the established hairline and placed 1 to 2 mm apart. Dilators are placed after removing the 18-gauge needle. A single graft is placed in each opening. Hair growth may continue immediately after surgery, but if telogen effluvium does occur, hair growth starts 3 months later.

TOBY G. MAYER

293-3. Four sessions are necessary to fill any area. All transplantations at each session are separated by width of one graft

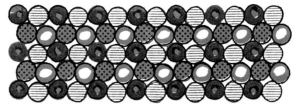

Punch graft sessions

1   3

2   4

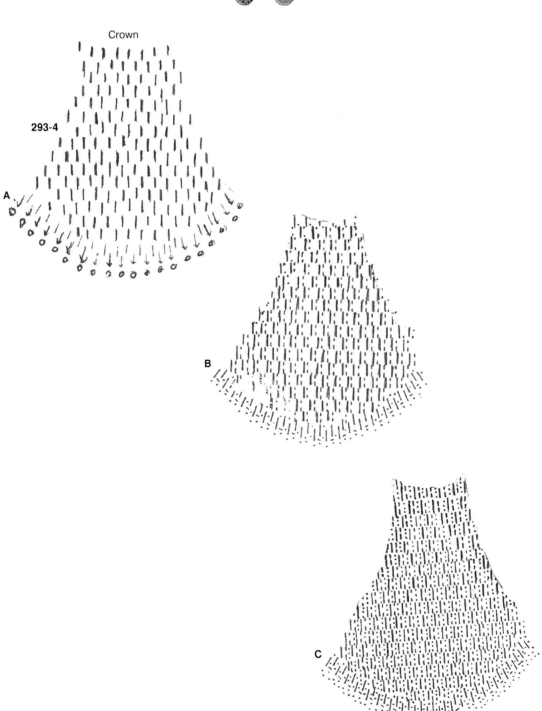

Crown

293-4

A

B

C

■ 294. FLEMING-MAYER FLAP PROCEDURE

Modification of the 4-cm-wide temporoparietoccipital flap described by Juri. Included in the modifications are variable widths, an irregular superior portion of the flap design, a frontotemporal recession that is not blunted, less curve in the flap design, and a straighter tail design. In the modified procedure, scalp reductions are often performed before flap rotation, tissue expansion commonly is used in conjunction with flap surgery, donor grafting is usual (when done without expansion), second flaps are delayed anteriorly at same time as the initial flap is delayed, forehead lifting is performed in conjunction with the flap procedure, and the dog-ear defect is placed anteriorly and the anterior portion grafted.

Indications

1. Male pattern baldness
2. Congenital alopecia or trauma
3. Diseased scalp, tumors, radiation therapy

Special Considerations

1. Age of patient and ultimate balding pattern
2. Height of donor area and width of crown baldness
3. Size of head and length of frontal hairline
4. Location of superficial temporal artery
5. Anterior temporal hair and hairline
6. Hair quality in posterior inferior triangle
7. Type of hairline to be created
8. Elasticity of scalp
9. Patient's desires
10. Scars or previously performed transplantations

Preoperative Preparation

1. Routine laboratory studies
2. Chest radiograph
3. Electrocardiogram if the patient is older than 40 years of age

(continued)

Operative Procedure

First Delay

The proposed hairline is drawn and shown to the patient preoperatively. The posterior branch of the superficial temporal artery is located with the Doppler flowmeter and drawn with dye (Fig. 294-1). The entire flap is drawn in a gentle curve, and the hair is tied. The artery within the flap creates an axial flap anteriorly. Because the occipital and posterior auricular arteries are severed with the delay process, the distal portion of the flap is random.

A #10 Bard-Parker blade is used to scratch the distal 25% of the flap along its tail. The scratching must be performed into the dermis so that the line can be seen 1 week later at the time of the second delay. The same blade is used to incise the inferior limb through the full thickness of the scalp, including the galea. Bleeding is controlled with electrocautery. A Penrose drain is placed distally, and the wound is closed with surgical staples.

The same procedure is then performed on the superior limb, which becomes the frontal hairline in an irregular pattern. A Penrose drain is placed in the incision distally, and the incision is closed (Fig. 294-2). The drains are removed 24 hours postoperatively.

Second Delay

The sutures are removed from the first delay. A #10 blade is used to make the incision around the distal 25% of the flap, beginning along the inferior limb. The superior border is incised next. A distal incision connecting the two limbs is made (Fig. 294-3). A plane of dissection is then started proximally that is begun along the inferior and superior margins and extends into the deep fat over the neck musculature. The tail of the flap is then elevated using Kahn scissors. Bleeding, including the occipital artery, is controlled by electrocautery. One or two Penrose drains are placed under the distal end of the flap, and the wound is closed using surgical staples. The drains are removed 24 hours postoperatively.

Transposition

The incision lines from the first and second delays are exposed by tying the hair back with rubber bands. The proposed hairline is drawn and shown to the patient before surgery is performed. The patient is given a general anesthetic, and areas to be undermined are injected with local anesthetic but no portion of the flap itself is injected.

A #15 blade is used to scratch the proposed hairline incision in case the dye is inadvertently removed during the procedure. The elevation of the flap is begun along the tail; the flap is elevated in a subgaleal plane. A finger can be used to separate the edges of the superior and inferior limbs and the tail of the flap, and a Kahn scissors is used to continue the dissection subgaleally to the base of the flap (Fig. 294-4). The entire flap is wrapped with a large lap sponge, placed in a plastic bag, and kept moist at all times with saline solution. Closure of the donor defect involves undermining in two separate areas. The first area involves the scalp inferior to the donor defect and extends onto the ear and into the neck. The second involves the scalp superior to the donor defect and extends to the distal frontal hairline.

The superior margin of the flap defect must be connected to the proposed hairline incision. The bevel must be posteriorly directed to avoid cutting any hair follicles while making this incision. This direction is the opposite of that used later for the hairline incision.

(continued)

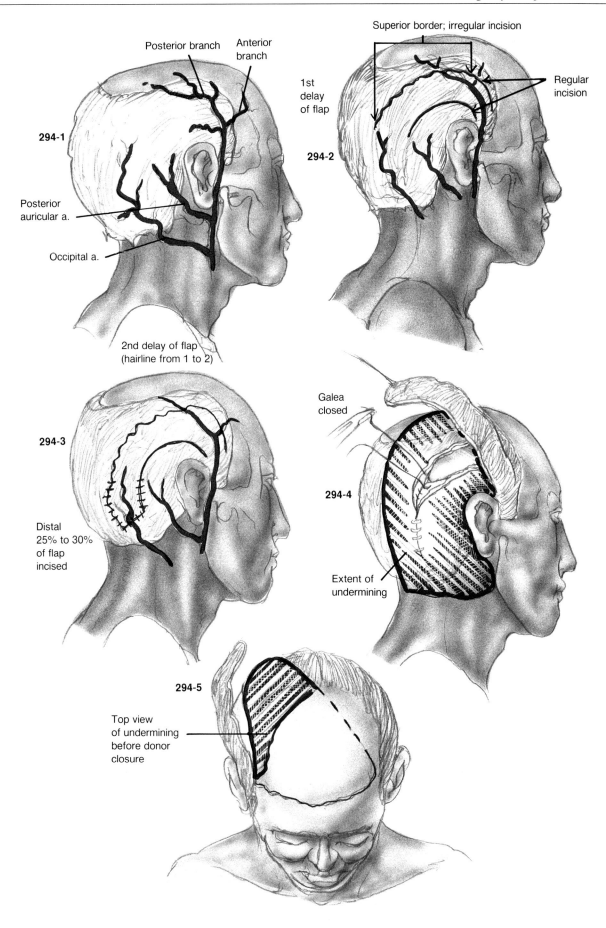

294-1

Posterior branch

Anterior branch

Posterior auricular a.

Occipital a.

Superior border; irregular incision

1st delay of flap

Regular incision

294-2

2nd delay of flap (hairline from 1 to 2)

294-3

Distal 25% to 30% of flap incised

Galea closed

294-4

Extent of undermining

294-5

Top view of undermining before donor closure

■ 294. FLEMING-MAYER FLAP PROCEDURE
(continued)

Special Instrumentation, Position, and Anesthesia

1. A 1% solution of lidocaine hydrochloride with a 1:100,000 concentration of epinephrine and a 0.5% solution of bupivacaine (Marcaine) in a 3:1 ratio of lidocaine to bupivacaine
2. First and second delays under local anesthesia; transposition under general anesthesia

Tips and Pearls

1. Creation of irregular trichophytic hairline
2. Micrografts after the Fleming-Mayer flap if hair is coarse to soften the hairline

Pitfalls and Complications

1. Temporary hair loss in the donor area or end of the flap is rare.
2. Bleeding is uncommon.
3. Infection is rare.
4. Folliculitis occasionally occurs with a hairline incision; treatment usually is unnecessary.
5. Spread of the posterior inferior donor wound closure
6. Altered sensation (ie, numbness and paresthesias)
7. Slight elevation of the posterior auricular hairline and the ear
8. Flap necrosis is rare.
9. Donor area necrosis and permanent hair loss are rare.
10. Smoking, prior extensive hair transplant surgery, and absent artery adversely affect flap procedure.

Postoperative Care Issues

1. Watch for hematoma first 2 to 3 hours
2. Patient placed on oral methylprednisolone, oxycodone, and antibiotics
3. All drains removed 24 to 48 hours postoperatively

References

Juri J. Use of parieto-occipital flaps in the surgical treatment of baldness. Plast Reconstr Surg 1975;55:456.

Kabaker S. Juri flap procedure for the treatment of baldness. Arch Otolaryngol 1979;105:509.

Mayer TG, Fleming RW. Aesthetic and reconstructive surgery of the scalp. St. Louis: Mosby Year Book, 1992.

A #10 blade is used to make an inferiorly directed bevel cut through the hairline along the line that was scratched before elevation of the flap. A #15 blade is used to make a small incision in the postauricular sulcus near the lobule; a Jackson-Pratt drain is placed at the most inferior portion of the wound and brought through this incision site.

A layered closure of the donor defect is performed. The galea is closed using 0 polydioxanone sutures. The skin edges are approximated with the surgical staple gun (see Fig. 294-4).

After closure of the donor wound, the flap is exposed, and the junction of the proximal temporal scalp and the frontal scalp is marked on the proximal portion of the flap (Fig. 294-5). A #15 blade is used to incise the anterior 2 mm of the flap through the epithelium into the superficial dermis. This anterior part is then de-eopithelialized along the anterior 2 mm, which maintains the irregular pattern of the new frontal hairline. The flap is stapled distally and at the proximal junction of the forehead and temporal hairline where the new frontal hairline will begin. The forehead skin is approximated to the flap beginning at the proximal portion of the hairline and continuing to the distal end. Hair will grow from the follicles buried beneath the skin closure and establish a new hairline to camouflage the scar (Fig. 294-6).

A dog-ear defect occurs at the anterior margin of the flap, because the flap skin is rotated back on itself to create the hairline. Closure of the dog-ear portion of the flap involves placing two or three 4-0 Prolene horizontal or vertical (or both) mattress sutures. The intervening spaces are then closed with the surgical staple gun.

The excess frontal scalp is draped over the posterior margin of the flap. Excess frontal scalp is excised to create a tension-free closure where the edges meet, and no tension is placed on the flap. This procedure is performed sequentially, beginning at the distal end of the flap and proceeding proximally. The surgical staple gun approximates the posterior edge of the flap to the frontal scalp (Fig. 294-7). Penrose drains are placed at the distal end of the flap, at the midpoint of the posterior portion of the flap, and under the proximal portion of the flap. The three drains are removed in 24 to 48 hours, the hairline suturing is removed in 6 days, and the staples are removed in 10 days.

The dog-ear defect is revised 6 or more weeks after transposition of the flap. The frontotemporal recession is marked at its apex, which is the junction of the frontal and temporal hairlines. A line perpendicular to the axis of the flap is drawn superiorly from this point. The incisions follow the shape of a small "h," and the frontotemporal recession and the proximal part of the flap are elevated. Bald skin is removed behind the dog-ear portion.

A second flap procedure can be performed after the baldness behind the front flap progresses. The design of the second flap and the surgical procedure are similar to those of the first flap procedure. Usually, an intervening space of 3 to 4 cm of bald skin is left between the flaps and later excised with scalp reductions (Fig. 294-8 and 294-9).

Crown baldness is often treated before using flaps with scalp reductions if the patient has or will have more than crown baldness alone. If the patient will never have more than crown baldness, a crown flap is used to remove this baldness (Fig. 294-10).

If the patient has or will have a narrow donor area or a tight scalp, tissue expanders are used in conjunction with flap surgery.

TOBY G. MAYER

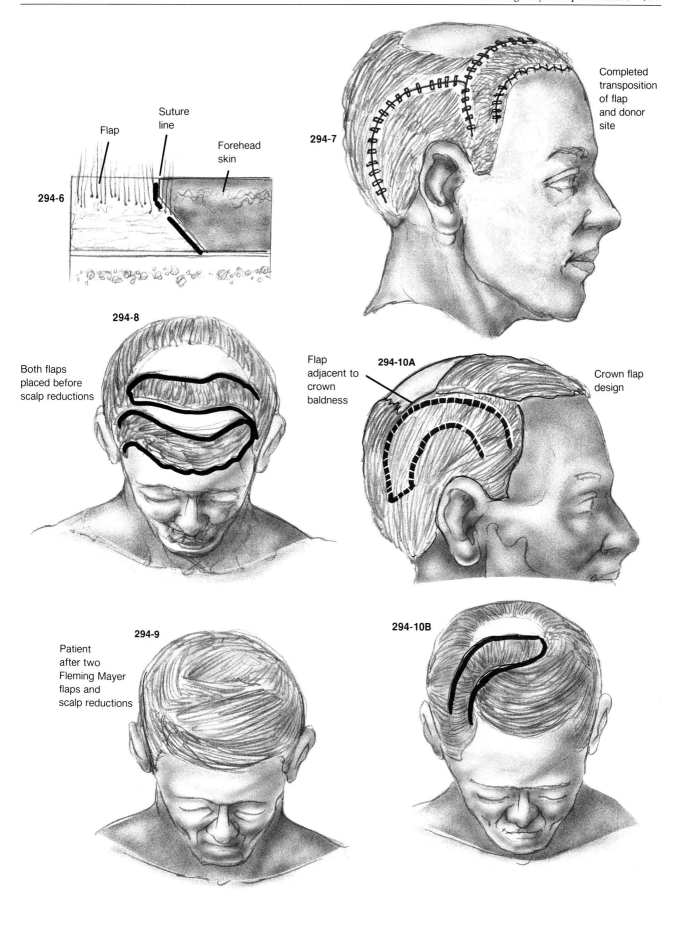

294-6
Flap
Suture line
Forehead skin

294-7
Completed transposition of flap and donor site

294-8
Both flaps placed before scalp reductions

294-10A
Flap adjacent to crown baldness
Crown flap design

294-9
Patient after two Fleming Mayer flaps and scalp reductions

294-10B

■ 295. SCALP REDUCTION

Serial excision of portions of a bald scalp

Indications

1. Before Fleming-Mayer flaps to increase the size of the donor area
2. After Fleming-Mayer flaps to increase the width of the flap or decrease the size of the remaining crown bald defect

Contraindications

1. Tight scalp
2. Patients older than 50 years of age with only frontal loss, young patients with only frontal loss and no loss in the midscalp or crown, and patients with very wide (12 to 14 cm in diameter) crown baldness may not be considered candidates.

Special Considerations

1. Surgical patterns include the midline ellipse, lateral (paramedian), and Y or double Y

(continued)

Operative Procedure

Types of Procedures

The easiest scalp reduction pattern for the novice to perform is the elliptic midline closure (Fig. 295-1A). However, this pattern has many significant disadvantages. No skin is removed in an anteroposterior direction (as with the Y closure), the remaining bald area is distorted, the posterior scar is lengthened and lowered instead of shortened and raised (as with the Y pattern), less bald skin is excised than with other procedures, and surgical exposure is limited.

The paramedian or lateral scalp reduction is more advantageous than the midline ellipse, but it is also less preferable than the Y-pattern scalp reduction (Fig. 295-1B). This approach also has disadvantages. Temporary anesthesia results over the top of the head, scalp circulation may be impaired if a central island is created, and impaired growth of subsequent grafts may occur. Distortion of the remaining bald area is the same as with a midline ellipse and greater than with the Y or double Y patterns. Less undermining is possible on the contralateral side than with the Y or double Y patterns.

My colleagues and I use the Y and double Y patterns for scalp reduction (Fig. 295-2). Occasionally, a different pattern is chosen, especially in revision surgery, when the patient's problem dictates a different approach. The Y or double Y patterns seem to have the greatest number of advantages and the fewest disadvantages. Excess scalp can be removed in the anteroposterior and lateral-to-lateral planes. More bald skin is removed than with the midline ellipse or paramedian reduction. Little distortion of the balding pattern occurs. The posterior dog-ear defect is distributed in two places instead of one. Undermining is easier than with other techniques. No central island of impaired circulation results. Because more bald skin is removed with each reduction, fewer reductions are necessary with this pattern than with the midline ellipse. There are several disadvantages of the Y and double Y patterns. These procedures may be more difficult than the midline ellipse. Tip necrosis of the apex of the posterior flap is a possible complication (although never seen). This procedure may take slightly longer to perform than the others.

(continued)

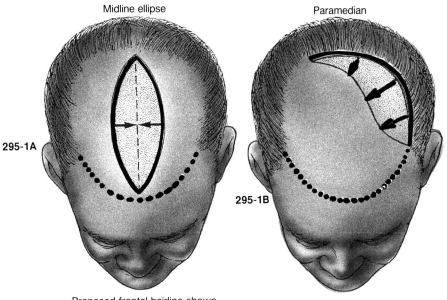

Midline ellipse

Paramedian

295-1A

295-1B

Proposed frontal hairline shown
with dotted line

295-2. Common scalp reduction patterns of excision

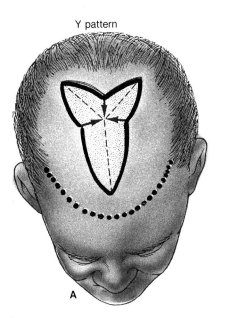

Y pattern

Double Y pattern
(designed to prevent elevation of frontotemporal
recessions, which would occur if midline
ellipse or Y pattern were used)

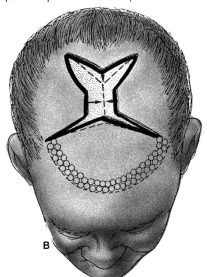

A

B

Stippled areas = areas of excision

■ *295.* SCALP REDUCTION *(continued)*

Tips and Pearls
1. Deep galeal sutures are placed to eliminate all tension on skin sutures
2. The Y pattern yields the most advantages and least disadvantages for almost all patients

Complications
1. Hematoma (rare)
2. Infection (rare)
3. Wide scarring (rare if properly done)

Postoperative Care Issues
1. Discomfort requires strong pain medication

References
Blanchard G, Blanchard B. Obliteration of alopecia by hair lifting: a new concept and technique. J Natl Med Assoc 1977;69:63.

Mayer TG, Fleming RW. Aesthetic and reconstructive surgery of the scalp. St. Louis: Mosby Year Book, 1992.

Unger MG. Scalp reductions. Facial Plast Surg 1985;2:253.

The double Y pattern is used in patients who have had grafting in the frontal region, when we do not want to elevate the frontotemporal recession (Fig. 295-3). The limbs of the anterior Y are placed posterior to the grafts. In this way, the temporal hair can be stretched without elevating the frontotemporal hairline.

Y and Double Y Techniques

The Y or double Y procedure is normally performed after local anesthesia has been given. Using an alcohol sponge, the areas to be injected are prepped. One-half percent lidocaine hydrochloride with 1:200,000 epinephrine is injected in all areas to be undermined. The same solution is then injected along the proposed lines of incision for hemostasis.

The left limb of the central ellipse is incised with a #10 blade through the galea, parallel to the hair follicles. The inferior limb of the Y incision is also completed at this time, and bleeding is controlled with electrocautery. The skin is elevated anteriorly with a double hook where the galea is loosely attached with Kahn scissors. I often use a Fleming-Mayer dissector to bluntly dissect the temporoparietal scalp. Posteriorly, the dissection is more difficult, because the galea becomes attached to the fascia over the neck musculature and the nuchal ridge. The dissection should extend to the hairline above the ear and posteriorly to the nuchal ridge (Fig. 295-4). After one side has been completely undermined, the same steps are repeated on the contralateral side.

After the excess skin has been removed and any residual bleeding controlled with electrocautery, the galea is approximated sequentially. Inverted interrupted sutures of 0 polydioxanone are used along the course of the incision, which usually proceeds from the midscalp forward. After this area has been closed at the galeal level, the skin edges are approximated with a surgical staple gun. The area next to the apex of the Y is similarly closed. Any excess tissue is trimmed, and the inferior triangular flap is elevated anteriorly so even more tissue in this plane can be removed. The galea and skin edges are closed in the fashion previously described.

I do not routinely use a drain. If much oozing occurs, a Penrose drain is placed in the most inferior portion of one limb of the Y before the final closure and sutured in place with a surgical staple gun. The hair is cleansed with normal saline and dried. The scalp is circumferentially blocked with bupivacaine hydrochloride, Telfa strips with K-Y jelly are placed over the incisions and secured with tape, and a fluff and cling–type dressing is applied. I have never found galeotomies (incisions in the galea) to be effective in significantly increasing the amount of tissue removed at each session. However, they can aid in closing an unusually tight wound after overzealous trimming of bald skin. The gain from this procedure is usually only a few millimeters, and my colleagues and I never use it.

Sutures are removed in 10 to 12 days, and subsequent reductions can be repeated every 3 months (Fig. 295-5).

TOBY G. MAYER

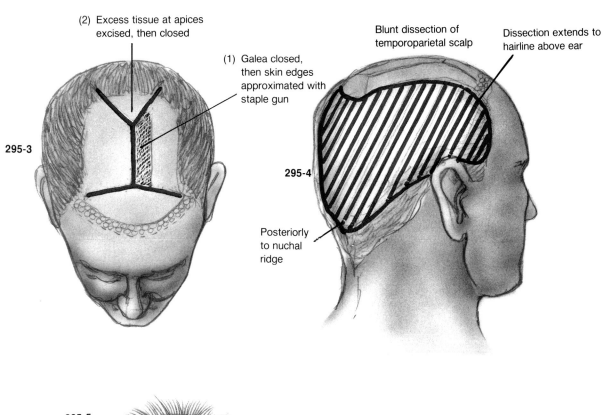

(2) Excess tissue at apices excised, then closed

(1) Galea closed, then skin edges approximated with staple gun

295-3

Blunt dissection of temporoparietal scalp

Dissection extends to hairline above ear

295-4

Posteriorly to nuchal ridge

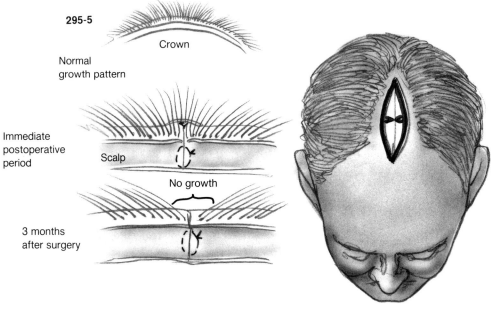

295-5

Crown

Normal growth pattern

Immediate postoperative period

Scalp

No growth

3 months after surgery

■ 296. TISSUE EXPANSION

Insertion of a silicone balloon with a self-sealing port used for injection

Indications

1. Used to assist scalp reduction of a tight scalp
2. Used in conjunction with Fleming-Mayer flaps for a tight scalp or narrow donor area
3. Reconstruction

Special Considerations

1. Type and size of expander
2. Type of injection port
3. Size and location of the defect or baldness compared with the remaining hair-bearing scalp
4. Morbidity and complications
5. Advantages in conjunction with a Fleming-Mayer flap
   a. Increased ease of donor area closure gained without undermining below the postauricular hairline
   b. Flap taken from the scalp with densest hair, thinned by approximately one third
   c. Postauricular hairline not raised
   d. Operating time, recovery time, and morbidity decreased
   e. Increased length and width of flap

Preoperative Preparation

1. Discussion with the patient about the cosmetic deformity involved with tissue expansion
2. Measuring the size of the expander to use, especially in reconstruction

Special Instruments, Position, and Anesthesia

1. Local or general anesthesia

Tips and Pearls

1. Creation of "new hair"
2. Procedure almost always improves the end result
3. Ability to repair a previously irreparable defect
4. Fewer operations
5. Specific area can be expanded
6. No donor defect or additional incisions, unless used with transposition flap
7. Minimal additional training required
8. Start patient on antibiotics two days before surgery to reduce risk of infection.

Pitfalls and Complications

1. Hematoma
2. Infection
3. Port or expander exposure
4. Port or expander leak
5. Flap failure (ie, partial necrosis)

References

Austad ED. Complications in tissue expansion. Clin Plast Surg 1987;14: 549.

Mayer TG, Fleming RW. Aesthetic and reconstructive surgery of the scalp. St. Louis: Mosby-Year Book, 1992.

Pasyk KA, Argenta LC, Austad ED. Histopathology of human expanded tissue. Clin Plast Surg 1987;14:435.

Operative Procedure

Preoperatively, tissue expansion is used as an adjunct to scalp reduction in patients with tight scalps, as an adjunct to transposition of Fleming-Mayer flaps, and in reconstructive surgery for the treatment of trauma, burns, tumors, and other such lesions.

Regardless of the ultimate goal or second procedure, placement follows a few general rules of tissue expansion technique. The hair is never shaved or clipped. The entire scalp and face are prepped using Phisohex. All areas to be undermined are infiltrated with a 0.5% solution of Xylocaine with 1:200,000 epinephrine. This solution is also placed as a ring block around the head and within the area of incision intradermally. Most expanders are placed with the use of local anesthesia only, except in children and anxious adults, for whom general anesthesia is used.

The incision used for placement of the tissue expander is approximately 4 cm long. The usual location of the injection port is over the bald area in the crown for patients receiving scalp reduction or Fleming-Mayer flaps. The port is placed under the area of the scar or skin graft, as long as this area is not atrophic and permits placement and prevents extrusion (Fig. 296-1).

After the incision is made, bleeding below the level of the hair follicles is controlled quickly with electrocautery. The Fleming-Mayer scalp dissector facilitates blunt dissection; occasionally, the Kahn scissors must be used to complete the pocket. The limits of dissection are drawn in ink before beginning the procedure and should allow the expander to be completely laid flat within the pocket.

The expander pocket should be located away from the site of the incision to prevent stretching of the scar and expander exposure. This can be accomplished by not bringing the entire pocket dissection superiorly up to the same plane as that of the incision itself. If multiple expanders are being used, a moist sponge is placed in the area of incision, and the other pocket is dissected in like fashion.

After insertion of the expander, the scalp incisions are closed using 0 polydioxanone sutures to approximate the galea and surgical staples for the skin. Drains are never used because of the risk of contaminating the expander. Before applying a dressing, the surgeon inflates the expander with saline and methylene blue; this inflation causes a slight pressure within the pocket, which minimizes the oozing of blood around the expander, and it will uncover any leaks.

The dressing consists of K-Y jelly, gauze, and a circumferential Kling dressing. Marcaine (0.5%) is administered before insertion of the expander to provide prolonged analgesia within the operative area. Injectable saline is used to inflate the expander after waiting 2 weeks. Expanders are filled twice each week until the designated expansion size is reached.

Most of the tissue expander removals that are combined with reductions, flaps, or reconstructions are performed under general anesthesia. Scalp reductions after tissue expansion can be done with local anesthesia (Fig. 296-2).

TOBY G. MAYER

Fleming-Mayer type A tissue expander in place and fully expanded

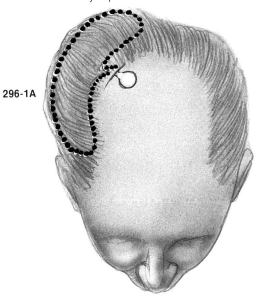

296-1A

Lateral view of the Fleming-Mayer tissue expander in place, showing incision for placement superiorly along the fringe and future design of a flap to be used in conjunction with expander

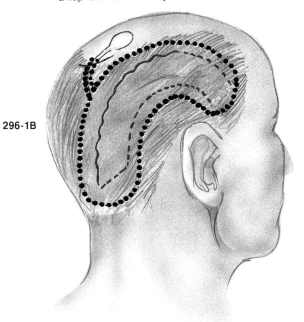

296-1B

Bilateral tissue expanders placed before scalp reduction. Standard port is marked (1), and a microport is marked (2). Dark line shows incisions for placement of expander.

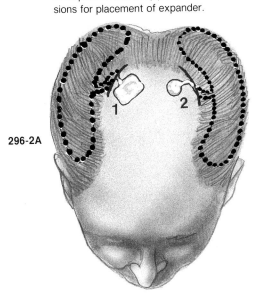

296-2A

After removal of the expanders, the patient has some divergence cí hair along the scar in the midscalp and crown, as well as complete frontal baldness, which is unchanged from its preoperative degree

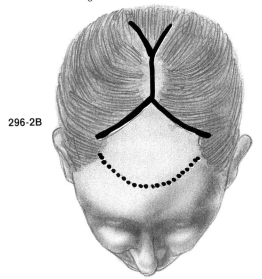

296-2B

Atlas of Head and Neck Surgery–Otolaryngology,
edited by Byron J. Bailey, J. Gail Neely, Karen H. Calhoun, and Amy R. Coffey.
Lippincott-Raven Publishers, Philadelphia © 1996.

Section Four
Endoscopy

Section Editor:

Amy R. Coffey

Laryngoscopy
Esophagoscopy
Bronchoscopy

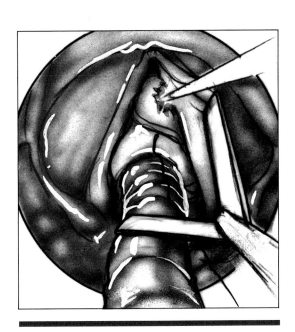

■ 297. DIRECT LARYNGOSCOPY WITH AND WITHOUT BIOPSY— Examination of the hypopharynx and larynx with the laryngoscope and biopsy of a lesion of the area

Indications

1. Change in voice, airway obstruction (eg, stridor)
2. Suspected malignancy, laryngeal mass
3. Persistent cough, hemoptysis
4. Tracheotomy decannulation
5. Persistent atelectasis, atypical asthma
6. Foreign body
7. Recurrent respiratory infection (eg, croup in a child)
8. Dysphagia

Special Considerations

1. C-spine abnormalities (especially Down syndrome in a child)
2. Immobility of mandible and craniofacial anomalies hinder exposure.

Preoperative Preparation

1. Routine laboratory studies; indicated labs
2. Anteroposterior (AP) and lateral chest radiographs, AP and lateral neck radiographs, barium swallow x-ray film, and computed tomography or magnetic resonance imaging, if indicated
3. Blood gases, if indicated
4. Anesthesia consult and planning

Special Instruments, Position, and Anesthesia

1. Laryngoscopes: vallecula scope, anterior commissure scope, sliding (Jackson) or slotted (Benjamin) scope for intubation or introduction of bronchoscope, and suspension laryngoscope and device for biopsy and instrumentation procedure
2. Bronchoscope for examination and establishment of emergency airway
3. Rigid metal suctions of various lengths
4. Biopsy and grasping forceps
5. Jet ventilation needle setup
6. Telescopes and microscopes for examinations
7. Tooth guard
8. Twin light sources and twin light cords
9. Tracheotomy set
10. Bronchoscopy sponges and vasoconstrictive solution (Afrin)
11. Xylocaine (1% to 2% concentration) spray bottle

Tips and Pearls

1. Position of patient and surgeon arranged for maximum easy exposure
2. Communication with anesthesiologist in reference to relaxation, intubation or no intubation, jet ventilation, and other matters
3. Choose and check all equipment before anesthesia induction.
4. Monitor temperature, especially in infants and children.

Pitfalls and Complications

1. Intraoperative airway compromise
2. Dental injury and mandibular dislocation
3. Pneumothorax from airway biopsy or jet ventilation at high pressure

Postoperative Care Issues

1. Maintain adequate ventilation.
2. Avoid postoperative respiratory depression drugs.
3. Observe for laryngospasm.
4. Monitor as appropriate: O_2 saturation, electrocardiogram, apnea and bradycardia monitor (infants).
5. Humidification with bedside humidifier, collar, shield, or tent
6. Postoperative steroids may be indicated to reduce edema.
7. Voice rest may be helpful for 24 to 72 hours.

References

Johns M, Price J, Mattox D. Atlas of head and neck surgery. Philadelphia: BC Decker, 1990.

Miller RH, Gianoli GJ. Airway evaluation and imaging. In: Bailey BJ, ed. Head and neck surgery—otolaryngology. Philadelphia: JB Lippincott, 1993;509.

Operative Procedures

Standard Adult Direct Laryngoscopy

The patient is positioned on the operating table with a slight shoulder roll and the head resting in a doughnut-shaped holder in the so-called sniffing position. Preoxygenation is accomplished with 100% oxygen and a mask. Anesthesia is induced, and paralysis accomplished with a short-acting muscle relaxant. A small endotracheal tube is inserted. The eyes are protected with Lacri-Lube and eye pads. Head drapes are applied, and a rubber mouth guard tooth protector is inserted.

The larynx is exposed with a suitable laryngoscope inserted into the vallecula (Fig. 297-1). The base of the tongue, both piriform fossae, the cricopharyngeal sphincter, the lateral and posterior pharyngeal walls, and postcricoid area are examined consecutively. The lingual and laryngeal surface of the epiglottis, both aryepiglottic folds, and the false vocal cords are inspected. The ventricles and true vocal cords are inspected. Using the anterior commissure laryngoscope, this area is inspected along with the immediate subglottic area (Fig. 297-2). The arytenoid cartilages are palpated to evaluate passive motion. The rod-lens telescope (0° and 30°) can be used during this examination to facilitate careful inspection of these areas (Fig. 297-3).

If vocal cord motion evaluation is indicated and has not been done previously with a flexible laryngoscope, it may be carried out at this point. The endotracheal tube is removed, and the anesthesia is reduced for sufficient time to completely evaluate vocal cord motion during inspiration and vocalization by the patient. This is best carried out with the laryngoscope blade in the vallecula so the vocal cord motion is not obscured or altered by the laryngoscope blade.

Biopsy

After complete examination of the larynx and hypopharynx, the suspension apparatus is attached and supported by a Mayo stand immediately above the patient's chest or attached to the operating room table if it is a self-retaining suspension apparatus (Fig. 297-4). The lesion is identified and grasped with cup forceps (Fig. 297-5). The lesion is then removed with a brief downward and then upward movement of the cup forceps to avoid stripping of tissue. An alternate method is carried out by grasping the lesion with a cup forceps, and with the microscissors or laryngeal knife, the lesion is removed under microscopic visualization. Bleeding points are controlled with a bronchoscopy sponge moistened with Afrin solution held in position over the biopsy site for 3 to 5 minutes. If the lesion is obscured by the endotracheal tube, the tube may be removed and anesthesia continued with Jet ventilation during the biopsy procedure. At the completion of the procedure, the patient is awakened, extubated, and taken to the recovery room.

Pediatric Laryngeal Evaluation

In infants and children, the most common technique is diagnostic laryngoscopy with spontaneous respiration using nitrous oxide, oxygen, and halothane administered with a face mask. Topical anesthesia up to 5 mg of Xylocaine per 1 kg of body weight is sprayed onto the epiglottis, larynx, and upper trachea. Anesthesia is then deepened. This technique allows careful, unhurried observation and assessment of vocal cord motion and of the dynamics of the larynx. Because there is no endotracheal tube, insufflation into the larynx of oxygen, nitrous oxide, and halothane may be continued through a side tube in the laryngoscope or passed through the nose into the hypopharynx to maintain stable anesthesia.

The examination is carried out as with adults, but congenital problems and foreign bodies are more likely findings than are the neoplasms of the adult population. In very young infants, it may be necessary to flex the head forward to allow the more anteriorly placed larynx to achieve a more posterior position for adequate visualization. The laryngoscope is placed in the posterior commissure to rule out congenital cleft of the larynx.

Bronchoscopy to complete the airway evaluation may be carried out from this point (see Procedures 310 through 314).

RONALD W. DESKIN

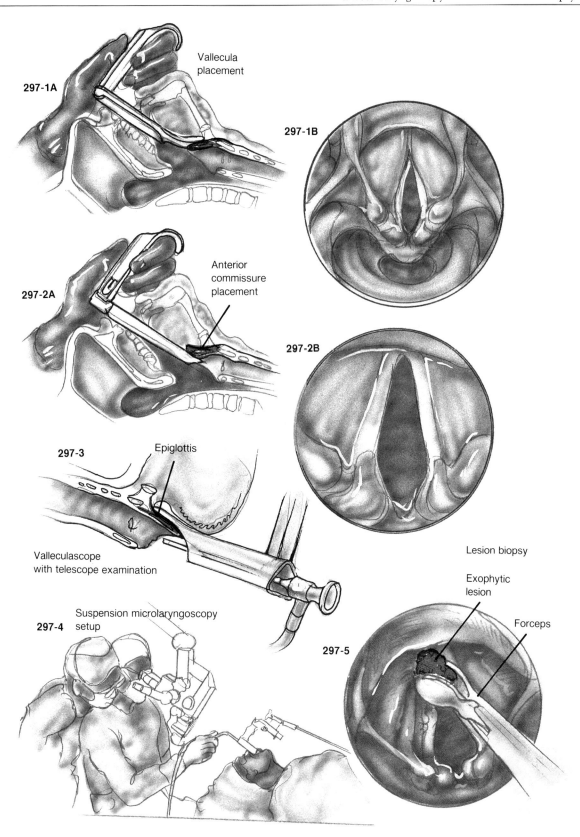

297-1A

Vallecula
placement

297-1B

297-2A

Anterior
commissure
placement

297-2B

297-3   Epiglottis

Valleculascope
with telescope examination

Lesion biopsy

Exophytic
lesion

Forceps

297-4   Suspension microlaryngoscopy
setup

297-5

■ 298. NASOPHARYNGOSCOPY

An examination of the nasopharynx that can be performed with or without a biopsy

Indications

1. Nasal obstruction, epistaxis, and unilateral hearing loss or otitis
2. Cranial nerve paralysis
3. Lymph nodes enlarged in the posterior cervical triangle or velopharyngeal insufficiency

Special Considerations

1. Before biopsy, if considering juvenile angiofibroma, obtain a computed tomography (CT) scan with contrast.
2. In preparation for a biopsy of a nasopharyngeal mass, the patient should be typed and crossmatched for transfusion in case a vascular tumor is found.
3. Nasopharyngeal biopsies should not be blind, but they can be performed in a random manner under direct visualization.
4. Biopsies should avoid area of the eustachian tube orifice to prevent scarring and permanent eustachian tube dysfunction.
5. This examination can be performed in the awake patient in the office with the use of topical anesthetic and topical hemostatic drops applied to the nares bilaterally.

Preoperative Preparation

1. Type and crossmatch the patient in case a vascular tumor is found.
2. Transoral palpation helps to estimate the size and location of the abnormality.
3. An awake patient should be sitting, and an anesthetized patient should be lying down.

Special Instruments

1. In the office, this examination can be performed with a headlight and nasopharyngeal mirror.
2. The 0°, 30°, or 70° sinus endoscope can provide panoramic views of the nasopharynx.
3. The flexible fiberoptic laryngoscope is also useful for examining this area.

References

Loré JM Jr. Nasopharyngoscopy. In: Loré JM Jr (ed). An atlas of head and neck surgery, 3rd ed. Philadelphia: WB Saunders, 1988:126.

Loré JM Jr. Rigid and flexible direct optical nasopharyngoscopy and rhinoscopy. In: Loré JM Jr (ed). An atlas of head and neck surgery, 3rd ed. Philadelphia: WB Saunders, 1988:130.

Operative Procedure

In the awake patient, this examination is performed in the sitting position. The anesthetized patient is usually supine. Topical decongestant, anesthetic, and hemostatic drops should be placed in both nares. When using the rigid sinus scope or the flexible laryngoscope, the scope should be lubricated to achieve the least traumatic entry and defogged to permit a clear view.

Introduce the scope along the floor of the nose, and rotate it past the posterior choanae bilaterally (Fig. 298-1). In the awake patient, the examiner can observe the dynamics of the soft palate by means of voicing tasks. Anatomic and functional abnormalities can be recognized.

In adults, a biopsy can be performed in the office under indirect view. A nasal cup forceps or sinus instrument can be used for biopsy (Fig. 298-2). All specimens should be sent for pathologic examination. Hemostasis usually is not problematic, but if finding a vascular lesion is possible, the biopsy is most safely performed in the operating room with the patient under general endotracheal anesthesia. Biopsy under general anesthesia is recommended if previous biopsy material was nondiagnostic. When the examination and biopsy are performed in the anesthetized patient, the nose should be topically decongested and anesthetized. The examination is most complete when the scope is passed twice: once through the right nares and once through the left to achieve visualization of the full nasopharynx. Biopsy sites are located with the sinus endoscope or the flexible nasopharyngoscope (Fig. 298-3). Specimens are obtained with a cup forceps transnasally or beneath the palate transorally. Efforts should be made to avoid the endotracheal orifice and possible permanent scarring in this area.

ELLEN M. FRIEDMAN

Introduce the nasopharyngoscope along floor of the nose;
rotate past posterior choanae bilaterally

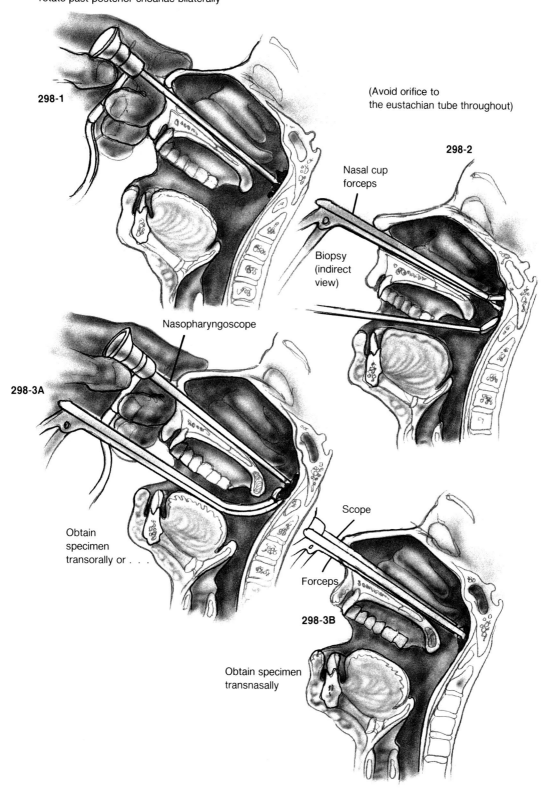

298-1

(Avoid orifice to
the eustachian tube throughout)

298-2

Nasal cup
forceps

Biopsy
(indirect
view)

Nasopharyngoscope

298-3A

Obtain
specimen
transorally or . . .

Scope

Forceps

298-3B

Obtain specimen
transnasally

■ 299. TRUE VOCAL CORD INJECTION FOR PARALYSIS—Medialization of a true vocal cord by injection of Teflon paste or Gelfoam paste

Indications
1. Unilateral paralysis of true vocal cord
   a. Hoarseness with air wasting
   b. Poor cough
   c. Aspiration
2. Partial vocal cord defects caused by excision of vocal cord lesions
3. Presbylarynx with bowing of the true vocal cords

Contraindications
1. Bilateral vocal cord paralysis
2. Risk of contralateral paralysis due to impending thyroid or anterior cervical disc surgery

Special Considerations
1. Teflon is used for permanent true vocal cord paralysis.
2. Gelfoam is used if the possibility of the return of true vocal cord function exists.
3. Unknown cause of paralysis should delay Teflon injection 6 to 12 months (possibility of the return of function).

Preoperative Preparation
1. Indirect or flexible fiberoptic laryngoscopy
2. Speech therapy consultation

Special Instruments, Position, and Anesthesia
1. Suspension laryngoscopy set with anterior commissure scope available
2. Arnold-Bruning intralaryngeal injection set with a No. 19 laryngeal needle
3. Teflon or Gelfoam paste
4. Supine position, with a foam doughnut
5. Local anesthesia with intravenous sedation

Tips and Pearls
1. Bruning syringe must be loaded and tested immediately before use and cleaned with ethyl alcohol after use.
2. Injection in the proper plane, not too deep or superficial, is aided by a guard on the needle.
3. Do not remove the Bruning needle immediately after clicking, because Teflon or Gelfoam continues to be extruded from the needle after each click.
4. Clear visualization of the paralyzed and normal cord is mandatory.
5. The first injection is made into the posterior portion of the true vocal cord at the level of the vocal process of the arytenoid.
6. Anesthesia should make the patient comfortable but able to vocalize on command.
7. Intraoperative steroid treatment

Pitfalls and Complications
1. Improper placement of the injection can cause airway obstruction, no improvement in the voice, or worsening of voice.
2. Overinjection or underinjection can result in airway obstruction and inadequate improvement of the voice or aspiration.
3. Aspiration may not be improved if other cranial nerves (eg, IX, X, XII) are also impaired.
4. The voice results in patients with superior and recurrent laryngeal nerve paralysis are not as good as the voice results in patients with recurrent laryngeal nerve paralysis alone.

Postoperative Care Issues
1. Speech pathology evaluation to compare results with preoperative function
2. Monitor the patient for airway obstruction due to overinjection, laryngeal edema, or both.

References
Dedo HH. Teflon injection of the vocal cord. In: Dedo HH, ed. Surgery of the larynx and trachea. Philadelphia: BC Decker, 1990:14.

Montgomery WW. Laryngeal paralysis. In: Montgomery W, ed. Surgery of the upper respiratory system, vol II. 2nd ed. Philadelphia: Lea & Febiger, 1989:623.

Operative Procedure
While the Bruning Teflon injection set is being loaded and tested, the patient is anesthetized by spraying Hurricane spray onto the floor of mouth and tongue. The patient is asked to swallow the spray, and the procedure is repeated two times. Intravenous sedation with Versed and Fentanyl is titrated so the patient is asleep or comfortable but arousable. Dexamethasone sodium phosphate (Decadron; 10 mg) is given intravenously. The Dedo laryngoscope is inserted (Fig. 299-1*A*), and Hurricane spray is used to anesthetize the tongue and vallecula as the instrument is advanced. After the cords are visualized (Fig. 299-1*B*), they and the cervical trachea are sprayed with 0.5 to 0.75 mL of 4% cocaine. The cocaine spray may be repeated three times or until the cough reflex is suppressed. On exposure of the vocal cords, the suspension apparatus is attached and the operating microscope is focused on the true vocal cords. If the patient is unable to tolerate suspension after maximal topical anesthesia, a superior laryngeal nerve block can be performed, with the understanding that voice quality may change after function of the superior laryngeal nerve returns.

With the patient's larynx suspended, the #19 Bruning needle is inserted such that the false vocal cord is displaced laterally (Fig. 299-2). The needle is aimed laterally, with the bevel facing medially, and inserted into the lateral thyroarytenoid muscle at the posterior portion of the vocal cord, just lateral to the vocal process (Fig. 299-3). Injection of the Teflon or Gelfoam is begun with one to two clicks. The needle should not be withdrawn immediately after clicking because Teflon or Gelfoam continues to be extruded from the needle for a short period after clicking. At first, conservative injection is suggested; this leaves the paralyzed cord slightly lateral to midline. The needle is removed and used to massage the cord to help distribute the injected material anteriorly. The patient is asked to vocalize, and the quality of the voice is assessed. Commonly, a second point of injection midway between the vocal process and the anterior commissure is necessary (Fig. 299-4).

Common errors of technique are to inject too deeply, too superficially, or too medially (Fig. 299-5). Deep injections do not medialize the cord but may narrow the subglottic airway. Superficial injections may cause obliteration of the laryngeal ventricle rather than medialize the cord. Medial injections can cause infiltration of the vibrating edge of the vocal cord or the medial thyroarytenoid muscle that does not result in medialization of the cord but does cause deterioration of the voice.

AMELIA F. DRAKE
WENDELL G. YARBROUGH

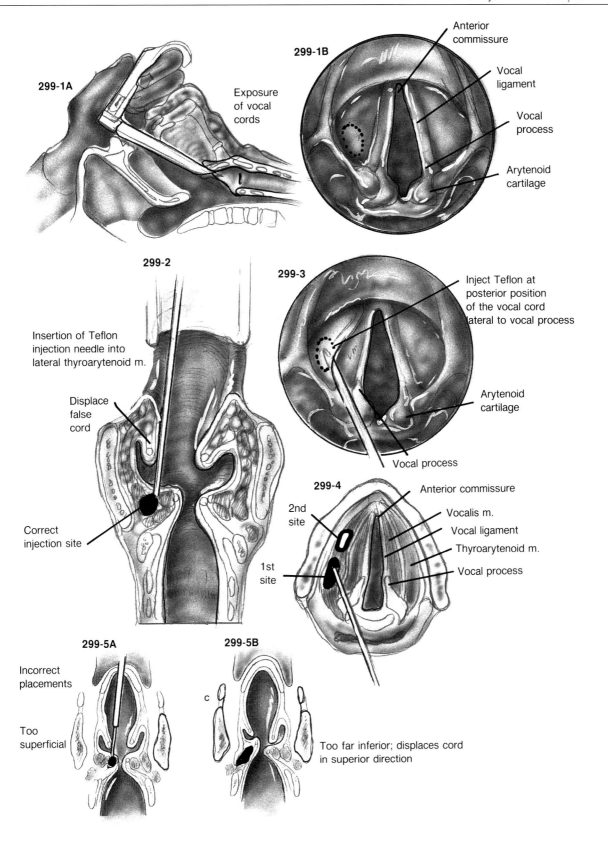

299-1A

Exposure of vocal cords

299-1B

Anterior commissure

Vocal ligament

Vocal process

Arytenoid cartilage

299-2

Insertion of Teflon injection needle into lateral thyroarytenoid m.

Displace false cord

Correct injection site

299-3

Inject Teflon at posterior position of the vocal cord lateral to vocal process

Arytenoid cartilage

Vocal process

299-4

2nd site

1st site

Anterior commissure

Vocalis m.

Vocal ligament

Thyroarytenoid m.

Vocal process

299-5A

Incorrect placements

Too superficial

299-5B

c

Too far inferior; displaces cord in superior direction

■ *300.* LASER LARYNGOSCOPY FOR PAPIL-
LOMA REMOVAL—Removal of recurrent respiratory papilloma with a laser

Indications
1. Recurrent respiratory papillomatosis
2. Other benign growths of the larynx

Special Considerations
1. C-spine abnormalities (especially Down syndrome in a child)
2. Immobility of the mandible and craniofacial anomalies may make exposure difficult.
3. The general medical status may make the patient a poor candidate for general anesthesia.
4. Correct a bleeding disorder before any anticipated procedure.

Preoperative Preparation
1. Routine laboratory studies
2. Bleeding and clotting studies if the patient's history is questionable
3. Anteroposterior (AP) and lateral chest radiographs, AP and lateral neck radiographs
4. Blood gases, if indicated
5. Anesthesia consultation and planning (Figs. 300-1 and 300-2)

Special Instruments, Position, and Anesthesia
1. Laryngoscopes: vallecula scope, anterior commissure scope, sliding (Jackson) or slotted (Benjamin) scope for intubation or introduction of bronchoscope, and suspension laryngoscope for use with a laser
2. Bronchoscope for examination and establishment of emergency airway
3. Rigid metal suctions of various lengths
4. Biopsy and grasping forceps
5. Jet ventilation needle setup
6. Telescopes and microscopes for examinations
7. Suspension setup
8. Tooth guard
9. Twin light source and twin light cords
10. Tracheotomy set
11. Bronchoscopy sponges and vasoconstrictive solution (Afrin)
12. Xylocaine (1% to 2% concentration) spray bottle
13. Appropriate-sized red rubber endotracheal tube
14. Aluminum foil wrapping for endotracheal tube
15. Bronchoscopy sponges or neuropledgets fastened to long wire applicator
16. Protective eye wear for operating room personnel
17. 50-mL syringe of water
18. Metal tracheotomy tubes if the patient has a tracheotomy
19. Carbon dioxide laser instrument
20. Laser bronchoscope with CO_2 laser coupler

(continued)

Operative Procedure
The patient is positioned on the operating room table with a slight shoulder roll and the head resting in a doughnut-shaped holder in the so-called sniffing position. A 20° reverse Trendelenburg position allows good exposure. Preoxygenation with 100% oxygen by mask is carried out, and then anesthesia is induced. At this point, several alternative types of anesthesia may be used. Jet ventilation anesthesia is a common safe method. After adequate plan of anesthesia has been reached, the larynx is sprayed with a 1% solution of Xylocaine.

The suspension laryngoscope (Jako-Pilling) is used to examine the larynx. If the papillomas are not significantly obstructing the airway, muscle relaxation is achieved, and the jet ventilation needle is attached to the proximal opening of the laryngoscope and ventilation begun (Fig. 300-3). This allows adequate exposure and visualization for laser operation without the disadvantage of a combustible endotracheal tube in the airway (Fig. 300-5). The eyes are protected by moistened eye pads, and the face is wrapped with moistened lap sponges and a moistened towel. Any exposed skin of the shoulders or chest area is also covered with moist towels.

The operating microscope with the CO_2 laser attached is brought into position, and the larynx is visualized, usually under low power. Cup forceps biopsy of the most easily obtained papilloma is carried out for histologic evaluation to rule out malignant transformation (Fig. 300-6). The papillomas may then be removed in an orderly fashion, starting at the level of the true vocal cord and continuing superiorly (Fig. 300-7). A 400-mm lens attachment on the microscope is used, and a power setting of 8 to 10 watts is used with 0.1-second exposure. The laser spot can be focused down to 0.5 mm for precise vaporization and up to about 2 mm for coagulation of vessels smaller than 0.5 mm. Intermittent laser application typically is used, although continuous mode may be used for larger gross vaporization in safe areas. The surgeon directs the laser beam with a micromanipulator "joystick," aiming with the helium-neon red beam. Both hands are then available for the joystick, cup forceps, grasping forceps, retractors, protectors, and suction. Removal of tissue "char" left from papilloma vaporization may be necessary from time to time with microcup forceps.

(continued)

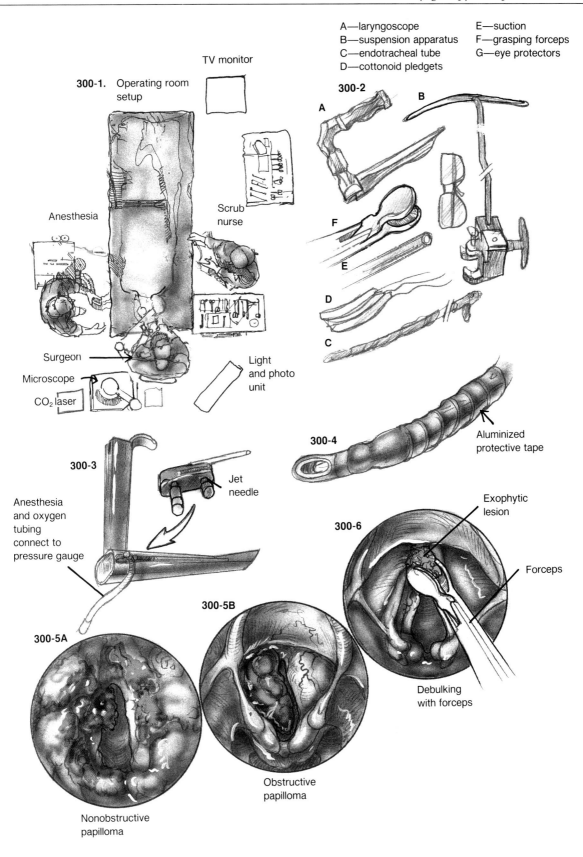

A—laryngoscope
B—suspension apparatus
C—endotracheal tube
D—cottonoid pledgets

E—suction
F—grasping forceps
G—eye protectors

300-1. Operating room setup

TV monitor

Anesthesia

Scrub nurse

Surgeon

Microscope

CO$_2$ laser

Light and photo unit

300-2

A

B

F

E

D

C

300-4

Aluminized protective tape

300-3

Anesthesia and oxygen tubing connect to pressure gauge

Jet needle

300-6

Exophytic lesion

Forceps

Debulking with forceps

300-5B

Obstructive papilloma

300-5A

Nonobstructive papilloma

■ 300. LASER LARYNGOSCOPY FOR PAPIL-LOMA REMOVAL (continued)

Tips and Pearls

1. Position of patient and surgeon arranged for maximum easy exposure
2. Communication with anesthesiologist in reference to relaxation, anesthesia technique (eg, intubation or no intubation, jet ventilation, wrapped red rubber tube), and special airway concerns and considerations
3. Choose and check all equipment before anesthesia induction.
4. Monitor temperature, especially in infants and children.
5. Have adequate operating room personnel to assist with the procedure and to operate laser equipment.

Pitfalls and Complications

1. Intraoperative airway compromise
2. Dental injury and mandibular dislocation
3. Pneumothorax from airway biopsy, laser penetration, or jet ventilation and high pressure
4. Eye injury
5. Burn of the skin, oral cavity, or airway
6. Endotracheal tube or other combustible material ignition and airway fire
7. Scaring or webbing of the airway from repeated or overly aggressive laser treatment

Postoperative Care Issues

1. Maintain adequate ventilation.
2. Avoid postoperative respiratory depression drugs.
3. Observe for laryngospasm.
4. Monitor as appropriate: O_2 saturation, electrocardiogram, apnea and bradycardia monitor (infants).
5. Humidification with bedside humidifier, collar, shield, or tent
6. Postoperative steroids may be indicated to reduce edema from instrumentation.
7. Voice rest may be helpful for 24 to 72 hours.

References

Benjamin B. Atlas of pediatric endoscopy. Oxford: Oxford University Press, 1981.

Healy GB. Congenital anomalies of the aerodigestive tract. In: Bailey BJ, ed. Head and neck surgery—otolaryngology. Philadelphia: JB Lippincott, 1993;848.

McGill T, Friedman E, Healy G. Laser surgery in the pediatric airway. Otolaryngol Clin North Am 1983;865.

It is essential to avoid bilateral or circumferential use of the laser in the area of the anterior commissure. Vocal cord retractors and protectors are used to protect the opposite vocal cord while using the laser (Fig. 300-9). Adequate smoke evacuation is carried out by suction, which may be used intermittently or attached through one of the light ports in a dual-light laryngoscope. The subglottic area and trachea are examined during the procedure with the microscope or the 0° rod-lens telescope to evaluate for possible distal spread of papilloma.

At the end of the procedure, the airway is carefully suctioned, and bleeding sites may be tamponaded with an Afrin-soaked sponge held against the bleeding area for 3 to 5 minutes. This is done carefully to ensure adequate ventilation through the jet ventilation needle. If adequate stability of the patient is obtained and spontaneous respiration is allowed to occur, the patient's anesthesia may be lightened, and the patient may then be taken to the recovery room at this point. Otherwise, the patient is intubated, the anesthesia lightened, and the patient then extubated before being taken to the recovery room. Adequate humidification in the recovery room is mandatory. Decadron (1 mg/kg, up to 10 mg) is given intravenously at the completion of procedure to reduce airway edema.

Other anesthetic techniques that may be useful, depending on the experience and desire of the surgeon and anesthesiologist, include foil-wrapped red rubber tubes, with the wrapping done from the distal end of the tube with overlapping folds and extending proximal to cover the tube adequately up into the pharynx (Fig. 300-4). Using this technique, the endotracheal tube cuff is filled with water. The area below the vocal cords where the tube is exposed is packed with moistened cotton sponges to protect the lower endotracheal tube and cuff (Fig. 300-8). This method has the advantage of adequate control of the airway, but the endotracheal tube limits the surgeon's field of vision, may traumatize the operative site, and produces the risk of endotracheal tube fire. Apneic techniques may be carried out with intermittent intubation, oxygenation, and removal of tube for brief periods of laser use, and reintubation intermittently to reoxygenate. Spontaneous ventilation with oxygen and anesthesia administered through a tube attached to the proximal laryngoscope or inserted to hypopharynx is limited by vocal cord motion during surgery. In patients with an existing tracheotomy, a metal tracheotomy tube may be inserted during the procedure to allow laser surgery to be carried out without the risk of ignition of the plastic tracheotomy tube.

RONALD W. DESKIN

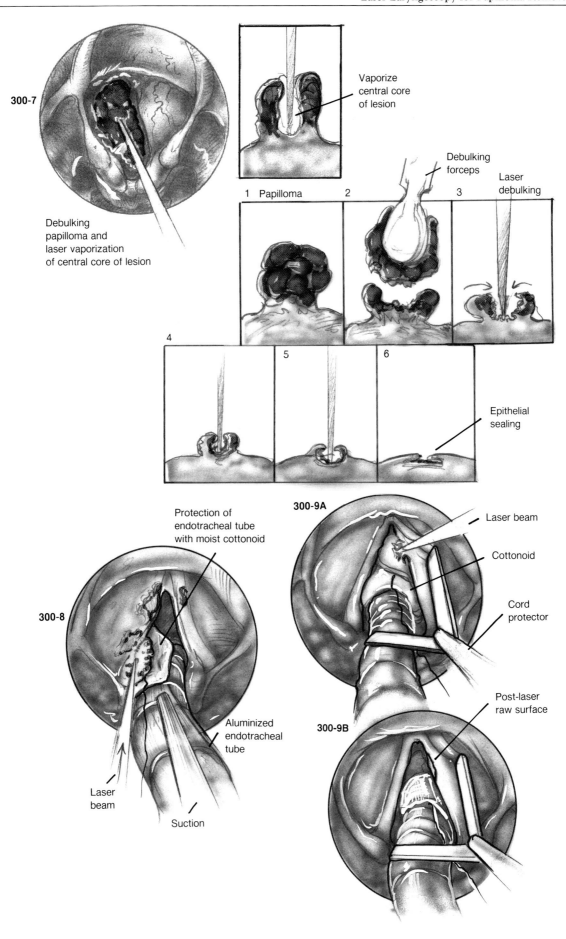

300-7

Debulking
papilloma and
laser vaporization
of central core of lesion

Vaporize
central core
of lesion

Debulking
forceps

Laser
debulking

1   Papilloma   2   3

4

5   6

Epithelial
sealing

Protection of
endotracheal tube
with moist cottonoid

300-8

Laser
beam

Suction

Aluminized
endotracheal
tube

300-9A

Laser beam

Cottonoid

Cord
protector

Post-laser
raw surface

300-9B

■ 301. LASER ARYTENOIDECTOMY

Laser vaporization of the corniculate and arytenoid cartilages

Indication

1. Bilateral vocal cord paralysis

Special Considerations

1. Bilateral vocal cord paralysis may be accompanied by posterior glottic web formation.
2. The fairly satisfactory voice produced with bilateral vocal cord paralysis usually worsens after this procedure.

Preoperative Preparation

1. Routine laboratory studies
2. Reflux precautions and H_2 blockers for patients with a history of reflux

Special Instruments, Position, and Anesthesia

1. CO_2 laser
2. Posterior commissure microlaryngoscope
3. Laser-safe endotracheal tube
4. Supine position, with shoulder roll
5. General anesthesia

Tips and Pearls

1. Protect eyes and all exposed skin and mucous membranes.
2. Minimize nonlaser instrumentation of the mucosa.
3. Avoid thermal injury to the interarytenoid area.

Pitfalls and Complications

1. Endotracheal fire
2. Laryngeal edema
3. Arytenoid granuloma
4. Loss of adequate voice production
5. Arytenoid perichondritis
6. Posterior laryngeal web

Postoperative Care Issues

1. Careful postoperative monitoring for airway compromise
2. Broad-spectrum antibiotics
3. Steroids to decrease edema
4. Overnight observation if laryngeal edema is suspected

References

Kashima HK. CO_2 Laser arytenoidectomy and transverse cordectomy. In: Johns ME, Price JC, Mattox DE, eds. Atlas of head and neck surgery. Philadelphia: BC Decker, 1990:41.

Lore JM. Carbon dioxide laser surgery. In: Lore JM, ed. An atlas of head and neck surgery, 3rd ed. Philadelphia: WB Saunders, 1988:874.

Ossoff RH, Sisson GA, Duncavage JA, Moselle HI, Andrews PE, McMillan WG. Endoscopic laser arytenoidectomy for the treatment of bilateral vocal cord paralysis. Laryngoscope. 1984;94:1293.

Operative Procedure

The patient is placed supine on the table, with a shoulder roll beneath the scapulae. The patient is intubated with a laser-safe endotracheal tube, and water, rather than air, is used to inflate the cuff. All operating room personnel should wear eye protection, and notices should be placed on operating room doors stating that a laser is in use. A posterior commissure microlaryngoscope is suspended for visualization of the larynx, with special attention to proper exposure of the posterior aspect of the arytenoids and interarytenoid cleft. A saline-saturated neurosurgical cottonoid may be placed below the level of the vocal cords to protect the endotracheal tube cuff. The patient's eyes should be protected with saline-saturated eye pads, and all exposed skin and mucous membranes must be covered with saline-moistened surgical towels.

Each arytenoid is gently palpated to identify the more mobile arytenoid. The Zeiss operating microscope coupled to the CO_2 laser is positioned to view the more mobile arytenoid. Initial laser settings include repeat mode (0.1 seconds) at 1990 watts/cm^2.

The mucoperichondrium overlying the corniculate cartilage is vaporized, exposing the corniculate cartilage, which is ablated (Fig. 301-1*A*). The mucoperichondrium overlying the exposed arytenoid cartilage is vaporized (see Fig. 301-1*B*). Laser settings are then increased to 3185 watts/cm^2 in the continuous mode, and the bulky upper portion of the arytenoid is ablated (see Fig. 301-1*C*). Laser settings are then changed to repeat mode at 1990 watts/cm^2, and the inferior body of the arytenoid cartilage is vaporized, working from lateral to medial aspects (Fig. 301-2). The lateral ligament is identified and transected, and the ablation is carried to the cricoid cartilage inferiorly and laterally, while the vocal and muscular processes remain intact.

The vocal process is ablated along with a small portion of the vocalis muscle (Fig. 301-3*A*). The muscular process is then vaporized up to, but not including, the interarytenoid muscle, with great care not to traumatize the mucosa of the interarytenoid cleft (see Fig. 301-3*B*). It may be necessary to switch laser settings to single-pulse mode to avoid injury to the critical adjacent tissues.

A small area lateral to the vocalis muscle is ablated with the laser to facilitate lateralization of the cord during healing (Fig. 301-4). The laser may be defocused so that the arytenoid defect can be treated with the laser for hemostasis. The surgeon must be careful not to leave excess carbonaceous debris, which may result in granuloma formation.

HAROLD C. PILLSBURY III
TIMOTHY L. SMITH

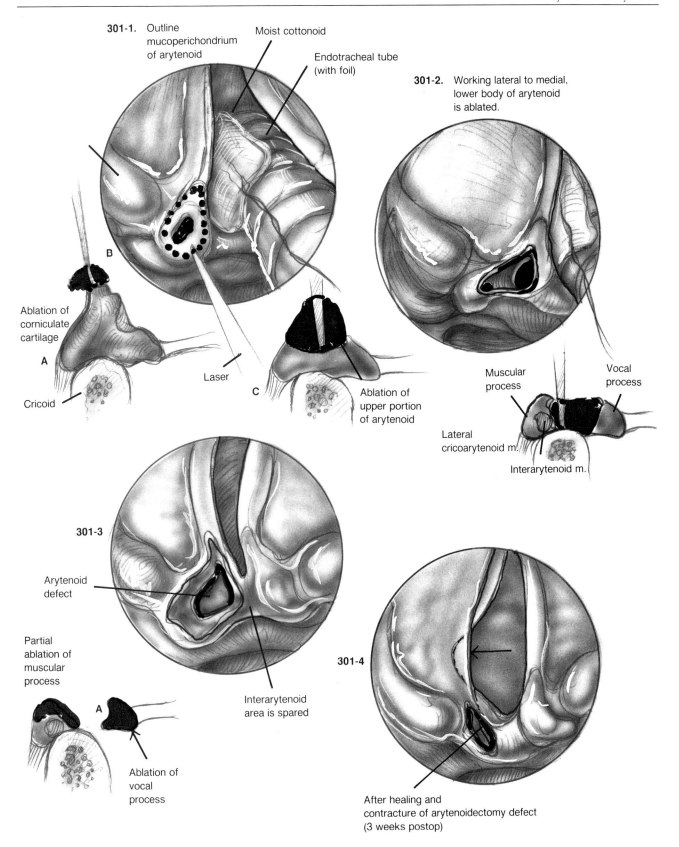

301-1. Outline mucoperichondrium of arytenoid

Moist cottonoid

Endotracheal tube (with foil)

B

Ablation of corniculate cartilage

A

Cricoid

Laser

C

Ablation of upper portion of arytenoid

301-2. Working lateral to medial, lower body of arytenoid is ablated.

Muscular process

Vocal process

Lateral cricoarytenoid m.

Interarytenoid m.

301-3

Arytenoid defect

Partial ablation of muscular process

A

Ablation of vocal process

Interarytenoid area is spared

301-4

After healing and contracture of arytenoidectomy defect (3 weeks postop)

■ *302.* MICROSUSPENSION LARYNGOSCOPY AND LASER EXCISION OF EARLY-STAGE VOCAL CORD CARCINOMA—Transglottic excision of T1 and some T2 carcinomas of the true vocal cord using CO_2 laser and laryngeal microsurgical instrumentation

Indications

1. T1 carcinoma of the true vocal cord in patients healthy enough to withstand a short period of general anesthesia
2. Verrucous carcinoma (ie, Ackerman's tumor)

Contraindications

1. T3 lesion (ie, cord fixation)
2. Inability to withstand anesthesia
3. Metastases
4. Involvement of the arytenoid, anterior commissure, or vocalis muscle may contraindicate endoscopic removal for cure.

Special Considerations

1. Tumor morphology; exophytic better than ulcerative
2. Tumor extent; must rule out cord fixation and cervical or distant metastasis
3. Patient must be available for close follow-up.

Preoperative Preparation

1. Complete history and physical examination
2. Routine preoperative studies, including chest radiograph
3. Computed tomography scans of the larynx and neck are advisable.
4. Consider pulmonary function testing if the respiratory reserve appears marginal.

Special Instruments, Position, and Anesthesia

1. Supine position, with a shoulder roll and the table turned 90°
2. Laser-safe endotracheal tube
3. Triple endoscopy before excision to rule out synchronous primary or unsuspected extension of laryngeal tumor
4. Dedo-Jako suspension laryngoscopes
5. Shapshay laryngeal microsurgical instruments
6. Operating microscope with 400-mm objective lens
7. CO_2 surgical laser with microspot micromanipulator

Tips and Pearls

1. Place saline-soaked pledgets around and behind the lesion to protect normal structures.
2. Constant endolaryngeal suction during laser use to clear smoke

Pitfalls and Complications

1. Hoarseness
2. Aspiration risk
3. Tumor-positive margins
4. Tracheal burn or perforation
5. Edema or hematoma producing airway compromise
6. Endotracheal tube fire
7. Vascular injury, bleeding, or death

Postoperative Care Issues

1. Frequently an outpatient procedure
2. Steroids can be used to minimize airway edema
3. Voice rest for 3 days to 1 week
4. Counsel the patient and family regarding bleeding, stridor, need for voice rest, and frequent follow-up visits.

References

Eckel HE, Thumfart WF. Laser surgery for the treatment of larynx carcinomas: indications, techniques, and preliminary results. Ann Otol Rhinol Laryngol 1992;101:113.

Shapshay SM. Issues in laser surgery. In: Pillsbury HC, Goldsmith MM, eds. Operative challenges in otolaryngology—head and neck surgery. Chicago: Yearbook Medical Publishers, 1990:764.

Operative Procedure

The patient is brought to the operating room and placed in a supine position on the operating table. After adequate anesthesia is obtained, the table is turned 90°, and a shoulder pad is placed, if desired. If staging procedures have not already been performed, the patient undergoes laryngoscopy, bronchoscopy, and esophagoscopy before addressing the the laryngeal lesion.

A laser-safe endotracheal tube is placed to secure the airway. After protecting the patient's dentition with an appropriate tooth guard, a Dedo-Jako laryngoscope is introduced into the vallecula, and the larynx is visualized by carefully lifting the tongue and the floor of the mouth upward. The laryngoscope can then be secured to the suspension arm, which rests on the patient's chest or on a Mayo stand placed over his or her chest. The operating microscope with its 400-mm objective lens and attached CO_2 laser microspot micromanipulator is then brought into position.

The surgeon, seated on a pump-up stool, sits at the head of the table. The lesion is visualized through the microscope, usually at 8 to $16\times$ magnification, and grasped with Shapshay side-biting endolaryngeal forceps. Saline-soaked pledgets are placed around and behind the lesion to protect normal tissue from stray laser energy (Fig. 302-1). The lesion is medialized with gentle traction applied with one hand, while the other directs the laser's output by means of the micromanipulator (Figs. 302-1 and 302-2). The laser is fired with a foot pedal and usually is set on 1 to 3 watts for a high-intensity, rapidly shuttered, 0.5-second pulse, which is called the superpulse mode. For larger spot sizes than those used with the microspot micromanipulator (300 μm), it is necessary to increase the laser's power output.

The margin of the excision is outlined with repeated pulses from the laser. With gentle traction directed medially, the lesion is progressively dissected free of the underlying vocal ligament or vocalis muscle, depending on the depth of the lesion (Figs. 302-3 through 302-6). Care is taken to not unduly damage the specimen with the forceps or the laser to allow an accurate frozen-section determination of tumor-free margins. Correct orientation of the specimen after removal necessitates close collaboration between the surgeon and pathologist. Positive margins can be addressed by additional laser excision or an alternate procedure.

Hemostasis usually is accomplished in the course of laser excision, but if sharp dissection is used to remove the tumor, hemostasis can be obtained with epinephrine-soaked pledgets or by the judicious use of defocused laser energy. Intravenous or intramuscular steroids and antibiotics can be given at the surgeon's discretion. After the laser excision is judged complete, the microscope and laser are removed, and the patient is taken out of suspension. The laryngoscope, tooth guards, and shoulder roll are removed, and the patient is returned to anesthesia.

HAROLD C. PILLSBURY III
JOHN E. BUENTING

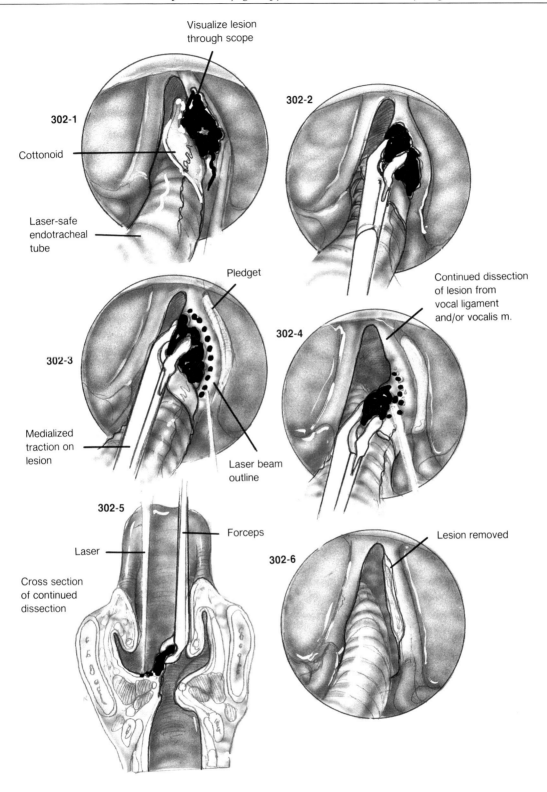

Visualize lesion
through scope

302-1

Cottonoid

Laser-safe
endotracheal
tube

302-2

Pledget

302-3

Medialized
traction on
lesion

Laser beam
outline

Continued dissection
of lesion from
vocal ligament
and/or vocalis m.

302-4

302-5

Forceps

Laser

Cross section
of continued
dissection

Lesion removed

302-6

■ 303. MICROSURGERY FOR VOCAL CORD POLYPS, CYSTS, AND NODULES—Microsurgical techniques to remove benign vocal cord lesions

Indications

1. Removal of symptomatic benign vocal cord tumors that have not responded to conservative (voice) therapy and that cause persistent poor voice quality or a foreign body sensation
2. Excision of lesions with features of neoplastic change
3. Excision of lesions with features of an infectious process

Special Considerations

1. Persistence of the lesion despite intense and prolonged voice therapy

Preoperative Preparation

1. Photodocumentation with videostroboscopy of the lesion preoperatively
2. Speech pathology consultation
3. Vital signs and appropriate laboratory studies

Special Instruments, Position, and Anesthesia

1. Complete suspension microlaryngoscopy instruments of various sizes
2. Laryngoscopes with built-in fiberoptic cables and smoke evacuation systems
3. Operating microscope
4. CO_2 laser equipment
5. Shoulder roll, if needed; sniffing position, with the head in a doughnut roll
6. Complete paralysis with jet ventilation, apnea technique, or a small endotracheal tube placed posteriorly

Tips and Pearls

1. Mucosal preservation is the key to good vocal results.
2. Do not excise redundant mucosa.
3. Overzealous excision is difficult to rectify.
4. Preservation of the anterior commissure

Pitfalls and Complications

1. Airway obstruction (eg, edema, laryngospasm, hematoma, mucous plugging)
2. Hemorrhage
3. Arytenoid dislocation and lacerations
4. Thermal injury from the laser or electrocautery
5. Epiglottic inversion
6. Contusion of the lip or tongue
7. Tooth fracture or dislocation
8. Endotracheal tube combustion
9. Resultant poor voice quality
10. Postoperative granuloma or scar formation
11. Postoperative anterior or posterior webbing
12. Postoperative subglottic stenosis or arytenoid fixation

Postoperative Care Issues

1. Complete voice rest for 1 week
2. Soft vocalization for the second week
3. Gradual return to normal vocalization by the third week
4. Cough suppression
5. Avoidance of tobacco smoke, gas fumes, chemical irritants, and known allergens
6. Minimize throat clearing
7. Moist mist inhalation to minimize mucosal drying
8. Adequate hydration

References

Carruth JAS. Laryngeal microsurgery with the carbon dioxide laser: techniques and instrumentation. J Laryngol Otol 1985;99:573.
Kashima HK. CO_2 laser excision of polyps, cysts, and nodules. In: Johns ME, Price JC, Mattox DE, eds. Atlas of head and neck surgery, vol 1. Philadelphia: BC Decker, 1990:20.
Shapshay SM, et al. Benign laryngeal lesions: should the laser be used? Laryngoscope 1990;100:953.

Operative Procedure

The patient is positioned supine on the operating table and monitored by pulse oximetry and electrocardiographic monitors throughout the procedure. A tooth guard is placed. Topical anesthesia or general anesthesia with jet ventilation is preferred. Suspension microlaryngoscopy is performed with the largest rigid fiberoptic laryngoscope that fits the patient's larynx. The operating microscope with a 400-mm lens at magnification powers of 10, 16, and 25 is used to examine the larynx. The dimension of the lesion is evaluated with a minimal amount of tension on the vocal cords. Photodocumentation is performed as necessary. The nodule or cyst can be palpated to determine the extent of the lesion and establish any infiltrative or indurative change. The remainder of the vocal cord and undersurface should be visualized to determine that no other epithelial lesion is present. Maximal mucosal preservation is the key objective. A moist sponge is placed immediately inferior to the operative site. Laser vaporization or cold techniques with microdissection instruments can be used.

The small-spot (3-mm) CO_2 laser is set at 1 to 3 watts with 0.1-second pulses. These settings minimize thermal damage to surrounding tissues. The beam is intermittently fired medially and slowly moved laterally until the nodule is encountered (Fig. 303-1). The nodule is then vaporized or excised with microspot technique until healthy mucosa and submucosa are seen. Steam is continuously evacuated with microlaryngeal suction. The hemostatic properties of the laser also facilitate precise treatment of polyps or polypoid vocal cords. The beam is directed to the superolateral aspect of the vocal cord, avoiding the free vibrating edge. The gelatinous fluid of the polyp is encountered and extracted with microsuction (Fig. 303-2A). A microflap is then meticulously raised using 1-mm cup forceps and probes. Healthy mucosa should not be violated. A small amount of polypoid material is deliberately left in place for lubrication. Excess mucosa is judiciously trimmed and spot welded in place using the CO_2 laser (see Fig. 303-2B).

Cold technique microdissection proceeds in a similar fashion for removal of nodules and polyps. Microflaps are carefully elevated, and the lesion is dissected from the healthy underlying mucosa or submucosa (Fig. 303-3). Any excess mucosa is conservatively trimmed, and the flaps are replaced (Fig. 303-4). Hydrostatic dissection can facilitate dissection of vocal cord cysts. Normal saline or a 1% solution of lidocaine with a 1:100,000 concentration of epinephrine can be injected with a 27-gauge needle just posterior to the cyst to develop a plane for dissection. An inferiorly based microflap is then elevated with microdissection techniques, and the cyst is carefully dissected from the surrounding submucosa. The flap is then replaced.

Regardless of which technique is used, mucosal conservation is the ultimate goal to optimize voice quality. Postoperative care proceeds as previously described.

DOUGLAS E. HENRICH
HAROLD C. PILLSBURY III

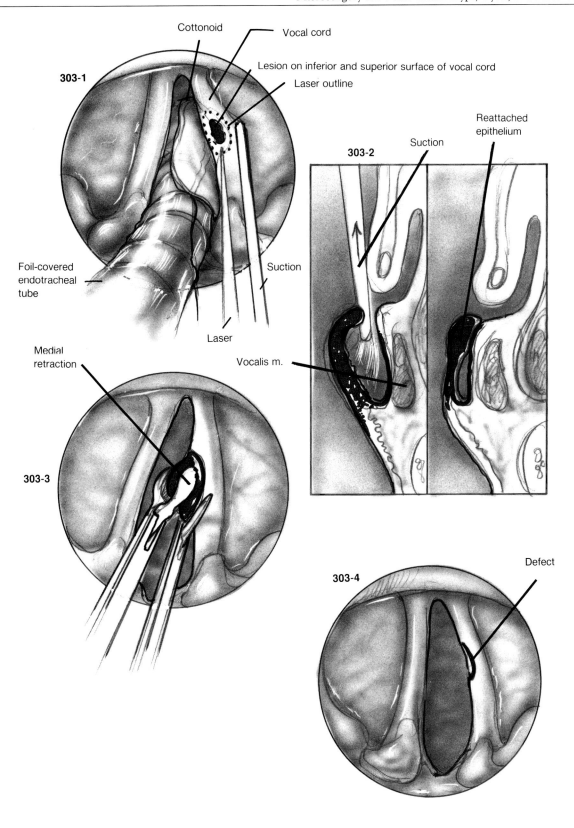

303-1

Cottonoid

Vocal cord

Lesion on inferior and superior surface of vocal cord

Laser outline

Foil-covered endotracheal tube

Suction

Laser

303-2

Suction

Reattached epithelium

Vocalis m.

Medial retraction

303-3

Defect

303-4

■ 304. ESOPHAGOSCOPY

The esophagoscope (rigid) is used for diagnosis of esophageal lesions.

Indications

1. Congenital anomalies: esophageal atresia, tracheoesophageal fistula, duplication cysts, congenital stenosis, vascular ring or sling
2. Neurologic or muscular diseases: achalasia of cricopharyngeus or esophagus, esophageal chalasia, hiatal hernia
3. Chemical trauma: gastroesophageal reflux, lye or other substance ingestion
4. Liver disease: esophageal varices

Special Considerations

1. Stable airway status
2. Adequate hemoglobin and hematocrit
3. Underlying medical conditions

Preoperative Evaluation

1. Routine complete blood counts

Special Instruments, Position, and Anesthesia

1. Anesthesia laryngoscope
2. Appropriate sized esophagoscopes and telescopes
3. Biopsy forceps, if indicated

Tips and Pearls

1. Use the anesthesia laryngoscope for oral cavity access.
2. Brace the esophagoscope on the thumb, with surgeon's middle finger braced on the palate. Never lever on the teeth.
3. Piriform sinuses may provide entry.
4. Never advance against resistance or without visualizing the lumen.
5. If mucosal folds obstruct the telescopic view, try the open tube method.
6. Be gentle.

Pitfalls and Complications

1. Avulsion of teeth
2. Hypopharyngeal or esophageal perforation is indicated by fever, neck or chest pain, elevated leukocyte count, and cervical or mediastinal emphysema.
3. Accidental extubation

Postoperative Care

1. Chest radiograph, if a perforation is suspected
2. Start oral intake with clear liquids, and progress as tolerated.

References

Benjamin B. Endoscopic esophageal atresia and trachea esophageal fistula. Ann Otol Rhinol Laryngol 1981;90:376–382.

Sieber WK. Functional abnormalities of the esophagus. In: Bluestone CD, Stool SE, eds. Pediatric Otolaryngology. Philadelphia: WB Saunders, 1990:985–997.

Operative Procedure

The patient is in the supine position on the operating table, and a small shoulder roll is under the shoulders. The head is extended, but not to the point where it can be difficult to introduce the esophagoscope or the esophagus is compressed against the cervical vertebral bodies by excessive head extension. The patient is draped, the eyes are taped, and a head drape covering the eyes is applied. The patient undergoes general anesthesia with intubation and control of the airway with an appropriately sized endotracheal tube.

Using the appropriate anesthesia laryngoscope (a Seward blade of appropriate size works best), the blade is advanced into the vallecula, and the oral cavity is opened (Fig. 304-1). Secretions are carefully suctioned. The posterior pharynx, piriform sinuses, and esophageal introitus are seen, and then a moistened gauze sponge is placed over the upper teeth. Holding the esophagoscope very much like a pistol, the instrument is advanced into the oral cavity and posterior to the endotracheal tube into the hypopharynx (Fig. 304-3). The esophagoscope is advanced very carefully, visualizing the pharynx and laryngeal structures (Fig. 304-2). The arytenoids and piriform sinuses should be seen. The esophagoscope is carefully advanced into the esophageal introitus directly posterior to the arytenoids or laterally down the piriform sinuses into the esophageal introitus. After the esophageal introitus is seen, entry is achieved very gently under direct visualization.

The body of the esophagoscope is braced on the surgeon's thumb. The surgeon holds the esophagoscope in the right hand like a pistol, and the left hand braces the esophagoscope off the patient's teeth (Fig. 304-4). The surgeon's middle and ring fingers are braced on the palate, with the thumb controlling the esophagoscope. This prevents damage to the teeth. Visualization may be accomplished with a telescope in place or using open tube technique with a prism and a lens cap on the esophagoscope (Fig. 304-5). If mucosal folds obstruct the view with a telescope in place, the telescope may be backed inside the lumen of the esophagoscope a few millimeters to clear the obstruction. The esophagoscope should not be advanced except under direct visualization.

The esophagoscope is very gently advanced to the area of the gastroesophageal junction, visualizing the anatomy along the way. A gentle circular motion can be used to completely visualize the mucosa.

In the case of lesions such as gastroesophageal reflux with Barrett's esophagus, for which a biopsy is indicated, or for tumors of the esophagus, a cup forceps is advanced through the lumen using the open tube technique and a prism. The area to be biopsied is carefully visualized, and small pieces of lesion mucosa and submucosa are removed with the cup forceps. Great care is taken not to perforate the esophagus.

In cases of anatomic defects, an esophagoscope is advanced until the blind pouch of an atresia or the anterior sinus of an tracheoesophageal fistula is seen. Congenital esophageal stenosis is seen as a circular narrowing in the esophagus. The esophagoscope is very gently placed at the lesion, and gentle pressure is used to carefully dilate the area. A vascular ring or sling can be seen as a pulsating intrusion into the lumen.

In the case of lye or other caustic ingestion, the esophagoscope is advanced until the mucosal burn is seen. Reddening without sloughing of the mucosa is safe to pass; after mucosal sloughing is seen, the esophagoscope is not advanced further.

Esophageal varices can be diagnosed and occasionally injected with sclerosing substances.

When the diagnostic or biopsy procedure is completed, the esophagoscope is carefully removed. The entire mucosa is evaluated with a careful circular sweeping motion of the esophagus during removal to detect any anatomic problems or lesions. After the esophagoscope has entered the hypopharynx, the instrument is rotated to a more vertical position and carefully removed from the oral cavity to prevent damage to teeth. Care is taken not to accidentally extubate the patient.

ORVAL E. BROWN

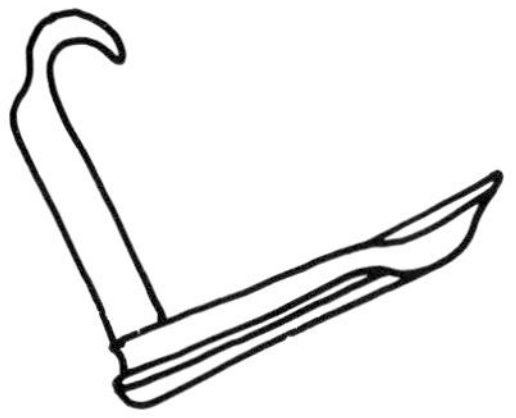

304-1A. Pediatric
laryngoscope

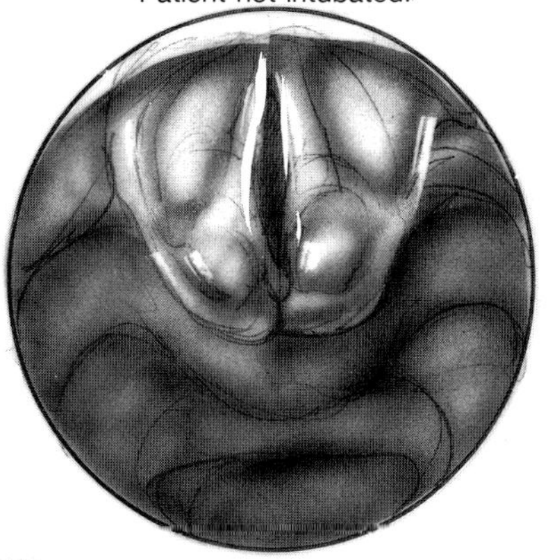

304-2. Normal cords and hypopharynx
(endoscopic view).
Patient not intubated.

304-3

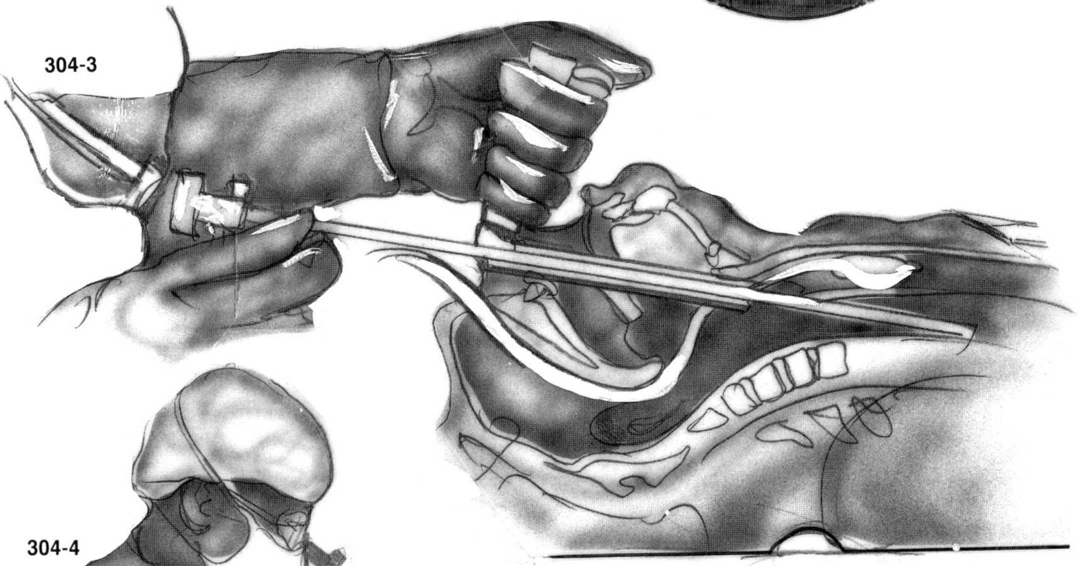

304-4

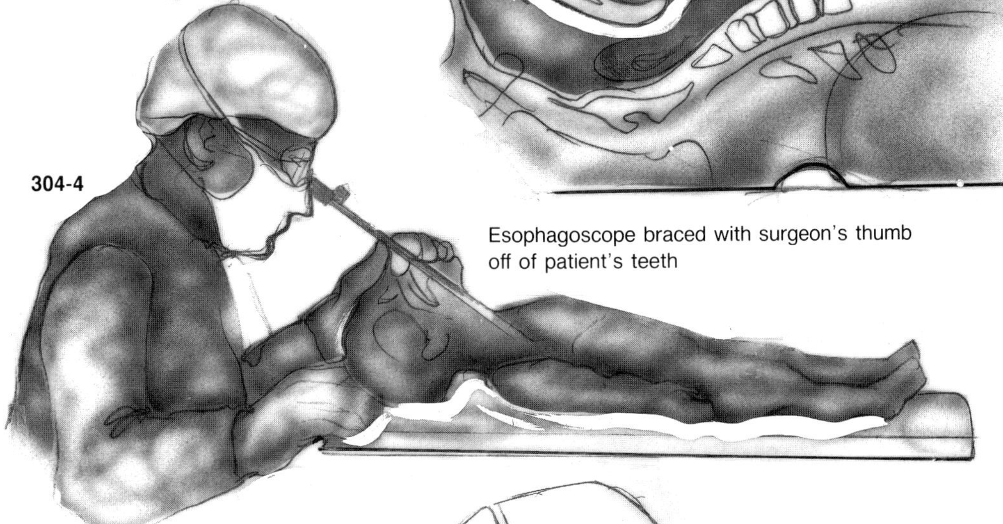

Esophagoscope braced with surgeon's thumb
off of patient's teeth

304-5

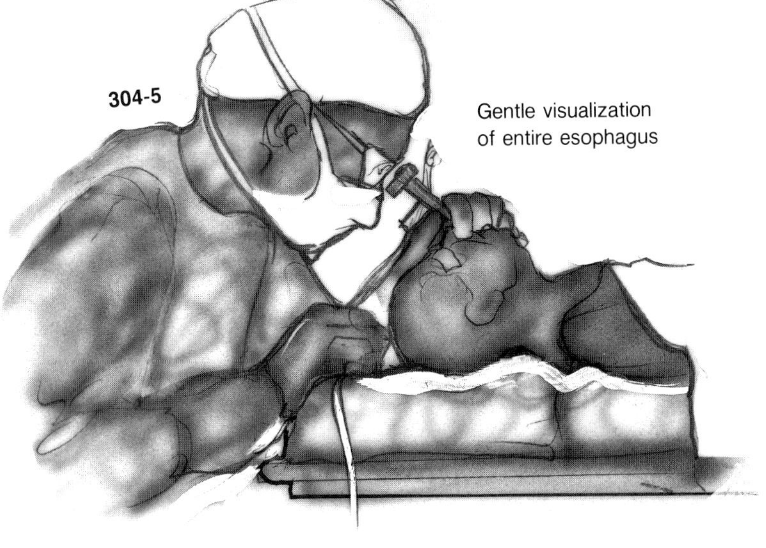

Gentle visualization
of entire esophagus

305. ESOPHAGOSCOPY FOR FOREIGN

BODY REMOVAL—Extraction of a foreign body from the digestive tract

Indications

1. Witnessed or suspected ingestion of foreign body
2. Unexplained airway distress in young children

Contraindications

1. Cervical neck fusion prohibits the use of the rigid esophagoscope.
2. Cervical extension should be limited in patients who are known to be at high risk for cervical spine subluxation (eg, Down syndrome children, achondroplastic dwarfs).
3. The use of papain to dissolve the foreign body may cause dissolution of the injured esophageal wall and result in esophageal perforation.

Special Considerations

1. Always look for a possible second foreign body after removing the first.
2. Especially in adults, look for an underlying esophageal lesion, such as a carcinoma or preexisting stricture, at the site of the impacted foreign body.
3. Button battery aspirations deserve special attention, because leakage of the alkaline contents may result in a caustic injury to the esophagus.
4. Never use force. If it is difficult to mobilize or extract the foreign body, it is better to displace the foreign body into the stomach than to perforate the esophagus.
5. Foreign bodies are most common in toddlers or edentulous adults.
6. The most common site for a foreign body impaction is at the cricopharyngeus or the other levels of normal anatomic narrowing, such as the aortic arch and left main stem bronchus take off and the esophagogastric junction.

Preoperative Preparations

1. Obtain a history, and consider the precise description, shape, and other characteristics of the foreign body to select the appropriate forceps preoperatively.
2. Check your own instruments on the instrument table and be familiar with the mechanism for the opening and closing action of the various foreign body extraction forceps.

Tips and Pearls

1. A negative radiograph does not rule out the possibility of a foreign body in the esophagus. If possible, avoid a barium swallow, because the barium makes endoscopic evaluation more difficult.
2. Esophageal foreign bodies may produce airway obstruction by compressing the membranous common wall of the trachea and esophagus.
3. Esophageal foreign body extraction is safest when performed with the patient under general anesthesia and with a protected airway.
4. Fogarty catheter removal and removal through the flexible esophagoscope have not been as successful in the retrieval of foreign bodies as other approaches.

Pitfalls and Complications

1. Complications include dental injuries, esophageal abrasions and perforation, pneumomediastinum, and inadvertent displacement of the foreign body into the airway.

References

Hollinger LD. Management of sharp and pediatric foreign bodies of the upper aerodigestive tract. Ann Otol Rhinol Laryngol 1990;99:684.

Jackson C, Jackson CL. Diseases of the aerodigestive and food passages of foreign body origin. Philadelphia: WB Saunders, 1950.

Operative Procedure

General endotracheal anesthesia is the safest option for esophageal foreign body removal. The use of a relatively small endotracheal tube enhances the surgeon's ability to pass the rigid scope. A small shoulder roll should be positioned to extend the neck somewhat.

The most common esophageal foreign body is a coin, and it is most commonly found at the level of the cricopharyngeus (Fig. 305-1). Proximal foreign bodies may be exposed most easily with a rigid laryngoscopy and retrieved with a McGill forceps. When the foreign body is beyond the cricopharyngeus, the rigid esophagoscope is necessary to locate the object (Fig. 305-2). The surgeon should proceed initially with slow movements to avoid sliding past or inadvertently advancing the foreign body. The esophagoscope should be moistened and inserted in the midline of the mouth and stabilized with the surgeon's left thumb.

The opening into the esophagus can be located in a variety of ways. The esophageal entrance can be exposed by the introducing laryngoscope, or the esophagoscope itself can be introduced in the midline, following posterior to the endotracheal tube to the level of the postcricoid region. The esophagoscope should be positioned in this region, with the tip slightly advanced to identify the cricopharyngeal sphincter. Only after identification of the esophageal lumen should the scope be passed more distally. If the surgeon encounters difficulty identifying the esophageal inlet by means of either of these approaches, the esophagoscope can be inserted laterally into the piriform sinus and gently moved to the midline of the postcricoid region to locate the esophageal opening. The esophagoscope should be advanced only if there is positive identification of the lumen.

When the foreign body is located, careful inspection of its size and orientation should be performed to assess the most appropriate forceps and the best approach for extraction. Slow, gentle advancement of the esophagoscope is critical; the esophagoscope should be positioned close enough to the foreign body to allow access without displacing the foreign body more distally (Figs. 305-3 through 305-6). Some metallic foreign bodies have sharp edges that can cause abrasions or lacerations of the esophageal mucosa. The foreign body should be grasped and, while maintaining gentle pressure, rotated to position the points distally. The lumen of the esophagoscope is extended beyond the foreign body, which is removed while being protected by the sheath of esophagoscope; the foreign body and esophagoscope are removed as a unit. If the foreign body is larger than the diameter of the esophagoscope, the foreign body should be positioned such that its largest dimension most readily passes through the cricopharyngeus, causing the least trauma.

If extraction becomes difficult because of anatomic considerations, duration of the impaction, or the size and shape of the foreign body, the surgeon can intentionally displace the foreign body into the stomach in a controlled manner. Persevering despite these obstacles could potentially cause a perforation.

If the foreign body extraction has not been traumatic, the esophagoscope should be passed again to rule out the possibility of additional foreign bodies and to evaluate the surrounding esophageal mucosa for a stricture or coexisting lesion.

ELLEN M. FRIEDMAN

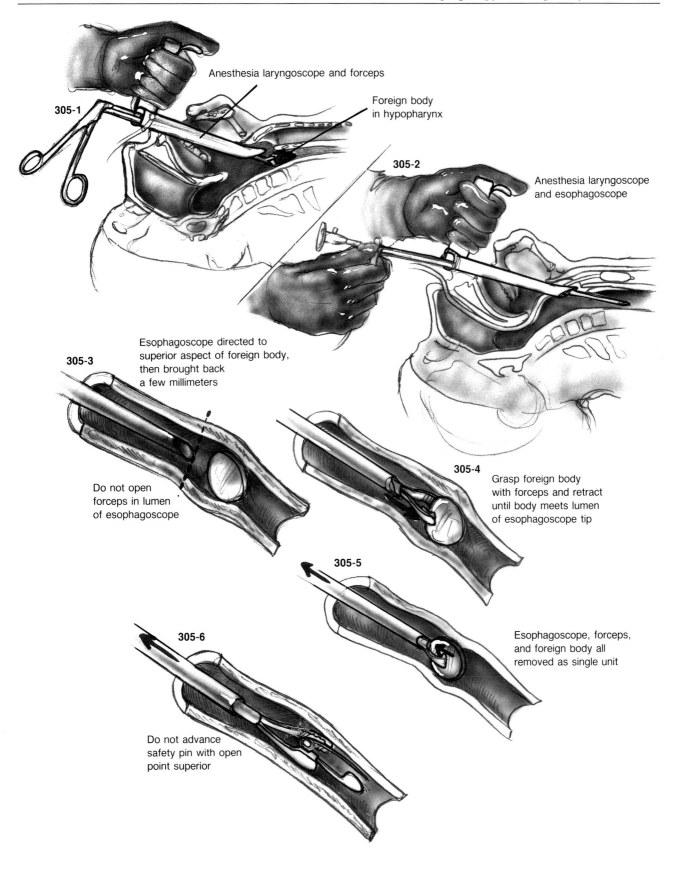

305-1

Anesthesia laryngoscope and forceps

Foreign body
in hypopharynx

305-2

Anesthesia laryngoscope
and esophagoscope

305-3

Esophagoscope directed to
superior aspect of foreign body,
then brought back
a few millimeters

Do not open
forceps in lumen
of esophagoscope

305-4

Grasp foreign body
with forceps and retract
until body meets lumen
of esophagoscope tip

305-5

Esophagoscope, forceps,
and foreign body all
removed as single unit

305-6

Do not advance
safety pin with open
point superior

◼ 306. ESOPHAGOSCOPY FOR CAUSTIC

INGESTION—Examination of the esophagus to determine the presence and extent of possible esophageal wall injury secondary to caustic ingestion

Indications
1. Dysphagia, hematemesis, or odynophagia
2. A suspected or confirmed history of accidental or intentional caustic or corrosive ingestion

Contraindications
1. Patients with retrogastric pain, tachycardia, hypotension, or progressive airway obstruction are at high risk for perforation.
2. Rigid esophagoscopy during the period of esophageal wall weakness should be avoided.
3. Emetics are contraindicated.

Special Considerations
1. If esophagoscopy is performed less than 12 hours after ingestion, there may not have been adequate time for evidence of the injury to develop.
2. If a rigid examination is performed soon after ingestion, there is a higher risk of iatrogenic esophageal perforation because of weakening of the wall.
3. The nasogastric tube has a limited role in the management of caustic injuries; total parental nutrition is available.
4. If a nasogastric tube is used, it should be passed under direct vision at the time of esophagoscopy.
5. The flexible scope can be passed more distally with caution.
6. A barium swallow should be obtained in approximately 4 weeks.

Preoperative Preparations
1. Rule out airway distress or involvement before proceeding.
2. Obtain as much information as possible about the quantity and specific agent ingested.
3. Check for acid-base and electrolyte imbalances preoperatively.
4. Control gastroesophageal reflux.
5. Check all instruments preoperatively.
6. If patient referral is delayed, the initial examination should be a barium swallow.

Tips and Pearls
1. Agents penetrate deeply and have a great impact on the oral cavity and upper esophagus.
2. Acids demonstrate limited initial penetration, with greater involvement occurring in the distal esophagus or stomach.
3. Bleach products are considered mild esophageal irritants and unlikely to have long-term sequelae. Esophagoscopy in cases of bleach ingestion is not mandatory.
4. The extent of injury depends on many factors, including the type and amount of agent and the duration of agent contact with the mucosa.
5. Do not be misled by the lack of obvious oral burns. Distal esophageal involvement is possible even without lip or mouth injury.

Pitfalls and Complications
1. Perforation, stricture, mediastinitis
2. Chronic anemia
3. Increased incidence of later esophageal carcinoma

Postoperative Care Issues
1. No oral intake for 6 to 8 hours after the examination
2. Endoscopic findings determine the postoperative treatment.
3. Because superficial injuries rarely progress to stricture, steroids are unnecessary.
4. Steroids are contraindicated for severe injuries.
5. Intermediate burns have a decreased likelihood of stricture formation when treated with steroids.
6. Barium swallow should be obtained 4 to 6 weeks after ingestion.

References
Cardona JC, Daly JF. Current management of corrosive esophagitis. Ann Otol Rhinol Laryngol 1971;80:521.

Friedman EM. Caustic ingestion and foreign body aspirations: an overlooked form of child abuse. Ann Otol 1987;96:709–712.

Operative Procedure
Esophagoscopy for caustic ingestion is similar to routine diagnostic esophagoscopy (see Procedure 305), but there are several important distinctions. When the rigid esophagoscope is used, it is introduced into the esophageal introitus in a similar manner to routine esophagoscopy, but certain technical considerations must be exercised. Particular care must be given to manipulation in the areas of natural anatomic narrowing of the esophagus, where pooling of the caustic agents may have had an increased impact (Fig. 306-1).

The goal of the examination is to assess the esophageal wall and to determine the extent and severity of the injury. The determination of the degree and depth of injury is subjective and usually characterized as superficial, moderate, or severe (ie, transmural; Fig. 306-2). This determination guides further medical or surgical management. Assessment of circumferential areas of involvement are important, because these also have a higher likelihood of stricture formation or actual perforation. If possible, the entire length of the esophagus should be examined. Classically, the rigid esophagoscope should not be passed beyond the first area of circumferential burns to avoid iatrogenic perforation. In some cases, flexible esophagoscopy (see Procedure 304) may provide a safer, more complete examination in experienced hands.

The assessment of esophageal wall integrity, including the degree and extent of involvement, has been beneficial in initiating early steroid therapy to decrease the likelihood of long-term complications. If it is determined that nasogastric tube feedings would be beneficial to a specific patient, the nasogastric tube can be inserted under direct visualization during the esophagoscopy.

ELLEN M. FRIEDMAN

306-1 Esophagoscopic and Gastroscopic Chart

Age (yrs)

Birth	1	3	6	10	14	Adults	
24	27	30	33	36	43	53	Greater curvature (cm)
21	23	25	26	27	34	40	Cardia (cm)
19	21	23	24	25	31	36	Hiatus (cm)
13	15	16	18	20	24	27	Left bronchus (cm)
12	14	15	16	17	21	23	Aorta (cm)
7	9	10	11	12	14	16	Cricopharyngeus (cm)

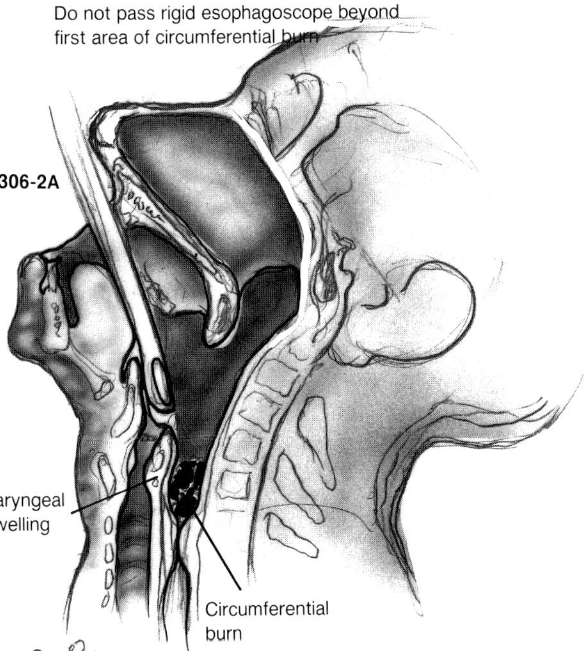

Do not pass rigid esophagoscope beyond first area of circumferential burn

306-2A

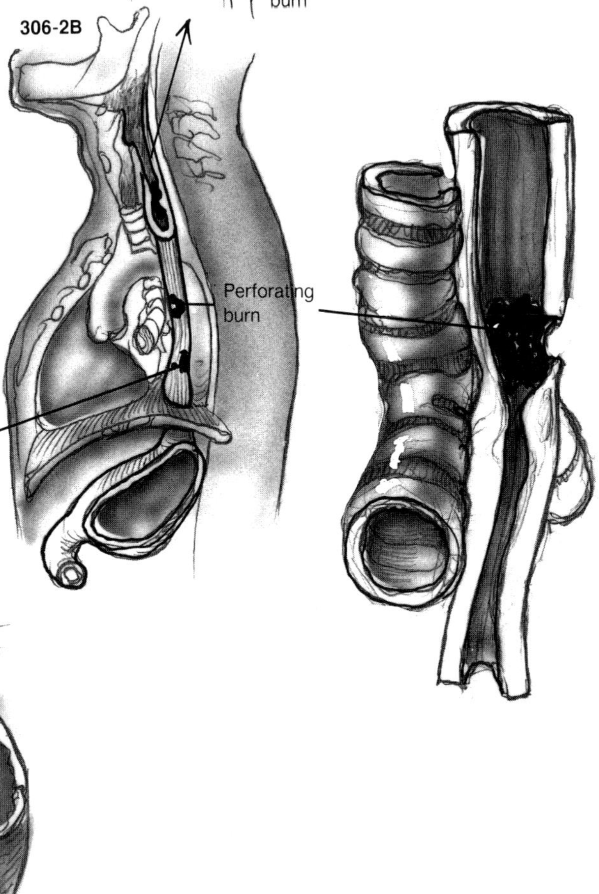

Laryngeal swelling

Circumferential burn

306-2B

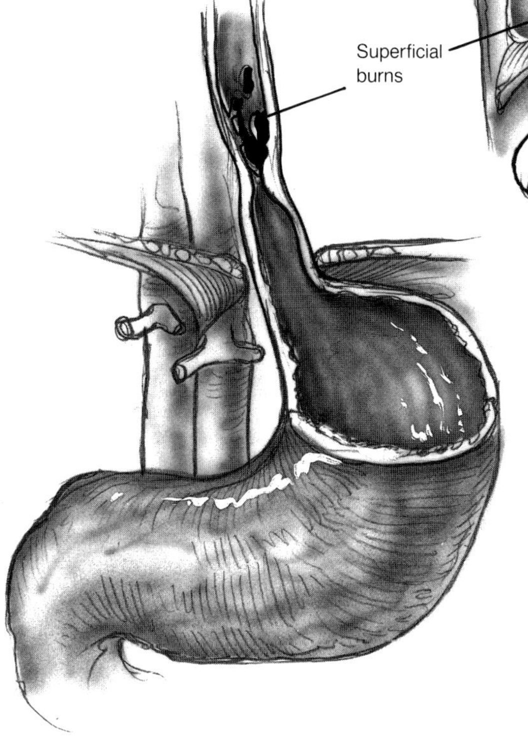

Perforating burn

306-2C

Superficial burns

■ *307.* ESOPHAGOSCOPIC DILATION UNDER DIRECT VISION— Dilation of the esophagus using rigid esophagoscopes and direct vision with an open-tube or telescopic technique

Indications
1. Esophageal stricture, benign or malignant
2. Esophageal atresia or stricture after repair
3. Congenital esophageal stenosis
4. Esophageal achalasia
5. Cricopharyngeal achalasia

Special Considerations
1. Requires general anesthesia
2. Stable upper airway
3. Adequate oral cavity access and mandibular range of motion
4. Loose or false teeth

Preoperative Preparation
1. Complete blood count
2. Barium swallow to document stricture length and the diameter of the lumen

Special Instruments, Position, and Anesthesia
1. General endotracheal anesthesia
2. Supine position
3. Graduated sizes of rigid esophagoscopes

Tips and Pearls
1. Be gentle to avoid esophageal perforation.
2. Start with a small, easily passed esophagoscope.

Pitfalls and Complications
1. Esophageal perforation because of overly aggressive endoscopy or an esophagoscope that is too large
2. Vision can be obscured at the tip of the optical telescope by esophageal mucosal folds.

Postoperative Care Issues
1. Chest radiographs if perforation is suspected

References
Benjamin B. Endoscopic esophageal atresia and tracheoesophageal fistula. Ann Otol Rhinol Laryngol 1981;90:376.

Holinger PH, Johnston KC. Post-surgical problems of congenital esophageal atresia. Ann Otol Rhinol Laryngol 1963;72:1035.

Mohr RM. Endoscopy foreign body removal. In: Paparella MM, Shumrick DA, Gluckman JL, Meyerhoff WL, eds. Otolaryngology. Philadelphia: WB Saunders, 1991:2399.

Operative Procedure
For dilation of the esophagus using rigid esophagoscopes and direct vision with an open-tube or telescopic technique, the patient is in the supine position on the operating table. A small shoulder roll may be used; this is less necessary for pediatric patients. The head is extended, and the mouth is opened. The head is draped, and the eyes are taped to prevent corneal abrasion.

Using an anesthesia laryngoscope such as a Seward blade, the oral cavity is opened to expose the hypopharynx (Fig. 307-1). The previously selected esophagoscope of the appropriate size is introduced into the oral cavity. The posterior pharynx, piriform sinuses, and the esophageal introitus are seen. The teeth are protected with a moistened gauze sponge. The esophagoscope is advanced into the esophageal introitus and into the esophageal lumen. Using open-tube technique, the lumen can be seen and suctioned if necessary. Using the Hopkins rod telescopic technique, it may necessary to slightly displace the tip of the telescope into the esophagoscope lumen so visualization is not obscured by the mucosal folds.

The esophagoscope is gently advanced to the area of stricture using a slightly circular motion to visualize the lumen at all times (Fig. 307-2). Initially, the esophagoscope is placed at the area of stricture such that the small lumen of the stricture is seen centrally in the esophagoscope lumen (Fig. 307-3). Using gentle but firm, continuous pressure, the esophagoscope is advanced through the area of stricture. The lumen should be visualized at all times, and after the stricture is passed, the inferior esophageal lumen is carefully assessed. The esophagoscope is then withdrawn. This procedure is repeated with increasing calibers of esophagoscopes until the stricture has been satisfactorily dilated (Fig. 307-4).

Pediatric patients are serially dilated with the Karl Storz esophagoscopes using the telescope. The preferred technique for adult patients is the Roberts-Jesberg esophagoscope with the Hopkins rod telescope. After the lesion has been dilated, the esophagoscope is carefully withdrawn, and the area of dilation is carefully observed for the possibility of esophageal perforation. It is not uncommon to see areas of mucosal splitting and some bleeding.

When the procedure is complete, the esophagoscope is carefully removed. The entire mucosa is evaluated with a careful circular sweeping motion of the esophagus on removal to look for any other lesions. After the esophagoscope has entered the hypopharynx, the instrument is rotated to a more vertical position on removal to prevent damage to the teeth and accidental extubation.

ORVAL E. BROWN

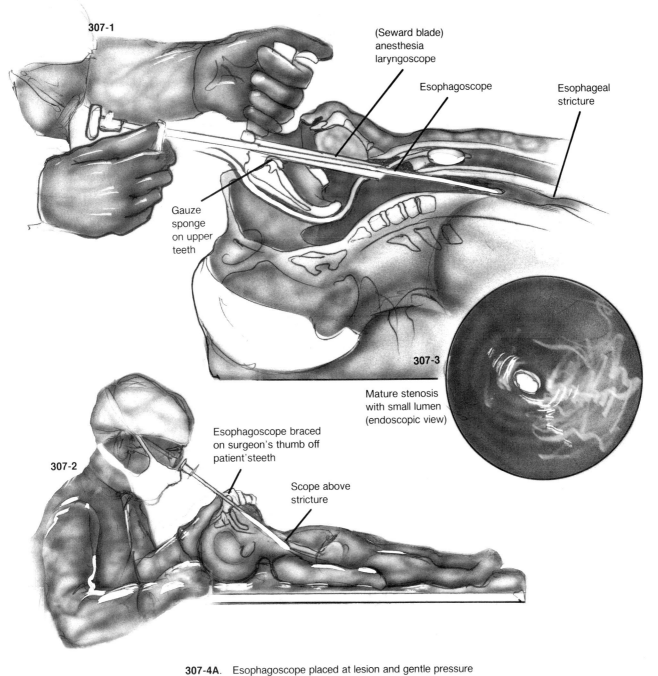

307-1

(Seward blade) anesthesia laryngoscope

Esophagoscope

Esophageal stricture

Gauze sponge on upper teeth

307-3

Mature stenosis with small lumen (endoscopic view)

307-2

Esophagoscope braced on surgeon's thumb off patient's teeth

Scope above stricture

307-4A. Esophagoscope placed at lesion and gentle pressure used to dilate stenosis

307-4B

Stenosis

■ 308. ANTEGRADE ESOPHAGEAL DILATION
Dilation of the esophagus through an oral or transnasal route

Indications
1. Esophageal stricture, benign or malignant esophageal atresia, or stricture after repair
2. Congenital esophageal stenosis
3. Esophageal achalasia
4. Cricopharyngeal achalasia

Special Considerations
1. Uncooperative patients, especially children may need general anesthesia.
2. Stable upper airway
3. Selection of dilator
   Hurst or Maloney for self-dilation or cooperative patient
   Plummer dilators used in operating room and under anesthesia
   Balloon dilation, with or without flexible gastrointestinal endoscope

Preoperative Preparation
1. Complete blood count
2. Barium swallow documentation of the length and lumen diameter of the stricture

Special Instruments, Position, and Anesthesia
1. Hurst or Maloney dilators are used with the patient in a sitting position; restraints are used for children.
2. Plummer dilators are used in anesthetized patients in the supine position in the operating room.
3. Balloon dilation is used in the operating room in pediatric patients under anesthesia and in sedated adults; fluoroscopy may be required, and a gastrointestinal endoscope may be needed for visualization.

Tips and Pearls
1. Hurst or Maloney dilation for lumen strictures greater than 12 mm
2. Be gentle and avoid esophageal perforation.
3. Simultaneous gastrointestinal endoscopy allows visualization for balloon dilation.

Pitfalls and Complications
1. Esophageal perforation
2. Postoperative bleeding (rarely severe)

Postoperative Care Issues
1. Chest radiograph if a perforation is suspected

References
Holinger PH, Johnston KC. Postsurgical endoscopic problems of congenital esophageal atresia. Ann Otol Rhino Laryngol 1963;72:1035.
Starck E, Paolucci U, et al. Esophageal stenosis; treatment with balloon catheters. Radiology 1989;153:637.

Operative Procedure
Pediatric patients under general anesthesia are placed in the supine position on the operative table. No shoulder roll is used. A bite block or mouth gag may be used to open the oral cavity. Being careful of the endotracheal tube, the Hurst and Maloney dilators are carefully introduced, beginning with small dilators and progressing to larger dilators (Fig. 308-1). Patients with tighter stenoses are candidates for Maloney dilators with more tapered tips, although the Hearst dilators begin at smaller French diameters (18 versus 24 Fr). The dilator is advanced into the hypopharynx and gently into the esophagus. It is advanced to a distance that would pass through the gastroesophageal junction and into the stomach (Fig. 308-2). The bougie is then removed, and a larger size is introduced. This is continued until appropriate resistance is met and dilation is appropriate for the patient's age and size. Care is taken not to perforate the esophagus. This procedure can be done by cooperative older patients and adults in the sitting position. The smaller dilators can be swallowed and the larger dilators passed with gentle assistance.

Plummer dilators are used in the operating room. These come in sizes of 15 to 45 Fr, and each tapered dilator has a shaft. The patient is placed in the supine position on the operating table, and endotracheal anesthesia is induced. Using an anesthesia laryngoscope, the oral cavity and hypopharynx are opened while being careful to avoid the endotracheal tube (Fig. 308-3). The esophageal introitus is identified, and starting with a small size, dilators are introduced into the esophageal introitus. These are gently, incrementally advanced until appropriate resistance is encountered, and dilation to the appropriate lumen size for the patient's age and size is performed.

Balloon dilation may be done in the operating room with the patient under anesthesia or in an outpatient facility with sedation or occasionally with no anesthesia (Fig. 308-4). In the operating room, the patient is intubated and placed in the supine position on the operating table. A guide wire is place initially through the oral cavity, through the esophageal stricture, and into the stomach. Initially, a nasal gastric tube may be placed, and the guide wire may be placed through this if necessary. The gastric tube may then be removed over the guide wire. The deflated balloon dilation catheter is then advanced with the guide wire to the stricture. Identification of the stricture may be done under fluoroscopic control with barium in the esophagus or may be done under direct vision using the gastrointestinal endoscope. The oral cavity is opened, and the gastrointestinal endoscope is placed in the esophagus to visualize a catheter and the stricture.

After the catheter is in proper position, the balloon is inflated under direct observation or fluoroscopic control. Dilation is maintained for 3 to 5 minutes, and the balloon may be deflated and reinflated as necessary. Total dilation time may be 7 to 10 minutes, depending on the response of the stricture to dilation. After the stricture has been dilated, the balloon catheter is deflated, and the balloon catheter, guide wire, and gastrointestinal endoscope are removed.

ORVAL E. BROWN

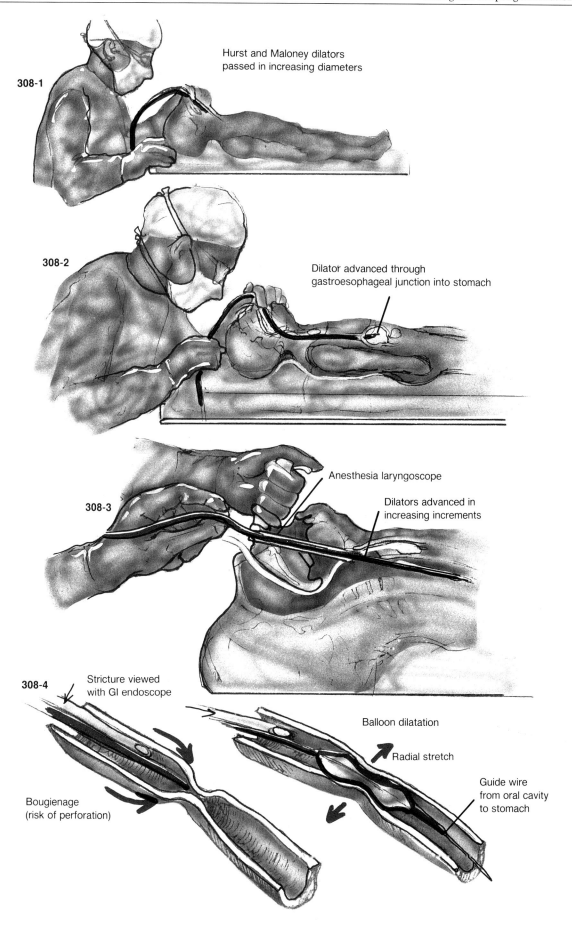

308-1

Hurst and Maloney dilators
passed in increasing diameters

308-2

Dilator advanced through
gastroesophageal junction into stomach

308-3

Anesthesia laryngoscope

Dilators advanced in
increasing increments

308-4

Stricture viewed
with GI endoscope

Balloon dilatation

Radial stretch

Guide wire
from oral cavity
to stomach

Bougienage
(risk of perforation)

■ 309. RETROGRADE ESOPHAGEAL DILA-TION—Esophageal dilation through a gastrostomy from the gastroesophageal sphincter

Indications
1. Severe esophageal stricture unable to be dilated with other means
2. Severe lye burn or stricture

Special Considerations
1. Consider general anesthesia in children
2. Stable upper airway

Preoperative Preparation
1. Complete blood count

Special Instruments, Position, and Anesthesia
1. Tucker dilators
2. Supine position
3. Afrin to decongest nasal cavity

Tips and Pearls
1. Dilate the gastrostomy site to allow bougie passage.
2. Tie a second string loop at the gastrostomy, and bring it out the oral cavity. Do not lose continuity of the gastrostomy-nasal string loop.
3. Use a second string for dilation, and maintain the original string loop.

Pitfalls and Complications
1. Esophageal perforation
2. Loss of string continuity

Postoperative Care Issues
1. Chest radiograph if a perforation is suspected

References
Riding KH, Bluestone CD. Burns and acquired strictures of the esophagus. In: Bluestone CD, Stool SE, eds. Pediatric otolaryngology. Philadelphia: WB Saunders, 1990:998.

Tucker G. Cicatricial stenosis of the esophagus with particular reference to treatment by continuous string, retrograde bougienage with the author's bougie. Ann Otol Rhinol Laryngol 1924;69:1180.

Operative Procedure
Children are treated under general anesthesia in the operating theater, and cooperative adults may be treated under sedation as outpatients. Initially, the circular, continuous string from the gastrostomy into the nasal cavity is cut, and a string loop is attached to the end of the string at the gastrostomy (Fig. 309-1). This is brought through into the oral cavity, and one end of the second string loop is brought out the oral cavity (Fig. 309-2). This is the string that is used for dilation. The gastrostomy-nasal loop is then brought back out the gastrostomy, and the continuity of this string is reestablished. This leaves two parallel strings in the esophagus; one is a loop from the gastrostomy to the nasal cavity, and one comes out the oral cavity and the gastrostomy (Fig. 309-3).

The gastrostomy site is dilated using the bougies or forceps. Bougies are attached to the second dilation string and are passed through the gastrostomy site and up to the gastroesophageal junction (Fig. 309-4). These are then brought through the esophageal stricture and out through the oral cavity. The bougies can be passed individually or can be tied together in sequence and brought through the stricture in sequence.

After a reasonable esophageal lumen has been established with retrograde bougienage, a change may be made to antegrade bougienage with Hurst or Maloney dilators or other techniques.

ORVAL E. BROWN

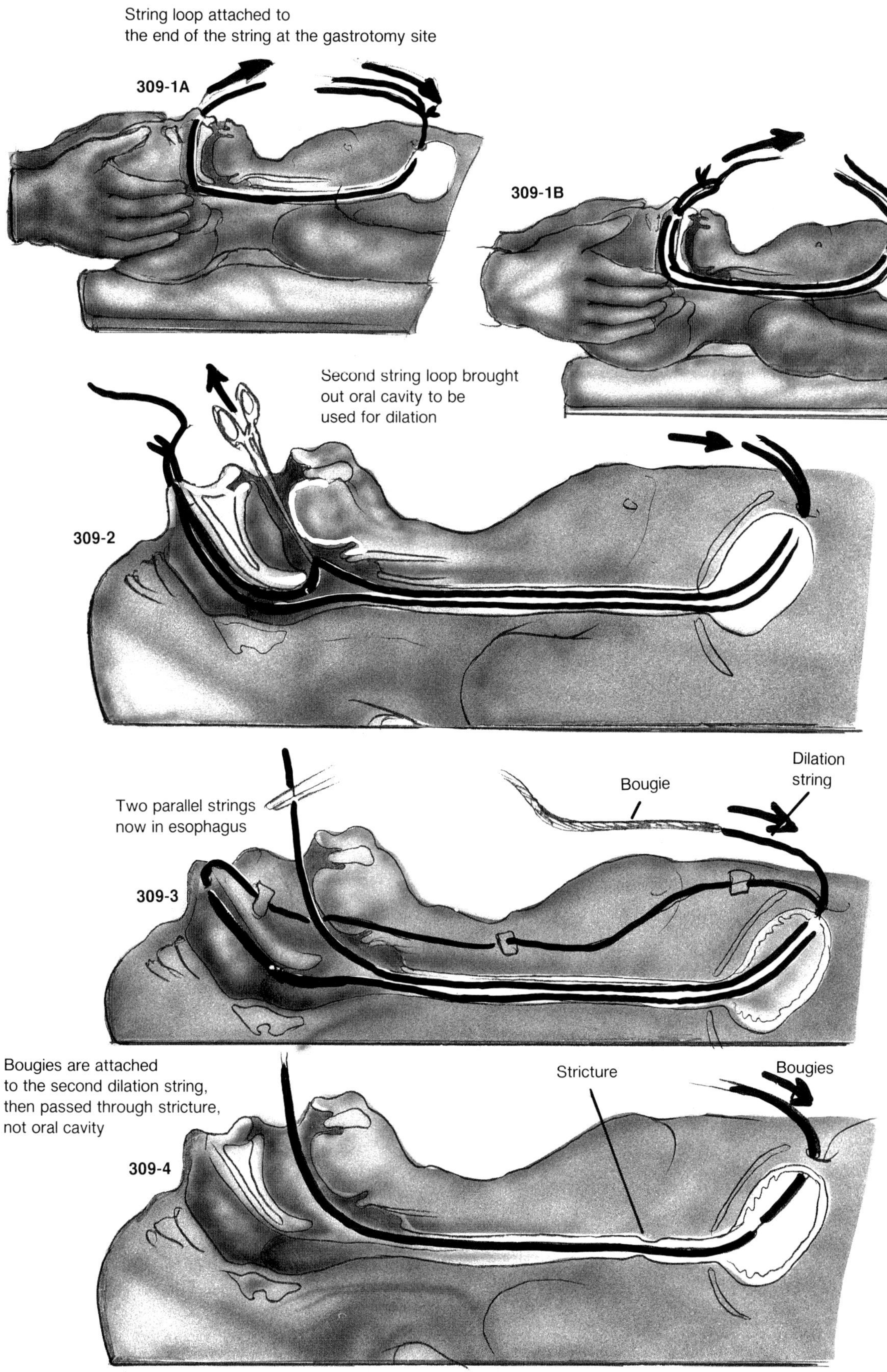

String loop attached to
the end of the string at the gastrotomy site

309-1A

309-1B

309-2

Second string loop brought
out oral cavity to be
used for dilation

309-3

Two parallel strings
now in esophagus

Bougie

Dilation
string

309-4

Bougies are attached
to the second dilation string,
then passed through stricture,
not oral cavity

Stricture

Bougies

■ *310.* DIAGNOSTIC BRONCHOSCOPY

Examination of the trachea and proximal bronchi with a rigid metal endoscope for diagnostic purposes or for removal of a foreign body

Indications

1. Suspected malignancy
2. Squamous cell carcinoma in another site in upper aerodigestive tract
3. Suspected foreign body
4. Airway obstruction

Special Considerations

1. Condition of the cervical spine
2. Airway compromise, preoperatively and intraoperatively
3. Position of suspected foreign body

Preoperative Preparation

1. Chest radiograph, posteroanterior and lateral views
2. No specific laboratory studies are required.
3. No oral intake status appropriate for age
4. Have the instruments ready before induction of anesthesia.
5. Check the function of light cables and sources.

Special Instruments, Position, Anesthesia

1. Bronchoscope in size anticipated and one size smaller
2. Adequate light source, with functioning suction apparatus
3. Biopsy forceps and various foreign body forceps
4. Small shoulder roll, if necessary; foam doughnut
5. Tooth guard

Tips and Pearls

1. Use an anesthesia laryngoscope to help view the glottis.
2. Topical lidocaine on the vocal cords to prevent laryngospasm
3. Intravenous Decadron to reduce laryngeal edema, if indicated.
4. Advise the anesthesiologist about the position of the scope at all times.

Pitfalls and Complications

1. Laryngeal edema or injury
2. Loss of airway
3. Dental injury

Postoperative Care Issues

1. Monitor for respiratory distress

References

Jackson C, Jackson CL. Bronchoesophagology. Philadelphia: WB Saunders, 1950:50.

Marsh BR. Removal of bronchial foreign bodies. In: Johns ME, Price JC, Mattox DE, eds. Atlas of head and neck surgery, vol. 1. Philadelphia: BC Decker, 1990:61.

Operative Procedure

Induction of anesthesia should begin only after the surgeon is present in the room and all equipment has been set up and checked. General anesthesia is begun using bag-mask ventilation with the patient in the supine position. A shoulder roll may be used but is usually not necessary. After preoxygenation, a rubber tooth guard is placed on the upper dentition, or in the edentulous patient, a moist gauze sponge is placed over the gingiva.

The bronchoscope may be introduced directly or with the aid of an anesthesia laryngoscope (Fig. 310-1). When introduced directly, the proximal portion of the bronchoscope is grasped firmly with the right hand while the left hand steadies the more distal end while retracting the upper lip. The bronchoscope is passed over the tongue, slightly toward the right angle of the mouth. As the tongue is lifted with the advancement of the instrument, the tip of the bronchoscope with the bevel down is used to lift the epiglottis. The bronchoscope is then passed through the glottis after rotating the scope 90 degrees so that the bevel is facing laterally (Fig. 310-2). The anesthesia laryngoscope may be used to identify the larynx before inserting the bronchoscope. With the bronchoscope in the trachea, the anesthesiologist then connects the ventilation tubing to a side port of the bronchoscope for continued manual ventilation and administration of inhalational anesthetic agents (Fig. 310-3).

In the trachea, the bronchoscope is anchored at the mouth, with the fingers of the left hand grasping the barrel of the scope above and below. The right hand is free to guide the advancement of the scope or for manipulation of other instruments through the scope. The anesthesiologist should be informed of the position of the bronchoscope at all times. Inspection of the tracheal mucosa is done by gently rotating the angle of the scope in all quadrants to examine the entire circumference of the lumen. The bronchoscope is gently advanced with the left hand still grasping the barrel at the level of the patient's mouth. The carina is identified, and the openings to the left and right main bronchi are inspected for lesions or foreign bodies (Fig. 310-4). The bronchoscope is then passed down each main bronchus for examination of the proximal bronchi. Passage is facilitated by turning the patient's head to the side opposite the main bronchus being examined.

After a lesion or foreign body has been identified, the appropriate forceps are selected for biopsy or removal. Various cupped forceps may be used for the biopsy of mucosal lesions. These are available in different sizes and angles. Various foreign body forceps are also available, with the selection based on the nature of the foreign body. A telescope-forceps combination permits a magnified view of the trachea and foreign body (Fig. 310-5). As with other forceps, this may be used through the rigid bronchoscope and is especially helpful in the pediatric patient. Generally, extraction of the foreign body requires removal of the bronchoscope along with it. The anesthesiologist should be informed of the impending removal so the airway may be safely managed. After the foreign body has been removed, a second-look bronchoscopy should be done to ensure that no other particles remain. The anesthesiologist may then manage the airway during awakening.

C. GAELYN GARRETT
AMELIA F. DRAKE

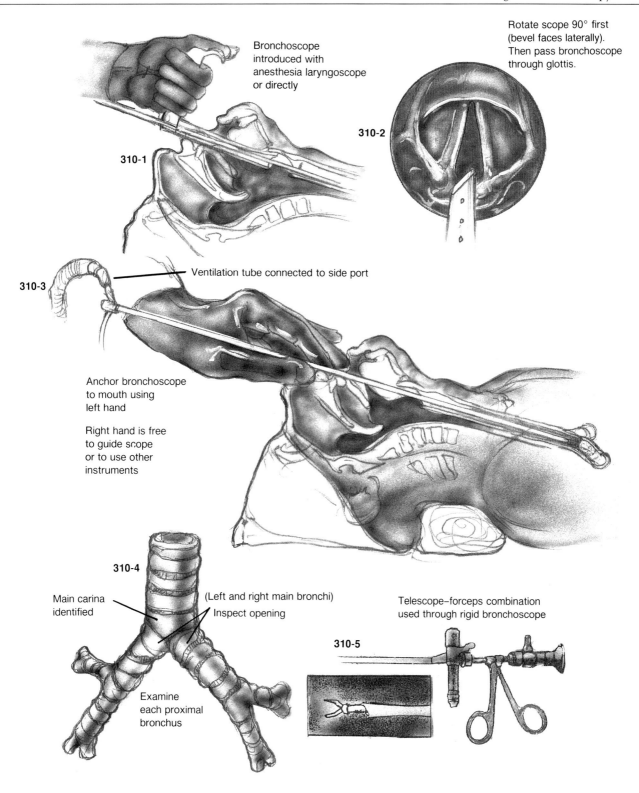

Bronchoscope
introduced with
anesthesia laryngoscope
or directly

310-1

Rotate scope 90° first
(bevel faces laterally).
Then pass bronchoscope
through glottis.

310-2

310-3

Ventilation tube connected to side port

Anchor bronchoscope
to mouth using
left hand

Right hand is free
to guide scope
or to use other
instruments

310-4

Main carina
identified

(Left and right main bronchi)
Inspect opening

Examine
each proximal
bronchus

Telescope–forceps combination
used through rigid bronchoscope

310-5

■ 311. BRONCHOSCOPY FOR A FOREIGN
BODY— Examination of the tracheobronchial tree because of suspicion of an aspirated foreign body

Indications
1. Witnessed aspiration
2. Wheezing, especially unilateral, in a child with no history of asthma, or with a poor response to treatment of asthma
3. Radiographic suspicion of foreign body

Special Consideration
1. Suspected foreign body aspiration in child (especially if younger than 4 years of age) with stridor, wheezing, respiratory distress, persistent or recurrent coughing
2. Witnessing of the foreign body aspiration may not occur.
3. The open tube (rigid) bronchoscope is the instrument of choice.
4. General anesthesia allows safe and comfortable removal of a foreign body.

Preoperative Preparation
1. History is important. Do not ignore the statement by a young patient that he has "swallowed something."
2. Auscultation of chest
3. Review the posteroanterior and lateral chest films during inspiration and expiration, and use videofluoroscopy for dynamic evaluation. If these are not available, use the right and left lateral decubitus films during expiration; the position allows the use of body weight to promote expiration. Partial obstruction in the bronchial tree causes unilateral overinflation of the obstructed side on expiration, with a shift of mediastinum to opposite side (Fig. 311-1). Total obstruction with a loss of air volume may cause atelectasis and decreased lung volume in the obstructed side.
4. Anesthesia consultation and careful planning (Fig. 311-2)
5. Duplicate foreign bodies (if known) should be obtained to facilitate the forceps choice and technique of extraction.
6. All foreign bodies in the airway (especially bronchial) are not urgent emergencies. If no urgent danger to the patient's life exists; the problem should be approached with careful consideration of the procedure, and endoscopic removal should be scheduled when trained personnel are available, after instruments have been chosen and checked, and after techniques have been tested.

Special Instruments, Position, and Anesthesia
1. Laryngoscopes: vallecula scope (slotted Benjamin scope), anterior commissure scope, and laryngeal suctions
2. Bronchoscopes: proximal lighted bronchoscopes with rod-lens telescopes. For most pediatric foreign bodies, a 3.5 mm × 26 mm or 4 mm × 30 cm bronchoscope is used (Fig. 311-3).
3. Passive-action forceps (Jackson type) offer the greatest range of blades and sizes (eg, forward grasping, rotation, bead, hollow object forceps). Positive-action (center or double) forceps are helpful when a foreign body is wedged in the distal bronchus, because the forceps blades can be used to dilate the bronchial wall when advancing over the foreign body. Pediatric optical forceps include the peanut, alligator, and cup forceps types.
4. Various lengths of rod-lens telescopes are chosen to fit bronchoscopes and optical forceps. Flexible microforceps fit down the suction channel of the ventilating bronchoscope.
5. Small Fogarty (arterial balloon) catheter (3 mm)

(continued)

Operative Procedure
Preoperative sedation is not used in patients with severe airway obstruction. Atropine (0.02 mg/kg of body weight) is given intramuscularly approximately one-half hour before the procedure. The patient is positioned on the operating room table, with a slight shoulder roll and the head resting in a doughnut holder in the sniffing position. Preoxygenation is carried out with 100% oxygen delivered by mask. Anesthesia is then continued with halothane and oxygen. All patients are monitored with an electrocardiogram, precardial stethoscope, blood pressure cuff, pulse oximeter, and thermometer. After 5 to 10 minutes of anesthesia induction, the endoscopist exposes and sprays the larynx with lidocaine (up to 5 mg/kg of body weight). Using the vallecular laryngoscope in the preepiglottic area, the larynx is inspected, and a foreign body in this area is ruled out. Spontaneous respiration is maintained throughout the procedure and is safer than apneic techniques in which the patient is completely paralyzed, because the patient can maintain adequate oxygenation through respiratory efforts in case temporary control of the airway is lost.

The bronchoscope is then inserted through the open slot in the laryngoscope and passed between the vocal cords with the bevel tip oriented vertically (Figs. 311-4 and 311-5). The tracheobronchial tree is inspected while the patient is ventilated and anesthetized through the side port of the bronchoscope. A closed system is used by maintaining an eye glass to occlude the proximal end of the bronchoscope. During the actual attempts at foreign body extraction, 100% oxygen is given through the bronchoscope. Positive-pressure ventilation (ie, bagging) tends to force the foreign body more distally and should be avoided. The foreign body is located, typically residing in the right main stem bronchus, although its location depends on many factors at the time of aspiration. Never try to force a scope, forceps, or foreign body. All manipulation is gentle and deliberate.

After adequate ventilation, the eye piece is removed, and the suction is used to remove any secretions hampering adequate visualization. The appropriate 0° telescope is then inserted and locked in position with the appropriate bridge adapter. A methodical inspection of the entire tracheobronchial tree begins with the anticipated normal lung if there is no airway obstruction at this point. All secretions are removed to promote optimal respiratory function in the normal side while the pathologic side is being inspected and manipulated. When the foreign body is located, its shape, its position, and space around it are evaluated. The suction is used to remove secretions around the foreign body, but suction usually should not be used for foreign body removal. The space around the foreign body may be obliterated by granulation tissue and edema. The granulations may need to be removed carefully, and bleeding may be controlled by topical epinephrine with a sponge carrier.

(continued)

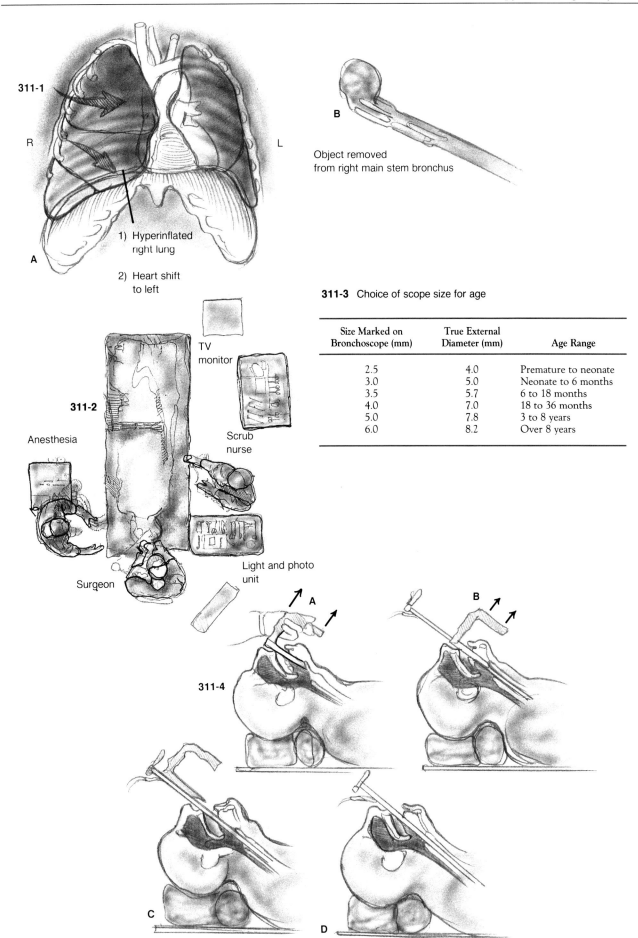

311-1

R

L

1) Hyperinflated right lung

2) Heart shift to left

A

B

Object removed from right main stem bronchus

311-2

Anesthesia

TV monitor

Scrub nurse

Surgeon

Light and photo unit

311-3 Choice of scope size for age

Size Marked on Bronchoscope (mm)	True External Diameter (mm)	Age Range
2.5	4.0	Premature to neonate
3.0	5.0	Neonate to 6 months
3.5	5.7	6 to 18 months
4.0	7.0	18 to 36 months
5.0	7.8	3 to 8 years
6.0	8.2	Over 8 years

311-4

A

B

C

D

■ *311.* BRONCHOSCOPY FOR A FOREIGN BODY *(continued)*

6. Twin light source and cords
7. Tooth guard
8. Xylocaine (1% to 2% concentration) spray
9. Tracheotomy set
10. Rigid metal suctions of various lengths

Tips and Pearls

1. Preoperative and intraoperative communication with anesthesiologist about anticipated technique and potential problems
2. Choose and check all equipment before anesthesia induction.
3. Practice on a duplicate foreign body if one is available and time permits.
4. Monitor temperature, especially in small infants and children.

Pitfalls and Complications

1. Intraoperative airway compromise
2. Dental injury and mandibular dislocation
3. Bleeding from foreign body irritation and manipulation
4. Distal lodging of foreign body
5. Inability to deliver foreign body through laryngeal opening
6. Laceration of the tracheobronchial tree from pointed objects during removal
7. Traumatic laryngitis and edema
8. Retained foreign body with chronic pulmonary infection and abscess
9. An esophageal foreign body may mimic an airway foreign body by compressing the trachea.
10. Possible bilateral foreign bodies

Postoperative Care Issues

1. Traumatic laryngitis and edema produced by foreign body or attempts at extraction can be treated by humidity, racemic epinephrine, and intravenous steroids (1 mg of dexamethasone/kg, up to 10-mg bolus) and elevation of the head of the bed.
2. Repetition of endoscopic procedure after an unsuccessful removal attempt should be avoided for 3 to 7 days. The waiting period also applies to patients who have had previous endoscopy elsewhere before presentation. An exception is made for severe respiratory obstruction.
3. Systemic antibiotics after bronchoscopy if the foreign body was present long enough to produce purulent secretions. Samples are cultured.
4. Postoperative chest physical therapy in cases of atelectasis and pneumonia from longstanding foreign bodies
5. Chest radiograph if pulmonary symptoms persist

References

Holinger LD. Foreign bodies of the larynx trachea and bronchi. In: Bluestone C, Stool S, eds. Pediatric otolaryngology. Philadelphia: Saunders, 1990:1205.

Marsh BR. Removal of bronchial foreign bodies. In: Johns ME, Price JC, Mattox DE, eds. Atlas of head and neck surgery, vol 1. Philadelphia: BC Decker, 1990:60.

Thompson JN, Browne JD. Caustic ingestions in foreign bodies in the aerodigestive tract. In: Bailey BJ, ed. Head and neck surgery—otolaryngology. Philadelphia: JB Lippincott, 1993:725.

Vegetable foreign bodies such as peanuts are grasped lightly to avoid fragmentation. For a round object such as a bead, the blades must pass beyond the axis of the foreign body before closing. If a pointed object is located, the point is sheathed within the scope by advancing the scope over the foreign body rather than by pulling the foreign body into the scope (see Fig. 311-6*A*). If the point cannot be sheathed, the foreign body may be manipulated and rotated to provide a trailing point. For all but very tiny foreign bodies it is best to remove the forceps, foreign body, and the scope as a unit. The foreign body is rotated to the largest diameter of the airway for removal; in the larynx, this is the sagittal plane. "Stripping off" of the foreign body can be avoided by adequate forceps application, choosing the correct forceps, and being sure the forceps close adequately. Failure to rotate the foreign body at the vocal cords also causes stripping off. A foreign body that is too large for the lumen of the larynx may need to be fragmented or a tracheotomy performed and the foreign body delivered through the tracheotomy site.

If a foreign body is stripped off in the larynx, the airway can be immediately reestablished by quickly relocating and removing the foreign body or pushing it down into the bronchus from which it was just removed. A foreign body lost in the trachea probably enters the opposite bronchus because there is more air moving in that side. A foreign body that has been stripped off and is difficult to locate may be found below the vocal cords, in the oral cavity, or in the pharynx or nasopharynx. Optical forceps that provide visualization, foreign body manipulation, and removal under direct magnified view may be used for this procedure (see Fig. 311-6*C*). A flexible microforceps may be passed through the auxiliary suction channel of the bronchoscope and, by inserting the telescope, provide magnification under direct visualization of the microforceps (see Fig. 311-6*D*).

After removal, a second look is taken to ensure that no fragments remain. If there are purulent secretions, washing with a culture trap can help antibiotic selection postoperatively.

If stable, the patient may be awakened from the general anesthesia after removal of the bronchoscope, or the patient may be intubated while the anesthesia is reduced and later extubated. Postoperative humidification, racemic epinephrine, and intravenous dexamethasone are used. Patients are usually discharged 24 hours after the procedure if the lungs are clear and the patient is a afebrile. A postoperative chest radiograph is obtained only if pulmonary symptoms do not resolve. Persistent symptoms of cough, fever, and respiratory obstruction require further investigation.

RONALD W. DESKIN

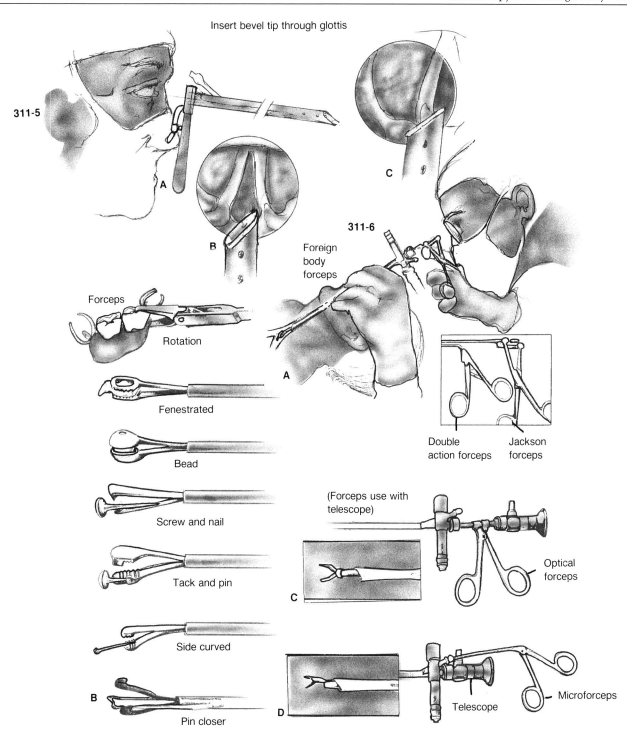

Insert bevel tip through glottis

311-5

A

B

C

311-6

Foreign body forceps

A

Forceps

Rotation

Fenestrated

Bead

Screw and nail

Tack and pin

Side curved

B

Pin closer

Double action forceps

Jackson forceps

(Forceps use with telescope)

C

Optical forceps

D

Telescope

Microforceps

■ *312.* BRONCHOSCOPIC STRICTURE DILATION—Bronchoscopic dilation of intraluminal cicatricial tracheobronchial strictures or stenosis

Indications
1. Intraluminal cicatricial tracheobronchial strictures or stenosis

Special Considerations
1. Patient may have minimal pulmonary reserve
2. All support equipment, including bronchoscopes of multiple sizes and suction, must be available.

Preoperative Preparation
1. Preoperative chest radiograph, posteroanterior and lateral views
2. Know the degree and position of the obstruction.
3. Pulmonary function tests, arterial blood gases, and routine laboratory studies
4. Preoperative anesthesia consultation, as needed
5. All equipment, including Jackson dilators, should be available.
6. Rule out other forms of stenosis, such as thymic or vascular compression

Special Instruments, Position, and Anesthesia
1. Appropriately sized bronchoscopes
2. Jackson tracheobronchial dilators
3. Supine or semirecumbent position, with the neck slightly flexed forward and with moderate hyperextension of head

Tips and Pearls
1. Second set of instruments and a bronchoscope smaller than anticipated
2. Knowledge of pulmonary anatomy
3. With the patient under general anesthesia, preoxygenate before bronchoscopy.
4. Never force a bronchoscope or dilator.

Pitfalls and Complications
1. Inadequate airway control before intubation
2. Damaged teeth
3. Lacerated oropharynx
4. Traumatized vocal cords
5. Hypoxemia or hypercapnia secondary to mainstem intubation with the bronchoscope
6. Tracheobronchial perforation
7. Pneumothorax or pneumomediastinum
8. Bradycardia with intubation secondary to vagal stimulation
9. Laryngospasm

Postoperative Care Issues
1. Supplemental oxygen for transportation to recovery room
2. Rule out pneumothorax and pneumomediastinum with a postoperative chest radiograph.
3. Postoperative bleeding with resultant pneumonitis
4. Edema of epiglottis, cords, and subglottic area, causing airway obstruction
5. Postoperative pneumonia or tracheitis secondary to contaminated instruments
6. High risk of restenosis

References
Gans SL. Bronchoscopy. In: Gans SL, ed. Pediatric endoscopy. New York: Grune & Stratton, 1983:37.

Jackson C. Bronchoesophagology. Philadelphia: WB Saunders, 1950: 111.

Marsh B. Removal of bronchial foreign bodies. In: Johns ME, Price JC, Mattox DE, eds. Atlas of head and neck surgery, vol. 1. Philadelphia: BC Decker, 1990:60.

Operative Procedure
Initially, the patient should be monitored by pulse oximetry and electrocardiography. An intravenous catheter should be placed with appropriate fluids running. Before general anesthesia, all pertinent bronchoscopy equipment is set up and available. The patient should be anesthetized with masking to an anesthetic level that laryngeal reflexes are absent. After general anesthesia has been administered, the patient may be placed in the supine or semireclining position, with the patient's airway simultaneously controlled by the anesthesiologist. At this time, a pillow or shoulder roll may be placed under the patient's lower neck or scapular region to slightly extend the neck while slightly flexing the head. This is accomplished with a foam doughnut or small pillow under the patient's head. The table then is turned 90°. All personnel are gowned and gloved, and the patient's head and neck are draped with sterile drapes. With the surgeon managing the airway, four or more breaths of 100% oxygen are delivered to help prevent desaturation. At this point, the anesthesiologist's laryngoscope can be used to visualize the vocal cords, and 1% lidocaine may be instilled on the cords to prevent laryngospasm. Before intubation with the bronchoscope, the patient's teeth are protected with a rubber tooth guard or a saline-soaked gauze sponge on the maxillary alveolar ridge if the patient is edentulous (Fig. 312-1).

The anesthesiologist's laryngoscope is used to visualize the glottis (Fig. 312-2). The bronchoscope may be introduced directly through the true vocal cords without the aid of the laryngoscope, but the laryngoscope allows a better view of glottis. With the glottis in view, the bronchoscope is passed between the cords. The trachea, down to the carina, is visualized to ensure both lungs will be adequately ventilated.

The bronchoscope is attached to the anesthesia tubing with a flexible connector to administer inhalational anesthesia and oxygen (Fig. 312-3). Suctioning may be needed if secretions prevent adequate inspection and assessment. The entire tracheobronchial tree is evaluated, with special attention to the region of stenosis (Fig. 312-4). The bronchoscope is positioned immediately proximal to the obstruction, and the surgeon observes for pulsations, a tumor, or foreign body. If none are present, he or she proceeds with dilation.

Using the Jackson tracheobronchial dilator appropriately sized for the stricture, the dilator is gently passed through (Fig. 312-5). Starting with a relatively small Jackson dilator allows serial dilation, reducing the risk of perforation. Special attention and communication with the anesthesiologist are required to prevent hypoxemia. Small amounts of bleeding can obstruct the narrow field of vision, and frequent suctioning may be required. After serial dilations have been done, the bronchoscope is removed. Usually, stricture dilation is done with a spontaneously breathing patient, and intubation with an endotracheal tube is not needed. Ventilation can be assisted with masking and high concentrations of inspired oxygen. At this point, the table is turned back to the original position, and the patient is turned over to the anesthesia staff for emergence from anesthesia.

Bronchoscopy and stricture dilation were formerly performed commonly, but this approach is being abandoned. Laser techniques and open surgical approaches can provide excellent results.

AMELIA F. DRAKE
TRACEY G. WELLENDORF

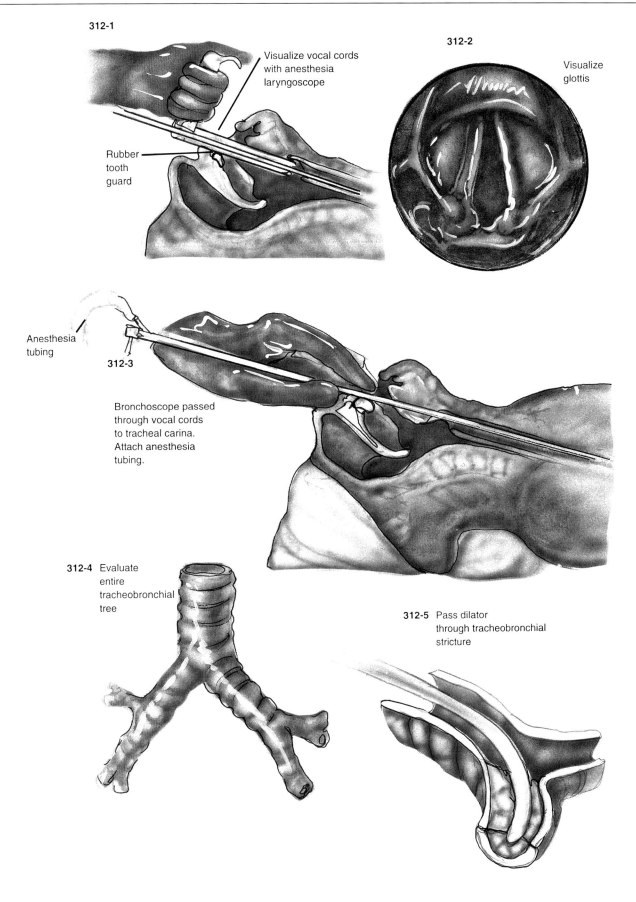

312-1

Visualize vocal cords with anesthesia laryngoscope

Rubber tooth guard

312-2

Visualize glottis

Anesthesia tubing

312-3

Bronchoscope passed through vocal cords to tracheal carina. Attach anesthesia tubing.

312-4 Evaluate entire tracheobronchial tree

312-5 Pass dilator through tracheobronchial stricture

■ *313.* LASER TECHNIQUES FOR BRONCHOS-COPY—Several types of lasers are used for treating assorted tracheobronchial lesions.

Indications

1. Recurrent respiratory papillomatosis, granulation tissue
2. Stenosis, adenoma, web
3. Palliation of obstructing carcinoma

Contraindications

1. Tumors causing extrinsic compression on airway (absolute)
2. Tracheomalacia and cartilage loss (absolute)
3. Circumferential stenosis or stenosis more than 1 cm wide (relative)

Special Considerations

1. Choice of endoscopic technique (rigid or flexible)
2. Choice of laser: CO_2, Nd:YAG, argon
3. Tumor location, pathology, and vascularity

Preoperative Preparation

1. Chest radiograph, CT scan, chest polytomograms
2. Pulmonary function tests, arterial blood gas
3. Discuss the anesthesia technique with the anesthesiologist.

Special Instruments, Position, and Anesthesia

1. Rigid laser bronchoscopes with CO_2 universal endoscopic coupler or Nd:YAG or argon delivered through a flexible fiber
2. Flexible bronchoscopes may also be used to deliver flexible quartz laser fibers through one of the ports. A 300-μm-diameter fiber can be used in a pediatric bronchoscope for treating infants.
3. Supine position, with a shoulder role and foam doughnut
4. Eye protection for the patient and everyone in the operating suite.
5. Rigid bronchoscopes allow room for ventilation, palpation, and suction with no endotracheal tube.

Tips and Pearls

1. The CO_2 laser is most useful for excision and ablation if no bleeding is anticipated (eg, stenosis, web, respiratory papillomatosis, granulation tissue).
2. The Nd:YAG laser is most useful with relatively vascular lesions (eg, transbronchial adenomas, obstructing carcinomas).
3. The argon laser is useful for pediatric endobronchial lesions.
4. The rigid bronchoscope is most useful for obstructions of the trachea and proximal bronchi.

Pitfalls and Complications

1. Hemorrhage is best controlled with a rigid bronchoscope and Nd:YAG laser.
2. Perforation of the airway is best prevented by avoiding firing the laser perpendicular to the wall and by using the lowest power setting possible (<50 watts). Continuous mode should not be used in the airway.
3. Fire is best prevented by keeping oxygen concentrations below 50% and keeping flammable materials out of the laser's path.
4. Eye protection for the patient includes taping the eyes closed, moistened cotton pads, and double-folded heavy aluminum foil.
5. Eye protection for the operating room personnel includes glasses that attenuate light at 1060 nm for the Nd:YAG laser and protective lenses for using the CO_2 laser.
6. The patient's skin should be double covered with moist towels.

Postoperative Care Issues

1. Hypoxemia is common in the postoperative period, and personnel should be trained in monitoring for this and providing care.
2. Postoperative complications include respiratory depression, retention of secretions and debris, and hemorrhage.
3. Emergent endotracheal intubation and bronchoscopy for tracheobronchial toilet should be readily available.
4. Observation for at least 24 hours postoperatively is recommended.

References

Ossoff RH. Bronchoscopic laser surgery: which laser when and why? Otolaryngol Head Neck Surg 1986;94:378.

Shapshay SM, Beamis JF Jr. Safety precautions for bronchoscopic Nd:YAG laser surgery. Otolaryngol Head Neck Surg 1986;94:175.

Operative Procedure

The patient is brought to the operating suite and placed in the supine position. Intravenous access is gained, and the patient is placed under general anesthesia. After a sufficient level of anesthesia is obtained, the table is turned 90°, and the patient is placed in the head hanging position by placing a role under the shoulders and a foam doughnut under the occiput.

The patient's eyes are taped closed, covered with wet cotton pads, and shielded with double-folded aluminum foil. Everyone in the room is provided with suitable eye protection, warning signs are posted outside, and all windows are covered. The universal CO_2 laser coupler is placed on the bronchoscope, and test firing is performed to check alignment. The coupler is removed, and the bronchoscope is placed in the trachea to the level of the lesion. Ventilation is attached to the bronchoscope, but the scope may need to be passed distal to the tumor if it is preventing adequate ventilation (Fig. 313-1).

The universal coupler is placed back on the bronchoscope, and suction is attached. A separate suction apparatus is attached to a long suction tip to allow palpation of lesions and the removal of debris and fragments of tissue (Fig. 313-2). The CO_2 laser is used to ablate or resect the lesion. Tissue fragments are removed by suction and by forceps. Hemostasis is obtained by placing Cottonoid pledgets soaked in epinephrine or phenylephrine in the bleeding areas.

After completion of the procedure and hemostasis is satisfactory, the CO_2 coupler is removed and the bronchoscope is removed from the airway. Control of the airway is returned to the anesthesiologist, and the table is returned to the original position. The patient is transferred to the postanesthesia care unit for observation. A chest radiograph is obtained to rule out pneumothorax.

The same procedure is used for Nd:YAG laser bronchoscopy, except the fiber is placed down the bronchoscope along with suction tubing and an optical telescope (Fig. 313-3). The laser fiber and suction tubing are positioned in view of the telescope, just distal to the bronchoscope. High power (40 to 50 watts) is used to resect tumor. Coagulation is obtained by using lower power settings. The thermal effects of the Nd:YAG laser in tissue may extend 4 mm. Care must be used to avoid perforation, especially posteriorly, where no cartilage is present.

The Nd:YAG laser offers the advantage of delivery through flexible bronchoscopes, which can be used with only topical anesthesia. This is useful in minor conditions and in upper lobe lesions. the disadvantages of flexible bronchoscopic laser surgery are a lack of control of the compromised airway, inability to palpate the lesion, less room for multiple suction ports, and inability to provide pressure on bleeding sites.

The argon laser offers the advantage of energy delivery through a very narrow quartz laser fiber. Fibers with a diameter of 300 μm have been used in combination with pediatric flexible bronchoscopes with outside diameters of 3 mm in infants with distal bronchial obstructions. The argon laser may be used in contact mode or held 1 mm away from tissue and produce a smaller amount of penetration than the Nd:YAG laser. This is a desirable feature for pediatric use.

AMELIA DRAKE
JEFFREY L. WILSON

313-1

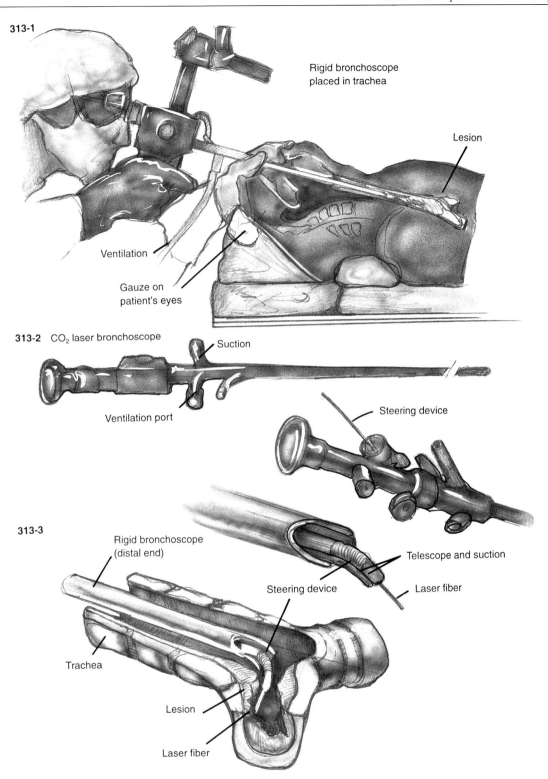

Rigid bronchoscope
placed in trachea

Lesion

Ventilation

Gauze on
patient's eyes

313-2 CO_2 laser bronchoscope

Suction

Ventilation port

Steering device

313-3

Rigid bronchoscope
(distal end)

Telescope and suction

Steering device

Laser fiber

Trachea

Lesion

Laser fiber

■ *314.* FLEXIBLE BRONCHOSCOPY

Examination of the upper and lower airway using the flexible bronchoscope for diagnostic or therapeutic purposes

Indications

1. Stridor
2. Persistent atelectasis
3. Persistent wheezing unresponsive to medical therapy
4. Recurrent or persistent pulmonary infiltrates
5. Pulmonary lesions of unknown cause
6. Chronic cough
7. Hemoptysis
8. Selective bronchography
9. Equivocal tracheobronchial foreign body
10. Assess airway damage related to the endotracheal tube
11. Assess inhalational injury
12. Sample lower airway secretions or cells by bronchoalveolar lavage.
13. Brush biopsy or transbronchial biopsy
14. Aid a difficult intubation
15. Removal of mucous plugs

Special Considerations

1. Coagulopathy
2. Massive hemoptysis
3. Severe airway obstruction
4. Refractory hypoxemia
5. Unstable hemodynamics

Preoperative Preparation

1. Vital signs
2. Routine laboratory studies, if appropriate
3. Bleeding and clotting studies, if history is questionable
4. Universal precautions for *Staphylococcus* infections

Special Instruments, Position, and Anesthesia

1. Flexible bronchoscopes
2. Resuscitation equipment, including oxygen, bag, and masks
3. Photographic equipment

Tips and Pearls

1. This approach may be helpful in combination with rigid bronchoscopy for foreign body removal.
2. Insufflation of oxygen through a suction port can be helpful, especially in infants with tracheostomies whose oxygen airway may be collapsed.

Pitfalls and Complications

1. Adverse effects of medication or sedation
2. Hypoxemia
3. Laryngospasm
4. Bradycardia
5. Epistaxis
6. Pneumothorax
7. Hemoptysis
8. Pneumonia

Postoperative Care Issues

1. Careful postoperative monitoring for airway obstruction

References

Green CG, Eisenberg J, Leong A, Nathanson I, Schnapf BM, Wood RE. Flexible endoscopy of the pediatric airway. Am Rev Respir Dis 1992;145:233.

Wood RE, Azizkhan RG, Lacey SR, Sidman J, Drake A. Surgical applications of ultrathin flexible bronchoscopes in infants. Ann Otol Rhinol Laryngol 1991;100:116.

Wood RE, Postma D. Endoscopy of the airway in infants and children. J Pediatr 1988;112:1.

Operative Procedure

Flexible bronchoscopy is best performed with the patient adequately sedated; general anesthesia is rarely necessary, but adequate sedation and topical anesthesia always are. The patient is in a supine position, with appropriate monitoring. Topical anesthesia is accomplished by instillation of 0.5 to 1 mL of 2% lidocaine (intravenous solution, without preservatives) into the nostril.

The bronchoscope is passed through each nostril to examine the nasal airway and choanae and then passed through the oropharynx and hypopharynx sequentially (Fig. 314-1*A, B*). Because the head is in a neutral position and no distorting forces are applied (as would be the case with a rigid laryngoscope), the dynamics of the airway and larynx may be observed in an almost natural state (Fig. 314-1*C*). Additional lidocaine is applied through the suction channel of the bronchoscope to the larynx and upper trachea, allowing the details of the subglottic space to be observed. It may be easier to see this area as the bronchoscope is withdrawn from the trachea than on entry into the trachea.

The bronchoscope is passed down the trachea, and the bronchi are examined systematically (Fig. 314-2). As in the upper airway, the dynamics of the trachea and bronchi can be observed with the patient breathing spontaneously; general anesthesia and positive-pressure ventilation may obscure the dynamics of the intrathoracic airways.

In patients with tracheostomies, the flexible bronchoscope can usually be passed through the glottis and along the tracheostomy tube; the tube can then be removed to observe the tracheal anatomy and dynamics around the stomal area. Alternatively, the flexible bronchoscope can be passed through the tracheostomy or endotracheal tube directly, if examination of the upper airway is unnecessary at that time (Fig. 314-3).

Great care must be taken to ensure adequate cleaning and sterilization of flexible bronchoscopes between patients. Great care must also be taken in the handling of flexible bronchoscopes, because they are made of glass, are fragile, and are quite expensive.

It is helpful to document endoscopic findings with videotape; parents and other physicians often understand much better what they have seen than what they have heard. Archiving the tapes and the pertinent data in a computerized database is useful, because it is often important to review the specific findings from a previous procedure.

AMELIA F. DRAKE
ROBERT E. WOOD

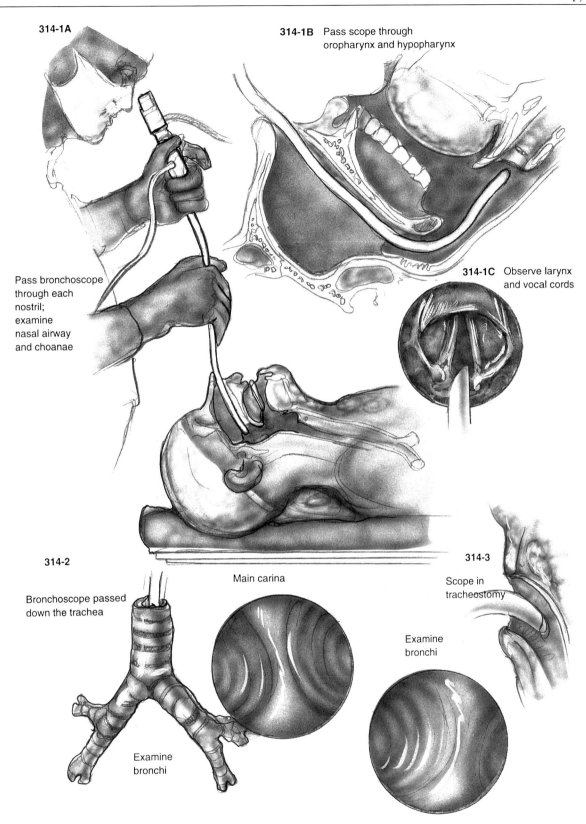

314-1A

Pass bronchoscope through each nostril; examine nasal airway and choanae

314-1B Pass scope through oropharynx and hypopharynx

314-1C Observe larynx and vocal cords

314-2

Bronchoscope passed down the trachea

Main carina

Examine bronchi

314-3

Scope in tracheostomy

Examine bronchi

Atlas of Head and Neck Surgery–Otolaryngology,
edited by Byron J. Bailey, J. Gail Neely, Karen H. Calhoun, and Amy R. Coffey.
Lippincott-Raven Publishers, Philadelphia © 1996.

Section Five

Pediatric and General Otolaryngology

Section Editors:

Byron J. Bailey and Amy R. Coffey

Tonsillectomy, Adenoidectomy, and UPPP
Nasal Polypectomy and Septal Surgery
Maxillary, Ethmoid, and Sphenoid Sinuses
Frontal Sinus
Miscellaneous

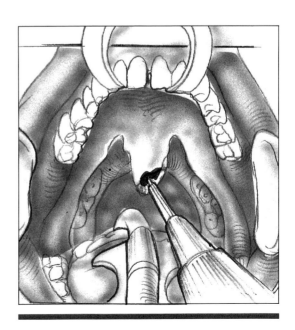

■ *315.* TONSILLECTOMY

Surgical removal of one or both palatine tonsils

Indications

1. Chronic infection: seven times in 1 year, five times annually for 2 years, or three times annually for 3 years
2. Cor pulmonale
3. Sleep apnea syndrome
4. Peritonsillar abscess
5. Suspected malignancy

Special Considerations

1. Submucosal cleft palate (if adenoidectomy is performed)
2. Hemoglobin less than 10 g/100 mL
3. Hematocrit less than 30
4. Bleeding, clotting abnormalities
5. Upper respiratory infection or asthma

Preoperative Preparation

1. Routine laboratory studies (per local hospital policy)
2. Bleeding and clotting studies if history questionable

Special Instruments, Position, and Anesthesia

1. Headlight
2. Head-hanging position
3. McIvor retractor
4. Dean and Fischer knives; foam doughnut

Tips and Pearls

1. Dissection in the plane of the tonsil capsule
2. Meticulous hemostasis

Pitfalls and Complications

1. Severe odynophagia may lead to dehydration
2. Postoperative bleeding
3. Velopharyngeal incompetence
4. Lymphoid tissue regrowth

Postoperative Care Issues

1. Careful postoperative monitoring for pulmonary edema or airway obstruction if the procedure was performed for chronic obstructive disease
2. Ensure postoperative hemostasis several hours after surgery if the patient is to be discharged to home.
3. Counsel the patient or parents regarding pain management, dietary restriction, adequate fluid intake, otalgia, fever, and bleeding.
4. Persistent or heavy bleeding may occur 7 to 10 days postoperatively and requires emergent attention.

References

Bluestone CD. Current indications for tonsillectomy and adenoidectomy. Ann Otol Rhinol Laryngol 1992;101(Suppl 155):58.

Keller C, Elliott W, Hubbell RN. Endotracheal tube safety during electrodesiccation tonsillectomy. Arch Otolaryngol Head Neck Surg 1992;118:643.

Operative Procedure

Tonsillectomy and adenoidectomy are frequently performed as a single surgical event. For a more complete discussion of adenoidectomy, see Chapter 317.

With the patient in the supine, head-hanging position on the operating table, exposure is obtained by opening the McIvor tongue retractor to expose the pharynx (Fig. 315-1). My colleagues and I prefer to pass a #8 red rubber catheter through each nostril and grasp it on each side. These catheters enable the surgeon to retract the soft palate and perform a mirror examination of the nasal pharynx to assess the volume and location of the hypertrophic adenoidal tissue.

An adenotome of appropriate size is selected and introduced into the nasopharynx in the midline to remove the bulk of the posterior and superior adenoidal pad. The remaining adenoidal tissue is removed by sweeping the roof and posterior wall of the nasal pharynx with a series of strokes, using gentle but firm pressure to curette the adenoidal tissue from the underlying muscle. Care is taken to avoid injury to the eustachian tube orifices. After the removal of adenoidal tissue is complete (we do not attempt to remove all vestiges of lymphoid tissue in these patients), the nasopharynx is packed with two gauze packs that have been moistened with a solution of 0.5% ephedrine. Light pressure is applied to these packs for 1 to 2 minutes; then the pressure is released, and the packs are left in place while the tonsillectomy is performed.

The superior pole of one tonsil is grasped with an Allis clamp and retracted toward the midline, placing the tonsillar pillars under some tension. The mucosa over the superior pole of the tonsil is incised using a curved knife blade at the junction of the tonsil and its muscular pillars. This incision is carried anteriorly and inferiorly toward the inferior pole of the tonsil (Fig. 315-2). The point of the knife blade is inserted just beneath the mucosa and then passed similarly along the margin of the posterior tonsillar pillar.

The next step in the operation is extremely important. The Dean knife is used to gently tease the muscles of the tonsillar pillars away from the capsule of the tonsil (Fig. 315-3). Developing this plane is important in terms of limiting blood loss and ensuring that all of the tonsil and its capsule have been removed. When the proper plane is created, the tonsil capsule is elevated from the muscular bed of the tonsillar fossa by exerting pressure against the tonsil with the edge of the Fischer knife (Fig. 315-4). As vessels are encountered, they may be electrocoagulated before they are divided or cauterized after they have been clamped with the hemostat (Fig. 315-5). The dissection is continued until the tonsil is attached only by a vascular and mucosal pedicle at the inferior pole. The loop of the wire snare is then passed around the tonsil and drawn tight at the inferior pole attachment using a slow, steady motion (Fig. 315-6). When the attachment of the inferior pole of the tonsil is transected, there is usually some bleeding, which is controlled by placing two gauze packs in the tonsillar fossa.

Meticulous hemostasis is achieved by leaving the packing in the side of the first tonsillectomy while the procedure is repeated on the contralateral side. After completing the second tonsillectomy, the packing is removed from the nasopharynx, and the area is irrigated with saline to remove any clots. Mirror inspection of the nasopharynx is accomplished as gentle traction is placed on the two rubber catheters to open the area for visualization. Bleeding can be controlled by further packing or by electrocoagulation. The packs are then removed from the side of the first tonsillectomy, and the tonsil bed is inspected carefully. Small bleeding points are electrocoagulated, and larger bleeding vessels are clamped and ligated using 2-0 or 3-0 catgut or Vicryl suture on a sturdy semicircular needle. It is common to see a vascular bundle near the superior pole and at the inferior pole of each tonsil. I prefer to place a superficial figure-of-8 suture around this area to avoid late hemorrhage. These sutures are not placed deeply, because they could injure larger vessels that are not visible beneath the muscular bed of the tonsil.

BYRON J. BAILEY

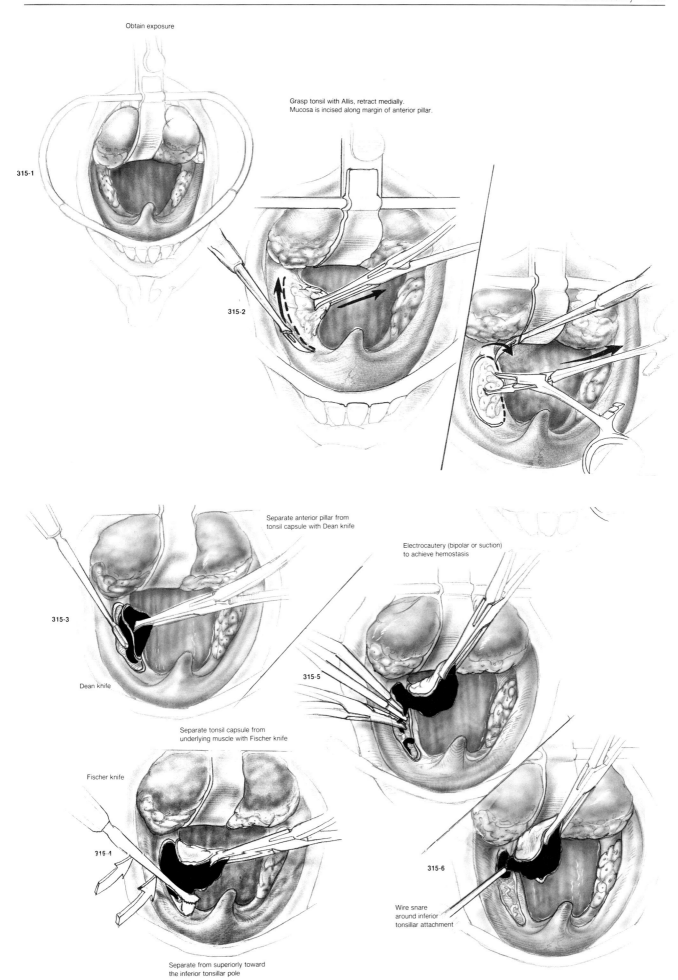

Obtain exposure

315-1

Grasp tonsil with Allis, retract medially.
Mucosa is incised along margin of anterior pillar.

315-2

Separate anterior pillar from
tonsil capsule with Dean knife

315-3

Dean knife

Electrocautery (bipolar or suction)
to achieve hemostasis

315-5

Separate tonsil capsule from
underlying muscle with Fischer knife

Fischer knife

315-4

315-6

Wire snare
around inferior
tonsillar attachment

Separate from superiorly toward
the inferior tonsillar pole

■ *316.* LINGUAL TONSILLECTOMY

Surgical removal of the lingual tonsils, consisting of the lymphoid tissue located at the base of the tongue

Indications

1. Clearly defined indications have not been established because this procedure is not commonly performed.
2. Obstructive sleep apnea secondary to obstructive lingual tonsillar hyperplasia
3. Chronic sore throat with evidence of lingual tonsillitis not directly attributable to other causes

Special Considerations

1. Patients at risk for C1–C2 subluxation (eg, Down syndrome)
2. Bleeding or clotting abnormalities

Preoperative Preparation

1. Routine laboratory testing as dictated by the patient's age or medical history
2. Bleeding and clotting studies as indicated by the patient's age and medical or surgical history

Special Instruments, Position, and Anesthesia

1. Headlight for dissection and electrocautery method
2. Suspension laryngoscope and CO_2 laser for suspension laryngoscopy
3. Rose position
4. If using the laser, anesthesia must prepare for fire-safe ventilation. Nasotracheal intubation is preferred for the dissection and electrocautery method.

Tips and Pearls

1. Be prepared to use either method in case the anatomy of the patient is not appropriate for the method first chosen.

Pitfalls and Complications

1. Postoperative bleeding
2. Postoperative edema with airway obstruction
3. Regrowth of lingual tonsils

Postoperative Care Issues

1. Intensive care unit monitoring may be needed for several days after the procedure, depending on the severity of the preoperative presentation and extent of the surgery.
2. Severe odynophagia may lead to decreased oral intake and dehydration.
3. Postoperative bleeding
4. Steroids may be used for 48 hours postoperatively to reduce edema.

References

Guarisco J, Littlewood SC, Butcher RB III. Severe upper airway obstruction in children secondary to lingual tonsil hypertrophy. Ann Otol Rhinol Laryngol 1990;99:621.

Joseph M, Reardon E, Goodman M. Lingual tonsillectomy: a treatment for inflammatory lesions of the lingual tonsil. Laryngoscope 1984;94:179.

Krespi YP, Har-El G, Levine TM, Ossoff RH, Wurster CF, Paulsen JW. Laser lingual tonsillectomy. Laryngoscope 1989;99:131.

Operative Procedures

Dissection and Electrocautery

The patient undergoes nasotracheal intubation and is then positioned with a shoulder roll to extend the shoulders and head (Fig. 316-1). With the patient in the supine, head-hanging (but supported) Rose position, a Jennings mouth gag is used to establish intraoral exposure. The tongue may be retracted by using a towel clip or a 00 silk suture through the anterior tongue. A large, cloverleaf tongue depressor is used to enhance exposure to the tongue base (Fig. 316-2). The lingual tonsil tissue is grasped with an Allis clamp, and an insulated Bovie tip set on coagulation between 15 and 20 (depending on the unit) is used to dissect the lingual tonsils from the underlying tongue (Fig. 316-3). Bleeding may be controlled with suction electrocautery or free 000 chromic ties.

Suspension Laryngoscopy With Laser Excision

The patient undergoes nasotracheal or orotracheal intubation with a laser-safe tube. A shoulder roll is placed for extension of the shoulders and head. Any wide-tipped laryngoscope that accommodates binocular vision and a suspension apparatus may be used (eg, Dedo, Ossoff-Karlan, Jako, Benjamin-Healy, Parsons). A tooth guard is placed on the upper teeth. The laryngoscope is placed into the vallecula toward one side (the second side is accomplished after repositioning the laryngoscope). The laryngoscope is suspended from an appropriate anchor.

After all laser safety rules governing patient draping and eye protection for the operating room personnel have been met, the laser attached to the operating microscope is brought into the field (Fig. 316-4). Some tissue is grasped with the forceps and sent for pathologic examination to rule out malignancy. The remainder is vaporized with the laser set at between 10 and 20 watts for ablation of the remaining tissue. Normal saline–soaked pledgets are used to shield other anatomic structures from thermal injury. On completion of both sides of the base of tongue and the vallecula, the laryngoscope is taken off suspension and withdrawn. The intraoral structures, lips, and teeth should be inspected before transferring the patient to the recovery room.

LINDA BRODSKY

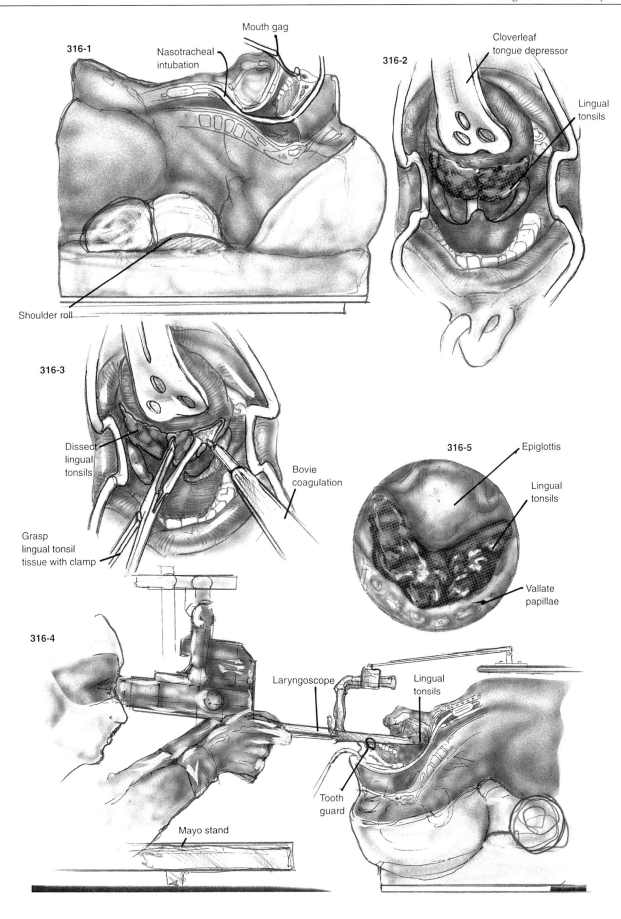

316-1

Mouth gag

Nasotracheal intubation

Shoulder roll

316-2

Cloverleaf tongue depressor

Lingual tonsils

316-3

Dissect lingual tonsils

Grasp lingual tonsil tissue with clamp

Bovie coagulation

316-5

Epiglottis

Lingual tonsils

Vallate papillae

316-4

Laryngoscope

Lingual tonsils

Tooth guard

Mayo stand

■ *317.* ADENOIDECTOMY

Surgical removal of the mass of lymphoid tissue in the nasopharynx known as the pharyngeal tonsils or adenoids

Indications

1. Chronic infection as evidenced by four or more episodes of adenoid infection (purulent rhiaorrhea) per year despite adequate medical therapy
2. Obstructive sleep apnea from obstructive adenoid hyperplasia
3. Orofacial growth abnormalities documented by an orthodontist secondary to obligate mouth breathing because of obstructing adenoids
4. Recurrent suppurative chronic or secretory otitis media

Special Considerations

1. Evaluation for palatal competence and an occult or overt submucous cleft palate
2. Bleeding or clotting abnormalities
3. C1–C2 stability (eg, Down syndrome)

Preoperative Preparation

1. Laboratory testing as dictated by the patient's age and medical or surgical history
2. Bleeding and clotting studies as indicated by the patient's age and medical or surgical history

Special Instruments, Position, and Anesthesia

1. Headlight
2. Rose position
3. McIvor mouth retractor
4. Laryngeal mirrors, sharp curet, adenotome, adenoid punch
5. Suction electrocautery

Tips and Pearls

1. Mirror visualization allows for precise, atraumatic removal.
2. Meticulous hemostasis

Pitfalls and Complications

1. Postoperative bleeding
2. Velopharyngeal incompetence
3. Peritubal scarring leading to chronic otitis media with effusion
4. Grisel's syndrome (ie, C1–C2 subluxation)

Postoperative Care Issues

1. Careful intraoperative and postoperative monitoring for postobstructive pulmonary edema if the procedure is performed for obstruction.
2. Ensure postoperative hemostasis for same-day surgery.
3. Normal diet and activity may be resumed as the patient's recovery permits.

References

Brodsky L. Modern assessment of the tonsils and adenoids. Pediatr Clin North Am 1989;36:1551.
Dana ST, et al. Clinical indicators compendium. Alexandria, VA: American Academy of Otolaryngology—Head and Neck Surgery, 1992.

Operative Procedure

After general orotracheal anesthesia is successfully established, anesthesia is positioned at the side of the patient. A shoulder roll is placed to extend the neck and head. A head drape and down sheet are placed. The orotracheal tube is centered on the tongue, and the McIvor mouth gag with the ring tongue depressor is used to anchor the tube against the tongue while the mouth gag is retracted open. The retractor is then suspended onto the Mayo stand on which the surgical instruments have been placed (Fig. 317-1).

A red rubber catheter is passed through one nares and brought out into the pharynx. The catheter is used to retract the soft palate, and a clamp on the red rubber catheter at the level of the tip of the nose helps to accomplish this. The nasopharynx is visualized indirectly with a defogged laryngeal mirror (Fig. 317-2). A sharp curet is passed to the caudal end of the septum (Fig. 317-3). At this level, the curet is pressed down until the posterior pharyngeal wall is met. It is then brought forward with a seesaw motion to remove the adenoid pad, usually in one piece (Fig. 317-4).

Dental roll packing is placed in the nasopharynx for several minutes. If tonsillectomy is being performed, it is done at this stage. If not, the packing is removed, and the nasopharynx is irrigated copiously with normal saline. Hemostasis is obtained under mirror visualization using suction-electrocautery, usually set at 20 to 25 watts, depending on the electrocautery unit (Fig. 317-5). If any residual tissue remains in the posterior choanae, it may be removed with a small, sharp curet, with an adenoid punch, or by ablation with the electrocautery. Care must be taken not to disturb adenoid tissue around Rosenmueller's fossae, or permanent eustachian tube damage may result. Adenotomes may be used to remove the bulk of the adenoid tissue with the first pass, but this usually is not as efficient or precise as a sharp adenoid curet.

After all bleeding is controlled, the mouth gag is released and removed, as is the red rubber catheter. The lips, teeth, and tongue are inspected for injury before taking the patient to the recovery room.

LINDA BRODSKY

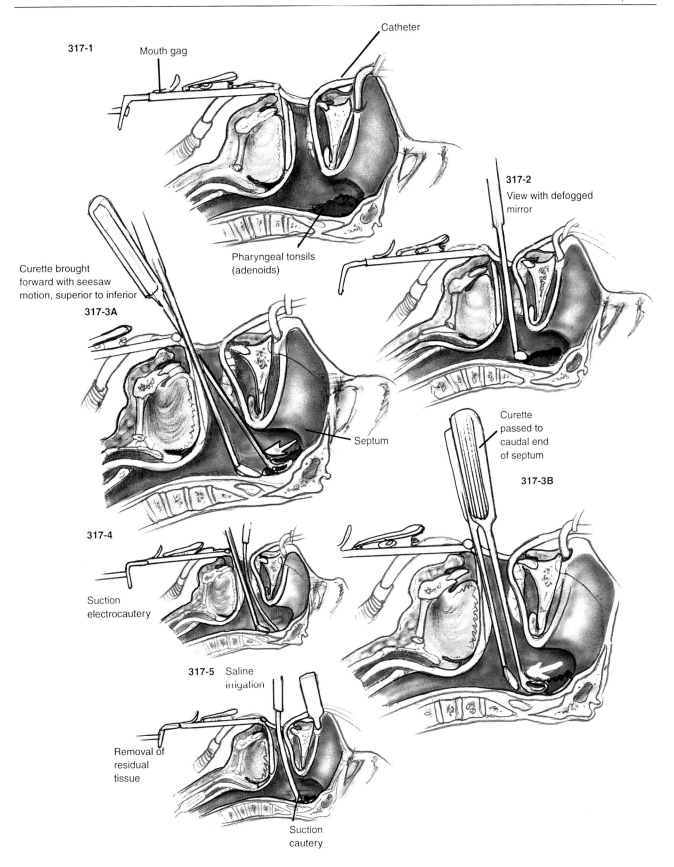

317-1

Mouth gag

Catheter

Pharyngeal tonsils (adenoids)

317-2
View with defogged mirror

Curette brought forward with seesaw motion, superior to inferior

317-3A

Septum

Curette passed to caudal end of septum

317-3B

317-4

Suction electrocautery

317-5 Saline irrigation

Removal of residual tissue

Suction cautery

■ *318.* UVULOPALATOPHARYNGOPLASTY

Enlargement of the airspace of the oropharynx by resection of redundant soft tissue in the palate and lateral pharyngeal walls, which may include tonsillectomy. Staged laser-assisted uvulopalatoplasty (LAUP) is the staged removal and reshaping of the redundant soft tissues of the palate to reduce snoring.

Indications

1. Obstructive sleep apnea syndrome (UP-3)
2. Socially disruptive snoring (UP-3 or LAUP)

Special Considerations

1. Preexisting velopharyngeal incompetence or clefts of palate
2. Bleeding or clotting disorders
3. Pulmonary function
4. Weight
5. Vocal performers or wind instrument players
6. Temporomandibular joint disorders
7. Soft palate not the source of obstruction
8. Neurologic dysfunction of the soft palate
9. Severity of apnea

Preoperative Preparation

1. Routine laboratory work
2. Clotting studies, if indicated by the patient's history
3. Polysomnogram
4. Multiple sleep latency test, if indicated
5. Electrocardiogram and chest radiograph
6. Subacute bacterial endocarditis prophylaxis, if indicated

Special Instruments, Position, and Anesthesia

1. Preoperative anesthesia evaluation is mandatory.
2. Headlight
3. Electrocautery unit
4. Davis retractor
5. Nasopharyngeal airway
6. Backstop hand piece for laser
7. Laser safety equipment

Tips and Pearls

1. Suture line not on leading edge of palate
2. Secure the airway postoperatively.
3. Postoperative steroids reduce pain.
4. Have the patient "snort" to judge the extent of vibratory tissue.
5. If pain is severe, reanesthetize the palate to relieve muscle splinting.

Pitfalls and Complications

1. Take too little, and the symptoms are not relieved.
2. Take too much, and velopharyngeal incompetence results.
3. Pain and possible dehydration
4. Postoperative bleeding
5. Postoperative infection
6. Nasopharyngeal stenosis
7. Change in taste or sensation in tongue
8. Swallowing "feels different" to the patient

Postoperative Care Issues

1. Careful postoperative monitoring for airway obstruction or post-obstructive pulmonary edema
2. Need for postoperative studies to ensure relief of apnea
3. Liberal use of topical anesthetics postoperatively
4. Care in the use of sedative analgesics postoperatively

References

Coleman JA. Laser assisted uvulopalatoplasty—method of Coleman. In: Fairbanks DNF, ed. Snoring and obstructive sleep apnea. New York: Raven Press, 1994.

Fujita S, Conway WA, Zoric F, et al. Surgical correction of anatomic abnormalities in obstructive sleep apnea syndrome: uvulopalatopharyngoplasty. Otolaryngol Head Neck Surg 1981;89:923.

Katsantonis GP, Friedman WH, Krebs FJ, et al. Nasopharyngeal complications following uvulopalatopharyngoplasty. Laryngoscope 1987;97:309.

Operative Procedures

The patient is brought into the operating room and placed on the table in a supine position. General anesthesia is administered. This can be a critical time in the procedure, because many of these patients have compromised airways. If needed, an awake intubation must be performed, or a nasopharyngeal airway should be placed before induction. The head is hanging, and a shoulder role is placed as for a tonsillectomy. A Davis tongue retractor is then passed, and opened.

To determine the optimal level of excision of redundant tissue, and notice what point it touches the posterior pharyngeal wall. The uvula is pulled anteriorly and superiorly. This movement gives an idea of the size of the airspace to be created and helps delineate the junction of the muscle of the soft palate and the mucosa of the soft palate by the formation of a crease. This junction marks the line of incision of the palate. This line of incision should not be more superior than the point at which the palate comes in contact with the posterior pharyngeal wall. An attempt should be made to spare the palatal muscle as much as possible. If the tonsils are intact, a tonsillectomy may be performed first.

The mucosal incision is started at the midline, superior to the uvula and extended along the crease already identified in a lateral direction and curving inferiorly to the base of tongue (Fig. 318-1). After incising the oral side of the mucosa, the incision is stepped inferiorly to create a flap of mucosa that can be rotated over the exposed edge of the palatal muscle (Fig. 318-2). The musculus uvulae is amputated at this level. The redundant mucosa in the lateral pharyngeal wall in the region of the posterior tonsil pillar is excised with the palatal mucosa. Hemostasis for this portion of the procedure is achieved with electrocautery.

The wound is closed by grasping the palatopharyngeus muscle and pulling it anteriorly to the palatoglossus muscle and suturing them together. The repair is then carried across the palate, rolling the mucosa over the cut edge to reduce the postoperative pain and to prevent scar contracture. The lateral pharyngeal wall mucosa over the posterior tonsil pillar is then pulled taught and sewn to the cut edge of the anterior tonsil pillar mucosa after trimming away any excess (Fig. 318-3).

After hemostasis has been achieved, the patient is awakened and taken to recovery. A nasopharyngeal airway should be placed until the patient is fully alert and able to protect his or her own airway. The airway should extend into the hypopharynx to prevent collapse of the base of the tongue against the posterior pharyngeal wall.

The staged uvulopalatoplasty is performed in the outpatient or clinic setting under local anesthesia.

This procedure may be performed with laser (ie, LAUP) or an electrocautery unit. We have had the greatest experience with the carbon dioxide laser for this procedure. With cautery, the tissues that would be vaporized by the laser are instead excised.

The first step in the operation is to make through-and-through incisions in the soft palate about 1 cm long in a vertical direction from the base of the uvula. This is done with a focused beam at 20 watts of power in a continuous mode. The laser is then defocused, and a crescent of tissue is vaporized from the apex of the incision laterally and inferiorly to the superior tonsil pole. This prevents side-to-side healing of the incision and promotes contraction of the palate (Fig. 318-4).

The uvula is shortened to a length of 1 cm (Fig. 318-5). In some individuals, the uvula may be very thick. The uvula can be trapped on a curved retractor and the laser used to vaporize the center of the uvula in a fish-mouth fashion (Fig. 318-6). This removes the bulky muscle but leaves the mucosa intact and allows faster healing with less pain.

The patient is sent home and allowed to heal for 4 weeks before being evaluated. The next stage is then performed. The endpoint is reached when the patient is satisfied, the snoring is gone, or no additional tissue should be removed for fear of causing velopharyngeal incompetence.

JACK A. COLEMAN, JR.
JAMES S. REILLY

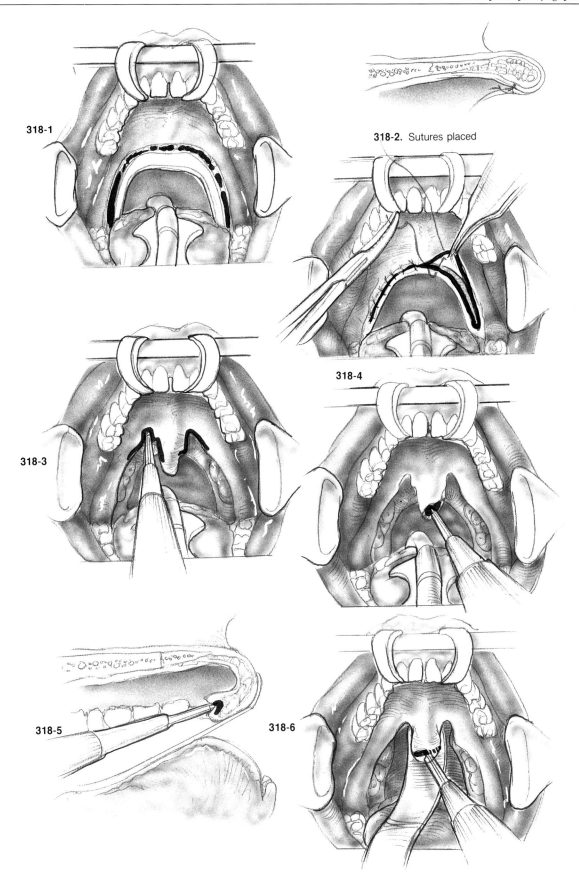

318-1

318-2. Sutures placed

318-3

318-4

318-5

318-6

■ *319.* EXTENDED UVULOPALATOPHARYN-GOPLASTY

—Enlargement of the airspace of the oropharynx by resection of redundant soft tissue in the palate and lateral pharyngeal walls. It may include tonsillectomy.

Indications

1. Obstructive sleep apnea syndrome
2. Socially disruptive snoring

Special Considerations

1. Preexisting velopharyngeal incompetence
2. Bleeding or clotting disorders
3. Pulmonary function
4. Infection
5. Weight
6. Severity of apnea
7. Obstruction in other parts of the upper airway

Preoperative Preparation

1. Routine laboratory studies
2. Clotting studies if history indicates
3. Polysomnogram
4. Multiple sleep latency test, if indicated
5. Electrocardiogram and chest radiograph

Special Instruments, Position, and Anesthesia

1. Preoperative anesthesia evaluation mandatory
2. Headlight
3. Electrocautery unit
4. Davis retractor
5. Nasopharyngeal airway

Tips and Pearls

1. Err on the side of conservative resection.
2. Suture line not on leading edge of palate
3. Hemostasis
4. Do not use too much tension on lateral pharyngeal wall closure. Mattress sutures may be needed to maintain intact suture line.
5. Secure the airway postoperatively.
6. Postoperative steroids can reduce pain, as does the use of Carbocaine.

Pitfalls and Complications

1. Take too little, and the symptoms are not relieved.
2. Take too much, and velopharyngeal incompetence results.
3. Pain and possible dehydration
4. Postoperative bleeding
5. Postoperative infection
6. Nasopharyngeal stenosis
7. Change in taste or sensation in tongue
8. Increased gag reflex
9. Thick pharyngeal secretions

Postoperative Care Issues

1. Careful postoperative monitoring for airway obstruction or post-obstructive pulmonary edema
2. Ensure postoperative hemostasis.
3. Discuss with patient issues of pain management, oral intake, possible temporary velopharyngeal reflux, change in taste, or numbness of tongue.
4. Watch for the onset of nasopharyngeal stenosis.
5. Postoperative studies to ensure relief of apnea

References

Koopmann CF, Moran WB. Surgical management of obstructive sleep apnea. Otolaryngol Clin North Am 1990;23:787.

Moran WB. Sleep apnea: the method of Willard B. Moran. In: Gates GA, ed. Current therapy in otolaryngology—head and neck surgery. 3rd ed. Philadelphia: BC Decker, 1987:317.

Strome M. Uvulopalatoplasty: surgical variations and results. Presented at the Tristate Otolaryngology Assembly, Destin, FL, 1994.

Operative Procedure

Uvulopalatopharyngoplasty has undergone some refinement and alteration of technique to maximize the benefits of the procedure while simultaneously reducing the morbidity. Some of these refinements are reviewed here. All of these techniques are aimed at creating a larger-diameter airway at the level of the oropharynx and reducing the redundant tissue of the soft palate while preserving palatal function.

In the method of Moran, the anterior pillars are almost totally excised by bringing the incision vertically along the lateral aspect of the anterior pillar to the musculocutaneous margin of the soft palate. This is the point at which the redundant mucosa of the soft palate joins with the muscle of the palate and is the level at which the horizontal incision should be made to avoid injury to the palatal muscle. The posterior pillar incision is made at the same level, and after excision of the tissue of the soft palate, a lateral mucosal flap is elevated over the muscle of the posterior pillar (Fig. 319-1). This is advanced to remove posterior pharyngeal corrugations and to remucosalize the tonsil fossa. The muscle of the posterior tonsil pillar is also excised from the juncture with the palate to the inferior tonsil pole to reduce closure at the level of the palate (Fig. 319-2). A few millimeters of tongue base is incised next to the tonsil fossa to promote scarring and decrease the tendency for the tongue to fall posteriorly into the airway during sleep.

In Koopmann's technique, the posterior superior aspect of the posterior tonsil pillar is pulled superiorly and laterally over the raw tonsil bed and held in place by a suture. The anterior tonsil pillar mucosa thus covered is resected, and the area is closed. The junction of the soft palate and anterior pillar is then incised at the point of the initial suture, and the posterior pillar is brought into this defect to make the repair at this point more of a right angle than a gentle curve. Z-plasty may be used to prevent a scar contracture.

Strome uses a procedure similar to that of Moran. In addition to excising the posterior tonsil pillar, he also removes a wedge of palatal tissue at the lateral aspect of the dissection to create more of an angle and reduce the chance of nasopharyngeal stenosis (Fig. 319-3).

Some surgeons leave a 1-cm remnant of uvula in the midline (Fig. 319-4). Besides giving a better cosmetic appearance to the palate, this may preserve some of the sweeping action of the uvula and cause less of a sensation of thick nasopharyngeal drainage in the postoperative period.

JACK A. COLEMAN, JR.
JAMES S. REILLY

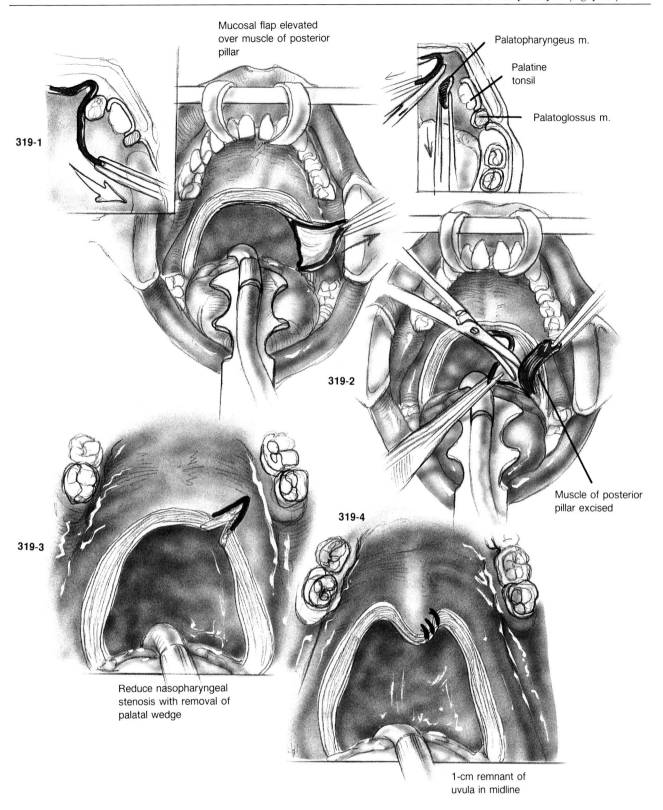

319-1

Mucosal flap elevated over muscle of posterior pillar

Palatopharyngeus m.

Palatine tonsil

Palatoglossus m.

319-2

Muscle of posterior pillar excised

319-3

Reduce nasopharyngeal stenosis with removal of palatal wedge

319-4

1-cm remnant of uvula in midline

■ *320.* HYOID MYOTOMY-SUSPENSION AND GENIOGLOSSUS ADVANCEMENT—Hyoid myotomy-suspension is the surgical release and anterior suspension of the hyoid bone and hyoglossus muscle. Genioglossus advancement is the surgical advancement of the origin of the genioglossus muscle from the poster aspect of the mandible to the anterior aspect.

Indications
1. Used in conjunction with other procedures to reconstruct the upper airway in patients with obstructive sleep apnea syndrome

Special Considerations
1. Size of the hypopharyngeal airspace
2. Bleeding disorders
3. Previous trauma to the neck or mandible
4. Preexisting aspiration or cord paralysis
5. Condition of dentition

Preoperative Preparation
1. Polysomnogram
2. Lateral cephalometric film and Panorex film
3. Routine preoperative laboratory studies
4. Preoperative anesthesia consultation

Special Instruments, Position, and Anesthesia
1. Headlight
2. Supine position
3. May be done under sedation and local anesthesia with fiberoptic monitoring of the base of the tongue's position
4. Oscillating saw and drill

Tips and Pearls
1. Mark the position of the midline of the hyoid before intubation.
2. Stay between the medial cornua of the hyoid.
3. Do not put too much tension on the sutures.
4. In about 15% of patients, a small thyroglossal duct cyst or remnant is encountered.
5. Warn patients to expect numbness in their lower teeth postoperatively.
6. The surgeon should see a window filled with muscle as the plug is advanced.
7. Make sure the patient is relaxed, because tension makes the plug difficult to advance.
8. The attachment of the muscle is very strong, and it will not avulse.

Pitfalls and Complications
1. Injury to the superior laryngeal nerve if dissection carried too far laterally
2. Sutures can saw through or tear through cartilage.
3. Hematoma in the neck causes airway obstruction and necessitates a tracheotomy.
4. Infection
5. Injury to mental nerves
6. Injury to the roots of the lower incisors
7. Hematoma of the floor of the mouth is not uncommon. This may cause some swelling and a temporary change in articulation postoperatively.
8. Violation of the floor of the mouth may make the patient more prone to infection.

Postoperative Care Issues
1. Postoperative monitoring in the intensive care unit for airway patency
2. Pulse oximetry postoperatively
3. Remove the drain the day after surgery.
4. Expect long-term edema of the neck superior to the incision.
5. Numbness of the lower lip and incisors postoperatively
6. The bone plug can be palpated, but the soft tissue over it should adequately camouflage it.

Reference
Riley RW, Powell NB. Obstructive sleep apnea syndrome: a review of 306 consecutively treated surgical patients. Otolaryngol Head Neck Surg 1993;108:2:117.

Operative Procedure

The patient is placed on the operating room table in a supine position, and a general anesthetic is administered. A shoulder role is placed, and the head is extended, exposing the neck. A horizontal incision line about 3 in (7.6 cm) long is marked on the anterior neck over the hyoid bone.

The neck incision is made. The hyoid bone is isolated at the midpoint and grasped with an Alice clamp. The attachments to the hyoid are then separated from the inferior, anterior, and superior aspects of the bone from middle cornu to middle cornu. Dissection is not carried laterally for fear of injuring the superior laryngeal nerve. The bone is then pulled anteriorly toward the thyroid cartilage without undue tension.

The inferior strap muscles are divided in the midline from the level of the hyoid to the notch of the thyroid cartilage (Fig. 320-1). The bursa over the superior thyroid cartilage is then entered through the anterior aspect. Six sutures of a #1 nonabsorbing, braided material on a round needle are placed just lateral to the thyroid notch, three on each side, about 5 mm inferior to the superior rim of the thyroid ala, between 0.5 and 1 cm apart and from posterior to anterior. The soft tissue posterior to the thyroid lamina is pushed inferiorly by the needle to the level at which the needle will pass, and then the needle is pushed through the cartilage.

These sutures are passed around the hyoid bone from the inferior posterior to superior anterior aspects (Fig. 320-2). They are tied down by having the assistant pull the hyoid bone down to the thyroid cartilage while a surgeon's knot is placed and tightened down. Care must be taken not to saw the suture back and forth or pull the knot too tightly, or the suture will tear through the cartilage. The knot is held gently in the jaws of a Webster needle holder while the next knot is thrown.

A local anesthetic with a vasoconstrictor is infiltrated in the lower labial-gingival sulcus and is used to block the inferior alveolar nerves bilaterally. A horizontal, sublabial incision is made canine to canine. The incision is placed so that there is an adequate cuff of tissue to close over the bone. The periosteum is elevated inferiorly to the inferior edge of the mandible and laterally to the mental nerves.

A finger is placed in the oral cavity, and the location of the genial tubercle is verified. A rectangular bone window is marked on the anterior face of the mandible overlying the genial tubercle.

An oscillating saw is used to make the osteotomies. The cuts are made parallel to each other, or the plug will not move in and out of the window. A 9-mm screw to be used for traction is screwed into the previously drilled hole, leaving about 3 mm of the shaft exposed. The osteotomies are then completed. The floor of the mouth should not be violated. The bone plug may be stabilized by grasping the traction screw with an Alice clamp (Fig. 320-3).

The bleeding from the marrow space is controlled with electrocautery and packing with a hemostatic agent or bone wax (Fig. 320-4). As the bone plug is pulled anteriorly, bleeding from the posterior soft tissues is tamponaded.

The plug is pulled anteriorly, rotated about 90° and rests on the anterior face of the mandible just off the midline. The anterior table, marrow space, and traction screw of the bone plug are then removed with a saw (Fig. 320-5). A hole is drilled from the lower edge of the plug and into the inferior edge of the window in the mandible. An 11-mm lag screw is placed to lock the plug in position, and a bur is used to smooth the edges of the bone plug (Fig. 320-6).

The wound is irrigated and closed in two layers using absorbable suture.

JACK A. COLEMAN, JR.
JAMES S. REILLY

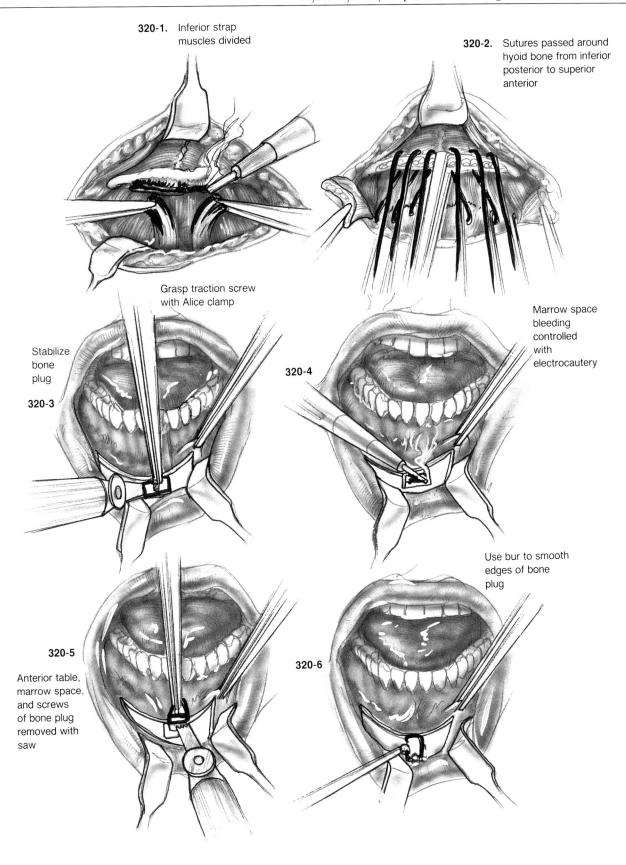

320-1. Inferior strap muscles divided

320-2. Sutures passed around hyoid bone from inferior posterior to superior anterior

Grasp traction screw with Alice clamp

Stabilize bone plug

320-3

320-4

Marrow space bleeding controlled with electrocautery

320-5

Anterior table, marrow space, and screws of bone plug removed with saw

Use bur to smooth edges of bone plug

320-6

■ *321*. NASAL POLYPECTOMY

Surgical removal of a polypoid intranasal mass

Indications

1. Presence of a mass, with or without nasal obstruction
2. Suspected malignancy
3. Bleeding
4. Lack of response to medical management, including antibiotics for infection and topical or intralesional steroids for inflammation

Special Considerations

1. Bleeding and clotting abnormalities
2. Cardiac instability
3. Full nasal examination with attention to the septum, nasal bones, and upper lateral cartilages for their possible role in obstruction

Preoperative Preparation

1. Routine laboratory studies
2. Bleeding and clotting studies, if the history is questionable
3. Axial and coronal computed tomography (CT) scans of the nasal cavity and paranasal sinuses

Special Instruments, Position, and Anesthesia

1. Headlight or fiberoptic endoscope
2. Nasal snare
3. Suction cautery
4. Supine position, with the head elevated 30°
5. Local or general anesthesia

Tips and Pearls

1. Careful preoperative determination of the origin of the polyp, including a meningocele, encephalocele, nasopharyngeal mass, or septal mass
2. Pathologic consultation with careful histologic examination
3. Meticulous hemostasis

Pitfalls and Complications

1. Incomplete removal may lead to recurrence
2. Mucosal damage may lead to synechiae or sinus ostial obstruction with secondary sinusitis
3. Vigorous bleeding may obscure the surgeon's vision and require cessation of the procedure.
4. Misdiagnosis of an intracranial polypoid mass may lead to intracranial complications or a cerebrospinal fluid leak.

Postoperative Care Issues

1. Packing, if any, should be completely removed within 3 days.
2. Ensure postoperative hemostasis before discharge.
3. Counsel the patient regarding bleeding, packing removal, nasal hygiene, and prevention of nasal abuse.

Reference

Donald PJ. Minor intranasal procedures. Otolaryngol Clin North Am 1973;6:715.

Operative Procedure

With the patient in the supine position and the head elevated 30°, the nasal cavities are inspected. The CT scan is in the operating room for comparison with clinical findings.

Local anesthesia is preferred over general anesthesia, but in either case, great care must be taken to achieve maximal vasoconstriction. The nasal cavity is sprayed with a 1% solution of phenylephrine. Topical anesthetic (up to 4 mL of 5% cocaine) is applied to 0.5-in (12-mm) plain cotton gauze or to cotton balls and used to anesthetize the sphenopalatine ganglion region at the posterior end of the middle turbinate, the anterior ethmoid nerve region superiorly, and the area in which the nasopalatine nerve comes into the floor of the nose through the incisive foramen (Fig. 321-1). Additional anesthetic is placed along the lateral wall of the nose in the region of the base of the polyp. For patients with evidence of cardiorespiratory instability, an anesthesiologist stands by to monitor and support the patient if necessary.

After a 10-minute wait to allow optimal levels of anesthesia and vasoconstriction, the nasal cavity is inspected again. The exact origin of the polyp is identified. The polyp should be presenting in the middle meatus from the maxillary or anterior ethmoid sinuses, in the superior meatus from the posterior ethmoid sinus, or in the sphenoethmoid recess from the sphenoid sinus (Fig. 321-2). If it originates in any other region, the diagnosis of benign inflammatory polyp must be questioned.

The base of the polyp is encircled with the nasal snare, and the snare is gently closed until the base is firmly grasped (Fig. 321-3). The snare is then withdrawn from the nose with the polyp in its grasp. The polyp is submitted for pathologic examination. The area from which the polyp has been removed is inspected for bleeding. Cotton gauze packing that was originally used to induce anesthesia and vasoconstriction can be reinserted temporarily and placed directly on any bleeding sites (Fig. 321-4). If necessary, the temporary packing can be replaced with petrolatum-impregnated gauze or Merocel gauze, which is left in the nose for 24 to 72 hours for hemostasis. A folded 2 × 2 gauze is taped to the upper lip, not to the nasal tip, to absorb any drainage.

A nasal polyp is rarely an isolated phenomenon. More commonly, it is part of a generalized condition known has hyperplastic polypoid rhinosinusitis, which requires more extensive therapy and is discussed elsewhere in this text.

FRANK E. LUCENTE

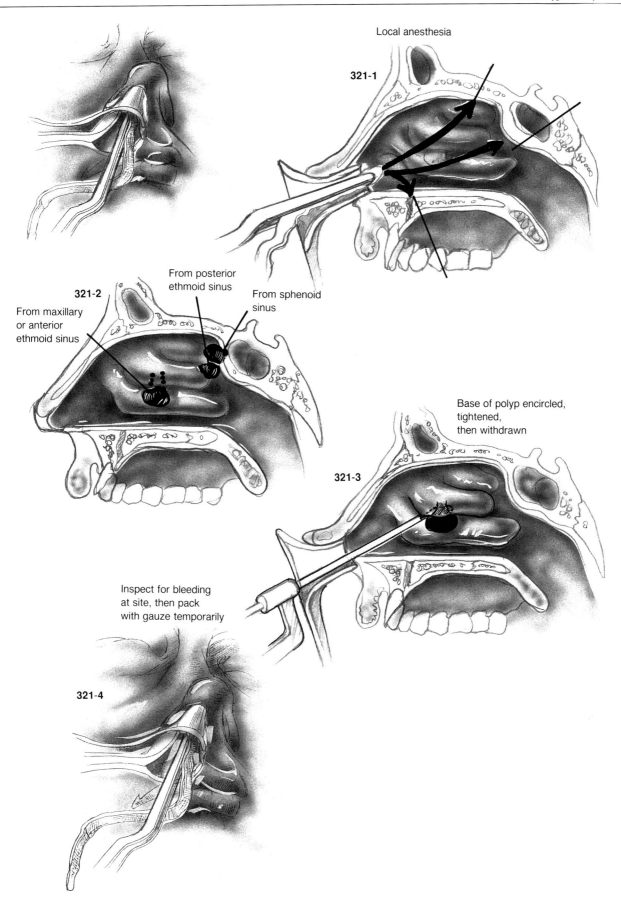

Local anesthesia

321-1

321-2

From maxillary
or anterior
ethmoid sinus

From posterior
ethmoid sinus

From sphenoid
sinus

321-3

Base of polyp encircled,
tightened,
then withdrawn

Inspect for bleeding
at site, then pack
with gauze temporarily

321-4

322. ENDOSCOPIC EXCISION OF ANTRO-CHOANAL POLYPS—The removal of inflammatory nasal polyps originating from the maxillary sinus and protruding into the nasal cavity

Indications

1. Nasal obstruction
2. Associated recurrent acute or chronic sinusitis
3. Associated obstructive sleep apnea

Special Considerations

1. Concomitant inflammatory sinus disease
2. Septal deflection limiting exposure and transnasal delivery of the polyp
3. Transoral delivery for large antrochoanal polyps
4. Bleeding diathesis
5. Nasal mass suspected to be an inverted papilloma or malignancy
6. Consider a Caldwell-Luc approach when the anatomy is poorly defined.

Preoperative Preparation

1. Antibiotics for treatment of associated sinusitis
2. Consider systemic steroids to reduce polyp size and nasal inflammation.

Special Instruments, Position, and Anesthesia

1. Nasal endoscopes and sinus instruments, including angled curets and malleable endoscopic biopsy forceps
2. Position the patient supine, with the surgeon sitting to the right or left of the patient's shoulder.
3. Local anesthesia with intravenous sedation or general anesthesia if transoral delivery is anticipated

Tips and Pearls

1. Antrochoanal polyps are often found in the absence of other sinus disease.
2. The anatomy may be significantly distorted by the polyp.
3. Do not strip the maxillary sinus mucosa; its function should be preserved.

Pitfalls and Complications

1. Incomplete removal of the uncinate process limits exposure.
2. Anterior dissection can jeopardize the nasolacrimal duct.
3. Inadequate antrostomy and polyp removal with resultant recurrent disease
4. Patient aspiration of the polyp
5. Postoperative hemorrhage
6. Orbital complications associated with maxillary sinus surgery
7. Paresthesias associated with infraorbital nerve injury

Postoperative Care

1. Meticulous postoperative debridement to prevent synechiae formation
2. Saline nasal irrigation helps to loosen crusts and evacuate dried blood.
3. Continuation of antibiotic coverage in the perioperative period

References

Crook PR, Davis WE, McDonald R, McKinsey JP. Antrochoanal polyposis: a review of 33 cases. ENT J 1993;72:401.

Loury MC, Hinkley DK, Wong W. Endoscopic transnasal antrochoanal polypectomy: an alternative to the transnasal approach. South Med J 1993;86:18.

Myers EN, Cunningham MJ. Modified Caldwell-Luc approach for the treatment of antral choanal polyps. Laryngoscope 1986;96:911.

Operative Procedure

Oxymetazoline (0.05%) is administered intranasally. While visualizing the nasal cavity with a 0° endoscope, a 1% solution of lidocaine with a 1:100,000 concentration of epinephrine is injected at the anterior root of the middle turbinate, anterior to the uncinate process, and at the superior aspect of the inferior turbinate, as in standard endoscopic sinus surgery. The polyp stalk can be injected to provide hemostasis if the nasal portion of the polyp is to be amputated. A greater palatine foramen block is also useful. This is performed with a 2-in (5-cm), 25-gauge needle attached to a 3-mL syringe. The needle is bent 60° to 80° at a position 2.5 cm from the tip. The hard palate is topically anesthetized if the patient is awake. The foramen is identified by palpation and visualization medial to the second molar. It is located approximately 5 mm anterior to the free border of the hard palate. The needle is inserted submucosally in the vicinity of the foramen, and 0.5 mL is administered. After identifying the foramen by probing along the hard palate, the needle is passed into the foramen no further than 2.5 cm; 1 to 2 mL of anesthetic is injected after aspiration. Air or blood return on aspiration signifies improper needle placement.

After the anesthetics and vasoconstrictive agents have had sufficient time to take effect, the nose is inspected using a 0° nasal endoscope. If necessary, the middle turbinate is medialized with a Freer elevator. An endoscopically guided uncinectomy is performed with a sickle knife and straight Weil-Blakesly forceps (Figs. 322-1 and 322-2). Alternatively, a backbiting forceps can be used for this maneuver. The stalk of the antrochoanal polyp may sufficiently widen the maxillary sinus ostium and result in atrophy of the uncinate process.

After the uncinate has been completely removed, the entry point of the antrochoanal polyp into the middle meatus is identified. The size and position of the polyp may prevent access for the creation of a middle meatal antrostomy, and it may be necessary to remove the nasal portion of the antrochoanal polyp to proceed. This can be achieved transnasally by grasping and avulsing the stalk with a large straight Weil-Blakesly forceps or polyp snare. Alternately, transoral removal may be performed by grasping the polyp in the nasopharynx with a curved Kelly or Crile clamp and transecting the polyp intranasally as it emerges from the sinus. Using a McIvor mouth gag facilitates transoral removal. If sufficient access is available, the polyp and stalk may be left intact until the antrostomy is created. This approach facilitates dissection of the antral portion by allowing gentle traction on the stalk.

The maxillary sinus natural ostium is identified with a 30° telescope and a ball-tipped Lusk seeker. Typically, the polyp protrudes into middle meatus through an accessory ostium in the posterior fontanel (Fig. 322-3). Care should be taken to create a wide antrostomy that includes the natural ostium of the maxillary sinus. The posterosuperior edge of the natural ostium is incised using a curved endoscopic scissors or forward-biting punch. The middle meatal antrostomy is widened with a backbiting forceps or forward-biting punch. The limits of the antrostomy are the basal lamella of the middle turbinate posteriorly; the attachment of the inferior turbinate inferiorly; and the orbit superiorly.

Wide access to the maxillary sinus is critical for complete removal of the antral portion of the polyp. The antral portion of the polyp usually has a cystic component that contains a straw-colored fluid. This cystic portion is decompressed during mobilization of the polyp (Fig. 322-4). The 70° telescope is helpful in visualizing the antral origin of the polyp, although an endoscope placed through a trocar in the canine fossa can also be used.

The polyp is grasped near its base with a large 70° giraffe forceps or a malleable endoscopic biopsy forceps and is delivered from the antrum. The point of attachment can be elevated from the underlying bone with frontal recess curets or giraffe forceps. At this point, the rough edges of the antrostomy are smoothed, and any other necessary sinus surgery can proceed.

ANDREW N. GOLDBERG
DONALD C. LANZA

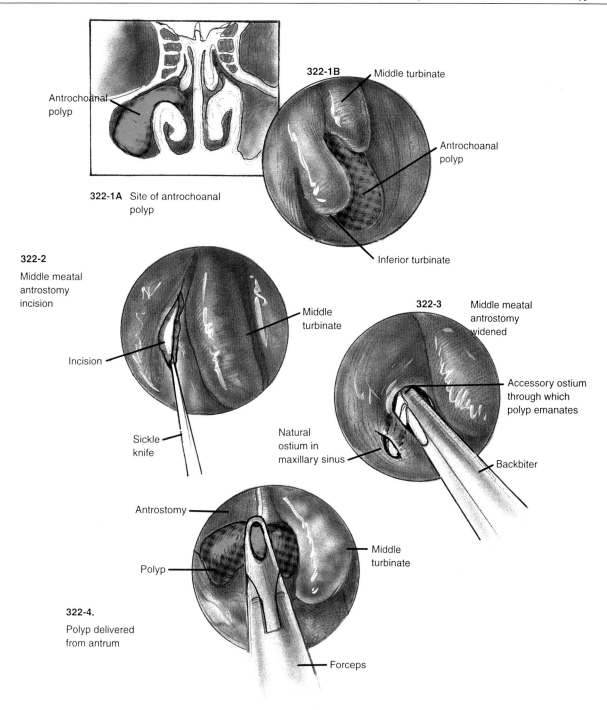

Antrochoanal polyp

322-1A Site of antrochoanal polyp

322-1B

Middle turbinate

Antrochoanal polyp

Inferior turbinate

322-2

Middle meatal antrostomy incision

Middle turbinate

Incision

Sickle knife

322-3 Middle meatal antrostomy widened

Accessory ostium through which polyp emanates

Natural ostium in maxillary sinus

Backbiter

Antrostomy

Polyp

Middle turbinate

322-4.

Polyp delivered from antrum

Forceps

■ 323. SUBMUCOUS RESECTION OF THE NASAL SEPTUM—Submucosal removal of a deviated portion of septal cartilage and bone

Indications

1. Deviation of the nasal septum, with partial or complete unilateral or bilateral obstruction of airflow
2. Persistent or recurrent epistaxis
3. Evidence of sinusitis secondary to septal deviation
4. Headaches secondary to septal deviation
5. Anatomic obstruction that makes indicated sinus procedures difficult to perform efficiently

Special Considerations

1. Nasal polyps
2. History of allergic rhinitis or nasal trauma
3. Bleeding or clotting abnormalities
4. Disorders of smell

Preoperative Preparation

1. Routine laboratory studies
2. Evaluation of nasal skeleton and turbinates for their possible role in nasal obstruction
3. Preoperative photography of the external and internal nose, if possible
4. Rhinomanometry, if possible

Special Instruments, Position, and Anesthesia

1. Headlight
2. Supine position, with the head elevated 30°
3. Local anesthesia (possibly general)
4. Cottle septal elevator, narrow Vienna speculum, Jansen-Middleton rongeur

Tips and Pearls

1. Hemitransfixion incision immediately behind caudal edge of septum
2. Dissection in subperichondrial and subperiosteal planes
3. Retention of 1 cm of dorsal and caudal struts
4. Adequate bone and cartilage resection
5. Quilting suture to reapproximate flaps
6. Provide a drainage site for any blood beneath the flaps.

Pitfalls and Complications

1. Excessive damage to flaps leading to perforation
2. Failure to elevate the perichondrium completely over the cartilage to be resected
3. Failure to resect adequate cartilage or bone
4. Failure to appreciate the role of external bony and cartilaginous skeleton in producing the obstruction

Postoperative Care Issues

1. Minimize the packing if quilting sutures are used.
2. Remove the packing within 72 hours.
3. Give thorough written instructions regarding postoperative care and expectations.
4. Remove any crusts cautiously.
5. Stress ongoing nasal health and protection.

References

Bernstein L. Submucous operations on the nasal septum. Otolaryngol Clin North Am 1973;6:675.

Kern EB. Nasal septal reconstruction versus submucous resection. In: Snow JB Jr, ed. Controversy in otolaryngology. Philadelphia: WB Saunders, 1980:335.

Operative Procedure

The nasal cavity is sprayed with a 1% solution of phenylephrine. Topical anesthetic is applied to 0.5-in (12-mm) plain cotton gauze or to cotton balls and used to anesthetize the sphenopalatine ganglion region at the posterior end of the middle turbinate, the anterior ethmoid nerve region superiorly, and the area in which the nasopalatine nerve comes into the floor of the nose through the incisive foramen (Fig. 323-1). After the cotton pledgets or gauze are removed and the anesthesiologist administers a short-acting barbiturate, the injections of 1% Xylocaine with a 1:100,000 concentration of epinephrine are used to complete the anesthesia.

The nasal speculum is inserted in the right nostril and used to displace the columella to the left. This move brings the septal mucosa a few millimeters anteriorly. In most instances, the hemitransfixion incision is made directly on the caudal tip of the septum (Fig. 323-2). The incision goes through the mucosa and perichondrium, directly down to the cartilage. If there is any doubt about the perichondrium being incised, the #15 blade is turned 90°, and the perichondrium is gently scraped off of the cartilage, which appears very pale or blue. The Cottle elevator is inserted in the submucoperichondrial plane and the perichondrium is completely elevated from one side of the septal cartilage by keeping the tip of the elevator against the cartilage and using the shaft for the elevation (Fig. 323-3).

As elevation proceeds posteriorly, the junction between the septal cartilage and the anterior edge of the ethmoid plate is encountered. I prefer to use the elevator to separate the bony-cartilaginous articulation. The mucoperiosteal flaps are elevated over both sides of the ethmoid plate and vomer. The last part of the elevation is from the lower edge of the septum to the floor. This part is often more difficult, because it is necessary to incise the decussating mucoperichondrial and mucoperiosteal fibers that envelope the septal cartilage and the bony maxillary-palatine crest.

Inspection of the septum determines exactly which portions of bone and cartilage are to be removed. I usually begin by partially incising the septal cartilage 1 cm behind the caudal edge and 1 cm below the articulation between the septal cartilage and the upper lateral cartilages (Fig. 323-4). This incision in then deepened by using the Cottle elevator. The mucoperichondrial flap is elevated from the opposite side of the central cartilaginous portion that is to be resected. The resection can be performed with the Ballenger swivel knife (Fig. 323-5) or with an angled or curved scissors. The Jansen-Middleton rongeur is used to remove deviated portions of the ethmoid plate and vomer (Fig. 323-6). Particular attention is paid to the inferior portion of the septum, where it is frequently found to be dislocated from the palatine-maxillary crest. The dislocated cartilage is resected, and if necessary, any deviated portions of bone are removed with the rongeur.

At this stage, I prefer to insert temporary packing moistened with the Xylocaine-epinephrine solution to reapproximate the flaps. After a few minutes, the packing is removed, and the patient's breathing is tested. If the patient still complains of obstruction, the adequacy of the resection of cartilage and bone is checked, and additional tissue is removed as needed. Because the elevation of the flaps is frequently accompanied by the creation of minor tears in them, creating a specific drainage site for blood that may accumulate usually is unnecessary.

The last stage of the procedure involves the use of a quilting suture of 3-0 chromic catgut to reapproximate the mucoperichondrial and mucoperiosteal flaps. A knot is placed at the distal end of the suture to anchor it in place, and the suture is woven from side to side and from the posterior to anterior aspects until it reaches the site of the hemitransfixion incision.

For packing, I prefer to use Telfa gauze, which is cut slightly larger than the septal cartilage and which is coated with antibiotic ointment. The gauze is placed along each side of the reconstructed septum for additional support. Minimal or no additional packing is used. An upper lip dressing of folded 2 × 2 in gauze is applied.

FRANK E. LUCENTE

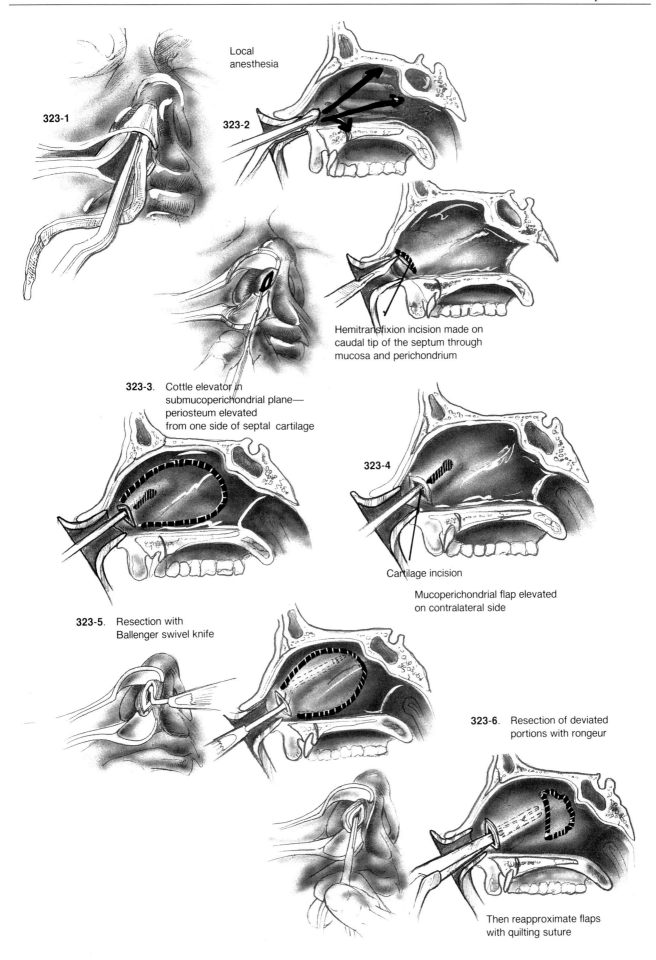

323-1

323-2   Local anesthesia

Hemitransfixion incision made on caudal tip of the septum through mucosa and perichondrium

323-3. Cottle elevator in submucoperichondrial plane— periosteum elevated from one side of septal cartilage

323-4

Cartilage incision

Mucoperichondrial flap elevated on contralateral side

323-5. Resection with Ballenger swivel knife

323-6. Resection of deviated portions with rongeur

Then reapproximate flaps with quilting suture

■ 324. SEPTOPLASTY

Repositioning of the bony and cartilaginous nasal septum while attempting to save as much of the cartilaginous septum as possible

Indications

1. Nasal obstruction
2. Epistaxis
3. Sinder's headache
4. Exposure for endoscopic sinus surgery
5. Obstructive sleep apnea

Contraindications

1. Severe underlying medical illness that increases the risk of surgery

Special Considerations

1. Must determine the degree of intrinsic deformity of the septal (quadrangular) cartilage

Preoperative Preparation

1. Coagulation studies
2. Helpful to have patient's nose sprayed with a topical decongestant in the preoperative holding area

Special Instruments, Position, and Anesthesia

1. Headlight, Cottle or Freer elevators, different lengths of nasal specula, a 4-mm chisel, and through-cutting and regular Jansen-Middleton bone rongeurs
2. Semi-Fowler position
3. Local or general anesthesia; careful topical and injected anesthesia to include the nasopalatine and sphenopalatine nerves, anterior and posterior ethmoid nerves, external branch of the anterior ethmoid nerve, incisive nerve, and infraorbital nerve

Tips and Pearls

1. Use hydrodissection at time of injection to elevate difficult convex surfaces.
2. Intrinsically deformed cartilage often requires bilateral submucoperichondrial elevation to avoid returning to the preoperative configuration.
3. Do not confuse the upper surface of the vomer with the floor of the nose.
4. Tunnels along the floor of the nose do not help with elevation from the maxillary crest.
5. A 4-0 mild chromic suture using a short Keith needle helps to prevent hematoma.

Pitfalls and Complications

1. Cerebrospinal fluid fistulas may result from too much traction on the perpendicular plate of the ethmoid bone. Use a cutting-type instrument in this area.
2. Avoid bilateral opposed perforations, and correct them if they occur with sutures and mucosal flaps.
3. Toxic shock syndrome is possible.

Postoperative Care Issues

1. Packing should be removed in 24 hours.
2. Leave the splints for 1 week if surgery of lateral nasal wall structures is performed concomitantly.
3. Watch for packing-related hypoxemia.

References

Haraldsson PO, Nordemar H, Anggard A. Long-term results after septal surgery—submucous resection versus septoplasty. ORL J Otorhinolaryngol Relat Spec 1987;49:218.

Larsen K, Oxhoj H. Spirometric forced volume measurements in the assessment of nasal patency after septoplasty. A prospective clinical study. Rhinology 1988;26:203.

Samad I, Stevens HE, Maloney A. The efficacy of nasal septal surgery. J Otolaryngol 1992;21:88.

Operative Procedures

Septoplasty can be performed under local or general anesthesia. The patient is placed in the semi-Fowler position, with the surgeon standing on the patient's right. Regardless of whether general anesthesia is used, proper injection with local anesthetic is critical, because this begins the mobilization of the submucosal flap. A topical decongestant should be sprayed in the patient's nose in the holding area before entering the operating theater. The surgeon should pack the nose with cocaine or a cocaine substitute before washing his or her hands. The packs should be positioned near the ethmoidal and nasopalatine nerves. Injection begins after the patient is adequately sedated or anesthetized. If the patient is under general anesthesia, the injection can be confined to the septum. The needle is bent toward the bevel at the septum's tip, which is insinuated under the mucosa. In response to slow, steady pressure, the mucosa should blanch and raise up from the underlying cartilage.

Inject over any convexities or concavities to aid with their later elevation. This hydrodissection can make later elevation much easier and safer. It is important to inject high and far posteriorly. Injections should be done bilaterally. A 1% solution of Xylocaine with a 1:100,000 dilution of epinephrine is used if the patient is anesthetized. A 1:1 mixture of 2% Xylocaine with 1:100,000 epinephrine and 0.5% bupivacaine with 1:200,000 epinephrine is used if the patient is awake. If the patient is merely sedated, more extensive injection is required. Both infraorbital nerves are injected sublabially. The base of the columella is injected. Although prophylactic antibiotics have not been definitively shown to be beneficial, they commonly are used intravenously, perioperatively, and orally for 10 days postoperatively.

The septoplasty operation is begun through a right hemitransfixion incision over the caudal end of the septal cartilage. Care is taken to find the proper plane between the cartilage and the perichondrium of the septum. Sharp instruments are helpful in getting started. There is a tendency to elevate too superficially between the perichondrium and the mucosa. After the proper plane is entered, the dissection proceeds easily posteriorly along the left side of the cartilaginous septum with blunt dissection (Fig. 324-1). The septal cartilage is fractured away from the perpendicular plate of the ethmoid and vomer, and dissection proceeds posteriorly on both sides of the bony septum.

The confluence of the quadrangular (septal) cartilage, the perpendicular plate of the ethmoid and the vomer, is the area most difficult to raise without perforating the mucosa. The leading edge of the bony septum and any other displaced bone are then resected (Fig. 324-2). Care must be taken superiorly where the perpendicular plate of the ethmoid inserts onto the cribriform plate to prevent creating a cerebrospinal fluid fistula. Cutting instruments that can cut the bone cleanly without pulling or great force are preferred for work in this area. The dissection proceeds along the floor of the nose (Fig. 324-3). The cartilage can be dissected free from the maxillary crest without too much difficulty. The cartilage commonly overrides the crest on one side or the other, and this redundant cartilage is resected.

Small mucosal perforations are generally of little concern as long as two such perforations on each side are not juxtaposed. Large perforations should be repaired with 4-0 catgut on a small needle. Releasing incisions laterally along the floor of the nose may aid in a tension-free closure.

The two leaves of mucoperichondrium can be quilted together using a 4-0 plain catgut suture on a small Keith needle. Septal splints of Silastic can aid in preventing synechiae, especially when septoplasty has been combined with some form of turbinate resection or endoscopic sinus surgery. The splints are held in place with one simple transseptal suture of 5-0 nylon. The hemitransfixion incision is closed with two mattress sutures of 4-0 chromic catgut on a Keith needle. The nose is packed with fingercot dressings impregnated with antibiotic ointment.

HAROLD PILLSBURY III
MARK C. WEISSLER

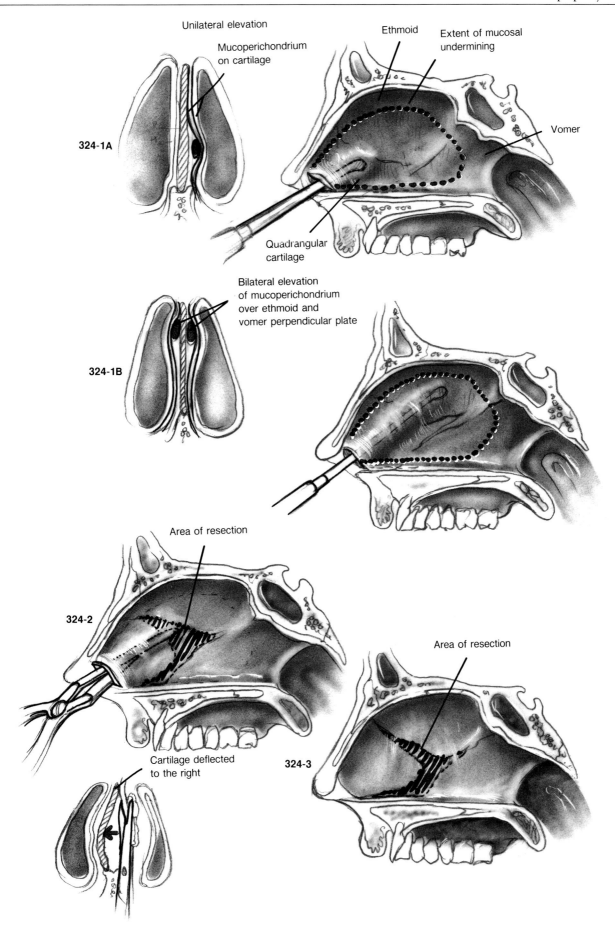

Unilateral elevation

Mucoperichondrium on cartilage

Ethmoid

Extent of mucosal undermining

Vomer

324-1A

Quadrangular cartilage

Bilateral elevation of mucoperichondrium over ethmoid and vomer perpendicular plate

324-1B

Area of resection

324-2

Cartilage deflected to the right

Area of resection

324-3

■ *325.* EXTRACRANIAL CLOSURE OF CERE-BROSPINAL FLUID RHINORRHEA USING A MUCOPERIOSTEAL FLAP—Intranasal closure of defects of the anterior cranial fossa or sphenoid using a pedicled flap of nasal mucoperiosteum from the septum or middle turbinate

Indications
1. Documented leakage of cerebrospinal fluid (CSF) from the nasal cavity, originating in the cribriform plate, ethmoid roof, or sphenoid sinus, that requires operative intervention

Contraindications
1. Lack of sufficient local tissue
2. Nasal inflammation or scarring, causing the flap to become unreliable
3. Active infection in the operative field

Special Considerations
1. Previous surgery on the nose or base of the skull
2. Adjunctive procedures and factors that affect the timing of surgery, such as increased intracranial pressure, fractures in need of reduction, intracranial infection, or residual tumor
3. Sphenoid sinus obliteration should be considered for defects of the sphenoid sinus.
4. Use of a mucoperiosteal flap for a previously irradiated recipient bed

Preoperative Preparation
1. Nasal endoscopy and computed tomography (CT) scanning
2. CT scan with intrathecal iohexol or metrizamide, when appropriate
3. Intrathecal radionuclide scan, when appropriate
4. Magnetic resonance imaging, as indicated
5. Preoperative neurosurgical consultation and availability during the procedure

(continued)

Operative Procedure
Identification of the Cerebrospinal Fluid Leak
The patient is prepared for surgery as described in Procedure 331. Intrathecal fluorescein, which causes the CSF to appear yellow-green, is helpful in localizing the leak and can be injected through a lumbar drain. Surgical access to the site of CSF leak is obtained through a nasal-orbital skin incision or endonasal approach. A complete ethmoidectomy is performed for leaks along the roof of the ethmoid, and a sphenoidotomy is added for defects in the sphenoid sinus (Fig. 325-1). A more limited dissection may be used for leaks along the cribriform plate, where an endonasal approach for medial skull base defects is preferred.

Mucosa surrounding the defect is removed by bipolar fulguration or stripping the bone for approximately 5 mm without widening the defect (Fig. 325-2). This allows the mucoperiosteal flap to adhere directly to bone; it does not adhere well to intervening mucosa. The mucosa is elevated for another 2 to 3 mm circumferentially beyond the bony defect, allowing the flap later to be tucked under the mucosal edge. Defects smaller than 1 cm^2 can be covered with a mucoperichondrial flap alone without placement of bone into the defect. If an ethmoid defect is larger than 1 cm^2, the dura can be elevated gently for a few millimeters on the intracranial side of the defect to accept a bone or cartilage graft (Fig. 325-3). A bone or cartilage free graft is harvested from the septum, turbinate, concha of the ear, canine fossa, or calvarium. If a graft is necessary, one of its dimensions is made slightly larger than the defect to prevent it from becoming dislodged. This graft is placed between the dura and bony cranium to support the intracranial structures and prevent their prolapse. In general, a graft is not used for sphenoid sinus defects.

The mucoperiosteal flap is then planned. The precise location of the defect and the nasal anatomy determine the configuration and size of the flap. After the defect has been exposed, the mucosa intervening between the defect and the proposed mucoperiosteal flap should be carefully removed to prevent it from becoming buried beneath the pedicle of the flap.

(continued)

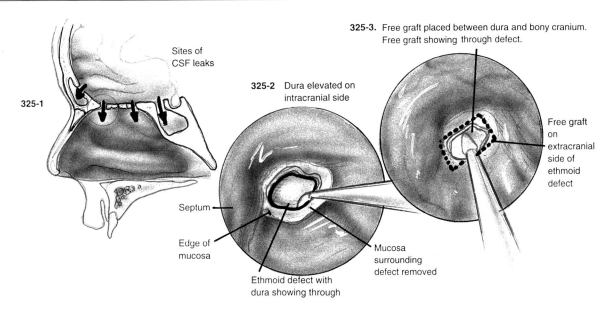

325-1

Sites of
CSF leaks

Septum

Edge of
mucosa

Ethmoid defect with
dura showing through

325-2   Dura elevated on
intracranial side

Mucosa
surrounding
defect removed

325-3. Free graft placed between dura and bony cranium.
Free graft showing through defect.

Free graft
on
extracranial
side of
ethmoid
defect

■ *325.* EXTRACRANIAL CLOSURE OF CERE-BROSPINAL FLUID RHINORRHEA USING A MUCOPERIOSTEAL FLAP *(continued)*

Special Instruments, Position, and Anesthesia

1. An endonasal or external approach, according to the surgeon's preference
2. Operating microscope or nasal endoscopes
3. Endoscopic sinus surgery set, otologic instruments, Landolt bipolar coagulation forceps (Aesculap 4), Beaver ear blade
4. Lumbar drain
5. General anesthesia

Tips and Pearls

1. Precise localization of the CSF leak is critical to success; a Valsalva maneuver may be helpful.
2. Provide a generous flap pedicle to prevent dislodgment, tenting, bridging, or tension.
3. Extubate patients deeply to avoid coughing.

Pitfalls and Complications

1. Inability to reach or adequately cover the defect with the pedicled flap
2. Flap failure with persistent CSF leak
3. Intracranial infection

Postoperative Care Issues

1. Control of intracranial pressure
2. Nasal sponges are removed on postoperative day 3 to 5.
3. Gradual endoscopic debridement of dissolvable packing over 4 weeks

References

Mattox DE, Kennedy DW. Endoscopic management of cerebrospinal fluid leaks and cephaloceles. Laryngoscope 1990;100:857.

Papay FA, Maggiano H, Dominquez S, Hassenbuxch SJ, Levine HL, Lavertu P. Rigid endoscopic repair of paranasal sinus cerebrospinal fluid fistulas. Laryngoscope 1989;99:1195.

Yessenow RS, McCabe BF. The osteo-mucoperiosteal flap in repair of cerebrospinal fluid rhinorrhea: a 20 year experience. Otolaryngol Head Neck Surg 1989;101:555.

Middle Turbinate Mucoperiosteal Flap

Defects lateral to the middle turbinate in the ethmoid roof can be effectively managed with a middle turbinate flap (Fig. 325-4*A*). The mucosa along the root of the turbinate adjacent to the defect is incised with a disposable sickle knife in a posterior to anterior direction. Care is used to prevent injury to the lateral lamella of the cribriform plate with this maneuver. An elevator is then used to develop a lateral mucoperiosteal flap, using the bone of the middle turbinate in the medial portion of the flap to reinforce the closure (Fig. 325-4*B*). To cover the defect, the root of the middle turbinate is mobilized by gently fracturing it laterally and superiorly. Typically, this necessitates a posterior vertical incision in the turbinate mucosa and bone to free the anterior portion of the middle turbinate (Fig. 325-4*C*).

Nasal Septal Mucoperiosteal Flap

Defects of the cribriform plate medial to the middle turbinate, portions of the ethmoid roof, or the sphenoid sinus may not be easily reached with a middle turbinate flap. In these situations, an anteriorly or posteriorly based flap can be fashioned from the mucoperiosteum of the nasal septum. For cribriform defects, some surgeons have used superiorly based septal flaps of contralateral mucoperiosteum and bone after removal of the mucoperiosteum of the ipsilateral septum. Posteriorly based flaps are more versatile and have the ability to reach all three areas described if designed appropriately (Fig. 325-5*A*).

A 1% solution of lidocaine with a 1:100,000 concentration of epinephrine is injected in a subperiosteal plane beneath the flap donor site. The flap is designed to rotate onto and lay easily across the defect without tension. Additional width and length is given to the flap to allow for postoperative contraction. A disposable sickle knife is used to make two parallel incisions from posterior to anterior through mucoperiosteum and down to bone. The anterior portion of the flap is then incised vertically with a Beaver ear blade. The mucoperiosteum is elevated from anterior to posterior with a Cottle elevator, taking care to prevent unnecessary suction on or trauma to the flap.

Defect Repair

The turbinate or septal flap is rotated over the defect and tucked under the previously elevated mucosa surrounding the defect (Fig. 325-5*B*). Care is taken to prevent any tension on the flap that can cause tenting across the defect. Allowances are also made for postoperative contracture of the flap, which causes it to pull away from the bone. The flap is secured in place using microfibrillar collagen (Avitene), Gelfoam coated in antibiotic ointment, and a Merocel sponge.

DONALD C. LANZA
ANDREW N. GOLDBERG

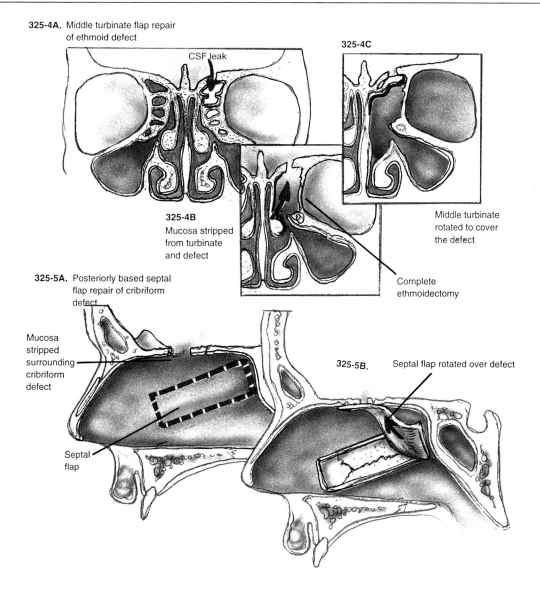

325-4A. Middle turbinate flap repair of ethmoid defect

CSF leak

325-4C

325-4B
Mucosa stripped from turbinate and defect

Middle turbinate rotated to cover the defect

Complete ethmoidectomy

325-5A. Posteriorly based septal flap repair of cribriform defect

Mucosa stripped surrounding cribriform defect

325-5B. Septal flap rotated over defect

Septal flap

■ *326.* SEPTAL DERMOPLASTY

Surgical removal of the mucous membranes of the nasal septum and turbinates and covering the denuded surfaces with split-thickness skin grafts or dermal grafts

Indications

1. Treatment of repeated epistaxis secondary to hereditary hemorrhagic telangiectasia (eg, Osler-Weber-Rendu disease).
2. Other nasal disorders (eg, CREST syndrome) that cause diffuse bleeding may also be an indication.
3. Diagnosis of hereditary hemorrhagic telangiectasia based on the "classic triad" of telangiectasia, recurrent epistaxis, and a family history of the disorder

Special Considerations

1. Anemia due to hemorrhage
2. Associated vascular abnormalities, such as pulmonary arteriovenous (AV) fistulas, central nervous system telangiectases, AV malformations, aneurysms, hepatic fibrotic AV malformations, aneurysms, systemic AV shunts, hepatic artery–portal vein shunts, intrahepatic portosystemic shunts, and retinal telangiectases
3. The viability of quadrangular cartilage should be assessed before removing the mucous membrane from both sides.

Preoperative Preparation

1. Routine laboratory studies
2. Coagulation screens and bleeding time (usually normal)

Special Instruments, Position, and Anesthesia

1. Headlight
2. Supine position, with the head elevated
3. General oral endotracheal anesthesia; local anesthesia is acceptable.
4. Dermatome

Tips and Pearls

1. Bleeding is controlled by the application of thrombin spray solution to the nasal cavity and the split-thickness skin graft (STSG) donor site.
2. Rolled Silastic splints provide protection to the STSG and a patent nasal conduit after removal of nasal packing.
3. The STSG may decrease recurrent epistaxis more than a dermal graft.
4. Exposure may be facilitated by a lateral alotomy incision.

Pitfalls and Complications

1. Excessive bleeding during the operation (ie, poor visualization)
2. Septal perforation
3. Nasal obstruction (eg, thick STSG)
4. Failure of the STSG to survive
5. Atrophic rhinitis and crusting
6. Recurrence of telangiectatic lesions
7. Postoperative infection and toxic shock syndrome

Postoperative Care Issues

1. Packing left in place for 7 to 10 days
2. Silastic splints left in place for 4 to 6 weeks
3. Nasal saline sprays used to decrease crusting
4. Necrotic areas of the skin graft that overlie nondenuded areas may be debrided gently.
5. Long-term nasal hygiene often includes debridement by the physician.
6. Indefinite follow-up to screen for recurrence

References

Goldsmith MM, Fry TL. Tips on septal dermoplasty. Laryngoscope 1987;97:994.

Lore JM. An atlas of head and neck surgery. Philadelphia: WB Saunders, 1988:192.

Peery WH. Clinical spectrum of hereditary hemorrhagic telangiectasia. Am J Med 1987;82:989.

Operative Procedure

The patient is brought to the operating suite and placed in the supine position. General anesthesia is administered, and endotracheal intubation with a cuffed endotracheal tube is performed. Local anesthesia is an acceptable alternative. The table is turned 90° away from the anesthesiologist, and the head is elevated and placed on a foam doughnut. Cottonoid pledgets soaked with topical decongestant (4% cocaine or 4% lidocaine with 0.5% phenylephrine) are placed in both sides of the nose. After topical decongestion, a 1% solution of lidocaine with a 1:100,000 concentration of epinephrine is infiltrated under the mucosa of the septum and the lateral sides of the nose.

Exposure with a nasal speculum is usually adequate when used with a headlight designed to allow vision parallel with the light beam. For patients with very small nasal vestibules, a lateral alotomy incision may be used to increase the exposure. Endoscopic examination of the nose before mucous membrane resection can ensure that all areas of diseased mucosa are identified. After the resection, endoscopic examination is impractical because of the significant hemorrhage usually encountered.

A ring curet is used to remove the mucous membrane of the septum and lateral portions of the nose. The mucosa of the inferior and middle meatus is left intact, but the mucosa of the medial portion of the inferior turbinate and floor of the nose is usually removed. Care must be used to preserve the underlying perichondrium and periosteum, because this surface provides the blood supply to the STSG. All mucosa must be removed in the diseased areas to ensure skin graft survival and prevent recurrence. A #15 blade is used to excise the mucosa at the mucocutaneous junction, which provides an anchor point for suturing the graft. Hemostasis is obtained by spraying both nasal cavities copiously with topical thrombin solution.

The STSG is then harvested. A thickness of about 0.012 in (0.3 mm) is usually acceptable. A graft of 9 × 15 cm is large enough to cover the mucosal defect on both sides. We generally use skin from the thigh for the donor site. The donor site is sprayed with topical thrombin and covered with gauze.

The harvested STSG is divided, with each half being placed in the nose in a sleeve-like fashion. The grafts are secured anteriorly to the vestibule with 4-0 absorbable sutures. Silastic sheeting (0.02 thickness) is sterilized, trimmed to approximately 5 × 5 cm, and rolled into a funnel configuration. Antibiotic ointment is generously applied to the Silastic sheeting, which is then gently inserted within the sleeve of the STSG and unrolled with the nasal speculum. The Silastic splints are secured to the nasal vestibule bilaterally with 4-0 nylon sutures. Antibiotic ointment–impregnated nasal packing is then placed within the Silastic splints.

Postoperatively, the nasal packing is left in place for about 10 days, and the splints are left in place for 4 to 6 weeks. The patient should be placed on a regimen of prophylactic antibiotics while foreign bodies are in the nose to prevent staphylococcal infection and possible toxic shock syndrome. Debridement of necrotic areas of the STSG must be done gently to prevent disrupting the graft. The patient is instructed on nasal hygiene, including daily irrigation with saline solution and periodic debridement by the physician. Follow-up assessment must be done at regular intervals to screen for recurrence of telangiectases.

HAROLD C. PILLSBURY III
JEFFREY L. WILSON

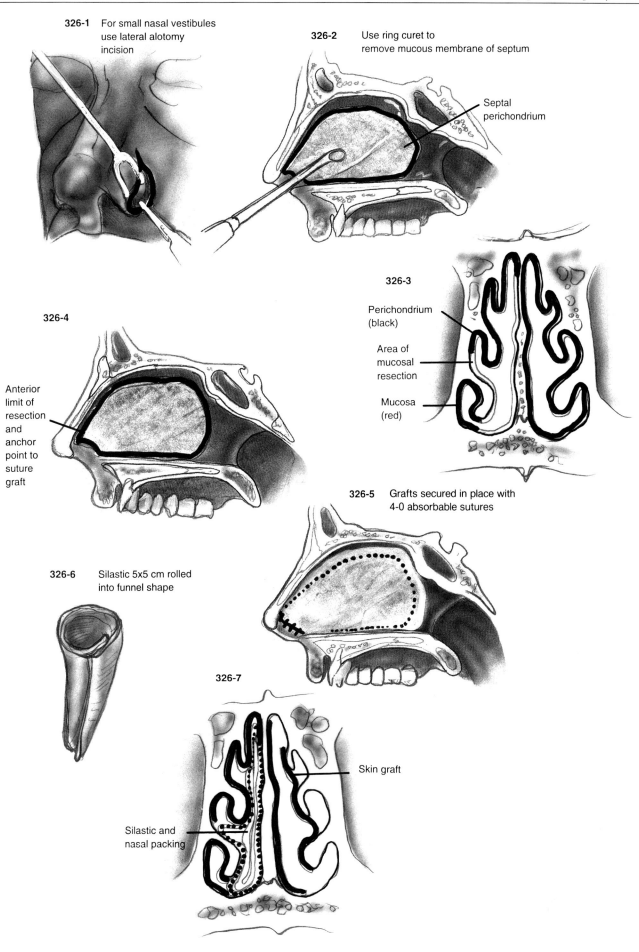

326-1 For small nasal vestibules use lateral alotomy incision

326-2 Use ring curet to remove mucous membrane of septum

Septal perichondrium

326-3

Perichondrium (black)

Area of mucosal resection

Mucosa (red)

326-4

Anterior limit of resection and anchor point to suture graft

326-5 Grafts secured in place with 4-0 absorbable sutures

326-6 Silastic 5x5 cm rolled into funnel shape

326-7

Skin graft

Silastic and nasal packing

■ 327. REPAIR OF SEPTAL PERFORATION

Repair of septal perforations to prevent excessive nasal crusting, nasal bleeding, and nasal whistling while maintaining adequate nasal airflow

Indications

1. Symptomatic perforations 1.5 cm or larger in diameter and usually located anteriorly
2. Symptoms include whistling, excessive crusting, recurrent bleeding, and excessive dryness of the nasal cavity.

Special Considerations

1. The cause of perforation must be identified.
2. Contraindications to surgical repair include collagen vascular disorders (eg, Wegener's granulomatosis, lupus erythematosus, polyarteritis nodosa, scleroderma) and habitual drug abuse.

Preoperative Preparation

1. Routine laboratory studies (eg, complete blood count, coagulation studies, chest radiograph if symptomatic or older than 35 years of age)
2. Biopsy or culture of perforated edges if a neoplasm or infection is suspected.
3. Careful screening for habitual drug abuse.

Special Instruments, Position, and Anesthesia

1. Routine nasal instruments and a Storz headlight
2. Surgeon's preference for local (1% lidocaine with 1:100,000 epinephrine) or general anesthesia
3. Topical anesthesia and decongestion is best achieved with a cotton pledget soaked with a 4% cocaine solution.
4. Semi-Fowler position

Tips and Pearls

1. The cause of the perforation must be identified to ensure the best chance of survival rate for the graft.
2. The septum should have minimal deviation to facilitate exposure and closure of flaps.
3. Closure of flaps on at least one side is ideal
4. Autogenous fascial or cartilaginous grafts are highly suitable.
5. Splints should be left in place until healing of the septal flap has been observed.
6. Decongestion of the turbinates is crucial to allow visualization of the septal structures for repair.

Pitfalls and Complications

1. Epistaxis may occur after either procedures.
2. Crusting around the repair may occur.
3. Postoperative infection requires antibiotics (usually antistaphylococcal) or removal of the button.
4. Ischemia caused by the tightness of the button may make the perforation larger.
5. Poor healing of the mucosal may lead to pain, crusting, and possibly exposed bone or cartilage.

Postoperative Care Issues

1. Systemic antistaphylococcal antibiotics are recommended for approximately 1 week postoperatively.
2. Antibiotic ointment–impregmented nasal packing is removed 24 to 48 hours after surgery, but septal splints are left in place until healing of the flaps is recognized, usually 1 to 3 weeks.
3. Care should be taken to explain to patients to avoid traumatic injury to the repair, as can be caused by nose picking or nasal sneezing.

References

Eviatar A, Myssiorek D. Repair of nasal septal perforations with tragal cartilage and perichondrium grafts. Otolaryngol Head Neck Surg 1989;100:300.

Fairbanks DNF. Closure of nasal septal perforations. Arch Otolaryngol 1980;106:509.

Kridel RWH, Appling D, Wright WK. Septal perforation closure utilizing the external septorhinoplasty approach. Arch Otolaryngol Head Neck Surg, 1986;112:168.

Operative Procedure

Repair of septal perforations is based on the size and location of the opening and the ability of the patient to avoid activity that may prevent healing of the repair.

Insertion of a Septal Button

Septal button insertion may be performed in the clinic or the operating room. With the patient in the semi-Fowler position, adequate decongestion is achieved with a cotton pledget soaked with a 4% cocaine solution. A 1% lidocaine solution with a 1:100,000 concentration of epinephrine is injected into the margins of the perforation. Septal buttons are available in one- or two-piece units. In either case, the flanges of the button are trimmed to fit the perforation; usually, a 3- to 5-mm overlap is left around the circumference of the perforation. Insertion of the one-piece button is achieved by compressing one of the flanges and placing a stay suture through this flange to form a rosette (Fig. 327-1A). The suture is then passed through the perforation and then through the compressed flange. The suture is released, allowing the flange to open and cover the perforation. The two-piece button is trimmed to fit the perforation. The male end of the button is inserted through the perforation, and the female end is fastened on the other side of the septum. Hemostats and a nasal speculum are used to hold the pieces for insertion. For the two-piece button, the distance between the flanges is adjustable, depending on how far the male end is pulled through the female portion. The remainder of the male tip is trimmed flush with the female flange (see Fig. 327-1B).

Surgical Closure

Surgical repair of septal perforations may be performed in patients under general anesthesia or using local anesthesia with intravenous sedation.

A hemitransfixion incision is used for the smaller perforations (<2 cm). Larger or more posterior perforations may be approached using the open rhinoplasty incision, which gives better exposure.

Bilateral mucoperichondrial flaps are elevated from the septum back to the perforation. These flaps are carried inferiorly to the maxillary crest, and subperiosteal flaps are elevated on the floor of the nose. These inferior floor flaps are elevated laterally up to the inferior meatus, just beneath the inferior turbinates bilaterally. The flaps are then taken posteriorly the entire length of the turbinate and, if needed, the length of the palate. Superiorly on the septum, the mucoperichondrial flaps are elevated to the nasal dorsum. These septal flaps are then taken posteriorly to the bony cartilaginous junction, where the flap extends as a subperiosteal flap along the perpendicular plate of the ethmoid. The posterior segment is carried to the anterior wall of the sphenoid sinus. Significant septal deviation is repaired at this time. Relaxing incisions are then made superiorly along the nasal dorsum and laterally just beneath the inferior turbinate to release the bipedicled flaps. These flaps are pedicled anteriorly and posteriorly (Fig. 327-2).

A graft is then designed and harvested to fit the perforation. I prefer a conchal cartilage graft. After injection of local anesthesia beneath the periosteum and into the conchal cartilage, a postauricular incision is made. With the size of the perforation predetermined, the conchal cartilage is harvested. A postauricular subperiosteal flap is elevated over the mastoid to match the size of the cartilage graft. This periosteum is left attached to the graft, because it is contiguous with the perichondrium on the graft. The anterior perichondrial surface is left in situ and is not harvested. The harvested graft is composed of cartilage exposed on one side and covered with perichondrium attached to periosteum on the other. The periosteal flap is then wrapped around the exposed side of the cartilage and sutured to the perichondrium, thus surrounding the free cartilage graft (Fig. 327-3). The graft is placed within the septal pocket, and the previously created flaps are closed using permanent sutures (Fig. 327-4).

Bilateral closure is ideal, but for large perforations, unilateral closure may have to suffice; at least one mucosal flap must be closed to facilitate healing.

HAROLD C. PILLSBURY III
CHAPMAN T. MCQUEEN

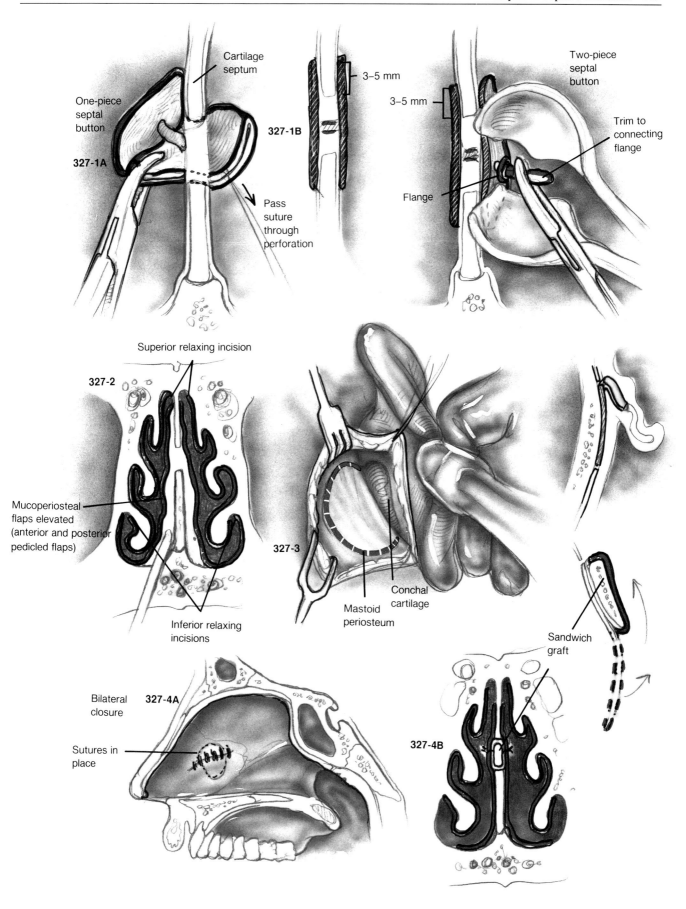

Cartilage septum

One-piece septal button

327-1A

Pass suture through perforation

327-1B

3–5 mm

Two-piece septal button

3–5 mm

Trim to connecting flange

Flange

Superior relaxing incision

327-2

Mucoperiosteal flaps elevated (anterior and posterior pedicled flaps)

Inferior relaxing incisions

327-3

Mastoid periosteum

Conchal cartilage

Bilateral closure   327-4A

Sutures in place

Sandwich graft

327-4B

■ *328.* SEPTAL RESECTION FOR BENIGN AND MALIGNANT NEOPLASIA— Surgical resection of a tumor-involved nasal septum

Indications
1. Documentation of malignancy

Contraindications
1. Extensive involvement of surrounding tissues, rendering resection impossible
2. Cranial nerve involvement or intracranial metastasis

Special Considerations
1. The mucocutaneous junction is the site of predilection for tumor occurrence.
2. Vestibular carcinomas are preponderantly squamous cell carcinomas.
3. The extent of malignancy beyond the superficial lesion, especially in the nasolabial fold, should be explored.
4. Prophylactic neck dissection is not warranted.
5. Detailed counseling regarding the postoperative defect

Preoperative Preparation
1. Routine laboratory studies, including coagulation assessment
2. Computed tomography scan to assess the extent of involvement

Special Instruments, Position, and Anesthesia
1. Headlight
2. Head stabilized in foam doughnut
3. Anatomic landmarks should be included in the field to assist in reconstruction.
4. Drape appropriately to include the specified donor site, if necessary.

Tips and Pearls
1. Microscopic examination of the surgical specimen
2. A larger resection site than initially expected may be required.
3. The advantage of early resection should not be lost in attempts to avoid disfigurement.
4. Prognosis is inversely proportional to the size of the tumor.

Pitfalls and Complications
1. Prolonged healing time is common.
2. Partial or complete loss of the graft
3. Saddling of the bridge of the nose
4. Unacceptable cosmetic result

Postoperative Care Issues
1. Perioperative antibiotics are indicated, especially when nasal packs are used.
2. Nasal dressing should be left in place for at least 1 week.
3. Elevate head of bed to 45°
4. Application of cold compresses over the nose and eyes in the immediate postoperative period
5. Follow-up examinations should be performed every 4 months.
6. Postoperative irradiation for control of disease at the primary site and the neck may be necessary for specific histopathology.

References
Batsakis JG. Tumors of the head and neck—clinical and pathological considerations, 2nd ed. Baltimore: Williams & Wilkins, 1979.

Deutsch HJ. Carcinoma of the nasal septum. Report of a case and review of the literature. Ann Otol 1966;75:1049.

Dickson RI, Flores AD. Nasopharyngeal carcinoma: an evaluation of 134 patients treated between 1971–1980. Laryngoscope 1985;95:276.

Lyons GD. Squamous cell carcinoma of the nasal septum. Arch Otol 1969;89:47.

Operative Procedure
Lateral Rhinotomy Approach to Septal Resection

After the patient is placed in the supine position, general anesthesia is initiated by means of endotracheal intubation. A solution of Xylocaine with a 1:100,000 concentration of epinephrine is infiltrated along the planned line of incision. Some surgeons suggest using a surgical marking pen or methylene blue to mark the line of incision. The face is prepped with povidone-iodine solution, and the drapes are placed in the standard fashion. Care should be taken to keep the eyes and upper lip within the surgical field. If the use of a graft or facial flap is indicated, care must be taken in positioning the head of the patient and in planning the extent of the surgical field. A tarsorrhaphy suture is placed for eye protection.

The incision begins just superior to the medial canthus, approximately midway between the canthus and the dorsum of the nose. The incision is extended along the deepest aspect of the nasofacial sulcus to the alar crease (Fig. 328-1). The lateral nasal and angular vessels should be identified and ligated. Following the contour of the nasal base, the incision extends into the floor of the nose. The ala nasi is mobilized and retracted upward and medially (Fig. 328-2). If exposure of the anterior septum is all that is required, only the inferior portion of the incision is made.

Additional exposure, if necessary, may be gained posteriorly by transecting the base of the nasal process of the maxilla and its superior attachment parallel to the nasal bone suture line. For more anterior lesions, the columella may be transected at its base. However, this latter technique may result in disruption of the nasal vestibule and should be reserved for specific needs.

With an electrocautery knife, the septal lesion is widely resected through and through (Fig. 328-3). Starting anteriorly, the incision is extended around the septal angle and upward along the dorsum of the nose. If margins permit, a strut of cartilage should be preserved along the bridge of the nose for support. If this is not possible, a bone graft is used to maintain structure for the dorsum to prevent a saddle nose deformity. The resection is continued posteriorly and inferiorly to the floor of the nose. Depending on the extent of the lesion, portions of the perpendicular plate of the ethmoid and the vomer may need to be included in the specimen. The resection is completed by using an osteotome to transect the crest of the maxilla (Fig. 328-4).

It is imperative to rely on the gross appearance and on frozen sections to ensure adequate margins of resection. If there is extension of tumor along the floor of the nose, which is the area most commonly involved, the central portion of the maxilla should be excised as well.

Reconstruction of the septum depends on the resultant defect. A small septal fistula usually causes little morbidity and therefore may be left unrepaired. Larger but superficial lesions may be resected to include perichondrium, sparing septal cartilage. These defects are treated with split- or full-thickness skin grafts, or they may be left to heal secondarily. If a significant portion of cartilage is removed, a full-thickness skin graft is employed to correct the defect (Fig. 328-5). The graft is sutured anteriorly to the vestibular skin and remaining portion of the columella. Supporting sutures may be applied around the circumference of the septal graft, but most support is derived from the packing. An anterior cartilage graft inserted into the columella may also be necessary to prevent saddling or ptosis of the tip.

Finger cots filled with petroleum gauze are then placed into each side, and the initial skin incision is approximated using a two-layer closure (Fig. 328-6). A light dressing is applied.

HAROLD C. PILLSBURY III
THOMAS C. LOGAN

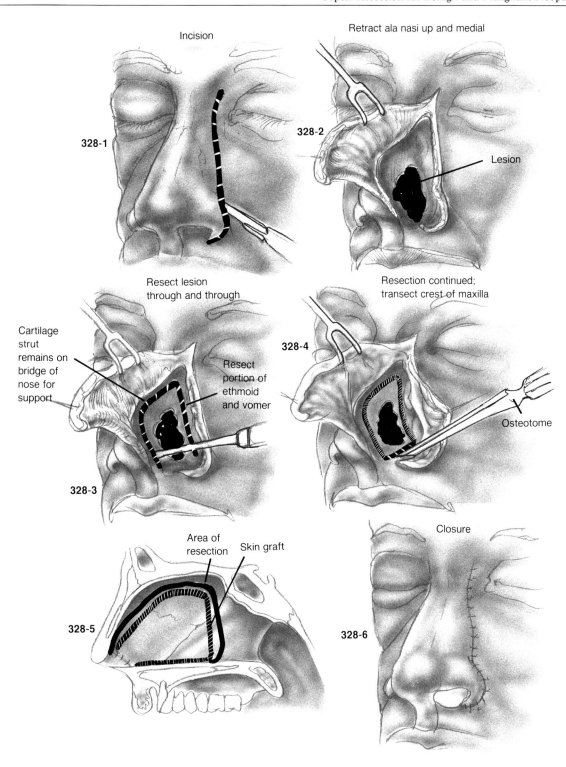

Incision

328-1

Retract ala nasi up and medial

328-2

Lesion

Resect lesion
through and through

Cartilage
strut
remains on
bridge of
nose for
support

Resect
portion of
ethmoid
and vomer

328-3

Resection continued;
transect crest of maxilla

328-4

Osteotome

Area of
resection   Skin graft

328-5

Closure

328-6

■ *329.* NASAL CAVITY EXAMINATION WITH NASAL BIOPSY OR FOREIGN BODY REMOVAL—Examination of the nasal cavity with surgical biopsy of tissue or removal of a foreign body

Indications
1. Presence of mass with or without nasal obstruction
2. Suspected malignancy
3. Suspicion of chronic infection, especially fungal infection in immune compromised patient
4. Evaluation of ciliary dyskinesia
5. Suspected or known foreign body

Special Considerations
1. Bleeding or clotting abnormalities
2. Local anesthesia for an adult patient, but may require general anesthesia for a small child
3. If considering congenital anomalies (eg, glioma, encephalocele), a computed tomography (CT) scan should be obtained before biopsy.

Preoperative Preparation
1. Routine laboratory studies
2. Bleeding and clotting studies
3. CT scan of the nasal cavity and paranasal sinuses, with axial and coronal views
4. Immunoglobulin evaluation, including IgG subclasses if an immunodeficiency is suspected

Special Instruments, Position, and Anesthesia
1. Headlight, nasal speculum, otoscope with large speculum, and nasal endoscopes (0, 30°, 70°)
2. Bronchoscopy brush
3. Flexible fiberoptic nasopharyngoscope
4. Nasal cup forceps
5. If local anesthesia is planned, have 2% Pontocaine, 0.25% and 0.5% Neo-Synephrine, a spray bottle, and cotton pledgets on hand.
6. Cotton-tip applicators, silver nitrate sticks, and nasal suction tips
7. For general anesthesia, preoperative planning with the anesthesiologist about the type of anesthesia and intubation techniques (usually oral)

Tips and Pearls
1. Careful preoperative determination and location of area for biopsy
2. Preoperative planning with the pathologist about the specimen fixative and the amount of tissue needed
3. Careful hemostasis at completion
4. Differential diagnosis of the nasal foreign body includes unilateral sinusitis and unilateral choanal stenosis or atresia.

Pitfalls and Complications
1. Bleeding from the biopsy site may compromise the view and airway.
2. The foreign body may be dislodged posteriorly and swallowed or aspirated if the procedure is done in an awake patient.
3. Intracranial extension of the nasal mass may lead to a cerebrospinal fluid leak.
4. A vascular lesion may produce brisk bleeding.
5. A second foreign body may be overlooked if it is posterior to or on the opposite side from the first.

Postoperative Care
1. Avoid packing if possible, especially in a child
2. Adequate postoperative hemostasis before discharge
3. Counsel the child and parent if the procedure was for foreign body removal to prevent a recurrence.

References
Potsic WP, Wetmore RF. Pediatric rhinology. In: Goldman JL, ed. The principles and practice of rhinology. New York: John Wiley & Sons, 1987:801.

Wood R, Jafek B, Eberhard R. Nasal obstruction. In: Bailey BJ, ed. Head and neck surgery—otolaryngology. Philadelphia: JB Lippincott, 1993: 302.

Operative Procedure

Depending on the circumstance and the age of the patient, several approaches may be employed to examine the nasal cavity (Figs. 329-1 through 329-3). For topical anesthesia, the patient is positioned sitting in an examination chair with the head resting comfortably against the head rest. The nasal cavity is inspected with a headlight and nasal speculum (see Fig. 329-1). Secretions are removed with a metal-tip suction device, carefully avoiding trauma to the nasal mucosa. Two percent Pontocaine spray is used to anesthetize the area. A cotton pledget with string attached is then soaked with 2% Pontocaine and Afrin solution and placed against the area to be biopsied. After 5 minutes, the pack is removed and the area inspected again, checking the adequacy of topical anesthesia.

The site of biopsy is carefully inspected, and a 0° rigid telescope is used to magnify and examine the area (Fig. 329-4). Using a nasal cup biopsy forceps, the lesion is biopsied, and pressure is held against the biopsy site with Afrin-moistened cotton gauze. If continuous oozing occurs, this area may be packed lightly with Gelfoam, or silver nitrate can be used to cauterize the base of the biopsy site. Careful examination of the rest of the nose and the opposite side is done to rule out a second lesion.

For foreign body removal, the preparation of the area is the same as for a biopsy. The foreign body is grasped with a nasal cup forceps, alligator forceps, or bayonet forceps (Fig. 329-5*A*). A cerumen loop or blunt, curved mastoid seeker may be used to roll a round foreign body from posterior to anterior locations (see Fig. 329-5*B*). For a foreign body of long duration, granulation tissue surrounding it may produce bleeding at this point. The foreign body is carefully delivered anteriorly and removed from the nose. Vegetable foreign bodies such as seeds or beans may fragment and be removed in fragments. Nonvegetable matter such as coins or small parts of toys are usually removed intact, and care should exercised to avoid laceration or further trauma to the nose from sharp edges. A common foreign body in the young child is sponge rubber from a seat cushion. This produces a lot of strong odor and copious secretion because of secondary infection and retention of the infectious material in the sponge rubber. Chronic foreign bodies may be encrusted and form hard, calcareous bodies. These rhinoliths usually are found along the nasal floor or between the inferior turbinate and in the septum. Careful removal is carried out to avoid posterior displacement of the foreign body into the nasopharynx.

An anterior nasal foreign body may be successfully removed in a young child with careful restraint in the parent's arms, with the parent sitting in a chair, or with the use of a papoose board while lying on the examination table. A nasal speculum and headlight may be used for this, but in a cooperative small child, the use of an otoscope or microscope with aural speculum may be better tolerated (see Figs. 329-2 and 329-3).

If the patient is awake, aspiration and or swallowing of the foreign body is a potential hazard. Because of this possibility and the typical uncooperative nature of the small child, general anesthesia is frequently required. After removal of the foreign body, the area is carefully suctioned to look for a second foreign body, and the other nasal cavity examined carefully for a potential foreign body.

For nasal ciliary biopsy, this technique may be carried out in the examination room in a cooperative child with good restraint and optimal lighting, as provided by a large otoscope speculum. A bronchial brush is used gently to brush the inferior turbinate midway back (Fig. 329-6). The thumb hole of the proximal end of the bronchial brush is worked forward and backward, causing the bronchoscopy brush to rotate on its axis and essentially peel off a superficial mucosal membrane lining for electron microscopy study of cilia. Two brushes are used for two specimens, and the tip of the brush is clipped off with scissors and dropped into the specimen jar before transport to the laboratory. One specimen is sent in glutaraldehyde for electron microscopic studies, and the second specimen is sent dry for evaluation of ciliary motility. This procedure is tolerated well in the office setting for children older than 5 years of age after careful preoperative counselling, but it may be carried out with the patient under general anesthesia in the operating room.

RONALD W. DESKIN

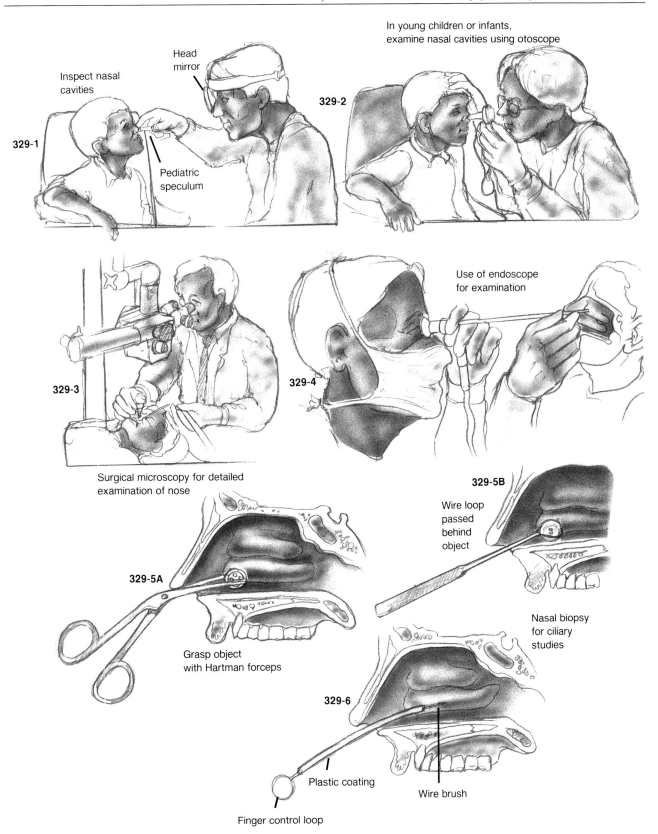

In young children or infants,
examine nasal cavities using otoscope

329-2

Inspect nasal
cavities

Head
mirror

329-1

Pediatric
speculum

329-3

Surgical microscopy for detailed
examination of nose

Use of endoscope
for examination

329-4

329-5B

Wire loop
passed
behind
object

329-5A

Grasp object
with Hartman forceps

Nasal biopsy
for ciliary
studies

329-6

Plastic coating

Wire brush

Finger control loop

■ *330.* SUBMUCOUS RESECTION OF THE TURBINATE—Surgical removal of the anterior two thirds of the inferior turbinate by a submucous approach

Indications

1. Unilateral or bilateral nasal obstruction due to enlargement of the inferior turbinate that does not respond to medical therapy or simpler surgical procedures

Special Considerations

1. Careful evaluation of the septum and nasal skeleton for their role in producing the obstruction
2. Control of allergy
3. Maximum trial of medical therapy before contemplating surgery

Preoperative Preparation

1. Routine laboratory studies
2. Rhinomanometry, if possible
3. Bleeding and clotting studies, if the history is questionable

Special Instruments, Position, and Anesthesia

1. Headlight
2. Supine position, with the head elevated 30°
3. Narrow Vienna speculum
4. Cottle elevator
5. Local or general anesthesia

Tips and Pearls

1. Maximal mucosal preservation
2. Minimal incision
3. Protect nasolacrimal duct opening
4. Preserve the posterior third of the turbinate

Pitfalls and Complications

1. Posterior bleeding
2. Inadequate resection
3. Persistent or recurrent obstruction
4. Synechia if the septal mucosa and turbinate mucosa are abraded

Postoperative Care Issues

1. Counsel the patient about postoperative expectations.
2. Cautious removal of crusts

References

House HP. Submucous resection of the inferior turbinal bone. Laryngoscope 1951;61:637.

Mabry RL. Inferior turbinoplasty. Laryngoscope 1982;92:459.

Operative Procedure

With the patient in the supine position and the head elevated 30°, the face is prepped and draped. In most instances, I prefer to begin anesthetizing the nasal cavity before scrubbing and gowning. Local anesthesia is preferred over general anesthesia, but in either case, great care must be taken to achieve maximal vasoconstriction. The nasal cavity is sprayed with a 1% solution of phenylephrine. Topical anesthetic (up to 4 mL of 5% cocaine) is applied to 0.5-in (12-mm) plain cotton gauze or to cotton balls and used to anesthetize the sphenopalatine ganglion region at the posterior end of the middle turbinate, the anterior ethmoid nerve region superiorly, and the area in which the nasopalatine nerve comes into the floor of the nose through the incisive foramen (Fig. 330-1). After the cotton pledgets or gauze are removed and the anesthesiologist administers a short-acting barbiturate, the injections of a 1% solution of Xylocaine with a 1:100,000 concentration of epinephrine are used to complete the anesthesia induction. After waiting 10 minutes for optimal levels of anesthesia and vasoconstriction to be achieved, the nose is reinspected.

An incision along the undersurface of the turbinate is made with a Bard-Parker #12 blade, moving the knife from posterior to anterior (Fig. 330-2). The incision goes through mucosa and stroma, down to the conchal bone. To reduce postoperative crusting, the incision should be only long enough to permit sufficient elevation of the mucosa and allow removal of the anterior two thirds of the turbinate bone. I prefer to limit the incision to the undersurface of the anterior third and the anterior face of the turbinate.

Using a sharp, pointed dissecting scissors and Cottle elevator, the mucoperiosteum is elevated from the medial, lateral, and inferior surfaces of the turbinate (Fig. 330-3). If the mucoperiosteum is very adherent, a #15 Bard-Parker blade can facilitate dissection. The upper surface of the blade acts as a microelevator when the blade is inserted beneath the periosteum, and the lower cutting edge of the blade separates periosteal attachments to the bone. If necessary, the turbinate can be fractured and displaced medially; however, fracturing the turbinate before adequate mucoperiosteal elevation makes this task more difficult.

The anterior two thirds of the turbinate is removed with the Jansen-Middleton rongeur or Takahashi forceps inserted beneath the mucoperiosteal flaps (Fig. 330-4). It is important to keep the flaps as intact as possible to facilitate healing and reduce crusting. It is also important to preserve the posterior one third of the turbinate to protect the vessels in this region. Some surgeons prefer to elevate mucosa from the entire turbinate, including the posterior aspect, and to resect the entire turbinate by inserting a polyp snare beneath the flaps and encircling the turbinate.

The disposable suction-cautery is used to electrocoagulate the raw surface of the remaining turbinate, which is frequently a source of bleeding. The remaining flaps of mucosa are reapproximated to each other and packed in place (Fig. 330-5). Although suturing the flaps together with absorbable sutures has been described, I have found it difficult, traumatic, and unnecessary. Telfa gauze covered with Bacitracin ointment is inserted along the medial and lateral surfaces of the turbinate and left in place for 24 to 48 hours (Fig. 330-6). When the packing is removed, the nose is sprayed with a 1% solution of phenylephrine, and any accumulated blood is removed. Subsequently, use of dilute phenylephrine solution or normal saline spray is encouraged to liquefy accumulated debris. Active removal of crusts is avoided to reduce the likelihood of bleeding. The crusts usually extrude spontaneously within 1 week.

FRANK E. LUCENTE

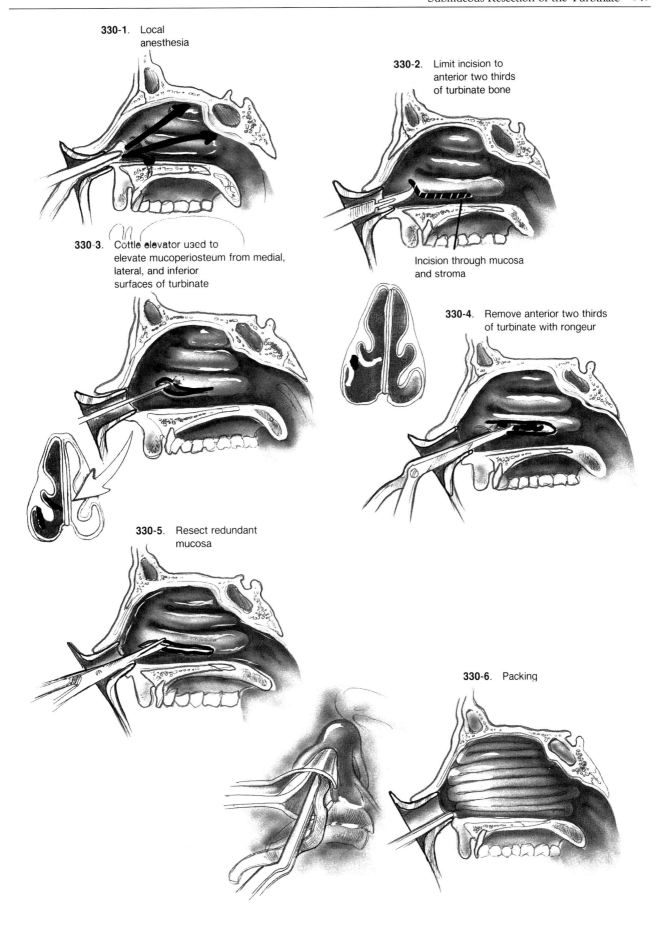

330-1. Local anesthesia

330-2. Limit incision to anterior two thirds of turbinate bone

Incision through mucosa and stroma

330-3. Cottle elevator used to elevate mucoperiosteum from medial, lateral, and inferior surfaces of turbinate

330-4. Remove anterior two thirds of turbinate with rongeur

330-5. Resect redundant mucosa

330-6. Packing

331. ENDOSCOPIC MANAGEMENT OF NASAL ENCEPHALOCELES AND MENINGOCELES—The endoscopic resection of brain and meninges herniating through the roof of the ethmoid and sphenoid sinuses and the repair of their associated skull base defects

Indications

1. Nasal encephalocele or meningocele
2. The urgency to repair increases when associated with frequent intranasal infections, cerebrospinal fluid (CSF) rhinorrhea, seizures, or intracranial infections
3. Modifications of this technique are used for endoscopic management of CSF rhinorrhea that is not associated with encephaloceles.

Special Considerations

1. Cause of the defect, such as intracranial hypertension, tumor, or trauma
2. Size of the defect, which may or may not require a bony or cartilaginous graft
3. Location of the defect and relation to vital structures
4. Vascular supply; may need angiography
5. Neurologic status
6. Concurrent sinonasal disease
7. Bleeding diathesis

Preoperative Preparation

1. Nasal endoscopy
2. Paranasal sinus coronal and axial computed tomography (CT) scans with 1.5-mm axial cuts
3. Magnetic resonance imaging to assess the extent of the lesion.
4. Magnetic resonance angiography or angiogram to determine vascular supply
5. Preoperative neurosurgical consultation and intraoperative availability

Special Instruments, Position, and Anesthesia

1. Full complement of endoscopic equipment and otologic instruments
2. Landolt bipolar coagulation forceps (eg, Aesculap 4 forceps), Beaver ear blade, 1-mm blunt nose punch (eg, Acufex)
3. General anesthesia is preferred.
4. Lumbar drain

(continued)

Operative Procedure

Identification and Resection of the Encephalocele

Lumbar puncture is performed, an opening pressure obtained, and the lumbar drain sewn into place. Intrathecal fluorescein is slowly infused, using 0.1 mL of 10% fluorescein for intravenous injection mixed with 10 mL of the patient's own CSF. The patient's nose is decongested with a 0.05% solution of oxymetazoline hydrochloride.

General anesthesia is typically selected. A Foley catheter is inserted, and pneumatic compression stockings are applied. The patient is prepped and draped in the usual sterile fashion with Betadine. The patient's head is positioned in a foam doughnut, slightly elevated, and rotated toward the surgeon.

Whether the patient is under general anesthesia or local anesthesia with sedation, the involved side of the nasal cavity is injected with a 1% solution of lidocaine with a 1:100,000 concentration of epinephrine in a fashion similar to that used during endoscopic total sphenoethmoidectomy (see Procedure 322). A transoral greater palatine foramen nerve block is also performed (see Procedure 322).

Wide exposure of the encephalocele and meticulous hemostasis are essential for surgical success. Typically, a complete endoscopic sphenoethmoidectomy is indicated if the lesion is within the sphenoid sinus. However, these lesions may be approached transnasally or transseptally in some patients. If the lesion is located in the roof of the ethmoid complex, an ethmoidectomy may suffice. Occasionally, it may be necessary to resect significant portions of the middle and superior turbinate. Septoplasty or even septal dislocation (in a narrow nose) may be required to ensure adequate access to the encephalocele. Portions of turbinate and septum serve as excellent donor grafts (Fig. 331-1).

After adequate exposure is obtained, encephalocele resection begins. Depending on the position of the encephalocele a 0°, 30°, or 70° endoscope may be used for the resection. If a mucosal capsule covers the lesion, it is incised with a sharp, disposable sickle knife. Fluorescein admixed with the CSF usually drains freely into the nose at this point. The mucosal capsule often bleeds and is gradually cauterized with a Landolt bipolar coagulation forceps. The encephalocele resection is best achieved through gradual fulguration with bipolar cautery (Fig. 331-2). The encephalocele is never grasped and torn as is done for a polyp, although portions of the lesion can be removed in sections after proximal control of its blood supply is obtained with cautery. Giraffe or Weil-Blakesly forceps are used for these maneuvers. Dissection is meticulous and slow to avoid intracranial hemorrhage.

The skull base is exposed for several millimeters around its defect. Two maneuvers are performed to allow any residual encephalocele to recede through the skull base defect. All intranasal connections with encephaloceles are meticulously separated, and 10 to 20 mL of CSF are withdrawn through the lumbar drain. A Rosen knife or similar otologic instrument can be used to lift the dura and encephalocele off the internal surface of the cranial vault.

Harvesting Free Grafts

The contralateral nose is prepared for harvesting two separate free grafts: a mucoperichondrial or mucoperiosteal free graft and a nasal septal bone graft. The contralateral side of the nose is injected with the lidocaine and epinephrine solution 10 minutes before harvesting the free grafts. After the local anesthetic and vasoconstrictor are have taken effect, the anterior and posterior septal donor beds are developed. The anterior donor bed is the source for the mucoperi-

(continued)

331-1. Site of encephalocele in cribriform region

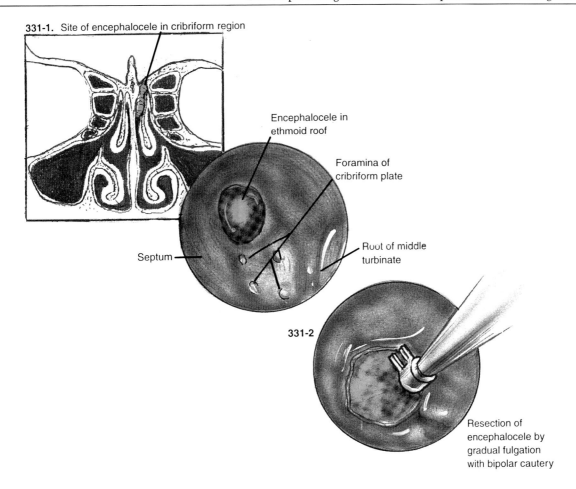

Encephalocele in ethmoid roof

Foramina of cribriform plate

Septum

Root of middle turbinate

331-2

Resection of encephalocele by gradual fulgation with bipolar cautery

■ *331.* ENDOSCOPIC MANAGEMENT OF NA-SAL ENCEPHALOCELES AND MENINGO-CELES *(continued)*

Tips and Pearls

1. Thoroughly identify the skull base defect, and maintain meticulous hemostasis.
2. Completely resect all mucosal attachments to the encephalocele.
3. The encephalocele is resected gradually and meticulously.
4. Soft tissue free grafts retract significantly.
5. If the sphenoid sinus is involved, rule out a carotid artery aneurysm.

Pitfalls and Complications

1. Death
2. Brain abscess or meningitis
3. Intracranial hemorrhage, stroke, or venous thrombosis
4. Pneumocephalus
5. Visual change, such as blindness or diplopia
6. Postoperative nasal crusting
7. Nasal septal perforation or nasal dorsal collapse
8. Donor site wound infection or hematoma

Postoperative Care Issues

1. Control intracranial pressure.
   a. Head of bed elevation of more than 30° for 1 week
   b. Bed rest for 3 to 5 days
   c. Stool softeners for 3 to 5 days
   d. Pain and blood pressure control as needed
   e. Lumbar drain for 2 to 3 days for large defects
   f. No strenuous activity for 4 to 6 weeks postoperatively
2. Postoperative CT scan of the head within 24 hours
3. Antibiotic prophylaxis for nasal packing
4. Nasal sponges are removed on postoperative day 3 to 5.
5. Gradual endoscopic debridement of dissolvable packing is achieved over the next 4 weeks. Debridement of the nasal septal donor site is done gently to avoid perforation.
6. Suture removal at all donor sites

Reference

Mattox DE, Kennedy DW. Endoscopic management of cerebrospinal fluid leaks and cephaloceles. Laryngoscope 1990;100:857.

chondrial or mucoperiosteal free graft. The posterior donor bed is the source for the bone graft (Fig. 331-3).

A rectangular mucoperichondrial or mucoperiosteal free graft from the anterior donor bed is easiest to harvest in the following sequence. First, a posterior, vertical incision is made just proximal to the anterior free border of the middle turbinate. The horizontal long axis of the rectangle is created with superior and inferior cuts that begin posteriorly and are drawn anteriorly. An anterior, vertical incision is the last incision and completes the rectangle. A Cottle elevator is used to elevate the mucoperiosteal free graft from the septum. An Alcon ophthalmic crescent knife or a disposable Beaver ear blade is ideal for the vertical incisions, and a #69 Beaver blade is excellent for the horizontal incisions.

The posterior donor bed is developed through the posterior edge of the anterior donor site. Here, at the posterior edge of the donor site, a Cottle knife is used to incise through the vomer or perpendicular plate of the ethmoid to the side of the nose involved with the encephalocele. A Cottle elevator is used endoscopically to create limited bilateral posterior mucoperiosteal tunnels. Typically, endoscopic scissors or a forward-biting, 1-mm, blunt nose punch (eg, Acufex punch) can be used to remove the bony graft from this posterior donor bed.

A sheet of Gelfilm coated with mupirocin ointment is placed over both donor beds. This protects the sites from crusting and averts localized infection. The exposed portion of the donor site remucosalizes in 3 to 4 weeks. The separation of donor beds minimizes any risk of nasal septal perforation. After harvesting the grafts, the anterior septal donor bed has exposed septal cartilage and bone, but the mucoperichondrium and mucoperiosteum are intact on the side of the encephalocele. The posterior septal donor site has mucoperiosteum juxtaposed to mucoperiosteum without intervening bone (ie, submucous resection).

A temporalis fascia graft or abdominal fat graft is harvested next.

Defect Repair

Typically, the defect is filled in three layers. The intracranial surface is supported by a fat or myofascial graft. Proper placement of this graft can be likened to placement of an underlay graft for tympanoplasty. Next, the bone or cartilage free graft is positioned on the intracranial side of the defect. A mucoperiosteal free graft is then positioned intranasally and extracranially with its mucosal surface facing the nasal cavity (Fig. 331-4). It is essential that this graft conform completely to the recipient bed. If it is tented or stretched across the defect, it is likely to retract away from the recipient bed during healing and lead to postoperatively CSF leakage. Alternatively, a pedicled septal graft can be endoscopically mobilized and positioned (see Procedure 325). Grafts are then held in position by microfibrillar collagen (eg, Avitene). The microfibrillar collagen can be delivered as a paste by mixing it with saline and filling a tuberculin syringe with the material. A 14-gauge Angiocath is positioned on the tuberculin syringe to allow the mixture to be delivered intranasally along side of the telescope.

Multiple layers of Gelfoam admixed with mupirocin ointment are applied. A Kennedy Merocel sponge is then placed within the nose to support the dissolvable packing. The Merocel sponge string is affixed with benzoin and Steri-Strips to the skin of the face. Anesthesia is reversed, and the lumbar drain is left in position. A postoperative CT scan is recommended for baseline assessment after the surgical manipulation and to detect intracranial bleeding or pneumocephalus.

Lateral sphenoid sinus encephaloceles pose a unique challenge, and under certain circumstances, it may be impossible to completely resect them. In this situation, a transseptal or transsphenoidal approach with sphenoidectomy and fat graft obliteration may be preferred. Reconstruction of the sphenoid sinus rostrum with bone helps maintain the fat graft position.

DONALD C. LANZA
DAVID W. KENNEDY

331-3. Region of free graft harvesting

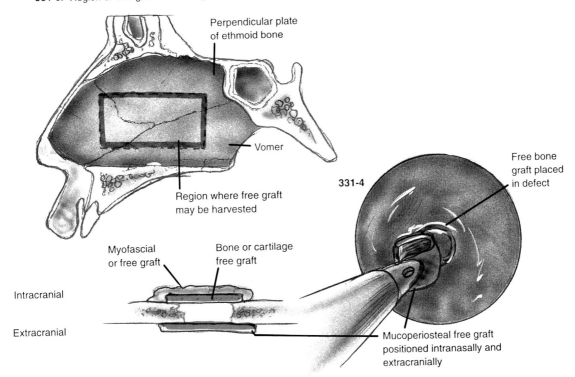

Perpendicular plate
of ethmoid bone

Vomer

Region where free graft
may be harvested

Myofascial
or free graft

Bone or cartilage
free graft

Intracranial

Extracranial

331-4

Free bone
graft placed
in defect

Mucoperiosteal free graft
positioned intranasally and
extracranially

■ *332.* NASAL CONGENITAL DERMOID CYST AND SINUS OPENING—Surgical resection of a skin-lined tract that sometimes extends from the nasal dorsal skin into the septum, occasionally to the dura, and rarely to the cerebral ventricles

Indications

1. The presence of a pit, fistula tract, or mass on the nasal dorsum causing cosmetic deformity
2. Infection of the lesion
3. Before expansion of the cyst causes permanent nasal deformity (before patient is 2 or 3 years of age).

Special Considerations

1. Need to establish whether there is intracranial involvement, for which computed tomography (CT) is useful, but MRI in the sagittal plane is better
2. Differentiate from glioma and encephalocele
3. If there is intracranial extension, a craniotomy is done first, followed by simultaneous or later removal of the extracranial portion.
4. It is best to operate when the cyst in not infected; it may need an initial incision and drainage before definitive removal.

Preoperative Preparation

1. Routine laboratory studies
2. Bleeding and clotting studies, if the history is questionable
3. Neurosurgical consultation in case of an unexpected intracranial extension
4. Perioperative antibiotics

Special Instruments, Position, and Anesthesia

1. Headlight
2. Loupes or surgical microscope
3. Rhinoplasty set
4. Otologic elevators (eg, Rosen, McCabe)
5. The patient's head slightly extended, with head of bed slightly elevated
6. A solution of 1% lidocaine with a 1:100,000 concentration of epinephrine for local anesthesia and vasoconstriction

Tips and Pearls

1. Most dermoids are extracranial and can be safely approached in a one-stage nasal procedure.
2. The surgeon must have adequate exposure of the nasal dorsum and continue deep to the nasal bones.
3. Superior to the pit, the dermis is often thinned by pressure from the cyst, and care must be taken not to "button hole" the skin of the dorsum.
4. Examine the specimen's blind end after its removal.
5. Consider frozen sections of the fibrous tract for epithelial elements if there is uncertainty about complete excision.
6. If there is an unsuspected intracranial extension, place a hemoclip at the distal end of sinus tract and include this as part of the intracranial resection.

Pitfalls and Complications

1. Incomplete resection with recurrence of the cyst
2. Unrecognized intracranial extension
3. Postoperative seroma
4. Postoperative infection
5. Transient cerebrospinal fluid leak after intracranial resection
6. Cosmetic nasal deformity

Postoperative Care Issues

1. Continue perioperative antibiotics for 7 to 10 days after intracranial resection.
2. Remove sutures on the fourth or fifth postoperative day.

References

Koltai PJ, Hoehn J, Bailey CM. The external rhinoplasty approach for rhinologic surgery in children. Arch Otolaryngol Head Neck Surg 1992;118:401.

Smith JD. Congenital anomalies of the nose and nasopharynx. In: Smith J, Bumstead R, eds. Pediatric facial plastic and reconstructive surgery. New York: Raven Press, 1993:13.

Operative Procedure

After orotracheal intubation, the child is positioned with the head slightly extended and the head of the table slightly elevated. The child is prepped and draped for a rhinologic procedure, which includes infiltration of the nose with a solution of 1% Xylocaine with a 1:100,000 concentration of epinephrine.

The traditional approach for exposing a dermoid cyst has been the vertical midline incision along the nasal dorsum (Fig. 332-1), but my preference for the approach for these lesions is a combination of the external rhinoplasty incision with a lateral rhinotomy (Fig. 332-2). A standard external rhinoplasty incision employing the inverted-V pattern on the columella is made, and the "elephant trunk" columella flap is raised onto the dome of the nose. The rim incision on one side is then extended into a lateral rhinotomy incision around the alar base. This is followed by careful elevation of the skin of the nasal dorsum, because it is vital to identify the tract from the punctum of the dermoid and excise it from below, flush with the skin (Fig. 332-3). If any of the tract is left behind, secondary infection will ensue, with the development of a discharging sinus. After the tract has been identified, for which middle ear dissectors such as Rosen and McCabe are useful, the skin elevation is completed. The tract is carefully preserved and usually is found to lead to a dip in the midline between the upper lateral cartilages, just under the caudal edge of the nasal bones (Fig. 332-4). The cyst extends into the nasal septum, deep to the nasal bone.

Using a 4-mm chisel, medial osteotomies are performed under direct vision, and the nasal bones are greenstick fractured laterally. The out fracture of the nasal bones gives a clear view of the cyst as it extends up toward the cribriform plate (Fig. 332-5). If the tract extends to the skull base, the surgical microscope and a small otologic drill can be useful in following the tract to its depth. If there is suspicion that the tract goes intracranially, it is amputated at the foramen cecum, and a hemoclip is placed across the proximal portion. The terminal end of the stalk is sent for frozen section to determine if any epithelial elements remain. If so, neurosurgical colleagues are notified, and a decision is made whether to perform an immediate craniotomy or do this as a secondary procedure.

After the cyst is removed, the nasal bones are replaced, the skin is redraped, and the columella and lateral rhinotomy incision are closed with interrupted 6.0 nylon sutures. The closure of the rim incision can be difficult in small children, but it can usually be tacked into position with one or two stitches of 5.0 chromic suture on each side of the nose. The nose is packed with Telfa splints for 24 hours, and the outside of the nose is dressed with Steri-Strips and an Aquaplast thermoplastic external splint. The sutures and the dressing are removed in 5 postoperative days in the office.

PETER J. KOLTAI

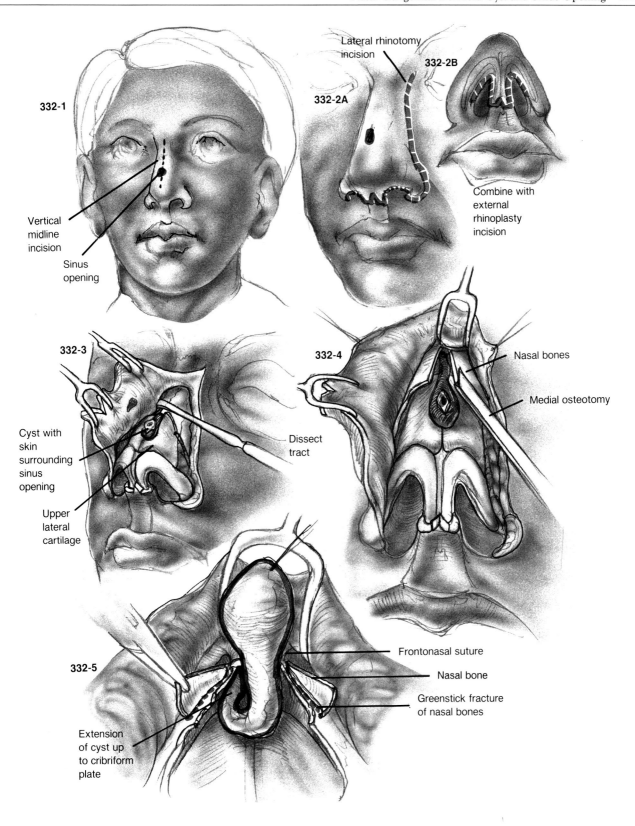

332-1

Vertical
midline
incision

Sinus
opening

Lateral rhinotomy
incision

332-2A

332-2B

Combine with
external
rhinoplasty
incision

332-3

Cyst with
skin
surrounding
sinus
opening

Upper
lateral
cartilage

Dissect
tract

332-4

Nasal bones

Medial osteotomy

332-5

Extension
of cyst up
to cribriform
plate

Frontonasal suture

Nasal bone

Greenstick fracture
of nasal bones

■ *333.* SUBLABIAL AND SEPTAL INCISIONS
Surgical approaches to the nasal septum

Indications
1. Nasal septoplasty and rhinoplasty
2. Nasal graft or implant placement
3. Septal fracture reduction
4. Drainage of an abscess or hematoma
5. Access to the sphenoid sinus
6. Transsphenoidal hypophysectomy

Special Considerations
1. Cosmesis
2. Influences on structural support
3. Adequacy of cover at closure
4. Nasal pathologies

Preoperative Preparation
1. Routine laboratory studies

Special Instruments, Position, and Anesthesia
1. Headlight
2. Local and topical vasoconstrictive agents for the mucosa

Tips and Pearls
1. Obtain good vasoconstriction of mucosa.
2. Minimize scar tissue formation in the distal portion of the nose.
3. Place the external columellar incision in the least obtrusive site, and use a broken-line design.

Pitfalls and Complications
1. Detractive external scar
2. Postoperative settling of nasal tip
3. Exposure and necrosis of septal cartilage

Postoperative Issues
1. Avoiding hemorrhage
2. Temporary supportive splinting
3. Suture removal with external incisions

References
Johns ME, Price JC, Mattox DE, eds. Atlas of head and neck surgery. Philadelphia: BC Decker, 1990.

Johnson CM, Toriumi DM. Open structure rhinoplasty. Philadelphia: WB Saunders, 1990.

Price JC, Holliday M, Kennedy D. The versatile midfacial degloving approach. Laryngoscope 1986;98:291.

Operative Procedure
Sublabial Incision
The sublabial incision offers access to the midfacial skeleton. It is made horizontally along the upper limit of the maxillary alveolar process, near the apex of the upper buccal sulcus. Lateral extension is most often made to approximately the plane of the molar teeth (Fig. 333-1).

Incision through mucosa and periosteum exposes the maxilla. Elevation of the soft tissues above this plane exposes the anterior nasal spine and septum. Dissection can be continued posteriorly along the nasal floor with elevation of the intranasal soft tissues. Access into the sphenoid sinus can be made by continuing dissection along the septum to the sphenoid rostrum and removing bone from the anterior sinus wall.

The sublabial incision can be extended laterally beyond the maxillary tuberosity and onto the palate to obtain access to the pterygomaxillary and adjacent spaces. Full midfacial degloving can be achieved with a combination of the sublabial approach and a complete anterior nasal release, which includes a full nasal transfixion incision along the caudal margin of the septum and bilateral complete circumnasal anterior marginal incisions along the anterior limit of the upper lateral cartilages and bony piriform aperture (Fig. 333-2).

Hemitransfixion (Killian) Incision
The hemitransfixion incision is designed vertically along the caudal margin of the septal cartilage on one side only (Fig. 333-3). Incision through the perichondrium is made at the caudal margin of the cartilage from which point access can be made to either or both sides of the septum. Greater exposure can be made from the base of the columella by extending the incision inferiorly, with a posterior angulation as it approaches the nasal floor.

There is greater adhesion to the skeleton at the point where the perichondrium and periosteum come together. Some surgeons favor elevating beneath the two separately and then connecting the two tunnels with careful lysis of this tight region to avoid a mucosal tear.

Transfixion Incision
The transfixion incision is a bilaterally approached and full separation of the soft tissues from the caudal margin of the septal cartilage (Fig. 333-4). The columella remains attached at the nasal base and tip. In rhinoplasty some prefer to perform a full "high" transfixion only in the upper region of the columella and a hemitransfixion only in the lower region to preserve some of the attachments of the columella to the septum.

Midseptal Incisions
Transmucosal incisions may be made at any desired point along the septum to gain direct access to specific sites. Most are directed either vertically or horizontally.

External Rhinotomy Incision
The external rhinotomy incision is designed transversely across the cutaneous surface of the columella. It is placed variously in the mid or upper third of the columella at a point that is felt to be the least conspicuous. An inverted V-shaped design is normally placed in the center third of the incision to cosmetically break up the transverse line (Fig. 333-5). As the transverse incision continues around the lateral margin of the columella it is continued bilaterally upward and then laterally as a "marginal" incision that outlines the anterior border of the lower lateral cartilage on both sides (Fig. 333-6). The soft tissues can then be raised up and allow exposure of the entire external nasal skeleton.

Access can be made to the septum through this approach anteriorly by separation of the paired mesial crura and dissection through the membranous columella, or superiorly with separation of the medial margin of the upper lateral cartilages from the dorsal margin of the septum. Some prefer to use a separate hemitransfixion approach to the septum to preserve more integrity of the tissue connections.

Columellar Incisions
Vertical incisions can be placed at various sites about the columella, either anterior or posterior to the mesial crura.

GREGORY RENNER

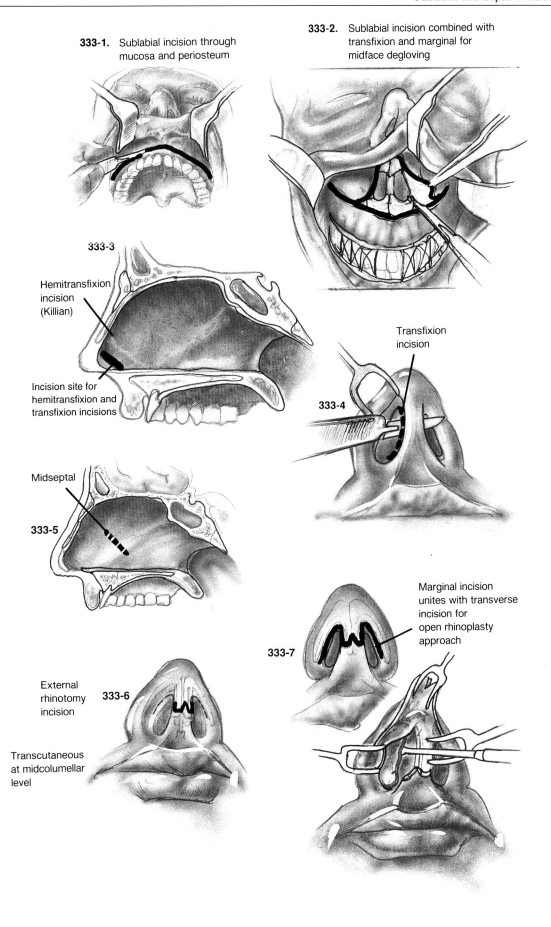

333-1. Sublabial incision through mucosa and periosteum

333-2. Sublabial incision combined with transfixion and marginal for midface degloving

333-3

Hemitransfixion incision (Killian)

Incision site for hemitransfixion and transfixion incisions

Transfixion incision

333-4

Midseptal

333-5

External rhinotomy incision

Transcutaneous at midcolumellar level

333-6

Marginal incision unites with transverse incision for open rhinoplasty approach

333-7

■ *334.* INTRANASAL ANTROSTOMY THROUGH THE INFERIOR MEATUS—Formation of a pathway between the maxillary sinus and nasal cavity through the inferior meatus to facilitate drainage and ventilation

Indications

1. The indications have varied during the past decade because of the introduction of the ostiomeatal complex concept and functional endoscopic sinus surgery.
2. Moderate chronic maxillary sinusitis unresponsive to medical therapy
3. Chronic maxillary sinusitis with systemic disease (eg, cystic fibrosis, immotile cilia syndrome)
4. Diagnostic biopsy or cultures

Contraindications

1. Aplastic or dysplastic maxillary sinus
2. Uncontrolled bleeding disorder

Special Considerations

1. Sinus radiographs displayed in the operating room
2. Good illumination and vasoconstriction

Preoperative Preparation

1. Control of active infection and inflammation
2. Oxymetazoline (0.05%, Afrin nasal spray) administered in the preoperative holding area 20 minutes before surgery

Special Instrumentation, Position, and Anesthesia

1. Nasal speculum, light source, bayonet forceps, Freer elevator, right-angle clamp, antral trocar, curved rasp, bone-cutting sponge, Kerrison forceps
2. Patient in the supine position, with the head elevated 30° and the eyes exposed
3. Local, general, or local and general anesthesia

Tips and Pearls

1. The inferior turbinate, floor of nose, floor of orbit, floor of maxillary sinus, anterior maxillary wall, and posterior maxillary wall are anatomic landmarks.
2. Direct the instruments horizontally or downward to avoid injury to the floor of the orbit.
3. Watch the patient's eyes closely when irrigating.
4. Stop irrigation if there is any resistance or increase in orbital volume or pressure.

Pitfalls and Complications

1. Injury to the orbital globe
2. Orbital hematoma
3. Subcutaneous emphysema: entering anterior to the anterior maxillary wall
4. Fracture of the floor of the orbit
5. Air embolism
6. Dependent, not physiologic, drainage of one sinus (eg, maxillary)
7. High failure and stenosis rates

Postoperative Care

1. Antibiotics, saline washes, and steroid spray for 2 to 3 weeks

References

Lore JM. The sinuses and maxilla. In: Lore JM, ed. The atlas of head and neck surgery. 3rd ed. Philadelphia: WB Saunders, 1988:134.

Montgomery WW. Surgery of the upper respiratory system antrostomy. 2nd ed. Philadelphia: Lea & Febiger, 1979:210.

Operative Procedure

The anterior edge of the inferior turbinate and the adjacent lateral nasal wall are injected with a 2% solution of Xylocaine with a 1:100,000 concentration of epinephrine. The nasal cavity is then packed for 10 minutes with 4% cocaine-soaked Cottonoid pledgets (Fig. 334-1).

The inferior turbinate is identified and then fractured medially using a Freer elevator or bayonet forceps. Using a long (Cottle) nasal speculum, the inferior turbinate is elevated superiorly, and the inferior meatus is visualized. An opening is made 1 to 2 cm posterior to the anterior edge of the inferior turbinate through the inferior meatus. A small, hollow antral trocar is used. Alternatively, a small right-angle clamp may be employed in children. No trocars or other instruments are used in children. The instruments are directed horizontally or downward to avoid orbital injury (Fig. 334-2).

A curved rasp (eg, Wien) may be inserted with a to and fro motion to enlarge the opening. This may help in removing bone at the base of the medial maxillary wall (Fig. 334-3).

A bone curet, bone punch, or both may be used to enlarge the opening anteriorly and posteriorly. This allows adequate drainage and ventilation. All instruments are directed downward to avoid injuring the floor of the orbit (Fig. 334-4).

A 4-mm, 30° or 70° Storz-Hopkins telescope may be introduced through the opening to visualize the area directly and inspect the maxillary cavity.

An olive-tip, curved suction device is introduced through the opening, and the maxillary sinus is irrigated with saline. The patient's eyes should always be exposed and under direct vision during surgery. If the floor of the orbit is injured, saline irrigation may lead to proptosis and increased orbital pressure. No packing is used (Fig. 334-5).

RANDE H. LAZAR
RAMZI T. YOUNIS

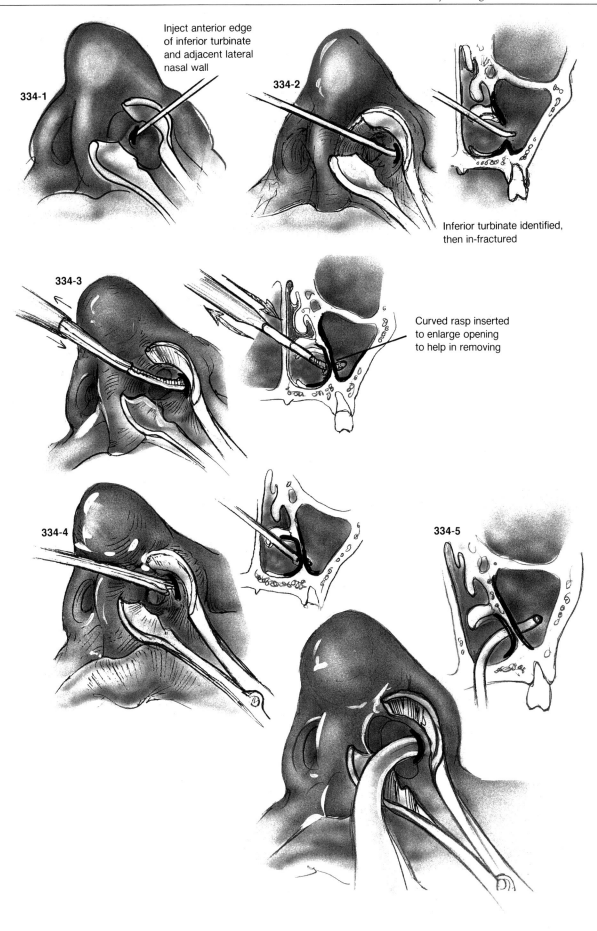

334-1   Inject anterior edge of inferior turbinate and adjacent lateral nasal wall

334-2   Inferior turbinate identified, then in-fractured

334-3   Curved rasp inserted to enlarge opening to help in removing

334-4

334-5

■ *335.* SUBLABIAL ANTROSTOMY (CALDWELL-LUC PROCEDURE)—Cleaning the maxillary sinus of diseased mucosa and forming an inferior meatal antrostomy

Indications
1. Chronic or recurrent maxillary sinusitis
2. Empyema of the maxillary sinus resistant to conservative therapy
3. Symptomatic maxillary mucocele
4. Maxillary sinus polyposis or antral choanal polyp
5. Maxillary sinus fracture
6. Fungal sinusitis
7. Maxillary sinus tumor
8. Maxillary sinus foreign bodies

Contraindications
1. Uncontrolled bleeding disorder
2. Usually not performed in pediatric patients
3. Aplastic maxillary sinus

Special Considerations
1. Optimal vasoconstriction
2. Eyes exposed
3. Radiographs displayed in the operating room

Special Instrumentation, Position, and Anesthesia
1. Osteotome, periosteal elevator, Kerrison forceps, and Coakley curet
2. Patient in the supine position, with the head elevated 30° and the eyes exposed
3. Local, general, or local and general anesthesia
   a. Solution of 2% Xylocaine plus 1:100,000 epinephrine or 2% Xylocaine plus 1:50,000 epinephrine
   b. 4% Cocaine-soaked Cottonoid pledgets

Tips and Pearls
1. The infraorbital rim, infraorbital nerve, gingivobuccal sulcus, canine fossa, floor of orbit, floor of sinus, inferior meatus, anterior maxillary wall, and posterior maxillary wall are anatomic landmarks.

Pitfalls and Complications
1. Infraorbital nerve injury
2. Check for hypoesthesia or paraesthesia
3. Subcutaneous emphysema
4. Bleeding
5. Globe injury
6. Orbital floor injury
7. Extraocular muscle injury
8. Orbital hematoma or proptosis and ecchymosis
9. Blindness
10. Internal maxillary artery injury
11. Injury to the roots of the teeth
12. Superior alveolar nerve injury
13. Facial swelling
14. Oroantral fistula

Postoperative Care
1. Antibiotics
2. Head remains elevated 45°, with packing, fluids, analgesia
3. Removal of packing 3 to 5 days after surgery

References
Lore JM. The sinuses and maxilla. In: Lore JM, ed. The atlas of head and neck surgery. 3rd ed. Philadelphia: WB Saunders, 1988:136.
Montgomery WW. Surgery of the upper respiratory system. 2nd ed. Philadelphia: Lea & Febiger, 1979:211.

Operative Procedure
The gingivobuccal sulcus and anterior edge of the inferior turbinate are injected with a 2% solution of Xylocaine plus a 1:100,000 concentration of epinephrine. The nose is then packed with 4% cocaine-soaked Cottonoid pledgets.

After 10 to 15 minutes, the gingivobuccal sulcus incision is performed in the mucosa and periosteum 2 to 3 cm lateral to the midline, well above the tooth socket. Sufficient mucosa is preserved inferiorly for closure (Fig. 335-1).

Using a periosteal or Freer elevator, the periosteum is elevated upward toward the infraorbital fossa. The infraorbital nerve is identified and carefully preserved. The anterior maxillary wall is identified. Using an osteotome, an opening is made through the canine fossa that is about 2 × 2 cm. This opening should be 1 to 2 cm inferior to the infraorbital rim and 1 to 2 cm superior to the gingivobuccal sulcus (Fig. 335-2). Using Kerrison forceps, the opening is enlarged to permit adequate exposure and cleaning of the maxillary sinus (Fig. 335-3).

Removal of a cyst, tumor, polyps, or diseased tissue is achieved using Blakesley forceps or Coakley curets. Normal mucosa is usually preserved. Temporary packing may be needed to control excessive intraoperative bleeding. Extreme care is taken while working posteriorly not to violate the posterior thin maxillary wall and injure the internal maxillary artery. Care is mandated when working superiorly to prevent injury to the floor of the orbit or to the infraorbital nerve (Fig. 335-4).

An intranasal antrostomy beneath the inferior turbinate is performed after the nasal packs are removed (see Procedure 334; Fig. 335-5). The intranasal antrostomy may be enlarged through the maxillary opening using forward and backward bone-cutting forceps (Fig. 335-6).

The maxillary sinus is irrigated with saline and packed with iodoform packing that is pulled through the inferior meatus antrostomy. The mucosal flap incision is closed with one layer of 4-0 chromic interrupted sutures.

RANDE H. LAZAR
RAMZI T. YOUNIS

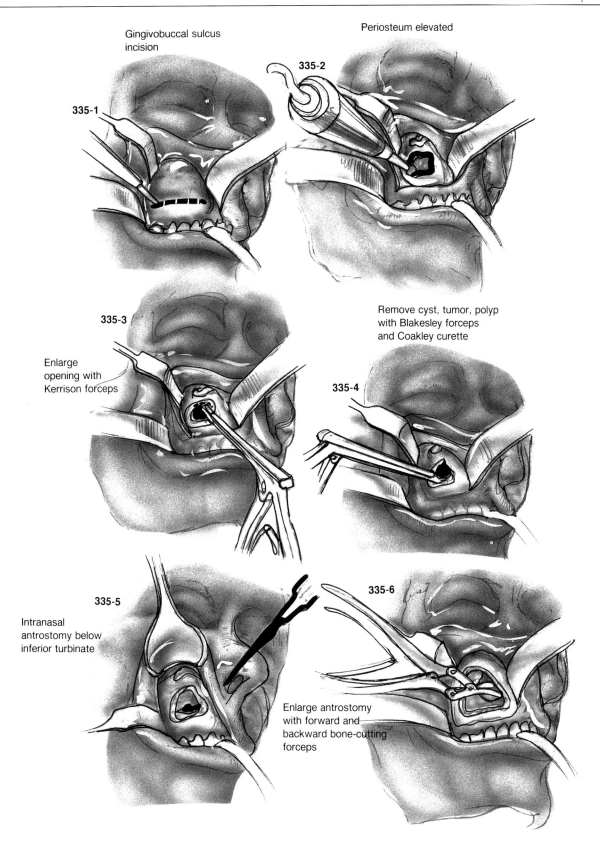

Gingivobuccal sulcus incision

335-1

Periosteum elevated

335-2

335-3

Enlarge opening with Kerrison forceps

Remove cyst, tumor, polyp with Blakesley forceps and Coakley curette

335-4

335-5

Intranasal antrostomy below inferior turbinate

335-6

Enlarge antrostomy with forward and backward bone-cutting forceps

■ *336.* TRANSANTRAL LIGATION OF THE INTERNAL MAXILLARY ARTERY—Surgical ligation of the internal maxillary artery to control posterior nasal bleeding from the sphenopalatine artery and the nasopalatine artery

Indications

1. Posterior epistaxis from the region of the sphenopalatine artery that has been refractory to nasal packing.
2. Recurrent epistaxis.

Special Considerations

1. Age of patient, hypertension, blood loss.
2. Atherosclerosis or cardiovascular disease
3. Central nervous system disease
4. Pulmonary disease
5. Aspirin use or coagulopathy

Preoperative Preparation

1. Electrocardiogram and chest radiograph
2. Arterial blood gas determination
3. Bleeding and coagulation studies
4. Radiographic studies, including a Waters view or CT scan
5. Localization of the bleeding site

Special Instruments, Position, and Anesthesia

1. A 1% solution of Xylocaine with a 1:100,000 concentration of epinephrine may be used for local anesthesia.
2. General anesthesia is preferred.
3. Bipolar cautery and headlight
4. Operating microscope with a 300-mm lens
5. Rotating bur drill, Kerrison rongeur, small osteotomes, and self-locking vascular clips
6. Pterygomaxillary fossa dissection instruments (eg, probes, spatula, hooks, cup and alligator forceps, curets)

Tips and Pearls

1. Localization of the bleeding site is imperative for the proper treatment of epistaxis.
2. Fiberoptic endoscopes may be useful in determining the bleeding site.
3. If bleeding persists after ligation of the internal maxillary artery, the surgeon must consider the presence of an unidentified collateral vessel or bleeding from another arterial distribution, such as the ethmoid arteries.
4. Meticulous hemostasis of the operative site is essential.

Pitfalls and Complications

1. Continued bleeding secondary to incomplete or inadequate ligation that allows collateral blood flow
2. Sinusitis
3. Oroantral fistula
4. Orbital or ocular injury
5. Infraorbital nerve injury
6. Vasomotor rhinitis or injury to vidian nerve

Postoperative Care Issues

1. Appropriate antibiotic coverage should be used to avoid infectious complications.
2. Elevation of the head or ice packs may decrease postoperative swelling.
3. Oxygen therapy and humidification should be used to maintain adequate O_2 saturation. Pulse oximetry is useful for postoperative monitoring.
4. Control of pain and blood pressure is necessary to prevent repeat bleeding.
5. Monitor ongoing blood loss and changes in the hemoglobin and hematocrit levels.

References

Montgomery WW, Reardon EJ. Early vessel ligations for control of severe epistaxis. In: Snow JB, ed. Controversy in otolaryngology. Philadelphia: WB Saunders, 1980:315.

Pearson BW, MacKenzie RG, Goodman WS. The anatomical basis of transantral ligation of the maxillary artery in severe epistaxis. Laryngoscope 1969;79:969.

Operative Procedure

The patient is placed in a supine position, with the head of the bed elevated 20° to 30°. The procedure is begun as for a Caldwell-Luc. The upper gingival-buccal sulcus is exposed and retracted by an assistant. The incision is made in the sulcus with electrocautery or a knife down to the bone. The tissues are elevated off the maxilla to expose the canine fossa. The infraorbital nerve and tooth roots are preserved. An antrostomy is made with the osteotome or rotating bur and enlarged with the Kerrison rongeur (Fig. 336-1). The posterior wall of the maxillary sinus is identified, and a laterally based mucosal flap is elevated (Fig. 336-2). Bone removal is begun with the osteotome and rongeur (or rotating bur) along the inferior lateral portion of the posterior sinus wall. The opening is enlarged toward the superomedial aspect of the posterior wall (Fig. 336-3).

The vasculature can be quite variable, and blunt dissection of the vessels within the adipose tissue is required for identification (Fig. 336-4). If the ligation is performed too far laterally, collateral blood flow is likely to occur, and the bleeding may persist. Bleeding from the adipose tissue is controlled with the bipolar cautery.

Removal of bone superiorly and medially over the orbital process of the palatine bone ensures exposure of the major vessels supplying the posterior nasal cavity. By placing clips more distally (medially), the surgeon is more likely to achieve control of the vascular supply and avoid collateral flow. The clips should be placed on the proximal maxillary artery, on the maxillary artery just proximal to the origin of the descending palatine artery, on the maxillary artery as high and medially as possible (ie, behind the orbital process of the palatine bone to ensure control of the sphenopalatine branch), and on the descending palatine artery as distally as possible (Fig. 336-5).

A single layer of Gelfoam and topical thrombin solution may be placed in the sinus if needed to control mucosal bleeding, and an antrostomy may be made for drainage of the sinus. Expansile packing should be avoided because of the possibility of bleeding with resulting ophthalmoplegia from a hematoma or pressure within the sinus.

Postoperative care includes antibiotics, elevation of the head of the bed, use of adequate oxygen therapy and humidification, control of hypertension and pain, and close monitoring of the hematocrit and any ongoing blood loss. Transfusions should be given if needed.

JOHN S. MAY

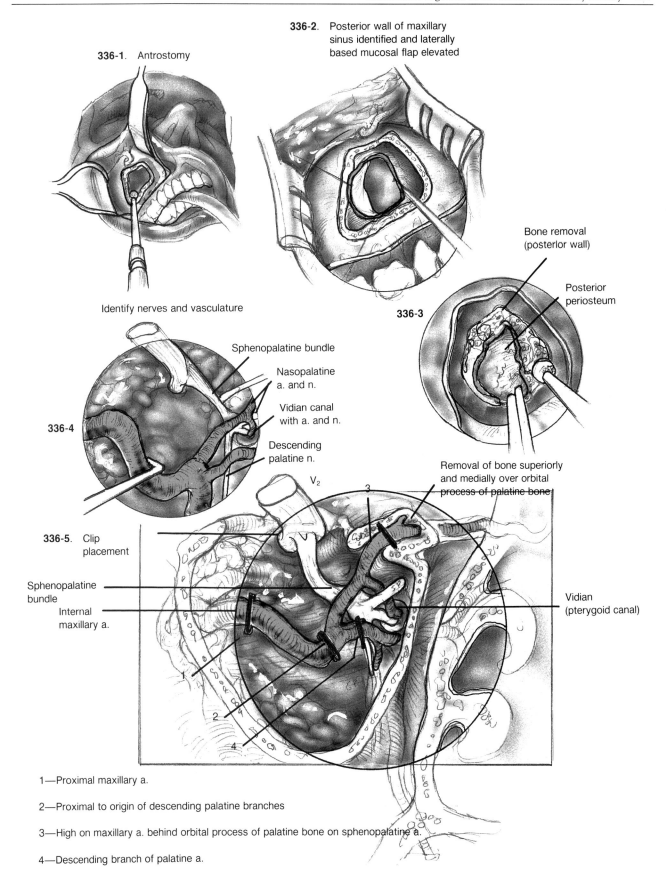

336-1. Antrostomy

336-2. Posterior wall of maxillary sinus identified and laterally based mucosal flap elevated

Identify nerves and vasculature

Bone removal (posterior wall)

Posterior periosteum

336-3

Sphenopalatine bundle

Nasopalatine a. and n.

Vidian canal with a. and n.

Descending palatine n.

V_2

336-4

Removal of bone superiorly and medially over orbital process of palatine bone

336-5. Clip placement

Sphenopalatine bundle

Internal maxillary a.

Vidian (pterygoid canal)

3

2

4

1—Proximal maxillary a.

2—Proximal to origin of descending palatine branches

3—High on maxillary a. behind orbital process of palatine bone on sphenopalatine a.

4—Descending branch of palatine a.

■ *337.* VIDIAN NEURECTOMY

Sectioning of the vidian nerve, which carries parasympathetic fibers from the greater superficial petrosal nerve and sympathetic fibers from the deep petrosal nerve around the internal carotid artery.

Indications

1. Vasomotor rhinitis resistant to medical therapy (ie, intractable secretomotor rhinopathy)
2. Severe senile rhinorrhea, chronic epiphora

Contraindications

1. Chronic maxillary sinusitis
2. Children with nonerupted secondary teeth

Special Considerations

1. Treatment of preexisting sinus disease
2. Need for additional or simultaneous procedures (eg, internal maxillary artery ligation)

Preoperative Preparation

1. Routine laboratory studies
2. Nasal smear, C & S, radiographic studies
3. Allergy testing, skin tests with or without radioallergosorbent tests

Special Instruments, Position, and Anesthesia

1. Zeiss microscope with 10× magnification and 300-mm objective lens
2. Sickle knife, curved scissors, small periosteal elevator, small chisel or bur, right-angled hook
3. Reverse Trendelenburg position, with the patient supine
4. General anesthesia with hypotension
5. For the endoscopic transnasal approach
   a. Rigid nasal endoscopes (0° and 30°)
   b. Sickle knife, curved probe, curved scissors, small periosteal elevator, curved suction tip, right-angled hook, and suction cautery

(continued)

Operative Procedures

Transantral Approach

The patient is placed on the operating table supine, in the reverse Trendelenburg position. Intravenous or inhalational techniques are used to induce general anesthesia, with placement of an oral endotracheal tube. Hypotensive anesthesia (systolic <90 mm Hg) is desirable.

Xylocaine (1%) with 1:100,000 epinephrine is injected intraorally into the sphenopalatine ganglion through the greater palatine foramen (posteromedial to the second molar), aspirating first to avoid intravascular injection. A volume of 2 mL is sufficient. For the initial incision, the buccogingival sulcus is infiltrated for hemostasis.

The upper lip is reflected, and a buccogingival incision is made with a scalpel, cautery, or both from the canine tooth to the second molar. Subperiosteal elevation of the tissue displays the anterior wall of the maxillary antrum. Care is taken to avoid injury or excessive stretching of the infraorbital nerve.

With high-speed drill or mallet and gouge, the antrum is entered at its thinnest point, and the opening is enlarged to remove the anterior wall to the infraorbital rim, preserving the infraorbital nerve and avoiding the cancellous bone of the upper alveolus and teeth roots (Fig 337-1).

Self-retaining retractors are inserted to provide exposure. A large inferiorly based U-shaped mucoperiosteal flap is elevated downward to the floor, and bleeding is controlled with electrocoagulation (Fig. 337-2).

The operating microscope is brought into place, and using the high-speed drill or mallet and gouge, the bone of the posterior antral wall is penetrated, taking care to preserve posterior periosteum. Bone removal is carried medially and superiorly with Kerrison rongeurs, drilling, or fragmentation and piecemeal removal.

Cautery is applied to coagulate the posterior periosteum, which is then incised in a U-shaped flap, avoiding the underlying vessels embedded in fat. The vessels are separated carefully using the nerve hook and pterygopalatine fossa instruments to identify the internal maxillary artery and its branches (Fig. 337-3).

The second division of the trigeminal nerve (V_2) is identified as it courses along the posterosuperior antral wall and crosses the pterygopalatine fossa superiorly. It is followed medially to the foramen rotundum.

The vessels of the fossa can often be retracted, but sometimes, the internal maxillary artery must be divided between clips (double clips on both sides) to permit adequate visualization (Fig. 337-4). A clip is always placed laterally on the internal maxillary artery before going posteriorly, whether it is retracted or divided.

One centimeter inferomedial to the foramen rotundum lies the vidian (pterygoid) canal and its nerve. This is located by following the sphenopalatine bundle downward and medially until the divergence of the descending palatine and nasal branches. The vidian nerve is cut with a sickle knife as it emerges from the canal while elevating and putting traction on its descending palatine and nasal branches with a nerve hook (Fig. 337-5). The stumps may be coagulated with special "shouldered" cautery tips (Golding-Wood tips), and the canal is packed with bone wax (Fig. 337-6).

(continued)

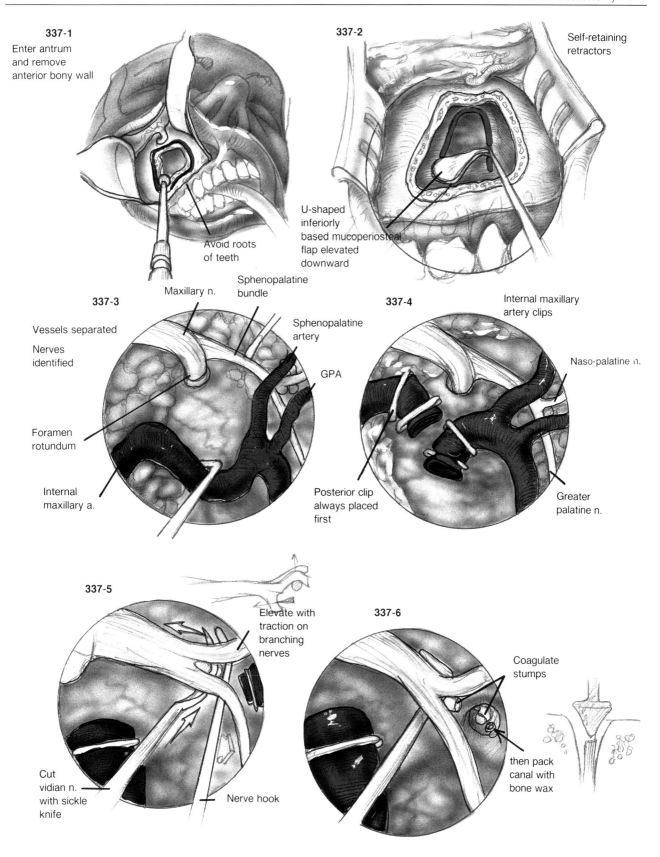

337-1
Enter antrum and remove anterior bony wall

Avoid roots of teeth

337-2

Self-retaining retractors

U-shaped inferiorly based mucoperiosteal flap elevated downward

337-3

Maxillary n.

Sphenopalatine bundle

Vessels separated

Sphenopalatine artery

Nerves identified

GPA

Foramen rotundum

Internal maxillary a.

337-4

Internal maxillary artery clips

Naso-palatine n.

Posterior clip always placed first

Greater palatine n.

337-5

Elevate with traction on branching nerves

Cut vidian n. with sickle knife

Nerve hook

337-6

Coagulate stumps

then pack canal with bone wax

■ *337.* VIDIAN NEURECTOMY *(continued)*

Tips and Pearls

1. If the medial antral wall bulges laterally into a sinus and impedes access, it may be mobilized and pushed medially with finger pressure or small chisel cuts. Restore the position of the wall at the end of case with outward pressure from within the nose.
2. Avoid overpenetration of the pterygoid canal with cautery by using a Golding-Wood shouldered cautery tip.
3. For the endoscopic transnasal approach, the superior turbinate, if present, acts as a pointer to the sphenopalatine foramen.

Pitfalls and Complications

1. Upper lip anesthesia
2. Cheek and palate neuralgia
3. Ophthalmoplegia from overpenetration of pterygoid canal
4. Internal maxillary artery hemorrhage
5. For the endoscopic transnasal approach
   a. Narrow field of surgery, which may necessitate lateral fracture of the posterior end of the middle turbinate or initial septoplasty for a grossly deviated septum or spur
   b. Bleeding at the posterior end of the middle turbinate

Postoperative Care Issues

1. Intraoperative and postoperative broad-spectrum antibiotics
2. For the endoscopic transnasal approach
   a. Gelfoam and pack intranasally for 6 hours
   b. Artificial tears, as needed

References

El Shazly MA. Endoscopic surgery of the vidian nerve (preliminary report). Ann Otol Rhinol Laryngol 1991;100:536.

Savard P, Stoney MB, Hawke M. An anatomical study of vidian neurectomy using an endoscopic technique: a potential new application. J Otolaryngol 1993;22:125.

The periosteal flap is then returned to its position and covered with Gelfoam, Surgicel, or Oxycel. Similarly, the antral mucoperiosteal flap is returned and covered. If the maxillary ostium is not widely patent, it should be enlarged or a nasoantral window created along the medial wall. The buccogingival incision is then closed with interrupted 3-0 chromic catgut sutures.

Endoscopic Transnasal Approach

Although we do not perform the endoscopic technique, it has been reported by many others in the literature. It allows transnasal vidian neurectomy under direct vision. The indications, contraindications, and preoperative preparation are the same as for other approaches. Special instrumentation, anesthesia, tips, and complications for the endoscopic approach are outlined in the preceding sections.

Packs saturated with 4% cocaine are placed intranasally to achieve topical anesthesia and vasoconstriction. Bilateral sphenopalatine nerve blocks are performed intraorally through the greater palatine canal with 2 mL of 1% Xylocaine with 1:100,000 epinephrine. With the aid of a 0° or 30° nasal endoscope, the posterior end of the middle turbinate, the superior meatus, and the middle meatus are infiltrated.

The sphenopalatine foramen is located just behind or slightly above the attachment of the posterior end of the middle turbinate, at the junction of the superior and lateral nasal walls, 12 mm superolateral to the superior border of the choana (Fig. 337-7). The foramen is carefully palpated and located with a blunt probe that pushes the intact mucosa before it (Fig. 337-8). A horizontal incision is placed 5 to 10 mm beneath the inferior rim of the sphenopalatine foramen to avoid damage to branches of the sphenopalatine artery (Fig. 337-9). Using the small periosteal elevator, a mucoperiosteal flap is elevated superiorly to the foramen. The elevator is advanced into the foramen posteriorly, separating the periosteum of the pterygopalatine fossa laterally away from the lateral wall of the sphenoid process of the palatine bone.

The mouth of the pterygoid (vidian) canal lies in the same plane as the sphenopalatine foramen, about 5 to 6 mm posterolaterally. If the sphenopalatine foramen is small, it may be widened carefully with a curette posteriorly and inferiorly (where the bone is thinner) to allow better visualization of the mouth of the vidian canal. The vidian nerve is found directly posterior to the sphenopalatine ganglion after it has been reflected laterally (Fig. 337-10). With anterior traction on the ganglion, the vidian nerve is stretched out of its canal (Fig. 337-11). It can then be isolated with a hook and cut with the curved scissors. Coagulation of the proximal stump is performed using the insulated suction cautery.

The mucoperiosteal flap of the posterolateral nasal wall is returned and covered with Gelfoam, Surgicel, or Oxycel that is held in place by a small pack.

ROBERT M. BUMSTED
NEAL M. LOFCHY

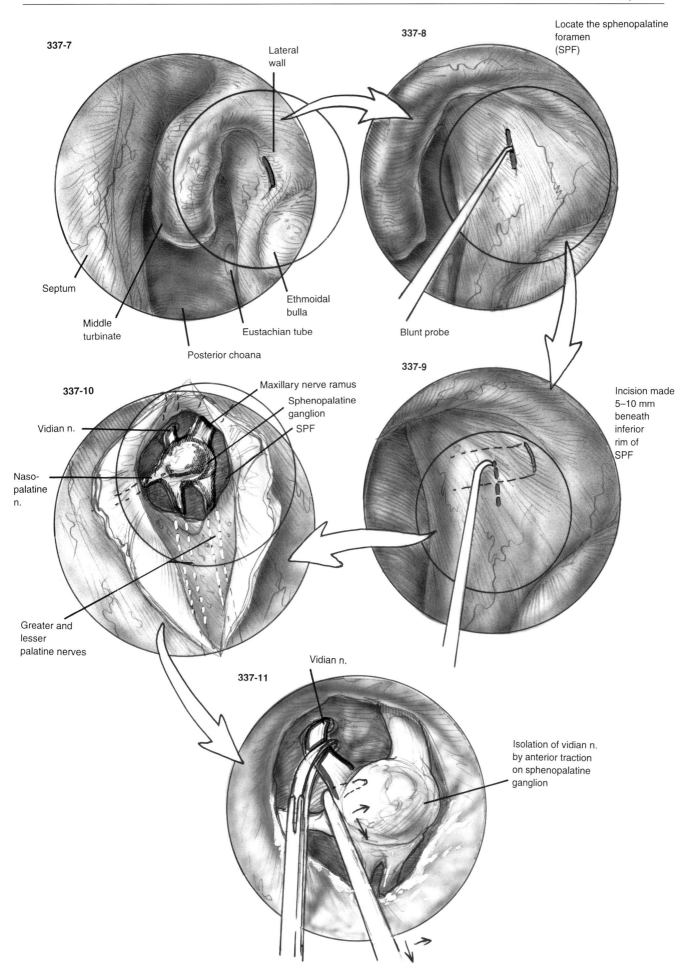

337-7

Lateral wall

Septum

Middle turbinate

Posterior choana

Eustachian tube

Ethmoidal bulla

337-8

Locate the sphenopalatine foramen (SPF)

Blunt probe

337-9

Incision made 5–10 mm beneath inferior rim of SPF

337-10

Vidian n.

Naso-palatine n.

Greater and lesser palatine nerves

Maxillary nerve ramus

Sphenopalatine ganglion

SPF

337-11

Vidian n.

Isolation of vidian n. by anterior traction on sphenopalatine ganglion

■ *338.* INTRANASAL ETHMOIDECTOMY

Intranasal drainage and cleaning of the anterior and posterior ethmoid sinuses

Indications

1. Chronic ethmoid sinusitis
2. Ethmoid polyposis
3. Ethmoid sinus tumor
4. Foreign bodies

Contraindications

1. Excessive ethmoid polyposis
2. Ethmoidal mucocele
3. Acute ethmoiditis plus orbital infections
4. Revision ethmoidal surgery

Special Considerations

1. Eyes should exposed and inspected during surgery
2. Optimal vasoconstriction
3. Good illumination

Preoperative Preparation

1. Afrin or Neo-Synephrine nose drops are administered in the preoperative holding area.
2. Control of acute or active infection

Special Instrumentation, Position, and Anesthesia

1. Freer elevator, blunt-tip curets, and ethmoidal blunt forceps
2. Patient in the supine position, with the head elevated 45° and the eyes exposed
3. Local, general, or local and general anesthesia

Tips and Pearls

1. Injury to the lamina papyracea, the paper-thin lateral border of dissection, can lead to orbital complications.
2. Injury to the cribriform plate, the superior border of dissection, can lead to intracranial complications.
3. The ethmoidal arteries can be the source of extensive bleeding or orbital hematoma.
4. The patient's eyes should remain exposed for frequent inspection
5. Always use curets in a downward and slightly medially motion; superior and lateral motion may lead to complications.
6. Slow and gentle dissection should be carried out with good illumination and visualization.

Complications

1. Bleeding intranasally or into the orbit
2. Violation of the lamina papyracea and orbit
   a. Blindness
   b. Extraocular muscle injury
   c. Globe injury
   d. Proptosis or orbital hematoma
3. Subcutaneous emphysema: lamina papyracea
4. Cerebrospinal fluid rhinorrhea may result from a cribriform plate injury or fovea ethmoidalis injury.
5. Meningitis may result from a cribriform plate injury or fovea ethmoidalis injury.
6. Death may result from injury to the cribriform plate and from an intracranial injury or complication.

Postoperative Care

1. Antibiotics, local or systemic decongestants, and steroid nasal spray
2. Removal of packing within 24 to 48 hours

References

Lore JM. The sinuses and maxilla. In: Lore JM, ed. Atlas of head and neck surgery. 3rd ed. Philadelphia: WB Saunders, 1988:146.

Montgomery WW. Surgery of the upper respiratory system. 2nd ed. Philadelphia: Lea & Febiger, 1979:41.

Operative Procedure

The anterior edge of the middle turbinate and lateral nasal wall are injected with a 2% solution of Xylocaine with a 1:100,000 concentration of epinephrine. The nose is packed with 4% cocaine-soaked Cottonoid pledgets for 10 minutes. The middle turbinate is identified and displaced medially with a Freer elevator. The turbinate is preserved unless it is found to be hypertrophic, cystic, or polypoid, in which case partial resection may be performed (Figs. 338-1 and 338-2).

The ethmoids are entered lateral to the middle turbinate using an asymmetric, oval, thin curet. The anterior ethmoids are opened with a downward and inward motion. Additional downward and backward dissection is performed until normal mucosa is reached or total ethmoidal exenteration is performed (Fig. 338-3).

A smaller curet may be needed as the operation progresses posteriorly or as the space narrows. The exenteration continues to the anterior wall of the sphenoid if extensive anterior and posterior ethmoidal disease is found. Alternatively, ethmoid-type blunt forceps may be used to remove diseased tissue. The superior turbinate may be removed with scissors if additional space is required (Fig. 338-4). However, minimal dissection and manipulation are advised for better postoperative healing and less scarring.

During the past decade, the importance of this procedure has decreased significantly because of the increased popularity and effectiveness of functional endoscopic sinus surgery.

RANDE H. LAZAR
RAMZI T. YOUNIS

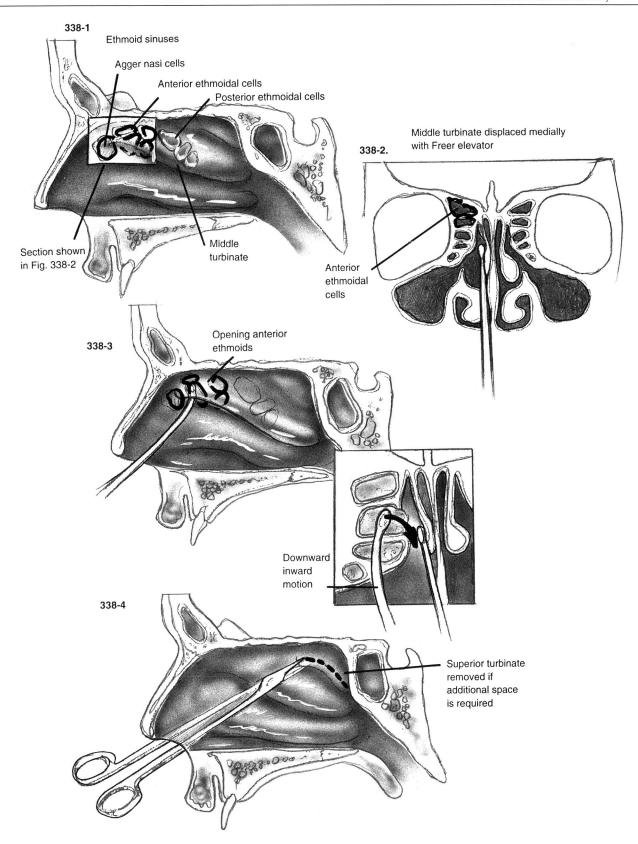

338-1

Ethmoid sinuses

Agger nasi cells

Anterior ethmoidal cells

Posterior ethmoidal cells

Section shown
in Fig. 338-2

Middle
turbinate

338-2.

Middle turbinate displaced medially
with Freer elevator

Anterior
ethmoidal
cells

338-3

Opening anterior
ethmoids

Downward
inward
motion

338-4

Superior turbinate
removed if
additional space
is required

■ *339.* EXTERNAL ETHMOIDECTOMY

Removal of the bony septa between the ethmoid cells through an external approach, resulting in the creation of an ethmoid cavity

Indications

1. Chronic ethmoid infection
2. Complications of acute ethmoid infection, including subperiosteal and retroorbital abscess
3. Tumor of the ethmoid sinus

Special Considerations

1. Visual acuity check
2. Bleeding tendency

Preoperative Preparation

1. Computed tomography scan of the sinuses
2. Routine laboratory tests

Special Instruments, Position, and Anesthesia

1. Headlight
2. Head elevated and turned, with the neck flexed
3. General anesthesia and an endotracheal tube

Tips and Pearls

1. Local infiltration to assist in hemostasis
2. Gentle retraction of the orbit
3. Use of the endoscope for intranasal assessment

Pitfalls and Complications

1. Difficult access to agger nasi and frontal recess
2. Bleeding at the posterior ethmoid artery
3. Intracranial extension with cerebrospinal fluid (CSF) leak
4. Postoperative retroorbital hematoma

Postoperative Care Issues

1. Visual acuity check
2. Wound care
3. Nasal hygiene

References

Arjmand EM, Lusk RP, Muntz HR. Pediatric sinusitis and subperiosteal orbital abscess formation: diagnosis and treatment. Otolaryngol Head Neck Surg 1993;109:886.

Fenton RA. Radical treatment of the ethmoid: intranasal. Ann Otol Rhinol Laryngol 1929;38:914.

Operative Procedure

General anesthesia is administered, and an endotracheal tube is placed. The table is positioned with the head elevated. A pillow is placed beneath the patient's head to gently flex the neck and turn the patient toward the operator. The patient's eyes are protected with lubricant and a tarsorrhaphy stitch. The area of the Lynch incision is injected with a lidocaine and epinephrine mixture, usually a 1% solution of lidocaine with a 1:100,000 concentration of epinephrine. The nose is packed with Afrin-soaked Cottonoid sponges. The face is prepped with antiseptic solution and draped in a standard fashion, exposing the nose, eye, and forehead.

After at least 5 minutes, the nasal packing is removed, and the nose is inspected with an endoscope. Attention is given to landmarks and signs of pathology. A Lynch incision (Fig. 339-1) is made at the lateral nose, through the skin and subcutaneous tissues to the periosteum. The supratrochlear nerve may be encountered.

The periosteum is elevated along the lateral aspect of the lacrimal and ethmoid bone (Fig. 339-2). A Sewald retractor gently retracts the periosteum and orbital contents laterally, allowing access to the ethmoid. If a subperiosteal orbital abscess is found, it should be drained at this time. If the abscess is retroorbital and within the orbital fat, the periosteum may be incised to allow drainage. Retraction of the orbit may cause reflex bradycardia and hypotension. If this happens, less aggressive retraction is needed. Pressure on the globe should be avoided.

Behind the lacrimal bone, the ethmoid bone thins at the laminae papyracea. The ethmoid labyrinth may be entered beneath the interpupillary line, a landmark for the cribriform plate.

Once into the ethmoid, dissection is carried out using Blakely or Takahashi forceps. Dissection of the ethmoid bullae and posterior ethmoid air cells can be evaluated through transnasal endoscopy. Tumor may be removed piecemeal or en bloc with adjacent bone. The mucosa is stripped from underlying bone. Cultures are taken of the tissue or mucus in the sinus.

After traversing the lamina behind the lacrimal bone, the instrument enters the anterior ethmoid sinus (Fig. 339-3). From the external approach, the middle turbinate is poorly visualized, and understanding the anatomy is essential because landmarks look different in this approach than in functional endoscopic sinus surgery. The agger nasi and frontal recess may be approached only with great difficulty, but the bullae ethmoidalis and anterior cells near the skull base are easily entered.

Identification of the basal lamella establishes the location of the posterior cells. The posterior cells are large and can help define the skull base. Care must be taken at the skull base. The frontal bone is thicker laterally, although the thinner cribriform plate drops beneath this level at the fovea ethmoidalis. The lateral lamella of fovea ethmoidalis is thin and easily penetrated, resulting in a CSF leak.

Closure is accomplished in multiple layers. The periosteum should be approximated, followed by the subcutaneous tissue and skin. Skin closure is best achieved by multiple interrupted sutures in cases of infection. Rapidly absorbing chromic or plain sutures with Steri-Strips can be used in other cases.

After the ethmoidectomy, drainage is established through the middle meatus. In cases of infections, it is helpful to place a catheter through the Lynch incision for irrigation with normal saline solution (Fig. 339-4). When the nasal irrigant is clear, the catheter may be removed.

Postoperative wound care may include cleaning and ointments to reduce the potential for a wide scar. Visual acuity should be assessed in the immediate postoperative period, documenting any change from the preoperative status. Although uncommon, increased lid edema and double vision may occur but should resolve quickly. Greater concern over extraocular movements would be warranted if the periosteum had been violated.

HARLAN MUNTZ

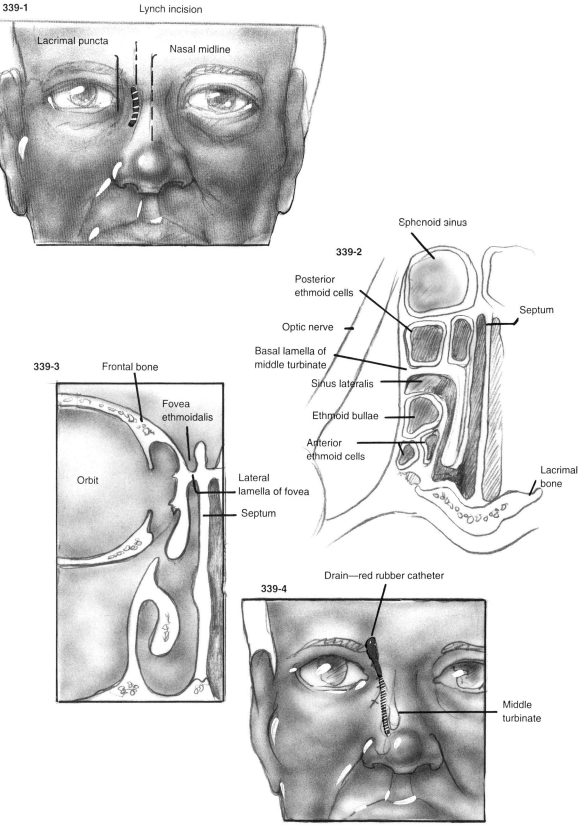

339-1 Lynch incision

Lacrimal puncta

Nasal midline

339-2

Sphenoid sinus

Septum

Posterior ethmoid cells

Optic nerve

Basal lamella of middle turbinate

Sinus lateralis

Ethmoid bullae

Anterior ethmoid cells

Lacrimal bone

339-3 Frontal bone

Fovea ethmoidalis

Orbit

Lateral lamella of fovea

Septum

Drain—red rubber catheter

339-4

Middle turbinate

Ethmoidal irrigation with external drain

■ *340.* EXTERNAL FRONTOETHMOIDECTOMY

Open approach to the removal of tumor, polyp, papilloma, or chronic mucosal disease in the frontal and ethmoid sinuses

Indications

1. Frontal and ethmoid mucoceles
2. Orbital complications of acute or chronic sinusitis
3. Frontocutaneous or ethmoidocutaneous fistula
4. Recurrent frontoethmoid sinusitis or polyposis after failure of endoscopic surgical management
5. Benign neoplasms of the superior nasal cavity, ethmoid or frontal sinuses, and anterior skull base
6. Malignant tumors (as part of a craniofacial resection)
7. Closure of cerebrospinal fluid rhinorrhea

Contraindications

1. No absolute contraindications
2. Relative contraindications
   a. Patient with a tendency to hypertrophic scarring
   b. Coagulopathy
   c. Trauma
   d. Previous failure of the same approach
   e. Suspected malignancy and metastatic cancer

Preoperative Preparation

1. Preoperative visual acuity assessment
2. Coronal and axial computed tomography to assess the extent of disease and the integrity of the skull base and lamina papyracea

Special Instruments, Position, and Anesthesia

1. Mayfield headrest (optional)
2. Bipolar cautery, periosteal elevators, osteotomes, rongeurs, cup forceps (eg, Takahashi forceps), retractors (eg, Sewall, malleable, hooks)
3. Supine position, general anesthesia

Tips and Pearls

1. Meticulous hemostasis
2. Establish wide frontoethmoid drainage into the nose
3. The frontoethmoid suture line contains anterior and posterior ethmoid arteries, which are landmarks for the optic nerve.

Pitfalls and Complications

1. Orbital injuries
   a. Hemorrhage, causing blindness
   b. Injury of the medial rectus or trochlea, causing diplopia
   c. Injury of the medial canthal ligament, causing telecanthus
2. Skull base or posterior table frontal sinus penetration
   a. Cerebrospinal fluid leak
   b. Central nervous system injury
3. Massive hemorrhage
4. Infection of the wound, orbit, meninges, or central nervous system
5. Epiphora due to lacrimal system injury
6. Forehead anesthesia due to supraorbital nerve injury
7. Stenosis of the frontonasal communication or synechiae
8. Recurrence or persistence of disease or symptoms, such as nasal obstruction, rhinorrhea, or anosmia
9. Hypertrophic or unacceptable scar, webbing, or keloid

Postoperative Care Issues

1. Visual assessment soon after surgery
2. Antibiotics as indicated by the results of cultures and Gram stains
3. Packing removal at 3 to 5 days after surgery
4. Nasal hygiene with saline irrigations every 4 to 6 hours
5. Stent removal in 1 to 6 months

References

Lynch RC. The technique of a radical frontal sinus operation which has given me the best results. Laryngoscope 1921;31:1.

Rubin JS, Lund VJ, Salmon B. Frontoethmoidectomy in the treatment of mucoceles (a neglected operation). Arch Otolaryngol Head Neck Surg 1986;112:434.

Operative Procedure

For vasoconstriction, the nasal cavity is packed with Cottonoid pledgets soaked with oxymetazoline. A throat pack is inserted, and 10 mg of Decadron is administered intravenously. The incision is injected with a 1:100,000 epinephrine solution, and the patient is then prepped with half-strength Betadine solution (not soap) and draped.

The incision is scored with a #15 blade and then carried immediately to bone medial to the canthal ligament (Fig. 340-1). Elevation is begun in a subperiosteal plane to identify the ligament. Using the bone and ligament as landmarks, the remaining incision can be performed superiorly, taking care to preserve the supraorbital neurovascular bundle. The orbicularis oculi muscle fibers must be divided and the angular vessels bipolar cauterized during this part of the procedure. The subperiosteal elevation is continued medially and posteriorly, preserving the trochlea and the medial canthal ligament. The lacrimal sac is usually elevated with the periosteum, leaving it intact; however, if the procedure is done for larger lesions, an osteotomy may be performed in the medial and inferior orbital walls, requiring division of the lacrimal apparatus (Fig. 340-2). If this is required, a dacryocystorhinostomy should be performed using Crawford stents (see Procedure 356). In this case, the canthal ligament can be left intact or divided. If it is divided, a wire pass drill should be used to make a hole in the bone for precise reattachment at the end of the procedure. Perforation of the periorbita is troublesome because of the herniation of orbital fat, which hinders exposure and may later result in orbital contents in the nasal cavity.

The dissection is continued until the anterior ethmoid artery is visualized in the frontoethmoid suture line and the entire inferior wall of the frontal sinus is exposed. The periosteum is rather adherent in the suture line, and care must be taken not to avulse the artery in the process. The anterior ethmoid artery is skeletonized and then cauterized. A long Stephens scissors is used to divide the vessel lateral to the cauterized area halfway through; if the cautery was inadequate, the artery can be recauterized without the risk of it retracting into the globe. The anterior ethmoid artery is located 24 mm posterior to the anterior lacrimal crest (Fig. 340-3). The posterior ethmoid artery is 12 mm posterior to the anterior ethmoid, and the optic nerve is not more than 6 mm further posterior. The posterior ethmoid artery should be identified, but only in rare cases does it require division. If it is necessary to divide it, there is higher risk of optic nerve injury.

At this point, the lamina papyracea is perforated with an osteotome, and bone (ie, lacrimal, frontal sinus floor, lamina, and nasal process of maxilla) is removed with a Kerrison rongeur to expose the ethmoid and frontal air cells (Fig. 340-4). The diseased mucosa, tumor, polyp, or papilloma are removed, and a wide nasofrontal connection is established to ensure mucociliary clearance. A mucosal flap from the superior ethmoid region may help to maintain patency. In the ethmoid, care is taken not to work above the plane of the frontoethmoid suture line to avoid injury to the cribriform plate. In most cases, the frontal sinus can be completely exenterated using this technique. If further exposure is needed, an osteoplastic flap can be created based superiorly (Fig. 340-5).

The frontonasal communication is stented with a large, fenestrated, indwelling Silastic tube that is secured with a suture superiorly (Fig. 340-6). The nose is packed with antibiotic-impregnated 0.5-in (12-mm) iodoform gauze. The periosteum is repaired with 3-0 chromic sutures, and the wound is closed with interrupted inverted 4-0 chromic deep dermal sutures and a simple running skin suture of 5-0 fast-absorbing catgut and Steri-Strips. A nasal drip pad dressing is taped in place, and the procedure is complete.

CHRISTOPHER H. RASSEKH

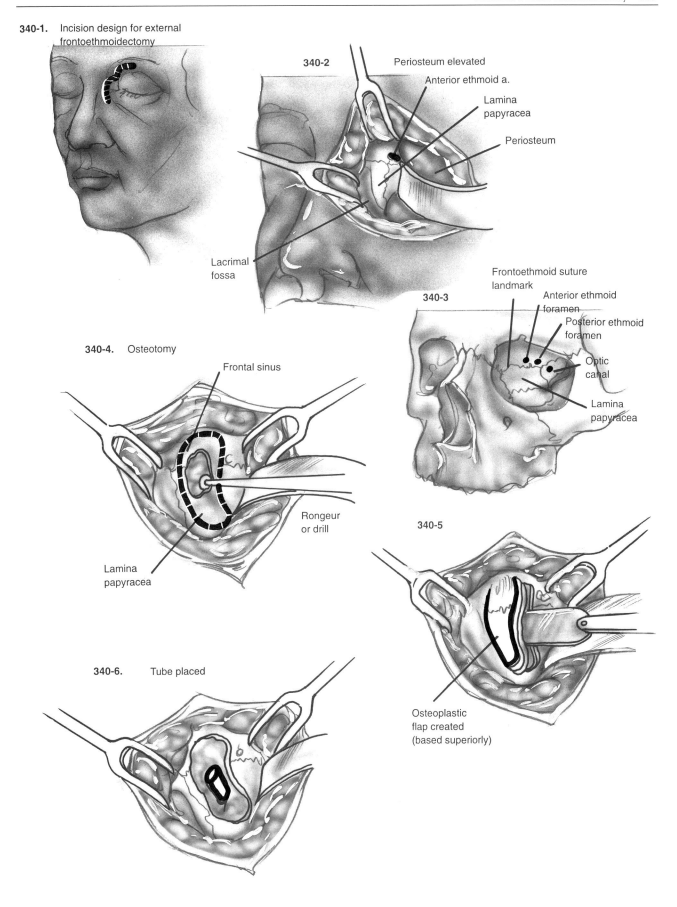

340-1.   Incision design for external frontoethmoidectomy

340-2
Periosteum elevated
Anterior ethmoid a.
Lamina papyracea
Periosteum
Lacrimal fossa

340-3
Frontoethmoid suture landmark
Anterior ethmoid foramen
Posterior ethmoid foramen
Optic canal
Lamina papyracea

340-4.   Osteotomy
Frontal sinus
Rongeur or drill
Lamina papyracea

340-5
Osteoplastic flap created (based superiorly)

340-6.   Tube placed

■ *341.* TRANSANTRAL ETHMOIDECTOMY

Operative approach to and removal of disease in the maxillary and ethmoid sinuses and in adjacent structures such as the sphenoid sinus, orbit, and pituitary fossa

Indications
1. Chronic, advanced hyperplastic sinusitis
2. Transantral removal of benign tumors
3. Transantral approach for sphenoid sinus disease, orbital wall decompression in Graves' disease, and transsphenoidal hypophysectomy
4. Transantral approach for removing foreign bodies

Contraindications
1. Children with unerupted permanent maxillary teeth

Special Considerations
1. Type and extent of previous sinus surgery
2. History of asthma or aspirin sensitivity
3. Preoperative status of ophthalmologic function

Preoperative Preparation
1. Coronal computed tomography scan without contrast

Special Instruments, Position, and Anesthesia
1. Headlight, surgical loupes, binocular operating microscope
2. A 15° reverse Trendelenburg position
3. General anesthesia
4. Drape the eyes into the operative field.
5. Turnbull self-retaining tractor, Gruenwald or Wilde straight and up-biting ethmoid forceps, Hajek sphenoid punch, Kerrison rongeur, monopolar or bipolar cautery

Tips and Pearls
1. Preserve a 1-cm cuff of mucosa above the gingivobuccal incision.
2. Preserve a bony rim around the infraorbital foramen while removing the anterior maxillary bony wall.
3. Enter the ethmoid labyrinth through the posterosuperior portion of the medial maxillary sinus wall.
4. If there is anterior ethmoid disease, it must be dealt with through an intranasal approach.
5. The roof of the ethmoid inclines inferiorly from anterior to posterior.
6. Preserve the middle turbinate if possible.
7. The attachment of the middle turbinate is the safe boundary for medial dissection and avoidance of the cribriform plate.

Pitfalls and Complications
1. Hemorrhage
2. Check for edema or ecchymosis.
3. Numbness in the distribution of the infraorbital nerve
4. Visual loss or blindness
5. Diplopia
6. Cerebrospinal fluid leak
7. Intracranial hemorrhage
8. Epiphora
9. Meningitis

Postoperative Care Issues
1. Postoperative vision checks.
2. Patient should be in semi-Fowler position postoperatively.
3. Cold compresses to the nose and cheek for 24 hours postoperatively
4. Continue antibiotics 3 to 5 days postoperatively.
5. Remove antral packing in 24 to 48 hours and nasal packs 3 to 5 days postoperatively.
6. The patient is instructed to use saline nasal spray several times each day until after the packs are out.
7. Resume steroid nasal spray postoperatively.

References
Friedman WK, Katsantonis GP. Intranasal and transantral ethmoidectomy: a 20-year experience. Laryngoscope 1990;100:343.

Malotte MJ, Petti GH, Chonkich GD, Rowe RP. Transantral sphenoethmoidectomy: a procedure for the 1990s? Otolaryngol Head Neck Surg 1991;104:358.

Operative Procedure

The patient is positioned supine on the operating table in a 10° to 15° reverse Trendelenburg position. Topical decongestion is obtained using a 4% solution of cocaine on cotton pledgets inserted into the nasal cavity. A 1% solution of Xylocaine with a 1:100,000 concentration of epinephrine is used to infiltrate the gingivobuccal sulcus, mucosa of the lateral nasal wall, middle turbinate, and ethmoid block mucosa. Two-inch (5-cm) saline-moistened gauze packing is placed intraorally to prevent blood from running into the hypopharynx.

A 3- to 5-cm incision is made in the gingivobuccal sulcus 1 cm above the fixed gingival margin in the canine fossa (Fig. 341-1). The periosteum of the anterior maxillary wall is elevated sharply until the infraorbital foramen is identified. The anterolateral bony wall of the maxilla is entered with a 4-mm chisel and mallet or with a cutting bur. The wall is removed generously with the cutting bur or Kerrison rongeur. It is helpful to remove bone as high as possible, especially superomedially, while preserving the bone around the infraorbital foramen (Fig. 341-2).

Using a headlight (with or without surgical loupes) or the binocular microscope, the maxillary sinus mucosa is inspected. Irreversibly diseased mucosa is removed with Coakley antral curets or Gruenwald forceps. Mucosa that appears normal or only slightly edematous is left in place. The middle and posterior ethmoid cells are entered by removing the posterosuperior portion of the medial wall of the antrum with a Gruenwald or Wilde forceps (Fig. 341-3). In patients with extensive polypoid ethmoid disease, there is frequently only a membranous wall between the maxillary and ethmoid sinuses. The ethmoid cells are cleaned of polyps and diseased mucosa using the straight and up-biting Gruenwald forceps in a stripping rather than a biting motion, working posteriorly until the anterior wall of the sphenoid sinus is reached.

The lateral extent of the dissection is indicated by the location of the superior extent of the medial wall of the antrum. If the middle turbinate is not involved by polypoid degeneration, it is preserved because it serves as a landmark for the medial extent of the dissection. If removal of the middle turbinate is necessary, it is removed with the Gruenwald forceps and a Knight nasal scissors, taking care to preserve the superior 0.5 to 1 cm to serve as a landmark for any later surgical approach. The cribriform plate is protected by not working medial to the attachment of the middle turbinate and not rocking the middle turbinate when removing the lower portion of it (Fig. 341-4).

The ethmoid cells are opened in a posterior direction until the anterior wall of the sphenoid sinus is reached. The average distance from the nasal spine to the anterior wall of the sphenoid sinus is 7 cm. The sphenoid sinus is entered only if it is involved by the disease.

The anterosuperior portion of the medial maxillary wall is removed with a Kerrison rongeur or Hajek sphenoid punch. To do a complete anterior ethmoidectomy, cells anterior to the nasolacrimal duct should be removed by an intranasal approach using an up-biting Gruenwald forceps to open the agger nasi and infundibular cells, as necessary (Fig. 341-5). After all ethmoid cells are opened and the bone fragments and diseased mucosa are removed, a nasoantral window is fashioned by removing the inferior medial antral wall with a Kerrison rongeur. Another option is to remove the entire medial antral bony wall, making one large communication with the nasal cavity (Fig. 341-6). The maxillary sinus is packed with antibiotic-impregnated 0.5-in (12-mm) gauze brought into the nose through the nasoantral window. The ethmoid cavity and nose are packed with additional 0.5-in (12-mm) antibiotic-impregnated packing. The pharynx is suctioned free of old blood, a 2 × 2 gauze pad is taped over the nostril, and the globe on the operated side is palpated for signs of excessive tension. In the recovery room, the eyes are checked for visual acuity and extraocular motion.

Postoperatively, elevate the head of bed and use iced saline gauze pads for the first 24 hours. The packs are left in place 3 to 5 days, and antibiotics are continued until the packs are removed. The patient is instructed to use saline nasal spray several times each day until the nasal crusting has subsided.

GEORGE D. CHONKICH

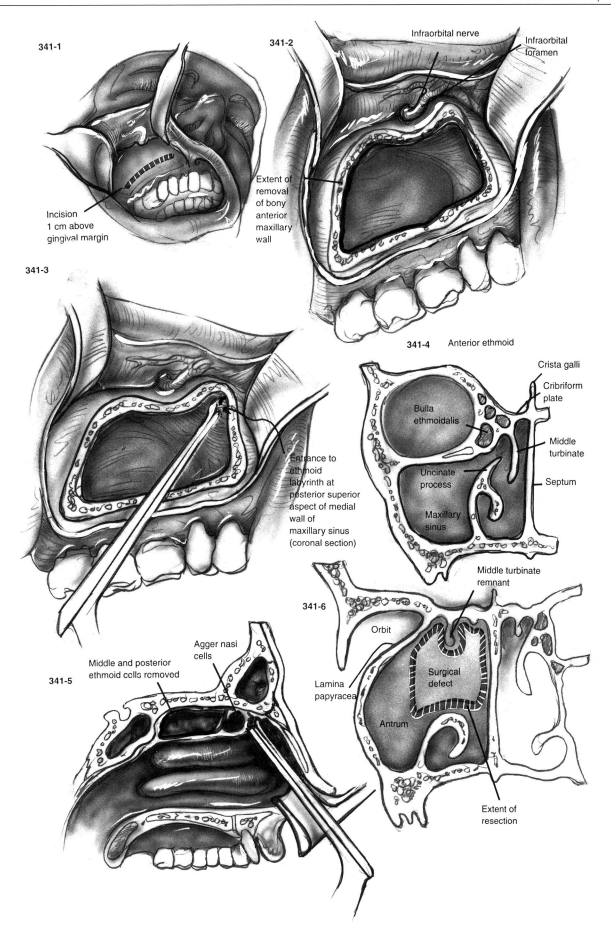

341-1

Incision
1 cm above
gingival margin

341-2

Infraorbital nerve

Infraorbital
foramen

Extent of
removal
of bony
anterior
maxillary
wall

341-3

Entrance to
ethmoid
labyrinth at
posterior superior
aspect of medial
wall of
maxillary sinus
(coronal section)

341-4   Anterior ethmoid

Crista galli

Cribriform
plate

Bulla
ethmoidalis

Middle
turbinate

Uncinate
process

Septum

Maxillary
sinus

341-6

Middle turbinate
remnant

Orbit

Lamina
papyracea

Surgical
defect

Antrum

Extent of
resection

341-5

Middle and posterior
ethmoid cells removed

Agger nasi
cells

■ *342.* INTRANASAL SPHENOIDECTOMY

Transnasal opening of the sphenoid sinus to promote drainage of its contents into the nasopharynx

Indications

1. Sphenoid sinusitis
2. Sphenoid mucocele
3. Neoplastic disease within the sphenoid sinus, such as inverting papilloma
4. Traumatic cerebrospinal fluid rhinorrhea originating in the sphenoid

Special Considerations

1. The sphenoid is the "silent sinus." The disease typically presents with unusual headaches of recent origin.
2. Acute sinusitis with impending neurologic complications, such as meningitis that requires immediate surgical drainage
3. Obtain appropriate imaging with computed tomography scans.
4. Previous septal surgery

Preoperative Preparation

1. Routine laboratory studies
2. Bleeding and clotting studies, if the patient's history is questionable
3. Trial of intravenous antibiotics for persistently symptomatic sinusitis if complications are not impending

Special Instruments, Positions, and Anesthesia

1. Headlight
2. Septoplasty set
3. Spurling rongeurs
4. Hardy speculum
5. Head slightly extended, with the head of the bed slightly elevated
6. Solution of 1% lidocaine with a 1:100,000 dilution of epinephrine and 0.05% oxymetazoline (Afrin) for nasal vasoconstriction

Tips and Pearls

1. Maintain the midline as a guide to the sphenoid.
2. Elevate the septal and nasal mucosa widely for adequate exposure.
3. The front face of the sphenoid sinus is typically 7 cm deep from the nasal spine at an angle of 30° from the floor of the nose.
4. The sphenoid septum is not always midline or singular, resulting in confusion about the completeness of the drainage. A computed tomography scan is a helpful guide.
5. Remove both sides of the posterior septal mucosa that covers the front face of the sphenoid for wide-open drainage.

Pitfalls and Complications

1. Loss of midline, resulting in injury to the carotid artery, cavernous sinus, or optic nerves
2. Laceration of the septal mucoperiosteum and chondrium, resulting in septal perforation
3. Postoperative epistaxis
4. Postoperative cerebrospinal fluid rhinorrhea
5. Loss of columellar skin
6. Numbness of the upper incisors

Postoperative Care Issues

1. Bilateral nasal packing of antibiotic impregnated ribbon gauze for 24 hours postoperatively
2. Perioperative systemic antibiotics
3. Attention to epistaxis after removal of packing
4. Removal of columellar sutures 5 days after surgery

References

Reese BR, Koltai PJ, Parnes SM, Decker JW. The external rhinoplasty approach for rhinologic surgery. Ear Nose Throat J 1992;71:408.

Sawyer R. Nasal approaches to the sphenoid sinus after prior septal surgery. Laryngoscope 1991;101:89.

Operative Procedures

Orotracheal intubation is used, and the patient is positioned in the usual fashion for rhinologic surgery, with the patient's head slightly extended and the head of the table slightly elevated. A pharyngeal pack is placed. Cottonoid pledgets are soaked in a solution of 0.05% oxymetazoline hydrochloride and placed into the nose for vasoconstriction. A solution of 1% lidocaine with a 1:100,000 dilution of epinephrine is infiltrated into the columellar skin, the intercrural area of the dome, both sides of the cartilaginous and bony septum, and the floor of the nose. A standard external rhinoplasty inverted-V incision is made (Fig. 342-1) and the "elephant trunk" is raised onto the dome of the nose (Fig. 342-2). The elevation is done midway over the lower lateral cartilages, because complete exposure of the lateral crura and the upper lateral cartilages is unnecessary. The intercrural ligaments between the medial crura are separated, exposing the caudal edge of the quadrilateral cartilage (Fig. 342-3). The mucoperichondral flap on one side of the quadrilateral cartilage is developed and continued over the perpendicular plate of the ethmoid and vomer.

The dissection proceeds onto the maxillary crest and the floor of the nose, connecting the medial and inferior tunnels. The quadrilateral cartilage is detached posteriorly at the bony cartilaginous junction, and the mucoperiosteum on the other side of the ethmoid and vomer is elevated. The quadrilateral cartilage is disarticulated from the maxillary crest (Fig. 342-4). The mucoperiosteal elevation is continued on the maxillary crest and the floor of the nose on the opposite side. The Hardy speculum is inserted, displacing the septal leaflets laterally. The perpendicular plate of the ethmoid is resected, taking care to preserve the vomer, which serves as an excellent midline guide to the anterior face of the sphenoid. The anterior sphenoid sinus wall is opened with a chisel, the opening is enlarged with a Spurling rongeur, and the intersinus septum is removed. The diseased sinus mucosa is exenterated (Fig. 342-5).

After drainage of the sinus has been completed, the Hardy speculum is removed using a long, hand-held nasal speculum. The mucosa that overlays what was the anterior face of the sphenoid is removed from one side and then from the other. This creates a large posterior and superior septal perforation, allowing the sphenoid contents to drain into the nasopharynx (Fig. 342-6). The septal flaps are then swung back into the midline and approximated with continuous mattress transfixion sutures of 4-0 plain catgut on a mini-Keith needle. Septal splints of Silastic sheeting are placed on either side of the septum and sewn into place with a 2-0 nylon suture. The medial crura are reapproximated with a transfixion suture of 4-0 chromic catgut. The columella incision is closed using 5-0 nylon. The nose is packed with antibiotic-coated ribbon gauze, which is removed the following morning. The sutures are removed from the columella 5 days after surgery.

PETER J. KOLTAI

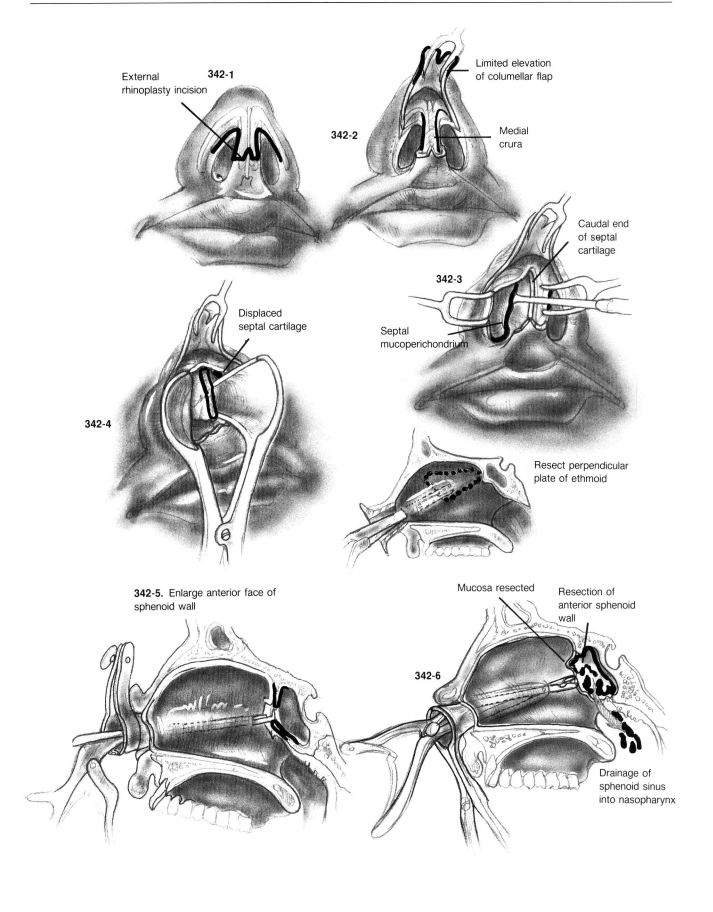

342-1

External rhinoplasty incision

342-2

Limited elevation of columellar flap

Medial crura

342-3

Caudal end of septal cartilage

Septal mucoperichondrium

342-4

Displaced septal cartilage

Resect perpendicular plate of ethmoid

342-5. Enlarge anterior face of sphenoid wall

342-6

Mucosa resected

Resection of anterior sphenoid wall

Drainage of sphenoid sinus into nasopharynx

■ *343.* TRANSETHMOIDAL SPHENOIDECTOMY

Removal of the ethmoidal bony septa and sphenoid sinus contents through an external approach, resulting in the creation of an ethmosphenoid cavity

Indications

1. Indications for external ethmoidectomy with extension of disease to the sphenoid sinus
2. Recurrent ethmosphenoid disease and a history of previous intranasal procedures resulting in a lack of intranasal landmarks
3. Pituitary tumor; an external transethmosphenoidal hypophysectomy is possible but not popular because of the increased risk of complications from its extraaxial approach

Special Considerations

1. Visual acuity check
2. Bleeding or clotting abnormalities
3. Confirmation of sphenoid pneumatization and the presence and location of an intersinus septum

Preoperative Preparation

1. Computed tomography scan of the paranasal sinuses
2. Routine laboratory tests, including bleeding and clotting studies (if the history is questionable)

Special Instruments, Position, and Anesthesia

1. Headlight
2. Beaded nasal measurement probe
3. Microscope with a 300-mm lens and fluoroscopy should be available.

Tips and Pearls

1. Local infiltration to assist in hemostasis
2. Gentle retraction of the orbit
3. Use of the endoscope for intranasal assessment
4. Careful assessment of the sphenoid lateral walls and roof

Pitfalls and Complications

1. Hemorrhage from the posterior ethmoid or internal carotid arteries
2. Intraoperative or postoperative retroorbital hematoma
3. Injury to optic nerve
4. Damage to the contents of the cavernous sinus
5. Intracranial extension with cerebrospinal fluid leak
6. Difficult access to the agger nasi cells and frontal recess

Postoperative Care Issues

1. Visual acuity check
2. Neurologic status
3. Wound care and nasal hygiene

References

Blitzer A, Lawson W, Friedman WH. Surgery of the paranasal sinuses. 2nd ed. Philadelphia: WB Saunders, 1991:219.

James JA. Transethmosphenoidal hypophysectomy. Arch Otolaryngol 1967;86:32.

Operative Procedure

After general endotracheal anesthesia has been established, the table is positioned with the patient's head elevated, slightly flexed, and turned toward the surgeon. The eyes are protected with lubricant and a tarsorrhaphy stitch. The area of the planned incision is injected with a lidocaine and epinephrine mixture, usually a 1% solution of lidocaine with a 1:100,000 concentration of epinephrine, as are other intranasal structures that are to be resected, such as the septum or turbinates. The nose is packed with cottonoid pledgets soaked in Neo-Synephrine or cocaine solution (usually 4c mL of a 4% solution). The face is prepped with antiseptic solution and draped in a standard fashion, exposing the nose, eye, and forehead.

The typical incision is curvilinear, extending from just below the eyebrow inferiorly along the lateral nasal wall, halfway between the inner canthus and the dorsum of the nose (Fig. 343-1). The incision can be extended laterally into the brow for frontal exposure to accomplish a frontoethmoidectomy and can be carried inferiorly into the melonasal and nostril margin for a lateral rhinotomy.

The periosteum is elevated along the lateral aspect of the lacrimal and ethmoid bone, gently retracting the orbital contents while not violating the periorbita (Fig. 343-2). For adequate exposure during the external approach, it may be necessary to mobilize the lacrimal sac from the surrounding anterior and posterior lacrimal crests and to incise the medial canthal ligament at its attachment to the anterior lacrimal crest. It is important to reattach the ligament at the completion of the procedure to prevent blunting or telecanthus. Blunt dissection is used to reveal the lamina papyracea and frontoethmoid suture line. Approximately 24 mm posterior to the adult posterior lacrimal crest, the anterior ethmoid artery is encountered. This artery is routinely clipped or electrocoagulated and divided. The posterior ethmoid artery (approximately 12 mm posterior to the anterior vessel) typically does not need to be ligated, and its preservation may help in avoiding damage to the optic nerve, which is approximately 6 mm posterior to the posterior ethmoid artery.

The operative field is then fully visualized, exposing the lacrimal bone, frontal process of maxilla, lamina papyracea, and orbital process of frontal bone. A mallet and gouge is used to enter the ethmoid cells through the lacrimal fossa and then widened with a rongeur (Fig. 343-3). The frontoethmoid suture line is an important landmark for identifying the level of the anterior cranial fossa. The ethmoid cells are removed sequentially, anteriorly and posteriorly, and the anterior wall of the sphenoid sinus is identified (Fig. 343-4). Medial cells are removed to expose the nasal cavity, and if the middle turbinate is diseased or obstructing the view, it can also be removed. If the middle turbinate is taken down, the cribriform plate mus not be disrupted.

If the entire anterior wall of the sphenoid sinus is to be exposed, the posterior one third of the septum is fenestrated to allow access to the opposite anterior sphenoid wall. Before entering the anterior wall, the exact position can be confirmed by fluoroscopy, if needed, and an operating microscope with 300-mm objective lens can be used. The anterior wall of the sphenoid sinus is thicker and harder than the bony lamellas of the ethmoidal cells and can be removed with a curet, chisel, or drill. After the sphenoid sinus has been entered, the diseased mucosa or tumor is removed carefully. Lateral and superior removal of tissue within the sinus should only be performed under good visualization to guard against possible neurologic and vascular complications. The intersinus septum may cause problems when using the transethmoidal approach, because with this extraaxial approach the heterolateral sinus cavity can be entered and the intersinus septum may be mistaken for the lateral wall of the sphenoid sinus. If a hypophysectomy is to be performed, the posterior wall of the sphenoid is carefully removed with the assistance of fluoroscopy.

After all diseased soft tissue and bone are resected, the nose is lightly packed with 0.5-in (12-mm) petrolatum gauze impregnated with antiseptic ointment. A drain is unnecessary. The periosteum and subcutaneous tissues are reapproximated with 3-0 absorbable sutures. Skin closure is accomplished with 6-0 nylon or mild chromic sutures, an ice pack is applied, and the head is kept elevated.

RAY L. WEISS

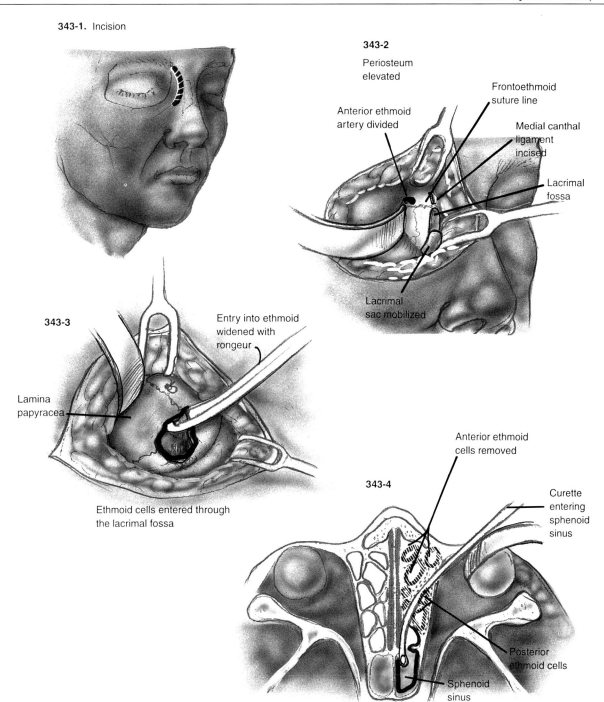

343-1. Incision

343-2
Periosteum
elevated

Anterior ethmoid
artery divided

Frontoethmoid
suture line

Medial canthal
ligament
incised

Lacrimal
fossa

Lacrimal
sac mobilized

343-3

Entry into ethmoid
widened with
rongeur

Lamina
papyracea

Ethmoid cells entered through
the lacrimal fossa

Anterior ethmoid
cells removed

343-4

Curette
entering
sphenoid
sinus

Posterior
ethmoid cells

Sphenoid
sinus

Entry into anterior
wall of sphenoid sinus

■ *344.* TRANSSPHENOIDAL HYPOPHYSEC-TOMY

—Surgical removal of the pituitary gland by a midline transnasal approach through the sphenoid sinus

Indications

1. Enlargement or dysfunction of the gland from pituitary adenoma, craniopharyngioma, or other neoplastic process

Special Considerations

1. Appropriate imaging with computed tomography and magnetic resonance imaging
2. Previous septal surgery
3. Nasal infection

Preoperative Preparation

1. Hormonal replacement
2. Routine laboratory studies
3. Bleeding and clotting studies, if the patient's history is questionable

Special Instruments, Position, and Anesthesia

1. Fluoroscopy unit with C-arm
2. Headlights
3. Septoplasty set
4. Spurling rongeurs
5. Hardy speculum
6. Surgical microscope for the neurosurgical team
7. Head slightly extended and secured with pins
8. Solution of 1% lidocaine with a 1:100,000 dilution of epinephrine and 0.05% oxymetazoline (Afrin) for nasal vasoconstriction

Tips and Pearls

1. Maintain the midline as a guide to the sphenoid
2. Elevate the septal and nasal mucosa as wide as the nose allows to prevent tearing.
3. The front face of the sphenoid sinus is typically 7 cm deep from the nasal spine at an angle of 30° from the floor of the nose.
4. Remove front face of the sphenoid intact, and use this bone later for closure.
5. The sphenoid septum is not always midline or singular, resulting in confusion about the position of the sella turcica. Use computed tomography scans as a guide.

Pitfalls and Complications

1. Loss of midline resulting in injury to the carotid artery, cavernous sinus or optic nerves
2. Laceration of the septal mucoperiosteum and perichondrium resulting in septal perforation
3. Postoperative epistaxis
4. Postoperative cerebrospinal fluid rhinorrhea
5. Loss of columellar skin
6. Numbness of the upper teeth

Postoperative Care Issues

1. Postoperative neurosurgical intensive care unit monitoring for 48 hours
2. Bilateral nasal packing of antibiotic-impregnated ribbon gauze for 4 days
3. Perioperative systemic antibiotics given while the nose is packed
4. After removal of the packing, careful attention to epistaxis and cerebrospinal fluid rhinorrhea
5. Endocrine management of the patient
6. Removal of the columellar sutures 5 days after surgery

References

Hardy J. Transsphenoidal hypophysectomy. J Neurosurg 1971;34:582.
Koltai PJ, Goufman DB, Parnes SM, Steiniger JR. Transsphenoidal hypophysectomy through the external rhinoplasty approach. Otolaryngol Head Neck Surg 1994;111:197.

Operative Procedures

Orotracheal intubation is used, and the patient is placed in the supine position, with the head slightly extended and secured with pins. The patient's face is prepared and draped with only the midfacial region exposed. The towels are sutured to the face, because towel clips tend to interfere with fluoroscopy. A pharyngeal pack is placed in the oropharynx. Saline-soaked cottonoid pledgets impregnated with a 0.05% solution of oxymetazoline (Afrin) are placed in the nose for vasoconstriction. A solution of 1% lidocaine with a 1:100,000 dilution of epinephrine is infiltrated into the columellar skin, intercrural area of the dome, both sides of the cartilaginous and bony septum, and the floor of the nose.

A standard external inverted-V rhinoplasty incision is made (Fig. 344-1) and the "elephant trunk" columella flap is raised. The elevation is done midway over the lower lateral cartilages, because complete exposure of the lateral crura and upper lateral cartilages is unnecessary (Fig. 344-2). The intercrural ligaments between the medial crura are sharply separated, exposing the caudal edge of the quadrilateral cartilage (Fig. 344-3). The mucoperichondrial flap on one side of the cartilage is developed and continued over the perpendicular plate of the ethmoid and vomer. The dissection proceeds onto the maxillary crest and the floor of the nose, connecting the medial and inferior tunnels. The quadrilateral cartilage is detached posteriorly at the bony cartilaginous junction, and the mucoperiosteum on the other side of the ethmoid and vomer is elevated. The quadrilateral cartilage is disarticulated from the maxillary crest (Fig. 344-4). The mucoperiosteal elevation is continued on the maxillary crest and the floor of the nose on the opposite side. The Hardy speculum is inserted, displacing the septal leaflets laterally. The perpendicular plate of the ethmoid is resected, taking care to preserve the vomer, which serves as an excellent midline guide to the anterior face of the sphenoid. The anterior sphenoid wall is removed using a 4-mm osteotome and mallet, and the opening is enlarged using a Spurling rongeur (Fig. 344-5). The intersinus septum, which is rarely in the midline, is removed, and the sinus mucosa is exenterated.

A neurosurgeon then performs the pituitary surgery with the use of the operating microscope. With the hypophysectomy completed, the sphenoid sinus is obliterated with fat, fascia, or muscle, and its anterior wall is reconstructed with the cartilage and bone previously harvested from the septum.

The septal flaps are swung into the midline and reapproximated with a continuous mattress transfixion suture of 4.0 plain catgut on a mini-Keith needle. Septal splints of Silastic sheeting are placed on either side of the septum and sewn into place with 2.0 nylon sutures. The medial crura are reapproximated with a transfixion suture of 4.0 chromic catgut, and the columellar incision is closed using 5.0 nylon suture. The nose is packed with antibiotic-impregnated gauze that is removed in 4 days.

PETER J. KOLTAI

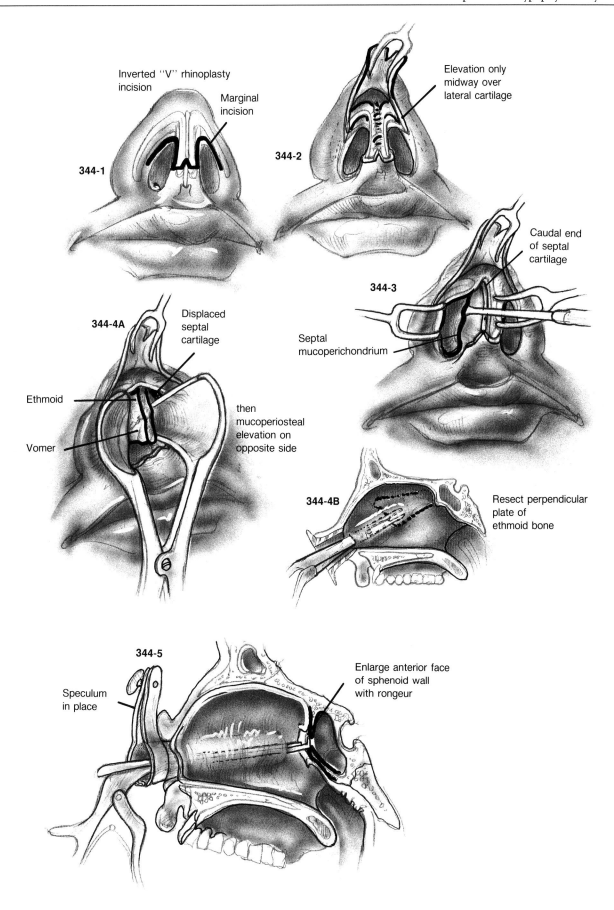

344-1

Inverted "V" rhinoplasty incision

Marginal incision

344-2

Elevation only midway over lateral cartilage

344-3

Caudal end of septal cartilage

Septal mucoperichondrium

344-4A

Displaced septal cartilage

Ethmoid

Vomer

then mucoperiosteal elevation on opposite side

344-4B

Resect perpendicular plate of ethmoid bone

344-5

Speculum in place

Enlarge anterior face of sphenoid wall with rongeur

■ *345.* LIGATION OF THE ANTERIOR ETHMOID ARTERY—Open surgical ligation of the anterior ethmoid artery to control bleeding in the superior aspect of the nose

Indications

1. Control of refractory bleeding coming from the superior portion of the nose in the distribution of the anterior ethmoid artery
2. Patients who are at risk for complications (eg, chronic pulmonary, cardiovascular, or central nervous system disease) from nasal packing

Special Considerations

1. Age of patient
2. Hypertension
3. Atherosclerosis or cardiovascular disease
4. Pulmonary disease
5. Aspirin use or coagulopathy
6. Visual acuity
7. Significant blood loss (eg, anemia, hypovolemia)

Preoperative Preparation

1. Visual acuity evaluation
2. Localization of the bleeding site
3. Bleeding and coagulation studies
4. Routine laboratory evaluations, as indicated
5. Electrocardiogram and chest radiograph

Special Instruments, Position, and Anesthesia

1. Headlight
2. Microsurgical loupes (optional)
3. Small malleable ribbon retractors, Sewall retractors
4. Bipolar cautery
5. Neurosurgical clips
6. Freer elevator
7. Corneal shield

Pitfalls and Complications

1. Postoperative bleeding
2. Orbital hematoma
3. Optic nerve injury
4. Corneal injury
5. Hypertrophic scarring

Tips and Pearls

1. Localization of the bleeding site is imperative for the proper treatment of epistaxis.
2. Fiberoptic endoscopes may be useful in determining the site of bleeding.
3. Recognize the proximity of the optic nerve to the posterior ethmoid artery.
4. Use a corneal shield or temporary tarsorrhaphy.
5. Meticulous hemostasis of the operative site is essential.
6. Elevation of the head, preoperative steroids, and a light compression dressing reduce swelling and ecchymosis.

Postoperative Care Issues

1. The patient should be watched closely and monitored for hypertension and recurrent bleeding.
2. Check visual acuity and evaluate for proptosis or development of an orbital hematoma in the postoperative period.
3. Consider ligation of the posterior ethmoid artery if bleeding persists after ligation of the anterior ethmoid artery.
4. Consider transantral ligation of the internal maxillary artery if bleeding persists after ethmoid artery ligation.
5. Supportive treatment should include monitoring of ongoing blood loss and hematocrit, maintenance of adequate oxygen tension, and blood pressure regulation.

References

Maris CR, Werth JL. Surgical management (epistaxis). Ear Nose Throat J 1981;60:463.

Montgomery WW, Reardon EJ. Early vessel ligations for control of severe epistaxis. In: Snow JB, ed. Controversy in otolaryngology. Philadelphia: WB Saunders, 1980:315.

Operative Procedure

The patient is placed in the supine position and general endotracheal anesthesia is established. A Lynch incision is delineated between the medial canthus and the midline of the nose (Fig. 345-1). The overlying tissue may be injected with a local anesthetic containing a 1:100,000 concentration of epinephrine.

An incision is made through the skin and subcutaneous tissue to the periosteum. The periosteum is elevated anteriorly and posteriorly. If the angular vein is encountered, it should be ligated and divided (Fig. 345-2). Focal bleeding may be controlled with bipolar cautery. The periosteum is elevated from the bone, and the lacrimal sac and orbital periosteum are retracted laterally. The lacrimal crest and lacrimal fossa are identified. The dissection is carried posteriorly, and the frontoethmoid suture line is identified (Fig. 345-3). This is followed posteriorly until the anterior ethmoid artery is identified.

The artery may be controlled with bipolar cautery, double ligation with suture material, or neurosurgical clips (Fig. 345-4). Larger vessels should be controlled by ligation. In most instances, it is not necessary to divide the posterior ethmoid artery. If it seems advisable to ligate the posterior ethmoid artery because of continued bleeding, the vessel may be located by dissecting further posteriorly, approximately 10 mm. The optic nerve lies only 5 mm posterior to the posterior ethmoidal foramen (Figs. 345-4 and 345-5). The periosteum is reapproximated with 4-0 chromic sutures and the skin with a 6-0 monofilament suture.

A moderate pressure dressing may be applied to prevent edema and ecchymosis around the eye. Postoperative elevation of the head of the bed also helps prevent postoperative swelling. A single intravenous dose of dexamethasone (20 to 30 mg) given preoperatively may also help prevent postoperative swelling and pain. If there is evidence of continued bleeding at the end of this procedure, ligation of the internal maxillary artery may be indicated. Localization of the bleeding site is essential to determine the optimal treatment, and fiberoptic endoscopes may be useful in identifying obscure bleeding sites.

JOHN S. MAY

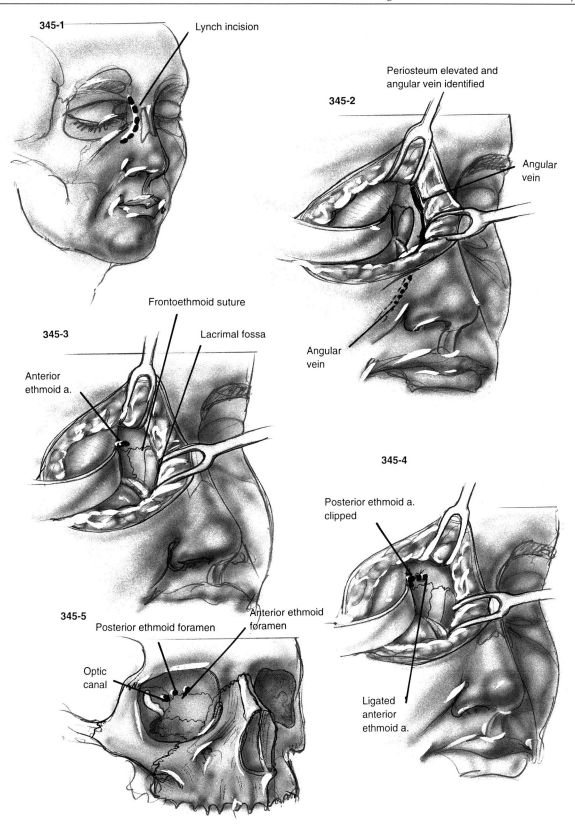

345-1 Lynch incision

345-2 Periosteum elevated and angular vein identified

Angular vein

Angular vein

345-3 Frontoethmoid suture

Lacrimal fossa

Anterior ethmoid a.

345-4 Posterior ethmoid a. clipped

Ligated anterior ethmoid a.

345-5 Posterior ethmoid foramen

Anterior ethmoid foramen

Optic canal

■ *346.* MAXILLARY DECOMPRESSION FOR EXOPHTHALMUS— Removal of the medial and inferior orbital walls through a transantral ethmoidectomy approach

Indications

1. Graves' ophthalmopathy with optic neuropathy
2. Proptosis with exposure keratopathy
3. Proptosis with severe cosmetic deformity and diplopia

Special Considerations

1. Optimal preoperative management of thyroid and cardiovascular status
2. Associated sinusitis
3. Previous sinus surgery

Preoperative Preparation

1. Ophthalmologic examination for optic neuropathy, including visual acuity, visual fields, color vision, and pupillary responses
2. Assessment of proptosis by means of exophthalmometry, ocular motility studies, and intraocular pressure measurement
3. Assessment of bony anatomy by computed tomography

Special Instruments, Position, and Anesthesia

1. Headlight
2. Sinus endoscopes may be used for better visualization
3. Small osteotomes and periosteal elevators
4. Small sickle knife

Tips and Pearls

1. Create an inferior meatus antrostomy to decrease the likelihood of sinusitis.
2. Avoid incising the periorbita until all bone removal is completed.
3. Perioperative steroids are administered to reduce surgical edema.

Pitfalls and Complications

1. Infraorbital nerve numbness and hypesthesia
2. Cerebrospinal fluid leak and meningitis
3. Oroantral fistula
4. Lacrimal sac injury and epiphora
5. Orbital hematoma and blindness

Postoperative Care Issues

1. Up to 50% rate of postoperative strabismus (medial entropion), which may require corrective surgery
2. Increased incidence of postoperative sinusitis; patients should be treated with antibiotics during the healing phase.
3. Patients should be told to expect temporary numbness in the distribution of the infraorbital nerve.

References

Girod DA, Orcutt JC, Cummings CW. Orbital decompression for preservation of vision in Graves' ophthalmopathy. Arch Otolaryngol Head Neck Surg 1993;119:229.

Warren JD, Spector JG, Burde R. Long-term follow-up and recent observations on 305 cases of orbital decompression for dysthyroidal orbitopathy. Laryngoscope 1989;99:35.

Operative Procedure

The patient is positioned in a semisitting attitude, and the nasal cavity is prepared with a topical decongestant (Fig. 346-1). The sublabial creases, both inferior meatus, and the uncinate processes are injected with a 1% solution of lidocaine with epinephrine.

Bilateral Caldwell-Luc procedures are carried out, including inferior meatus antrostomies. The infraorbital nerves are carefully preserved. Bilateral transantral ethmoidectomies are then performed (Fig. 346-2). Sinus endoscopes may be used to ensure complete exenteration of all ethmoid cells and to better define and preserve anatomic boundaries, such as the fovea ethmoidalis.

A small, sharp osteotome is used to crack the inferomedial orbital wall. Using the infraorbital nerve as a lateral limit, bone fragments are carefully removed using small periosteal elevators, curved curets, and sinus forceps. The lateral wall of the ethmoid sinus (lamina papyracea) is removed in a similar fashion, keeping intact the underlying periorbita (Fig. 346-4). The thicker bony strut between the orbital floor and lateral ethmoid wall may require further use of an osteotome or drill for removal (Fig. 346-3). Some surgeons advocate preserving this strut for cases with mild or no optic neuropathy to lessen the incidence of postoperative medial entropion.

Beginning at the most posterosuperior aspect of the medial orbit, a small sickle knife is used to make longitudinal periosteal incisions from back to front along the axis of the orbit (Fig. 346-5). Several incisions are made, proceeding inferiorly and laterally until orbital fat is seen to prolapse into the ethmoid and maxillary sinuses. Gentle pressure on the orbits, while observing fat prolapse into the sinuses (Fig. 346-6), helps to demonstrate areas where further periosteal division is necessary. Starting the periosteal incisions medially and superiorly helps to ensure that prolapsing orbital fat does not block visualization as the operation progresses. The overall fat prolapse and decompression on each side is based on judgments made from orbital palpation, visual inspection for symmetry, and further exophthalmometry (if desired).

Intraoperative hemostasis is maintained with intermittent use of oxymetazoline-soaked cotton pledgets and with careful use of cautery. Gauze packing is avoided unless absolutely necessary for hemostasis. Postoperatively, the patient is maintained in a head-elevated position, and steroids are continued for a few days to minimize edema.

SCOTT C. MANNING

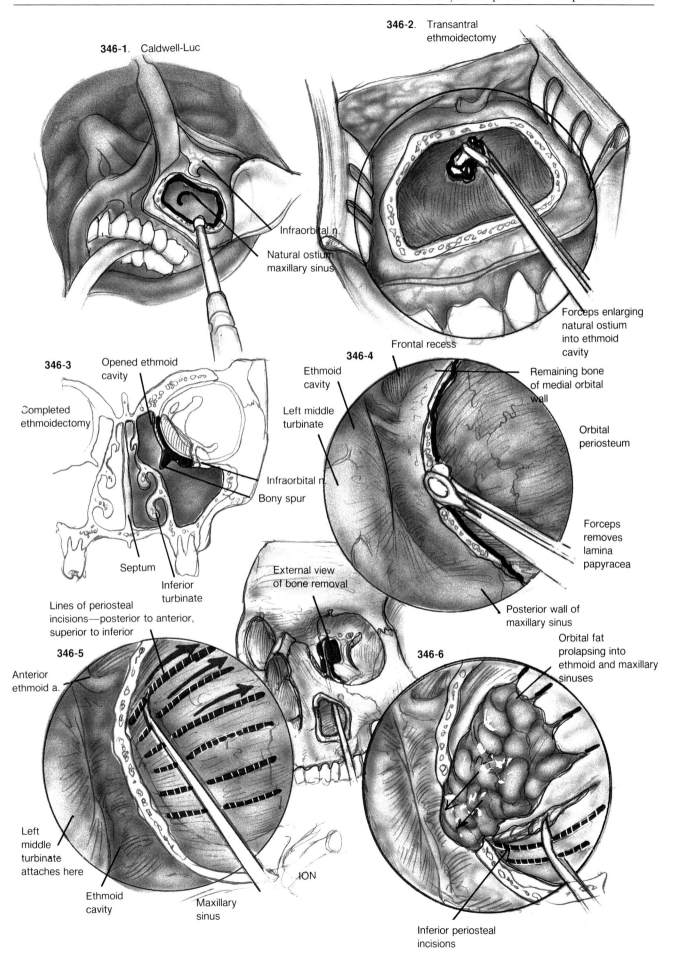

346-1. Caldwell-Luc

Infraorbital n.

Natural ostium maxillary sinus

346-2. Transantral ethmoidectomy

Forceps enlarging natural ostium into ethmoid cavity

346-3

Opened ethmoid cavity

Completed ethmoidectomy

Infraorbital n.

Bony spur

Septum

Inferior turbinate

Lines of periosteal incisions—posterior to anterior, superior to inferior

346-4

Frontal recess

Ethmoid cavity

Left middle turbinate

Remaining bone of medial orbital wall

Orbital periosteum

Forceps removes lamina papyracea

Posterior wall of maxillary sinus

Orbital fat prolapsing into ethmoid and maxillary sinuses

External view of bone removal

346-5

Anterior ethmoid a.

Left middle turbinate attaches here

Ethmoid cavity

Maxillary sinus

ION

346-6

Inferior periosteal incisions

■ 347. MIDFACIAL DEGLOVING PROCE-
DURE—Surgical exposure of the midface region and anterior midline skull base, including the nasal fossae, nasal and perinasal bone and soft tissue, nasopharynx, maxillary, ethmoid and sphenoid sinuses, and clivus

Indications

1. Selected cases of extensive infectious or allergic paranasal sinus disease
2. Extensive paranasal sinus fungal infection (eg, *Mucor, Aspergillus*)
3. Inverted papilloma
4. Selected cases of nasopharyngeal angiofibroma
5. Selected benign neoplasms accessible by this approach, such as minor salivary gland tumors, fibrous dysplasia, glioma, schwannoma and neurofibroma, aggressive fibromatosis, chondroma, and benign vascular neoplasms such as hemangioma and hemangiopericytoma
6. When adequate margins are attainable, selected low-grade malignant neoplasms, such as adenoid cystic carcinoma, mucoepidermoid carcinoma and other minor salivary gland malignant neoplasms, fibrosarcoma, and chondrosarcoma
7. When adequate margins are attainable, selected high-grade malignant neoplasms, such as squamous cell carcinoma of the nasal septum, anterior and inferior maxillary sinus, and hard palate; mucoepidermoid carcinoma; adenocarcinoma and other minor salivary gland neoplasms; mucosal melanoma and various soft tissue sarcomas
8. Selected clivus chordomas without lateral extension
9. Selected facial fractures
10. Cranial bone graft reconstruction of bony defects of the midface

Contraindications

1. This approach alone is not adequate for malignant neoplasms involving the orbits or lateral skull base.
2. Tumor extension to the temporal fossa, infratemporal fossa, lateral pharyngeal space, and possibly pterygopalatine fossa
3. For adequate tumor removal, this approach may be combined with other standard approaches such as the extended bicoronal approach to the anterior skull base, lateral transparotid approach, temporal and infratemporal fossa procedures, maxillary osteotomies, mandibular osteotomies, the transpalatal approach, and craniotomy.

Special Considerations

1. Appropriate patient selection, with careful consideration of tumor location, size, and anatomic extent and of tumor histology
2. Avoidance of a facial scar in a child
3. Use of a marginal incision instead of an intercartilaginous incision in children
4. Creation of a small Z-plasty or triangle cut in the floor of the nose to break the main incision line and help prevent postoperative stenosis

(continued)

Operative Procedure

General anesthesia is induced, and a curved RAE endotracheal tube is secured to the midline of the chin. The head is positioned on a foam doughnut or towel rolled at both ends, allowing the head to be rotated from side to side during the operative procedure. As for a standard rhinoplasty, neurosurgical pledgets soaked in a 1% solution of oxymetazoline are placed in both nasal fossae. The nasal septum, columella, dorsum, alar base, gingivobuccal sulcus, and infraorbital regions are injected with a 1% solution of lidocaine with a 1:100,000 concentration of epinephrine. The surgeon's preferred surgical scrub, head drape, and body drape are completed. Suture tarsorrhaphies are placed bilaterally.

Using head illumination and preferably using loupe magnification, the intranasal incisions are scored with a #63 Beaver blade. In adults and adolescents, a standard hemitransfixion incision is completed first, bisecting the caudal cartilaginous septum and membranous septum (Fig. 347-1). An intercartilaginous incision is scored next, with a meticulous connection created with the hemitransfixion incision in the area of the nasal valve. The intercartilaginous incision is continued laterally, following the cephalic border of the lower lateral cartilage and curving inward toward the junction of the vestibule skin and intranasal mucosa. The incision is continued across the floor of the nose, opposite the piriform aperture, and just anterior to the junction of the vestibule skin and intranasal mucosa.

Medially and just before joining the hemitransfixion incision, a small Z-plasty or triangle cut is created to break the incision and help to prevent postoperative stenosis (Fig. 347-2). Identical incisions are scored in the contralateral nostril. Using fine scissors, the soft tissue separating the two hemitransfixion incisions is incised, creating a transfixion incision (Fig. 347-3). Through the the intercartilaginous incisions, Joseph scissors are used to elevate the nasal dorsum soft tissues and the nasal tip, identical to the required step in a standard rhinoplasty (Fig. 347-4). This dissection and elevation should be relatively wide, anticipating future connection to the gingivobuccal dissection. In children, I prefer to maintain the soft tissue connection between the upper and lower lateral cartilages to minimize the possibility of future facial growth disturbance, and the approach is done with marginal incisions (as for external rhinoplasty) instead of intercartilaginous incisions.

(continued)

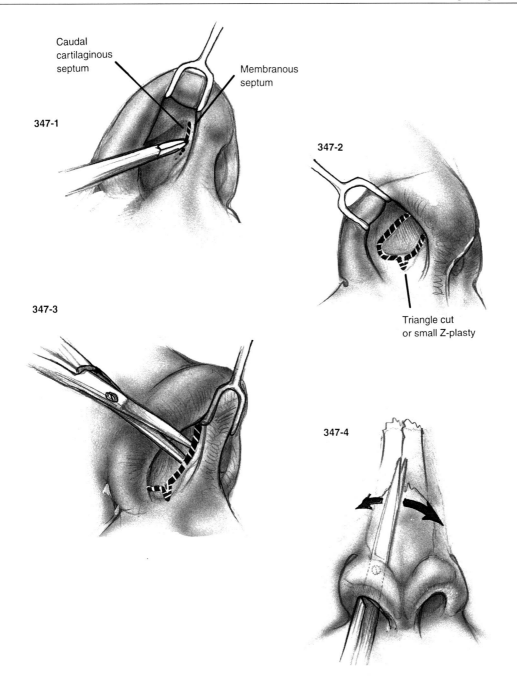

347-1

Caudal
cartilaginous
septum

Membranous
septum

347-2

Triangle cut
or small Z-plasty

347-3

347-4

■ *347.* MIDFACIAL DEGLOVING PROCEDURE
(continued)

Preoperative Preparation

1. Routine laboratory studies
2. Optional computed tomography scan
3. Optional magnetic resonance scan
4. Fiberoptic endoscopy

Special Instruments, Position, and Anesthesia

1. Headlight
2. Loupe magnification
3. Operating microscope
4. Small, delicate plastic or rhinoplasty instruments for intranasal incisions
5. Head stabilized in a foam doughnut or by a rolled towel
6. Bipolar cautery

Tips and Pearls

1. If visualization or exposure becomes inadequate for tumor removal, do not hesitate to add any other facial incisions, such as Sewell, subciliary, subconjunctival, and lateral rhinotomy, that are judged necessary or to use another approach.
2. The plane of dissection over the face of the maxilla may be subperiosteal or supraperiosteal.
3. The infraorbital nerve may be freed from the foramen through osteotomies for improved flap mobility and retraction.
4. Repositioning of the nose and nasal tip and closure of the nasal incisions should be as meticulous and anatomic as possible to achieve the best cosmetic result.

Pitfalls and Complications

1. Possibility of infraorbital or anterior maxillary tooth anesthesia or paresthesia
2. Possibility of stenosis of the nasal vestibule
3. Excessive deposition of healing fibrous tissue over the nose or maxilla that causes a "sneer deformity," which usually resolves
4. Other complications, depending on the anatomic extent or histology of the tumor removed
5. Possible future facial growth disturbance in children

Postoperative Care Issues

1. Packing is removed on the third to fifth postoperative day.
2. Adequate nasal cleaning with nasal saline irrigations and removal of crusts in the postoperative period
3. Intravenous antibiotics are continued until the packing is removed.

References

Manigila AJ. Indications and techniques of midfacial degloving; a 15-year experience. Arch Otolaryngol Head Neck Surg 1986;112:750.
Price JC, Holliday M, Kennedy D, et al. The versatile midfacial degloving approach. Laryngoscope 1986;98:291.

A needlepoint cautery is used to create a gingivobuccal sulcus incision across the midline from maxillary tuberosity to maxillary tuberosity (Fig. 347-5). The incision can be extended past the maxillary tuberosity into the lateral soft palate if more lateral access is required. Working simultaneously from above through the intranasal incisions and below through the gingivobuccal sulcus incisions, soft tissue is dissected to create a free connection between the floor of the nose incisions and the gingivobuccal incision (Fig. 347-6). The soft tissue overlying the anterior maxilla is completed elevated (Fig. 347-7). The dissection may be in the supraperiosteal plane or subperiosteal plane; the choice depends on the lesion or neoplasm to be removed. Dissection is completed superiorly to the infraorbital rims and laterally over the malar buttress and lateral maxilla, with exposure of the pterygomaxillary fissure (ie, entrance to the pterygopalatine fossa). The infraorbital neurovascular bundle is preserved if possible and may be freed from its foramen with osteotomies; this maneuver allows increased flap mobility and easier retraction.

The final dissection involves the release of soft tissue attachments along the lateral border of the piriform aperture, which allows free connection between the nasal dorsum and anterior maxilla; if the dissection over the maxilla has been in the subperiosteal plane, an incision of the periosteum is required (Fig. 347-8). Dissection along the lateral border of the piriform aperture is continued until limited superiorly by the medial canthus and lacrimal apparatus. After the dissection is completed, the nasal tip (including the columella and alae), upper lip, and facial soft tissues may be retracted superiorly over the bony nasal dorsum to the level of the intercanthal line (Fig. 347-9).

After the basic surgical exposure is completed, the remaining portion of the operative procedure depends on the lesion type, tumor histology, and the size and anatomic extent of disease. the possibilities include any or a combination of the following:

- Removal of the anterior wall of the maxillary sinus
- Medial maxillectomy, with preservation or removal and replacement of the anterior medial face of the maxilla that borders the piriform aperture, a maneuver that is accomplished with superior and inferior oblique microsaw cuts and replacement of bone with microplates and screws after tumor resection
- Partial maxillectomy
- Transnasal or transantral ethmoidectomy
- Septoplasty, including partial or complete nasal septum resection with preservation of a dorsal caudal strip or septal release and mobilization for posterior access
- Sphenoidotomy or partial sphenoidectomy
- Exposure of the planum ethmoidale or cribriform plate, visualizing from below
- Removal of the posterior medial wall of the maxillary sinus and the vertical part of the palatine bone and medial pterygoid plate for exposure of the nasopharynx and clivus
- Removal of the posterior wall of the maxillary sinus for access to the pterygopalatine fossa
- Use of the operating microscope and diamond bur drill for resection of the midline clivus

Appropriate patient selection for the midfacial degloving approach is paramount and mandates careful consideration of tumor location, size, extent, and histology. For example, an angiofibroma involving the anterior skull base often can be "peeled off" the dura using the midfacial degloving approach alone, but an ethmoid sinus adenocarcinoma in the same location may require the addition of a craniotomy for adequate margins.

DENNIS M. CROCKETT

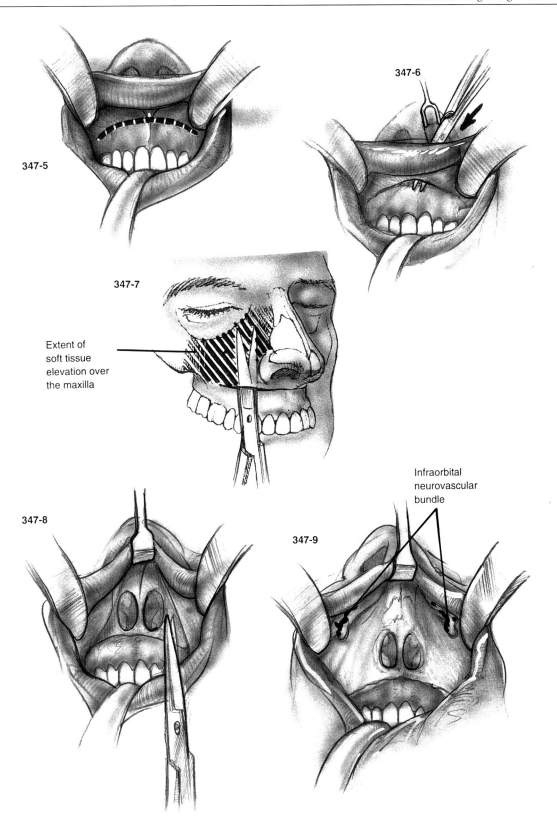

347-5

347-6

347-7

Extent of
soft tissue
elevation over
the maxilla

347-8

347-9

Infraorbital
neurovascular
bundle

■ *348.* ENDOSCOPIC MAXILLARY, ETHMOID, SPHENOIDECTOMY—Removal of diseased mucosa and drainage of the ethmoid, maxillary, and sphenoid sinuses is accomplished under direct endoscopic visualization.

Indications

1. Absolute indications
   a. Chronic or recurrent sinusitis with ostiomeatal unit stenosis or obstruction refractory to medical therapy
   b. Chronic or recurrent sinusitis with nasal polyposis
   c. Chronic sinusitis with symptomatic mucocele, except for frontal sinus mucocele
   d. Fungal sinusitis
   e. Chronic or recurrent sinusitis that persists for more than 6 months despite optimal medical therapy
   f. Sinusitis with complications
   g. Diagnosis of sinus tumor
   h. Drainage of subperiosteal abscess
2. Relative indications
   a. Repair of a cerebrospinal fluid leak
   b. Sinus-mediated headache
   c. Persistent sinusitis with abnormal computed tomography (CT) findings (eg, concha bullosa, paradoxical turbinate)
   d. Orbital decompression and bilateral exophthalmus
   e. Orbital nerve decompression
   f. Revision sinus surgery with extensive polyposis or systemic disease

Special Considerations

1. Thorough and explicit knowledge of paranasal sinus anatomy and physiology
2. Close review of the CT scan
3. Training includes special course work and supervised training
4. Office nasal endoscopy
5. Simultaneous septoplasty or partial turbinectomies
6. The CT scan must be in the operating room for guidance.

Preoperative Preparation

1. Control of acute infection and inflammation
2. Oxymetazoline (0.05% solution, Afrin nasal spray) 20 minutes before surgery
3. Allergy evaluation

(continued)

Operative Procedure

The anterior edge of the middle turbinate, the lateral nasal wall, and the superior aspect of the inferior turbinate are injected with a solution of 2% Xylocaine and 1:100,000 epinephrine. The nose is packed for 10 minutes with 4% cocaine-soaked cotton pledgets.

The nose is inspected using a 4-mm, 0° Storz-Hopkins telescope (Fig. 348-1). The septum, turbinate, posterior choana, and adenoids are visualized. Holding the 0° Storz-Hopkins telescope in the left hand and applying suction with the right hand, the nasal cavity is examined. The middle turbinate is identified and then medially displaced using a Freer elevator. The uncinate process is delineated (Fig. 348-2).

An infundibulectomy is performed by placing a sickle knife as close as possible to the superior attachment of the uncinate process. With a sawing action, the knife is moved firmly from the antero-superior to the posteroinferior position, taking care not to violate the lamina papyracea. The cut is extended posteriorly in a line parallel to the lower borders of the middle turbinate. The uncinate process is displaced toward the middle turbinate. Using a small Blakesley ethmoid forceps, the uncinate process is grasped at its superior attachment and twisted medially while pushing posteroinferiorly (ie, articulating the blade toward the orbit).

Keeping the 4-mm, 0° Storz-Hopkins telescope in the left hand, the ethmoid bulla is visualized (Fig. 348-3). It is entered by gentle, blunt dissection using a suction tip or a Blakesley forceps in the inferior medial aspect. The anterior ethmoidal artery may be just anterosuperior to the bulla. Under direct visualization using the telescope, the ethmoidal cavity is exenterated. The basal lamella is identified. It is the bony layer that defines the posterior extension of the anterior ethmoids and the insertion of the middle turbinate to the lateral nasal wall. The lamella is opened in the inferomedial aspect by Blakesley forceps to enter the posterior ethmoids (Fig. 348-4). Any diseased mucosa or polyps are cleaned from the posterior ethmoids. The roof of the ethmoid sinus (ie, fovea ethmoidalis) may be identified at this stage. Similarly, the lamina papyracea is identified to expose the lateral wall of the ethmoid complex (see Fig. 348-4).

(continued)

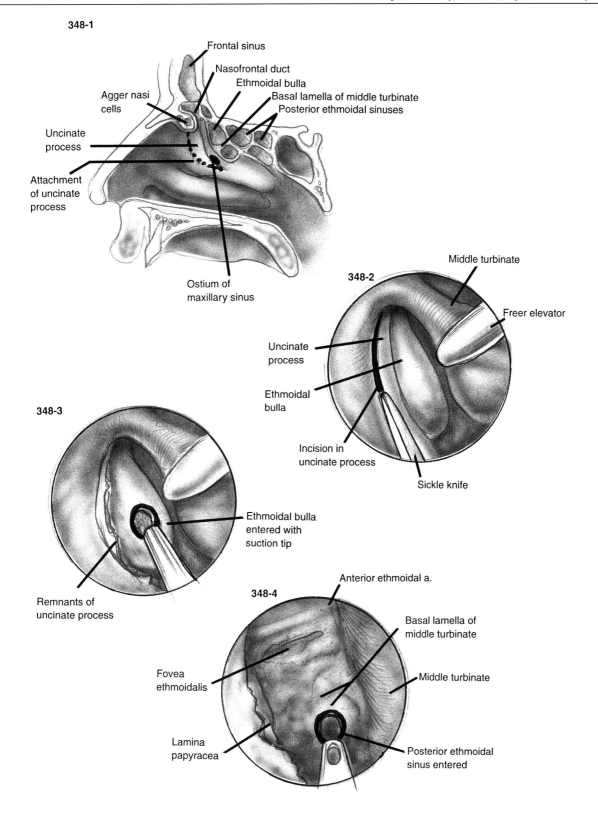

348-1

Frontal sinus

Nasofrontal duct

Ethmoidal bulla

Basal lamella of middle turbinate

Posterior ethmoidal sinuses

Agger nasi cells

Uncinate process

Attachment of uncinate process

Ostium of maxillary sinus

348-2

Middle turbinate

Freer elevator

Uncinate process

Ethmoidal bulla

Incision in uncinate process

Sickle knife

348-3

Ethmoidal bulla entered with suction tip

Remnants of uncinate process

348-4

Anterior ethmoidal a.

Basal lamella of middle turbinate

Middle turbinate

Fovea ethmoidalis

Lamina papyracea

Posterior ethmoidal sinus entered

■ 348. ENDOSCOPIC MAXILLARY, ETHMOID, SPHENOIDECTOMY (continued)

Special Instruments, Position, and Anesthesia

1. Patient in the supine position, with the head elevated 30°
2. Local, general, or local and general anesthesia
3. Blakesley ethmoid forceps, sickle knife, curved Eicken cannula, double-ended maxillary sinus ostium seeker, Gruenwald cutting forceps, side-biting or backbiting cutting forceps, up-biting forceps, giraffe forceps; 0°, 30°, and 70° Storz-Hopkins telescopes

Tips and Pearls

1. Anatomic landmarks include the middle turbinate, uncinate process, inferior turbinate, septum, fovea ethmoidalis, basal lamella, anterior wall of the sphenoid, maxillary ostium, anterior and posterior ethmoid arteries, nasal lacrimal duct and sac, sphenopalatine artery, cribriform plate, lamina papyracea, optic nerve, internal carotid artery.
2. Maximal vasoconstriction and illumination
3. No blind dissection
4. Minimal instrumentation and manipulation
5. Television monitor
6. Blunt dissection and delicate handling of tissue
7. When in doubt, stop.
8. Do not hesitate to ask for help.
9. Vasoconstriction with 1:100,000 epinephrine–soaked cottonoid pledgets for temporary packing, if needed to control bleeding and secure visualization during surgery

Pitfalls and Complications

1. Limited mucosal bleeding
2. Arterial bleeding from the anterior ethmoidal artery, sphenopalatine artery, or internal carotid artery
3. Adhesion or stenosis (most common)
4. Blindness resulting from violation of the lamina papyracea and globe, optic nerve injury, optic neuritis, or orbital hematoma
5. Violation of the lamina papyracea and injury of the extraocular muscles
6. Intracranial injury, meningitis, or cerebrospinal fluid leak resulting from violation of the fovea ethmoidalis and dura, violations of cribriform plate, or aggressive fracture of the middle turbinate
7. Subcutaneous emphysema resulting from violation of the lamina papyracea
8. Epiphora resulting from lacrimal duct injury caused by excessive anterior widening of the ethmoidal ostium
9. Toxic shock syndrome, especially likely if packing is used

Postoperative Care Issues

1. Office nasal endoscopic examination every 7 to 10 days for 3 months and periodically thereafter, depending on the symptoms
2. Antibiotics and steroid spray for 3 to 6 weeks after surgery
3. Nasal endoscopic examination and cleaning under general anesthesia for children 2 to 3 weeks after surgery

References

Lazar RH, Younis RT. Functional endonasal sinus surgery in pediatrics. In: Practical endoscopic sinus surgery. New York: McGraw-Hill, 1992: 107.

Levine HL, May M. Rhinology and sinusology—endoscopic sinus surgery. New York: Thieme, 1993.

Using the same 4-mm, 0° Storz-Hopkins telescope, a sphenoidotomy may be performed if required. Blunt, gentle dissection with a suction tip or Blakesley forceps is performed in the inferomedial aspect of the posterior wall of the posterior ethmoids (Fig. 348-5). The posterior attachment of the middle turbinate, the arch of the posterior choana, and the posterior aspect of the nasal septum are important landmarks (Fig. 348-6).

After the anterior wall of the sphenoid is entered, it can be enlarged using down-biting and up-biting Kerrison forceps. Lateral or superior dissection is avoided, but superomedial or inferior dissection is considered safe.

It is advisable not to perform any dissection within the sphenoid sinus or remove any material. Extreme caution is warranted when inserting instruments into the sphenoid sinus. Gentle suction may be used to remove polyps, debris, or fungal material. The sphenopalatine artery lies inferior to the front face of the sphenoid sinus. The internal carotid artery and optic nerve are prominent and vital structures in the lateral wall of the sphenoid sinus. Dehiscence in this area or surgical dissection may result in serious or fatal complications.

Maxillary antrostomy may then be performed if indicated. A 4-mm, 30° Storz-Hopkins telescope is used for visualization . This telescope is introduced medially and parallel to the inferior border of the middle turbinate with the instrument's beveled surface facing the lateral nasal wall. The maxillary sinus ostium can usually be visualized after the uncinate process has been removed. After the ostium is identified, it is cannulated with an olive-tip, 3-mm, short, curved Eicken antrum sinus cannula (Fig. 348-7). Alternatively, if the ostium is not readily identified, a double-ended maxillary sinus ostium seeker can be inserted gently inferoanteriorly, behind the uncinate process remnant and above the superior border of the inferior turbinate, under direct visualization using the same scope.

The ostium is enlarged posteriorly into the posterior fontanel using the Gruenwald cutting forceps. Anterior enlargement is performed using side-biting or backbiting cutting forceps. The ostium is enlarged eight to ten times its normal size. Care should be taken to avoid injury of the sphenopalatine artery posteriorly and the nasal lacrimal duct or sac anteriorly.

The maxillary sinus is inspected using 30° and 70° Storz-Hopkins telescopes (Fig. 348-7). Any polyps, cysts, or diseased mucosa may be removed using up-biting forceps or giraffe forceps. The maxillary sinus is irrigated with saline.

No packs are left in place (Fig. 348-8). The surgical site may be covered by Bactroban antibiotic ointment.

RANDE H. LAZAR
RAMZI T. YOUNIS

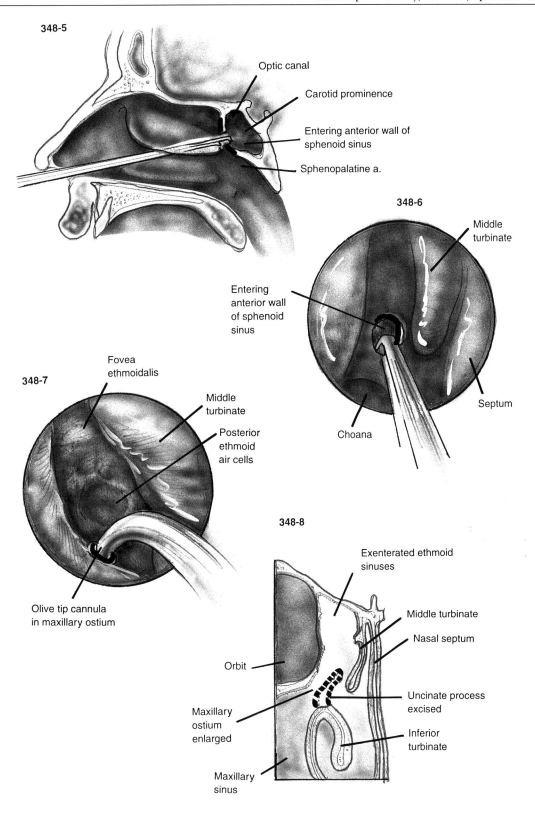

348-5

Optic canal

Carotid prominence

Entering anterior wall of sphenoid sinus

Sphenopalatine a.

348-6

Middle turbinate

Entering anterior wall of sphenoid sinus

Septum

Choana

348-7

Fovea ethmoidalis

Middle turbinate

Posterior ethmoid air cells

Olive tip cannula in maxillary ostium

348-8

Exenterated ethmoid sinuses

Middle turbinate

Nasal septum

Uncinate process excised

Inferior turbinate

Orbit

Maxillary ostium enlarged

Maxillary sinus

■ *349.* ENDOSCOPIC FRONTAL SINUSEC-
TOMY—Endoscopic widening of the nasofrontal isthmus to promote drainage of the frontal sinus

Indications

1. Symptomatic, chronic frontal sinusitis with nasofrontal ductal obstruction refractory to endoscopic sinus surgery and medical therapy
2. Chronic frontal sinusitis and an extensively pneumatized frontal sinus
3. Limited nasofrontal recess obstruction
4. Patients who object strongly to the external approach
5. Biopsy of a frontal sinus tumor
6. Foreign body removal

Contraindications

1. Frontal sinus tumor or osteoma
2. Displaced fracture of the anterior or posterior wall of the frontal sinus
3. Osteomyelitis of the anterior or posterior table of the frontal sinus
4. Cerebrospinal fluid leak through the frontal sinus
5. Disease of the lateral most recess of the frontal sinus, which is inaccessible endoscopically

Special Considerations

1. Axial and coronal computed tomography scans of the frontal sinus provide detailed information about the dimensions and anatomic associations of the frontal sinus, nasofrontal recess, nasofrontal isthmus, and rest of the sinonasal system.

Preoperative Preparation

1. Control of acute infection and inflammation
2. Oxymetazoline (0.05% solution, Afrin nasal spray) 20 minutes before surgery
3. Allergy evaluation

Special Instruments, Position, and Anesthesia

1. Functional endoscopic sinus surgery instruments
2. Microslim drill for functional endoscopic sinus surgery
3. Operating microscope (optional)
4. C-arm fluoroscopy
5. Patient in the supine position, with the head elevated 30°

(continued)

Operative Procedure

The anterior edge of the middle turbinate, the lateral nasal wall, and the superior aspect of the inferior turbinate are injected with a 2% solution of Xylocaine and 1:100,000 epinephrine. The nose is packed for 10 minutes with cotton pledgets soaked with a 4% solution of cocaine.

Endoscopic ethmoidectomy is performed if not already done (see Procedure 348). Using a 4-mm, 30° Storz-Hopkins telescope, the middle turbinate, frontal recess, agger nasi cells, junction of the middle turbinate and lateral nasal wall, cribriform plate, lamina papyracea, and fovea ethmoidalis are identified (Fig. 349-1). Alternatively, a binocular operating microscope may be used for visualization, as reported by Draf.

If the frontal recess is difficult to identify because of scarring or diffuse polyposis, a double-ended maxillary seeker and a C-arm fluoroscope are used for visualization. This procedure may aid in identifying the nasofrontal isthmus at the different stages of the procedure.

Using a microslim diamond bur, the frontonasal duct isthmus may be widened anteriorly and laterally. The agger nasi cells are identified and drilled out, and then the nasolacrimal duct isthmus is widened laterally (Fig. 349-2). Special care is taken not to injure the nasolacrimal system or the orbit (Fig. 349-3). Drilling medially can be extended toward the nasal septum, but extreme care should be taken not to violate the cribriform plate. The main enlargement can be achieved by drilling anteriorly and removing the nasofrontal "beak" and bone of the anterior floor of the frontal sinus (Fig. 349-4).

(continued)

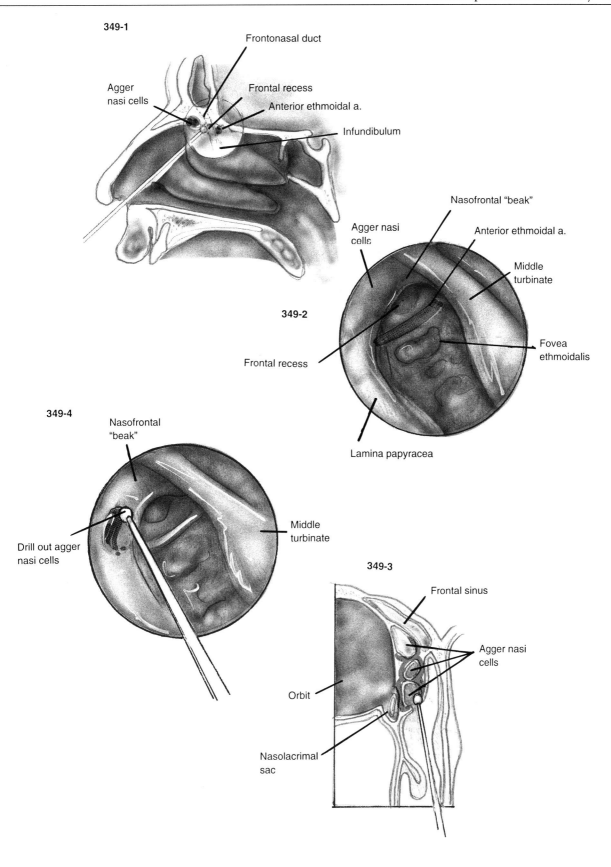

349-1

Frontonasal duct

Agger nasi cells

Frontal recess

Anterior ethmoidal a.

Infundibulum

Nasofrontal "beak"

Agger nasi cells

Anterior ethmoidal a.

Middle turbinate

349-2

Frontal recess

Fovea ethmoidalis

Lamina papyracea

349-4

Nasofrontal "beak"

Drill out agger nasi cells

Middle turbinate

349-3

Frontal sinus

Agger nasi cells

Orbit

Nasolacrimal sac

■ 349. ENDOSCOPIC FRONTAL SINUSEC-TOMY *(continued)*

Tips and Pearls

1. Explicit knowledge of frontal sinus anatomy and its relation to the orbit, brain, and nasal cavity
2. Maximal vasoconstriction
3. Optimal illumination and visualization

Pitfalls and Complications

1. Limited mucosal bleeding
2. Arterial bleeding from the anterior ethmoidal artery, sphenopalatine artery, or internal carotid artery
3. Adhesion or stenosis (most common)
4. Blindness resulting from violation of the lamina papyracea and globe, optic nerve injury, optic neuritis, or orbital hematoma
5. Violation of the lamina papyracea and injury of the extraocular muscles
6. Intracranial injury, meningitis, or cerebrospinal fluid leak resulting from violation of the fovea ethmoidalis and dura, violations of cribriform plate, or aggressive fracture of the middle turbinate
7. Subcutaneous emphysema resulting from violation of the lamina papyracea
8. Epiphora resulting from lacrimal duct injury caused by excessive anterior widening of the ethmoidal ostium
9. Toxic shock syndrome, especially likely if packing is used

Postoperative Care Issues

1. Office nasal endoscopic examination every 7 to 10 days for 3 months and periodically thereafter, depending on the symptoms
2. Antibiotics and steroid spray for 3 to 6 weeks after surgery
3. Nasal endoscopic examination and cleaning under general anesthesia for children 2 to 3 weeks after surgery

References

Draf. Endonasal micro-endoscopic frontal sinus surgery, the fulda concept. Op Tech Otolaryngol Head Neck Surg 1991;2:234.

May M. Frontal sinus surgery: endonasal endoscopic osteoplasty rather than external osteoplasty. Op Tech Otolaryngol Head Neck Surg 1991;2:247.

The following anatomic landmarks form the limits of surgical widening:

The bulge of the anterior ethmoidal artery forms the posterior limit (Fig. 349-5).

The medial lamella of the middle turbinate after its insertion to the roof of the ethmoid forms the medial limit. It marks the lateral limit of the cribriform plate (Fig. 349-6).

The medial orbital wall (ie, lamina papyracea) forms the lateral limit. In the case of bilateral disease, the intrasinus septum may also be drilled out.

In addition to a drill, a curved curet or Kerrison forceps may be used for removing bone.

The sinus is inspected by using a 4-mm, 30° or 70° Storz-Hopkins telescope (Fig. 349-7). Any diseased tissue or polyps should be removed. The sinus is then irrigated with saline (Fig. 349-8). No packs or stents are used.

RAMZI T. YOUNIS
RANDE H. LAZAR

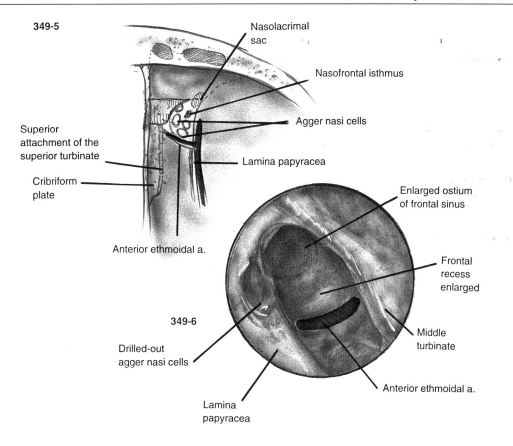

349-5

Nasolacrimal sac

Nasofrontal isthmus

Agger nasi cells

Superior attachment of the superior turbinate

Lamina papyracea

Cribriform plate

Anterior ethmoidal a.

Enlarged ostium of frontal sinus

Frontal recess enlarged

349-6

Drilled-out agger nasi cells

Middle turbinate

Anterior ethmoidal a.

Lamina papyracea

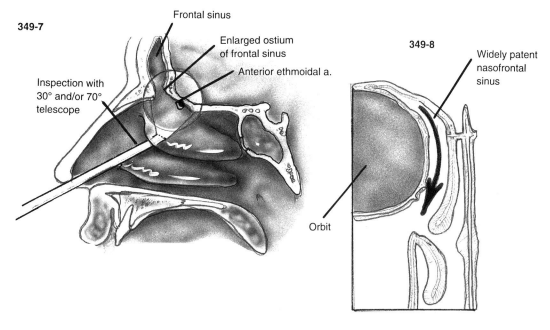

349-7

Frontal sinus

Enlarged ostium of frontal sinus

Anterior ethmoidal a.

Inspection with 30° and/or 70° telescope

349-8

Widely patent nasofrontal sinus

Orbit

■ *350.* MANAGEMENT OF ORBITAL HEMOR-
RHAGE WITH LATERAL CANTHOTOMY
AND CANTHOLYSIS—Incision of the lateral canthal skin
and tendon

Indications
1. Compromise of the central retinal artery perfusion
2. Compression of the optic nerve
3. Vision-threatening intraocular pressure elevation (>30 mm Hg in patient with normal optic nerve; >20 mm Hg in patient with large optic cup)

Special Considerations
1. Clotting abnormalities
2. Susceptibility to mild intraocular pressure elevation (eg, sickle cell anemia, preexisting glaucoma)

Preoperative Preparation
1. Complete ophthalmic examination
2. Optional axial and coronal computed tomography (CT) scans of the orbit; delay CT scan until vision not threatened

Special Instruments
1. Small, straight hemostat
2. Straight Stevens scissors

Tips and Pearls
1. Identify the inferior crus of the lateral canthal tendons by strumming it, not by visualization.

Pitfalls and Complications
1. If vision loss is suspected, do not be tentative in proceeding with a lateral canthotomy and cantholysis, because it is usually a benign procedure.

Postoperative Care Issues
1. Until the patient is stable, evaluate the visual acuity, afferent pupillary defect, intraocular pressure, and central retinal artery perfusion daily.

References
Khan JA. Blunt trauma to orbital soft tissues. In: Shingleton BJ, Hersh PS, Kenyon KR, eds. Eye trauma. St. Louis: Mosby Year Book, 1991:287.

Spoor TC. Orbital hemorrhages. In: Spoor TC, Nesi FA, eds. Management of ocular, orbital, and adnexal trauma. New York: Raven Press, 1988: 351.

Operative Procedures

The most important step in treatment of orbital hemorrhage is identifying the emergent situation. A patient with a significant orbital hemorrhage may present with progressive proptosis, reduced retropulsion, diffuse subconjunctival hemorrhage, spreading eyelid ecchymosis, elevated intraocular pressure, or extraocular motility restriction. Evaluate the visual acuity, pupillary reaction, intraocular pressure, and central retinal artery perfusion to decide if a procedure is warranted. If these tests are abnormal or cannot be carried out and visual loss is suspected, lateral canthotomy and cantholysis should be performed.

A solution of 2% lidocaine with epinephrine (1:100,000) is injected into the lateral canthus for anesthesia and hemostasis (Fig. 350-1). The blades of a small, straight hemostat are inserted anterior and posterior to the lateral canthal tendon, 1 cm lateral to the canthal skin margin (Fig. 350-2). The hemostat is clamped for at least 1 minute to help provide hemostasis. After removal of the hemostat, a small, straight Stevens scissors is placed around the crush mark, and the canthus is incised (ie, canthotomy; Fig. 350-3). Although not usually needed, bipolar cautery may be used to stop bleeding.

The inferior crus of the lateral canthal tendon is identified by strumming it with the scissors. The skin and conjunctiva are dissected away from the inferior crus. The blades of the scissors are inserted around the inferior crus in a inferolateral direction until the scissors tips abut the orbital rim. The tendon is then incised with one firm cut (ie, cantholysis; Fig. 350-4).

The lateral lower eyelid should easily come away from the orbital rim, and the eye should feel less tense with ballottement (Fig. 350-5). If this is not the case, an incomplete cantholysis was performed. Repeat the tendon incision until a release of orbital pressure is attained.

Intraocular pressure is remeasured to verify its reduction, and the fundus is reexamined to determine if central retinal artery perfusion has been reestablished. In most instances, a lateral canthotomy with cantholysis lowers the orbital pressure, preventing damage to the eye.

Severe and diffuse orbital hemorrhage that does not respond to lateral canthotomy with cantholysis may require two- or three-wall orbital decompression (see Procedure 346). Ophthalmic consultation should be requested as soon as possible, preferably at the time the orbital hemorrhage is first recognized.

BRIAN R. WONG

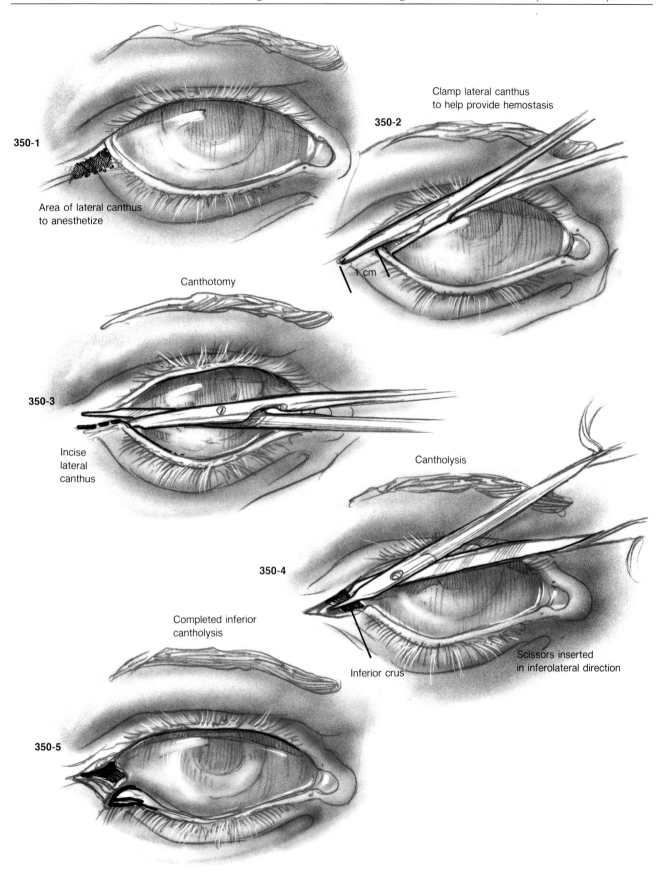

350-1

Area of lateral canthus
to anesthetize

350-2   Clamp lateral canthus
to help provide hemostasis

1 cm

Canthotomy

350-3

Incise
lateral
canthus

Cantholysis

350-4

Completed inferior
cantholysis

Inferior crus

Scissors inserted
in inferolateral direction

350-5

■ *351.* FRONTAL SINUS TREPHINATION

Formation of an opening in the floor of the frontal sinus to facilitate drainage and ventilation

Indications

1. Symptomatic, acute, purulent frontal sinusitis that is unresponsive to maximal medical therapy
2. Frontal sinus pain and tenderness, with or without swelling, that persists despite conservative treatment
3. Frontal sinus exploration
4. Biopsy of frontal sinus tumor

Special Considerations

1. Radiographically confirm that the anterior and posterior walls of the frontal sinus are intact preoperatively and postoperatively.
2. Avoid injury to the globe, medial canthal ligament, extraocular muscle, and orbital roof.
3. Avoid injury to the anterior wall of the frontal sinus to prevent osteomyelitis secondary to the spread of infection through cancellous bone.
4. Irrigation in cases of orbital roof dehiscence may cause blindness.
5. Continue conservative treatment.

Preoperative Preparation

1. Broad-spectrum oral and intravenous antibiotics
2. Local and systemic decongestants
3. X-ray evaluation

Special Instruments, Position, and Anesthesia

1. Freer elevator, curets, bur, Storz-Hopkins telescope (optional)
2. Patient in the supine position, with the head elevated 45° and the eyes exposed
3. Local, general, or local and general anesthesia

Tips and Pearls

1. Anatomic landmarks include the intraorbital rim, floor of the orbit, floor of the frontal sinus, anterior wall, roof of the orbit, and medial canthal ligament.

Complications

1. Osteomyelitis of the frontal bone
2. Blindness
3. Globe injury
4. Extraocular muscle injury
5. Medial canthal ligament injury
6. Dural injury
7. Frontal lobe injury and intracranial complications

Postoperative Care Issues

1. Continue preoperative treatment, and tailor the antibiotic to the culture and sensitivity results.
2. Postoperative x-ray films to assess the integrity of the anterior and posterior walls.
3. Irrigation of the frontal sinus cavity four times daily with antibiotic solution
4. Drain removal within 48 hours or when drainage subsides

References

Loré JM. The sinuses and maxilla. In: Loré JM, ed. The atlas of head and neck surgery. 3rd ed. Philadelphia: WB Saunders, 1988:150.

Montgomery WW. Surgery of the upper respiratory system. 2nd ed. Philadelphia: Lea & Febiger, 1979:120.

Operative Procedure

The superomedial aspect of the orbit is injected with a 2% solution of Xylocaine and 1:100,000 epinephrine (Fig. 351-1). After 10 minutes, a slightly curved, 2- to 3-cm incision is made in the superomedial aspect of the orbit immediately below the eyebrow and supraorbital rim. It is carried through all layers. The periosteum is elevated, and the floor of the frontal sinus is exposed (Fig. 351-2).

The anteromedial aspect of the frontal sinus floor below the prominence of the frontal sinus is opened using a small curet or a drill. Cultures of any purulent material are obtained (Fig. 351-3), and gentle irrigation with saline is performed. A 4-mm, 0° or 30° Storz-Hopkins telescope may be inserted through the trephine to explore the frontal sinus.

Two small plastic or rubber tubes are inserted into the frontal sinus and held in place using 4-0 silk sutures (Fig. 351-4). One tube can be used for daily irrigation, and the other releases the irrigation fluid. Methylene blue stain may be delivered through the tube to assess the patency of the nasofrontal duct. The duct should not be probed, because this may result in stenosis.

This procedure has been used far less frequently during the past 5 years because of the introduction of functional endoscopic sinus surgery, which achieves excellent results by draining the frontal sinus endoscopically through the nose.

RAMZI T. YOUNIS
RANDE H. LAZAR

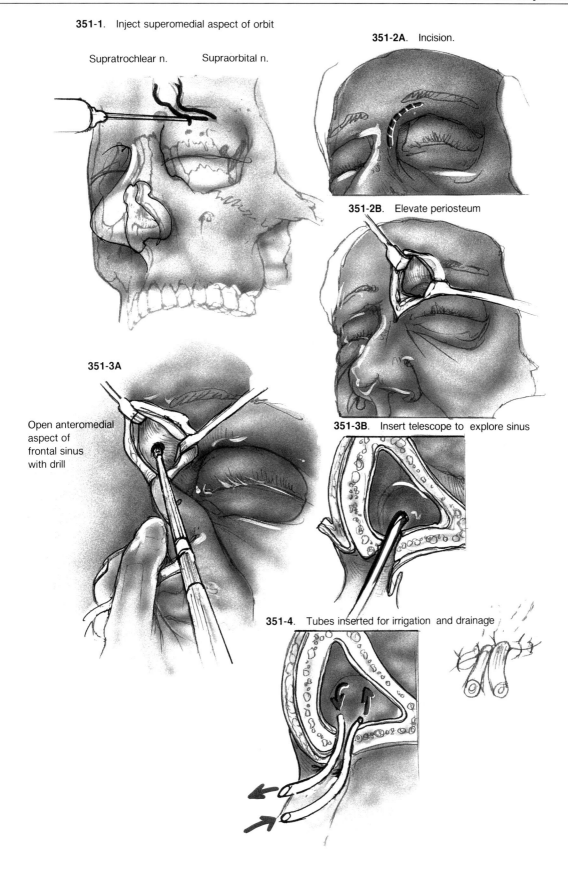

351-1. Inject superomedial aspect of orbit

Supratrochlear n.   Supraorbital n.

351-2A. Incision.

351-2B. Elevate periosteum

351-3A

Open anteromedial
aspect of
frontal sinus
with drill

351-3B. Insert telescope to explore sinus

351-4. Tubes inserted for irrigation and drainage

■ 352. OSTEOPLASTIC FRONTAL SINUSEC-TOMY PROCEDURE AND FAT OBLITERA-TION— External frontal sinus surgery that allows direct access to the frontal sinus with total exenteration of any disease process and complete sinus obliteration

Indications

1. Chronic symptomatic frontal sinusitis unresponsive to conservative therapy
2. Symptomatic frontal osteoma
3. Symptomatic frontal sinus mucocele or pyocele
4. Frontal sinusitis with orbital or cranial complications
5. Frontal sinus fracture
6. Frontal sinus tumor
7. Frontal sinus osteomyelitis
8. Revision surgery for chronic frontal sinusitis

Special Considerations

1. This procedure provides direct access to the frontal sinuses.
2. Except for the scar, there is no facial deformity, as with other external surgeries of the frontal sinuses.
3. The procedure has a high success rate with a relatively low rate of morbidity.
4. The two frontal sinuses may be explored and treated simultaneously.
5. Adipose tissue can provide complete sinus obliteration and has been shown to resist infection.
6. Most adipose tissue can survive and become revascularized; otherwise, it may be replaced by fibrous tissue.

Preoperative Preparation

1. Preoperative computed tomography scans of the sinuses are required to assess the exact pathology and dimensions of the frontal sinuses.
2. A 6-foot (1.8-m) Caldwell view of the sinuses is obtained.
3. A template of the frontal sinuses is mandatory. This is done by placing an exposed transparent x-ray film over the Caldwell view. The cutout may be made smaller than the actual dimensions of the sinuses to ensure that the bone cut lies within the limits of the sinus.
4. The template should be available and sterilized before surgery.
5. Preoperative antibiotic therapy is required.
6. Consultation with an ophthalmologist is advisable.

(continued)

Operative Procedure

Unilateral Procedure

The eyebrow is injected with a solution of 2% Xylocaine and 1:100,000 epinephrine (Fig. 352-1). Tarsorrhaphy may be preformed using 5-0 silk sutures (Fig. 352-2).

An incision is made along the upper margin of the entire length of the eyebrow: this is carried through subcutaneous tissue and the frontalis muscle, and the periosteum is preserved. A superiorly based forehead flap is raised in a plane between the periosteum and frontalis muscle, exposing the anterior surface of the frontal sinus. The frontal flap is retracted using 2-0 silk sutures (Fig. 352-3).

The x-ray template is used to outline the location of the frontal sinus. This could be fixed in place using an 18-gauge needle. The periosteum is cut along the lateral superior and medial margins of the template. Carefully preserve the inferior supraorbital rim of periosteum to ensure the blood supply to the periosteum and bone. The periosteum is elevated a few millimeters superiorly to facilitate cutting and suturing after surgery is completed. While elevating the flap and performing the periosteal cut, take care to preserve the supraorbital nerve that arises though the supraorbital fossa (Fig. 352-4).

Using a Stryker saw, an inward beveled bone incision is made along the periosteal incision. Make sure that the supraorbital rim is cut medially and laterally. This is essential to provide a hinging effect across the floor of the frontal sinus (Fig. 352-5).

An osteotome and mallet are used to inspect the completion of the bone cutting. The osteoplastic flap is then elevated downward and forward by inserting the osteotome in the superior aspect of the cut and pushing gently (Fig. 352-6).

The sinus is inspected, and the decision is made about whether to obliterate the sinus or not. If an osteoma is found and the rest of the mucosa is normal, the osteoma is removed, and no obliteration or mucosa removal is needed. If polyps, cysts, or diffuse infection exist, cultures are taken, and the sinus should be obliterated. The entire mucosal lining of the frontal sinus is removed by curets, Freer elevators, or Blakesley forceps. A diamond bur is then used over the inner surface of all the walls of the frontal sinus. The entire inner surface of the frontal sinus is cleaned, and the inner cortex is removed to make sure that all mucosa is removed and to secure adequate revascularization of the adipose tissue obliteration. The nasofrontal duct is also inspected and cleaned (Fig. 352-7B).

Subcutaneous adipose tissue may be obtained from the left abdominal wall by a left rectus incision. The abdomen is usually shaved and prepped before surgery. After removal of the adipose tissue, hemostasis is secured by electrocautery or 3-0 silk suture ties. A drain is placed, and the incision is closed using 4-0 chromic interrupted sutures for the subcutaneous tissue and 4-0 nylon interrupted suture for the skin. The drain is removed 48 hours later.

The sinus is then totally obliterated with adipose tissue (Fig. 352-8) that is fashioned to fit and obliterate the entire sinus (Fig. 352-9A). The flap is replaced and fixed in place by using 4-0 chromic

(continued)

352-1. Eyebrow injection

352-2. Tarsorrhaphy

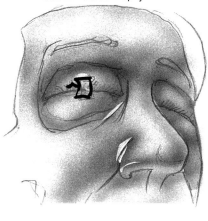

352-4. Use x-ray template to outline location of frontal sinus; incise periosteum

Preserve inferior supraorbital rim to ensure blood supply to bone and periosteum

352-3. Incision along margin of entire length of eyebrow

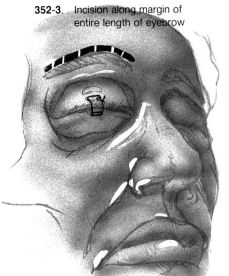

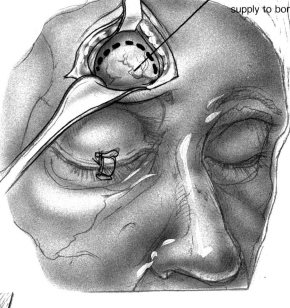

Make inward beveled bone incision along periosteal incision

352-5

■ *352.* OSTEOPLASTIC FRONTAL SINUSECTOMY PROCEDURE AND FAT OBLITERATION *(continued)*

Special Instruments, Position, and Anesthesia

1. Freer elevator, Stryker saw, mallet, osteotome, chisel, curets, cutting bur
2. Patient in the supine position, with the head elevated 30° and the face exposed
3. General anesthesia

Tips and Pearls

1. Use an eyebrow incision in men, especially for bald patients; use a coronal incision in women.
2. The periosteum of the supraorbital rim should remain intact at all times to secure adequate flap vascularization.
3. For bone cutting, bevel the cut inward to secure adequate closure and avoid intracranial injury.
4. If the mucous membrane is diseased or polypoid, remove it totally with a bur along with inner surface of the cortex to secure revascularization of the adipose tissue. If the mucosa is normal, it is preserved, and no adipose obliteration is required.
5. The eyebrows should not be shaved.
6. Temporary tarsorrhaphy using 5-0 silk suture (optional)

Pitfalls and Complications

1. Fracture or injury of the posterior wall of the frontal sinus
2. Cerebrospinal fluid leak
3. Frontal lobe injury
4. Fracture of the roof of the orbit
5. Globe injury
6. Extraocular muscle injury
7. Supraorbital nerve injury
8. Forehead paraesthesia or hypoesthesia

Postoperative Care Issues

1. Pressure dressing is applied over the forehead and eyes for 48 hours.
2. Drains are removed after 48 hours.
3. Intravenous antibiotics are given. The antibiotics should be selected according to sensitivity reports for the intraoperative cultures.

References

Loré JM. The sinuses and maxilla. In: Loré JM, ed. The atlas of head and neck surgery. 3rd ed. Philadelphia: WB Saunders, 1988:154.

Montgomery WW. Surgery of the upper respiratory system. 2nd ed. Philadelphia: Lea & Febiger, 1979:127.

interrupted sutures to close the periosteum (see Fig. 352-9B). Hemostasis is secured by electrocautery. A Penrose drain is inserted. The frontalis muscle is approximated using 4-0 chromic interrupted suture. The subcutaneous tissue is approximated using 4-0 chromic interrupted sutures, and the skin is closed using 5-0 continuous nylon suture or 5-0 Vicryl subcuticular sutures.

A pressure dressing is applied using Telfa gauze over the incision and an eye pad over the eye, with fluffed 4 × 4 gauze overlying the whole forehead and the dressings held in place with gauze wrapped around the head. This is usually removed along with the drain 48 hours after the surgery.

Bilateral Procedure

A coronal or eyebrow incision can be used. The eyebrow incision extends over the entire length of both eyebrows along the nasal process in a butterfly fashion. If a coronal incision is selected, it is performed about 2 to 3 cm behind the anterior hairline. The hair is shaved 4 to 5 cm behind the anterior hairline.

The incision site (coronal or eyebrow) is injected with a solution of 2% Xylocaine and 1:100,000 epinephrine. The eye lids may be closed using 5-0 silk sutures. With an eyebrow incision, the frontal flap is raised superiorly between the frontalis muscle and periosteum. With a coronal incision, the flap is raised inferiorly in a similar fashion until the supraorbital rim and nasal process are identified.

The template is obtained as previously described and is applied over the frontal sinus and nasal process. It may be held in place using an 18-gauge needle or a knife. The periosteum is transected along the lateral superior and medial margin of the template using a #15 blade.

The periosteum is elevated a few millimeters superiorly. The bone is cut, beveling downward and inward toward the sinus cavity. The supraorbital rim is cut on each side laterally. The nasal process also should be transected using an osteotome. This helps in the flap elevation and in avoiding trauma and fracture to the anterior wall of the frontal sinus. The periosteum overlying the supraorbital rim should always remain intact.

An osteotome is used along the entire length of the bone incision to inspect the completeness of the bone cutting. If an intrafrontal septum is present, it is transected using an osteotome and mallet. The bone and periosteum are then elevated inferiorly and forward by applying gentle pressure with an osteotome, starting at the midline. Gradual elevation with gentle pressure at different locations of the flap may be required to avoid fracture of the anterior table.

After the flap is reflected inferiorly, the sinus is inspected. The diseased tissue and mucosal membrane may be removed using curets, a Freer elevator, and Blakesley forceps. A diamond bur is used to remove the remaining mucosa and inner cortical layer of the walls of the frontal sinus, as described previously.

After the subcutaneous fat is obtained from a left rectus incision as described previously, it is fashioned to obliterate both sinuses. After the fat is employed in both sinuses, the flap is replaced. The flap is fixed in place using 4-0 chromic interrupted sutures through the periosteum. Hemostasis is secured with electrocautery. A Penrose drain is placed subcutaneously. The frontalis muscle is closed using 4-0 chromic interrupted sutures. The subcutaneous tissue is closed using 4-0 chromic interrupted sutures, and the skin is closed using 4-0 or 5-0 continuous nylon skin sutures for the eyebrow or the coronal incision. However, 5-0 Vicryl subcuticular sutures may sometimes be used to close the eyebrow incision. A pressure dressing is applied consisting of Telfa gauze over the incision, with pads over the eyes, and fluffed 4 × 4 inch gauze overlying the eyes and the forehead. The dressing is held in place for 48 hours with gauze wrapped around the head. Thereafter, the dressing is changed, the drain is removed, and the eyes are exposed.

Functional endoscopic sinus surgery may also be performed with unilateral or bilateral osteoplastic frontal sinusectomy. Using a 4-mm, 30° or 70° Storz-Hopkins telescope, the nasofrontal duct can be inspected and identified intranasally during surgery.

RAMZI T. YOUNIS
RANDE H. LAZAR

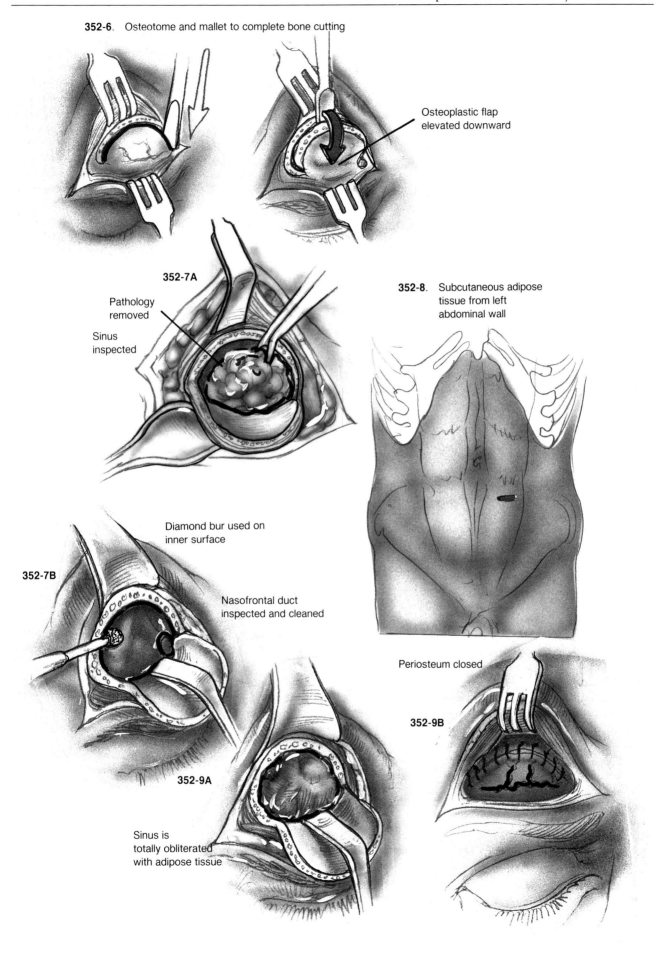

352-6. Osteotome and mallet to complete bone cutting

Osteoplastic flap elevated downward

352-7A

Pathology removed

Sinus inspected

352-8. Subcutaneous adipose tissue from left abdominal wall

Diamond bur used on inner surface

352-7B

Nasofrontal duct inspected and cleaned

Periosteum closed

352-9B

352-9A

Sinus is totally obliterated with adipose tissue

■ *353.* FRONTAL SINUS ABLATION AND COLLAPSE
—Removing the anterior wall and floor of the frontal sinus, obliterating the sinus

Indications
1. Osteomyelitis of the frontal sinus
2. Frontal sinus tumor
3. Chronic frontal sinusitis with a small frontal sinus

Preoperative Preparation
1. Preoperative computed tomography scans of the sinuses are required to assess the exact pathology and dimensions of the frontal sinuses.
2. A 6-foot (1.8-m) Caldwell view of the sinuses is obtained.
3. A template of the frontal sinuses is mandatory.
4. The template should be available and sterilized before surgery.
5. Preoperative antibiotic therapy is required.
6. Consultation with an ophthalmologist is advisable.

Special Instruments, Position, and Anesthesia
1. Freer elevator, Stryker saw, mallet, osteotome, chisel, curettes, cutting bur
2. Patient in the supine position, with the head elevated 30° and the face exposed
3. General anesthesia

Tips and Pearls
1. Use an eyebrow incision in men, especially if the patients are bald; use a coronal incision in women.
2. For bone cutting, bevel the cut inward to secure adequate closure and avoid intracranial injury.
3. If the mucous membrane is diseased or polypoid, remove it totally with a bur along with inner surface of the cortex to secure revascularization of the adipose tissue. If the mucosa is normal, it is preserved, and no adipose obliteration is required.
4. The eyebrows should not be shaved.
5. Temporary tarsorrhaphy using 5-0 silk suture (optional)

Pitfalls and Complications
1. This procedure should be avoided because of its many drawbacks. It causes severe disfiguring, producing a flattened deformity of the forehead, and it requires a second procedure using an implant for reconstruction.
2. The cure rates are no higher than for other open procedures used for the frontal sinuses.
3. The frontal sinus may not be completely obliterated if the anteroposterior dimensions are large.
4. Other complications associated with osteoplastic frontal sinusectomy may be encountered:
   a. Fracture or injury of the posterior wall of the frontal sinus
   b. Cerebrospinal fluid leak
   c. Frontal lobe injury
   d. Fracture of the roof of the orbit
   e. Globe injury
   f. Extraocular muscle injury
   g. Supraorbital nerve injury
   h. Forehead paraesthesia or hypoesthesia

Postoperative Care Issues
1. A pressure dressing is applied over the forehead and eyes for 48 hours.
2. Drains are removed after 48 hours.
3. The intravenous antibiotics given should be selected according to the sensitivity reports for the intraoperative cultures.

References
Ritter FN. Surgical management of paranasal sinusitis—Riedel procedure. In: Cummings C, Fredrickson JM, Harke LA, Krause CJ, eds. Otolaryngology—Head and Neck Surgery. St. Louis: CV Mosby, 1986:943.

Montgomery WW. Surgery of the upper respiratory system. 2nd ed. Philadelphia: Lea & Febiger, 1979:128.

Operative Procedure
This procedure can be unilateral or bilateral. The eyebrow is injected with a 2% solution of Xylocaine with a 1:100,000 concentration of epinephrine. Tarsorrhaphy may be preformed using 5-0 silk sutures.

After 10 minutes, an incision is made along the upper margin of the entire length of the eyebrow (Fig. 353-1). This is carried through subcutaneous tissue and the frontalis muscle, and the periosteum is preserved. A forehead flap is raised in the plane between the periosteum and the frontalis muscle in a fashion similar to the creation of a frontal osteoplastic flap (see Procedure 352) (Fig. 353-2).

Using an x-ray template, the periosteum is incised and marked, and the bone is cut in a fashion similar to that described in Procedure 352 (Fig. 353-3). The periosteum and the bone are elevated as described in Procedure 352 (Fig. 353-4A), but they are totally removed along with the floor of the frontal sinus using a chisel or a Stryker saw and a cutting bur. The remaining cavity of the frontal sinus is cleaned of any diseased mucosa using a Freer elevator, curets, and Blakesley forceps. The entire cavity of the frontal sinus is drilled using a cutting bur to ensure that any remaining mucosa is removed (Fig. 353-4B). Hemostasis is secured with electrocautery. The frontal flap is then put back in place and left to occupy the cavity that is produced after removing the anterior wall and the floor of the frontal sinus (Fig. 353-4C). A Penrose drain is placed.

A pressure dressing is applied using Telfa gauze over the incision and an eye pad over the eye, with fluffed 4 × 4 cm gauze overlying the whole forehead and with the dressings held in place by gauze wrapped around the head. This is usually removed along with the drain 48 hours after the surgery.

RAMZI T. YOUNIS
RANDE H. LAZAR

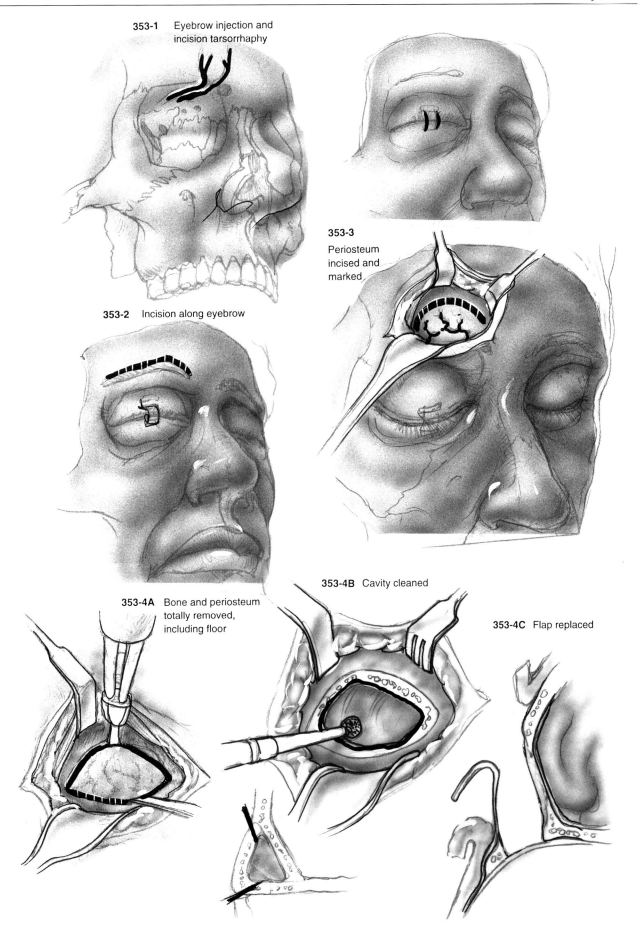

353-1 Eyebrow injection and incision tarsorrhaphy

353-2 Incision along eyebrow

353-3 Periosteum incised and marked

353-4A Bone and periosteum totally removed, including floor

353-4B Cavity cleaned

353-4C Flap replaced

◼ *354.* ENDOSCOPIC SINUS SURGERY IN CHILDREN

— Removal of the lower portion of the uncinate process, verification of an adequate natural ostium of the maxillary sinus or its enlargement if necessary, and inspection of the interior mucosa of the bulla ethmoidalis

Indications
1. Medically recalcitrant chronic sinusitis
2. Unremitting recurrent sinusitis

Special Considerations
1. Hematologic abnormalities
2. Recent aspirin or ibuprofen ingestion
3. Use of vasoconstrictive and hemostatic agents in the preoperative staging area
4. Injection of no more than 7 mg/kg of lidocaine with 1:100,000 epinephrine into the greater palatine foramen and root of the middle turbinate
5. Placement of oxymetazoline-soaked cottonoids in the middle meatus

Preoperative Preparation
1. Extensive hematologic history
2. Tests for bleeding time, hemoglobin, and hematocrit, as indicated

Special Instruments, Position, and Anesthesia
1. Back biter or side biter
2. Ball-tipped seeker
3. Pediatric endoscopes, if needed
4. Pediatric functional endoscopic surgery instruments
5. Pediatric microdebrider

Tips and Pearls
1. Careful examination of the ostiomeatal unit, palpating with a ball-tipped seeker
2. Use the back biter to remove the uncinate.
3. Enlargement of the natural ostium is seldom required.
4. If accessory ostia are present, enlarge only the natural ostium posteriorly to include these.
5. For verifying natural ostia
   a. Natural sinus ostia do not lie in the same plane as the lateral nasal wall; they lie in an oblique plane.
   b. Accessory ostia tend to be perfectly circular, but natural ostia are ovoid.
   c. Natural ostia usually are anterior or superior to accessory ostia. If an opening is identified into the maxillary sinus that is in the same plane as the lateral wall, perfectly circular, or away from the anterior insertion of the uncinate, this is an accessory ostium and not the natural ostium.

Pitfalls and Complications
1. Using the sickle knife to remove the uncinate in children may cause damage to the lacrimal drainage system and increase bleeding.
2. The most common cause of functional endoscopic sinus surgery (FESS) failure is creating a middle meatus antrostomy that is not in continuity with the natural ostium. An inadequately resected lower uncinate frequently conceals the intact natural ostium in failed FESS cases.

Postoperative Care Issues
1. A rolled Gelfilm stent is placed in the middle meatus and left for 2 weeks postoperatively.
2. No nasal packing is used.
3. Stents are removed after 2 weeks.

References
Bolger WE, Butzin CA, Parsons DS. Paranasal sinus bony anatomic variations and mucosal abnormalities: CT analysis for endoscopic sinus surgery. Laryngoscope 1991;101:56.

Parsons DS, Pransky SM, Functional endoscopic sinus surgery in infants and young children. Instruct Course Lect 1992;5:159.

Parsons DS, Setliff RC, Chambers D. Innovative techniques: special considerations in pediatric functional endoscopic sinus surgery. Op Tech Otolaryngol Head Neck Surg 1994;5:40.

Operative Procedure

The steps of this procedure are the removal of the lower portion of the uncinate process, verification of an adequate natural ostium of the maxillary sinus or its enlargement if necessary, and inspection of the interior mucosa of the bulla ethmoidalis (Fig. 354-1). Although conceptually simple, precise surgical technique is critical for an optimal outcome.

The uncinate process is approached with a back biter, not a sickle knife (Fig. 354-2*A*). The use of a sickle knife is discouraged in children, because the cut is made from medial to lateral, toward the lacrimal drainage system and orbit. The action of the back biter blade is from lateral to medial, which dramatically reduces the potential for injury and bleeding. A ball-tipped seeker, which is used to explore the infundibulum, may also be used to displace the uncinate medially so the back biter may be positioned more easily.

The lower one half of the uncinate process is removed to its anterior limit (Figs. 354-3 and 354-4). The posteroinferior pathway of the infundibulum or final common pathway for drainage from the frontal, agger nasi, and maxillary sinus is identified and followed anteriorly. The natural ostium is found within this pathway 1 to 2 mm posterior to the anterior extent of the uncinate bone as it inserts into the lateral nasal wall. The natural ostium is in the anterior superior-most portion of the fontanelle. Identification of the natural ostium may be further facilitated with palpation using a ball-tipped seeker (Fig. 354-5). The anterior-most uncinate bone covers the natural ostium and prevents the surgeon from identifying this critical structure. It is essential that all of the inferior uncinate be removed to the limits of its anterior insertion.

The most common cause of FESS failure is a created middle meatus antrostomy that is not contiguous with the natural ostium. Residual lower uncinate is frequently found anteriorly, hiding an intact natural ostium in revision cases. The created antrostomy is nothing more than an accessory ostium. Mucociliary flow continues to advance toward the tiny, diseased natural ostium. This situation has been called the "recirculatory phenomenon," in which purulence escaping through the diseased natural ostium reenters the ineffective, larger, surgically created accessory ostium.

After the natural ostium is uncovered by removing the uncinate and identified, the decision regarding the need for enlargement is made. Enlargement usually is unnecessary. When required, it should only be enlarged posteriorly, not anteriorly. Anterior enlargement may injure the lacrimal duct. Enlarging the natural ostium posteriorly is accomplished by incising the posterior fontanelle, staying as close to the roof of the maxillary sinus as possible. This incision should incorporate any accessory ostium.

The posterior fontanelle is then sharply removed to create the middle meatus antrostomy. The anterior edge of the middle meatus antrostomy is always the anterior lip of the natural ostium. A thorough examination of the maxillary antrum is performed with a 30° or 70° telescope.

A 0° telescope is used to identify the bulla ethmoidalis and its lower medial portion is removed. A functional opening is created when the dissection includes the posteriorly located natural ostium of the bulla (Fig. 354-5). If the anterior ethmoid mucosa is normal, the procedure is terminated and a Gelfilm middle meatal stent is placed. The surgery may be extended to include other anterior or posterior ethmoid cells if severe disease is present.

The benefit of this limited procedure is that modest disease extending beyond the ostiomeatal complex usually heals with medical therapy after ventilation and drainage are restored. For those who fail the this approach, a more extensive procedure may be undertaken with all the important landmarks still intact. The potential for surgical complications in children are markedly reduced by using this operative technique.

DAVID S. PARSONS
PAUL R. COOK

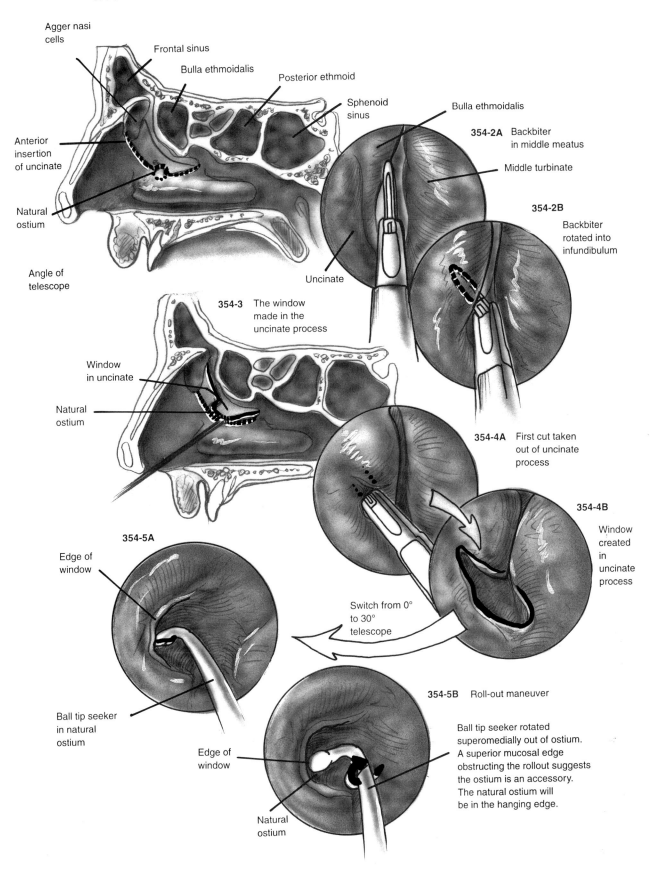

354-1

Agger nasi cells

Frontal sinus

Bulla ethmoidalis

Posterior ethmoid

Sphenoid sinus

Bulla ethmoidalis

354-2A Backbiter in middle meatus

Middle turbinate

Anterior insertion of uncinate

Natural ostium

354-2B

Backbiter rotated into infundibulum

Angle of telescope

Uncinate

354-3 The window made in the uncinate process

Window in uncinate

Natural ostium

354-4A First cut taken out of uncinate process

354-4B

Window created in uncinate process

354-5A

Edge of window

Switch from 0° to 30° telescope

Ball tip seeker in natural ostium

Edge of window

354-5B Roll-out maneuver

Ball tip seeker rotated superomedially out of ostium. A superior mucosal edge obstructing the rollout suggests the ostium is an accessory. The natural ostium will be in the hanging edge.

Natural ostium

■ *355.* FRONTAL DEFECT RECONSTRUCTION

Restoration of the osseous contours of the frontal cranial vault and the orbital roof using either alloplastic or autogenous materials

Indications

1. Posttraumatic or postsurgical defects.

Contraindications

1. Lack of well vascularized, supple scalp for a tension-free closure
2. For methylmethacrylate, history of any infectious symptoms within the proposed operative field in the prior year, or no intact bony separation from the nose or any paranasal sinus
3. For bone, ongoing osteomyelitis in the margin of the defect if the infected bone cannot be removed and replaced.
4. Relative contraindication: the only seeing eye.

Special Considerations

1. Proximity of the defect to the nasal cavity and sinuses
2. Visual status of both eyes
3. Hairline recession

Preoperative Preparation

1. Axial and coronal CT scans to define exact size of the defect and its relationship to the brain, eyes, optic nerves and sinuses
2. Antibiotics (cephalosporin) and steroids (Decadron 10–12 μg).
3. Head shaving not mandatory even if intracranial approach

Special Instruments, Position, and Anesthesia

1. Orotracheal intubation with anesthesia to side at waist or beyond
2. 15° to 20° reverse Trendelenburg
3. Head stabilized in a foam doughnut
4. If acrylic is being used, the face must be draped to isolate the nose and mouth from the operative field.
5. Tarsorrhaphies
6. Oscillating or reciprocating power saws, drills
7. Microplating system

Tips and Pearls

1. The frontal bone (including both orbital rims) should be totally exposed so symmetry can be evaluated.
2. The supraorbital neurovascular bundles should be released from their foramina to allow maximum inferior flap retraction.
3. The temporalis muscles should not be detached from the lateral orbital rims or temporal fossa unless the bony defect involves the site of attachment.
4. Avoid using local soft tissue (pericranial, galeal flaps) for skull base reconstruction if at all possible.
5. Direct bone-to-bone contact (even along craniotomy bone cuts) should be reestablished in non–hair-bearing areas if possible.

Pitfalls and Complications

1. Dural and cortical injuries may occur at both the defect site and the cranial bone graft site if the osteotomies or outer table harvesting are performed incorrectly.
2. Cerebrospinal fluid may accumulate under the skin if a watertight closure of all dural violations is not obtained.

Postoperative Care Issues

1. Steroids (Decadron 4 to 6 mgm) are given every 6 hours during surgery and for 24 hours postoperatively.
2. Antibiotics are continued for 3 days postoperatively.
3. One drain (bulb suction) is placed under the flap across the forehead and a second over the bone graft donor site. These are removed as soon as possible, ideally within 48 hours.

References

Crewley WA. Problems and complications of cranioplasty. In Manson PN (ed). Cranio-maxillofacial trauma. Philadelphia: JB Lippincott, 1991:458.

Stuzin JM, Wagstrom L, Kawamoto HK, Wolfe SA. Anatomy of the frontal branch of the facial nerve: the significance of the temporal fad pad. Plast Reconstr Surg 1989;265.

Operative Procedure

The forehead flap (Fig. 355-1) is elevated in the subgaleal plane down to approximately 1.5 cm above the lateral end of the eyebrow. The pericranium is then elevated as a second U-shaped flap, following the superior temporal lines to the same level as the previous subgaleal dissection. The pericranial flap is available to be rotated intracranially if unanticipated findings necessitate use of vascularized soft tissue for repair of the skull base.

At 1.5 cm above the lateral end of the brow, the pericranium is further elevated to the superior orbital rims, with the supraorbital neurovascular bundles identified and removed from their foramina. Lateral to the superior temporal line at the same level, the superficial layer of the deep temporal fascia is incised over the temporalis muscle to the root of the zygomatic arch and this layer of fascia is elevated with the forehead flap to the arch and lateral orbital rim. The subperiosteal and subfascial dissections are then connected by sharply dissecting their junction free from the superior temporal line, staying on bone down to the zygomatic process of the frontal bone. The temporal fascia is then incised at its attachment to the arch and rim in an inside-out fashion and the periosteum is elevated over the those structures to allow necessary rotation of the flap for maximum exposure. The anterior branches of the superficial temporal vessels and the frontal branch of the facial nerve are therefore elevated with the flap and protected from irreversible injury.

Simple contour problems of the forehead, glabella, or supraorbital rims are usually treated with onlay grafts to correct depressions or inlay grafts to correct bone loss. Large defects can be treated with methylmethacrylate if limited donor bone is available. Also, methylmethacrylate is more contourable into an exact reproduction of anatomic detail, particularly in the area of the superior orbital rims and frontonasal angle, the most technically demanding areas of contour cranioplasty. An onlay acrylic implant can be fixed to the underlying bone using microplates and screws or simply micro lag screws. The micro drills used for the screw holes must have drill stops to prevent inadvertent intracranial intrusion. An inlay acrylic implant can be reinforced with metallic mesh (usually titanium) and the acrylic or mesh can be locked into bony undercuts for stability.

Methylmethacrylate can be used to repair small or large defects with no donor site morbidity. However, it cannot be used in immediate or even close proximity to the nose or paranasal sinuses and it should not be used for at least one year from the time of the most recent local or regional infection. Split cranial bone grafts, however, are highly resistant to infection and can be placed into immediate contact with the sinuses and can be grafted into a recently infected field as long as the defect margins are free of osteomyelitis. These grafts can also be placed as onlay or inlay grafts and stabilized with microplates and screws or micro lag screws (Fig. 355-2). However, they cannot be contoured as readily as methylmethacrylate.

Inlay bone grafts may be necessary to fill small gaps created by the osteotomies. Unfortunately, complex defects tend to have a fronto-orbital unit that is anatomically disrupted in addition to being displaced. This would be expected following trauma that produces fragmentation or actual loss of bone following tumor extirpation. Segmental osteotomies might allow for repositioning of some of the unit, but most likely the distorted bone is best discarded and replaced with inlay and onlay bone grafts to totally reconstruct the unit. The orbital roof must be reconstructed to prevent downward displacement of the globe by the brain (Fig. 355-3). Because of the difficulty with recreating the upward convexity of the roof, a flat bone graft must be cantilevered from the reconstructed frontal bar area at a level approximating the highest point of the normal convexity, not at the reconstructed orbital rim itself.

ROBERT B. STANLEY, JR.

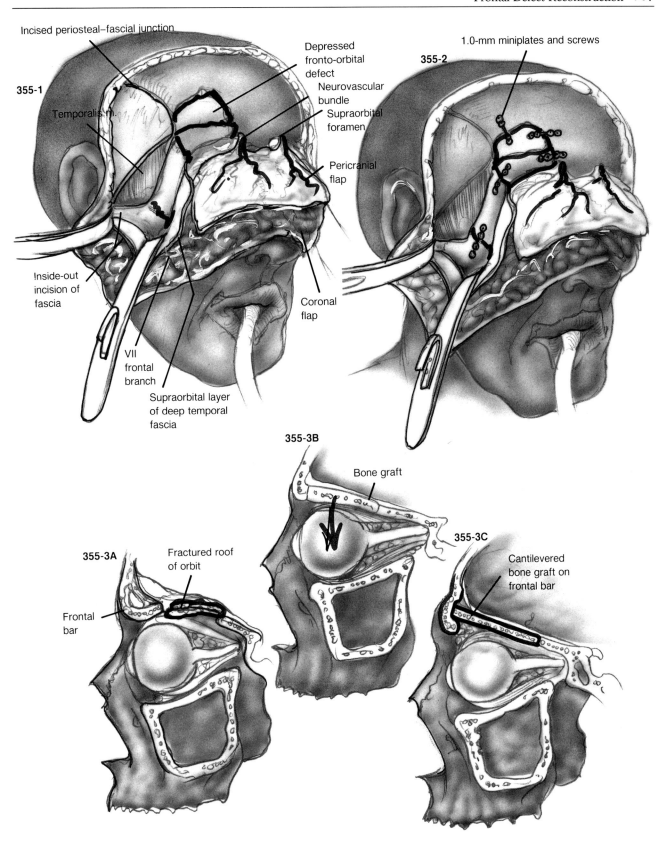

Incised periosteal–fascial junction

355-1

Temporalis m.

Inside-out incision of fascia

VII frontal branch

Supraorbital layer of deep temporal fascia

Depressed fronto-orbital defect

Neurovascular bundle

Supraorbital foramen

Pericranial flap

Coronal flap

355-2

1.0-mm miniplates and screws

355-3B

Bone graft

355-3A

Fractured roof of orbit

Frontal bar

355-3C

Cantilevered bone graft on frontal bar

■ 356. DACRYOCYSTORHINOSTOMY

Creation of an anastomosis between the nasal cavity and the lacrimal sac

Indications

1. Nasolacrimal duct obstruction
   a. Epiphora
   b. Acute or chronic dacryocystitis
   c. Lacrimal sac mucocele
   d. Dacryolith

Special Considerations

1. Bleeding or clotting abnormalities
2. Nasal abnormalities

Contraindications

1. Lacrimal sac malignancy
2. Punctal obstruction
3. Canalicular obstruction

Preoperative Preparation

1. Nasal examination
2. Optional computed tomography scan (eg, trauma)
3. Optional dacryocystography (eg, congenital abnormalities)

Special Instruments, Position, and Anesthesia

1. Headlight
2. Hall or Stryker drill
3. Medium-sized olive-tip bur, 4 mm long
4. Small blunt rakes
5. Rongeur forceps
6. Kerrison punch
7. Punctal dilator
8. Lacrimal probe (0/00)
9. Lacrimal cannula
10. Freer periosteal elevator
11. Bard-Parker #12 blade

Tips and Pearls

1. Discourage nasal mucosal bleeding by packing the middle meatus with cottonoid pledgets soaked in 4% cocaine.
2. Prevent an unsightly scar by avoiding a skin incision that is excessively curved and positioned too close to the medial commissure.
3. Avoid damage to the angular vessels by bluntly dissecting down to periosteum.
4. Place a probe into the canaliculus and lacrimal sac to confirm the exact location of the sac.
5. Confirm that the lacrimal sac is open by irrigating with a cannula.
6. Liberally grease antibiotic-steroid ointment on the nasal packing to prevent bleeding when it is removed.

Pitfalls and Complications

1. Immature bony anatomy in infants and small children
2. Nasal polyps or markedly deviated nasal septum
3. Postoperative bleeding
4. Late obstruction

Postoperative Care Issues

1. Antibacterial ointment to skin incision
2. Light pressure dressing for the first day to minimize the risk of postoperative bleeding
3. Remove the nasal packing after 2 days, and irrigate to confirm the patency of the dacryocystorhinostomy.
4. Systemic antibiotics for 1 week
5. Patients should not blow their noses for the first few days after surgery.

References

Quickert MH. Lacrimal drainage surgery. In: Soll DB, ed. Management of complications in ophthalmic plastic surgery. Birmingham: Aesculapius Publishing Company, 1976:100.

Wilkins RB, Berris CE, Dryden RM, et al. Lacrimal drainage system disorders: diagnosis and treatment. In: McCord CD, Tanenbaum M, eds. Oculoplastic surgery. 2nd ed. New York: Raven Press, 1987:387.

Operative Procedure

Before the the patient is prepped and draped, a local anesthetic consisting of a solution of 2% lidocaine with epinephrine mixed with a solution of 0.5% Marcaine with epinephrine is injected into the operative site. The middle meatus is packed with two neurosurgical Cottonoid pledgets soaked in a 4% solution of cocaine.

A 3-cm, oblique, straight line is marked on the skin just below the medial canthal tendon and 4 mm nasal to the medial commissure, extending over the inferior nasal rim of the orbit (Fig. 356-1). The skin is incised with a #15 Bard-Parker blade. The subcutaneous tissue down to periosteum is bluntly dissected with a sharp iris scissors. Care should be taken not to lacerate the angular vessels.

Periosteum about 5 mm medial to the anterior lacrimal crest is incised with a #15 Bard-Parker blade. Visualization for this step is improved by retracting with two small rakes. The lacrimal sac is reflected laterally by lifting the periosteum from the lacrimal fossa with a Freer elevator (Fig. 356-2). The periosteum is also loosened anteriorly over the nasal bone to allow easier reapposition of the periosteum at the end of the procedure. Before removing the lacrimal fossa bone, the Cottonoid strips should be removed from the nose to help prevent nasal mucosal trauma from the bur. The anterior lacrimal crest is then carefully removed using a medium-sized olive-tip bur. Trauma to the nasal mucosa should be avoided by placing only light pressure on the bone by the bur. The lacrimal sac is protected by inserting the Freer elevator between the bone and sac (Fig. 356-3). Once into the nose, the rest of the lacrimal fossa is extracted with rongeurs and kerrison punches to form a 0.8 × 1.5 cm opening. Bone wax and cautery may be used to acquire hemostasis:

The lacrimal sac is identified by placing a 00 nasolacrimal probe into the canaliculus and tenting the sac. The periosteum and tear sac are cut with a #12 Bard-Barker blade that is wrapped with Steri-Strips such that only the tip remains clear. The anterior lacrimal sac flap is formed by making a semicircular incision, taking care not to go too deep and thereby pierce the other side of the sac and enter the orbital fat. A posterior lacrimal sac flap is removed with Wescott scissors to widen the opening. The nasolacrimal probe should be seen coming through the sac (Fig. 356-4). If not, the sac was not completely incised, or there is an obstruction at the common internal punctum. The blocked common internal punctum is opened by tenting it up with the nasolacrimal probe and snipping it with Wescott scissors. Water is injected with a lacrimal cannula into the canaliculus.

The anterior lacrimal sac flap is isolated with 4-0 Vicryl on a small half-circle needle. The suture is placed through once and left long. The two ends are held together with a seraphine. The suture is used later to appose the lacrimal sac and nasal mucosal flaps.

Attention is then focused on creating an anterior nasal mucosal flap with a #12 Bard-Parker blade in a semicircular fashion. A small hemostat inserted in the nose to tent the nasal mucosa laterally aids in making the flap (see Fig. 356-4). The posterior flap is excised with Wescott scissors. Hemorrhage is common at this point because nasal mucosa is quite vascular. Gelfoam soaked in thrombin may be placed in the nose and allowed to remain there permanently.

If the common internal punctum was occluded, a Crawford tube should be inserted. One of the Crawford probes is inserted through the superior punctum and into the nose. The probe is removed from the nose with a Crawford crochet-type hook (Fig. 356-5). The other Crawford probe is inserted through the inferior punctum and removed from the nose.

Umbilical tape greased in antibiotic-steroid ointment is placed through the nostril in the surgical site for hemostasis. Approximately 20 cm is packed in the site and then cut at the nostril; it is removed on postoperative day 2. The Crawford probes are pulled off, and the tubes are tied together in a single square knot. The seraphine is released from the 4-0 Vicryl, and interrupted sutures are placed to appose the lacrimal sac and nasal mucosal flaps (Fig. 356-6). Care is taken not to include the umbilical tape. The periosteum is reapposed with the 4-0 Vicryl. Subcutaneous tissue is sutured with buried interrupted 5-0 Vicryl. The skin is closed with interrupted 6-0 mild chromic sutures. Antibiotic ointment is placed on the incision, and a folded eye pad is taped over the surgical site.

BRIAN R. WONG

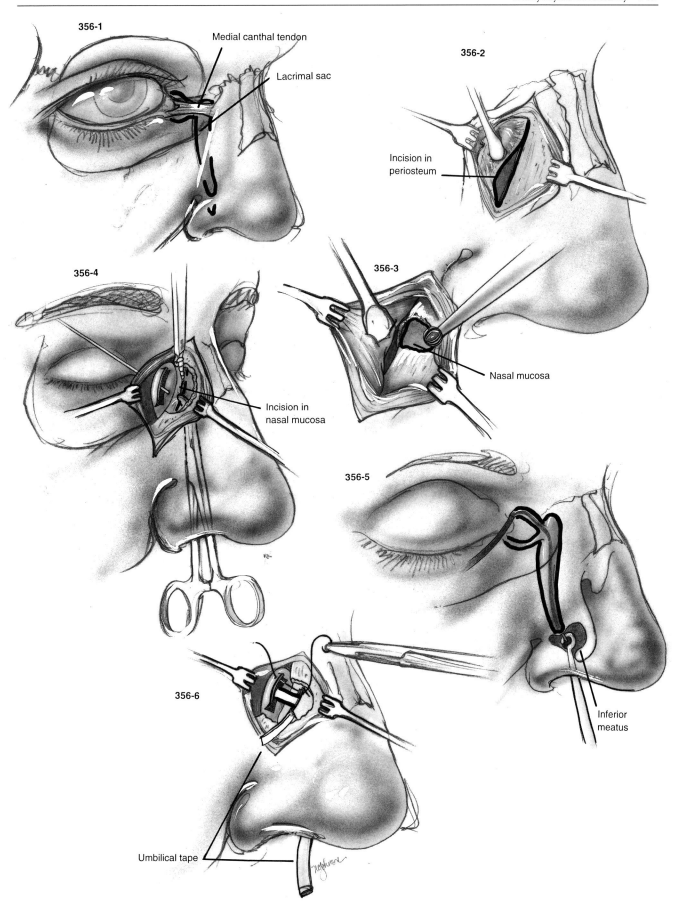

356-1

Medial canthal tendon

Lacrimal sac

356-2

Incision in periosteum

356-4

356-3

Nasal mucosa

Incision in nasal mucosa

356-5

356-6

Inferior meatus

Umbilical tape

■ 357. INCISIONAL AND EXCISIONAL

BIOPSY—Procedures for obtaining tissue for histopathologic diagnosis or culture

Indications

1. Head or neck mass that may be a tumor or infection
2. Systemic lymphadenopathy of unknown cause

Special Considerations

1. Cranial nerves
2. Great vessels

Preoperative Preparation

1. PPD with control
2. Complete inspection of the upper aerodigestive tract
3. Chest x-ray examination (posteroanterior and lateral views)
4. Esophagogram and thyroid scan (optional)

Special Instruments, Position, and Anesthesia

1. Nerve stimulator available
2. Position depends on location of the mass
3. Local or general anesthesia

Tips and Pearls

1. Complete excision is preferable.
2. If multiple nodes are involved, resection of a smaller node may be adequate.
3. Consideration of future neck dissection or resection may dictate the ideal incision for biopsy.
4. The pathologist should be called to handle the fresh specimen.

Pitfalls and Complications

1. Detailed attention to hemostasis helps prevent hematoma.
2. Early identification and dissection of cranial nerves prevents injury.

References

Lee YN, Terry R, Lukes RJ. Lymph node biopsy for diagnosis: a statistical study. J Surg Oncol 1980;14:53.
Slap GB, Connor JL, Wigton RS, Schwartz JS. Validation of a model to identify young patients for lymph node biopsy. JAMA 1986;255: 2768.

Operative Procedure

When a patient presents with a mass in the head or neck, a biopsy may be necessary to obtain the diagnosis through histopathologic analysis or culture. Before biopsy, a complete evaluation of the upper aerodigestive tract, PPD and chest film should be done. A thyroid scan and esophagogram are indicated in many circumstances. A primary tumor may be detected in one of these locations, and a biopsy of the primary tumor may preclude the need for a biopsy of the mass. If an infectious process is considered, the workup must include the described tests, and in certain clinical situations, serologic analysis may be necessary for tularemia, toxoplasmosis, histoplasmosis, or other conditions. In some cases, excisional biopsy is diagnostic and the only needed treatment.

The incision is planned to be camouflaged within the relaxed skin tension lines (Figs. 357-1 and 357-2). If a neck dissection is contemplated, the incision may be a portion of the incision planned for the later dissection (see Fig. 357-2). The approximate location of the nearby cranial nerves should be kept in mind (Fig. 357-3).

After the skin incision is made, the mass should be identified. If superficial, it may be encountered just beneath the skin. If deep, the overlying soft tissue should be dissected until the mass is identified. The nearby cranial nerves must be identified and dissected to ensure their integrity. The great vessels are also at risk if the mass is adjacent. Careful dissection using magnification, if necessary, helps safe excision. The surgeon may find the use of a nerve stimulator helpful in defining the cranial nerve and protecting it from harm.

If the mass is small or medium sized, an excisional biopsy is usually done without much difficulty. If the mass is very large or if cranial nerves or vessels are encased by the mass, or if the mass is likely to be treated only with radiation and chemotherapy, an incisional biopsy may be appropriate. The disadvantages include tumor spillage and leaking of residual disease.

If an incisional biopsy is chosen, the surgeon should dissect the lateral portion of the mass so it is well exposed. If there may be underlying vessels or nerves, a portion of the mass should be selected to avoid their injury. A wedge resection of the mass is mapped out. On either side, a large silk suture is placed and tied, leaving long tags. The wedge is removed. The long tags on either side of the wedge are then quickly tied together, reducing tumor spillage and helping with hemostasis (Fig. 357-4).

The pathologist should take the specimen from the operative field for special handling. If indicated, a portion of the mass should be submitted for cultures for anaerobic and aerobic organisms, for acid-fast *Bacillus*, and for any other suspected pathogens. A touch preparation can be done of the node to assist in diagnosing lymphoma. A portion of the specimen should be fixed in glutaraldehyde for electron microscopy.

A multilayer closure should be accomplished, leaving a drain in place if the wound is at risk for bleeding. The skin may be closed with nonabsorbable sutures, fast-absorbing chromic sutures, or plain sutures to reduce scarring. A Barton dressing or neck wrap may be used.

Postoperative wound care includes prompt removal of any existing drains and inspection to rule out hematoma, seroma, or infection. Early cleaning and ointment use may help to keep the scar from broadening. Sutures may be removed 5 to 7 days after surgery.

HARLAN R. MUNTZ

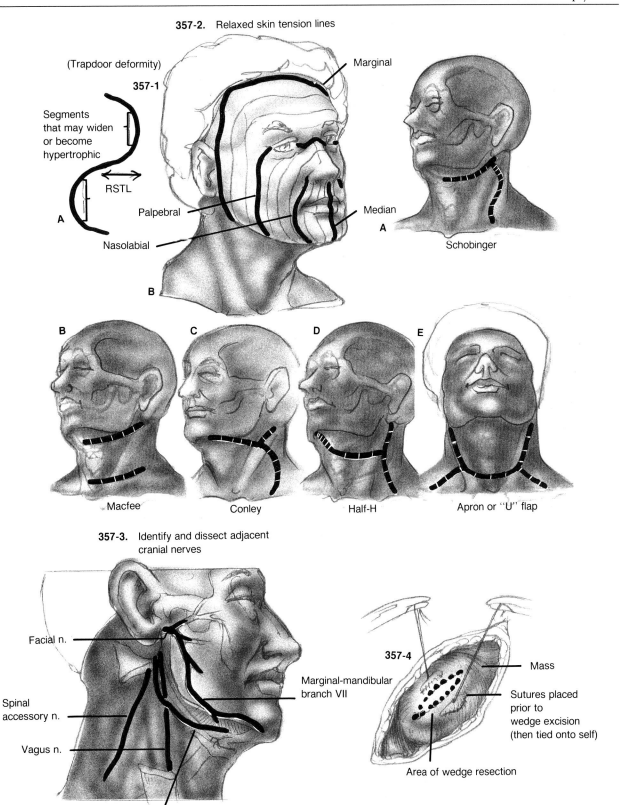

357-2. Relaxed skin tension lines

(Trapdoor deformity)

357-1

Segments
that may widen
or become
hypertrophic

RSTL

A

Marginal

Palpebral

Median

Nasolabial

A

Schobinger

B

B

C

D

E

Macfee

Conley

Half-H

Apron or "U" flap

357-3. Identify and dissect adjacent
cranial nerves

Facial n.

Spinal
accessory n.

Vagus n.

Marginal-mandibular
branch VII

Hypoglossal n.

357-4

Mass

Sutures placed
prior to
wedge excision
(then tied onto self)

Area of wedge resection

358. NEEDLE BIOPSY

A sampling of tissue from a palpable mass using a fine-needle aspiration technique to differentiate benign from malignant lesions and to classify neoplasms and other pathologic processes

Indications

1. A persistent, enlarged lymph node
2. A neck mass of unknown origin
3. Salivary gland masses (to assist in advance planning of the proper therapeutic procedure)
4. Thyroid "cold" nodule or cyst

Contraindications

1. Bleeding disorders, especially for deep neck masses and thyroid masses
2. Suspected carotid body tumor

Preoperative Preparation

1. Explain the procedure and possible side effects to the patient.
2. Disinfection of the skin with alcohol-soaked swab or Betadine.

Special Instruments, Position, and Anesthesia

1. Hypodermic needle with long bevel, 22 to 27 gauge.
2. Slip-tip syringe for easy needle removal; 3 to 10 mL, based on comfort, convenience, and availability (difference in suction is trivial)
3. Syringe holder that allows easy access to needle and plunger for slide preparation
4. Position the patient so that the neck muscles are relaxed and there is optimal access to the target mass.
5. Anesthesia is rarely required. Sedation or topical anesthetic may be needed in children who are anxious about needles.

Tips and Pearls

1. A successful procedure depends in large part on the experience and training of the operator in obtaining and preparing the samples and on the expertise of the observer interpreting the case.
2. Results improve with adequate target immobilization and proper needle tip placement and movement.

Pitfalls and Complications

1. Discomfort is comparable to a venipuncture lasting for 5 to 10 seconds.
2. Hematoma is the most common complication.
3. Infection is extremely rare.
4. False-negative results can result in cases of fibrosis, well-differentiated tumor cells mimicking normal cells, and geographic misses caused by inexperience, tumor size, or tumor location.
5. False-positive results can be attributed to pregnancy; contamination; heterotopia, which can be secondary to changes caused by inflammatory conditions, radiation, and chemotherapy; and attempts by the observer to interpret scant material containing only a few abnormal cells.
6. Seeding is a rare problem that is usually limited to patients with carcinomatosis.

Postoperative Care Issues

1. Firm, accurate pressure for 5 minutes after procedure
2. Simple dressing (Band-Aid)
3. Results must correlate with clinical appearance, or reaspiration may be indicated. If the biopsy is used to confirm a benign lesion, the lesion must be followed clinically.

References

1. Koss LG, Woyke S, Olszewski W. Aspiration biopsy: cytologic interpretation and histologic bases. New York: Igaku Shoin, 1992:12.
2. Stanley MW, Lowhagen T. Fine needle aspiration of palpable masses. Boston: Butterworth-Heinemann, 1993:6.
3. Nguyen GK, Kline TS. Essentials of aspiration biopsy cytology. New York: Igaku Shoin, 1991:2

Operative Procedure

The length of the needle should reach the center of the mass. The larger-bore needles may be necessary to remove viscous fluid, and they tend to get more material from loosely structured tumors, such as melanomas and lymphomas. Smaller-bore needles are more effective in tissue with few epithelial cells and extensive fibrosis, allowing easier penetration of the fibrous stroma. The size of the syringe should allow easy handling with a short distance from the operator's hand to the mass. Larger needles do not obtain larger samples. If a holder is to be used, it should hold the syringe firmly and allow removal of the needle and retraction of the plunger without having to remove the entire syringe from the holder. Injected local anesthesia can mask small masses. Some anxious children may benefit from prior sedation and topical anesthetic.

Carefully palpate the target mass, and localize anatomic landmarks that may be at risk during the procedure, such as the carotid artery. Immobilize the target mass by holding it closely between two fingers and stretching the overlying skin tightly across the lesion. Very small lesions can be palpated with the tips of the fingers held tightly together. Push the mass as far as possible in one direction in the subcutaneous space. Without lifting the fingertips, retract the overlying skin. The pressure causes the lesion to "pop up" under the skin surface in front of the fingertips (Fig. 358-1). Without moving the fingers, clean the skin before aspiration.

Thyroid or other deep-seated neck masses often are located deep to the sternocleidomastoid muscle, which must be avoided because it can add discomfort to the procedure, makes needle placement more difficult and uncertain, and may plug the needle with muscle tissue. Position the patient so the skin and muscles of the neck are relaxed, turning the head toward the side of the mass. Immobilize the mass by pushing the lesion against the trachea, then push the sternocleidomastoid muscle laterally with the thumb, accomplishing adequate exposure of the mass (Fig. 358-2). Aspiration should be in a tangential plane to the trachea or neighboring vessel to lower the chance of complications.

Insert the needle tip in the target mass, and then apply suction by retracting the syringe plunger to a position that is comfortable (Fig. 358-3A and B). Only 1 to 2 mL of suction is needed for an adequate sample. Keep the suction at this level throughout the sampling period and avoid pumping the plunger during the procedure. Move the needle tip back and forth within the boundaries of the target as many as 15 to 20 times in approximately the same plane, which lessens the chance of bleeding (see Fig. 358-3C). If blood appears immediately, stop after only four or five times.[1] The first sample from a given area usually contains the least amount of blood. Perform two standard aspirations in different areas of a mass measuring more than 1.5 cm. The needle should be aimed for the center of a mass that is smaller than 1 cm, the edge of a mass that is larger than 5 cm, or sampled from two mirror-image areas if the mass is 2 to 4 cm.[1]

If the mass is very fibrous or ill defined and requires more than one sample, the direction of the needle can be changed while in the skin. Release the suction, and withdraw the needle from the target mass, leaving the tip of the needle under the skin. The angle is then changed before the needle is reintroduced into the mass and suction reapplied.[1] Cysts should be completely evacuated. If diagnostic amounts of epithelial cells cannot be obtained, microscopic evaluation is impossible.

Withdraw the needle by first releasing the suction (see Fig. 358-3D and E). The collected material stays within the needle and syringe tip. To prepare the slides, remove the needle, and pull back on the plunger (see Fig. 358-3F and G). Reattach the needle and expel the material onto a glass slide by pushing the plunger swiftly through the syringe, with the tip of the needle resting on the slide with the bevel pointing down to avoid splattering (see Fig. 358-3H). The slide can then be prepared for fixation and Papanicolaou staining with hematoxylin and eosin, or it can be air dried for Romanovsky staining.

AMY R. COFFEY

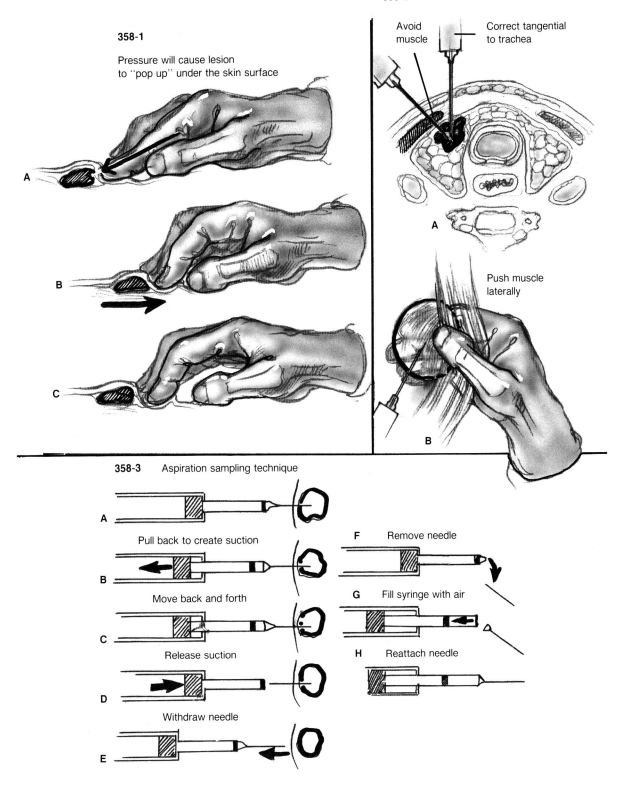

358-1

Pressure will cause lesion to "pop up" under the skin surface

A

B

C

358-2

Avoid muscle

Correct tangential to trachea

A

Push muscle laterally

B

358-3   Aspiration sampling technique

A

Pull back to create suction

B

Move back and forth

C

Release suction

D

Withdraw needle

E

F   Remove needle

G   Fill syringe with air

H   Reattach needle

■ *359.* ENDOSCOPIC BIOPSY
Sampling of tissue within the nose guided by a nasal endoscope

Indications
1. Pathologic diagnosis of a nasal mass
2. Olfactory epithelium sampling for evaluation of anosmia

Contraindications
1. Bleeding or clotting abnormalities
2. Encephalocele, meningocele, or meningoencephalocele
3. Arteriovenous malformation

Preoperative Preparation
1. Physical examination, looking for an increase in size with crying and straining or with compression of the jugular veins (ie, Furstenberg's test)
2. Consider computed tomography (CT) or magnetic resonance imaging (MRI) if information regarding the origin, nature, or vascularity of the mass is needed.

Special Instruments, Position, and Anesthesia
1. Nasal endoscope (2.7 mm, 30°)
2. Olfactory biopsy instrument, giraffe forceps, or nasal snare
3. Local anesthesia using 0.5% ephedrine sulfate and 2% Pontocaine spray, followed by 4% cocaine solution on cotton-tipped nasal applicators
4. General anesthesia if other procedures are planned

Tips and Pearls
1. Success rates are higher with endoscopic guidance.
2. An experienced operator improves the quality of the specimen.

Pitfalls and Complications
1. Cerebrospinal fluid leak and meningitis
2. Bleeding
3. Inadequate sample
4. Vasovagal reactions

Postoperative Care Issues
1. Nonaspirin pain medications to lessen risk of bleeding
2. Limitation of activity and straining

References
1. Myers EN, Carrau RL. Neoplasms of the nose and paranasal sinuses. In: Bailey BJ, ed. Head and neck surgery—otolaryngology, vol 2. Philadelphia: JB Lippincott, 1993:1096.
2. Lanza DC, Moran DT, Doty RL, et al. Endoscopic human olfactory biopsy technique: a preliminary report. Laryngoscope 1993;103:815–819.
3. Lovell MA, Jafek BW, Moran DT, Rowley JC III. Biopsy of human olfactory mucosa: an instrument and a technique. Arch Otolaryngol 1982;108:247–249.

Operative Procedure
Any mass in the nose should be approached with caution. Preoperative imaging is advised to prevent inadvertent sampling of a vascular tumor or an encephalocele.[1] A CT scan can confirm the bony integrity of the skull base. MRI should be done if a vascular tumor or encephalocele is suspected. Biopsy of vascular tumors should be performed under general anesthesia in the operating suite after preparations for control of bleeding and blood replacement have been made. Removal of simple masses or biopsies of the olfactory epithelium may be performed under local anesthesia. Endoscopic sinus surgery instruments may be used for the biopsy.

The patient is placed in a comfortable, upright position. Nasal endoscopy is performed using a 2.7-mm, 30° nasal endoscope, looking for signs of infection and the best access to the mass or olfactory cleft. The nasal cavity is anesthetized using 0.5% ephedrine sulfate and 2% Pontocaine spray applied by atomizer. Pledgets or cotton-tipped nasal applicators soaked in a 4% solution of cocaine are placed in the area to be sampled.

After adequate anesthesia has been obtained, the mass is visualized with the endoscope and grasped with the biopsy forceps (Fig. 359-1). A nasal snare may be helpful for retrieving pedunculated masses such as nasal polyps (Fig. 359-2).

Olfactory neuroepithelium is found along the roof of the nose overlying the cribriform plate and extending onto the superior septum and superior turbinates. The superior septum is the preferred target because of the vertical orientation and smooth surface (Fig. 359-3). The cribriform plate should be avoided because it could be fractured during the procedure. Although the success of olfactory epithelium biopsies improves with the use of the nasal endoscope, the biopsy site usually is not directly visualized during the biopsy procedure. Endoscopic identification of the superior turbinate is carried out routinely.

Several methods and instruments for harvesting have been described. The most successful have been the Stortz olfactory biopsy instrument and the giraffe forceps routinely used in endoscopic sinus surgery (Fig. 359-4). The olfactory biopsy instrument is 120 mm long and 1 mm in diameter, with a cutting edge bent 150° in a U shape toward the shaft. The U-shaped trough is 1.5 mm wide, 0.5 mm deep, and 1 mm long. The sharp cutting edge was designed to give a higher-quality tissue sample, but the narrow shaft can slip and rotate between the fingers during use.[2] The volume of the specimen obtained is approximately 3 mm³.[3] The 70° forward-biting giraffe forceps are thought to be easier to manipulate with greater control. The 3-mm round biting cup at the distal end gave a specimen of equal quality to the that of the olfactory biopsy instrument in one study.[2]

The instrument selected is introduced into the nose under endoscopic guidance. The olfactory biopsy instrument is introduced to a depth of 60 to 70 mm along the septum. It should be withdrawn slightly if resistance is encountered to prevent fracture of the cribriform plate. It is rotated medially, pressing the cutting edge against the septum and then carefully withdrawn.[3] Alternatively, the giraffe forceps are introduced to the skull base and then slightly withdrawn and rotated toward the septal side of the olfactory cleft, which may result in fracturing the superior turbinate. The giraffe forceps is then opened and closed, and a bite of tissue is removed.[2]

The tissue sample is immediately removed and placed in appropriate fixative for processing for electron microscopic and immunohistochemical analysis. A fresh sample is required for these tests, especially if a lymphoreticular tumor is suspected.

AMY R. COFFEY

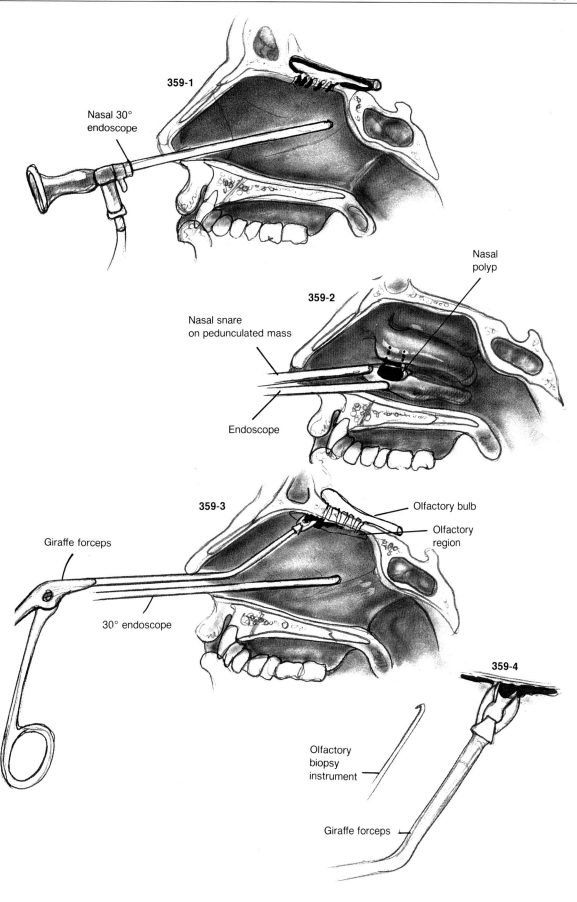

359-1

Nasal 30° endoscope

359-2

Nasal polyp

Nasal snare on pedunculated mass

Endoscope

359-3

Giraffe forceps

30° endoscope

Olfactory bulb

Olfactory region

359-4

Olfactory biopsy instrument

Giraffe forceps

■ 360. PUNCH BIOPSY

A biopsy technique that produces a cylinder of tissue from the skin surface to the underlying subcutaneous fat

Indications

1. Superficial benign or malignant lesions
2. Lesions that require information about depth of involvement
3. Lupus erythematosus, granulomatous conditions, vasculitis

Contraindications

1. Bleeding or clotting abnormalities
2. Lesions located deep beneath the dermis

Special Considerations

1. Plan the closure according to the location of the lesion for the best cosmetic result.
2. Avoid injection of anesthetic directly into lesion.

Preoperative Preparation

1. Clean the skin with chlorhexidine, povidone iodine, or alcohol.
2. Sterile drape

Special Instruments, Position, and Anesthesia

1. Sterile punch of 3 mm (range, 2 to 6 mm) with pencil grip
2. Iris scissors, fine skin hook, toothed (Adson) forceps
3. Relaxed, comfortable position that gives adequate exposure of the lesion
4. Local anesthesia using a solution of 1% lidocaine with 1:100,000 epinephrine

Tips and Pearls

1. Careful orientation of the biopsy is important. Apply skin tension at a right angle to the relaxed skin tension line to result in an elliptical defect along this line giving a more cosmetic closure.
2. Avoid electrocautery; use pinpoint cautery only if necessary.
3. This procedure cannot be used for staging based on the depth of invasion, because the sample may miss the area of deepest tumor penetration.

Pitfalls and Complications

1. Bleeding
2. Scarring, which becomes worse if allowed to granulate
3. Inadequate or damaged sample caused by poor technique or handling
4. Hypertension from local anesthetic

Postoperative Care Issues

1. Use pressure hemostasis; use pinpoint electrocautery only if necessary.
2. Suture closure gives a better cosmetic result.
3. Hydrogen peroxide, antibiotic ointment

Reference

Zachary CB. Basic cutaneous surgery: a primer in technique. New York: Churchill Livingstone, 1991:17.

Operative Procedure

The skin surrounding the biopsy site should be cleaned with chlorhexidine (Hibiclens), povidone iodine (Betadine), or alcohol. Local anesthesia of 1% lidocaine with 1:100,000 epinephrine is injected, using a 27- to 30-gauge needle, circumferential to the lesion (Fig. 360-1). Injections directly in the lesion can cause distortions of the architecture. A delay of 5 to 10 minutes should be allowed for the epinephrine to take effect. The area may be draped using sterile drapes.

The skin should be held taut by the thumb and forefinger of the nondominant hand. The orientation of skin tension by the fingers should be perpendicular to the relaxed skin tension lines. This allows an elliptical defect that is easier to close (Fig. 360-2). Grasp the punch between the thumb and fingers, pressing the sharp steel cutting edge of the cylinder down firmly against the biopsy site. As pressure is applied, the punch should be twisted back and forth until there is a slight give, indicating that subcutis deep to the dermis has been reached (Fig. 360-3).

The specimen should be handled delicately. The punch is removed and the sight inspected. The skin sample is in the punch or still attached at the base. If attached, the sample is caught with a fine skin hook and retracted until the base can be reached with the iris scissors. Use the scissors to divide the sample from the base.

Hemostasis is accomplished with pressure for 5 to 10 minutes. Pinpoint electrocoagulation can be used if necessary. The wound may be allowed to heal by granulation, but a better cosmetic result is obtained with one or two wound-everting sutures placed immediately.

The wound should be cleaned once or twice daily with hydrogen peroxide and antibiotic ointment applied. The sutures are removed from the facial lesions in 3 to 5 days and from neck or other lesions in approximately 7 to 14 days. If the wound is allowed to granulate, it can be cared for in the same fashion but will take longer to heal completely.

AMY R. COFFEY

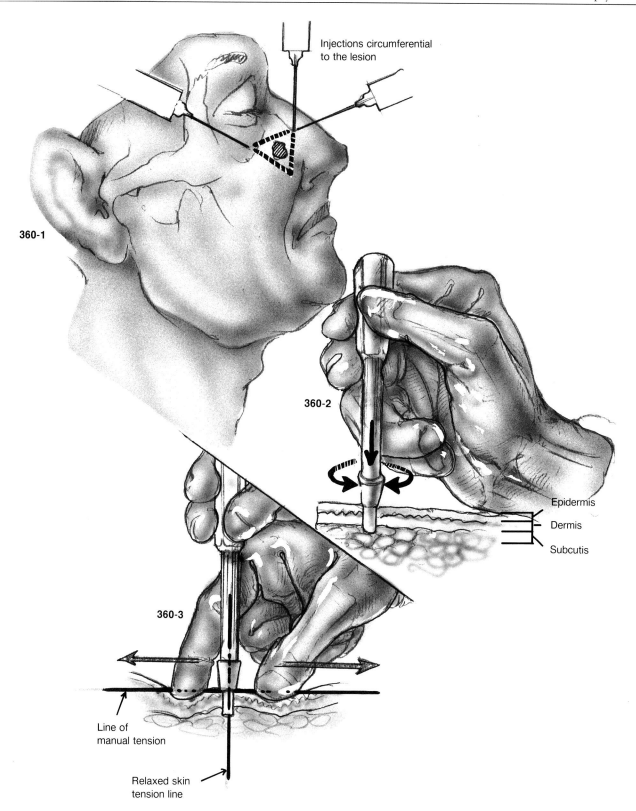

Injections circumferential to the lesion

360-1

360-2

Epidermis

Dermis

Subcutis

360-3

Line of manual tension

Relaxed skin tension line

■ *361.* COMMON INJECTION SITES FOR LO-CAL ANESTHESIA—Injection of a local anesthetic to achieve anesthesia of the specified anatomic region or structure sufficient to perform a desired surgical or therapeutic procedure without pain to the patient; common sites are the face, external auditory canal, oral cavity, tonsil, and neck.

Indications

1. Anesthesia for procedures not requiring general anesthesia
2. Anesthesia in patients at risk for general anesthesia
3. Local vasoconstriction for control of bleeding

Special Considerations

1. History of allergic reactions to local anesthetics must be reviewed.
2. Local anesthetics may be less effective and have a slower onset of action in the presence of a local inflammatory process.
3. Underlying medical conditions may be affected by local injections.
4. The length of the proposed procedure must be included in the decision about the type of anesthetic used.
5. Vasoconstrictors may be added to local anesthetics to prolong the duration of anesthesia and to control local bleeding. Epinephrine is most commonly used for this purpose.

Tips and Pearls

1. Commercially prepared anesthetics containing epinephrine require lowering of the pH to promote stability of the solution. This results in slower onset of action and sometimes more discomfort for the patient.
2. Adding the epinephrine just before use alleviates the need for the stabilizing agent and lowering the pH.
3. The use of a control type syringe with aspiration before injection helps avoid the complication of intravascular injection.
4. The maximum safe dose of anesthetic should be determined before the start of the procedure, and the quantity used should be documented. Because of the rich vascular supply to the head and neck, rapid toxicity may be reached if the toxic threshold is exceeded.
5. Pediatric patients have a lower toxic dose and tend to have a greater blood supply to the mucous membranes than adults. This may result in a more rapid absorption of topical anesthetics than seen in adults.
6. Toxicity is usually manifested by allergic reactions or systemic toxicity, including tremors, agitation, seizures, respiratory suppression, hypotension, and myocardial depression.

References

Eriksson E, ed. Illustrated handbook of local anaesthesia. Philadelphia: WB Saunders, 1980.

Raj P, ed. Clinical practice of regional anesthesia. New York: Churchill Livingstone, 1991.

Technique

Local anesthesia is generally obtained by local infiltration of the anesthetic around the operative site and the region of the sensory nerve supplying the area. The sensory distribution to the head and neck is illustrated in Figures 361-1 through 361-6.

Face

Local anesthesia of the face is accomplished by local infiltration of the area involved or by blocking the appropriate division of the trigeminal nerve. Blocking of the supratrochlear and supraorbital nerves provides anesthesia over the forehead and scalp as far posterior as the lambdoid suture. The supraorbital notch is palpated, and a 27-gauge needle is advanced medial to the notch to block the supraorbital nerve and directly on the notch to block the supraorbital nerve. No more than 5 mL of anesthetic should be used to avoid swelling of the eyelids (Fig. 361-1).

The infraorbital nerve is the terminal branch of the maxillary division of the trigeminal nerve. It arises from the infraorbital foramen and divides into four branches: inferior palpebral, external nasal, internal nasal, and superior labial. Infiltration of local anesthetic in the infraorbital foramen produces anesthesia to the areas supplied by the nerve, which include the lower eyelid, lateral inferior portion of the nose and the vestibule, and the upper lip and its mucosa. The injection may be made through an intraoral or extraoral approach. The notch is palpated, and the needle positioned within the foramen. The infraorbital canal lies at a 45° angle backward and upward as it exits from the maxilla. The needle should not be advanced more than 0.5 cm into the foramen, and no more than 3 mL of solution should be injected to avoid the possibility of orbital complications (Fig. 361-3).

Anesthesia for the lower one third of the face is accomplished by blocking the mental nerve, which is a terminal branch of the mandibular division of the trigeminal nerve. The inferior alveolar nerve passes through the mandibular canal and exits through the mental foramen to give rise to the mental nerve (Fig. 361-4). Blocking the mental nerve as it exits the foramen results in anesthesia of the skin and mucous membrane of the lower lip and the skin covering the anterior portion of the mandible.

Ear and External Auditory Canal

Local anesthesia of the ear may be necessary for closing lacerations or formal otologic surgery. The great auricular nerve is blocked by injection of local anesthetic along the mastoid process. The auriculotemporal nerve is blocked by injection into the bony-cartilaginous junction of the anterior canal wall and infiltration of the skin and periosteum around the auditory canal in front of the ear (Fig. 361-5).

Oral Cavity and Tonsil

The region of the tonsil is innervated by the tonsilar branches of the glossopharyngeal nerve. The trunk of the nerve runs along the stylopharyngeus muscle. Anesthesia is obtained by first spraying the pharynx and palatal arches with a topical anesthetic containing a solution of 4% lidocaine (Xylocaine) or 14% benzocaine (Cetacaine). This technique is contraindicated in children younger than 15 years of age and in anxious or unpredictable adults (Fig. 361-6).

Injection of the greater palatine foramen is useful in the control of bleeding during functional endoscopic sinus surgery. After induction of anesthesia, the greater palatine foramen is located at the level of the second molar and about 1 cm above the gingival margin. A 45° angle is made in a 2-inch (5-cm), 25-gauge needle 25 mm from the tip. The tip is advanced into the foramen, and 0.75 to 1 mL of 1% lidocaine with a 1:100,000 concentration of epinephrine is injected in adults; 0.5 to 0.75 mL is used in children.

Neck

Local anesthesia of the neck for minor procedures is best aimed at blocking of the superficial cervical nerves supplying the area. If the planned surgery involves the deeper structures of the neck, a physician who is not experienced in cervical nerve blocks should consider having this performed by a qualified anesthesiologist.

JOHN S. MAY

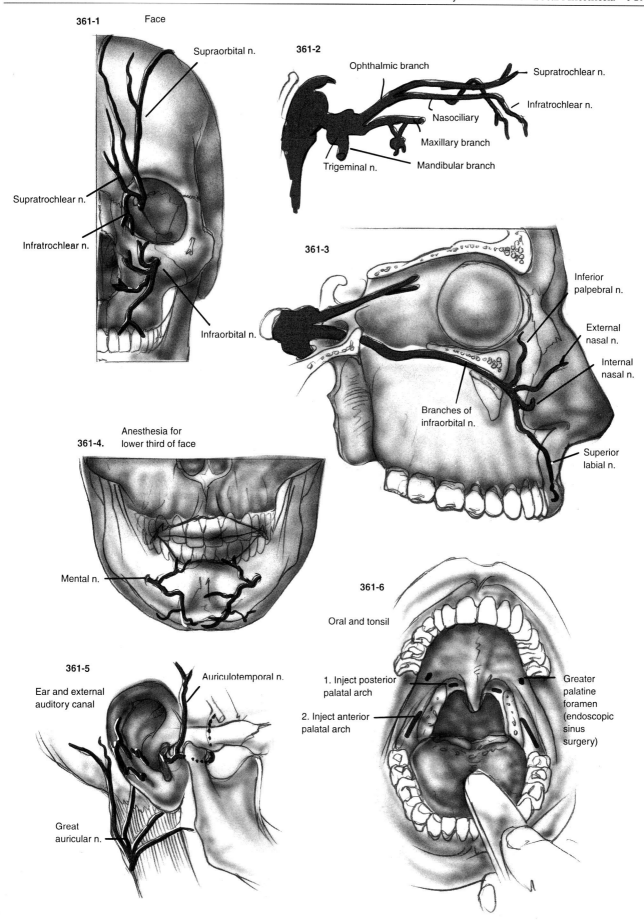

361-1   Face

Supraorbital n.

Supratrochlear n.

Infratrochlear n.

Infraorbital n.

361-2

Ophthalmic branch

Supratrochlear n.

Infratrochlear n.

Nasociliary

Maxillary branch

Trigeminal n.

Mandibular branch

361-3

Inferior palpebral n.

External nasal n.

Internal nasal n.

Branches of infraorbital n.

Superior labial n.

361-4.   Anesthesia for lower third of face

Mental n.

361-5   Ear and external auditory canal

Auriculotemporal n.

Great auricular n.

361-6   Oral and tonsil

1. Inject posterior palatal arch

2. Inject anterior palatal arch

Greater palatine foramen (endoscopic sinus surgery)

Figure Credits

The authors and publisher wish to acknowledge the contribution of materials from the following sources:

Figures 45-1, 45-2, 45-3, and 45-4: modified by A. Pazos after D. Factor, from Gacek RR. Pathophysiology and management of cupulolithiasis. Am J Otolaryngol 1985;6:66–74.

Figures 57-1, 57-2, 57-3, 57-4, 57-5, 57-6, 57-7, and 57-8: modified by A. Pazos after T. Allen and L. Lyons, from Shockley WW and Pillsbury HC. The neck: diagnosis and surgery. St. Louis: Mosby, 1994.

Figures 58-1, 58-2, 58-3, and 58-4: modified by A. Pazos after T. Allen and L. Lyons, from Shockley WW and Pillsbury HC. The neck: diagnosis and surgery. St. Louis: Mosby, 1994.

Figures 59-1, 59-2, 59-3 and 59-4: modified by A. Pazos after T. Allen and L. Lyons, from Shockley WW and Pillsbury HC. The neck: diagnosis and surgery. St. Louis: Mosby, 1994.

Figures 60-1, 60-2, 60-3, 60-4, 60-5, 60-6, 60-7, and 60-8: modified by A. Pazos after T. Allen and L. Lyons, from Shockley WW and Pillsbury HC. The neck: diagnosis and surgery. St. Louis: Mosby, 1994.

Figures 64-1, 64-2, 64-3, 64-4, 64-5, and 64-6: modified by A. Pazos after T. Allen and L. Lyons, from Shockley WW and Pillsbury HC. The neck: diagnosis and surgery. St. Louis: Mosby, 1994.

Figures 68-1, 68-2, 68-3, 68-4, 68-5, and 68-6: from Shapiro J, Zeitels SM, and Fried MP. Laser surgery for laryngeal cancer. Operative techniques in otolaryngology—head and neck surgery, 1992;3:84–92.

Figures 77-1, 77-2, 77-3, 77-4, 77-5, 77-6, 77-7, 77-8, 77-9, 77-10, 77-11, and 77-12: modified by Pazos after Balich, from Pearson BW, De Santo LW. Near-total laryngectomy. Operative techniques in otolaryngology—head and neck surgery, 1990;1:28–41.

Figures 114-2, 114-3, 114-4, and 114-5: modified by A. Pazos after R. Galla, from Nadol JB and Schuknecht HJ. Surgery of the ear and temporal bone. New York: Raven, 1993.

Figures 119-7, 119-8, and 119-9: modified by A. Pazos after L. Tackett, from Schwaber, MK. Medial graft tympanoplasty: the "swinging door" technique. Operative techniques in otolaryngology—head and neck surgery, 1992;3:232–238.

Figures 121-1, 121-2, 121-3, 121-4, 121-5, 121-6, 121-7, and 121-8: adapted from Brackmann DE, ed. Otologic surgery. Philadelphia: WB Saunders, 1994.

Figures 123-1, 123-2, 123-3, and 123-4: modified by A. Pazos after L. Cook.

Figures 124-1, 124-2, 124-3, 124-4, 124-5, 124-6, 124-7, 124-8, 124-9, 124-10, 124-11, and 124-12: modified by A. Pazos after D. Slaughton (Project HEAR).

Figures 133-1, 133-2, 133-3, 133-4, 133-5, 133-6, 133-7, 133-8, 133-9, and 133-10: adapted from Brackmann DE, ed. Otologic surgery. Philadelphia: WB Saunders, 1994.

Figures 134-1, 134-2, 134-3, 134-4, 134-5, and 134-6: adapted from Brackmann DE, ed. Otologic surgery. Philadelphia: WB Saunders, 1994.

Figure 138-7: adapted from Coker NJ. Management of traumatic injuries to the facial nerve. Otolaryngol Clin North Am, 1991;24:215–227. Figure 138-8: adapted from Fisch U. Facial paralysis in fractures of the petrous bone. Laryngoscope 1974;84:2141–2154.

Figures 143-1, 143-2, 143-3, 143-4, 143-5, 143-6, 143-7, and 143-8: adapted from Brackmann DE, ed. Otologic surgery. Philadelphia: WB Saunders, 1994.

Figures 144-1, 144-2, 144-3, 144-4, 144-5, and 144-6: adapted from Brackmann DE, ed. Otologic surgery. Philadelphia: WB Saunders, 1994.

Figures 145-2, 145-3, 145-4, 145-5, and 145-6: Pillsbury HC and Goldsmith MM III. Operative challenges in otolaryngology—head and neck surgery. Chicago: Year Book, 1990.

Figures 146-1, 146-2, 146-3, and 146-4: from Gacek RR. Transection of the posterior ampullary nerve for the relief of benign paroxymal positional nystagmus. Ann Otol Rhinol, 1974;83:596–605; and from Brackmann DE, ed. Otologic surgery. Philadelphia: WB Saunders, 1994.

Figures 147-1, 147-2, 147-3, and 147-4: modified by A. Pazos after D. Factor, from Brackmann DE, ed. Otologic surgery. Philadelphia: WB Saunders, 1994; and Gacek RR. Pathophysiology and management of cupulolithiasis. Am J Otolaryngol 1985;6:66–74.

Figures 150-1, 150-2, 150-3, 150-4, 150-5, 150-6, 150-7, and 150-8: adapted from Brackmann DE, ed. Otologic surgery. Philadelphia: WB Saunders, 1994.

Figures 151-1, 151-2, 151-3, 151-4, 151-5, 151-6, 151-7, and 151-8: adapted from Brackmann DE, ed. Otologic surgery. Philadelphia: WB Saunders, 1994.

Figures 152-1, 152-2, 152-3, 152-4, 152-5, 152-6, 152-7, and 152-8: modified by A. Pazos after R Margulies, from Cohen NL. Acoustic neuroma resection. Otolaryngol Clin North Am 1992;25:302.

Figures 154-1, 154-2, 154-3, 154-4, 154-5, 154-6, 154-7, and 154-8: modified by A. Pazos after G. Card, from Brackmann DE, ed. Otologic surgery. Philadelphia: WB Saunders, 1994.

Figures 171-1, 171-2, 171-3, and 171-4: modified by A. Pazos from Burget GC and Menick FJ. Nasal support and lining: the marriage of beauty and blood supply. Plast Reconstr Surg 1989;84:189–203.

Figures 298-1, 298-2, 298-3, and 298-4: modified by A. Pazos after T. C. Hengst, from Mayer TG and Fleming RW. Aesthetic and reconstructive surgery of the scalp. St. Louis: Mosby–Year Book, 1992.

Index

A

Abbe flap, lip reconstruction and, 48–49
Abscesses. *See* Infections; *specific sites*
Acne, chemical peels for. *See* Chemical peels
Acoustic neuromas, 394–405
  resection of
    middle fossa, 398–401
    retrosigmoid approach to, 402–405
    translabyrinthine approach to, 394–397
Actinic changes, chemical peels for. *See* Chemical peels
Adenoidectomy, 816–817
Adenomas
  parathyroid
    mediastinal exploration and dissection and, 258–261
    parathyroidectomy for, 242–245
    subtotal, autotransplantation and, 240–241
    total parathyroidectomy for, 236–241
  pituitary, hypophysectomy for, transsphenoidal, 876–877
  pleomorphic, total parotidectomy with nerve resection and graft for, 10–11
  thyroid lobectomy and isthmusectomy for, 218–221
  tracheobronchial, laser techniques for, 806–807
Adenopathy, mediastinal exploration and dissection and, 258–261
Advancement flaps, 626–627
  bipedicle, 626–627
  with modified Burow's technique, for upper lip reconstruction, 62–63
  rotation-advancement, oral, for oronasal and oroantral fistula repair, 732–733
  simple, 626–627
  single pedicle, 626–627
Aging, chemical peels for. *See* Chemical peels
Airway obstruction, supraglottic swelling causing, endoscopic partial laryngectomy for, 170–171
Alar procedures. *See* Rhinoplasty
Alar to lobule proportion, 442–443
Alloplastics, for vocal cord paralysis, 604
Alopecia
  hair transplantation for. *See* Hair transplantation
  tissue expansion for, 632–635

Alveolar bone, resorption of, vestibuloplasty for, 116–117
Alveolar ridge resection, 94–95
Amplitude, stroboscopy and, 592
Anastomosis, of nerves, 674–676
Anatomic lines, alignment of, Z-plasty for, 624–625
Androphonia, thyroplasty for, type IV, 602–603
Anesthesia
  for laser laryngoscopy, 776, 778–779
  local, 918–919
    of ear and external auditory canal, 918–919
    of face, 918–919
    for nasal surgery, 444–445
    of oral cavity and tonsil, 918–919
Angiofibromas, nasopharyngeal
  facial translocation for, 38–41
  midfacial degloving procedure for, 882–885
Antrostomy, 854–857
  intranasal, through inferior meatus, 854–855
  maxillary, 888
  sublabial, 856–857
Aphonia, tracheoesophageal shunt for, 210–211
Apicectomy, petrous, 356–357
Apnea. *See* Sleep apnea
Apron incision
  for exploration and repair of penetrating injuries to neck, 168–169
  modified, for neck surgery, 138–139
Aryepiglottic fold
  resection of, 170–171
  tumors of
    extended supraglottic partial laryngectomy for, 194–195
    near-total laryngectomy for, 196
    vertical partial laryngectomy with extension for, 188–189
Aryepiglottis, tumors of, near-total laryngopharyngectomy for, 196
Arytenoid(s)
  displaced, laryngeal fracture and, repair of, 606–607
  impaired motion of, laryngeal fracture and, repair of, 606–607
  tumors of
    extended supraglottic partial laryngectomy for, 194–195

    vertical partial laryngectomy with extension for, 188–189
Arytenoidectomy, 216–217
  endoscopic, 216
  external, 216–217
  laser, 780–781
Ascending ramus, mandibular osteotomy and, 102–103
Asians
  blepharoplasty of upper lid for, 518–519
  rhinoplasty for, 478–479
Aspiration
  cricopharyngeal myotomy and myectomy for, 262–263
  laryngeal diversion for, 214–215
  laryngeal fracture and, repair of, 606–607
  vocal cord injection for, 604–605
A to T flaps, 622–623
Audiant bone conduction hearing device, implantation of, 352–353
Auditory canal, external. *See* External auditory canal; Otitis externa
Auditory nerve, vestibular neurectomy and. *See* Vestibular neurectomy
Auricle
  auriculectomy and, 124–125
  avulsion of. *See* Otoplasty, for auricular avulsions
  hematomas of, drainage of, 440–441
  local auricular excision and skin graft and, 132–133
  reconstruction of, 124–125
Auricular nerve
  great, for nerve grafts, 10–11
  greater, as grafts, 674, 677
Auriculectomy, 124–125
Autograft fat injections, 506–507
Autotransplantation, of parathyroid gland, 238–241
Avascular necrosis, of ear, auriculectomy for, 124–125

B

Balance disorders. *See also* Vertigo
  perilymphatic fistula repair for, 332–335
Baldness
  hair transplantation for. *See* Hair transplantation
  scalp reduction for. *See* Scalp reduction
  tissue expansion for, 632–635

Barotrauma, otic, myringotomy tube placement for, 302–303
Bernard technique, for lip reconstruction, Webster modification of, 54–55
Bilobed flaps, 610–611
Biodegradable cribs, for mandibular reconstruction, 118–119
Biopsy. See also specific sites
  endoscopic, 914–915
  incisional and excisional, 910–911
  needle, 912–913
  punch, 916–917
Birth trauma, septal dislocation due to, 532–533
Bite, open, anterior, LeFort I osteotomy for, 712–713
Blacks, rhinoplasty for, 478–479
Blair procedure, Ivy modification of, 472, 474–475
Blepahrochalasia, blepharoplasty for, 512–513
Blepharoplasty, 512–529
  facial analysis and, 500
  for laceration repair, 520–521
  lower lid, 514–517
    for repair of defects, 526–527
      cartilaginous-perichondral grafts for, 526
      Mustarde cheek flaps for, 526–527
      skin-only pedicle or transposition flaps for, 526–527
    skin and muscle flap, 514–517
    skin flap, 516–517
    transconjunctival, 514, 516–517
  lower lid malposition after, surgical treatment of, 528–529
    full-thickness skin grafting for ectropion and, 528
    lateral canthopexy in conjunction with levator recession for, 528–529
  upper lid, 512–513
    for Asian eye, 518–519
    for repair of defects, 522–525
      cartilaginous-perichondral grafts for, 524–525
      skin-only pedicle or transposition flaps for, 522, 524–525
Bolus grafting, for intraoral skin grafting, 106
Bone flaps
  free, vascularized, for mandibular reconstruction, 118–123
  scapular, 680–683
Bone grafts
  harvesting
    from calvarium, 672–673
    from rib, 670–671
    for temporomandibular joint reconstruction, 740–741
    iliac crest, for mandibular reconstruction, 118–119
Bone loss, mandibular, mandibular reconstruction for, 118–123
Brain herniation, management of, 360–361
Brain stem implants, placement of, translabyrinthine approach to acoustic neuromas for, 394–395
Branchial cleft
  cysts of, excision of, 276–277, 312–313
  fistulas of, excision of, 312–313
Brauer-Foerster columellar lengthening technique, 472–473
Bronchoscopy, 798–809
  diagnostic, 798–799
  flexible, 808–809
  for foreign bodies, 800–803
  laser techniques for, 806–807
  stricture dilation using, 804–805

Brow, 744–745
  browlifts and, 502–505
    coronal, trichophytic, and pretrichial, 502–503
    direct, indirect, midforehead, and temporal, 504–505
    endoscopic, 502–504
Buccal mucosa
  intraoral skin grafting for defects of, 106–107
  resection of, 106–107
  tongue flaps for reconstruction of, 104–105
Buccal resection, partial- and full-thickness, 100–101
Burns, contractures due to, radial forearm flaps for, 688–689
Burow's technique, modified, advancement flaps for upper lip reconstruction with, 62–63

C
Caldwell-Luc procedure, 856–857
Calvarial grafts, harvesting, 672–673
Canaloplasty, 296–297
Cancellous marrow, for mandibular reconstruction, 118–119
Canthal tendons, medial
  fracture of, frontal sinus fractures and, 558–559
  repair of, 552–553
Cantholysis, lateral, 894–897
Canthopexy, lateral, with levator recession, for lower lid malposition following blepharoplasty, 528–529
Canthotomy, lateral, 894–897
  for lower lid malposition following blepharoplasty, 528–529
Canthus, medial, defects of, glabellar flaps for, 614–615
Carcinoma. See specific types and sites
Carotid arteries
  coverage of, superior trapezius myocutaneous flaps for, 640–641
  external, ligation of, 286–287
  injury of
    exploration and repair of, 168–169
    repair of, 292–293
  interior, exposure of, mandibular osteotomy for, 102–103
  lymphangiomas and, excision of, 278–279
  resection of, access to nasopharynx and, 416–417
Carotid body tumors
  carotid vessel repair and, 292–293
  paragangliomas, resection of, 284–285
Carotid veins, injury to, repair of, 292–293
Cartilage grafts
  from ear, 666–667
  from septum, 664–665
Caustic ingestions
  esophageal dilation for, retrograde, 796–797
  esophagoscopy for, 790–791
Cavernous sinus, facial translocation for nasopharyngeal angiofibroma resection and, 38–41
Cephalometric analysis, 480–481
Cerebrospinal fluid leaks
  endoscopic maxillary, ethmoid, sphenoidectomy for, 886–889
  frontal sinus fractures and
    anterior wall, 558–559
    posterior wall, 560–561
  repair of, 360–361

Cerebrospinal fluid otorrhea, mastoidectomy for, simple, 340–343
Cerebrospinal fluid rhinorrhea
  extracranial closure of, mucoperiosteal flaps for, 832–835
    defect repair and, 834–835
    identification of cerebrospinal fluid leak and, 832–833
    middle turbinate, 834–835
    nasal septal, 834–835
  frontoethmoidectomy for, external, 868–869
  nasal encephaloceles and meningoceles causing. See Nose, encephaloceles and meningoceles of
  sphenoidectomy for, intranasal, 872–873
Cervical node biopsy, 158–159
Cheek, 744–745
  defects of
    bilobed flaps for, 610–611
    cheek-neck rotation flaps for, 616–617
    malar implants and, 488–489
Cheek advancement flaps, for lip reconstruction, 54–57
  McHugh flap, 56–57
  Webster flap, 54–55
Cheek-neck rotation flaps, 616–617
Cheilitis, actinic, vermilionectomy for, 42–43
  with wedge resection, 44–45
Chemical peels, 510–511
  light, 510–511
  medium, supplemented, 510
  phenol, 510–511
Chest, cutaneous loss over, latissimus dorsi myocutaneous flaps for, 648–651
Children
  endoscopic sinus surgery in, 904–905
  esophageal dilation in
    antegrade, 794
    retrograde, 796
  facial fractures in, 566–567
  mandibular fractures in, 580–581
  nasal ciliary biopsy in, 842–843
Chin, 744–745. See also Mentoplasty
  augmentation of, nasal-facial analysis for, 442–443
  genioplasty and, 484–487
    horizontal position changes and, 484–485
    vertical position changes and, 486–487
  implants and, 482–483
Choanal atresia
  transnasal repair of, 714–715
  transpalatal repair of, 716–719
Cholesteatomas
  facial recess approach for, 358–359
  mastoidectomy for
    radical, modified, 344–347
    simple, 340–343
  of middle ear, removal of, 328–329
  pearls and, exploratory tympanotomy for, tympanomeatal flaps for, 304–307
  repair of congenital aural atresia and, 422–425
Chondrocutaneous advancement flaps, for pinna reconstruction, 128–131
Chordomas, clivus, midfacial degloving procedure for, 882–885
Ciliary dyskinesia, nasal cavity examination for, 842–843
Cleft lip, repair of, 720–725
  Abbe-Estlander reconstruction for, 48–49
  bilateral, 724–725
  nasal, 472–475
  unilateral, rotation-advancement technique for, 720–723

Cleft palate, repair of, 726–731
    of complete secondary cleft palate, 726–727
    of complete unilateral cleft palate, 730–731
    of incomplete secondary cleft palate, 728–729
    two-flap palatoplasty with intravelar veloplasty for, 726–727, 730–731
Clivus
    facial translocation for nasopharyngeal angiofibroma resection and, 38–41
    inferior, lateral transcondylar approach to, extreme, 410–413
Cochlea, 384–387
    cochlear implants and, 380–381
        facial recess approach for, 358–359
    posterior semicircular canal occlusion and, 384–385
    singular neurectomy and, 386–387
Collagen injections, 506–507
    for vocal cord paralysis, 604–605
Collateral arteries, radial, posterior, lateral arm free flaps and, 690–691
Columellar incisions, 852–853
Commissures
    anterior
        anterolateral vertical partial laryngectomy and, 180–183
        partial laryngectomy and, 186–187
    lateral, repair of, 64–65
Composite grafts, from ear, 668–669
Compression plating, for mandibular fractures, 570–571
Contractures, in burn patients, radial forearm flaps for, 688–689
Cordectomy, 174–175
Coronoidectomy, temporomandibular joint reconstruction and, 740–741
Cor pulmonale, tonsillectomy for, 812–813
Costochondral grafts, harvesting, 740
Cranial base. See Skull base
Cranial fossa, defects of, pericranial flaps for, 630–631
Cranialization, for frontal sinus fractures, posterior wall, 560
Cranial neuropathies. See also specific nerves
    glomus tumor excision for, 406–407
Cranial vault, frontal defects of, reconstruction of, 906–907
Craniectomy
    access to nasopharynx and, 414
    middle and posterior fossa, intermediate or lateral temporal bone resection and, 134, 136–137
Craniofacial dysjunction, LeFort II fracture repair for, 544–547
Craniofacial resection, including ethmoid labyrinth and cribriform plate, 34–37
Craniofacial skeleton, facial translocation for nasopharyngeal angiofibroma resection and, 38–41
Craniomaxillofacial defects, bone grafts for, harvesting, 670–671
Cranioplasty, tissue expansion for, 632–635
Craniotomy
    access to nasopharynx and, 414–417
    bifrontal, craniofacial resection including ethmoid labyrinth and cribriform plate and, 34–35
    frontotemporal, facial translocation for nasopharyngeal angiofibroma resection and, 38
Cribriform plate, craniofacial resection including ethmoid labyrinth and cribriform plate and, 34–37

Cricoid ring, midline division of, anterior, 582–583
Cricopharyngeal achalasia, esophageal dilation for. See Esophagus, dilation of
Cricopharyngeal stenosis, cricopharyngeal myotomy and myectomy for, 262–263
Cricothyroid muscles, paralysis of, thyroplasty for, type IV, 602–603
Cutaneous nerve, lateral femoral, for nerve grafts, 10–11
Cyst(s). See specific sites
Cystic hydromas, excision of, 278–279
Cystic hygromas, of supraclavicular space, excision of, 164–165

D
Dacryocystitis, dacryocystorhinostomy for, 908–909
Dacryocystorhinostomy, 908–909
Dacryoliths, dacryocystorhinostomy for, 908–909
Dedo laryngoscope, 172
Deltopectoral flaps, 620–621
    for lip reconstruction, 58–59
Dental appliance method, for intraoral skin grafting, 106–107
Dentures, for mandibular fractures, 578–579
Dermabrasion, 508–509
Dermatochalasia, blepharoplasty for, 512–517
    lower eyelid, 514–517
    upper eyelid, 512–513
Dermoid cysts
    nasal, 850–851
    of neck, excision of, 280–281
Dermoplasty, septal, 836–837
Dingman technique, 474–475
Diplopia, maxillary decompression for, 880–881
Diverticulopexy, myotomy and, for Zenker's diverticulum, 256
Dog-ear defects, cheek-neck rotation flaps for, 616
Drooling, tympanic neurectomy for, 338–339
Dufourmental flaps, 618–619
Durotomy, curvilinear, 412–413
Dysphagia
    branchial cleft cyst excision for, 276–277
    cricopharyngeal myotomy and myectomy for, 262–263
    dermoid cyst excision for, 280–281
    lymphangioma excision for, 278–279
    oropharyngeal, 256–257
    thyroglossal duct cyst excision for, 274–275
    vocal cord injection for, 604–605
Dysphonia
    laryngeal fracture and, repair of, 606–607
    recurrent laryngeal nerve section and avulsion for, 212–213
    stroboscopy and, 592–593
    thyroplasty for. See Thyroplasty
    vocal cord injection for, 604–605
Dysplasia
    laryngeal, endoscopic partial laryngoscopy for, 172–173
    of lip, vermilionectomy for, 42–43
        with wedge resection, 44–45
Dyspnea
    branchial cleft cyst excision for, 276–277
    laryngeal fracture and, repair of, 606–607
    lymphangioma excision for, 278–279

thyroglossal duct cyst excision for, 274–275

E
Ear(s), 124–137, 295–340, 428–441, 744–745
    atresia of, congenital, repair of, 422–425
    auricle of. See Auricle
    barotrauma and, myringotomy tube placement for, 302–303
    bleeding from, glomus tumor excision for, 406–407
    cartilage grafts from, 666–667
    cochlear implants and, 380–381
    composite grafts from, 668–669
    facial recess approach for, 358–359
    glomus tympanicum and, excision of, 354–355
    hearing loss and. See Hearing loss
    hematomas of, drainage of, 440–441
    labyrinthectomy and, 376–379
        transcanal, 376–377
        transmastoid, 378–379
    local anesthesia of, 918–919
    Meniere's disease and. See Meniere's disease
    middle, 322–329, 332–339
        cerebrospinal fluid leaks into, management of, 360–361
        cholesteatomas of, removal of, 328–329
        obliteration of, 348–351
        otitis media and. See Otitis media
        paragangliomas of, excision of, 354–355
        tumors of, facial recess approach for, 358–359
        tympanic membrane and. See Tympanic membrane; Tympanoplasty
    myringoplasty and, 308–309
    myringotomy tube placement and removal and, 302–303
    ossicular chain of. See Ossicular chain
    otitis and. See Otitis externa; Otitis media
    otoplasty and. See Otoplasty
    perilymphatic fistulas of, repair of, 332–335
    petrous apicectomy and, 356–357
    pinna reconstruction and
        with composite grafts, 130–131
        following regional, wedge, and stellate excision, 126–129
    reconstruction of
        bone grafts for, harvesting, 670–671
        pericranial flaps for, 630–631
    temporal bone and. See Temporal bone, resection of
    tinnitus and
        glomus tumor excision for, 406–407
        paraganglioma excision for, 354–355
    tympanic membrane and. See Tympanic membrane; Tympanoplasty
    tympanic neurectomy and, 338–339
    tympanotomy and, exploratory, tympanomeatal flaps for, 304–307
Ectropion, full-thickness skin grafting for, 528
Emphysema, subcutaneous, cervical, laryngeal fracture and, repair of, 606–607
Empyema, of maxillary sinus, antrostomy for, sublabial, 856–857
Encephaloceles, nasal. See Nose, encephaloceles and meningoceles of

Endolymphatic hydrops, endolymphatic sac exposure, decompression, or shunt for, 382–383
Endoscopy, 769–809. *See also* Bronchoscopy; Esophagoscopy; Laryngoscopy
  antrochoanal polyp excision using, 826–827
  arytenoidectomy using, 216
  biopsy using, 914–915
  browlifts using, 502–504
  frontal sinusectomy using, 890–893
  laryngeal web surgery using, 590–591
  laryngectomy using, partial
    glottic, 172–173
    for supraglottic disease, 170–171
  maxillary, ethmoid, sphenoidectomy using, 886–889
  resection of nasal encephaloceles and meningoceles using. *See* Nose, encephaloceles and meningoceles of
Enophthalmos, traumatic, late repair of, 564–565
Enteral feeding, cervical esophagostomy for, 254–255
Epiglottic resection, 170–171
Epiphora
  dacryocystorhinostomy for, 908–909
  nasolacrimal system evaluation and repair for, 554–557
  vidian neurectomy for, 860–863
    endoscopic transnasal approach for, 862–863
    transantral approach for, 860–862
Epistaxis
  anterior ethmoid artery ligation for, 878–879
  septal dermoplasty for, 836–837
  septoplasty and submucous resection for. *See* Rhinoplasty, septoplasty and submucous resection and; Septoplasty; Submucous resection
  transantral ligation of internal maxillary artery for, 858–859
Esophagoscopy, 786–793
  for caustic ingestion, 790–791
  dilation under direct vision using, 792–793
  for foreign body removal, 788–789
Esophagostomy, cervical, 254–255
Esophagus
  cervical
    defects of, trapezius myocutaneous flaps for
      lateral island, 642–643
      lower island, 644–647
    esophagostomy and, 254–255
    reconstruction of, deltopectoral flaps for, 620–621
    strictures of, free jejunal transfer for, 696–697
    tumors of, free jejunal transfer for, 696–697
    upper, tumors of, total pharyngolaryngectomy for, 206–209
  dilation of
    antegrade, 794–795
      balloon dilation and, 794–795
      in children, 794
      Plummer dilators for, 794–795
    esophagoscopic, under direct vision, 792–793
    retrograde, 796–797
      in children, 796
Estlander flap, lip reconstruction and, 48–49
Ethmoid artery, anterior, ligation of, 878–879

Ethmoid bone, fracture of, frontal sinus fractures and, anterior wall, 558–559
Ethmoidectomy, 864–871
  endoscopic, 886–889, 890
  external, 866–867
  frontoethmoidectomy, external, 868–869
  intranasal, 864–865
  with total maxillectomy, 28
  transantral, 870–871
Ethmoid labyrinth
  craniofacial resection including ethmoid labyrinth and cribriform plate and, 34–37
  radical maxillectomy with orbital exenteration and, 30–33
Ethmoidocutaneous fistulas, frontoethmoidectomy for, external, 868–869
Ethmoid plate, superior, craniofacial resection including ethmoid labyrinth and cribriform plate and, 34–37
Ethmoid sinus
  ethmoidectomy and. *See* Ethmoidectomy
  medial maxillectomy and, 24–25
Eustachian tube, nonfunctioning, mastoidectomy for, radical, modified, 344–347
Exophthalmos, maxillary decompression for, 880–881
Exostoses
  canaloplasty for, 296–297
  of external auditory canal, excision of, 298–299
External auditory canal, 296–301, 312–313
  branchial cleft fistula and cyst excision and, 312–313
  canaloplasty and, 296–297
  exostoses of, excision of, 298–299
  local anesthesia of, 918–919
  meatoplasty and, 296–297
  osteomas of, excision of, 298–299
  otitis externa and. *See* Otitis externa
  preservation of, auriculectomy and, 124–125
  soft tissue canal stenosis and, 300–301
External rhinotomy incision, 852–853
Eye(s)
  enophthalmos and, traumatic, late repair of, 564–565
  orbit of. *See* Orbit
Eyebrows
  browlifts and, 502–505
  defects of, forehead flaps for, median, 612–613
  facial analysis and, 500
Eyelids
  blepharoplasty and. *See* Blepharoplasty
  defects of
    cartilage grafts for, 666–667
    composite grafts for, 668–669
  reanimation techniques for, 374–375
    gold weight implantation and, 374–375
    spring implantation and, 374
  retraction of, composite grafts for, 668–669
  tarsorrhaphy and, 372–373

F

Face. *See also* Facial *entries; specific sites*
  aesthetic subunits of, 744–745
  local anesthesia of, 918–919
  tumors of, supraomohyoid neck dissection for, 144–147

Facial analysis
  for mentoplasty, 480–481
  upper one-third, 500–501
Facial defects. *See also specific sites*
  augmentation of, pericranial flaps for, 630–631
  bone graft reconstruction of, midfacial degloving procedure for, 882–885
  cheek-neck rotation flaps for, 616–617
  deltopectoral flaps for, 620–621
  pectoralis major myocutaneous flaps for, 636–639
  platysma flaps for, 656–657
  scapular free flaps for, 680–683
  superior trapezius myocutaneous flaps for, 640–641
  temporalis myocutaneous flaps for, 654–655
  A to T flaps for, 622–623
Facial injuries, 530–581
  fractures. *See also specific sites*
    LeFort I, repair of, 540–541
    midfacial degloving procedure for, 882–885
    pediatric, 566–567
  lacerations, complex, repair of, 752–753
    Gilles corner stitch for, 752–753
    of stellate lacerations, 752–753
    subcutaneous skin eversion sutures for, 752–753
    of trap door defects, 752–753
Facial nerve, 362–375
  cross grafts and, 698–699
  decompression of, 368–371
  eyelid reanimation techniques and, 374–375
    gold weight implantation and, 374–375
    spring implantation and, 374
  grafting of, 362–365
    of intracranial segment, 362–365
    of labyrinthine segment, 364–365
    of tympanic and mastoid segment, 364–365
  hypoglossal-facial crossover techniques for, 366–367
    classic technique for, 366–367
    interpositional-jump technique for, 366–367
  injury of
    facial recess approach for, 358–359
    management of, 16–17
    mastoidectomy for, simple, 340–343
  partial- and full-thickness buccal resection and, 100
  tarsorrhaphy and, 372–373
  total parotidectomy and
    with nerve resection and graft, 10–11
    with nerve sparing, 8–9
  tumors of, facial recess approach for, 358–359
Facial paralysis, 698–709
  cross facial nerve grafts for, 698–699
  dynamic temporalis and masseter muscle transposition for, 706–709
  facial reanimation for. *See* Facial reanimation
  nasal valve surgery for. *See* Rhinoplasty, for nasal valve collapse or incompetence
  nerve-muscle pedicle for, 700–701
  static slings for, 702–705
  tarsorrhaphy for, 372–373
  temporalis myocutaneous flaps for, 654–655
Facial reanimation, eyelid reanimation procedures for, 374–375

gold weight implantation and, 374–375
spring implantation and, 375
Facial recess approach
extended, glomus tumor excision and,
406–407
to mesotympanum, 358–359
Facial translocation, for nasopharyngeal
angiofibroma resection, 38–41
Facial triangle, lower, 480–481
Farrior repair, 474–475
Fasciaform grafts, for reconstruction of large
tympanic membrane perforations,
326–327
Fat injections, 506–507
Fat obliteration, of frontal sinus, 898–901
bilateral procedure for, 900
unilateral procedure for, 898–901
Fibula osseocutaneous free flaps, 692–693
Fistulas. *See also specific sites*
draining, branchial cleft cyst excision for,
276–277
Flaps
deltopectoral, 620–621
for lip reconstruction, 58–59
forehead, median, 612–613
free, 24–125. *See* Free flaps
local and regional. *See* Advancement flaps;
Local and regional flaps
myocutaneous. *See* Myocutaneous flaps
pharyngeal, superiorly based, 734–735
rotation-advancement, oral, for oronasal
and oroantral fistula repair, 732–
733
skin
free composite, for pharyngeal
reconstruction, 270–271
regional, for pharyngeal reconstruction,
270–271
tongue, for oropharyngeal reconstruction,
104–105
posteriorly based flaps and, 104–105
turnover, for oronasal and oroantral fistula
repair, 732–733
Fleming-Mayer flap procedure, 758–761
Foramen magnum, inferior, lateral
transcondylar approach to,
extreme, 410–413
Forehead, 744–745
defects of, A to T flaps for, 622–623
Forehead flaps, median, 612–613
Foreign bodies
bronchoscopy for, 800–803
ethmoidectomy for, intranasal, 864–865
of maxillary sinus, antrostomy for,
sublabial, 856–857
removal of
esophagoscopy for, 788–789
form nasal cavity, 842–843
stripping off of, 802–803
Fovea ethmoidalis, craniofacial resection
including ethmoid labyrinth and
cribriform plate and, 34–37
Fractures. *See specific sites*
Frankfurt horizontal line, 480
Free flaps
for auriculectomy, 124–125
fibula osseocutaneous, 692–693
iliac crest, internal oblique, 684–687
inferior rectus abdominis, 694–695
lateral arm, 690–691
in microvascular surgery, 678–679
radial forearm, 688–689
scapular, with and without bone, 680–683
Free grafts, for nasal encephalocele and
meningocele repair, harvesting of,
846, 848–849
Free jejunal transfer, 696–697

Frey's syndrome
sternocleidomastoid flaps for, 658–659
tympanic neurectomy for, 338–339
Frontal sinus
ablation and collapse of, 902–903
fractures of
anterior wall, 558–559
frontal sinusectomy and fat obliteration
for, 898–901
bilateral procedure, 900
unilateral procedure, 898–901
posterior wall, 560–561
trephination of, 896–897
Frontal sinusectomy
endoscopic, 890–893
osteoplastic, fat obliteration and, 898–901
bilateral procedure for, 900
unilateral procedure for, 898–901
Frontocutaneous fistulas,
frontoethmoidectomy for, external,
868–869
Frontoethmoidectomy, external, 868–869
Frontonasal duct, injury of, 562–563

G

Gastric pullup, for pharyngeal
reconstruction, 272–273
Gender reassignment, thyroplasty for, type
IV, 602–603
Genioglossus advancement, 822–823
Genioplasty, 484–487
horizontal position changes and, 484–485
nasal-facial analysis for, 442–443
vertical position changes and, 486–487
Geometric broken line closure, 750–751
Gilles corner stitch, 752–753
Gilles fan flap, 50–51
Gilles technique, for lateral commissure
repair, 64–65
Glabellar flaps, 614–615
Glenn technique, for lateral commissure
repair, 64–65
Glomus tumors
excision of, 406–409
exploratory tympanotomy for,
tympanomeatal flaps for, 304–307
Glomus tympanicum, excision of, 354–355
Glossectomy
anterior, partial, 70–71
iliac crest internal oblique free flaps for
reconstruction following, 684–687
midline, partial, of tongue base, 76–77
near-total, 78–81
posterior, partial, of tongue base, 72–75
radial forearm flaps for reconstruction
following, 688–689
total, 82–83
pectoralis major myocutaneous flaps for
reconstruction following, 82
Glossotomy, labiomandibular, median, 68–
69
Glottal closure, stroboscopy and, 592
Glottic split, posterior, with cartilage graft,
584–585
Glottic web, laryngotracheal decompression
for, anterior, 582–583
Glottis
asymmetric, laryngeal fracture and, repair
of, 606–607
incompetent, thyroplasty for, type I, 594–
597
insufficiency, vocal cord injection for,
604–605
shortening of, laryngeal fracture and,
repair of, 606–607

Goiters
mediastinal, excision of, 224–227
multinodular, total thyroidectomy for,
228–229
Gold weights, for eyelid reanimation,
placement of, 374–375
Gonzalez-Ulloa approach, to facial analysis,
480–481
Goode approach, to facial analysis, 480–481
Goode technique, for lateral commissure
repair, 64–65
Gore-Tex graft augmentation, 506–507
Grafts
bone. *See* Bone grafts
cartilage
for ear, 666–667
from septum, 664–665
composite, for ear, 668–669
free, for nasal encephalocele and
meningocele repair, harvesting of,
846, 848–849
for hair transplantation. *See* Hair
transplantation, grafts for
in microvascular surgery, 678–679
mucosal, 660, 662–663
nerve. *See* Nerve grafts
skin. *See* Skin grafts
Granulation tissue, laser techniques for, 806–
807
Granulomatous disease, midline, cartilage
grafts for, 664–665
Graves' disease
ethmoidectomy for, transantral, 870–871
maxillary decompression for, 880–881
total thyroidectomy for, 228–229
Guerin's fracture repair, 540–541

H

Hair transplantation
Fleming-Mayer flap procedure for, 758–
761
first delay and, 758–759
second delay and, 758–761
grafts for, 754–757
micrografts, 756
minigrafts, 754
punch grafts, 754–756
slit grafts, 756–757
Hard palate
fistulas of, anterior, repair of, 732–733
intraoral skin grafting for defects of, 106–
107
resection of, 96–97
Head. *See also specific sites*
defects of, lateral arm free flaps for, 690–
691
Headaches
endoscopic maxillary, ethmoid,
sphenoidectomy for, 886–889
septoplasty for, 830–831
submucous resection of nasal septum for,
828–829
Hearing loss
Audiant bone conduction hearing device
implantation for, 352–353
cochlear implants for, 380–381
endolymphatic sac exposure,
decompression, or shunt for, 382–
383
exostosis excision for, 298–299
exploratory tympanotomy for,
tympanomeatal flaps for, 304–307
glomus tumor excision for, 406–407
myringoplasty for, 308–309
osteoma excision for, 298–299

Hearing loss (*continued*)
  paraganglioma excision for, 354–355
  perilymphatic fistula repair for, 332–335
  soft tissue canal stenosis and, 300–301
  stapedotomy and stapedectomy for, 330–331
  translabyrinthine approach to acoustic neuromas for, 394–395
  tympanoplasty for, type I, 308–311
Hematomas, auricular, drainage of, 440–441
Hemifacial microsomia, skeletal correction of, 742–743
Hemilaryngectomy, 184, 186–187
  horizontal (supraglottic laryngectomy), 190–193
Hemilaryngopharyngectomy, radial forearm flaps for reconstruction following, 688–689
Hemitransfixion incision, 852–853
Hemorrhage
  into lymphangiomas, excision for, 278–279
  neck surgery and, mediastinal exploration and dissection and, 258–261
  orbital, lateral canthotomy and cantholysis for, 894–897
Hennebert's sign (symptom), perilymphatic fistula repair for, 332–335
Hockey stick incision
  for exploration and repair of penetrating injuries to neck, 168–169
  inverted, for neck surgery, 138–139
  for neck surgery, 138–139
Holinger laryngoscope, modified, 172
Hydromas, cystic, excision of, 278–279
Hydrops, endolymphatic, endolymphatic sac exposure, decompression, or shunt for, 382–383
α-Hydroxy acid peels, 510
Hygromas, cystic, of supraclavicular space, excision of, 164–165
Hyoid myotomy-suspension, 822–823
Hyperparathyroidism, parathyroidectomy for, 242–245
Hypoglossal nerve
  hypoglossal-facial crossover techniques and, 366–367
    classic technique for, 366–367
    interpositional-jump technique for, 366–367
  injury of, management of, 16–17
Hypopharynx
  defects of
    latissimus dorsi myocutaneous flaps for, 648–651
    trapezius myocutaneous flaps for
      lateral island, 642–643
      superior, 640–641
  mucosal herniation of, 256–257
  tumors of
    pharyngectomy for, 266–269
    total pharyngolaryngectomy for, 206–209
Hypophysectomy
  transethmosphenoidal, 874–875
  transsphenoidal, 876–877
    transantral approach for, 870–871

I

Iliac crest bone grafts, for mandibular reconstruction, 118–119
Iliac crest internal oblique free flaps, 684–687
Immunocompromised hosts, invasive mucormycosis in, radical

maxillectomy with orbital exenteration for, 30–33
Incus. *See* Ossicular chain
Infections
  adenoidectomy for, 816–817
  branchial cleft cyst excision for, 276–277, 312–313
  branchial cleft fistula excision for, 312–313
  of deep neck space, drainage of, 166–167
  dermoid cyst excision for, 280–281
  of ear, auriculectomy for, 124–125
  laryngocele excision for, 282–283
  of lip, Gilles fan flap for, 50–51
  lymphangioma excision for, 278–279
  mandibular bone loss from, mandibular reconstruction due to, 118–123
  of maxillary sinus, radical maxillectomy with orbital exenteration for, 30–33
  midfacial degloving procedure for, 882–885
  nasal cavity examination for, 842–843
  of petrous apex, petrous apicectomy for, 356–357
  thyroglossal duct cyst excision for, 274–275
  tonsillectomy for, 812–813
Inferior rectus abdominis free flaps, 694–695
Infratrichial incision, for rhytidectomy, 490–491
Infundibulectomy, 886
Injuries. *See specific sites*
Intermaxillary fixation, 568–569
Intraoral salivary gland tumor removal, 6–7
Intratrichial incision
  hidden, for rhytidectomy, 490–491
  for rhytidectomy, 490–491
Isthmusectomy, 218–221

J

Jejunal autografts, free, for pharyngeal reconstruction, 270–271, 273
Jejunal transfer, free, 696–697
Jones dysfunction tests, 554–555
Jugular foramen, glomus tumor excision and, 406–407
Jugular vein
  internal, preservation of, modified radical neck dissection and, 150–153
  lymphangiomas and, excision of, 278–279

K

Karapandzic flap reconstruction, 52–53, 62
Keratopathy, exposure, maxillary decompression for, 880–881
Keratoses, chemical peels for. *See* Chemical peels
Killian incision, 664–665, 852–853

L

Labyrinth
  endolymphatic hydrops and, endolymphatic sac exposure, decompression, or shunt for, 382–383
  ethmoid, craniofacial resection including ethmoid labyrinth and cribriform plate and, 34–37
  labyrinthectomy and. *See* Labyrinthectomy
  streptomycin perfusion of, 388–389
  traumatic labyrinthitis and, vestibular neurectomy for. *See* Vestibular neurectomy

Labyrinthectomy, 376–379
  transcanal, 376–377
  translabyrinthine approach to acoustic neuromas and, 394–395
  transmastoid, 378–379
Labyrinthitis, traumatic, vestibular neurectomy for. *See* Vestibular neurectomy
Lacerations, facial. *See* Facial injuries
Lag screws, for mandibular fractures, 574–575
Laryngeal webs, lysis of, 590–591
  endoscopic keel approach to, 590–591
  microlaryngal, 590
Laryngectomy
  endoscopic, partial, glottic, 172–173
  near-total, 196–199
  partial
    endoscopic, for supraglottic disease, 170–171
    supraglottic, extended, 194–195
    vertical, 184–187
      anterior commissure, 186–187
      anterolateral, 180–183
      extended (frontolateral), 184
      with extension (subtotal or three-quarter), 188–189
      hemilaryngectomy procedure for, 186–187
      including thyroid cartilage, 176–179
      laryngofissure and cordectomy and, 174–175
      laryngofissure procedure for, 185–187
  stomal recurrence following
    mediastinal exploration and dissection and, 258–261
    transsternal mediastinal node dissection for, 154–157
  supraglottic (horizontal hemilaryngectomy), 190–193
  total, 200–203
    aphonia following, tracheoesophageal shunt for, 210–211
    with extension, 204–205
Laryngoceles, excision of, 282–283
Laryngofissure, 174–175, 185–187
Laryngopharyngectomy, near-total, 196
  extended, 196
Laryngopharyngoesophagectomy, mediastinal exploration and dissection and, 258–261
Laryngoplasty
  anterolateral vertical partial laryngectomy and, 182–183
  imbrication, after cordectomy, 174–175
  vertical partial laryngectomy and, 184–186
    including thyroid cartilage, 178
Laryngoscopy
  direct
    near-total laryngectomy and, 196
    with and without biopsy, 770–771
      adult, 770–771
      pediatric, 770
    laser, for papilloma removal, 776–779
    microsuspension, laser excision of early-stage vocal cord carcinoma and, 782–783
    suspension, with laser excision of lingual tonsils, 814–815
Laryngotracheal decompression, anterior, 582–583
Laryngotracheal-esophageal stenosis, sternocleidomastoid flaps for, 658–659
Laryngotracheal reconstruction, anterior and posterior, 586–589

Larynx, 170–217. *See also* Laryngectomy
  aryepiglottic fold resection and, 170–171
  arytenoidectomy and, 216–217
    endoscopic, 216
    external, 216–217
  biopsy of, 196
  combined resection and, 170–171
  diversion of, 214–215
  epiglottic resection and, 170–171
  foreign bodies in, stripping off of, 802–803
  fracture of, repair of, 606–607
  laryngocele excision and, 282–283
  reconstruction of, with composite shunt,
      198–199
  recurrent laryngeal nerve and
    section and avulsion of, 212–213
    subtotal thyroidectomy and, 222
  total pharyngolaryngectomy and, 206–209
  tracheoesophageal shunt and, 210–211
  tumors of, free jejunal transfer for, 696–
      697
  vestibular fold resection and, 170–171
Laser techniques
  arytenoidectomy, 780–781
  bronchoscopy, 806–807
  for excision of early-stage vocal cord
      carcinoma, 782–783
  for excision of lingual tonsils, 814–815
  for granulation tissue, 806–807
  laryngoscopy, for papilloma removal, 776–
      779
  for respiratory papillomatosis, 806–807
  for tracheobronchial adenomas, 806–807
  for tracheobronchial stenosis, 806–807
Lateral arm free flaps, 690–691
Latissimus dorsi myocutaneous flaps, 648–
    651
LeFort I fracture repair, 540–541
LeFort II fracture repair
  for craniofacial dysjunction, 544–547
  of pyramidal fractures, 542–543
LeFort I osteotomy, 712–713
  facial translocation for nasopharyngeal
      angiofibroma resection and, 38–39
Legan's angle, 480–481
Lids. *See* Eyelids
Lingual nerve, injury of, management of,
    16–17
Lip(s), 42–65, 744–745
  Abbe-Estlander reconstruction of, 48–49
  cheek advancement flaps for
      reconstruction of, 54–57
    McHugh flap, 56–57
    Webster flap, 54–55
  cleft. *See* Cleft lip
  deltopectoral flap reconstruction of, 58–59
  Gilles fan flap and, 50–51
  injury of
    deltopectoral flap reconstruction for,
        58–59
    lateral commissure repair for, 64–65
    nasolabial flap for, 60–61
    pectoralis major flap reconstruction for,
        58–59
  Karapandzic flap reconstruction of, 52–53,
      62
  lower, reconstruction of, radial forearm
      flaps for, 688–689
  mandibular deformity of, lateral
      commissure repair for, 64–65
  paralytic distortion of, lateral commissure
      repair for, 64–65
  pectoralis major flap reconstruction of,
      58–59
  pentagonal shield excision and, 46–47
  reconstruction of, nasolabial flaps for,
      608–609

as reference points for facial analysis, 480–
    481
  tumors of, supraomohyoid neck dissection
      for, 144–147
  upper
    advancement flaps with modified
        Burow's technique for
        reconstruction of, 62–63
    nasolabial flap for reconstruction of, 60–
        61
    vermilionectomy and, 42–43
      with wedge resection, 44–45
    W-excision of, 46–47
Lipomas, of neck, excision or liposuction of,
    288–289
Liposuction
  of lipomas, of neck, 288–289
  of neck, with facelift pretunneling, 496–
      497
Lip-splitting incision, for resection of tonsils
    and retromolar trigone, 112–113
Lip switch flap, 48–49
Lobectomy, parotid
  deep lateral, with nerve sparing, 4–5
  superficial, 2–3
Local and regional flaps, 608–659
  advancement. *See* Advancement flaps
  bilobed, 610–611
  deltopectoral, 620–621
  forehead, median, 612–613
  glabellar, 614–615
  myocutaneous. *See* Myocutaneous flaps
  nasolabial, 608–609
    subcutaneous pedicle, 608–609
  pericranial, 630–631
  rhomboid, 618–619
    triple, 628–629
  rotation, cheek-neck, 616–617
    A to T, 622–623
  temporoparietal fascia, 652–653
  tissue expansion and, 632–635
  Z-plasty, 624–625
Ludwig's angina, drainage of, 166–167
Lymphangiomas, excision of, 278–279
Lymph nodes. *See* specific nodes and sites
Lymphomas, staging of, cervical node biopsy
    for, 158–159

M

McFee-type incisions, 66–67, 72
McGregor modification, of Gilles fan flap,
    50–51
McHugh cheek flap, 56–57
Macrogenia, genioplasty for, 484–487
  horizontal position changes and, 484–485
  vertical position changes and, 484–485
Malar implants, 488–489
Malleolus. *See* Ossicular chain
Mandible. *See also* Mandibulectomy;
    Mandibulotomy
  cysts and tumors of, segmental resection
      for, 108–109
  defects of
    anterior, microvascular surgery for,
        678–679
    of archiliac crest internal oblique free
        flaps for, 684–687
    fibula osseocutaneous free flaps for,
        692–693
  fractures of
    in children, 566–567
    dentures and splints for, 578–579
    external fixation with biphase apparatus
        for, 576–577
    intermaxillary fixation for, 568–569

open reduction and internal fixation for
    with compression plating, 570–571
    with lag screws, 574–575
    with noncompression plating, 572–
        573
  pediatric, 580–581
mandibular osteotomy and, 102–103
  midline, paramedian, lateral, and
      ascending ramus, 102–103
  tongue flaps for oropharyngeal
      reconstruction and, 104–105
ramus of, sagittal osteotomy of, 710–711
reconstruction of, 118–123
  near-total glossectomy and, 80
  primary, 120–123
    pectoralis flap with mandibular
        reconstruction plate for, 120
    vascular free bone flaps for, 120–123
  secondary, 118–119
    biodegradable cribs for, 118–119
    solitary iliac crest block for, 118–119
    titanium tray with particular bone
        and cancellous marrow for, 118–
        119
    vascularized free bone flaps for, 118–
        119
resection of tonsils and retromolar trigone
    and
  mandibular, segmental, 112, 114–115
  with mandibular sparing, 112–113
squamous cell carcinoma of, floor of
    mouth resection for. *See* Oral
    cavity, floor of mouth resection and
Mandibular shave, 108–109
Mandibulectomy
  marginal, 108–109
    anterior floor of mouth resection and, 84
    floor of mouth resection and, posterior,
        marginal, 92–93
    lateral floor of mouth resection and, 86–
        87
  segmental
    near-total glossectomy and, 78, 80
    total glossectomy and, 82–83
Mandibulotomy, 66–68
  ascending ramus, mandibular osteotomy
      and, 102–103
  for exploration and repair of penetrating
      injuries of neck, 168–169
  lateral, resection of tonsils and retromolar
      trigone and, 114
  midline
    mandibular osteotomy and, 102
    resection of tonsils and retromolar
        trigone and, 114
    near-total glossectomy and, 78–79
  paramedian, mandibular osteotomy and,
      102
  partial posterior glossectomy of tongue
      base and, 72–74
  pharyngectomy and, 268–269
  segmental, mandibular osteotomy and,
      102–103
  total parotidectomy with seventh nerve
      sparing and, 8–9
Masseter muscle, dynamic temporalis and
    masseter muscle transposition and,
    706–709
Mastoid, 340–361. *See also* Mastoidectomy
  contracted, mastoidectomy for, radical,
      modified, 344–347
  removal of tip of, glomus tumor excision
      and, 406–407
Mastoidectomy, 340–351
  canal wall, intact, 360–361
  canal wall-down, meatoplasty and, 296–
      297

Mastoidectomy (*continued*)
canal wall-up, petrosal approach to posterior cranial fossa and, 418–419
endolymphatic sac exposure, decompression, or shunt and, 382–383
glomus tumor excision and, 406–407
paraganglioma excision and, 354
posterior semicircular canal occlusion and, 384–385
radical, 348–351
grafting and, 346–347
meatoplasty and, 346–347
modified, 344–347
bone work and, 344–347
postoperative care for, 346–347
simple, 340–343
transcortical, facial nerve decompression and, 368–371
translabyrinthine approach to acoustic neuromas and, 394–395
tympanoplasty and, type III, 318–321
Mastoiditis, mastoidectomy for, simple, 340–343
Maxilla. *See also* Maxillectomy
decompression of, for exophthalmos, 880–881
deficiency of, LeFort I osteotomy for, 712–713
excess of, LeFort I osteotomy for, 712–713
exenteration of, Weber-Ferguson approach for, 26–27
mucocele of, antrostomy for, sublabial, 856–857
reconstruction of
fibula osseocutaneous free flaps for, 692–693
scapular free flaps for, 680–683
total maxillectomy with orbital preservation and, 28–29
Maxillary artery, internal, transantral ligation of, 858–859
Maxillary sinus
antrostomy for, sublabial, 856–857
endoscopic surgery of, in children, 904–905
medial maxillectomy and, 24–25
Maxillectomy
endoscopic, 886–889
medial, 24–25
partial, nasolacrimal system evaluation and repair following, 554–557
radical, with orbital exenteration, 30–33
subtotal, Weber-Ferguson approach for, 26–27
total, with orbital preservation, 28–29
Meatoplasty, 296–297
mastoidectomy and, radical, modified, 346–347
Mediastinum
exploration and dissection of, 258–261
lymph nodes of, superior, dissection of, total thyroidectomy with, 230–231
mediastinal (retrosternal) goiter excision and, 224–227
transsternal mediastinal node dissection and, 154–157
Melasma, chemical peels for. *See* Chemical peels
Meniere's disease
endolymphatic sac exposure, decompression, or shunt for, 382–383
streptomycin perfusion of labyrinth for, 388–389

vestibular neurectomy for. *See* Vestibular neurectomy
Meningoceles, nasal. *See* Nose, encephaloceles and meningoceles of
Meningoencephaloceles, management of, 360–361
Mentoplasty, facial analysis for, 480–481
Mesotympanum, facial recess approach to, 358–359
Microgenia
chin implants for, 482–483
genioplasty for, 484–487
horizontal position changes and, 484–485
vertical position changes and, 484–485
Micrognathia, chin implants for, 482–483
Micrografts, for hair transplantation, 756
Microlaryngoscopes, 172
Microsomia, hemifacial, skeletal correction of, 742–743
Microsurgery, for vocal cord polyps, cysts, and nodules, 784–785
Microvascular surgery, 678–679
Middle ear. *See* Ear(s), middle; Otitis media; Tympanic membrane; Tympanoplasty
Midface fractures, pediatric, 566–567
Midfacial degloving, 882–885
Midline granulomatous disease, cartilage grafts for, 664–665
Midseptal incisions, 852–853
Minigrafts, for hair transplantation, 754
Mondini deformity, intralabyrinthine repair of, 360–361
Mouth. *See* Glossectomy; Oral cavity; Tongue
Mucoceles
of ethmoid sinus, frontoethmoidectomy for, external, 868–869
of floor of mouth, excision of, 110–111
of frontal sinus
frontal sinusectomy and fat obliteration for, 898–901
bilateral procedure, 900
unilateral procedure, 898–901
frontoethmoidectomy for, external, 868–869
of lacrimal sac, dacryocystorhinostomy for, 908–909
maxillary, antrostomy for, sublabial, 856–857
sinusitis with, endoscopic maxillary, ethmoid, sphenoidectomy for, 886–889
sphenoid, sphenoidectomy for, intranasal, 872–873
Mucoperiosteal flaps, for cerebrospinal fluid rhinorrhea closure. *See* Cerebrospinal fluid rhinorrhea
Mucormycosis, of maxillary sinus, radical maxillectomy with orbital exenteration for, 30–33
Mucosal grafts, 660, 662–663
Mucosal waves, stroboscopy and, 592
Multiple endocrine neoplasia syndrome, total parathyroidectomy and autotransplantation for, 240–241
Mustarde cheek flaps, 526–527
Myectomy, cricopharyngeal, 262–263
Myocutaneous flaps
for auriculectomy, 124–125
latissimus dorsi, 648–651
for partial- and full-thickness buccal resection, 100–101
pectoralis major, 636–639
platysma, 656–657

sternocleidomastoid, 658–659
superior trapezius, 640–641
temporalis, 654–655
trapezius
lateral island, 642–643
lower island, 644–647
Myotomy
cricopharyngeal, 262–263
partial midline glossectomy of tongue base and, 76
supraglottic laryngectomy and, 192–193
vertical partial laryngectomy with extension and, 188–189
for Zenker's diverticulum, 256
diverticulopexy and, for Zenker's diverticulum, 256
hyoid, 822–823
for Zenker's diverticulum, 256–257
Myringoplasty, 308–309
fat, for tympanic membrane perforations, 336–337
Myringotomy tubes, placement and removal of, 302–303

N
Nasal allergic disease, nasolacrimal system evaluation and repair for, 554–557
Nasal ciliary biopsy, 842–843
Nasal-facial analysis, for rhinoplasty, 442–443
Nasal obstruction
nasal valve surgery for. *See* Rhinoplasty, for nasal valve collapse or incompetence
septoplasty and submucous resection for. *See* Rhinoplasty, septoplasty and submucous resection and; Septoplasty; Submucous resection
Nasal polyps, 886–889
nasolacrimal system evaluation and repair for, 554–557
polypectomy for, 824–827
endoscopic, of antrochoanal polyps, 824–827
Nasal profile, 442–443
Nasal septum
craniofacial resection including ethmoid labyrinth and cribriform plate and, 34–37
dermoplasty and, 836–837
perforation of, 838–839
cartilage grafts for, 664–665
lateral-rhinotomy for, 22–23
septal button insertion for, 838–839
surgical closure and, 838–839
resection of, for tumors, 840–841
lateral rhinotomy approach to, 840–841
submucous resection of, 828–829
of turbinate, 844–845
Nasal tip
projection of, 442–443
rotation of, 442–443
Nasoethmoid fractures, 550–551
Nasofacial angle, 442–443
Nasofrontal angle, 442–443
Nasolabial flaps, 608–609
subcutaneous pedicle, 608–609
for upper lip reconstruction, 60–61
Nasolacrimal system
evaluation and repair of, 554–557
obstruction of, dacryocystorhinostomy for, 908–909
Nasopharyngoscopy, 772–773

Nasopharynx
    access to, 414–417
    facial translocation for nasopharyngeal
        angiofibroma resection and, 38–41
Neck, 138–169
    abscesses of, drainage of, 166–167, 290
    analysis of, 500–501
    biopsy of, radical neck dissection
        following, 140–143
    cervical node biopsy and, 158–159
    defects of
        deltopectoral flaps for, 620–621
        lateral arm free flaps for, 690–691
        latissimus dorsi myocutaneous flaps for,
            648–651
        pectoralis major myocutaneous flaps
            for, 636–639
        platysma flaps for, 656–657
        scapular free flaps for, 680–683
        superior trapezius myocutaneous flaps
            for, 640–641
        A to T flaps for, 622–623
        trapezius myocutaneous flaps for, lateral
            island, 642–643
    dermoid cysts of, excision of, 280–281
    dissection of
        floor of mouth resection and, posterior,
            marginal, 92
        modified radical
            preserving internal jugular vein, 150–
                153
            preserving spinal accessory nerve,
                148–153
            preserving sternocleidomastoid
                muscle, 150–153
        near-total laryngectomy and, 196
        posterolateral, 162–163
            with spinal accessory nerve
                preservation, 162–163
        radical, 140–143
            inferior, 142–143
            medial, 142–143
            posterior, 140, 143
            submandibular gland excision with,
                12–13
            of submandibular triangle, 140–141
            upper, 140–141
        supraomohyoid, 144–147
        upper, intermediate or lateral temporal
            bone resection and, 134–135
    hemorrhage associated with surgery of,
        mediastinal exploration and
        dissection and, 258–261
    incisions for surgery of, 138–139
    lipomas of, excision or liposuction of,
        288–289
    liposuction of, with facelift pretunneling,
        496–497
    penetrating injuries of, exploration and
        repair of, 168–169
    scalene node biopsy and, 160–161
    submental tuck for, 498–499
    supraclavicular space mass excision and,
        164–165
    transsternal mediastinal node dissection
        and, 154–157
Needle biopsy, 912–913
NEET areas, 744–745
Nerve grafts, 674–677
    facial nerve, cross, 698–699
    greater auricular nerve, 674, 677
    nerve technique of anastomosis for, 674–
        676
    sural nerve, 674–675, 677
    total parotidectomy with nerve resection
        and graft and, 10–11

vascularized, lateral arm free flaps for,
        690–691
Neurectomy
    tympanic, 338–339
    vidian, 860–863
        endoscopic transnasal approach for,
            862–863
        transantral approach for, 860–862
Neuromas, acoustic. See Acoustic neuromas
Newborns, septal dislocation in, 532–533
NOCH areas, 744
Nose, 18–23, 744–745. See also Nasal
        entries; Rhinoplasty
    congenital dermoid cyst and sinus opening
        of, 850–851
    defects of
        cartilage grafts for, 666–667
        composite grafts for, 668–669
        forehead flaps for, median, 612–613
        glabellar flaps for, 614–615
    encephaloceles and meningoceles of,
        endoscopic resection of, 846–849
        defect repair and, 848–849
        free graft harvest and, 846, 848–849
        identification and resection of
            encephaloceles and, 846–847
    epistaxis and. See Epistaxis
    injury of
        fractures and, 530–533
            closed reduction of, 530–531
            septal fracture-dislocations, 532–533
        midline forehead flap nasal
            reconstruction for, 20–21
        lateral rhinotomy and, 22–23
        nasal cavity examination with nasal biopsy
            or foreign body removal and, 842–
            843
    reconstruction of
        bone grafts for, harvesting, 670–673
        midline forehead flap, 20–21
        nasal-facial analysis for, 442–443
        nasolabial flaps for, 608–609
    septum of. See Nasal septum
    sublabial and septal incisions for, 852–853
    total rhinectomy and, 18–19

O

Olfactory tracts, craniofacial resection
        including ethmoid labyrinth and
        cribriform plate and, 34–37
Onlay cartilage grafts, for cleft-lip nasal
        repair, 474
Optic neuropathy, maxillary decompression
        for, 880–881
Oral cavity, 66–123
    alveolar ridge resection and, 94–95
    buccal resection and, partial- and full-
        thickness, 100–101
    defects of
        deltopectoral flaps for, 620–621
        mucosal, radial forearm flaps for, 688–
            689
        pericranial flaps for, 630–631
        platysma flaps for, 656–657
        sternocleidomastoid flaps for, 658–659
        temporalis myocutaneous flaps for,
            654–655
    floor of mouth abscesses and, drainage of,
        166–167
    floor of mouth defects and
        intraoral skin grafting for, 106–107
        reconstruction of, nasolabial flaps for,
            608–609
        tongue flaps for reconstruction of, 104–
            105

floor of mouth resection and
    anterior, 84–85
    with anterior mandibular invasion, 88–
        89
    lateral, 86–87
    with lateral mandibular invasion, 90–92
    marginal, with posterior mandibular
        invasion, 92–93
intraoral skin grafting and, 106–107
local anesthesia of, 918–919
mandible and. See Mandible
oropharynx and. See Oropharynx
palate and. See Cleft palate; Hard palate;
    Palate; Soft palate
ranulas of, superficial and plunging,
    excision of, 110–111
retromolar trigone and. See Retromolar
    trigone
surgical approaches to, 66–69
tongue and. See Glossectomy; Tongue
tonsils and. See Tonsil(s); Tonsillectomy
tumors of, posterior, mandibular
    osteotomy for, 102–103
vestibuloplasty and, 116–117
Oral rotation-advancement flaps, for
        oronasal and oroantral fistula
        repair, 732–733
Orbicularis oculi muscle, hypertrophy of,
        blepharoplasty for, 514–517
Orbit
    blowout fractures of, 548–549
    decompression of, endoscopic maxillary,
        ethmoid, sphenoidectomy for, 886–
        889
    frontal defects of, reconstruction of, 906–
        907
    hemorrhage of, lateral canthotomy and
        cantholysis for, 894–897
    radical maxillectomy with orbital
        exenteration and, 30–33
    reconstruction of
        fibula osseocutaneous free flaps for,
            692–693
        temporalis myocutaneous flaps for,
            654–655
    total maxillectomy with orbital
        preservation and, 28–29
Orbital nerve, decompression of, endoscopic
        maxillary, ethmoid,
        sphenoidectomy for, 886–889
Oroantral fistulas, repair of, 732–733
Orocutaneous fistulas
    closure of, sternocleidomastoid flaps for,
        658–659
    creation of, superior trapezius
        myocutaneous flaps for, 640–641
Orofacial growth abnormalities,
        adenoidectomy for, 816–817
Oromandibular defects
    iliac crest internal oblique free flaps for,
        684–687
    scapular free flaps for, 680–683
Oronasal fistulas, repair of, 732–733
Oropharynx
    defects of
        latissimus dorsi myocutaneous flaps for,
            648–651
        pericranial flaps for, 630–631
        trapezius myocutaneous flaps for
            lateral island, 642–643
            lower island, 644–647
            superior, 640–641
    intraoral skin grafting for defects of, 106–
        107
    tongue flaps for reconstruction of, 104–
        105

Oropharynx (*continued*)
tumors of, mandibular osteotomy for, 102–103
Orthognathic surgery
genioplasty and, 484–487
horizontal position changes and, 484–485
vertical position changes and, 484–485
nasal-facial analysis for, 442–443
Ossicular chain
ankylosis of, tympanoplasty for, type I, 308–311
destruction of, tympanoplasty for, type IV, 322–323
discontinuity of
exploratory tympanotomy for, tympanomeatal flaps for, 304–307
tympanoplasty for
type I, 308–311
type II, 314–317
fixation of
exploratory tympanotomy for, tympanomeatal flaps for, 304–307
tympanoplasty for, type II, 314–317
missing malleus handle and, tympanoplasty for, type III, 318–321
necrosis of, tympanoplasty for, type I, 308–311
stapedotomy and stapedectomy and, 330–331
Ossoff-Pilling laryngoscope, 172
Osteomas
canaloplasty for, 296–297
of external auditory canal, excision of, 298–299
frontal, frontal sinusectomy and fat obliteration for, 898–901
bilateral procedure, 900
unilateral procedure, 898–901
Osteomyelitis, of frontal sinus
frontal sinus ablation and collapse for, 902–903
frontal sinusectomy and fat obliteration for, 898–901
bilateral procedure, 900
unilateral procedure, 898–901
Osteomyocutaneous free flaps, microvascular, for mandibular resection, 108–109
Osteotomy
LeFort I, 712–713
mandibular. *See* Mandible, mandibular osteotomy and
for rhinoplasty, 452–453
sagittal, of mandibular ramus, 710–711
for skeletal correction of hemifacial microsomia, 742–743
Otalgia, paraganglioma excision for, 354–355
Otitis externa
canaloplasty for, 296–297
exostosis excision for, 298–299
osteoma excision for, 298–299
soft tissue canal stenosis and, 300–301
Otitis media
adenoidectomy for, 816–817
facial recess approach for, 358–359
mastoidectomy for, simple, 340–343
myringotomy tube placement for, 302–303
tympanoplasty for, type I, 308–311
Otoplasty, 428–435
for antihelical fold, 430–433
for auricular avulsions
partial, 436–437
fenestrations for, 436

pocket procedure for, 436–437
tunnel procedure for, 436–437
total, 436, 438–439
microvascular technique for, 438
for deep conchal bowl, 428–429
for deficient helical folds, 434–435
for reduction of helical prominences, 434–435
for reduction of large ear lobes, 434–435
for reduction of large scapha, 434–435
Otorrhea, mastoidectomy for
radical, modified, 344–347
simple, 340–343
Otosclerosis
exploratory tympanotomy for, tympanomeatal flaps for, 304–307
stapedotomy and stapedectomy for, 330–331

P

Palate
cleft. *See* Cleft palate
fractures of, wiring and plating of, 538–539
hard. *See* Hard palate
soft. *See* Soft palate
Palatoplasty, two-flap, with intravelar veloplasty, 726–727, 730–731
Paper patches, for tympanic membrane perforations, 336–337
Papillary carcinoma, laryngeal, laryngofissure and cordectomy for, 174–175
Papillomas
inverted, midfacial degloving procedure for, 882–885
laser laryngoscopy for removal of, 776–779
Papillomatosis, respiratory, laser techniques for, 806–807
Paragangliomas
of carotid body, resection of, 284–285
of jugular foramen, lateral transcondylar approach to, extreme, 410–413
of middle ear, excision of, 354–355
Paranasal sinuses. *See also specific sinuses*
craniofacial resection including ethmoid labyrinth and cribriform plate and, 34–37
draining, branchial cleft fistula and cyst excision for, 312–313
Paraneoplastic syndromes, glomus tumor excision for, 406–407
Parapharyngeal space, abscesses of, drainage of, 166–167
Parathyroidectomy, 236–239
for recurrent hyperparathyroidism and cancer of parathyroid, 242–245
subtotal, 236
total, 240–241
Parathyroid gland, 236–245. *See also* Parathyroidectomy
autotransplantation of, 238–241
hyperplasia of, parathyroidectomy for
subtotal, 236, 242, 244–245
total, 236–239, 242, 244–245
autotransplantation and, 240–241
mediastinal exploration and dissection and, 258–261
tumors of, mediastinal exploration and dissection and, 258–261
Paratracheal lymph nodes, dissection of, total thyroidectomy with, 230–231
Parotidectomy
incisions for, 138
partial- and full-thickness buccal resection and, 100

superficial, intermediate or lateral temporal bone resection and, 134–135
total
with nerve resection and graft, 10–11
with seventh nerve sparing, 8–9
Parotid gland. *See also* Parotidectomy
deep lateral lobectomy with nerve sparing and, 4–5
Frey's syndrome following surgery of, tympanic neurectomy for, 338–339
injury of, management of, 16–17
intraoral deep-lobe tumor excision and, 6–7
superficial lobectomy and, 2–3
Parotid space, abscesses of, drainage of, 166–167
Particulate bone, for mandibular reconstruction, 118–119
Pectoralis major flaps, 636–639
for glossectomy defect reconstruction, 82
for lip reconstruction, 58–59
for mandibular reconstruction, 120
Pentagonal shield excision, of lip, 46–47
Pericranial flaps, 630–631
Perilymphatic fistulas
exploratory tympanotomy for, tympanomeatal flaps for, 304–307
repair of, 332–335
Periodicity, stroboscopy and, 592
Perioral area, 744–745
Periorbit, 744–745
Peritonsillar abscesses, tonsillectomy for, 812–813
Petrous apicectomy, 356–357
Pharyngeal flaps, superiorly based, 734–735
Pharyngeal pouches, 256–257
cricopharyngeal myotomy and myectomy for, 262–263
Pharyngectomy, 266–269
pharyngeal reconstruction following, 270–273
free composite skin flaps for, 270–271
free jejunal autografts for, 270–271, 273
regional skin flaps for, 270–271
posterior and limited lateral wall resections and, 266–269
subtotal, 268–269
total, 268–269
Pharyngocutaneous fistulas, free jejunal transfer for, 696–697
Pharyngolaryngectomy, total, 206–209
Pharyngomaxillary space, tumors of, mandibular osteotomy for, 102–103
Pharyngotomy
cricopharyngeal, 76
transhyoid, 68–69
Pharynx, 266–273. *See also* Hypopharynx; Oropharynx; Pharyngectomy
defects of
circumferential, microvascular surgery for, 678–679
mucosal, radial forearm flaps for, 688–689
reconstruction of, 270–273
deltopectoral flaps for, 620–621
tumors of
free jejunal transfer for, 696–697
near-total laryngopharyngectomy for, 196
wall of, tumors of, total pharyngolaryngectomy for, 206–209
Phenol peels. *See* Chemical peels
Phonosurgery. *See* Thyroplasty

Pinna, reconstruction of
  with composite grafts, 130–131
  following regional, wedge, and stellate
    excision, 126–129
Piriform fossa, tumors of, near-total
    laryngopharyngectomy for, 196
  extended, 196
Piriform sinus, tumors of
  extended supraglottic partial laryngectomy
    for, 194–195
  total laryngectomy for, with extension,
    204–205
Pituitary gland
  removal of. See Hypophysectomy
  tumors of, sphenoidectomy for,
    transethmoidal, 874–875
Plating
  compression, for mandibular fractures,
    570–571
  noncompression, for mandibular fractures,
    572–573
Platysma flaps, 656–657
Polypectomy, nasal, 824–827
  endoscopic, of antrochoanal polyps, 826–
    827
Polyposis
  frontoethmoid, frontoethmoidectomy for,
    external, 868–869
  nasal. See Nasal polyps
  sinus, endoscopic maxillary, ethmoid,
    sphenoidectomy for, 886–889
Polytef paste, for vocal cord paralysis, 604–
    605
Postauricular skin flap of Dieffenbach, for
    pinna reconstruction, 130–131
Postcricoid tumors, total
    pharyngolaryngectomy for, 206–
    209
Posttragal incision, for rhytidectomy, 490–
    491
Pretracheal lymph nodes, dissection of, total
    thyroidectomy with, 230–231
Pretragal incision, for rhytidectomy, 490–
    491
Prognathism, mandibular, sagittal osteotomy
    of mandibular ramus for, 710–711
Prominauris, otoplasty for, 430–433
Proptosis, maxillary decompression for, 880–
    881
Ptosis, blepharoplasty for, 512–513
Punch biopsy, 916–917
Punch grafts, for hair transplantation, 754–
    756
Pyoceles, of frontal sinus, frontal
    sinusectomy and fat obliteration
    for, 898–901
  bilateral procedure, 900
  unilateral procedure, 898–901
Pyramidal fractures, LeFort II repair of,
    542–543

Q
Quilted grafts, for intraoral skin grafting, 106

R
Radial forearm flaps, 688–689
Ranulas, of floor of mouth, superficial and
    plunging, excision of, 110–111
Recurrent laryngeal nerve
  section and avulsion of, 212–213
  subtotal thyroidectomy and, 222
Regional flaps. See Advancement flaps;
    Local and regional flaps;
    Myocutaneous flaps

Respiratory disorders, following
    tracheostomy, revision of stenotic
    tracheostomy and, 264–265
Respiratory papillomatosis, laser techniques
    for, 806–807
Resting skin tension lines, 746–747
Retrognathia
  chin implants for, 482–483
  sagittal osteotomy of mandibular ramus
    for, 710–711
Retromolar trigone, tumors of, resection for
  lateral mandibulotomy for, 114
  mandibular, segmental, 112, 114–115
    with mandibular sparing, 112–113
  midline mandibulotomy and, 114
  transoral, 114
Retroorbital abscesses, ethmoidectomy for,
    external, 866–867
Rhinectomy, total, 18–19
Rhinitis, vasomotor, vidian neurectomy for,
    860–863
  endoscopic transnasal approach for, 862–
    863
  transantral approach for, 860–862
Rhinophyma, 476–477
Rhinoplasty, 442–479
  for black and Asian populations, 478–479
  for cleft lip repair, 472–475
  dorsal augmentation and, 462–463
  dorsal reduction and, 462–463
  intercartilaginous approach to, 450–451
  local anesthesia for, 444–445
  major nasal reconstruction and, 464–465
  nasal base procedures for, 458–461
    alar wedge excision, 459–461
    internal nostril floor reduction, 460–461
    sheen alar flap, 460–461
    sliding alar flap, 460–461
    wedge excision nostril floor and sill,
      460–461
  nasal-facial analysis for, 442–443
  nasal tip procedures for, 454–457
    delivery, 455–456
    nondelivery, 454–455
      transcartilaginous, 454
    open (external), 455–456
    tip-refinement techniques and, 455–456
  for nasal valve collapse or incompetence,
    470–471
    inadequate cartilage and, 470–471
    inadequate vestibular skin and, 470–471
    inadequate vestibular skin and cartilage
      and, 470–471
  osteotomies for, 452–453
  outline revision, 466–469
    for alar retraction, 466–467
    for bossa, 466–467
    for columella retraction, 466, 468–469
    for excessive reduction, 466
    for midnasal deformities, 468–469
    for pinching, 466–467
    for supratip fullness, 468–469
  for rhinophyma, 476–477
  septoplasty and submucous resection and,
    446–449
    for anterior deflections, 446–449
    for deviations of bony perpendicular
      plate of septum, 448
    for nasal spine deviations, 448
    for posterior deflections, 448–449
Rhinorrhea
  cerebrospinal fluid. See Cerebrospinal fluid
    rhinorrhea
  senile, vidian neurectomy for, 860–863
    endoscopic transnasal approach for,
      862–863
    transantral approach for, 860–862

Rhinotomy
  external, incision for, 852–853
  lateral, 22–23
    craniofacial resection including ethmoid
      labyrinth and cribriform plate and,
      36–37
    for septal resection, 840–841
Rhomboid flaps, 618–619
  triple, 628–629
Rhytid(s), 500. See also Rhytidectomy
  chemical peels for. See Chemical peels
  dermabrasion for, 508–509
Rhytidectomy, 490–495
  incisions for, 490–491
  superficial musculoaponeurotic system
    plication and short or long flap for,
    492–495
Rib grafts, harvesting, 670–671
Rinne test, negative, stapedotomy and
    stapedectomy for, 330–331
Rotation-advancement flaps
  for cleft lip repair, 720–723
  oral, for oronasal and oroantral fistula
    repair, 732–733

S
Salivary glands, 2–17. See also specific
    glands
  intraoral deep-lobe tumor excision and,
    6–7
  parotid. See Parotid gland
  sublingual, excision of, 14–15
  submandibular
    excision of, 12–13
    injury of, management of, 16–17
  tumors of
    alveolar ridge resection for, 94–95
    midfacial degloving procedure for, 882–
      885
    partial anterior glossectomy for, 70–71
Scalene node biopsy, 160–161
Scalp. See also Hair transplantation; Scalp
    reduction
  cutaneous defects of, scapular free flaps
    for, 680–683
  tight, tissue expansion for, 766–767
Scalp reduction, 762–765
  elliptic midline closure for, 762–763
  paramedian (lateral), 762–763
  Y and double Y patterns for, 762–765
Scapular free flaps, 680–683
Scarring
  dermabrasion for, 508–509
  scar excision for, 748–751
    geometric broken line closure for, 750–
      751
    simple closure for, 748–749
    W-plasty for, 750–751
    Z-plasty for, 624–625, 748–751
Schirmer I test, 554–555
Schwannomas, transcranial, lateral
    transcondylar approach to,
    extreme, 410–413
Semicircular canals
  posterior, occlusion of, 384–385
  singular neurectomy and, 386–387
Septal dermoplasty, 836–837
Septal incisions, 852–853
Septicemia
  branchial cleft cyst excision for, 276–277
  thyroglossal duct cyst excision for, 274–
    275
Septoplasty, 830–831. See also Rhinoplasty,
    septoplasty and submucous
    resection and

Septoplasty (*continued*)
    anesthesia for, local, 444–445
    cleft-lip nasal repair and, 472
    for septal fracture-dislocations, 532–533
Septum, cartilage grafts from, 664–665
Shoulder, cutaneous loss over, latissimus
        dorsi myocutaneous flaps for, 648–
        651
Sialadenitis
    deep lateral lobectomy with nerve sparing
        for, 4–5
    submandibular gland excision for, 12–13
    superficial lobectomy for, 2–3
    total parotidectomy with seventh nerve
        sparing for, 8–9
Sialolithiasis
    submandibular gland excision for, 12–13
    superficial lobectomy for, 2–3
Sialosis, superficial lobectomy for, 2–3
Sinusitis
    antrostomy for
        intranasal, through inferior meatus,
            854–855
        sublabial, 856–857
    endoscopic surgery for
        in children, 904–905
        maxillary, ethmoid, sphenoidectomy,
            886–889
    ethmoidectomy for. *See* Ethmoidectomy
    frontal sinus ablation and collapse for,
        902–903
    frontal sinusectomy and fat obliteration
        for, 898–901
        bilateral procedure, 900
        unilateral procedure, 898–901
    frontal sinus trephination for, 896–897
    midfacial degloving procedure for, 882–
        885
    nasolacrimal system evaluation and repair
        for, 554–557
    septoplasty and submucous resection for.
        See Rhinoplasty, septoplasty and
        submucous resection and
    sphenoidectomy for, intranasal, 872–873
    submucous resection of nasal septum for,
        828–829
Skin flaps
    free composite, for pharyngeal
        reconstruction, 270–271
    regional, for pharyngeal reconstruction,
        270–271
Skin grafts
    dermal, 660–662
    full-thickness, 662–663
    intraoral, 106–107
    split-thickness, 660–662
Skin lesions, local excision and primary
        closure of, 746–747
Skull base
    anterior, defects of, pericranial flaps for,
        630–631
    defects of, temporalis myocutaneous flaps
        for, 654–655
    lateral, 406–421
        access to nasopharynx and, 414–417
        defects of, trapezius myocutaneous flaps
            for, lower island, 644–647
        glomus tumor excision and, 406–409
        lateral transcondylar approach to,
            extreme, 410–413
        petrosal approach to, 418–421
    occipital, defects of, trapezius
        myocutaneous flaps for, lower
        island, 644–647
    resection of, craniofacial resection
        including ethmoid labyrinth and
        cribriform plate and, 34–37

transtemporal, 390–405
    acoustic neuromas and. *See* Acoustic
        neuromas
    vestibular neurectomy and. *See*
        Vestibular neurectomy
    tumors of, mandibular osteotomy for,
        102–103
Sleep apnea
    adenoidectomy for, 816–817
    hyoid myotomy-suspension and
        genioglossus advancement for,
        822–823
    septoplasty and submucous resection for.
        See Rhinoplasty, septoplasty and
        submucous resection and
    septoplasty for, 830–831
    tonsillectomy for, 812–815
    uvulopalatopharyngoplasty for. *See*
        Uvulopalatopharyngoplasty
Slit grafts, for hair transplantation, 756–757
Snoring, uvulopalatopharyngoplasty for. *See*
        Uvulopalatopharyngoplasty
Soft palate
    intraoral skin grafting for defects of, 106–
        107
    resection of, 98–99
    tongue flaps for reconstruction of, 104–
        105
Spasm, cricopharyngeal, myotomy and
        myectomy for, 262–263
Sphenoidectomy, 872–875
    endoscopic, 886–889
    intranasal, 872–873
    transethmoidal, 874–875
Spinal accessory nerve, preservation of
    modified radical neck dissection and, 148–
        153
    posterolateral neck dissection with, 162–
        163
Splints, for mandibular fractures, 578–579
Springs, for eyelid reanimation, placement
        of, 374
Squamous cell carcinoma
    of floor of mouth. *See also* Oral cavity,
        floor of mouth resection and
    anterior, sublingual gland excision for,
        14–15
    of gingiva, alveolar ridge resection for, 94–
        95
    laryngeal, endoscopic partial laryngoscopy
        for, 172–173
    of tongue, partial anterior glossectomy for,
        70–71
Stair-step incisions, 68, 72–73
Stapedectomy, 330–331
Stapedotomy, 330–331
Stapes. *See* Ossicular chain
Stapes reflex, negative, stapedotomy and
        stapedectomy for, 330–331
Static slings, for facial reanimation, 702–705
Stellate lacerations, repair of, 752–753
Stenson's duct, injury of, management of,
        16–17
Sternoclavicular grafts, harvesting, 740–741
Sternocleidomastoid flaps, 658–659
Sternocleidomastoid muscle, preservation of,
        modified radical neck dissection
        and, 150–153
Sternotomy, median, mediastinal
        (retrosternal) goiter excision and,
        226–227
Stomal recurrence, following laryngectomy
    mediastinal exploration and dissection
        and, 258–261
    transsternal mediastinal node dissection
        for, 154–157

Stridor
    branchial cleft cyst excision for, 276–277
    laryngeal fracture and, repair of, 606–607
    lymphangioma excision for, 278–279
Stroboscopy, 592–593
Subcutaneous skin eversion sutures, 752–753
Subglottic stenosis, laryngotracheal
        decompression for, anterior, 582–
        583
Sublabial incisions, 852–853
    for palatal fracture wiring and plating,
        538–539
Sublingual gland excision, 14–15
Submandibular gland
    excision of, 12–13
    injury of, management of, 16–17
Submental tuck, for neck, 498–499
Submucous resection
    nasal. *See also* Rhinoplasty, septoplasty
        and submucous resection and
    anesthesia for, local, 444–445
    of nasal septum, 828–829
Subperiosteal abscesses
    drainage of, endoscopic maxillary,
        ethmoid, sphenoidectomy for, 886–
        889
    ethmoidectomy for, external, 866–867
    mastoidectomy for, simple, 340–343
Subtrichial incision, for rhytidectomy, 490–
        491
Supraclavicular space, masses of, excision of,
        164–165
Sural nerve
    as grafts, 674–675, 677
    for nerve grafts, 10–11
Swallowing difficulty, laryngeal fracture and,
        repair of, 606–607
Symmetry, stroboscopy and, 592

T

Tarsorrhaphy, 372–373
Temple, defects of
    cheek-neck rotation flaps for, 616–617
    A to T flaps for, 622–623
Temporal bone
    defects of, trapezius myocutaneous flaps
        for, lateral island, 642–643
    resection of, 134–137
        facial recess approach for, 358–359
        intermediate or lateral, 134–135
        radical, 134, 136–137
        superficial, 136–137
    tumors of, mastoidectomy for, simple,
        340–343
Temporalis muscle, dynamic temporalis and
        masseter muscle transposition and,
        706–709
Temporalis muscle flaps, 654–655
    harvest of, 32–33
Temporomandibular joint
    ankylosis of, temporalis myocutaneous
        flaps for, 654–655
    reconstruction of, bone grafts for, 740–741
        harvesting, 670–671
    reposition of articular disc of, 738–739
    surgical approaches to, 736–737
        endaural, 736–737
        hemicoronal, 736–737
        postauricular, 736–737
        preauricular, 736–737
Temporoparietal fascia flaps, 652–653
30° transposition flaps, 618–619
Thoracic inlet, exploration of, 258–259
Three-quarters H-incision, 78–79
Thyroglossal duct cysts, excision of, 274–275

Thyroid cartilage, vertical partial laryngectomy including, 176–179
Thyroidectomy
    subtotal, 222–223
    total, 228–235
        with paratracheal and superior mediastinal node dissection, 230–231
        with tracheal resection for malignant invasion, 232–235
            sleeve resection and, 232–235
            wedge resection and, 234–235
        total parathyroidectomy and, 238
Thyroid gland, 218–235. *See also* Thyroidectomy
    cysts of, thyroid lobectomy and isthmusectomy for, 218–221
    enlargement of, thyroid lobectomy and isthmusectomy for, 218–221
    lobectomy and isthmusectomy and, 218–221
    mediastinal (retrosternal) goiter excision and, 224–227
    substernal extension of, mediastinal exploration and dissection and, 258–261
    thyroglossal duct cyst excision and, 274–275
    tumors of, mediastinal exploration and dissection and, 258–261
Thyroplasty
    type I, 594–597
    type II, 598–599
    type III, 600–601
    type IV, 602–603
Thyrotomy, midline, laryngofissure and cordotomy and, 174–175
Tinnitus
    glomus tumor excision for, 406–407
    paraganglioma excision for, 354–355
Tissue expansion, 632–635, 766–767
Tongue. *See also* Glossectomy
    base of
        tongue flaps for reconstruction of, 104–105
        tumors of
            near-total laryngopharyngectomy for, 196
            total laryngectomy for, 200–203
        intraoral skin grafting for defects of, 106–107
        median labiomandibular glossotomy and, 68–69
        tumors of, extended supraglottic partial laryngectomy for, 194–195
Tongue flaps, for oropharyngeal reconstruction, 104–105
    posteriorly based flaps and, 104–105
Tonsil(s). *See also* Tonsillectomy
    local anesthesia of, 918–919
    tongue flaps for reconstruction of, 104–105
    tumors of, resection for
        lateral mandibulotomy and, 114
        mandibular, segmental, 112, 114–115
        with mandibular sparing, 112–113
        midline mandibulotomy and, 114
        transoral, 114
Tonsillectomy, 812–815
    lingual, 814–815
        dissection and electrocautery and, 814–815
        suspension laryngoscopy with laser excision and, 814–815
Trachea, 246–253. *See also* Tracheostomy
    defects of, cartilage grafts for, 666–667
    reconstruction of, 248–249

mediastinal exploration and dissection for, 258–261
    resection of
        reanastomosis and, 250–253
        total thyroidectomy with, 232–235
            sleeve resection and, 232–235
            wedge resection and, 234–235
Tracheobronchial stenosis
    bronchoscopic dilation of, 804–805
    laser techniques for, 806–807
Tracheobronchial strictures, bronchoscopic dilation of, 804–805
Tracheoesophageal shunt, 210–211
Tracheoesophageal stenosis, cricopharyngeal myotomy and myectomy for, 262–263
Tracheostoma, permanent, total laryngectomy and, 202–203
Tracheostomy, 246–247
    flexible bronchoscopy and, 808–809
    floor of mouth resection and, posterior, marginal, 92
    partial posterior glossectomy of tongue base and, 74
    stenotic, revision of, 264–265
    total pharyngolaryngectomy and, 208
    tracheal reconstruction and, 248
    tracheal resection and reanastomosis and, 250
Tracheotomy
    laryngeal diversion and, 214–215
    laryngocele excision and, 282
    laryngofissure and cordotomy and, 174–175
    near-total laryngectomy and, 196
    partial midline glossectomy of tongue base and, 76
    pharyngectomy and, 266
    in total maxillectomy, 28
Transfixion incision, 852–853
Transhyoid approach, 68–69
Transoral approach, 66–67
Trap door defects, repair of, 752–753
Trapezius myocutaneous flaps
    lateral island, 642–643
    lower island, 644–647
    superior, 640–641
Trauma. *See specific sites*
Trephination, of frontal sinus, 896–897
Trichloroacetic acid peels, 510
T-shaped incision, 72
Tuberculosis, cervical node biopsy and, 158–159
Tumors. *See specific tumors and sites*
Tunnel technique, for pinna reconstruction, 130–131
Turnover flaps, for oronasal and oroantral fistula repair, 732–733
Tympanic membrane, 302–311, 314–322. *See also* Tympanoplasty
    destruction of, tympanoplasty for, type IV, 322–323
    homograft, placement of, 326–327
    perforation of
        large, reconstruction of, 324–327
        office repair of, 336–337
            fat myringoplasty for, 336–337
            paper patches for, 336–337
        tympanoplasty for, type I, 308–311
        tympanomeatal flaps for exploratory tympanotomy and, 304–307
Tympanic neurectomy, 338–339
Tympanomastoiditis, tympanoplasty for, type IV, 322–323
Tympanomeatal flaps, for exploratory tympanotomy, 304–307

Tympanoplasty
    canal wall, tympanoplasty and, type III, 318–321
    type I, 308–311
        postauricular, 308–311
            closure for, 310
            incisions and grafts for, 308–309
            lateral or overlay technique for, 310–311
            medial or underlay graft technique for, 308, 310–311
        transcanal approach for, 308–309
    type II, 314–317
    type III, 318–321
    type IV, 322–323
Tympanostomy tubes, removal of, myringoplasty for, 308–309
Tympanotomy, exploratory, tympanomeatal flaps for, 304–307

U

Uvulopalatopharyngoplasty, 818–821
    extended, 820–821
        Koopmann's technique for, 820
        Moran's method for, 820–821
        Strome's method for, 820–821

V

Vagus nerve, lymphangiomas and, excision of, 278–279
Vascular coverage, sternocleidomastoid flaps for, 658–659
Vasomotor rhinitis, vidian neurectomy for, 860–863
    endoscopic transnasal approach for, 862–863
    transantral approach for, 860–862
Velopharyngeal insufficiency, superiorly based pharyngeal flaps for, 734–735
Veloplasty, intravelar, with two-flap palatoplasty, 726–727, 730–731
Vermilionectomy, 42–43
    with wedge resection, 44–45
Verrucous carcinoma, laryngeal
    endoscopic partial laryngoscopy for, 172–173
    laryngofissure and cordectomy for, 174–175
Vertebral artery, aneurysms of, lateral transcondylar approach to, extreme, 410–413
Vertical facial folds of Leonardo Dopamine Vinci, 500
Vertical phase difference, stroboscopy and, 592
Vertigo
    endolymphatic sac exposure, decompression, or shunt for, 382–383
    labyrinthectomy for, 376–379
        transcanal, 376–377
        transmastoid, 378–379
    posterior semicircular canal occlusion for, 384–385
    singular neurectomy for, 386–387
    streptomycin perfusion of labyrinth for, 388–389
    translabyrinthine approach to acoustic neuromas for, 394–395
    vestibular neurectomy for. *See* Vestibular neurectomy
Vestibular disorders. *See also* Vertigo
    perilymphatic fistula repair for, 332–335

Vestibular folds
    carcinoma of, vertical partial laryngectomy
        with extension for, 188–189
    resection of, 170–171
Vestibular neurectomy
    combined retrolabyrinthine-retrosigmoid
        approach for, 390, 392–393
    middle fossa approach for, 392
    retrolabyrinthine approach for, 390, 391–
        393
    transcochlear approach for, 390
    translabyrinthine approach for, 390
Vestibular neuronitis, vestibular neurectomy
    for. *See* Vestibular neurectomy
Vestibular sulcus, shallow, vestibuloplasty
    for, 116–117
Vestibuloplasty, 116–117
Videostroboscopy, 592–593
Vidian neurectomy, 860–863
    endoscopic transnasal approach for, 862–
        863
    transantral approach for, 860–862
Visor flaps, 68–69, 88–89
Visual field loss, blepharoplasty for, 512–513
Vocal cords
    carcinoma of, microsuspension

        laryngoscopy and laser excision of,
        782–783
    inadequate closure of, thyroplasty for, type
        I, 594–597
    microsurgery for polyps, cysts, and
        nodules of, 784–785
    paralysis of
        injection for, 604–605, 774–775
        laser arytenoidectomy for, 780–781
        stroboscopy and, 592–593
        thyroplasty for, type I, 594–597
Vocal folds, impaired mobility of
    glottic split for, posterior, with cartilage
        graft, 584–585
    laryngotracheal reconstruction for,
        anterior and posterior, 586–589
Voice rehabilitation, 210–211
V-Y advancement flaps, for cleft-lip nasal
    repair, 472–473

W

Weber-Ferguson incision
    with subtotal maxillectomy, 26–27
    with total maxillectomy, 28

Webster sliding cheek flap, 54–55
Webster-type subcutaneous everting 5–0
    PDS sutures, 750–751
Wedge resection, vermilionectomy with, 44–
    45
Weir resections, 478
W-excision, of lip, 46–47
Wharton's duct, injury of, management of,
    16–17
W-plasty, 750–751
Wullstein's tympanoplasty, 322–323

Z

Zenker's diverticulum, 256–257
    cricopharyngeal myotomy and myectomy
        for, 262–263
Z-plasty, 624–625, 748–751
Zygoma
    anterior, radical maxillectomy with orbital
        exenteration and, 30–33
    fractures of
        zygomatic arch reduction and, 534–535
        zygomatic-trimalar reduction and
            fixation for, 536–537